Thompson & Thompson

GENETICS GENOMICS IN MEDICINE

NINTH EDITION

Ronald Doron Cohn, MD, FACMG

President and CEO
Senior Scientist
The Hospital for Sick Children;
Professor
Department of Paediatrics and Molecular Genetics
University of Toronto
Toronto, Ontario, Canada

Stephen W. Scherer, PhD

Chief of Research
Hospital for Sick Children;
Professor
Department of Molecular Genetics
University of Toronto
Toronto, Ontario, Canada

Ada Hamosh, MD, MPH

Dr. Frank V. Sutland Professor of Pediatric Genetics
McKusick-Nathans Department of Genetic Medicine and Department of Pediatrics,
Clinical Director
Department of Genetic Medicine,
Scientific Director, OMIM
Johns Hopkins University
Baltimore, Maryland, USA

ELSEVIER

Elsevier
1600 John F. Kennedy Blvd.
Ste 1800
Philadelphia, PA 19103-2899

THOMPSON & THOMPSON GENETICS AND GENOMICS IN MEDICINE,
NINE EDITION

ISBN: 978-0-323-54762-8

Notice

Practitioners and researchers must always rely on their own experience and knowledge in evaluating and using any information, methods, compounds or experiments described herein. Because of rapid advances in the medical sciences, in particular, independent verification of diagnoses and drug dosages should be made. To the fullest extent of the law, no responsibility is assumed by Elsevier, authors, editors or contributors for any injury and/or damage to persons or property as a matter of products liability, negligence or otherwise, or from any use or operation of any methods, products, instructions, or ideas contained in the material herein.

Previous editions copyrighted 2016, 2007, 2004, 2001, 1991, 1986, 1980, 1973.

Content Strategist: Alexandra Mortimer
Content Development Specialist: Kayla Jarman
Publishing Services Manager: Shereen Jameel
Project Manager: Beula Christopher
Design Direction: Bridget Hoette

Printed in India.

Last digit is the print number: 9   8   7   6   5   4   3   2

ELSEVIER Book Aid International Working together to grow libraries in developing countries

www.elsevier.com • www.bookaid.org

Chapter Contributors

Gonçalo R. Abecasis, DPhil
Department of Biostatistics
University of Michigan School of Public Health
Ann Arbor, Michigan, USA

Carolyn Dinsmore Applegate, MGC, CGC
Genetic Counselor Manager
Department of Genetic Medicine
Johns Hopkins University School of Medicine
Baltimore, Maryland, USA

Laura Arbour, MSc, MD FRCPC FCCMG
Professor
Department of Medical Genetics, Faculty of Medicine
University of British Columbia
Vancouver, British Columbia, Canada
Medical Genetics Services, Island Health,
Victoria, BC, Canada

Christine R. Beck, PhD
Assistant Professor
The University of Connecticut Health Center and
The Jackson Laboratory for Genomic Medicine
Farmington, Connecticut, USA

Iris Cohn, MSc (Pharm), RPh
Clinical Specialist/Pharmacogenomics Pharmacist
Division of Clinical Pharmacology and Toxicology
The Hospital for Sick Children;
Assistant Professor
Department of Paediatrics
Temerty Faculty of Medicine
University of Toronto
Toronto, Ontario, Canada

Ronald Doron Cohn, MD, FACMG
President and CEO
Senior Scientist
The Hospital for Sick Children;
Professor
Department of Paediatrics and Molecular
Genetics
University of Toronto
Toronto, Ontario, Canada

Gregory Costain, MD, PhD, FRCPC
Staff Physician
Division of Clinical and Metabolic Genetics
The Hospital for Sick Children
Toronto, Ontario, Canada

Cheryl Cytrynbaum, MS
Genetic Counsellor
Division of Clinical and Metabolic Genetics
The Hospital for Sick Children;
Assistant Professor
Department of Molecular Genetics
University of Toronto;
Project Investigator
Genetics and Genome Biology Program
Research Institute, The Hospital for Sick Children
Toronto, Ontario, Canada

Wei Q. Deng, PhD
Assistant Professor
Psychiatry & Behavioural Neuroscience, Faculty of
Health Sciences
McMaster University
Hamilton, Ontario, Canada

Sarah Goodman, PhD
Research Fellow
Genetics and Genome Biology Program
Research Institute, The Hospital for Sick Children
Toronto, Ontario, Canada

Ada Hamosh, MD, MPH
Dr. Frank V. Sutland Professor of Pediatric Genetics
McKusick-Nathans Department of
Genetic Medicine and Department of Pediatrics,
Clinical Director
Department of Genetic Medicine,
Scientific Director, OMIM
Johns Hopkins University
Baltimore, Maryland, USA

Angie Child Jelin, MD
Associate Professor
Department of Gynecology and Obstetrics
Johns Hopkins Hospital
Baltimore, Maryland, USA

Ophir Klein, MD, PhD
Executive Director of Cedars-Sinai Guerin Children's,
Vice Dean for Children's Services,
David and Meredith Kaplan Distinguished Chair in
Children's Health,
Professor of Pediatrics,
Adjunct Professor of Orofacial Sciences and Pediatrics
UC San Francisco
San Francisco, California, USA

Bartha Maria Knoppers, PhD
Professor
Department of Human Genetics,
Faculty of Medicine and Health Sciences
McGill University
Montreal, Quebec, Canada

Charles Lee, PhD, FACMG
Director and Professor
The Jackson Laboratory for Genomic Medicine
Farmington, Connecticut, USA

Christian R. Marshall, PhD
Clinical Laboratory Director
Division of Genome Diagnostics
Department of Paediatric Laboratory Medicine
The Hospital for Sick Children;
Assistant Professor
Laboratory Medicine and Pathobiology
University of Toronto
Toronto, Ontario, Canada

Philipp G. Maass, PhD
Scientist
Genetics and Genome Biology
The Hospital for Sick Children
Assistant Professor
Department of Molecular Genetics
University of Toronto
Toronto, Ontario, Canada

Alice B. Popejoy, PhD
Assistant Professor
Department of Public Health Sciences,
Division of Epidemiology
University of California, Davis
Davis, California, USA

Stephen W. Scherer, PhD
Chief of Research
Hospital for Sick Children;
Professor
Department of Molecular Genetics
University of Toronto
Toronto, Ontario, Canada

Neal Sondheimer, MD, PhD
Associate Professor
Paediatrics and Molecular Genetics
University of Toronto;
Staff Physician
Clinical and Metabolic Genetics
The Hospital for Sick Children
Toronto, Ontario, Canada

Dimitri J. Stavropoulos, PhD, FCCMG
Clinical Laboratory Director
Genome Diagnostics, Department of Pediatric
Laboratory Medicine
The Hospital for Sick Children;
Assistant Professor
Department of Laboratory Medicine and
Pathobiology
University of Toronto
Toronto, Ontario, Canada

Lei Sun, PhD
Professor
Department of Statistical Sciences, Faculty of
Arts and Science
Division of Biostatistics, Dalla Lana School of
Public Health
University of Toronto,
Toronto, Ontario, Canada

Ignatia B. Van den Veyver, MD
Professor
Department of Obstetrics and Gynecology,
Professor
Department of Molecular and Human Genetics
Baylor College of Medicine
Houston, Texas, USA

Jodie Marie Vento, MGC, LCGC
Assistant Professor, Program Director
Department of Human Genetics
University of Pittsburgh
Pittsburgh, Pennsylvania, USA

Michael F. Walsh, MD, FAAP, FACMG, DABMG
Associate Member
Department of Pediatrics and Medicine, Divisions of
Solid Tumor and Clinical Genetics
Memorial Sloan Kettering Cancer Center
New York City, New York, USA

Rosanna Weksberg, MD, PhD
Senior Associate Scientist
Genetics and Genome Biology Program
Hospital for Sick Children,
Clinical Geneticist
Division of Clinical and Metabolic Genetics
The Hospital for Sick Children;
Professor
Department of Molecular Genetics
Institute of Medical Science;
Department of Paediatrics
University of Toronto
Toronto, Ontario, Canada

Cristen J. Willer, DPhil
Professor
Department of Internal Medicine
Division of Cardiovascular Medicine
University of Michigan
Ann Arbor, Michigan, USA

Anthony Wynshaw-Boris, MD, PhD
Professor and Chair
Genetics and Genome Sciences
CWRU School of Medicine;
Chair and Director
Genetics and Genome Sciences and Center for Human
Genetics
University Hospitals Cleveland Medical Center
Cleveland, Ohio, USA

Feyza Yilmaz, PhD
Associate Computational Scientist
The Jackson Laboratory for Genomic Medicine
Farmington, Connecticut, USA

Ryan Yuen, PhD
Senior Scientist
Genetics and Genome Biology Program
The Hospital for Sick Children
Toronto, Ontario, Canada

Ma'n H. Zawati, BCL, LLM, DCL (PhD)
Assistant Professor
Department of Human Genetics,
Faculty of Medicine and Health Sciences
McGill University
Montreal, Quebec, Canada

Case Study Contributors

Carolyn Dinsmore Applegate, MGC, CGC
Genetic Counselor Manager
Department of Genetic Medicine
Johns Hopkins University School of Medicine
Baltimore, Maryland, USA

Leslie G. Biesecker, MD
Distinguished Investigator,
Director
Center for Precision Health Research
National Human Genome Research Institute
National Institutes of Health
Bethesda, Maryland, USA

Janet A. Buchanan, MSc, PhD, FCCMG
Molecular Geneticist
The Centre for Applied Genomics
The Hospital for Sick Children
Toronto, Ontario, Canada

Manuel Carcao, MD, MSc, FRCPC
Professor
Division of Haematology/Oncology
Department of Paediatrics
Hospital for Sick Children
Toronto, Ontario, Canada

John Christodoulou, AM, MB, BS, PhD
Director
Genomic Medicine Research Theme
Murdoch Children's Research Institute;
Chair of Genomic Medicine
University of Melbourne
Melbourne, Victoria, Australia

Iris Cohn, MSc (Pharm), RPh
Clinical Specialist/Pharmacogenomics
Pharmacist
Division of Clinical Pharmacology and
Toxicology
The Hospital for Sick Children;
Assistant Professor
Department of Paediatrics
Temerty Faculty of Medicine
University of Toronto
Toronto, Ontario, Canada

Ronald Doron Cohn, MD, FACMG
President and CEO
Senior Scientist
The Hospital for Sick Children;
Professor
Department of Paediatrics and Molecular Genetics
University of Toronto
Toronto, Ontario, Canada

Jill A. Fahrner, MD, PhD
Director
Epigenetics and Chromatin Clinic;
Assistant Professor of Genetic Medicine and
Pediatrics
Johns Hopkins School of Medicine
Baltimore, Maryland, USA

Amy Finch, PhD, CGC
Post-Doctoral Fellow
Women's College Research Institute
Toronto, Ontario, Canada

Peter St George-Hyslop, OC, MD, FRCPC, FRS
Professor of Experimental Neuroscience
Cambridge Neuroscience
University of Cambridge
Cambridge, United Kingdom

Ashima Gulati, MD, PhD
Attending Nephrologist
Children's National Hospital
Washington, District of Columbia, USA

Kelsey Guthrie, MGC, CGC
Pediatric Genetic Counselor
The Johns Hopkins University School of Medicine
Baltimore, Maryland, USA

Robert Hamilton, MD, FRCPC
Department of Paediatrics
Hospital for Sick Children (SickKids)
Toronto, Ontario Canada

Ada Hamosh, MD, MPH
Dr. Frank V. Sutland Professor of Pediatric Genetics
McKusick-Nathans Department of Genetic Medicine
and Department of Pediatrics,
Clinical Director
Department of Genetic Medicine,
Scientific Director, OMIM
John Hopkins University
Baltimore, Maryland, USA

Robert A. Hegele, MD, FRCPC, FACP
Distinguished University Professor
Department of Medicine and Biochemistry
Schulich School of Medicine, University of Western
Ontario
London, Ontario, Canada

Johann Hitzler, MD, FRCP(C), FAAP
Professor
Department of Pediatrics
University of Toronto;
Division of Hematology/Oncology
The Hospital for Sick Children;
Senior Scientist
Developmental and Stem Cell Biology
The Hospital for Sick Children Research Institute
Toronto, Ontario, Canada

Julie Hoover-Fong, MD, PhD, FACMG
Professor
Department of Genetic Medicine
Johns Hopkins University
Baltimore, Maryland, USA

Alexander Y. Kim, MD
Medical Biochemical Geneticist
Division of Genetics
Department of Pediatric Medicine
Johns Hopkins All Children's Hospital
Saint Petersburg, Maryland, USA

Paul Kruszka, MD, MPH
Chief Medical Officer
Department of Medical Affairs
GeneDx
Gaithersburg, Maryland, USA

David Lillicrap, MD, FRCPC
Professor
Department of Pathology and Molecular Medicine
Queen's University
Kingston, Ontario, Canada

James R. Lupski, MD, PhD, DSc (Hon)
Cullen Professor of Genetics and Genomics and
Professor of Pediatrics
Baylor College of Medicine
Houston, Texas, USA

Farid Mahmud, MD, FRCPC
Staff Physician
Division of Endocrinology
The Hospital for Sick Children and University of
Toronto
Toronto, Ontario, Canada

David Malkin, MD, FRCPC, FRSC
CIBC Children's Foundation Chair in Child Health
Research
Staff Oncologist and Director, Cancer Genetics
Program
Division of Hematology/Oncology,
Senior Scientist, Genetics and Genome Biology
Program
The Hospital for Sick Children;
Department of Pediatrics
University of Toronto
Toronto, Ontario, Canada

Ashwin Mallipatna, MD
Head of Retinoblastoma Program
Hospital for Sick Children;
Assistant Professor
Department of Ophthalmology and Vision
Sciences
University of Toronto
Toronto, Ontario, Canada

Donna Martin, MD, PhD
Chair
Department of Pediatrics,
Professor of Pediatrics and Human Genetics
Ravitz Foundation Endowed Professor of
Pediatrics
The University of Michigan
Ann Arbor, Michigan, USA

Kristen Miller, MSPH, DrPH
Scientific Director
National Center for Human Factors in Healthcare
MedStar Health;
Associate Professor
Department of Emergency Medicine
Georgetown University School of Medicine
Washington, District of Columbia, USA

Weiyi Mu, ScM
Assistant Professor of Genetic Medicine
Johns Hopkins University
Baltimore, Maryland, USA

Steven Narod, MD, FRCPC, FRSC
Senior Scientist
Women's College Research Institute
Toronto, Ontario, Canada

Isaac Odame, MB ChB, MRCP (UK), FRCPCH,
FRCPath, FRCPC
Haematology Section Head
Division of Haematology/Oncology,
Professor
Department of Paediatrics,
Faculty of Medicine
University of Toronto;
Director
Division of Haematology
Departments of Medicine and Paediatrics
University of Toronto
Toronto, Ontario, Canada

Christopher A. Ours, MD, MHS
Assistant Research Physician
National Human Genome Research Institute
National Institutes of Health
Bethesda, Maryland, USA

Christopher Pearson, PhD
Senior Scientist
Department of Genetics and Genome Biology,
Professor
Department of Molecular Genetics
The Hospital for Sick Children
Toronto, Ontario, Canada

Xiao P. Peng, MD, PhD
Director
Genetics of Blood and Immunity Clinic;
Clinical Advisor
JHG DNA Diagnostics Lab;
Assistant Professor
Department of Genetic Medicine
Johns Hopkins University School of Medicine
Baltimore, Maryland, USA

Karen Raraigh, MGC
Certified Genetic Counselor
McKusick-Nathans Department of Genetic Medicine
Johns Hopkins University
Baltimore, Maryland, USA

Heidi L. Rehm, PhD, FACMG
Professor of Pathology
Center for Genomic Medicine
Massachusetts General Hospital and Harvard Medical
School;
Co-Director
Medical and Population Genetics
Broad Institute of MIT and Harvard Medical;
Clinical Laboratory Director
Broad Clinical Labs
Boston, Massachusetts, USA

Miriam Reuter, MD
Senior Scientific Manager
CGEn, The Hospital for Sick Children
Toronto, Ontario, Canada

Maian Roifman, MD
Clinical Geneticist
Division of Clinical and Metabolic Genetics
Department of Pediatrics
The Hospital for Sick Children, University of Toronto;
Clinical Geneticist
The Prenatal Diagnosis and Medical Genetics Program
Department of Obstetrics and Gynecology
Mount Sinai Hospital
Toronto, Ontario, Canada

Chaim M. Roifman, MD, FRCPC, FCACB
Director, Canadian Centre for Primary
Immunodeficiency
Director, Fellowship Program in Immunology/Allergy
Director, Fellowship Program in Immunodeficiency and
Transplantation
Staff Physician, Immunology and Allergy, Department
of Paediatrics
Hospital for Sick Children;
Senior Scientist, Molecular Medicine
Hospital for Sick Children Research Institute;
Professor of Paediatrics and Immunology
University of Toronto
Toronto, Ontario, Canada

Krista Schatz, MS, CGC
Certified Genetic Counselor
Department of Genetic Medicine
Johns Hopkins University School of Medicine
Baltimore, Maryland, USA

Eric Shoubridge, PhD, FRSC
Professor and Chair
Department of Human Genetics
The Neuro (Montreal Neurological Institute-Hospital)
McGill University
Montreal, Quebec, Canada

Mandeep Singh, MBBS, MD, PhD
Associate Professor of Ophthalmology
Wilmer Eye Institute
Johns Hopkins University
Baltimore, Maryland, USA

David Skuse, MD, FRCP, FRCPsych, FRCPCH
Professor
Great Ormond Street Institute of Child Health
University College London
London, United Kingdom

Marisa Gilstrop Thompson, BA, MD
Physician
Gynecology and Obstetrics - Maternal Fetal Medicine
Johns Hopkins Hospital
Baltimore, Maryland, USA

Cynthia J. Tifft, MD, PhD
Deputy Clinical Director
Office of the Clinical Director,
Senior Clinician
Medical Genetics Branch,
Head
Glycosphingolipid Disorders Unit
Pediatric Undiagnosed Diseases Program
National Human Genome Research Institute
Bethesda, Maryland, USA

Christopher B. Toomey, MD, PhD
Assistant Professor of Ophthalmology
Shiley Eye Institute, Viterbi Family Department of
Ophthalmology
UC San Diego
La Jolla, California, USA

Jacob A.S. Vorstman, MD, PhD
Professor
Department of Psychiatry
University of Toronto;
SickKids Psychiatry Associates Chair in Developmental
Psychopathology,
Senior Scientist
Genetics and Genome Biology Program
Sickkids Research Institute;
Department of Psychiatry
The Hospital for Sick Children
Toronto, Ontario, Canada

Terry J. Watnick, MD
Joan B. and John H. Sadler, MD Professor of
Nephrology
University of Maryland, School of Medicine
Baltimore, Maryland, USA

Rosanna Weksberg, MD, PhD
Senior Associate Scientist
Genetics and Genome Biology Program
Research Institute, The Hospital for Sick Children,
Clinical Geneticist
Division of Clinical and Metabolic Genetics
The Hospital for Sick Children;
Professor
Department of Molecular Genetics
Institute of Medical Science;
Department of Paediatrics
University of Toronto
Toronto, Ontario, Canada

Jeanne Wolstencroft, PhD
Great Ormond Street Institute of Child Health
University College London
London, United Kingdom

Changrui Xiao, MD
Assistant Clinical Professor, Neurology
School of Medicine
University of California
Irvine, California, USA

Shira G. Ziegler, MD, PhD
McKusick-Nathans Department of Genetic Medicine
Johns Hopkins University School of Medicine
Baltimore, Maryland, USA

We agreed somewhat reluctantly to take on the assignment to be three new editors for the 9th Edition of the acclaimed *Genetics in Medicine*, which has been in circulation since 1966. Our hesitancy had nothing to do with a looming pandemic, about to throw up major obstacles (work and life) along the way. Nor did it have to do with the scope of work sure to be involved. Our uncertainty really had to do with doubts that we could ever deliver a book to the standards of the founding authors, James S. Thompson (1919-1982) (Editions 1-3) and Margaret W. Thompson ("Peggy") (1920-2014) (Editions 1-5), and their successors (Editions 6-8), Roderick McInnes (Edition 5 with Peggy Thompson) and later Editions 6-8), Robert Nussbaum (Editions 6-8), and Huntington Willard (Editions 5-8). We also worried how we three alone could cover the immense body of literature in medical genetics and genomics that had arisen over the period since the 8th Edition was released.

We took the time-tested approach of "standing on shoulders", changing little of the book's well-covered and well-written core principles of medical genetics. Technologies have been more of an evolving component. When we did make edits, we drew from our own knowledge in the field, scrutinized the literature and databases (some of which we oversee), and consulted experts. Even as we ourselves had done, some of these experts had contributed to earlier editions, but for many it was a new experience. The expressions of gratitude at being asked to be part of the initiative spoke to the status this book still holds in the professional community. For the first time, we credit these contributions through co-authorship or specific acknowledgement—something we thought was right to do. At the same time, we and they acknowledge the foundations laid out by the contributors to earlier editions.

To this version of what the field endearingly calls "Thompson and Thompson", we have amended some evolving content, including: (1) moving from the study of genes to genomes in biology and testing, (2) increasing awareness of copy number and structural genomic variation in both the population and medical genomic context, (3) novel discoveries and application of the functional roles of non-coding RNAs, chromatin-regulation and epigenetics, and how their dysregulation can affect gene expression in disease, (4) genetic variation in worldwide populations, (5) latest technologies (e.g., genome sequencing) and statistical/informatics approaches, such as polygenic risk scores, used to resolve and interpret them, and (6) the many new genetic diagnoses arising

from application of these new principles and technologies (for example, genomic syndromes and ciliopathies). Each chapter still closes with questions that challenge the reader to consolidate the material into practice, perhaps in preparation for exams, along with comprehensive answers.

The highly popular Clinical Cases—first introduced in the sixth edition to demonstrate the general principles of inheritance, pathogenesis, diagnosis, management, and counseling—were entirely updated or expanded with input from yet more experts. They capture the challenges of variable expression, pleiotropy, and complex disorders as they present to medical genetics practitioners in the field.

We are most proud of our efforts to portray this edition of *Genetics in Medicine*, now *Genetics and Genomics in Medicine* through the lens of a society that has changed drastically in how it accesses, interprets, and communicates information. Simply put, genetics is an information science: the DNA, RNA and proteins, and their networks and combinations, underlie our biology in health and disease. We made every attempt to capture the new knowledge from beyond the central dogma, but perhaps more importantly, we strove to contextualize the information as both medicine and society now want it to be applied.

For example, to update some of the illustrations of genetic conditions, we asked the not-for-profit organization, *Positive Exposure*, to contribute photographs from their portfolio of volunteers. The organization works with various genetics support groups to present individuals living with their genetic differences in ways that are respectful, inclusive, and frankly beautiful. Where names are used, it is at their request. We also incorporated updated guidelines for language and terminology, notably for words such as race, ethnicity, polymorphism, and mutation (the term "mutation" at time of writing was used ~590 times in this edition and over 1000 in the last!). We also included new sections describing the use (and need for) genetic information in the study of unique indigenous and founder populations. The publishers have also continued to enhance the accompanying eBook version which by expanding the search options of all the text, figures, and references on a variety of devices

As stated by our editorial predecessors, "*any medical genetic counseling student, advanced undergraduate, graduate student in genetics or genomics, resident in any field of clinical medicine, practicing physician, or allied medical professional in nursing or physical therapy should find this book to be a thorough but not exhaustive (or exhausting!) presentation of the fundamentals of human genetics and genomics as applied to health and disease*".

We gratefully acknowledge Dr. Janet Buchanan (PhD, FCCMG) who helped us in all aspects of development, editing and writing of the book. Having been tutored by Peggy Thompson for exam preparation, she ensured that all of us involved lived up the high standards established by her mentor. We also thank Jennifer Howe, Jo-Anne Herbrick, Allison Gignac and Dr. Richard Wintle for proofing final versions of the book.

We wish to dedicate this book to the millions of people around the world who succumbed to the SARS-CoV-2 RNA coronavirus that ravaged and continues to ravage the earth, while we tried to focus our attention to the very different task of this book. We also acknowledge the front-line health workers, diagnostic laboratory personnel, and researchers—some of whom also pivoted to co-author this book—whose efforts have left the rest of us in a better place.

In the end, even genetic data of the highest quality still need to be interpreted and applied in the best possible way to benefit the patient, the family, and society. If we get the presentation right, as we hope we did in this 9th Edition, we may retain the respect of those who follow us, having learned from the communication of our experiences (and perhaps some wisdom). In such a rapidly evolving field as medical genetics and genomics, however, we recognize the need to update this book again soon.

Ronald D. Cohn, MD
Stephen W. Scherer, PhD
Ada Hamosh, MD

Contents

Clinical Cases

Abbreviations

1000GP, 1000 Genomes Project

2D/3D/4D, two-dimensional/three-dimensional/
four-dimensional

AAVs, adeno-associated viruses

ACAT, A:cholesterol acyltransferase

ACMG, American College of Medical Genetics and
Genomics

ACOG, American College of Obstetricians and
Gynecologists

AD, autosomal dominant

AD, Alzheimer disease

ADA, adenosine deaminase

ADHD, attention-deficit hyperactivity disorder

AFAFP, amniotic fluid α-fetoprotein

AFP, α-fetoprotein

AHH, aryl hydrocarbon hydroxylase

AI, artificial intelligence

AIMs, ancestry informative markers

AIP, acute intermittent porphyria

A1AT, α1-Antitrypsin

ALA, δ-aminolevulinic acid

AMD, age-related macular degeneration

AML, acute myeloid leukemia

AMP, American Molecular Pathology

APOE, apolipoprotein E

AR, androgen receptor

AR, autosomal recessive

ART, assisted reproductive technologies

AS, Angelman syndrome

ASD, autism spectrum disorder

ASO, antisense oligonucleotide

AZF, azoospermia factors

βAPP, β-amyloid precursor protein

BCG, bacillus Calmette-Guérin

BEFAHRS, Beck-Fahrner syndrome

BH$_4$, tetrahydrobiopterin

β-hCG, human chorionic gonadotropin β subunit

BMD, Becker muscular dystrophy

BMI, body mass index

bp, base pair

CAD, coronary artery disease

CAH, congenital adrenal hyperplasia

CBAVD, congenital bilateral absence of the vas deferens

CBP, CREBB-binding protein

CCMG, Canadian College of Medical Geneticists

CDM1, congenital myotonic dystrophy

cDNA, copy of the mRNA; complementary DNA

CDG, congenital disorders of glycosylation

CES, cat-eye syndrome

CF, cystic fibrosis

CFH, complement factor H

CFTR, cystic fibrosis transmembrane conductance
regulator

CGD, complete gonadal dysgenesis

CGH, comparative genomic hybridization (also
array-CGH)

CHD, congenital heart defect

CI, confidence interval

CL, cleft lip

CL(P), cleft lip without a palate

cM, centimorgans

CMA, chromosome microarray analysis

CML, chronic myelogenous leukemia

CMMRD, constitutional mismatch repair deficiency

CNS, central nervous system

CNV, copy number variation (or variants)

CODIS, Combined DNA Index System

CPIC, Clinical Pharmacogenetics Implementation
Consortium

CPM, confined placental mosaicism

CREBBP, CREB-binding protein

CRISPR, *c*lustered *r*egularly *i*nterspaced *s*hort *p*alindromic *r*epeats

CSS, Coffin-Siris syndrome

CVS, chorionic villus sampling

CVT, cerebral vein thrombosis

dbSNP, Single Nucleotide Polymorphism Database

dbVar, Structural Variation Database

DGC, dystrophin glycoprotein complex

DGS, DiGeorge syndrome

DM1/2, myotonic dystrophy 1/2

DMD, Duchenne muscular dystrophy

DMR, differentially methylated region

DNA, Deoxyribonucleic Acid

DNAm, DNA methylation

DOHaD, developmental origins of health and disease

DPWG, Royal Dutch Association for the Advancement
of Pharmacy–Pharmacogenetic Working Group

DRP1, dynamin-related protein 1

DS, deletion syndrome

DSBs, double-strand breaks

DSDs, disorders of sex development

DTC, direct-to-consumer

DVT, deep venous thrombosis

DZ, dizygotic

EGFR, epidermal growth factor receptor

ENCODE Project, *Enc*yclopedia *of D*NA *E*lements
ER, endoplasmic reticulum
ERT, enzyme replacement therapy
ES, exome sequencing
ESN, Esan in Nigeria
EUR, European ancestry
EWAS, epigenome-wide association analysis
FAP, familial adenomatous polyposis
FBI, Federal Bureau of Investigation
FDA, US Food and Drug Administration
FEV$_1$, forced expiratory volume after 1 second
FISH, fluorescence in situ hybridization
FMRP, fragile X mental retardation protein
FoSTeS, fork stalling or template switching
FVL, factor V Leiden
FXTAS, fragile X tremor/ataxia syndrome
GALT, galactose-1-phosphate uridyltransferase
GCPS, Greig cephalopolysyndactyly syndrome
GDC, Genomic Data Commons
GDPR, General Data Protection Regulation
GENIE, Genomics Evidence Neoplasia Information Exchange
GF2, insulin-like growth factor 2
GINA, Genetic Information Nondiscrimination Act
GnomAD, Genome Aggregation Database
GTP, guanosine triphosphate
GWAS, genome-wide association studies
Hb F, fetal hemoglobin
Hb A, adult hemoglobin
hCG, human chorionic gonadotropin
HD, Huntington disease
HDAC, histone deacetylase
HDR, homology-directed repair
HELLP, *h*emolysis, *e*levated *l*iver enzymes, and *l*ow *p*latelets
HER2, human epidermal growth factor receptor 2
hESCs, human embryonic stem cells
HGSVC, Human Genome Structural Variation Consortium
HIPAA, Health Insurance Portability and Accountability Act
Histone types: H2A, H2B, H3, and H4
HLA, human leukocyte antigen
hmC, hydroxymethylcytosine
HMG CoA, 3-hydroxy-3-methylglutaryl coenzyme A
HOX, homeobox (gene)
HPFH, hereditary persistence of fetal hemoglobin
HSCs, hematopoietic stem cells
HSCR, Hirschsprung disease
HSCR-L, Hirschsprung disease with a long aganglionic segment
HSCR-S, Hirschsprung disease with a short aganglionic segment
HSPCs, hematopoietic stem and progenitor cells
HSRs, hypersensitivity reactions
HWE, Hardy-Weinberg equilibrium
H3K4me2, dimethylation of histone H3 at lysine 4
H3K4me3, trimethylation of histone H3 at lysine 4

H3K9 methylation, histone H3 methylated at lysine position 9
H3K27acetylation, histone H3 acetylated at lysine position 27
IAP, intracisternal A-particle
IBD, identical by descent
IBS, identical by state
IC, imprinting center
IDDM, insulin dependent diabetes mellitus
IGSR, International Genome Sample Resource
iPSCs, induced pluripotent stem cells
IVF, in vitro fertilization
1KG, 1000 Genomes
KS, Kabuki syndrome
LCA, Leber congenital amaurosis
LCR, locus control region
LD, linkage disequilibrium
LDL, low-density lipoprotein
LFS, Li-Fraumeni syndrome
LHON, Leber hereditary optic neuropathy
LINE, long interspersed nuclear element
LINE-1, long interspersed element 1
lncRNA, long noncoding RNA
LOD, logarithm of the odds
LOH, loss of heterozygosity
LR, long-read
LS, Lynch syndrome
MAF, minor allele frequency
Mb, megabase pair (million base pairs)
MBD, methyl-CpG-binding domain
mC, methylcytosine
MCAD, medium-chain acyl-CoA dehydrogenase
MCC, maternal cell contamination
MeCP2, methyl-CpG-binding protein 2
MELAS, mitochondrial encephalomyopathy with lactic acidosis and stroke-like episodes
MEN2A, multiple endocrine neoplasia, type 2A
MEN2B, multiple endocrine neoplasia, type 2B
MH, microhomology
MHC, major histocompatibility complex
MI, myocardial infarction
miRNA, microRNA
MLID, multilocus imprinting disorder
MLPA, Multiplex Ligation-Dependent Probe Amplification
MMA, methylmalonic acidemia
MMBIR, microhomology-mediated break-induced replication
MME, Matchmaker Exchange
MMR, mismatch repair
MODY, maturity-onset diabetes of the young
MoM, multiples of the median
MOMS, Management of Myelomeningocele Study
MRCA, most recent common ancestor
MRI, magnetic resonance imaging
mRNA, messenger RNA
MS, multiple sclerosis

MSAFP, maternal serum α-fetoprotein
MSI+, microsatellite instability-positive
MSL, Mende in Sierra Leone
MSMD, mendelian susceptibility to mycobacterial disease
MLPA, multiple ligation-dependent probe amplification
mtDNA, mitochondrial genome DNA
MZ, monozygotic
NAHR, nonallelic homologous recombination
NCBRS, Nicolaides-Baraitser syndrome
ncRNA, noncoding RNA
NF1, neurofibromatosis type 1
NGS, next generation sequencing
NHEJ, nonhomologous end joining
NIDDM, non–insulin dependent diabetes mellitus
NIPS, noninvasive prenatal screening
NIPT, noninvasive prenatal testing
NMD, nonsense-mediated mRNA decay
NPV, negative predictive value
NT, nuchal translucency
NTD, neural tube defect
OI, osteogenesis imperfecta
OMIM, *Online Mendelian Inheritance in Man*
OR, odds ratio
OR, olfactory receptor
PAGE, Population Architecture Using Genomics and
    Epidemiology
PAGN, phenylacetylglutamine
PAH, phenylalanine hydroxylase
PAPP-A, pregnancy-associated plasma protein A
PARP, poly-ADP ribose polymerase
PBG, porphobilinogen
PC, principal component
PCA, principal component analysis
PCGP, Pediatric Cancer Genome Project
PCR, polymerase chain reaction
PD, Parkinson disease
PEG, polyethylene glycol
PGC, Psychiatric Genomics Consortium
PGD, preimplantation genetic diagnosis
PGL, paraganglioma
PGT, preimplantation genetic testing
PGT-A, preimplantation genetic testing aneuploidy
PGT-M, preimplantation genetic testing for monogenic
    disorders
PGT-SR, preimplantation genetic testing structural
    rearrangements
PKU, phenylketonuria
PML, promyelocytic leukemia
PMP22, peripheral myelin protein 22
POAD, postaxial acrofacial dysostosis
POLG, polymerase γ
PPV, positive predictive value
PRS, polygenic risk score
PTC, premature termination codon
PWS, Prader-Willi syndrome
RB1, retinoblastoma (gene)
RNA, Ribonucleic Acid

ROH, region of homozygosity
RNAi, RNA interference
rRNA, ribosomal RNA
RP, retinitis pigmentosa
RPE, retinal pigment epithelium
RR, relative risk
RTS, Rubinstein-Taybi syndrome
RUSP, Recommended Universal Screening Panel
SCAD, short-chain acyl-CoA dehydrogenase
SCD, sickle cell disease
SCID, severe combined immunodeficiency
scRNAseq, single-cell RNA sequencing technologies
SD, segmental duplication
SD, standard deviation
SHH, Sonic hedgehog
SINE, short interspersed element
siRNA, small interfering RNAs
SJS, Stevens-Johnson syndrome\
SMA, spinal muscular atrophy
SMN, survival motor neuron
snoRNA, small nucleolar RNA
SNP, single nucleotide polymorphism
SNV, single nucleotide variant
SR, short-read
SR, structural rearrangements
STR, short tandem repeat
SV, structural variant
T1D, type 1 diabetes; also IDDM, insulin dependent
    diabetes mellitus
T2D, type 2 diabetes; also NIDDM, non–insulin
    dependent diabetes mellitus
TAD, topologically associating domain
TBRS, Tatton-Brown-Rahman syndrome
TDT, transfusion-dependent β-thalassemia
TEN, toxic epidermal necrolysis
TGFβ, transforming growth factor β
TGFβ1, transforming growth factor β1
TMS, tandem mass spectrometry
tRNA, transfer RNA
TSG, tumor suppressor gene
U, uracil
UBE3A, ubiquitin-protein ligase E3A gene
uE3, unconjugated estriol
UPD, uniparental disomy
UTR, untranslated region
VCFS, velocardiofacial syndrome
VNTR, variable number of tandem repeats
VUS, variant of uncertain significance
WBS, Williams-Beuren syndrome
WGS, whole genome sequencing
WHO, World Health Organization
WWII, World War II
Xi, inactive X
XIC, X inactivation center
XIST, inactive X [Xi]–specific transcripts
XXX, triple X syndrome

CHAPTER 1

Introduction

Ada Hamosh • Stephen W. Scherer • Ronald Doron Cohn

THE BIRTH AND DEVELOPMENT OF GENETICS AND GENOMICS

It may surprise students today to learn that an appreciation of the role of genetics in medicine dates back to the recognition by Archibald Garrod and others, in the early 20th century, that Mendel's laws of inheritance could explain the recurrence of certain clinical disorders in families. During the ensuing years, with developments in molecular biology, the field of medical genetics grew from a small clinical subspecialty concerned with a handful of rare hereditary disorders to a recognized medical specialty whose concepts and approaches are integral to diagnosis and management across the spectrum of disease.

At the dawn of the 21st century, the international **Human Genome Project** generated a virtually complete **sequence** of human DNA—our **genome** (the suffix *-ome* coming from the Greek for "all" or "complete"). This now serves as the foundation of efforts to catalogue all human genes (both DNA and RNA based), understand their structure and regulation, determine the extent of their variation in different populations, and uncover how **genetic** variation contributes to disease. Driven by advances in technology and analytics and the ensuing databases, the human genome of any individual can now be studied in its entirety (**genomics**) rather than one **gene** at a time (genetics). This paradigm shift of testing "genome first"—compared to gene (or gene panel) or **phenotype** first—arises often throughout the remaining chapters in this book. In the research realm there are already more than 1 million human genome sequences completed; we predict by the next edition of this book, or sooner, whole **genome sequencing** will be fully adopted as the first-tier diagnostic test for most heritable conditions.

GENETICS AND GENOMICS IN MEDICINE
The Practice of Genetics

The medical geneticist is usually a physician who works as part of a team of health care providers, including many other physicians, nurses, laboratory geneticists, genetic counselors, and (more recently) genome informaticists, to evaluate patients for possible hereditary diseases. They characterize the patient's illness through careful history taking and physical examination, assess possible modes of inheritance, arrange for diagnostic testing, develop treatment and surveillance plans, and participate in outreach to other family members at **risk** for the disorder.

However, genetic principles and approaches are not restricted to any one medical specialty or subspecialty; they permeate many, and perhaps all, areas of medicine. We provide 49 case studies of how genetics and genomics are applied to medicine today. For example,

- A psychiatrist, developmental pediatrician, or medical geneticist evaluates a child with autism; **microarray** or genome sequencing reveals the 16p11.2 **microdeletion** associated with a **syndrome** exhibiting variable **expressivity** with diverse outcomes (Case 5).

- A genetic counselor specializing in hereditary breast cancer offers education, testing, interpretation, and support to a young woman with a family history of hereditary breast and ovarian cancer (Case 7).

- A hematologist combines family and medical history with gene panel sequencing of a young adult with deep venous thrombosis to assess the benefits and risks of initiating and maintaining anticoagulant therapy (Case 46).

- An immunologist suspecting a rare **congenital** disorder, including antibody deficiency, uses genome sequencing to reveal compound pathogenic **splicing** variants in the *RNU4ATAC* small nuclear RNA gene, thus confirming a diagnosis of Roifman syndrome (Case 35).

- A teenager with a diagnosis of type 1 diabetes was not doing well on insulin treatment. His mother felt that diabetes "ran in the family," and the local medical team referred them to Genetics, where a multigene sequencing panel for monogenic diabetes revealed a **variant** consistent with maturity-onset diabetes of the young (MODY). With the revised diagnosis, the young man's insulin treatment was discontinued in favor of other low-dose medication, and he was soon back on the soccer field (Case 15).

Categories of Genetic Disease

Virtually any disease is the result of the combined action of genes and environment, but the relative effect of the genetic component may be large or small. Among disorders caused wholly or partly by genetic factors, three main types are recognized: **chromosome** disorders, single-gene disorders, and multifactorial disorders. At the time of writing this chapter (1 May 2022) 7160 phenotypes were catalogued as caused by variants in 4629 genes. Many others remain to be defined. There have also been phenomenal advances in cataloguing genetic variation in online databases, to be used in **genotype** and phenotype correlations; we point to many of the most-used ones throughout the book.

In **chromosome disorders**, the defect is due not to a single alteration in the genetic blueprint but to a change in dosage of genes located on entire **chromosomes** or chromosome segments. For example, an extra copy (**trisomy**) of chromosome 21 underlies a specific disorder, Down syndrome, even though no individual gene on that chromosome is abnormal. Duplication or **deletion** of smaller segments of chromosomes—called copy number variations (CNVs), ranging in size from submicroscopic to a few percent of a chromosome's length—can cause complex birth defects such as 22q11.2 deletion syndrome or isolated phenotypes such as autism without obvious physical abnormalities. Along with 22q11.2 deletion syndrome, a list of identified recurrent genomic disorders is growing. These arise frequently due to illegitimate recombination catalyzed by flanking duplicated repeat segments; the resulting CNVs involving genes are associated with multiple phenotypes (see Chapter 6). As a group, chromosome disorders are common, with a prevalence of 3% in liveborn infants and accounting for approximately half of all spontaneous losses within the first trimester of pregnancy. These types of disorders are discussed in Chapter 6.

Monogenic disorders are caused by pathogenic mutations in individual genes. The resulting variants may be present on both chromosomes of a pair (one of paternal and one of maternal origin) or on only one chromosome of a pair (matched with a normal copy of that gene on the other copy of that chromosome). Single-gene defects, also called **mendelian** conditions, often cause diseases that follow one of the classic inheritance patterns in families (autosomal recessive, autosomal **dominant**, or X linked). In a few cases, the **mutation** occurs in the mitochondrial rather than in the nuclear genome. In any case, the cause is a critical error in the genetic information carried by a single gene. Monogenic disorders, such as cystic fibrosis (**Case 12**), Huntington disease (**Case 24**), or Marfan syndrome (**Case 30**), usually exhibit obvious and characteristic **pedigree** patterns. Most such defects are rare, with a frequency that may be as high as 1 in 500 to 1000 individuals but is usually much less. Although individually rare,

monogenic disorders as a group are responsible for a significant proportion of disease and death. Overall, the incidence of serious monogenic disorders in the pediatric population has been estimated to be approximately 1 per 300 liveborn infants; over an entire lifetime, the prevalence of these disorders is 1 in 50. They are discussed in Chapter 7.

Multifactorial disease with **complex inheritance** encompasses most diseases in which there is a genetic contribution. The category is characterized by increased incidence of disease in identical twins or other close relatives of affected individuals, compared to that in the general population, yet the family history does not fit the inheritance patterns typical of monogenic disorders. Multifactorial diseases include congenital malformations—such as Hirschsprung disease, cleft lip and palate, or congenital heart defects—as well as many common disorders of adult life—such as breast and ovarian cancer (**Case 7**), diabetes and inflammatory bowel disease (**Case 11**). There appears to be no single pathogenic genetic variant in many of these conditions. Rather, disease results from the combined impact of variants in many different genes; each variant may cause, protect from, or predispose to a serious defect, often in concert with or triggered by environmental factors. Estimates of the impact of multifactorial disease range from 5% in the pediatric population to more than 60% in the entire population. Aspects of qualitative and quantitative traits, relative risks, and heritability are the subjects of Chapter 9.

Another remarkable expansion is our understanding of the regulation of gene expression and the role of epigenetics in rare monogenic conditions, in common complex diseases, and in cancer (see Chapter 8).

EVOLUTION OF GENETICS IN MEDICINE

In the 6 years since the previous edition of this book, our understanding of the role of genetics in medicine has increased dramatically. Sometimes genetic interpretations have become clearer with enhanced knowledge, but not always. Terms such as **variant of uncertain significance**, variable expression, **penetrance**, and **pleiotropy** prevail, reflecting the residual challenges. There are still roughly 20,000 protein-coding genes, but many more of their transcriptional isoforms are now characterized, and an equal number of noncoding RNA genes and regulatory elements must also be considered. To capture all of these, the medical geneticist now regularly relies on **genome-wide testing**, sometimes sequencing of the whole genome. The genome reference build (most recent sequence) used for comparison has already changed twice in less than a decade. Indeed, these newer reference genomes and the accompanying population genomic databases better capture the extent of sequence-level and structural variation used in medical genetic interpretations; we discuss their use.

As an adaptation to changing norms, we have endeavored to update certain terminology for this edition. The rationale is that the terms *mutation* and *polymorphism* have gradually taken on meanings that can be ambiguous, value laden, or confusing. Instead, *variant* is more neutral and can be readily modified for precision and clarity. Thus we generally limit use of *mutation* to a genetic change that gives rise to heritable variation or to the process by which such change arises. Polymorphism refers to having two or more alleles at one **locus**, each with appreciable frequency. The outcome of mutation is a variant, which may have any number of characteristics, such as pathogenic (disease causing), loss of function, exonic, common, of uncertain significance, etc. Judicious use of relevant modifiers for *variant* is an essential part of the transition; some existing nomenclature remains entrenched.

We have also tried to emphasize the need for dignity, inclusion, respect, and privacy in genetics practice. To such ends, we have (respectively) updated picture formats of individuals with genetic conditions, undertaken new discussion of the importance of studies of diverse populations, been mindful of our word choices in reference to individuals and groups, and advocated proper delivery of genetic information through **genetic counseling**.

This introduction to the ever-evolving language and concepts of human and medical genetics, along with appreciation of the genetic and genomic perspectives on health and disease, will serve to frame the lifelong learning that comprises every health professional's career.

CHAPTER 2

Introduction to the Human Genome

Ada Hamosh • Stephen W. Scherer

Understanding the organization, variation, and transmission of the human **genome** is central to appreciating the role of genetics in medicine, as well as the emerging principles of genomic and individualized medicine. With the availability of the **sequence** of the human genome and a growing awareness of the role of genome variation in disease, it is now possible to begin to interpret the impact of that variation on human health on a broad scale. The comparison of individual genomes underscores the first major take-home lesson of this book—*every individual has a unique constitution of gene products, produced in response to the combined inputs of the genome sequence and one's particular set of environmental exposures and experiences.* As pointed out in the previous chapter, this realization reflects what Garrod termed "**chemical individuality**" over a century ago and provides a conceptual foundation for the practice of genomic and individualized medicine.

Advances in genome technology and the resulting explosion in knowledge and information stemming from the **Human Genome Project** are thus playing an increasingly transformational role in integrating and applying concepts and discoveries in genetics to the practice of medicine.

THE HUMAN GENOME AND THE CHROMOSOMAL BASIS OF HEREDITY

Appreciation of the importance of genetics to medicine requires an understanding of the nature of the hereditary material, how it is packaged into the human genome, and how it is transmitted from cell to cell during cell division and from generation to generation during reproduction. The human genome consists of large amounts of the chemical **deoxyribonucleic acid (DNA)** that contains within its structure the **genetic** information needed to specify all aspects of embryogenesis, development, growth, metabolism, and reproduction—essentially all aspects of what makes a human being a functional organism. Every nucleated cell in the body carries its own copy of the human genome, which contains, depending on how one defines the term, approximately 20,000 to 50,000 **genes** (see Box 2.1). Genes,

BOX 2.1 CHROMOSOME AND GENOME ANALYSIS IN CLINICAL MEDICINE

Chromosome and genome analysis has become important diagnostic procedures in clinical medicine. As described more fully in subsequent chapters, these applications include the following:
- *Clinical diagnosis.* Numerous medical conditions, including some that are common, are associated with changes in chromosome number or structure and require chromosome or genome analysis for diagnosis and **genetic counseling** (see Chapters 5 and 6).
- *Disease gene identification.* A major goal of medical genetics and genomics today is the identification of the role of specific genes in health and disease. This topic is referred to repeatedly but is discussed in detail in Chapter 11.
- *Cancer genomics.* Genomic and chromosomal changes in **somatic cells** are involved in the initiation and progression of many types of cancer (see Chapter 16).
- *Disease treatment.* Understanding the exact molecular basis of each individual's monogenic disorder allows for targeted therapies to address the condition (see Chapter 14).
- *Prenatal diagnosis.* Chromosome and genome analysis are essential procedures in prenatal diagnosis (see Chapter 18).

which at this point we consider simply and most broadly as functional units of genetic information, are encoded in the DNA of the genome, organized into a number of rod-shaped organelles called **chromosomes** in the nucleus of each cell. The influence of genes and genetics on states of health and disease is profound, and its roots are found in the information encoded in the DNA that makes up the human genome.

Each species has a characteristic chromosome complement (**karyotype**) in terms of the number, morphology, and content of the chromosomes that make up its genome. The genes are in linear order along the chromosomes, each gene having a precise position or **locus**. A **gene map** is the map of the genomic location of the genes and is characteristic of each species and the individuals within a species.

The study of chromosomes, their structure, and their inheritance is called **cytogenetics**. The science of human cytogenetics dates from 1956, when it was first established that the normal human chromosome number is 46. Since that time, much has been learned about human chromosomes, their normal structure and composition, and the identity of the genes that they contain, as well as their numerous and varied abnormalities.

With the exception of cells that develop into **gametes** (the **germline**), all cells that contribute to one's body are called **somatic cells** (*soma*, "body"). The genome contained in the nucleus of human somatic cells consists of 46 chromosomes, made up of 24 different types and arranged in 23 pairs (Fig. 2.1). Of those 23 pairs, 22 are alike in males and females and are called **autosomes**, originally numbered in order of their apparent size from the largest to the smallest. The remaining pair comprises the two different types of **sex chromosomes:** an X and a Y chromosome in males and two **X chromosomes** in females. Central to the concept of the human genome, each chromosome carries a different subset of genes arranged linearly along its DNA (see Box 2.2). Members of a pair of chromosomes (referred to as homologous chromosomes or **homologues**) carry matching genetic information; that is, they typically have the same genes in the same order.

At any specific locus, however, the homologues either may be identical or may vary slightly in sequence; these different forms of a gene are called **alleles**. One member of each pair of chromosomes is inherited from the father, the other from the mother. Normally, the members of a pair of autosomes are microscopically indistinguishable from each other. In females, the sex chromosomes, the two **X chromosomes**, are likewise largely indistinguishable. In males, however, the sex chromosomes differ. One is an X, identical to the Xs of the female, inherited by a male from his mother and transmitted to his daughters; the other, the **Y chromosome**, is inherited from his father and transmitted to his sons. In Chapter 6, as we explore the chromosomal and genomic basis of disease, we will look at some exceptions to the simple and almost universal rule that human biological females are XX and human biological males are XY.

In addition to the nuclear genome, a small but important part of the human genome resides in mitochondria in the cytoplasm (see Fig. 2.1). The mitochondrial chromosome, to be described later in this chapter, has a number of unusual features that distinguish it from the rest of the human genome.

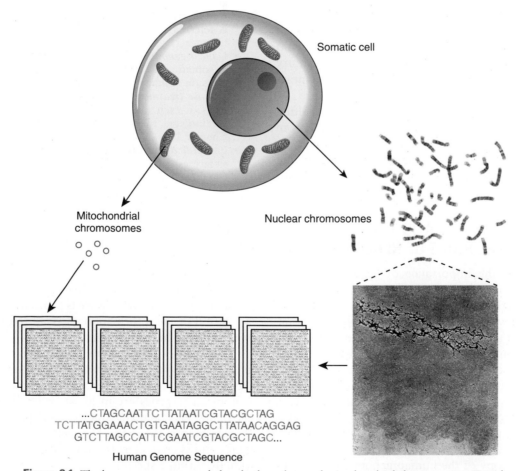

Somatic cell

Mitochondrial chromosomes

Nuclear chromosomes

...CTAGCAATTCTTATAATCGTACGCTAG
TCTTATGGAAACTGTGAATAGGCTTATAACAGGAG
GTCTTAGCCATTCGAATCGTACGCTAGC...

Human Genome Sequence

Figure 2.1 The human genome, encoded on both nuclear and mitochondrial chromosomes. (Based on Brown TA: *Genomes,* ed 2, New York, 2002, Wiley-Liss. Inset from Paulson JR, Laemmli UK: The structure of histone-depleted metaphase chromosomes, *Cell* 12:817–828, 1977. Reprinted with permission of the authors and Cell Press.)

BOX 2.2 GENES IN THE HUMAN GENOME

What is a gene? And how many genes do we have? These questions are more difficult to answer than they might seem.

The word *gene*, first introduced in 1908, has been used in many different contexts since the essential features of heritable "unit characters" were first outlined by Mendel over 150 years ago. To physicians (and indeed to Mendel and other early geneticists), a gene can be defined by its observable impact on an organism and on its statistically determined transmission from generation to generation. To medical geneticists, a gene is recognized clinically in the context of an observable **variant** that leads to a characteristic clinical condition, and today we recognize over 7000 such conditions (see Chapter 7).

The Human Genome Project provided a more systematic basis for delineating human genes, relying on DNA sequence analysis rather than clinical acumen and family studies alone; indeed, this was one of the most compelling rationales for initiating the project in the late 1980s. However, even with the finished sequence product in 2003, it was apparent that our ability to recognize features of the sequence that point to the existence or identity of a gene was sorely lacking. Interpreting the human genome sequence and relating its variation to human biology in both health and disease is thus an ongoing challenge for biomedical research.

Although the ultimate catalogue of human genes remains an elusive target, we recognize two general types of gene, those whose product is a protein and those whose product is a functional **RNA**.

- The number of protein-coding genes—recognized by features in the genome that will be discussed in Chapter 3—is estimated to be somewhere between 20,000 and 25,000. In this book, we typically use approximately 20,000 as the number, and the reader should recognize that this is both imprecise and perhaps an underestimate.
- In addition, however, it has been clear for several decades that the ultimate product of some genes is not a protein at all, but an RNA transcribed from the DNA sequence. There are many different types of such RNA genes (typically called **noncoding genes** to distinguish them from protein-coding genes), and it is currently estimated that there are at least another 20,000 to 25,000 **noncoding RNA** genes around the human genome.

Thus overall—and depending on what one means by the term—the total number of genes in the human genome is on the order of approximately 20,000 to 50,000. However, the reader will appreciate that this remains a moving target, subject to evolving definitions, increases in technological capabilities and analytical precision, advances in informatics and digital medicine, and more complete genome annotation. Recent efforts to complete the sequencing of the highly repetitive **heterochromatin** segments of chromosomes in the centromeres, on the short arms of the **acrocentric** chromosomes, in **segmental duplications** and in subtelomeric and telomeric regions, accounting for 8% of the human genome, has identified 200 million bp of DNA, and thousands of new genes, hundreds of them protein coding.

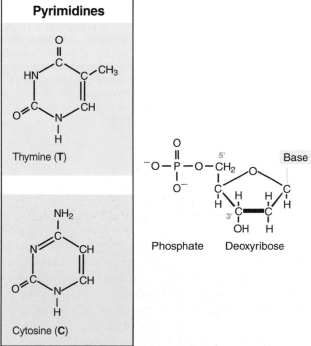

Figure 2.2 **The four bases of DNA and the general structure of a nucleotide in DNA.** Each of the four bases bonds with deoxyribose (through the nitrogen shown in *magenta*) forming a nucleoside which bonds with a phosphate group to form the corresponding nucleotides.

DNA Structure: A Brief Review

Before the organization of the human genome and its chromosomes are considered in detail, it is necessary to review the nature of the DNA that makes up the genome.

DNA is a polymeric nucleic acid macromolecule composed of three types of units: a five-carbon sugar, deoxyribose; a nitrogen-containing base; and a phosphate group (Fig. 2.2). The bases are of two types, **purines** and **pyrimidines**. In DNA, there are two **purine** bases, adenine

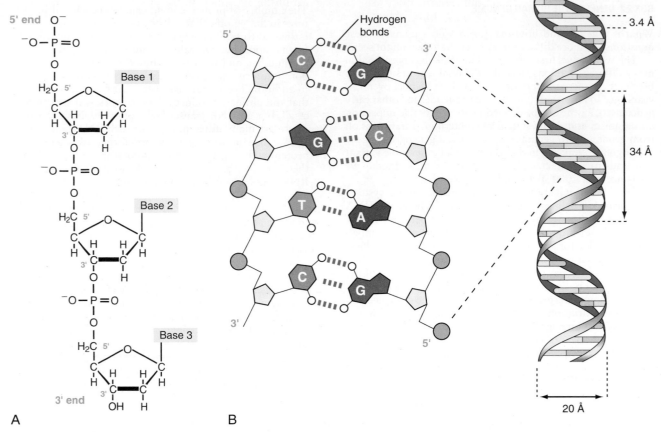

Figure 2.3 **The structure of DNA.** (A) A portion of a DNA polynucleotide chain, showing the 5'-3' phosphodiester bonds that link adjacent nucleotides. (B) The double-helix model of DNA, as proposed by Watson and Crick. The horizontal "rungs" represent the paired bases. The helix is said to be right-handed because the strand going from lower left to upper right crosses over the opposite strand. The detailed portion of the figure illustrates the two complementary strands of DNA, showing the AT and GC base pairs. Note that the orientation of the two strands is antiparallel. (Based on Watson JD, Crick FHC: Molecular structure of nucleic acids: a structure for deoxyribose nucleic acid, *Nature* 171:737–738, 1953.)

(A) and guanine (G), and two **pyrimidine** bases, thymine (T) and cytosine (C). Nucleotides, each composed of a base, a phosphate, and a sugar moiety, polymerize into long polynucleotide chains held together by 5'-3' phosphodiester bonds formed between adjacent deoxyribose units (Fig. 2.3A). In the human genome, these polynucleotide chains exist in the form of a double helix (see Fig. 2.3B) that can be hundreds of millions of nucleotides long in the case of the largest human chromosomes.

The anatomic structure of DNA carries the chemical information that allows the exact transmission of genetic information from one cell to its daughter cells and from one generation to the next. At the same time, the primary structure of DNA specifies the amino acid sequences of the polypeptide chains of proteins, as described in the next chapter. DNA has elegant features that give it these properties. The native state of DNA, as elucidated by James Watson and Francis Crick in 1953, is a double helix (see Fig. 2.3B). The helical structure resembles a right-handed spiral staircase in which its two polynucleotide chains run in opposite directions, held together by hydrogen bonds between

pairs of bases: T of one chain paired with A of the other, and G with C. The specific nature of the genetic information encoded in the human genome lies in the sequence of Cs, As, Gs, and Ts on the two strands of the double helix along each of the chromosomes, both in the nucleus and in mitochondria (see Fig. 2.1). Because of the complementary nature of the two strands of DNA, knowledge of the sequence of **nucleotide** bases on one strand automatically allows one to determine the sequence of bases on the other strand. The double-stranded structure of DNA molecules allows them to replicate precisely by separation of the two strands, followed by synthesis of two new complementary strands, in accordance with the sequence of the original template strands (Fig. 2.4). Similarly, when necessary, the base complementarity allows efficient and correct repair of damaged DNA molecules.

Structure of Human Chromosomes

The composition of genes in the human genome, as well as the determinants of their expression, is specified in the

DNA of the 46 human chromosomes in the nucleus plus the mitochondrial chromosome. *Each human chromosome consists of a single, continuous DNA double helix;* that is, each chromosome is one long, double-stranded DNA molecule, and the nuclear genome consists therefore of 46 linear DNA molecules, totaling more than 6 billion nucleotide pairs (see Fig. 2.1).

Chromosomes are not naked DNA double helices, however. Within each cell, the genome is packaged as **chromatin**, in which **genomic DNA** is complexed with several classes of specialized proteins. Except during cell division, chromatin is distributed throughout the nucleus and is relatively homogeneous in appearance under the microscope. When a cell divides, however, its genome condenses to appear as microscopically visible chromosomes. Chromosomes are thus visible as discrete structures only in dividing cells, although they retain their integrity between cell divisions.

The DNA molecule of a chromosome exists in chromatin as a complex with a family of basic chromosomal proteins called **histones**. This fundamental unit interacts with a heterogeneous group of nonhistone proteins, which are involved in establishing a proper spatial and functional environment to ensure normal chromosome behavior and appropriate gene expression.

Five major types of histones play a critical role in the proper packaging of chromatin. Two copies each of the four core histones H2A, H2B, H3, and H4 constitute an octamer, around which a segment of DNA double helix winds, like thread around a spool (Fig. 2.5). Approximately 140 base pairs (bp) of DNA are associated with each histone core, making just under two turns around the octamer. After a short (20- to 60-bp) "spacer" segment of DNA, the next core DNA complex forms, and so on, giving chromatin the appearance of beads on a string. Each complex of DNA with core histones is called a **nucleosome** (see Fig. 2.5), which is the basic structural unit of chromatin, and each of the 46 human chromosomes contains several hundred thousand to well over 1 million nucleosomes. A fifth histone, H1, appears to bind to DNA at the edge of each nucleosome, in the internucleosomal spacer region.

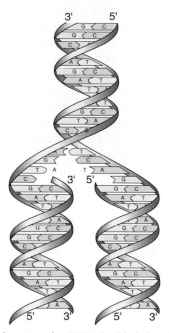

Figure 2.4 Replication of a DNA double helix, resulting in two identical daughter molecules, each composed of one parental strand and one newly synthesized strand.

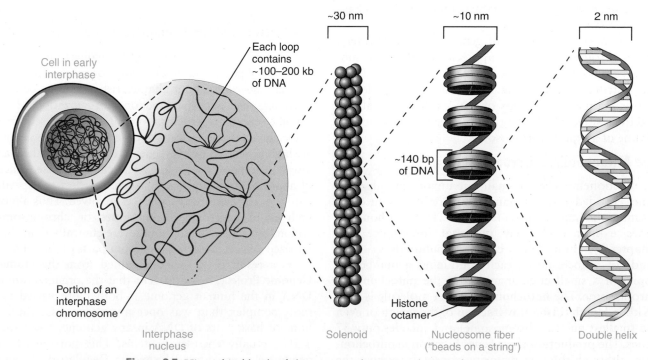

Figure 2.5 Hierarchical levels of chromatin packaging in a human chromosome.

The amount of DNA associated with a core nucleosome, together with the spacer region, is approximately 200 bp.

In addition to the major histone types, a number of specialized histones can substitute for H3 or H2A and confer specific characteristics on the genomic DNA at that location. Histones can also be modified by chemical changes, and these modifications can change the properties of nucleosomes that contain them. As discussed further in Chapter 3, the pattern of major and specialized histone types and their modifications can vary from cell type to cell type and is thought to specify how DNA is packaged and how accessible it is to regulatory molecules that determine gene expression or other genome functions.

During the **cell cycle**, as we will see later in this chapter, chromosomes pass through orderly stages of condensation and decondensation. However, even when chromosomes are in their most decondensed state, in a stage of the cell cycle called **interphase**, DNA packaged in chromatin is substantially more condensed than it would be as a native, protein-free, double helix. Further, the long strings of nucleosomes are themselves compacted into a secondary helical structure, a cylindrical **solenoid** fiber (from the Greek *solenoeides*, "pipe shaped") that appears to be the fundamental unit of chromatin organization (see Fig. 2.5). The solenoids are themselves packed into **loops** or domains attached at intervals of approximately 100,000 bp (equivalent to 100 kilobase pairs [kb] because 1 kb = 1000 bp) to a protein **scaffold** within the nucleus. It has been speculated that these loops are the functional units of the genome and that the attachment points of each loop are specified along the chromosomal DNA. As we shall see, one level of control of gene expression depends on how DNA and genes are packaged into chromosomes and on their **association** with chromatin proteins in the packaging process.

The enormous amount of genomic DNA packaged into a chromosome can be appreciated when chromosomes are treated to release the DNA from the underlying protein scaffold (see Fig. 2.1). When DNA is released in this manner, long loops of DNA can be visualized, and the residual scaffolding can be seen to reproduce the outline of a typical chromosome.

The Mitochondrial Chromosome

As mentioned earlier, a small but important subset of genes encoded in the human genome resides in the cytoplasm in the mitochondria (see Fig. 2.1). Mitochondrial genes exhibit exclusively **maternal inheritance** (see Chapter 7). Human cells can have hundreds to thousands of mitochondria, each containing a number of copies of a small circular molecule, the mitochondrial chromosome. The **mitochondrial DNA** molecule is only 16 kb in length (just a tiny fraction of the length of even the smallest nuclear chromosome) and encodes only 37 genes. The products of these genes function in mitochondria, although the vast majority of proteins within the

mitochondria are, in fact, the products of nuclear genes. Pathogenic variants in mitochondrial genes have been demonstrated in several maternally inherited as well as **sporadic** disorders (Case 33) (see Chapters 7 and 13).

The Human Genome Sequence

With a general understanding of the structure and clinical importance of chromosomes and the genes they carry, scientists turned attention to the identification of specific genes and their location in the human genome. From this broad effort emerged the Human Genome Project, an international consortium of hundreds of laboratories around the world, formed to map and determine the sequence of the 3.3 billion bp of DNA located among the 24 types of human chromosomes.

Over the course of 15 years, powered by major developments in DNA-sequencing technology, large sequencing centers collaborated to assemble sequences of each chromosome. The genomes actually being sequenced came from several different individuals, and the **consensus sequence** that resulted at the conclusion of the Human Genome Project was reported in 2003 as a "reference" sequence assembly, to be used as a basis for later comparison with sequences of individual genomes. This reference sequence is maintained in publicly accessible databases to facilitate scientific discovery and its **translation** into useful advances for medicine. Genome sequences are typically presented in a 5′ to 3′ direction on just one of the two strands of the double helix because—owing to the complementary nature of DNA structure described earlier—if one knows the sequence of one strand, one can infer the sequence of the other strand (Fig. 2.6).

Organization of the Human Genome

Chromosomes are not just a random collection of different types of genes and other DNA sequences. Regions of the genome with similar characteristics tend to be clustered together, and the functional organization of the genome reflects its structural organization and sequence. Some chromosome regions, or even whole chromosomes, are high in gene content ("gene rich"), whereas others are low ("gene poor") (Fig. 2.7). The clinical consequences of abnormalities of genome structure reflect the specific nature of the genes and sequences involved. Thus abnormalities of gene-rich chromosomes or chromosomal regions tend to be much more severe clinically than similar-sized defects involving gene-poor parts of the genome.

As a result of knowledge gained from the Human Genome Project, it is apparent that the organization of DNA in the human genome is both more varied and more complex than was once appreciated. Of the billions of base pairs of DNA in any genome, fewer than 1.5% actually encodes proteins. This portion of the genome is referred to as the **exome**. Regulatory elements

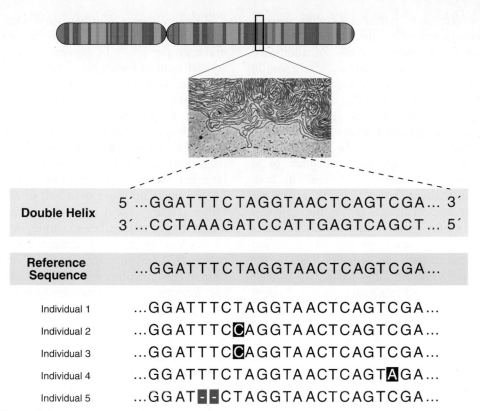

Figure 2.6 A portion of the reference human genome sequence. By convention, sequences are presented from one strand of DNA only, because the sequence of the complementary strand can be inferred from the double-stranded nature of DNA (shown above the reference sequence). The sequence of DNA from a group of individuals is similar but not identical to the reference, with single nucleotide changes in some individuals and a small deletion of two bases in another.

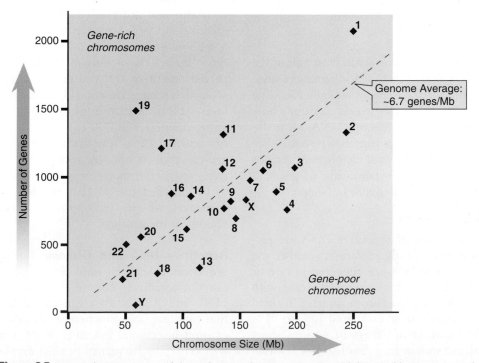

Figure 2.7 Size and gene content of the 24 human chromosomes. Dotted diagonal line corresponds to the average density of genes in the genome, approximately 6.7 protein-coding genes per megabase (Mb). Chromosomes that are relatively gene rich are above the diagonal and trend to the upper left. Chromosomes that are relatively gene poor are below the diagonal and trend to the lower right. (Based on data from European Bioinformatics Institute and Wellcome Trust Sanger Institute: *Ensembl release 70*, January 2013. Available from http://www.ensembl.org, v37.)

that influence or determine patterns of gene expression during development or in tissues were believed to account for only approximately 5% of additional sequence, although more recent analyses of chromatin characteristics suggest that a much higher proportion of the genome may provide signals that are relevant to genome functions. Only approximately half of the total linear length of the genome consists of so-called **single-copy** or unique DNA, that is, DNA whose linear order of specific nucleotides is represented only once (or at most a few times) around the entire genome. This concept may appear surprising to some, given that there are only four different nucleotides in DNA. But consider even a tiny stretch of the genome that is only 10 bases long; with four types of bases, there are over 1 million possible sequences. Although the order of bases in the genome is not entirely random, any particular 16-base sequence would be predicted by chance alone to appear only once in any given genome.

The rest of the genome consists of several classes of repetitive DNA and includes DNA whose nucleotide sequence is repeated, either identically or with some variation, hundreds to millions of times in the genome. Whereas most (but not all) of the estimated 20,000 protein-coding genes in the genome (see box earlier in this chapter) are represented in single-copy DNA, sequences in the repetitive DNA fraction contribute to maintaining chromosome structure and are an important source of variation between different individuals; some of this variation can predispose to pathologic events in the genome, as we will see in Chapters 5 and 6.

Single-Copy DNA Sequences

Although single-copy DNA makes up at least half of the DNA in the genome, much of its function remains a mystery because, as mentioned, sequences actually encoding proteins (i.e., the coding portion of genes) constitute only a small proportion of all the single-copy DNA. Most single-copy DNA is found in short stretches (several kilobase pairs or less), interspersed with members of various repetitive DNA families. The organization of genes in single-copy DNA is addressed in depth in Chapter 3.

Repetitive DNA Sequences

Several different categories of repetitive DNA are recognized. A useful distinguishing feature is whether the repeated sequences ("repeats") are clustered in one or a few locations or whether they are interspersed with single-copy sequences along the chromosome. Clustered repeated sequences constitute an estimated 10% to 15% of the genome and consist of arrays of various short repeats organized in tandem in a head-to-tail fashion. The different types of such **tandem repeats** are collectively called **satellite DNAs**, so named because many of the original tandem repeat families could be separated by biochemical methods from the bulk of the genome as distinct ("satellite") fractions of DNA.

Tandem repeat families vary with regard to their location in the genome and the nature of sequences that make up the array. In general, such arrays can stretch several million base pairs or more in length and constitute up to several percent of the DNA content of an individual human chromosome. Some tandem repeat sequences are important as tools that are useful in clinical cytogenetic analysis (see Chapter 5). Long arrays of repeats based on repetitions (with some variation) of a short sequence such as a pentanucleotide are found in large genetically inert regions on chromosomes 1, 9, and 16 and make up more than half of the Y chromosome. Other tandem repeat families are based on somewhat longer basic repeats. For example, the α-satellite family of DNA is composed of tandem arrays of an approximately 171-bp unit, found at the **centromere** of each human chromosome, which is critical for attachment of chromosomes to microtubules of the spindle apparatus during cell division.

In addition to tandem repeat DNAs, another major class of repetitive DNA in the genome consists of related sequences that are dispersed throughout the genome rather than clustered in one or a few locations. Although many DNA families meet this general description, two in particular warrant discussion because together they make up a significant proportion of the genome and because they have been implicated in genetic conditions. Among the best-studied dispersed repetitive elements are those belonging to the so-called *Alu* **family**. The members of this family are approximately 300 bp in length and are related to each other although not identical in DNA sequence. In total, there are more than 1 million *Alu* family members in the genome, making up at least 10% of human DNA. A second major dispersed repetitive DNA family is called the long interspersed nuclear element (**LINE**, sometimes called L1) family. LINEs are up to 6 kb in length and are found in approximately 850,000 copies per genome, accounting for nearly 20% of the genome. Both of these families are plentiful in some regions of the genome but relatively sparse in others—regions rich in GC content tend to be enriched in *Alu* elements but depleted of **LINE sequences**, whereas the opposite is true of more AT-rich regions of the genome.

Repetitive DNA and Disease. Both *Alu* and LINE sequences have been implicated as the cause of mutations in hereditary disease. At least a few copies of the LINE and *Alu* families generate copies of themselves that can integrate elsewhere in the genome, occasionally causing insertional inactivation of a medically important gene. The frequency of such events causing genetic disease in humans is unknown, but they may account for as many as 1 in 500 mutations. In addition, aberrant recombination events between different LINE repeats or *Alu* repeats can also be a cause of variants in some genetic diseases.

An important additional type of repetitive DNA found in many different locations around the genome includes sequences that are duplicated, often with extraordinarily high sequence conservation. Duplications involving substantial segments of a chromosome, called **segmental duplications**, can span hundreds of kilobase pairs and account for at least 5% of the genome. When the duplicated regions contain genes, genomic rearrangements involving the duplicated sequences can result in the **deletion** of the region (and the genes) between the copies and thus give rise to disease (see Chapters 5 and 6).

VARIATION IN THE HUMAN GENOME

With completion of the reference human genome sequence, much attention has turned to the discovery and cataloging of variation in sequence among different individuals (including both healthy individuals and those with various diseases) and among different populations around the globe. As we will explore in much more detail in Chapter 4, there are many tens of millions of common sequence variants that are seen at significant frequency in one or more populations; any given individual carries millions of these sequence variants. In addition, there are countless very rare variants, many of which probably exist in only a single or a few individuals. In fact, given the number of individuals in our species, *essentially each and every base pair in the human genome is expected to vary in someone somewhere around the globe.* It is for this reason that the original human genome sequence is considered a reference sequence for our species, and not one that is actually identical to any individual's genome.

Early estimates were that any two randomly selected individuals would have sequences that are 99.9% identical or, put another way, that an individual genome would carry two *different* versions (**alleles**) of the human genome sequence at some 3 to 5 million positions, with different bases (e.g., a T or a G) at the maternally and paternally inherited copies of that particular sequence position (see Fig. 2.6). Although many of these allelic differences involve simply one nucleotide, much of the variation consists of insertions or deletions of (usually) short sequence stretches, variation in the number of copies of repeated elements (including genes), or inversions in the order of sequences at a particular position (**locus**) in the genome (see Chapter 4). These copy number variations account for at least 12 million bp of difference between any two unrelated individuals.

The total amount of the genome involved in such variation is now known to be substantially more than originally estimated and approaches 2% between any two randomly selected individuals. As will be addressed in future chapters, any and all of these types of variation can influence biologic function and thus must be accounted for in any attempt to understand the contribution of genetics and genomics to human health.

TRANSMISSION OF THE GENOME

The chromosomal basis of heredity lies in the copying of the genome and its transmission from a cell to its progeny during typical cell division and from one generation to the next during reproduction, when single copies of the genome from each parent come together in a new embryo.

To achieve these related but distinct forms of genome inheritance, there are two kinds of cell division, mitosis and meiosis. **Mitosis** is ordinary **somatic cell** division by which the body grows, differentiates, and effects tissue regeneration. Mitotic division normally results in two daughter cells, each with chromosomes and genes identical to those of the parent cell. There may be dozens or even hundreds of successive mitoses in a lineage of somatic cells. In contrast, **meiosis** occurs only in cells of the germline. Meiosis results in the formation of reproductive cells (**gametes**), each of which has only 23 chromosomes—one of each kind of autosome and either an X or a Y. Thus, whereas somatic cells have the **diploid** (*diploos*, "double") or the 2n chromosome complement (i.e., 46 chromosomes), gametes have the **haploid** (*haploos*, "single") or the n complement (i.e., 23 chromosomes). Abnormalities of chromosome number or structure, which are usually clinically significant, can arise either in somatic cells or in cells of the germline by errors in cell division.

The Cell Cycle

A human being begins life as a fertilized ovum (**zygote**), a diploid cell from which all the cells of the body (estimated to be ~100 trillion in number) are derived by a series of dozens or even hundreds of mitoses. Mitosis is obviously crucial for growth and **differentiation**, but it takes up only a small part of the life cycle of a cell. The period between two successive mitoses is called **interphase**, the state in which most of the life of a cell is spent.

Immediately after mitosis, the cell enters a **phase**, called G_1, in which there is no DNA synthesis (Fig. 2.8). Some cells pass through this stage in hours; others spend a long time, days or years, in G_1. In fact, some cell types, such as neurons and red blood cells, do not divide at all once they are fully differentiated; rather, they are permanently arrested in a distinct phase known as G_0 ("G zero"). Other cells, such as liver cells, may enter G_0 but, after organ damage, return to G_1 and continue through the cell cycle.

The cell cycle is governed by a series of **checkpoints** that determine the timing of each step in mitosis. In addition, checkpoints monitor and control the accuracy of DNA synthesis as well as the assembly and attachment of an elaborate network of microtubules that facilitate chromosome movement. If damage to the genome is detected, these mitotic checkpoints halt cell cycle progression until repairs are made or, if the

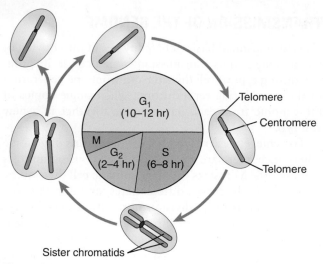

Figure 2.8 **A typical mitotic cell cycle, described in the text.** The telomeres, the centromere, and sister chromatids are indicated.

damage is excessive, until the cell is instructed to die by programmed cell death (a process called **apoptosis**).

During G_1, each cell contains one diploid copy of the genome. As the process of cell division begins, the cell enters S phase, the stage of programmed DNA synthesis, ultimately leading to the precise replication of each chromosome's DNA. During this stage, each chromosome, which in G_1 has been a single DNA molecule, is duplicated and consists of two sister **chromatids** (see Fig. 2.8), each of which contains an identical copy of the original linear DNA double helix. The two sister chromatids are held together physically at the **centromere**, a region of DNA that associates with a number of specific proteins to form the **kinetochore**. This complex structure serves to attach each chromosome to the microtubules of the **mitotic spindle** and to govern chromosome movement during mitosis. DNA synthesis during S phase is not synchronous throughout all chromosomes or even within a single chromosome; rather, along each chromosome, it begins at hundreds to thousands of sites, called **origins of DNA replication**. Individual chromosome segments have their own characteristic time of replication during the 6- to 8-hour S phase. The ends of each chromosome (or chromatid) are marked by **telomeres**, which consist of specialized repetitive DNA sequences that ensure the integrity of the chromosome during cell division. Correct maintenance of the ends of chromosomes requires a special enzyme called **telomerase**, which ensures that the very ends of each chromosome are replicated.

The essential nature of these structural elements of chromosomes and their role in ensuring genome integrity is illustrated by a range of clinical conditions that result from defects in elements of the telomere or kinetochore or cell cycle machinery or from inaccurate replication of even small portions of the genome (see Box 2.3). Some of these conditions will be presented in greater detail in subsequent chapters.

BOX 2.3 CLINICAL CONSEQUENCES OF ABNORMALITIES AND VARIATION IN CHROMOSOME STRUCTURE AND MECHANICS

Medically relevant conditions arising from abnormal structure or function of chromosomal elements during cell division include the following:

- A broad spectrum of **congenital** abnormalities in children with inherited defects in genes encoding key components of the mitotic spindle checkpoint at the kinetochore
- A range of **birth defects and developmental disorders** due to anomalous **segregation** of chromosomes with multiple or missing centromeres (see Chapter 6)
- A variety of cancers associated with overreplication (amplification) or altered timing of replication of specific regions of the genome in S phase (see Chapter 16)
- Roberts **syndrome** of short stature, limb shortening, and microcephaly in children with abnormalities of a gene required for proper sister chromatid alignment and cohesion in S phase
- Premature ovarian failure as a major cause of female infertility due to deleterious variants in a meiosis-specific gene required for correct sister chromatid cohesion
- The so-called telomere syndromes, a number of degenerative disorders presenting from childhood to adulthood in patients with abnormal telomere shortening due to defects in components of telomerase (see Case 49)
- At the other end of the spectrum, common gene variants that correlate with the number of copies of the repeats at telomeres and with life expectancy and longevity

By the end of S phase, the DNA content of the cell has doubled, and each cell now contains two copies of the diploid genome. After S phase, the cell enters a brief stage called G_2. Throughout the whole cell cycle, the cell gradually enlarges, eventually doubling its total mass before the next mitosis. G_2 is ended by mitosis, which begins when individual chromosomes begin to condense and become visible under the microscope as thin, extended threads, a process that is considered in greater detail in the following section.

The G_1, S, and G_2 phases together constitute interphase. In typical dividing human cells, the three phases take a total of 16 to 24 hours, whereas mitosis lasts only 1 to 2 hours (see Fig. 2.8). There is great variation, however, in the length of the cell cycle, which ranges from a few hours in rapidly dividing cells, such as those of the dermis of the skin or the intestinal mucosa, to months in other cell types.

Mitosis

During the mitotic phase of the cell cycle, an elaborate apparatus ensures that each of the two daughter cells receives a complete set of genetic information. This result is achieved by a mechanism that distributes one chromatid of each chromosome to each daughter cell (Fig. 2.9). The process of distributing a copy of each chromosome to each daughter cell is called **chromosome segregation**. The importance of this process for normal

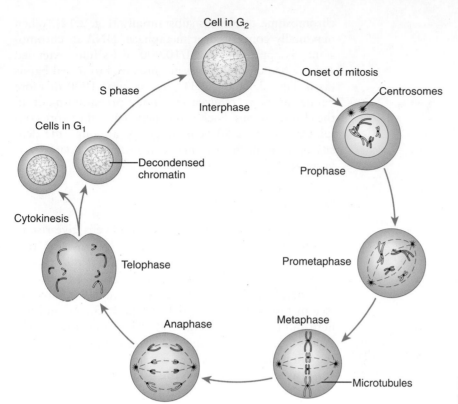

Figure 2.9 **Mitosis.** Only two chromosome pairs are shown. For details, see text.

cell growth is illustrated by the observation that many tumors are invariably characterized by a state of genetic imbalance resulting from mitotic errors in the distribution of chromosomes to daughter cells.

The process of mitosis is continuous, but five stages (see Fig. 2.9) are distinguished: **prophase, prometaphase, metaphase, anaphase,** and **telophase**.

- *Prophase*. This stage is marked by gradual condensation of the chromosomes, formation of the mitotic spindle, and formation of a pair of **centrosomes**, from which microtubules radiate and eventually take up positions at the poles of the cell.
- *Prometaphase*. Here, the nuclear membrane dissolves, allowing the chromosomes to disperse within the cell and to attach, by their kinetochores, to microtubules of the mitotic spindle.
- *Metaphase*. At this stage, the chromosomes are maximally condensed and line up at the equatorial plane of the cell.
- *Anaphase*. The chromosomes separate at the centromere, and the sister chromatids of each chromosome now become independent **daughter chromosomes**, which move to opposite poles of the cell.
- *Telophase*. Now, the chromosomes begin to decondense from their highly contracted state, and a nuclear membrane begins to re-form around each of the two daughter nuclei, which resume their interphase appearance. To complete the process of cell division, the cytoplasm cleaves by a process known as **cytokinesis**.

There is an important difference between a cell entering mitosis and one that has just completed the process. A cell in G_2 has a fully replicated genome (i.e., a 4n complement of DNA), and each chromosome consists of a pair of sister chromatids. In contrast, after mitosis, the chromosomes of each daughter cell have only one copy of the genome. This copy will not be duplicated until a daughter cell in its turn reaches the S phase of the next cell cycle (see Fig. 2.8). The entire process of mitosis thus ensures the orderly duplication and distribution of the genome through successive cell divisions.

The Human Karyotype

The condensed chromosomes of a dividing human cell are most readily analyzed at metaphase or prometaphase. At these stages, the chromosomes are visible under the microscope as a so-called **chromosome spread;** each chromosome consists of its sister chromatids, although in most chromosome preparations, the two chromatids are held together so tightly that they are rarely visible as separate entities.

As stated earlier, there are 24 different types of human chromosomes, each of which can be distinguished cytologically by a combination of overall length, location of the centromere, and sequence content, the latter reflected by various staining methods. The centromere is apparent as a **primary constriction**, a narrowing or pinching-in of the sister chromatids due to formation of the kinetochore. This is a recognizable cytogenetic

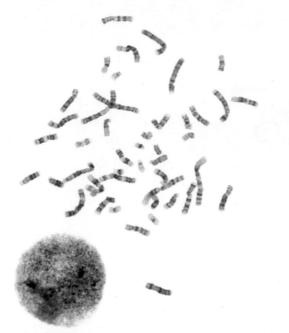

Figure 2.10 A chromosome spread prepared from a lymphocyte culture that has been stained by the Giemsa-banding (G-banding) technique. The darkly stained nucleus adjacent to the chromosomes is from a different cell in interphase, when chromosomal material is diffuse throughout the nucleus. (Courtesy Stuart Schwartz, University Hospitals of Cleveland, Ohio.)

landmark, dividing the chromosome into two arms, a short arm designated **p** (for *petit*) and a long arm designated **q**.

Fig. 2.10 shows a prometaphase cell in which the chromosomes have been stained by the Giemsa-staining (**G-banding**) method (also see Chapter 5). Each chromosome pair stains in a characteristic pattern of alternating light and dark bands (G bands) that correlates roughly with features of the underlying DNA sequence, such as base composition (i.e., the percentage of base pairs that are GC or AT) and the distribution of repetitive DNA elements. With such banding techniques, all of the chromosomes can be individually distinguished, and the nature of many structural or numerical abnormalities can be determined, as we examine in greater detail in Chapters 5 and 6.

Although experts can often analyze metaphase chromosomes directly under the microscope, a common procedure is to cut out the chromosomes from a digital image or photomicrograph and arrange them in pairs in a standard classification (Fig. 2.11). The completed picture is called a **karyotype**. The word *karyotype* is also used to refer to the standard chromosome set of an individual ("a normal male karyotype") or of a species ("the human karyotype") and, as a verb, to the process of preparing such a standard figure ("to karyotype").

Unlike the chromosomes seen in stained preparations under the microscope or in photographs, the chromosomes of living cells are fluid and dynamic structures. During mitosis, the chromatin of each interphase

chromosome condenses substantially (Fig. 2.12). When maximally condensed at metaphase, DNA in chromosomes is approximately 1/10,000 of its fully extended state. When chromosomes are prepared to reveal bands (as in Figs. 2.10 and 2.11), as many as 1000 or more bands can be recognized in stained preparations of all the chromosomes. Each cytogenetic band therefore contains as many as 50 or more genes, although the density of genes in the genome, as mentioned previously, is variable.

Meiosis

Meiosis, the process by which diploid cells give rise to haploid gametes, involves a type of cell division that is unique to germ cells. In contrast to mitosis, meiosis consists of one round of DNA replication followed by *two* rounds of chromosome segregation and cell division (see meiosis I and meiosis II in Fig. 2.13). As outlined here and illustrated in Fig. 2.14, the overall sequence of events in male and female meiosis is the same; however, the timing of gametogenesis is very different in the two sexes, as we will describe more fully later in this chapter.

Meiosis I is also known as the **reduction division** because it is the division in which the chromosome number is reduced by half through the pairing of homologues in prophase and by their segregation to different cells at anaphase of meiosis I. Meiosis I is also notable because it is the stage at which genetic recombination (also called meiotic **crossing over**) occurs. In this process, as shown for one pair of chromosomes in Fig. 2.14, **homologous** segments of DNA are exchanged between nonsister chromatids of each pair of homologous chromosomes, thus ensuring that none of the gametes produced by meiosis will be identical to another. The conceptual and practical consequences of recombination for many aspects of human genetics and genomics are substantial and are outlined in the box at the end of this section.

Prophase of meiosis I differs in a number of ways from mitotic prophase, with important genetic consequences, because homologous chromosomes need to pair and exchange genetic information. The most critical early stage is called **zygotene**, when homologous chromosomes begin to align along their entire length. The process of meiotic pairing—called **synapsis**—is normally precise, bringing corresponding DNA sequences into alignment along the length of the entire chromosome pair. The paired homologues—now called **bivalents**—are held together by a ribbonlike proteinaceous structure called the **synaptonemal complex**, which is essential to the process of recombination. After synapsis is complete, meiotic crossing over takes place during **pachytene**, after which the synaptonemal complex breaks down.

Metaphase I begins, as in mitosis, when the nuclear membrane disappears. A spindle forms, and the paired

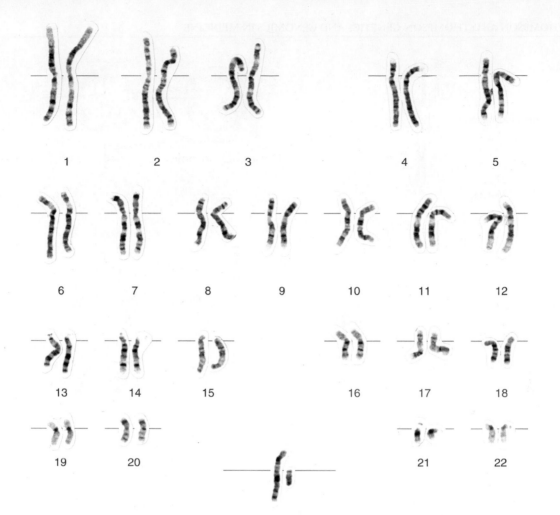

1 2 3 4 5

6 7 8 9 10 11 12

13 14 15 16 17 18

19 20 21 22

SEX CHROMOSOMES

Figure 2.11 A human male karyotype with Giemsa banding (G-banding). The chromosomes are at the prometaphase stage of mitosis and are arranged in a standard classification, numbered 1 to 22 in order of length, with the X and Y chromosomes shown separately. *Courtesy Stuart Schwartz, University Hospitals of Cleveland, Ohio.*

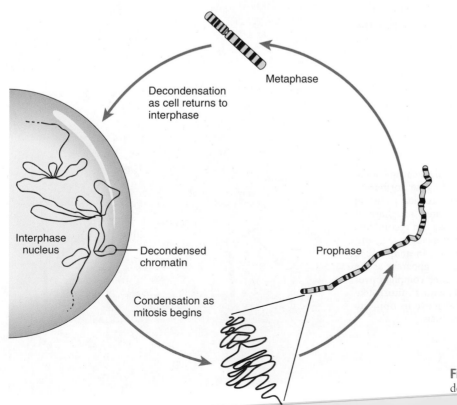

Metaphase

Decondensation as cell returns to interphase

Interphase nucleus

Decondensed chromatin

Prophase

Condensation as mitosis begins

Figure 2.12 Cycle of condensation and decondensation as a chrom...

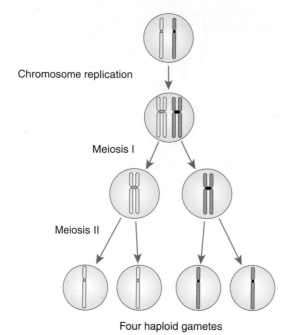

Chromosome replication

Meiosis I

Meiosis II

Four haploid gametes

Figure 2.13 A simplified representation of the essential steps in meiosis, consisting of one round of DNA replication followed by two rounds of chromosome segregation, meiosis I and meiosis II.

chromosomes align themselves on the equatorial plane with their centromeres oriented toward different poles (see Fig. 2.14).

Anaphase of meiosis I again differs substantially from the corresponding stage of mitosis. Here, it is the two members of each bivalent that move apart, not the sister chromatids (contrast Fig. 2.14 with Fig. 2.9). The homologous centromeres (with their attached sister chromatids) are drawn to opposite poles of the cell, a process termed disjunction. Thus the chromosome number is halved, and each cellular product of meiosis I has the haploid chromosome number. The 23 pairs of homologous chromosomes assort independently of one another, and as a result the original paternal and maternal chromosome sets are sorted into random combinations. The possible number of combinations of the 23 chromosome

Figure 2.14 Meiosis and its consequences. A single chromosome pair and a single crossover are shown, leading to formation of four distinct gametes. The chromosomes replicate during interphase and begin to condense as the cell enters prophase of meiosis I. In meiosis I, the chromosomes synapse and recombine. A crossover is visible as the homologues align at metaphase I, with the centromeres oriented toward opposite poles. In anaphase I, the exchange of DNA between the homologues is apparent as the chromosomes are pulled to opposite poles. After completion of meiosis I and cytokinesis, meiosis II proceeds with a mitosis-like division. The sister kinetochores separate and move to opposite poles in anaphase II, yielding four haploid products.

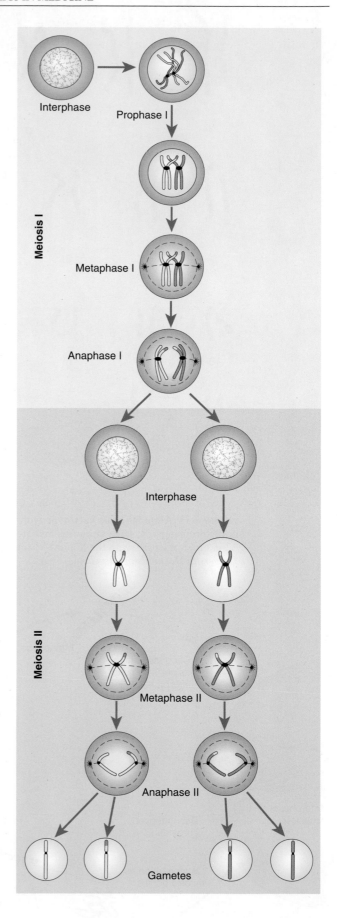

Interphase

Prophase I

Meiosis I

Metaphase I

Anaphase I

Interphase

Meiosis II

Metaphase II

Anaphase II

Gametes

pairs that can be present in the gametes is 2^{23} (>8 million). Owing to the process of crossing over, however, the variation in the genetic material that is transmitted from parent to child is actually much greater than this (see Box 2.4). As a result, each chromatid typically contains segments derived from each member of the original parental chromosome pair, as illustrated schematically in Fig. 2.14. For example, at this stage, a typical large human chromosome would be composed of three to five segments, alternately paternal and maternal in origin, as inferred from DNA sequence variants that distinguish the respective parental genomes (Fig. 2.15).

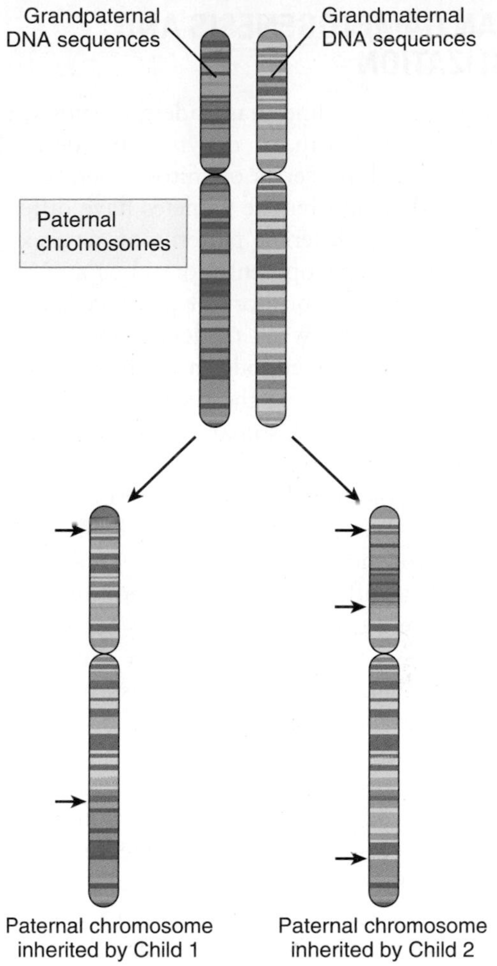

BOX 2.4 GENETIC CONSEQUENCES AND MEDICAL RELEVANCE OF HOMOLOGOUS RECOMBINATION

The take-home lesson of this portion of the chapter is a simple one: the genetic content of each gamete is unique because of random **assortment** of the parental chromosomes to shuffle the combination of sequence variants *between* chromosomes and because of homologous recombination to shuffle the combination of sequence variants *within* each and every chromosome. This has significant consequences for patterns of genomic variation among and between different populations around the globe and for diagnosis and counseling of many common conditions with complex patterns of inheritance (see Chapters 9 and 10).

The amounts and patterns of meiotic recombination are determined by sequence variants in specific genes and at specific "hot spots" and differ between individuals, between the sexes, between families, and between populations (see Chapter 10).

Because recombination involves the physical intertwining of the two homologues until the appropriate point during meiosis I, it is also critical for ensuring proper chromosome segregation during meiosis. Failure to recombine properly can lead to chromosome missegregation (**nondisjunction**) in meiosis I and is a frequent cause of pregnancy loss and of chromosome abnormalities such as Down syndrome (see Chapters 5 and 6).

Major ongoing efforts to identify genes and their variants responsible for various medical conditions rely on tracking the inheritance of millions of sequence differences within families or the sharing of variants within groups of even unrelated individuals affected with a particular condition. The utility of this approach, which has uncovered thousands of gene-disease associations to date, depends on patterns of homologous recombination in meiosis (see Chapters 6, 11, and 12).

Although homologous recombination is generally precise, areas of repetitive DNA in the genome and genes of variable copy number in the population are prone to occasional unequal **crossing over** during meiosis, leading to variations in clinically relevant traits such as drug response, to common disorders such as the thalassemias or autism, or to abnormalities of sexual differentiation (see Chapters 6, 11, and 12).

Although homologous recombination is a normal and essential part of meiosis, it also occurs, albeit more rarely, in somatic cells. **Anomalies** in **somatic recombination** are one of the causes of genome instability in cancer (see Chapter 16).

Figure 2.15 The effect of homologous recombination in meiosis. In this example, representing the inheritance of sequences on a typical large chromosome, an individual has distinctive homologues, one containing sequences inherited from his father *(blue)* and one containing homologous sequences from his mother *(purple)*. After meiosis in spermatogenesis, he transmits a single complete copy of that chromosome to his two offspring. However, as a result of crossing over *(arrows)*, the copy he transmits to each child consists of alternating segments of the two grandparental sequences. Child 1 inherits a copy after two crossovers, whereas child 2 inherits a copy with three crossovers.

After telophase of meiosis I, the two haploid daughter cells enter meiotic interphase. In contrast to mitosis, this interphase is brief, and meiosis II begins. The notable point that distinguishes meiotic and mitotic interphase is that there is no S phase (i.e., no DNA synthesis and duplication of the genome) between the first and second meiotic divisions.

Meiosis II is similar to an ordinary mitosis, except that the chromosome number is 23 instead of 46; the chromatids of each of the 23 chromosomes separate, and one chromatid of each chromosome passes to each daughter cell (see Fig. 2.14). However, as mentioned earlier, because of crossing over in meiosis I, the chromosomes of the resulting gametes are not identical (see Fig. 2.15).

HUMAN GAMETOGENESIS AND FERTILIZATION

The cells in the germline that undergo meiosis, primary spermatocytes or primary oocytes, are derived from the zygote by a long series of mitoses before the onset of meiosis. Male and female gametes have different histories, marked by different patterns of gene expression that reflect their developmental origin as an XY or XX embryo. The human primordial germ cells are recognizable by the fourth week of development outside the embryo proper, in the **endoderm** of the yolk sac. From there, they migrate during the sixth week to the genital ridges and associate with somatic cells to form the primitive gonads, which soon differentiate into testes or ovaries, depending on the cells' sex chromosome constitution (XY or XX), as we examine in greater detail in Chapter 6. Both spermatogenesis and oogenesis require meiosis but have important differences in detail and timing that may have clinical and genetic consequences for the offspring. Female meiosis is initiated once, early during fetal life, in a limited number of cells. In contrast, male meiosis is initiated continuously in many cells from a dividing cell population throughout the adult life of a male.

In the female, successive stages of meiosis take place over several decades—in the fetal ovary before the female in question is even born, in the oocyte near the time of ovulation in the sexually mature female, and after fertilization of the egg that can become that female's offspring. Although postfertilization stages can be studied *in vitro*, access to the earlier stages is limited. Testicular material for the study of male meiosis is less difficult to obtain, inasmuch as testicular biopsy is included in the assessment of many men attending infertility clinics. Much remains to be learned about the cytogenetic, biochemical, and molecular mechanisms involved in normal meiosis and about the causes and consequences of meiotic irregularities.

Spermatogenesis

The stages of spermatogenesis are shown in Fig. 2.16. The seminiferous tubules of the testes are lined with **spermatogonia**, which develop from the primordial germ cells by a long series of mitoses and are in different stages of differentiation. Sperm (spermatozoa) are formed only after sexual maturity is reached. The last cell type in the developmental sequence is the primary spermatocyte, a diploid germ cell that undergoes meiosis I to form two haploid secondary spermatocytes. Secondary spermatocytes rapidly enter meiosis II, each forming two spermatids, which differentiate without further division into sperm. In humans, the entire process takes approximately 64 days. The enormous number of sperm produced, typically approximately 200 million per ejaculate and an estimated 10^{12} in a lifetime, requires several hundred successive mitoses.

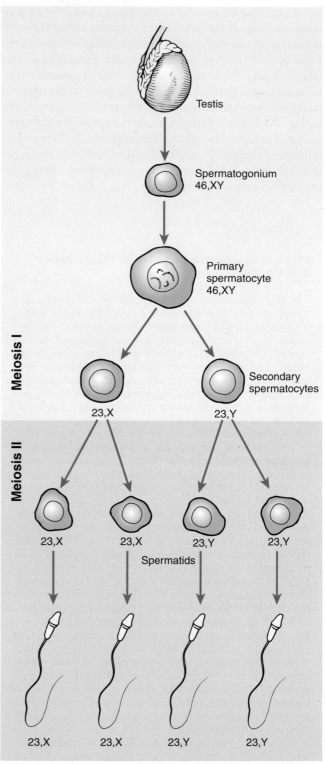

Figure 2.16 Human spermatogenesis in relation to the two meiotic divisions. The sequence of events begins at puberty and takes approximately 64 days to be completed. The chromosome number (46 or ɟ23) and the sex chromosome constitution (X or Y) of each cell are shown. (Modified from Moore KL, Persaud TVN: *The developing human: clinically oriented embryology*, ed 6, Philadelphia, 1998, WB Saunders.)

As discussed earlier, normal meiosis requires pairing of homologous chromosomes followed by recombination. The autosomes and the X chromosomes in females present no unusual difficulties in this regard; but what of the X and Y chromosomes during spermatogenesis? Although the X and Y chromosomes are different and are not homologues in a strict sense, they do have relatively short identical segments at the ends of their respective short arms (Xp and Yp) and long arms (Xq and Yq) (see Chapter 6). Pairing and crossing over occurs in both regions during meiosis I. These homologous segments are called **pseudoautosomal** to reflect their autosome-like pairing and recombination behavior, despite being on different sex chromosomes.

Oogenesis

Whereas spermatogenesis is initiated only at the time of puberty, oogenesis begins during a female's development as a fetus (Fig. 2.17). The ova develop from **oogonia**, cells in the ovarian cortex that have descended from the primordial germ cells by a series of approximately 20 mitoses. Each oogonium is the central cell in a developing follicle. By approximately the third month of fetal development, the oogonia of the embryo have begun to develop into primary oocytes, most of which have already entered prophase of meiosis I. The process of oogenesis is not synchronized, and both early and late stages coexist in the fetal ovary. Although there are several million oocytes at the time of birth, most of these degenerate; the others remain arrested in prophase I (see Fig. 2.14) for decades. Only approximately 400 eventually mature and are ovulated as part of a woman's menstrual cycle.

After a woman reaches sexual maturity, individual follicles begin to grow and mature, and a few (on average one per month) are ovulated. Just before ovulation, the oocyte rapidly completes meiosis I, dividing in such a way that one cell becomes the secondary oocyte (an egg or ovum), containing most of the cytoplasm with its organelles; the other cell becomes the first polar body (see Fig. 2.17). Meiosis II begins promptly and proceeds to the metaphase stage during ovulation, where it halts again, only to be completed if fertilization occurs.

Fertilization

Fertilization of the egg usually takes place in the fallopian tube within a day or so of ovulation. Although many sperm may be present, the penetration of a single sperm into the ovum sets up a series of biochemical events that usually prevent the entry of other sperm.

Fertilization is followed by the completion of meiosis II, with the formation of the second polar body (see Fig. 2.17). The chromosomes of the now-fertilized egg and sperm form **pronuclei**, each surrounded by its own

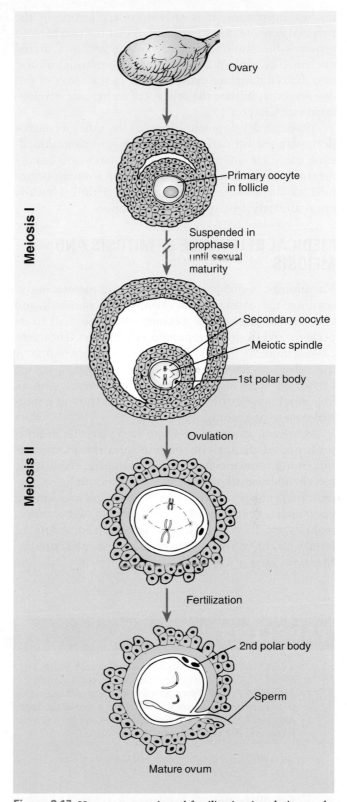

Figure 2.17 Human oogenesis and fertilization in relation to the two meiotic divisions. The primary oocytes are formed prenatally and remain suspended in prophase of meiosis I for years until the onset of puberty. An oocyte completes meiosis I as its follicle matures, resulting in a secondary oocyte and the first polar body. After ovulation, each oocyte continues to metaphase of meiosis II. Meiosis II is completed only if fertilization occurs, resulting in a fertilized mature ovum and the second polar body.

nuclear membrane. It is only upon replication of the parental genomes after fertilization that the two haploid genomes become one diploid genome within a shared nucleus. The diploid **zygote** divides by mitosis to form two diploid daughter cells, the first in the series of cell divisions that initiate the process of embryonic development (see Chapter 15).

Although development begins at the time of conception, with the formation of the zygote, in clinical medicine the stage and duration of pregnancy are usually measured as the "menstrual age," dating from the beginning of the mother's last menstrual period, typically approximately 14 days before conception.

MEDICAL RELEVANCE OF MITOSIS AND MEIOSIS

The biologic significance of mitosis and meiosis lies in ensuring the constancy of chromosome number—and thus the integrity of the genome—from one cell to its progeny and from one generation to the next. The medical relevance of these processes lies in errors of one or the other mechanism of cell division, leading to the formation of an individual or of a cell lineage with an abnormal number of chromosomes and thus an abnormal dosage of genomic material.

As we see in detail in Chapter 5, meiotic nondisjunction, particularly in oogenesis, is the most common mutational mechanism in our species, responsible for chromosomally abnormal fetuses in at least several percent of all recognized pregnancies. Among pregnancies that survive to term, chromosome abnormalities are a leading cause of developmental defects, failure to thrive in the newborn period, and intellectual disability.

Mitotic nondisjunction in somatic cells also contributes to genetic disease. Nondisjunction soon after fertilization, either in the developing embryo or in extraembryonic tissues like the placenta, leads to chromosomal **mosaicism** that can underlie some medical conditions, such as a proportion of patients with Down syndrome. Further, abnormal chromosome segregation in rapidly dividing tissues, such as in cells of the colon, is frequently a step in the development of chromosomally abnormal tumors, and thus evaluation of chromosome and genome balance is an important diagnostic and prognostic test in many cancers.

GENERAL REFERENCES

Gates, AJ, et al: A wealth of discovery built on the Human Genome Project - by the numbers, *Nature*, 590, 212–215, 2021.

Green ED, et al: Mapping genomic loci implicates genes and synaptic biology in schizophrenia, *Nature* 604:502–508, 2022.

Miga KH, et al: Telomere-to-telomere assembly of a complete human X chromosome, *Nature*, 585, 79-84, 2020

Moore KL, Presaud TVN, Torchia MG: *The developing human: clinically oriented embryology*, ed 9, Philadelphia, 2013, WB Saunders.

REFERENCES FOR SPECIFIC TOPICS

Deininger P: Alu elements: know the SINES, *Genome Biol* 12:236, 2011.

Frazer KA: Decoding the human genome, *Genome Res* 22:1599–1601, 2012.

International Human Genome Sequencing Consortium: Initial sequencing and analysis of the human genome, *Nature* 409:860–921, 2001.

International Human Genome Sequencing Consortium: Finishing the euchromatic sequence of the human genome, *Nature* 431:931–945, 2004.

Nurk S, Koren S, Rhie A, et al: The complete sequence of a human genome, *Science* 376:44–53, 2022. https://doi.org/10.1126/science.abj6987. Epub 2022 Mar 31. PMID: 35357919.

Venter J, Adams M, Myers E, et al: The sequence of the human genome, *Science* 291:1304–1351, 2001.

PROBLEMS

1. At a certain locus, a person has two alleles, *A* and *a*.
   a. What alleles will be present in this person's gametes?
   b. When do *A* and *a* segregate (1) if there is no crossing over between the locus and the centromere of the chromosome? (2) if there is a single crossover between the locus and the centromere?

2. What is the main cause of numerical chromosome abnormalities in humans?

3. Disregarding crossing over, which increases the amount of genetic variability, estimate the probability that all your chromosomes have come to you from your father's mother and your mother's mother. Would you be male or female?

4. A chromosome entering meiosis is composed of two sister chromatids, each of which is a single DNA molecule.
   a. In our species, at the end of meiosis I, how many chromosomes are there per cell? How many chromatids?
   b. At the end of meiosis II, how many chromosomes are there per cell? How many chromatids?
   c. When is the diploid chromosome number restored? When is the two-chromatid structure of a typical metaphase chromosome restored?

5. From Fig. 2.7, estimate the number of genes per million base pairs on chromosomes 1, 13, 18, 19, 21, and 22. Would a chromosome abnormality of equal size on chromosome 18 or 19 be more likely to have clinical impact? On chromosome 21 or 22?

The Human Genome
Gene Structure and Function

Stephen W. Scherer

Since the discovery of the structure of DNA and the development of technologies in molecular biology, remarkable progress has been made in our understanding of the structure and function of genes and chromosomes. The development of even newer methods to globally study the entire **genome** provides additional tools for a distinctive new approach to medical genetics. In this chapter we present an overview of **gene** structure and function and the aspects of molecular genetics required for an understanding of the principles underlying **genomic medicine**. We provide additional material online.

The increased knowledge of genes and of their organization in the genome has had an enormous impact on medicine and on our perception of human physiology. As 1980 Nobel laureate Paul Berg stated presciently at the dawn of this new era:

> *Just as our present knowledge and practice of medicine relies on a sophisticated knowledge of human anatomy, physiology, and biochemistry, so will dealing with disease in the future demand a detailed understanding of the molecular anatomy, physiology, and biochemistry of the human genome.... We shall need a more detailed knowledge of how human genes are organized and how they function and are regulated. We shall also have to have physicians who are as conversant with the molecular anatomy and physiology of chromosomes and genes as the cardiac surgeon is with the structure and workings of the heart.*

INFORMATION CONTENT OF THE HUMAN GENOME

How does the approximately 3-billion-letter digital code of the human genome guide the intricacies of human anatomy, physiology, and biochemistry to which Berg referred? The answer lies in the enormous amplification and integration of information content that occurs as one moves from genes in the genome to their products in the cell and to the observable expression of that **genetic** information as cellular, morphologic, clinical, or biochemical traits—that is, the **phenotype** of the individual. This hierarchic expansion of information from the genome to phenotype includes a wide range of structural and regulatory **RNA** products, as well as protein products that orchestrate the many functions of cells, tissues, organs, and the entire organism, in addition to their interactions with the environment. Even with the essentially complete **sequence** of the human genome in hand, we still do not know the precise number of genes in the genome. Our traditional definition of genes has also expanded. Current estimates are that the genome contains ~20,000 protein-coding genes (see Box in Chapter 2), but this figure only begins to hint at the levels of complexity that emerge from the decoding of this digital information (Fig. 3.1).

As introduced briefly in Chapter 2, the product of protein-coding genes is a protein whose structure ultimately determines its particular function(s) in the cell. But if there were a simple one-to-one correspondence between genes and proteins, we could have at most ~20,000 different proteins. This number is insufficient to account for the vast array of functions that occur in human cells over the life span. The answer to this dilemma is found in two features of gene structure and function. First, many genes are capable of generating multiple different products, not just one (see Fig. 3.1). This process, discussed later in this chapter, is accomplished through the use of alternative coding segments in genes and through the subsequent biochemical modification of the encoded protein; these two features of complex genomes result in a substantial amplification of information content. Indeed, it has been estimated that in this way, these 20,000 human genes can encode many hundreds of thousands of different proteins, collectively referred to as the **proteome**. Second, individual proteins do not function by themselves. They form networks, often involving many different proteins and regulatory RNAs that respond in a coordinated and integrated fashion to many different genetic, developmental, or environmental signals. The combinatorial nature of protein networks results in an even greater diversity of possible cellular functions.

Genes are located throughout the genome but tend to cluster in particular regions on particular chromosomes

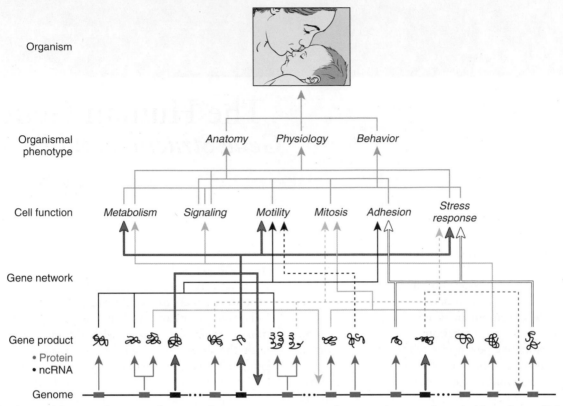

Figure 3.1 **The amplification of genetic information from genome to gene products to gene networks and ultimately to cellular function and phenotype.** The genome contains both protein-coding genes *(blue)* and noncoding RNA (ncRNA) genes *(red)*. Many genes in the genome use alternative coding information to generate multiple different products. Both small and large ncRNAs participate in gene regulation. Many proteins participate in multigene networks that respond to cellular signals in a coordinated and combinatorial manner, thus further expanding the range of cellular functions that underlie organismal phenotypes.

and to be relatively sparse in other regions or on other chromosomes. For example, chromosome 11, an ~135 million-bp (**megabase pairs [Mb]**) chromosome, is relatively gene-rich with ~1300 protein-coding genes (see Fig. 2.7). These genes are not distributed randomly along the chromosome, and their localization is particularly enriched in two chromosomal regions with gene density as high as one gene every 10 kb (Fig. 3.2). Some of the genes belong to families of related genes, as we will describe more fully later in this chapter. Other regions are gene-poor, and there are several so-called gene deserts of 1 million bp or more without any identified protein-coding genes. There are two caveats here: first, the process of gene identification and genome annotation remains an ongoing process despite the apparent robustness of recent estimates. It is virtually certain that there are some genes, including clinically relevant genes, that are currently undetected or that display characteristics that we do not currently recognize as being associated with genes. Second, as mentioned in Chapter 2, many genes are not protein coding; their products are functional RNA molecules (**noncoding RNAs [ncRNAs]**) (see Fig. 3.1) that play a variety of roles in the cell, many of which are only just being uncovered.

For genes located on the autosomes, there are two copies of each gene, one on the chromosome inherited from the mother and one on the chromosome inherited from the father. For most autosomal genes, both copies are expressed and generate a product. There are, however, a growing number of genes in the genome that are exceptions to this general rule and are expressed at characteristically different levels from the two copies, including some that, at the extreme, are expressed from only one of the two homologues. These examples of **allelic imbalance** are discussed in greater detail later in this chapter, as well as in Chapters 6 and 7. In addition, many genes are present in variable numbers at a particular location on a chromosome. One example is the variability in the copy number of the genes for amylase, an enzyme important in starch digestion; *AMY1* exists in two to eight copies per chromosome and is expressed in the salivary glands.

THE CENTRAL DOGMA: DNA → RNA → PROTEIN

How does the genome specify the functional complexity and diversity evident in Fig. 3.1? As we saw in the previous chapter, genetic information is contained in DNA in the chromosomes, within the cell nucleus. However, protein synthesis, the process through which information encoded in the genome is used to specify cellular

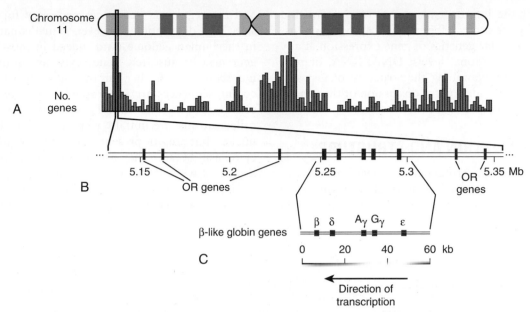

Figure 3.2 Gene content on chromosome 11, which consists of 135 Mb of DNA. (A) The distribution of genes is indicated along the chromosome and is high in two regions of the chromosome and low in other regions. (B) An expanded region from 5.15 to 5.35 Mb (measured from the short-arm telomere), which contains 10 known protein-coding genes, five belonging to the olfactory receptor (OR) gene family and five belonging to the globin gene family. (C) The five β-like globin genes expanded further. (Data from European Bioinformatics Institute and Wellcome Trust Sanger Institute: Ensembl release 70, January 2013. Available from http://www.ensembl.org).

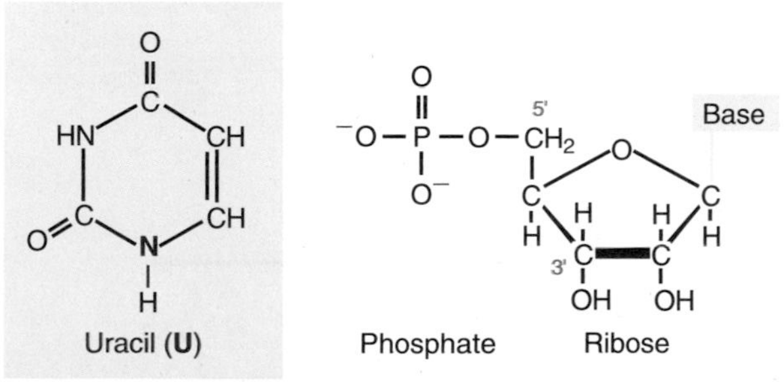

Figure 3.3 The pyrimidine uracil and the structure of a nucleotide in RNA. Note that the sugar ribose replaces the sugar deoxyribose of DNA. Compare with **Fig. 2.2.**

functions, takes place in the cytoplasm. This compartmentalization reflects the fact that the human organism is a **eukaryote**. This means that human cells have a nucleus containing the genome, which is separated by a nuclear membrane from the cytoplasm. In contrast, in prokaryotes like the intestinal bacterium *Escherichia coli*, DNA is not enclosed within a nucleus. Because of the compartmentalization of eukaryotic cells, information transfer from the nucleus to the cytoplasm is a complex process that has been a focus of much attention among molecular and cellular biologists.

The molecular link between these two related types of information—the DNA code of genes and the amino acid code of protein—is ribonucleic acid (RNA). The chemical structure of RNA is similar to that of DNA, except that each **nucleotide** in RNA has a ribose sugar component instead of a deoxyribose; in addition, uracil (U) replaces thymine as one of the **pyrimidine** bases of

RNA (Fig. 3.3). An additional difference between RNA and DNA is that RNA in most organisms exists as a single-stranded molecule, whereas DNA, as we saw in Chapter 2, exists as a double helix.

The informational relationships among DNA, RNA, and protein are intertwined: **genomic DNA** directs the synthesis and sequence of RNA, RNA directs the synthesis and sequence of polypeptides, and specific proteins are involved in the synthesis and metabolism of DNA and RNA. This flow of information is referred to as the central dogma of molecular biology.

Genetic information is stored in the DNA of the genome by means of a code (the **genetic code**, discussed later) in which the sequence of adjacent bases ultimately determines the sequence of amino acids in the encoded polypeptide. First, RNA is synthesized from the DNA template through the process of **transcription**. The RNA, carrying the coded information in a form called **messenger RNA (mRNA)**, is then transported from the nucleus to the cytoplasm, where the RNA sequence is decoded, or translated, to determine the sequence of amino acids in the protein being synthesized. The process of **translation** occurs on **ribosomes**, which are cytoplasmic organelles with binding sites for all of the interacting molecules, including the mRNA, involved in protein synthesis. Ribosomes are themselves made up of many different structural proteins in **association** with specialized types of RNA known as ribosomal RNA (rRNA). Translation involves yet a third type of RNA, **transfer RNA (tRNA)**, which provides the molecular link between the code contained in the base sequence of each mRNA and the amino acid sequence of the protein encoded by that mRNA.

Because of the interdependent flow of information represented by the central dogma, one can begin discussion of the molecular genetics of gene expression at any of its three informational levels: DNA, RNA, or protein. We begin by examining the structure of genes in the genome as a foundation for discussion of the genetic code, transcription, and translation.

GENE ORGANIZATION AND STRUCTURE

In its simplest form, a protein-coding gene can be visualized as a segment of a DNA molecule containing the code for the amino acid sequence of a polypeptide chain and the regulatory sequences necessary for its expression. This description, however, is inadequate for genes in the human genome (and indeed in most eukaryotic genomes) because few genes exist as continuous coding sequences. Rather, in the majority of genes, the coding sequences are interrupted by one or more noncoding regions (Fig. 3.4). These intervening sequences, called **introns**, are initially transcribed into RNA in the nucleus but are not present in the mature mRNA in the cytoplasm because they are removed ("spliced out") by a process we will discuss later. Thus information from the intronic sequences is not normally represented in the final protein product. Introns alternate with **exons**, the

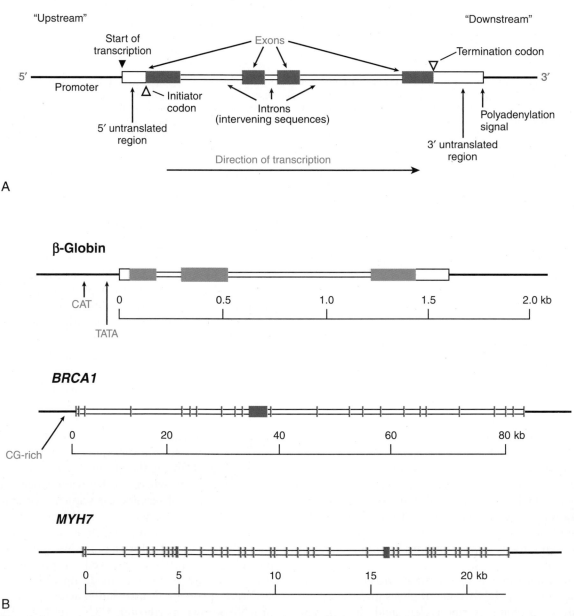

Figure 3.4 (A) General structure of a typical human gene. Individual labeled features are discussed in the text. (B) Examples of three medically important human genes. Different deleterious variants in the β-globin gene, with three exons, cause a variety of important disorders of hemoglobin (Case 25). Mutations in the *BRCA1* gene (24 exons) are responsible for many cases of inherited breast or breast and ovarian cancer (Case 7). Mutations in the β-myosin heavy chain (*MYH7*) gene (40 exons) lead to inherited hypertrophic cardiomyopathy.

segments of genes that ultimately determine the amino acid sequence of the protein. In addition, the collection of coding exons in any particular gene is flanked by additional sequences that are transcribed but untranslated, called the 5′ and 3′ untranslated regions (see Fig. 3.4). Although a few genes in the human genome have no introns, most genes contain at least one, with nine exons spanning ~25 kb found in an average gene. In many genes, the cumulative length of the introns makes up a far greater proportion of a gene's total length than do the exons. Whereas some genes are only a few kilobase pairs in length, others stretch on for hundreds of kilobase pairs. Also, a few genes are exceptionally large (e.g., the *CTNAP2* gene on **chromosome** 7 and the dystrophin gene on the **X chromosome** [pathogenic variants that lead to Duchenne/Becker muscular dystrophy (Case 14)] span >2 Mb, of which, remarkably, <1% consists of coding exons). The *KCNIP4* potassium channel gene has a single intron that is over 1 Mb in size.

Structural Features of a Typical Human Gene

A range of features characterize human genes (see Fig. 3.4). In Chapters 1 and 2, we briefly defined gene in general terms. At this point, we can provide a molecular definition of a gene as a sequence of DNA that specifies production of a functional product, be it a polypeptide or a functional RNA molecule. A gene includes not only the actual coding sequences but also adjacent nucleotide sequences required for the proper expression of the gene—that is, for the production of normal mRNA or other RNA molecules in the correct amount, in the correct place, and at the correct time during development or during the **cell cycle**.

The adjacent nucleotide sequences provide the molecular start and stop signals for the synthesis of mRNA transcribed from the gene. Because the primary RNA transcript is synthesized in a 5′ to 3′ direction, the transcriptional start is referred to as the 5′ end of the transcribed portion of a gene (see Fig. 3.4). By convention, the genomic DNA that precedes the transcriptional start site in the 5′ direction is referred to as the upstream sequence, whereas DNA sequence located in the 3′ direction past the end of a gene is the downstream sequence. At the 5′ end of each gene lies a **promoter** region that includes sequences responsible for the proper initiation of transcription. Within this region are several DNA elements whose sequence is often conserved among many different genes; this conservation, together with functional studies of gene expression, indicates that these particular sequences play an important role in gene regulation. Importantly, only a subset of genes in the genome is expressed in any given tissue or at any given time during development. Several different types of promoter are found in the human genome, with different regulatory properties that specify the patterns as well as the levels of expression of a particular gene in different tissues

and cell types, both during development and throughout the life span. Some of these properties are encoded in the genome, whereas others are specified by features of **chromatin** associated with those sequences, as discussed later in this chapter. Both promoters and other **regulatory elements** (located either 5′ or 3′ of a gene or in its introns) can be sites of variation causing genetic disease that can interfere with the normal expression of a gene. These regulatory elements, including **enhancers**, insulators, and **locus control regions**, are discussed more fully later in this chapter. Some of these elements lie a significant distance away from the coding portion of a gene, thus reinforcing the concept that the genomic environment in which a gene resides is an important feature of its evolution and regulation.

The 3′ untranslated region contains a signal for the addition of a sequence of adenosine residues (the so-called polyA tail) to the end of the mature RNA. Although it is generally accepted that such closely neighboring regulatory sequences are part of what is called a gene, the precise dimensions of any particular gene will remain somewhat uncertain until the potential functions of more distant sequences are fully characterized.

Gene Families

Many genes belong to gene families, which share closely related DNA sequences and encode polypeptides with closely related amino acid sequences.

Members of two such gene families are located within a small region on chromosome 11 (see Fig. 3.2) and illustrate a number of features that characterize gene families in general. One small and medically important **gene family** is composed of genes that encode the protein chains found in hemoglobins. The β-globin gene cluster on chromosome 11 and the related α-globin gene cluster on chromosome 16 are believed to have arisen by duplication of a primitive precursor gene ~500 million years ago. These two clusters contain multiple genes coding for closely related globin chains expressed at different developmental stages, from embryo to adult. Each cluster is believed to have evolved by a series of sequential gene duplication events within the past 100 million years. The exon-intron patterns of the functional globin genes have been remarkably conserved during evolution; each of the functional globin genes has two introns at similar locations (see the β-globin gene in Fig. 3.4), although the sequences contained within the introns have accumulated far more nucleotide base changes over time than have the coding sequences of each gene. The control of expression of the various globin genes, in the normal state as well as in the many inherited disorders of hemoglobin, is considered in more detail both later in this chapter and in Chapter 12.

The second gene family shown in Fig. 3.2 is the family of olfactory receptor (OR) genes. There are estimated to be as many as 1000 OR genes in the genome

(390 putatively functional genes and 465 pseudogenes). ORs are responsible for our acute sense of smell that can recognize and distinguish thousands of structurally diverse chemicals. OR genes are found throughout the genome on nearly every chromosome, although more than half are found on chromosome 11, including a number of family members near the β-globin cluster.

Pseudogenes

Within both the β-globin and OR gene families are sequences that are related to the functional globin and OR genes but that do not produce any functional RNA or protein product. DNA sequences that closely resemble known genes but are nonfunctional are called **pseudogenes**, and there are ~20,000 pseudogenes related to many different genes and gene families located all around the genome. Pseudogenes are of two general types, processed and nonprocessed. Nonprocessed pseudogenes are thought to be byproducts of evolution, representing "dead" genes that were once functional but are now vestigial, having been inactivated by **variants** in critical coding or regulatory sequences. In contrast to nonprocessed pseudogenes, processed pseudogenes are pseudogenes that have been formed, not by **mutation**, but by a process called **retrotransposition**, which involves transcription, generation of a DNA copy of the mRNA (a so-called **cDNA**) by reverse transcription, and finally integration of such DNA copies back into the genome at a location usually quite distant from the original gene. Because such pseudogenes are created by retrotransposition of a DNA copy of processed mRNA, they lack introns and are usually not on the same chromosome (or chromosomal region) as their progenitor gene. In many gene families there are as many or even more pseudogenes as there are functional gene members.

Noncoding RNA Genes

Many genes are protein coding and are transcribed into mRNAs that are ultimately translated into their respective proteins; their products comprise the enzymes, structural proteins, receptors, and regulatory proteins that are found in various human tissues and cell types. However, as introduced briefly in Chapter 2, there are additional genes whose functional product appears to be the RNA itself (see Fig. 3.1). These so-called **noncoding RNAs (ncRNAs)** have a range of functions in the cell, although many do not as yet have any identified function. By current estimates, there are some 15,000 to 20,000 ncRNA genes in addition to the ~20,000 protein-coding genes that we introduced earlier. Thus the collection of ncRNAs represents approximately half of all identified human genes.

Some of the types of ncRNA play largely generic roles in cellular infrastructure, including the tRNAs and rRNAs involved in translation of mRNAs on ribosomes, other RNAs involved in control of **RNA splicing**, and small nucleolar RNAs (snoRNAs) involved in modifying rRNAs. Additional ncRNAs can be quite long (thus sometimes called long ncRNAs [**lncRNAs**]) and play roles in gene regulation, gene silencing, and human disease, as we explore in more detail later in this chapter and in Case Report 35.

A particular class of small RNAs of growing importance are the **microRNAs (miRNAs)**, ncRNAs of only ~22 bases in length that suppress translation of target genes by binding to their respective mRNAs and regulating protein production from the target transcript(s). Well over 1000 miRNA genes have been identified in the human genome; some are evolutionarily conserved, whereas others appear to be of quite recent origin. Some miRNAs have been shown to down-regulate hundreds of mRNAs each, with different combinations of target RNAs in different tissues; combined, the miRNAs are thus predicted to control the activity of as many as 30% of all protein-coding genes in the genome.

Although this is a fast-moving area of genome biology, pathogenic variants in several ncRNA genes have already been implicated in human diseases, including cancer, developmental disorders, and various diseases of both early and adult onset (see Box 3.1).

BOX 3.1 NONCODING RNAS AND DISEASE

The importance of various types of ncRNAs for medicine is underscored by their roles in a range of human diseases, from early developmental syndromes to adult-onset disorders.

- **Deletion** of a cluster of miRNA genes on chromosome 13 leads to a form of Feingold syndrome, a developmental syndrome of skeletal and growth defects, including microcephaly, short stature, and digital **anomalies**.
- Pathogenic variants in the miRNA gene *MIR96*, in the region of the gene critical for the **specificity** of recognition of its target mRNA(s), can result in progressive hearing loss in adults.
- Aberrant levels of certain classes of miRNAs have been reported in a wide variety of cancers, central nervous system disorders, and cardiovascular disease (see Chapter 15).
- Deletion of clusters of snoRNA genes on chromosome 15 results in Prader-Willi syndrome, a disorder characterized by obesity, hypogonadism, and cognitive impairment (see Case 38).
- Abnormal expression of a specific lncRNA on chromosome 12 has been reported in patients with a pregnancy-associated disease called HELLP (*h*emolysis, *e*levated *l*iver enzymes, and *l*ow *p*latelets) syndrome.
- Deletion, abnormal expression, and/or structural abnormalities in different lncRNAs with roles in long-range regulation of gene expression and genome function underlie a variety of disorders involving **telomere** length maintenance, monoallelic expression of genes in specific regions of the genome, and X chromosome dosage (see Chapter 6).

FUNDAMENTALS OF GENE EXPRESSION

For genes that encode proteins, the flow of information from gene to polypeptide involves several steps (Fig. 3.5). Initiation of transcription of a gene is under the influence of promoters and other regulatory elements, as well as specific proteins known as **transcription factors**, which interact with specific sequences within these regions and determine the spatial and temporal pattern of expression of a gene. Transcription of a gene is initiated at the transcriptional start site on chromosomal DNA at the beginning of a 5′ transcribed but *un*translated *region* (called the 5′ UTR), just upstream from the coding sequences, and continues along the chromosome for anywhere from several hundred **base pairs** to more than a million base pairs, through both introns and exons and past the end of the coding sequences. After modification at both the 5′ and 3′ ends of the primary RNA transcript, the portions corresponding to introns are removed, and the segments corresponding to exons are spliced together, a process called RNA splicing. After splicing, the resulting mRNA (containing a central segment that is now colinear with the coding portions of the gene) is transported from the nucleus to the cytoplasm, where the mRNA is finally translated into the amino acid sequence of the encoded polypeptide. Each of the steps in this complex pathway is subject to error, and DNA variations that interfere with the individual steps have been implicated in a number of inherited disorders (see Chapters 12 and 13).

Transcription

Transcription of protein-coding genes by **RNA polymerase** II (one of several classes of RNA polymerases) is initiated at the transcriptional start site, the point in the 5′ UTR that corresponds to the 5′ end of the final RNA product (see Figs. 3.4 and 3.5). Synthesis of the primary RNA transcript proceeds in a 5′ to 3′ direction, whereas the strand of the gene that is transcribed and that serves as the template for RNA synthesis is read in a 3′ to 5′ direction with respect to the direction of the deoxyribose phosphodiester backbone (see Fig. 3.5). Because the RNA synthesized corresponds both in polarity and in base sequence (substituting U for T) to the 5′ to 3′ strand of DNA, this 5′ to 3′ strand of nontranscribed DNA is sometimes called the coding, or **sense**, DNA strand. The 3′ to 5′ strand of DNA that is used as a template for transcription is then referred to as the noncoding, or **antisense**, strand. Transcription

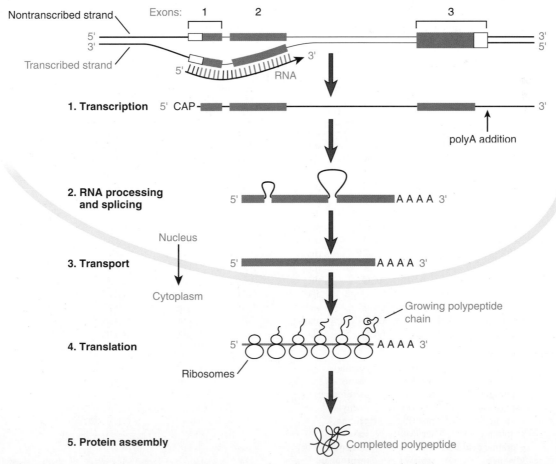

Figure 3.5 Flow of information from DNA to RNA to protein for a hypothetical gene with three exons and two introns. Within the exons, *purple* indicates the coding sequences. Steps include transcription, RNA processing and splicing, RNA transport from the nucleus to the cytoplasm, and translation.

continues through both intronic and exonic portions of the gene, beyond the position on the chromosome that eventually corresponds to the 3′ end of the mature mRNA. Whether transcription ends at a predetermined 3′ termination point is unknown.

The primary RNA transcript is processed by addition of a chemical cap structure to the 5′ end of the RNA and cleavage of the 3′ end at a specific point downstream from the end of the coding information. This cleavage is followed by addition of a polyA tail to the 3′ end of the RNA; the polyA tail appears to increase the stability of the resulting polyadenylated RNA. The location of the **polyadenylation** point is specified in part by the sequence AAUAAA (or a variant of this), usually found in the 3′ untranslated portion of the RNA transcript. All of these posttranscriptional modifications take place in the nucleus, as does the process of RNA splicing. The fully processed RNA, now called mRNA, is then transported to the cytoplasm, where translation takes place (see Fig. 3.5).

Translation and the Genetic Code

In the cytoplasm, mRNA is translated into protein by the action of a variety of short RNA adaptor molecules, the tRNAs, each specific for a particular amino acid. These remarkable molecules, each only 70 to 100 nucleotides long, have the job of bringing the correct amino acids into position along the mRNA template, to be added to the growing polypeptide chain. Protein synthesis occurs on ribosomes, macromolecular complexes made up of rRNA (encoded by the 18 S and 28 S rRNA genes), and several dozen ribosomal proteins (see Fig. 3.5).

The key to translation is a code that relates specific amino acids to combinations of three adjacent bases along the mRNA. Each set of three bases constitutes a **codon**, specific for a particular amino acid (Table 3.1). In theory, almost infinite variations are possible in the arrangement of the bases along a polynucleotide chain. At any one position, there are four possibilities (A, T, C, or G); thus, for three bases, there are 4^3, or 64, possible triplet combinations. These 64 codons constitute the **genetic code**.

Because there are only 20 amino acids and 64 possible codons, most amino acids are specified by more than one codon; hence the code is said to be degenerate. For instance, the base in the third position of the triplet can often be either **purine** (A or G) or either pyrimidine (T or C) or, in some cases, any one of the four bases, without altering the coded message (see Table 3.1). Leucine and arginine are each specified by six codons. Only methionine and tryptophan are each specified by a single, unique codon. Three of the codons are called stop (or nonsense) codons because they designate termination of translation of the mRNA at that point.

TABLE 3.1 The Genetic Code

First Base	Second Base								Third Base
	U		C		A		G		
U	UUU	phe	UCU	ser	UAU	tyr	UGU	cys	U
	UUC	phe	UCC	ser	UAC	tyr	UGC	cys	C
	UUA	leu	UCA	ser	UAA	stop	UGA	stop	A
	UUG	leu	UCG	ser	UAG	stop	UGG	trp	G
C	CUU	leu	CCU	pro	CAU	his	CGU	arg	U
	CUC	leu	CCC	pro	CAC	his	CGC	arg	C
	CUA	leu	CCA	pro	CAA	gln	CGA	arg	A
	CUG	leu	CCG	pro	CAG	gln	CGG	arg	G
A	AUU	ile	ACU	thr	AAU	asn	AGU	ser	U
	AUC	ile	ACC	thr	AAC	asn	AGC	ser	C
	AUA	ile	ACA	thr	AAA	lys	AGA	arg	A
	AUG	met	ACG	thr	AAG	lys	AGG	arg	G
G	GUU	val	GCU	ala	GAU	asp	GGU	gly	U
	GUC	val	GCC	ala	GAC	asp	GGC	gly	C
	GUA	val	GCA	ala	GAA	glu	GGA	gly	A
	GUG	val	GCG	ala	GAG	glu	GGG	gly	G

Abbreviations for Amino Acids

ala (A)	alanine	leu (L)	leucine
arg (R)	arginine	lys (K)	lysine
asn (N)	asparagine	met (M)	methionine
asp (D)	aspartic acid	phe (F)	phenylalanine
cys (C)	cysteine	pro (P)	proline
gln (Q)	glutamine	ser (S)	serine
glu (E)	glutamic acid	thr (T)	threonine
gly (G)	glycine	trp (W)	tryptophan
his (H)	histidine	tyr (Y)	tyrosine
ile (I)	isoleucine	val (V)	valine

Stop, Termination codon. Codons are shown in terms of mRNA, which are complementary to the corresponding DNA codons.

Translation of a processed mRNA is always initiated at a codon specifying methionine. Methionine is therefore the first encoded (amino-terminal) amino acid of each polypeptide chain, although it is usually removed before protein synthesis is completed. The codon for methionine (the **initiator codon**, AUG) establishes the **reading frame** of the mRNA; each subsequent codon is read in turn to predict the amino acid sequence of the protein.

The molecular links between codons and amino acids are the specific tRNA molecules. A particular site on each tRNA forms a three-base **anticodon** that is complementary to a specific codon on the mRNA. Bonding between the codon and anticodon brings the appropriate amino acid into the next position on the ribosome for attachment, by formation of a peptide bond, to the carboxyl end of the growing polypeptide chain. The ribosome then slides along the mRNA exactly three bases, bringing the next codon into line for recognition by another tRNA with the next amino acid. Thus proteins are synthesized from the amino terminus to the carboxyl terminus, which corresponds to translation of the mRNA in a 5′ to 3′ direction.

As mentioned earlier, translation ends when a **stop codon** (UGA, UAA, or UAG) is encountered in the same reading frame as the initiator codon. (Stop codons in either of the other unused reading frames are not read, and therefore have no effect on translation.) The completed polypeptide is then released from the ribosome, which becomes available to begin synthesis of another protein.

BOX 3.2 INCREASING FUNCTIONAL DIVERSITY OF PROTEINS

Many proteins undergo extensive posttranslational packaging and processing as they adopt their final functional state (see Chapter 13). The polypeptide chain that is the primary translation product folds on itself and forms intramolecular bonds to create a specific 3D structure that is determined by the amino acid sequence itself. Two or more polypeptide chains, products of the same gene or of different genes, may combine to form a single multiprotein complex. For example, two α-globin chains and two β-globin chains associate noncovalently to form a tetrameric hemoglobin molecule (see Chapter 12). The protein products may also be modified chemically by, for example, addition of methyl groups, phosphates, or carbohydrates at specific sites. These modifications can have significant influence on the function or abundance of the modified protein. Other modifications may involve cleavage of the protein, either to remove specific amino-terminal sequences after they have functioned to direct a protein to its correct location within the cell (e.g., proteins that function within mitochondria) or to split the molecule into smaller polypeptide chains. For example, the two chains that make up mature insulin, one 21 and the other 30 amino acids long, are originally part of an 82–amino acid primary translation product called proinsulin. The SSH gene involved in holoprosencephaly (see Case Report 23) encodes a protein that also goes through a series of processing steps before being secreted from the cell.

Transcription of the Mitochondrial Genome

The previous sections described fundamentals of gene expression for genes contained in the nuclear genome. The mitochondrial genome has its own transcription and protein-synthesis system. A specialized RNA polymerase, encoded in the nuclear genome, is used to transcribe the 16-kb mitochondrial genome, which contains two related promoter sequences, one for each strand of the circular genome. Each strand is transcribed in its entirety, and the mitochondrial transcripts are then processed to generate the various individual mitochondrial mRNAs, tRNAs, and rRNAs.

GENE EXPRESSION IN ACTION

The flow of information outlined in the preceding sections can best be appreciated by reference to a particular well-studied gene, the β-globin gene. The β-globin chain is a 146–amino acid polypeptide, encoded by a gene that occupies ~1.6 kb on the short arm of chromosome 11. The gene has three exons and two introns (see Fig. 3.4). The β-globin gene, as well as the other genes in the β-globin cluster (see Fig. 3.2), is transcribed in a centromere-to-telomere direction. The orientation, however, is different for different genes in the genome and depends on which strand of the chromosomal double helix is the **coding strand** for a particular gene.

DNA sequences required for accurate initiation of transcription of the β-globin gene are located in the promoter within ~200 bp upstream from the transcription start site (see Box 3.2). The double-stranded DNA sequence of this region of the β-globin gene, the corresponding RNA sequence, and the translated sequence of the first 10 amino acids are depicted in Fig. 3.6 to illustrate the relationships among these three information levels. As mentioned previously, it is the 3′ to 5′ strand of the DNA that serves as the template and is transcribed, but it is the 5′ to 3′ strand of DNA that directly corresponds to the 5′ to 3′ sequence of the mRNA (and, in fact, is identical to it except that U is substituted for T). Because of this correspondence, the 5′ to 3′ DNA strand of a gene (i.e., the strand that is not transcribed) is the strand generally reported in the scientific literature or in databases.

In accordance with this convention, the complete sequence of ~2.0 kb of chromosome 11 that includes the β-globin gene is shown in Fig. 3.7. (It is sobering to reflect that a printout of the entire human genome at this scale would require >300 books the size of this textbook!) Within these 2.0 kb are contained most, but not all, of the sequence elements required to encode and regulate the expression of this gene. Indicated in Fig. 3.7 are many of the important structural features of the β-globin gene, including conserved promoter sequence elements, intron and exon boundaries, 5′ and 3′ UTRs, RNA splice sites, the initiator and termination codons, and the polyadenylation signal, all of which are

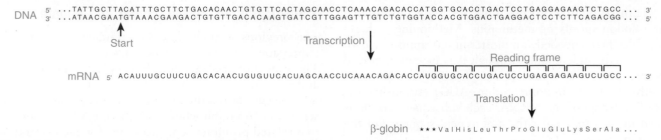

Figure 3.6 **Structure and nucleotide sequence of the 5′ end of the human β-globin gene on the short arm of chromosome 11.** Transcription of the 3′ to 5′ *(lower)* strand begins at the indicated start site to produce β-globin messenger RNA (mRNA). The translational reading frame is determined by the AUG initiator codon (★★★); subsequent codons specifying amino acids are indicated in *blue*. The other two potential frames are not used.

known to be mutated in various inherited defects of the β-globin gene (see Chapter 12).

Initiation of Transcription

The β-globin promoter, like many other gene promoters, consists of a series of relatively short functional elements that interact with specific regulatory proteins (generically called transcription factors) that control transcription, including, in the case of the globin genes, those proteins that restrict expression of these genes to erythroid cells, the cells in which hemoglobin is produced. There are well over a thousand sequence-specific, DNA-binding transcription factors in the genome, some of which are ubiquitous in their expression, whereas others are cell type or tissue specific.

One important promoter sequence found in many but not all genes is the **TATA box,** a conserved region rich in adenines and thymines that is ~25 to 30 bp upstream of the start site of transcription (see Figs. 3.4 and 3.7). The TATA box appears to be important for determining the position of the start of transcription, which in the β-globin gene is ~50 bp upstream from the translation initiation site (see Fig. 3.7). Thus in this gene, there are ~50 bp of sequence at the 5′ end that are transcribed but are not translated; in other genes, the 5′ UTR can be much longer and can even be interrupted by one or more introns. A second conserved region, the so-called CAT box (actually CCAAT), is a few dozen base pairs farther upstream (see Fig. 3.7). Both experimentally induced and naturally occurring variants in either of these sequence elements, as well as in other regulatory sequences even farther upstream, lead to a sharp reduction in the level of transcription, thereby demonstrating the importance of these elements for normal gene expression. Many variants in these regulatory elements have been identified in individuals with the hemoglobin disorder β-thalassemia (see Chapter 12).

Not all gene promoters contain the two specific elements just described. Importantly, genes that are constitutively expressed in most or all tissues (so-called **housekeeping genes**) often lack the CAT and TATA boxes, which are more typical of tissue-specific genes. Promoters

of many housekeeping genes contain a high proportion of cytosines and guanines in relation to the surrounding DNA (see the promoter of the *BRCA1* breast cancer gene in Fig. 3.4). Such CG-rich promoters are often located in regions of the genome called **CpG islands,** so named because of the unusually high concentration of the dinucleotide 5′-CpG-3′ (the *p* representing the phosphate group between adjacent bases) (see Fig. 2.3) that stands out from the more general AT-rich genomic landscape. Some of the CG-rich sequence elements found in these promoters are thought to serve as binding sites for specific transcription factors. CpG islands are also important because they are targets for **DNA methylation.** Extensive DNA methylation at CpG islands is usually associated with repression of gene transcription, as we will discuss later in the context of chromatin and its role in the control of gene expression (see Chapter 8).

Transcription by RNA polymerase II (RNA pol II) is subject to regulation at multiple levels, including binding to the promoter, initiation of transcription, unwinding of the DNA double helix to expose the template strand, and elongation as RNA pol II moves along the DNA. Although some silenced genes are devoid of RNA pol II binding altogether, consistent with their inability to be transcribed in a given cell type, others have RNA pol II poised bidirectionally at the transcriptional start site, perhaps as a means of fine-tuning transcription in response to particular cellular signals.

In addition to the sequences that constitute a promoter itself are other sequence elements that can markedly alter the efficiency of transcription. The best characterized of these activating sequences are called enhancers. Enhancers are sequence elements that can act at a distance from a gene to stimulate transcription. Enhancers can be located several or even hundreds of kilobases away from a gene, and in the case of the Sonic hedgehog (*SHH*) gene there can be many, with some being 1 million bp away, acting in different tissues. Unlike promoters, enhancers are both position and orientation independent and can be located either 5′ or 3′ of the transcription start site. Specific enhancer elements function only in certain cell types and thus appear to be involved in establishing the tissue specificity or level of

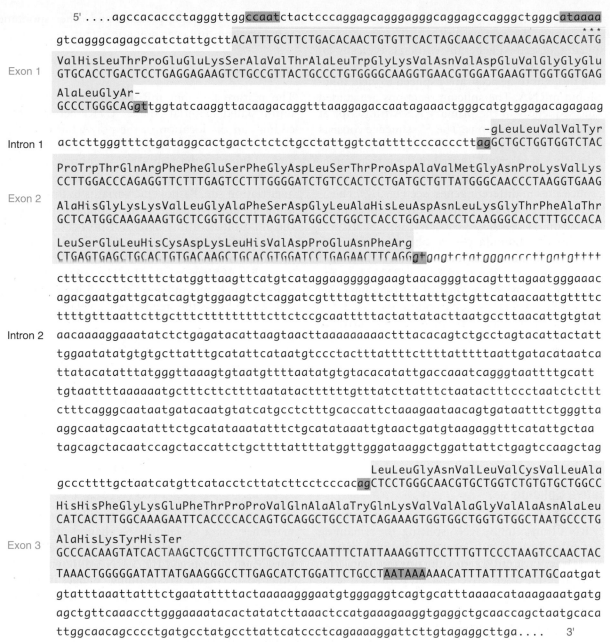

Figure 3.7 Nucleotide sequence of the complete human β-globin gene. The sequence of the 5′ to 3′ strand of the gene is shown. *Tan* areas with capital letters represent exonic sequences corresponding to mature mRNA. Lowercase letters indicate introns and flanking sequences. The CAT and TATA box sequences in the 5′ flanking region are indicated in *brown*. The GT and AG dinucleotides important for RNA splicing at the intron-exon junctions and the AATAAA signal important for addition of a polyA tail are also highlighted. The ATG initiator codon (AUG in mRNA) and the TAA stop codon (UAA in mRNA) are shown in *red* letters. The amino acid sequence of β-globin is shown above the coding sequence; the three-letter abbreviations in Table 3.1 are used here. (Original data from Lawn RM, Efstratiadis A, O'Connell C, et al: The nucleotide sequence of the human β-globin gene. *Cell* 21:647–651, 1980.)

expression of many genes, in concert with one or more transcription factors. In the case of the β-globin gene, several tissue-specific enhancers are present both within the gene itself and in its flanking regions. The interaction of enhancers with specific regulatory proteins leads to increased levels of transcription.

Normal expression of the β-globin gene during development also requires more distant sequences called the locus control region (LCR), located upstream of the ε-globin gene (see Fig. 3.2), which is required for

establishing the proper chromatin context needed for appropriate high-level expression. As expected, variants that disrupt or delete either enhancer or LCR sequences interfere with or prevent β-globin gene expression (see Chapter 12).

RNA Splicing

The primary RNA transcript of the β-globin gene contains two introns, ~100 and 850 bp in length, that need to be removed and the remaining RNA segments joined together to form the mature mRNA. The process of RNA splicing, described generally earlier, is typically an exact and highly efficient one; 95% of β-globin transcripts are thought to be accurately spliced to yield functional globin mRNA. The splicing reactions are guided by specific sequences in the primary RNA transcript at both 5′ and 3′ ends of introns. The 5′ sequence consists of nine nucleotides, of which two (the dinucleotide GT [GU in the RNA transcript] located in the intron immediately adjacent to the splice site) are virtually invariant among splice sites in different genes (see Fig. 3.7). The 3′ sequence consists of approximately a dozen nucleotides, of which, again, two—the AG located immediately 5′ to the intron-exon boundary—are obligatory for normal splicing. The splice sites themselves are unrelated to the reading frame of the particular mRNA. In some instances, as in the case of intron 1 of the β-globin gene, the intron actually splits a specific codon (see Fig. 3.7).

The medical significance of RNA splicing is illustrated by the fact that variants within the conserved sequences at the intron-exon boundaries commonly impair RNA splicing, with a concomitant reduction in the amount of normal, mature β-globin mRNA; alterations in the GT or AG dinucleotides mentioned earlier invariably eliminate normal splicing of the intron containing the variant. Representative splice site variants identified in patients with β-thalassemia are discussed in detail in Chapter 12.

Alternative Splicing

As just discussed, when introns are removed from the primary RNA transcript by RNA splicing, the remaining exons are spliced together to generate the final, mature mRNA. However, for most genes, the **primary transcript** can follow multiple alternative splicing pathways, leading to the synthesis of multiple related but different mRNAs, each of which can be subsequently translated to generate different protein products (see Fig. 3.1). Some of these alternative events are tissue or cell type specific, and, to the extent that such events are determined by primary sequence, they are subject to allelic variation between different individuals. Nearly all human genes undergo alternative splicing to some degree, and it has been estimated that there are an average of two or three alternative transcripts per gene in the human genome, thus greatly expanding the information content of the human genome beyond the ~20,000 protein-coding genes. The regulation of alternative splicing appears to play a particularly impressive role during brain development, where it may contribute to generating the high levels of functional diversity needed in the nervous system. The reason for this may be because genes expressed in the brain tend to be larger in size and have more exons than those expressed in other tissues. Consistent with this, susceptibility to a number of neurodevelopmental conditions has been associated with shifts or **disruption** of alternative splicing patterns and other spontaneous, rare **germline**, and even somatic events.

Polyadenylation

The mature β-globin mRNA contains ~130 bp of 3′ untranslated material (the 3′ UTR) between the stop codon and the location of the polyA tail (see Fig. 3.7). As in other genes, cleavage of the 3′ end of the mRNA and addition of the polyA tail is controlled, at least in part, by an AAUAAA sequence ~20 bp before the polyadenylation site. Pathogenic variants in this polyadenylation signal in patients with β-thalassemia document the importance of this signal for proper 3′ cleavage and polyadenylation (see Chapter 12). The 3′ UTR of some genes can be up to several kb in length. Other genes have a number of alternative polyadenylation sites, **selection** among which may influence the stability of the resulting mRNA and thus the steady-state level of each mRNA.

RNA Editing and RNA-DNA Sequence Differences

Recent findings suggest that the conceptual principle underlying the central dogma—that RNA and protein sequences reflect the underlying genomic sequence—may not always hold true. RNA editing to change the nucleotide sequence of the mRNA has been demonstrated in a number of organisms, including humans. This process involves deamination of adenosine at particular sites, converting an A in the DNA sequence to an inosine in the resulting RNA; this is then read by the translational machinery as a G, leading to changes in gene expression and protein function, especially in the nervous system. More widespread RNA-DNA differences involving other bases (with corresponding changes in the encoded amino acid sequence) have also been reported, at levels that vary among individuals. Although the mechanism(s) and clinical relevance of these events remain controversial, they illustrate the existence of a range of processes capable of increasing transcript and proteome diversity.

EPIGENETIC AND EPIGENOMIC ASPECTS OF GENE EXPRESSION

Given the range of functions and fates that different cells in any organism must adopt over its lifetime, it is apparent that not all genes in the genome can be actively expressed in every cell at all times. As important as completion of the Human Genome Project has been for contributing to our understanding of human biology and disease, identifying the genomic sequences and features that direct developmental, spatial, and temporal aspects of gene expression remains a formidable challenge. Several decades of work in molecular biology have defined critical regulatory elements for many individual genes, as we saw in the previous section, and more recent attention has been directed toward performing such studies on a genome-wide scale.

In Chapter 2 we introduced general aspects of chromatin that package the genome and its genes in all cells. Here, we explore the specific characteristics of chromatin that are associated with active or repressed genes as a step toward identifying the regulatory code for expression of the human genome. Such studies focus on reversible changes in the chromatin landscape as determinants of gene function rather than on changes to the genome sequence itself and are thus called *epigenetic* or, when considered in the context of the entire genome, *epigenomic* (Greek *epi-*, over or upon).

The field of epigenetics is growing rapidly and is the study of heritable changes in cellular function or gene expression that can be transmitted from cell to cell (and even generation to generation), as a result of chromatin-based molecular signals (Fig. 3.8). Complex epigenetic states can be established, maintained, and transmitted by a variety of mechanisms: modifications to the DNA, such as DNA methylation; numerous **histone** modifications that alter chromatin packaging or access; and substitution of specialized histone variants that mark chromatin associated with particular sequences or

regions in the genome. These chromatin changes can be highly dynamic and transient, capable of responding rapidly and sensitively to changing needs in the cell, or they can be long lasting, capable of being transmitted through multiple cell divisions or even to subsequent generations. In either instance, the key concept is that epigenetic mechanisms do *not* alter the underlying DNA sequence, and this distinguishes them from genetic mechanisms, which are sequence based. Together, the epigenetic marks and the DNA sequence make up the set of signals that guide the genome to express its genes at the right time, in the right place, and in the right amounts. These topics are covered in detail in Chapter 8.

DNA Methylation

DNA methylation involves the modification of cytosine bases by methylation of the carbon at the fifth position in the pyrimidine ring (Fig. 3.9). Extensive DNA methylation is a mark of repressed genes and is a widespread mechanism associated with the establishment of specific programs of gene expression during cell **differentiation** and development. Typically, DNA methylation occurs on the C of CpG dinucleotides (see Fig. 3.8)

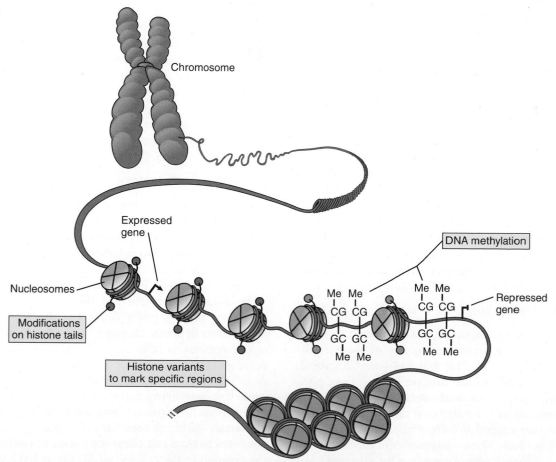

Figure 3.8 Schematic representation of chromatin and three major epigenetic mechanisms: DNA methylation at CpG dinucleotides, associated with gene repression; various modifications *(indicated by different colors)* on histone tails, associated with either gene expression or repression; and various histone variants that mark specific regions of the genome, associated with specific functions required for chromosome stability or genome integrity. Not to scale.

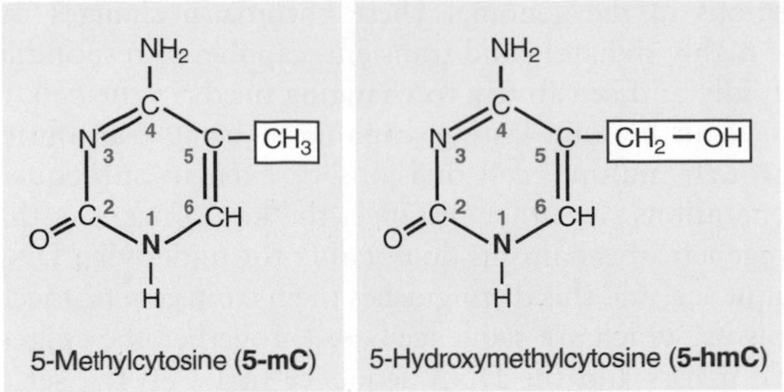

Figure 3.9 The modified DNA bases, 5-methylcytosine and 5-hydroxymethylcytosine. Compare to the structure of cytosine in Fig. 2.2. The added methyl and hydroxymethyl groups are boxed in *purple*. The atoms in the pyrimidine rings are numbered 1–6 to indicate the 5-carbon.

and inhibits gene expression by recruitment of specific methyl-CpG–binding proteins that, in turn, recruit chromatin-modifying enzymes to silence transcription. The presence of 5-methylcytosine (5-mC) is considered to be a stable epigenetic mark that can be faithfully transmitted through cell division; however, altered methylation states are frequently observed in cancer, with hypomethylation of large genomic segments or with regional hypermethylation (particularly at CpG islands) in others (see Chapter 16).

Extensive demethylation occurs during germ cell development and in the early stages of embryonic development, consistent with the need to reset the chromatin environment and restore totipotency or pluripotency of the **zygote** and of various **stem cell** populations. Although the details are still incompletely understood, these reprogramming steps appear to involve the enzymatic conversion of 5-mC to 5-hydroxymethylcytosine (5-hmC) (see Fig. 3.9), as a likely intermediate in the demethylation of DNA. Overall, 5-mC levels are stable across adult tissues (~5% of all cytosines), whereas 5-hmC levels are much lower and much more variable (0.1–1% of all cytosines). Interestingly, although 5-hmC is widespread in the genome, its highest levels are found in known regulatory regions, suggesting a possible role in the regulation of specific promoters and enhancers.

Histone Modifications

A second class of epigenetic signals consists of an extensive inventory of modifications to any of the core histone types: H2A, H2B, H3, and H4 (see Chapter 2). Such modifications include histone methylation, phosphorylation, acetylation, and others at specific amino acid residues, mostly located on the N-terminal tails of histones that extend out from the core **nucleosome** itself (see Fig. 3.8). These epigenetic modifications are believed to influence gene expression by affecting chromatin compaction or accessibility and by signaling protein complexes that—depending on the nature of the signal—activate or silence gene expression at that site.

There are dozens of modified sites that can be experimentally queried genome-wide by using antibodies that recognize specifically modified sites—for example, histone H3 methylated at lysine position 9 (H3K9 methylation, using the one-letter abbreviation K for lysine; see Table 3.1) or histone H3 acetylated at lysine position 27 (H3K27 acetylation). The former is a repressive mark associated with silent regions of the genome, whereas the latter is a mark for activating regulatory regions.

Histone Variants

The histone modifications just discussed involve modification of the core histones themselves, which are all encoded by multigene clusters in a few locations in the genome. In contrast, the many dozens of histone variants are products of entirely different genes located elsewhere in the genome, and their amino acid sequences are distinct from, although related to, those of the canonical histones.

Different histone variants are associated with different functions, and they replace—all or in part—the related member of the core histones found in typical nucleosomes to generate specialized chromatin structures (see Fig. 3.8). Some variants mark specific regions or loci in the genome with highly specialized functions (e.g., the CENP-A histone is a histone H3-related variant that is found exclusively at functional **centromeres** in the genome and contributes to essential features of centromeric chromatin that mark the location of kinetochores along the chromosome fiber). Other variants are more transient and mark regions of the genome with particular attributes (e.g., H2A.X is a histone H2A variant involved in the response to DNA damage to mark regions of the genome that require DNA repair).

Chromatin Architecture

In contrast to the impression one gets from viewing the genome as a linear string of sequence (see Fig. 3.7), the genome adopts a highly ordered and dynamic arrangement within the space of the nucleus, correlated with and likely guided by the epigenetic and epigenomic signals just discussed. This three-dimensional (3D) landscape is highly predictive of the map of all expressed sequences in any given cell type (the **transcriptome**) and reflects dynamic changes in chromatin architecture at different levels (Fig. 3.10). First, large chromosomal domains (up to millions of base pairs in size) can exhibit coordinated patterns of gene expression at the chromosome level, involving dynamic interactions between different intrachromosomal and interchromosomal points of contact within the nucleus. At a finer level, technical advances to map and sequence points of contact around the genome in the context of 3D space have pointed to ordered **loops** of chromatin that position and orient genes precisely, exposing or blocking critical regulatory regions for access by RNA pol II, transcription factors,

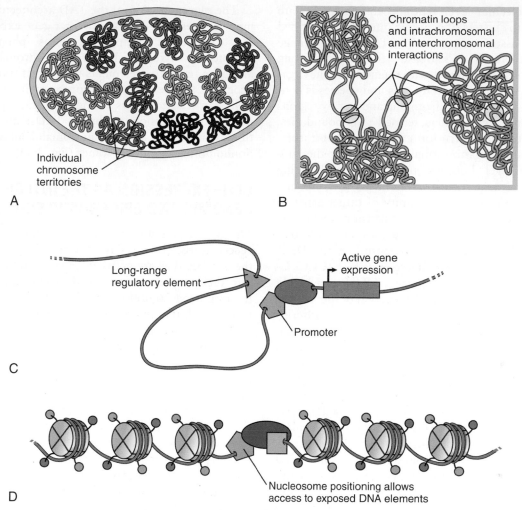

Figure 3.10 **Three-dimensional architecture and dynamic packaging of the genome, viewed at increasing levels of resolution.** (A) Within interphase nuclei, each chromosome occupies a particular territory, represented by the different colors. (B) Chromatin is organized into large subchromosomal domains within each territory, with loops that bring certain sequences and genes into proximity with each other, with detectable intrachromosomal and interchromosomal interactions. (C) Loops bring long-range regulatory elements (e.g., enhancers or locus-control regions) into association with promoters, leading to active transcription and gene expression. (D) Positioning of nucleosomes along the chromatin fiber provides access to specific DNA sequences for binding by transcription factors and other regulatory proteins.

and other regulators (see Chapter 2). Lastly, specific and dynamic patterns of nucleosome positioning differ among cell types and tissues in the face of changing environmental and developmental cues (see Fig. 3.10). The biophysical, epigenomic, and/or genomic properties that facilitate or specify the orderly and dynamic packaging of each chromosome during each cell cycle, without reducing the genome to a disordered tangle within the nucleus, remain a marvel of landscape engineering.

Topologically Associating Domains

Philipp Maass

Chromosomes are organized in the 3D space of the nucleus to fulfill gene regulation. Within this 3D genome organization, chromosomes are spatially segregated in A- and B-type genomic compartments that represent active (**euchromatin** = open chromatin) and inactive (**heterochromatin** = repressive chromatin) domains, respectively. Euchromatin is typically associated with higher gene density and early replication, while repressive chromatin—which tends to be transcriptionally silent—is densely packed and protects chromosome integrity. Genomic compartmentalization can comprise multiple subcompartments with specific histone marks, which contribute to the general organization of the genome in the nucleus by establishing subnuclear domains with various functions. For example, the nucleolus is the largest subnuclear compartment and forms at the site of hundreds of ribosomal genes of the five **acrocentric** chromosomes (13, 14, 15, 21, and 22) for the preassembly of the ribosomal subunits. Splicing or nuclear speckles are nuclear domains enriched for splicing machinery; Cajal bodies relate to mRNA processing, and promyelocytic leukemia (PML) bodies are involved in cell cycle processes and DNA repair. Collectively, these 3D organizational hubs in the nuclei regulate gene expression and posttranscriptional processing of RNAs, and facilitate tissue-specific gene regulation.

On the molecular level genomic compartments are subdivided into clusters of genomic interactions, termed topologically associating domains (TADs). They range from several hundred kilobase- to megabase-long genomic regions that interact with themselves. The organization of TADs between cell types and species is consistent. TADs are separated from one another by regions with less frequent interactions, termed TAD boundaries. A model called loop-extrusion can explain the formation of TADs as organizational structures at the subchromosomal level. Loop-extrusion suggests bringing otherwise distal gene-regulatory elements (i.e., enhancers and silencers) into 3D proximity of target genes to regulate their expression. Loop extrusion forms the majority of TADs by two cohesin/condensin molecules sliding toward each other while extruding the DNA from in between, until two convergent CTCF (CCCTC-binding factor) sites are recognized. CTCF is a highly conserved zinc finger protein, considered the master regulator of the genome because it acts as a transcriptional repressor to regulate the communication between gene-regulatory elements and genes. TAD boundaries often show enrichment of CTCF, cohesion, and mediator proteins, which contribute to the 3D topology of the genome by establishing chromatin loops and the TAD structure. Weaker TAD boundaries may allow for interactions between different TADs (inter-TAD) to regulate genes at larger genomic distances; however, this occurs less frequently than interactions within the same TAD (intra-TAD). Most gene-regulatory processes occur by intra-TAD chromatin loops; an enhancer with bound transcription factors reaches spatial proximity with the target gene's promoter site and its core transcriptional machinery (i.e., polymerase II), just upstream of its transcription start site. The analysis of intra-TAD interactions in different cell types and single cell studies showed high variability, indicating that tissue-specific gene expression can be partially explained by specific cells and by genomic contacts within TADs.

The reorganization of the TAD architecture by chromosomal **rearrangements** can alter gene expression and may cause clinically apparent disease phenotypes (see Chapter 6). Disrupting higher-order chromatin features and gene-regulatory elements may affect transcriptional programs and development. For example, genomic deletions can lead to TADs fusing; duplications may form neo-TADs; inversions reshuffle TADs; and translocations could alter interchromosomal contacts between nonhomologous chromosomes (Fig. 3.11).

GENE EXPRESSION AS THE INTEGRATION OF GENOMIC AND EPIGENOMIC SIGNALS

The gene expression program of a cell encompasses the specific subset of the ~20,000 protein-coding genes in the genome that are actively transcribed and translated into their respective functional products, the subset of the estimated 20,000 to 25,000 ncRNA genes that are transcribed, the amount of product produced, and the particular sequence (alleles) of those products. The gene **expression profile** of any particular cell or cell type in a given individual at a given time (whether in the context of the cell cycle, early development, or one's entire life span) and under a given set of circumstances (as influenced by environment, lifestyle, or disease) is thus the integrated sum of several different but interrelated effects, including the following:

- The primary sequence of genes, their allelic variants, and their encoded products
- Regulatory sequences and their epigenetic positioning in chromatin
- Interactions with the thousands of transcriptional factors, ncRNAs, and other proteins involved in the control of transcription, splicing, translation, and posttranslational modification
- Organization of the genome into subchromosomal domains
- Programmed interactions between different parts of the genome

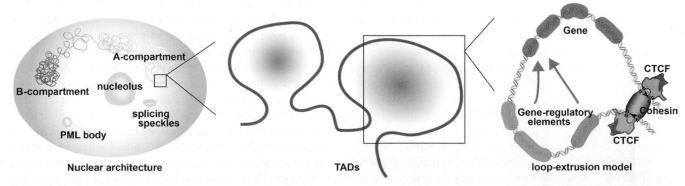

Figure 3.11 Topologically associating domains (TADs). The genome is organized in the three-dimensional architecture of the nucleus, with A and B compartments representing open chromatin and heterochromatin, respectively. Further functional nuclear subdomains are the nucleolus, splicing speckles, and promyelocytic leukemia (PML) bodies. The next organization level of chromatin involves TADs that are formed by the loop-extrusion model, with CCCTC-binding factor (CTCF) and cohesion to facilitate spatial proximity of gene-regulatory elements (enhancers), and gene promoters to regulate gene expression. (Courtesy Philipp Maass.)

- Dynamic 3D chromatin packaging in the nucleus

All of these orchestrate in an efficient, hierarchic, and highly programmed fashion. Disruption of any—due to genetic variation, to epigenetic changes, and/or to disease-related processes—would be expected to alter the overall cellular program and its functional output (see Box 3.3).

BOX 3.3 THE EPIGENETIC LANDSCAPE OF THE GENOME AND MEDICINE

- Different chromosomes and chromosomal regions occupy characteristic territories within the nucleus. The probability of physical proximity influences the incidence of specific chromosome abnormalities (see Chapters 5 and 6).
- The genome is organized into megabase-sized domains with locally shared characteristics of base pair composition (i.e., GC rich or AT rich), gene density, timing of replication in the S phase, and presence of particular histone modifications (see Chapter 5).
- Modules of coexpressed genes correspond to distinct anatomic or developmental stages in, for example, the human brain or the hematopoietic lineage. Such coexpression networks are revealed by shared regulatory networks and epigenetic signals, by clustering within genomic domains, and by overlapping patterns of altered gene expression in various disease states.
- Although **monozygotic twins** share virtually identical genomes, they can be quite **discordant** for certain traits, including susceptibility to common diseases. Significant changes in DNA methylation occur during the lifetime of such twins, implicating epigenetic regulation of gene expression as a source of diversity.

ALLELIC IMBALANCE IN GENE EXPRESSION

It was once assumed that genes present in two copies in the genome would be expressed from both homologues at comparable levels. However, it has become increasingly evident that there can be extensive imbalance between alleles, reflecting both the amount of sequence variation in the genome and the interplay between genome sequence and epigenetic patterns that were just discussed.

In Chapter 2, we introduced the general finding that any individual genome carries two different alleles at a minimum of 3 to 5 million positions around the genome, thus distinguishing by sequence the maternally and paternally inherited copies of that sequence position (see Fig. 2.6). Here we explore ways in which those sequence differences reveal allelic imbalance in gene expression, both at autosomal loci and at X chromosome loci in females.

By determining the sequences of all the RNA products—the transcriptome—in a population of cells, one can quantify the relative level of transcription of all the genes (both protein coding and noncoding) that are transcriptionally active in those cells. Consider, for example, the collection of protein-coding genes.

Although an average cell might contain ~300,000 copies of mRNA in total, the abundance of specific mRNAs can differ over many orders of magnitude; among genes that are active, most are expressed at low levels (estimated to be <10 copies of that gene's mRNA per cell), whereas others are expressed at much higher levels (several hundred to a few thousand copies of that mRNA per cell). Only in highly specialized cell types are particular genes expressed at very high levels (many tens of thousands of copies) that account for a significant proportion of all mRNA in those cells.

Now consider an expressed gene with a sequence variant that allows one to distinguish between the RNA products (whether mRNA or ncRNA) transcribed from each of two **alleles**, one allele with a T that is transcribed to yield RNA with an A and the other allele with a C that is transcribed to yield RNA with a G (Fig. 3.12). By sequencing individual RNA molecules and comparing the number of sequences generated that contain an A or G at that position, one can infer the ratio of transcripts from the two alleles in that sample. Although most genes show essentially equivalent levels of biallelic expression, recent analyses of this type have demonstrated widespread unequal allelic expression for 5% to 20% of autosomal genes in the genome (Table 3.2). For most of these genes, the extent of imbalance is twofold or less, although up to tenfold differences have been observed for some genes. This allelic imbalance may reflect interactions between genome sequence and gene regulation; for example, sequence changes can alter the relative binding of various transcription factors or other transcriptional regulators to the two alleles or the extent of DNA methylation observed at the two alleles (see Table 3.2).

Monoallelic Gene Expression

Some genes, however, show a much more complete form of allelic imbalance, resulting in monoallelic gene expression (see Fig. 3.12). Several different mechanisms have been shown to account for allelic imbalance of this type for particular subsets of genes in the genome: DNA rearrangement including copy number variation, random monoallelic expression, parent-of-origin **imprinting**, and, for genes on the X chromosome in females, X chromosome inactivation. Their distinguishing characteristics are summarized in Table 3.2.

Somatic Rearrangement

A highly specialized form of monoallelic gene expression is observed in the genes encoding immunoglobulins and T-cell receptors, expressed in B cells and T cells, respectively, as part of the immune response. Antibodies are encoded in the germline by a relatively small number of genes that, during B-cell development, undergo a unique process of somatic rearrangement that involves the cutting and pasting of DNA sequences in lymphocyte precursor cells (but not in any other cell lineages)

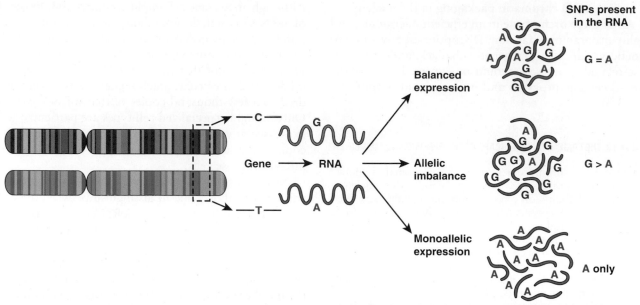

Figure 3.12 Allelic expression patterns for a gene sequence with a transcribed DNA variant (here, a C or a T) to distinguish the alleles. As described in the text, the relative abundance of RNA transcripts from the two alleles (here, carrying a G or an A) demonstrates whether the gene shows balanced expression *(top)*, allelic imbalance *(center)*, or exclusively monoallelic expression *(bottom)*. Different underlying mechanisms for allelic imbalance are compared in Table 3.2. *SNP,* Single nucleotide polymorphism.

TABLE 3.2 Allelic Imbalance in Gene Expression

Type	Characteristics	Genes Affected	Basis	Developmental Origin
Unbalanced expression	Unequal RNA abundance from two alleles due to DNA variants and associated epigenetic changes; usually < twofold difference in expression	5–20% of autosomal genes	Sequence variants cause different levels of expression at the two alleles	Early embryogenesis
Monoallelic expression				
• Somatic rearrangement	Changes in DNA organization to produce functional gene at one allele, but not other	Immunoglobulin genes, T-cell receptor genes	Random choice of one allele	B- and T-cell lineages
• Random allelic silencing or activation	Expression from only one allele at a locus, due to differential epigenetic packaging at locus	Olfactory receptor genes in sensory neurons; other chemosensory or immune system genes; up to 10% of all genes in other cell types	Random choice of one allele	Specific cell types
• Genomic imprinting	Epigenetic silencing of allele(s) in imprinted region	>100 genes with functions in development	Imprinted region marked epigenetically according to parent of origin	Parental germline
• X chromosome inactivation	Epigenetic silencing of alleles on one X chromosome in females	Most X-linked genes in females	Random choice of one X chromosome	Early embryogenesis

to rearrange genes in somatic cells to generate enormous antibody diversity. The highly orchestrated DNA rearrangements occur across many hundreds of kilobases but involve only one of the two alleles, which is chosen randomly in any given B cell (see Table 3.2). Thus expression of mature mRNAs for the immunoglobulin heavy or light chain subunits is exclusively monoallelic.

This mechanism of somatic rearrangement and random monoallelic gene expression is also observed at the T-cell receptor genes in the T-cell lineage. However, such behavior is unique to these gene families and cell lineages; the rest of the genome, even DNA segments bearing genomic repeats, remains surprisingly stable throughout development and differentiation.

Random Monoallelic Expression

In contrast to this highly specialized form of DNA rearrangement, monoallelic expression typically results from differential epigenetic regulation of the two alleles. One well-studied example of random monoallelic expression involves the OR gene family described earlier (see Fig. 3.2). In this case, only a single allele of one OR gene is expressed in each olfactory sensory neuron; the many hundred other copies of the OR family remain repressed in that cell. Other genes with chemosensory or immune system functions also show random monoallelic expression, suggesting that this mechanism may be a general one for increasing the diversity of responses for cells that interact with the outside world. However, this mechanism is apparently not restricted to the immune and sensory systems because a substantial subset of all human genes (5–10% in different cell types) has been shown to undergo random allelic silencing; these genes are broadly distributed on all autosomes, have a wide range of functions, and vary in terms of the cell types and tissues in which monoallelic expression is observed.

Parent-of-Origin Imprinting

For the examples just described, the choice of which allele is expressed is not dependent on parental origin; either the maternal or paternal copy can be expressed in different cells and their clonal descendants. This distinguishes random forms of monoallelic expression from **genomic imprinting**, in which the choice of the allele to be expressed is nonrandom and is determined solely by parental origin. Imprinting is a process involving the introduction of epigenetic marks (see Fig. 3.8) in the germline of one parent, but not the other, at specific locations in the genome. These lead to monoallelic expression of a gene or, in some cases, of multiple genes within the imprinted region.

Imprinting takes place during gametogenesis, before fertilization, and marks certain genes as having come from the mother or father (Fig. 3.13). After conception, the parent-of-origin imprint is maintained in some or all of the somatic tissues of the embryo and silences gene expression on allele(s) within the imprinted region; whereas some imprinted genes show monoallelic expression throughout the embryo, others show tissue-specific imprinting, especially in the placenta, with biallelic expression in other tissues. The imprinted state persists postnatally into adulthood through hundreds of cell divisions so that only the maternal or paternal copy of the gene is expressed. Yet, imprinting must be reversible: a paternally derived allele, when it is inherited by a female, must be converted in her germline so that she can then pass it on with a maternal imprint to her offspring. Likewise, an imprinted maternally derived allele, when it is inherited by a male, must be converted in his germline so that he can pass it on as a paternally imprinted allele to his offspring (see Fig. 3.13). Control over this conversion process appears to be governed by specific DNA elements called imprinting control regions or **imprinting centers** that are located within imprinted regions throughout the genome; although their mechanism

of action is not fully known, many appear to involve ncRNAs that initiate the epigenetic change in chromatin, which then spreads outward along the chromosome over the imprinted region. Notably, although the imprinted region can encompass more than a single gene, this form of monoallelic expression is confined to a delimited genomic segment, typically a few hundred kilobase pairs to a few megabases in overall size; this distinguishes genomic imprinting both from the more general form of random monoallelic expression described earlier (which appears to involve individual genes under locus-specific control) and from X chromosome inactivation, described in the next section (which involves genes along the entire chromosome).

To date, ~100 imprinted genes have been identified on many different autosomes. The involvement of these genes in various chromosomal disorders is described more fully in Chapter 6. For clinical conditions due to a single imprinted gene, such as Prader-Willi syndrome (Case 38) and Beckwith-Wiedemann syndrome (Case 6), the effect of genomic imprinting on inheritance patterns in pedigrees is discussed in Chapter 8.

X Chromosome Inactivation

The chromosomal basis for sex **determination**, introduced in Chapter 2 and discussed in more detail in Chapter 6, results in a dosage difference between typical males and females with respect to genes on the X chromosome. Here we discuss the chromosomal and molecular mechanisms of X chromosome inactivation, the most extensive example of random monoallelic expression in the genome and a mechanism of **dosage compensation** that results in the epigenetic silencing of most genes on one of the two X chromosomes in females.

In normal female cells, the choice of which X chromosome is to be inactivated is a random one that is then maintained in each clonal lineage. Thus females are mosaic with respect to X-linked gene expression; some cells express alleles on the paternally inherited X but not the maternally inherited X, whereas other cells do the opposite (Fig. 3.14). This mosaic pattern of gene expression distinguishes most X-linked genes from imprinted genes, whose expression, as we just noted, is determined strictly by parental origin.

Although the inactive X chromosome was first identified cytologically by the presence of a heterochromatic mass (called the **Barr body**) in interphase cells, many epigenetic features at the molecular level distinguish the active and inactive X chromosomes, including DNA methylation, histone modifications, and a specific histone variant, macroH2A, that is particularly enriched in chromatin on the inactive X. As well as providing insights into the mechanisms of **X inactivation**, these features can be useful diagnostically for identifying inactive X chromosomes in clinical material, as we will see in Chapter 6.

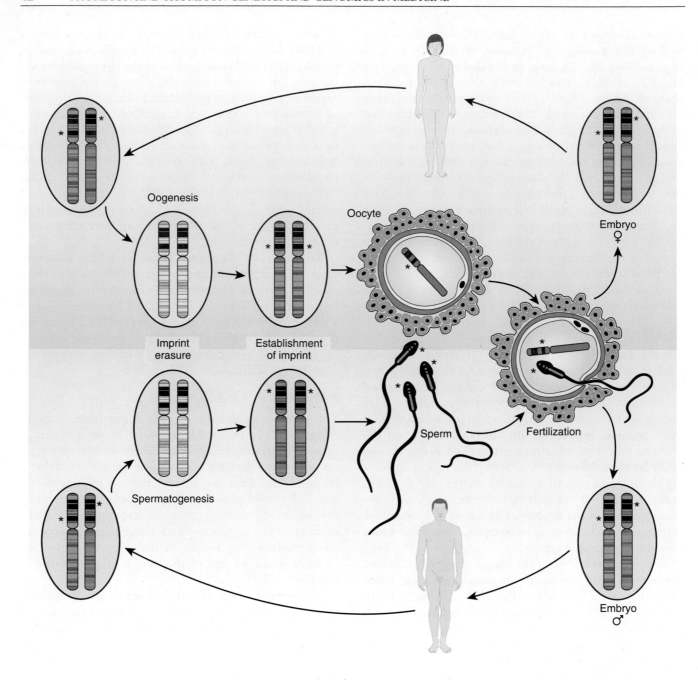

Figure 3.13 **Genomic imprinting and conversion of maternal and paternal imprints during passage through male or female gametogenesis.** Within a hypothetical imprinted region on a pair of homologous autosomes, paternally imprinted genes are indicated in *blue*, whereas a maternally imprinted gene is indicated in *red*. After fertilization, both male and female embryos have one copy of the chromosome carrying a paternal imprint and one copy carrying a maternal imprint. During oogenesis *(top)* and spermatogenesis *(bottom)*, the imprints are erased by removal of epigenetic marks, and new imprints determined by the sex of the parent are established within the imprinted region. Gametes thus carry a monoallelic imprint appropriate to the parent of origin, whereas somatic cells in both sexes carry one chromosome of each imprinted type.

Although X inactivation is clearly a chromosomal phenomenon, not all genes on the X chromosome show monoallelic expression in female cells. Extensive analysis of expression of nearly all X-linked genes has demonstrated that at least 15% of the genes show biallelic expression and are expressed from both active and inactive X chromosomes, at least to some extent; a proportion of these show significantly higher levels of mRNA production in female cells compared to male cells and are interesting candidates for a role in explaining sexually dimorphic traits.

A special subset of genes is located in the pseudoautosomal segments, which are essentially identical on the X and Y chromosomes and undergo recombination during

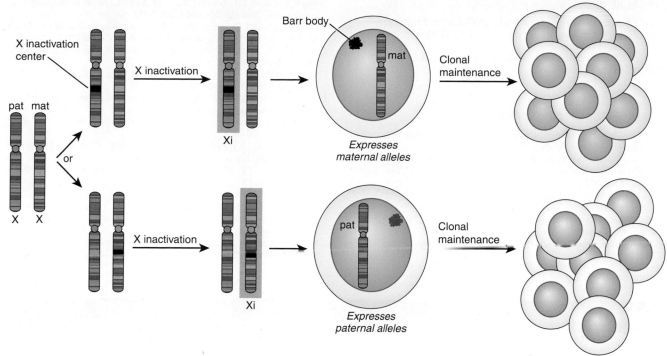

Figure 3.14 **Random X chromosome inactivation early in female development.** Shortly after conception of a female embryo, both the paternally and maternally inherited X chromosomes (pat and mat, respectively) are active. Within the first week of embryogenesis, one or the other X is chosen at random to become the future inactive X, through a series of events involving the X inactivation center *(black box).* That X then becomes the inactive X (Xi, indicated by the *shading*) in that cell and its progeny and forms the Barr body in interphase nuclei. The resulting female embryo is thus a clonal mosaic of two epigenetically determined cell types: one expresses alleles from the maternal X (*pink* cells), whereas the other expresses alleles from the paternal X (*blue* cells). The ratio of the two cell types is determined randomly but varies among normal females and among females who are carriers of X-linked disease alleles (see Chapters 6 and 7).

spermatogenesis (see Chapter 2). These genes have two copies in both females (two X-linked copies) and males (one X-linked and one Y-linked copy) and thus do not undergo X inactivation; as expected, these genes show balanced biallelic expression, as one sees for most autosomal genes.

The X Inactivation Center and the XIST Gene. X inactivation occurs very early in female embryonic development, and determination of which X will be designated the inactive X in any given cell in the embryo is a random choice under the control of a complex locus called the X inactivation center. This region contains a unique ncRNA gene, *XIST*, that appears to be a key master regulatory locus for X inactivation. *XIST* (an acronym for inactive X [*Xi*]–specific *t*ranscripts) has the novel feature that it is expressed only from the allele on the inactive X; it is transcriptionally silent on the active X in both male and female cells. Although the exact mode of action of *XIST* is unknown, X inactivation cannot occur in its absence. The product of *XIST* is a long ncRNA that stays in the nucleus in close association with the inactive X chromosome.

Additional aspects and consequences of X chromosome inactivation will be discussed in Chapter 6, in the context of individuals with structurally abnormal X chromosomes or an abnormal number of X chromosomes, and in Chapter 7, in the case of females carrying deleterious mutant alleles for X-linked disease.

VARIATION IN GENE EXPRESSION AND ITS RELEVANCE TO MEDICINE

The regulated expression of genes in the human genome involves a set of complex interrelationships among different levels of control, including proper **gene dosage** (controlled by mechanisms of chromosome replication and **segregation**), gene structure, chromatin packaging and epigenetic regulation, transcription, RNA splicing, and, for protein-coding loci, mRNA stability, translation, protein processing, and protein degradation. For some genes, fluctuations in the level of functional gene product, due either to inherited variation in the structure of a particular gene or to changes induced by nongenetic factors such as diet or the environment, are of relatively little importance. For other genes, even relatively minor changes in the level of expression can have dire clinical consequences, reflecting the importance of those gene products in particular biologic pathways. The nature of inherited variation in the structure and function of chromosomes and the genes they contain, combined with the influence of this variation on the expression of specific traits, is the very essence of medical genetics and is dealt with in subsequent chapters.

GENERAL REFERENCES

Brown TA: *Genomes,* ed 3, New York, 2007, Garland Science.
Lodish H, Berk A, Kaiser CA, et al: *Molecular cell biology,* ed 9, New York, 2021, WH Freeman.
Strachan T, Read A: *Human molecular genetics,* ed 5, New York, 2018, Garland Science.

REFERENCES FOR SPECIFIC TOPICS

Bartolomei MS, Ferguson-Smith AC: Mammalian genomic imprinting, *Cold Spring Harbor Perspect Biol* 3:1002592, 2011.
Beck CR, Garcia-Perez JL, Badge RM, et al: LINE-1 elements in structural variation and disease, *Annu Rev Genomics Hum Genet* 12:187–215, 2011.
Berg P: Dissections and reconstructions of genes and chromosomes (Nobel Prize lecture), *Science* 213:296–303, 1981.
Chess A: Mechanisms and consequences of widespread random mono-allelic expression, *Nat Rev Genet* 13:421–428, 2012.
Dekker J: Gene regulation in the third dimension, *Science* 319:1793–1794, 2008.

Djebali S, Davis CA, Merkel A, et al: Landscape of transcription in human cells, *Nature* 489:101–108, 2012.
ENCODE Project Consortium: An integrated encyclopedia of DNA elements in the human genome, *Nature* 489:57–74, 2012.
Gerstein MB, Bruce C, Rozowsky JS, et al: What is a gene, post-ENCODE? *Genome Res* 17:669–681, 2007.
Guil S, Esteller M: Cis-acting noncoding RNAs: friends and foes, *Nat Struct Mol Biol* 19:1068–1074, 2012.
Heyn H, Esteller M: DNA methylation profiling in the clinic: applications and challenges, *Nature Rev Genet* 13:679–692, 2012.
Hubner MR, Spector DL: Chromatin dynamics, *Annu Rev Biophys* 39:471–489, 2010.
Li M, Wang IX, Li Y, et al: Widespread RNA and DNA sequence differences in the human transcriptome, *Science* 333:53–58, 2011.
Nagano T, Fraser P: No-nonsense functions for long noncoding RNAs, *Cell* 145:178–181, 2011.
Willard HF: The human genome: a window on human genetics, biology and medicine. In Ginsburg GS, Willard HF, editors: *Genomic and personalized medicine,* ed 2, New York, 2013, Elsevier.
Zhou VW, Goren A, Bernstein BE: Charting histone modifications and the functional organization of mammalian genomes, *Nat Rev Genet* 12:7–18, 2012.

PROBLEMS

1. The following amino acid sequence represents part of a protein. The wild-type sequence and four variant forms are shown. By consulting Table 3.1, determine the double-stranded sequence of the corresponding section of the normal gene. Which strand is the strand that RNA polymerase "reads"? What would be the sequence of the resulting mRNA? What kind of variation is each altered protein most likely to represent?

Normal	-lys-arg-his-his-tyr-leu-
Mutant 1	-lys-arg-his-his-cys-leu-
Mutant 2	-lys-arg-ile-ile-ile-
Mutant 3	-lys-glu-thr-ser-leu-ser-
Mutant 4	-asn-tyr-leu-

2. The following items are related to each other in a hierarchic fashion: chromosome, base pair, nucleosome, kilobase pair, intron, gene, exon, chromatin, codon, nucleotide, promoter. What are these relationships?

3. Describe how a variant in each of the following might alter or interfere with gene function and thus cause human disease: promoter, initiator codon, splice sites at intron-exon junctions, one base-pair deletion in the coding sequence, stop codon.

4. Most of the human genome consists of sequences that are not transcribed and do not directly encode gene products. For each of the following, consider ways in which these genome elements might contribute to human disease: introns, *Alu* or LINE repetitive sequences, locus control regions, pseudogenes.

5. Contrast the mechanisms and consequences of RNA splicing and somatic rearrangement.

6. Contrast the mechanisms and consequences of genomic imprinting and X chromosome inactivation.

CHAPTER 4

Human Genetic Diversity
Genomic Variation

Stephen W. Scherer • Ada Hamosh

The study of DNA variation is the conceptual cornerstone for genetics in medicine and for the broader field of human genetics. During the course of evolution, the steady influx of new variation has ensured a high degree of genetic diversity and individuality, and this theme extends through all fields in human and medical genetics. Genetic diversity may manifest as differences in the organization of the genome, as nucleotide changes in the genome sequence, as variation in the copy number of segments of DNA or entire chromosomes, as balanced or unbalanced alterations, as alterations in the structure or amount of proteins found in various tissues, or as any of these in the context of clinical disease.

This chapter is one of several in which we explore the nature of genetically determined differences among individuals. Considering all classes of genetic variation, the sequence of nuclear DNA is ~99% identical between any two unrelated humans. Yet it is precisely the small fraction of DNA sequence difference among individuals that is responsible for the genetically determined variability evident both in one's daily existence and in clinical medicine. Many DNA sequence differences have little or no effect on outward appearance, whereas other differences are directly responsible for disease. Between these two extremes is the variation responsible for genetically determined variability in anatomy, physiology, dietary intolerances, susceptibility to infection, predisposition to cancer, therapeutic responses or adverse reactions to medications, and perhaps even variability in various personality traits, athletic aptitude, and artistic talent.

One of the important concepts of human and medical genetics is that diseases with a clearly inherited component are only the most obvious and often the most extreme manifestation of genetic differences: one end of a continuum of variation that extends from rare deleterious variants that cause illness, sometimes representing a spectrum of clinical phenotypes, through more common variants that can increase susceptibility to disease, to the most common variation in the population that is of uncertain relevance with respect to disease.

THE NATURE OF GENETIC VARIATION

As described in Chapter 2, a segment of DNA occupying a particular position or location on a chromosome is a locus (plural loci). A locus may be large, perhaps containing many genes, such as the major histocompatibility complex locus involved in the response of the immune system to foreign substances; it may be a single gene, such as the β-globin locus we introduced in Chapter 3; or it may be just a single base in the genome, as in the case of a single nucleotide variant (SNV) (see Fig. 2.6 and later in this chapter). Alternative versions of the DNA sequence at a locus are called alleles. For many genes, there is a single prevailing allele, usually present in more than half of the individuals in a population, that geneticists call the wild-type or common allele. (In lay parlance, this is sometimes referred to as the normal allele; however, because genetic variation is itself very much normal, the existence of different alleles in normal individuals is commonplace. Thus one should avoid using normal to designate the most common or major allele.) The other versions of the gene are variant alleles that differ from the wild-type allele because of the effect of a mutation having changed the nucleotide sequence or arrangement of DNA. Note that the terms *mutation* and *mutant* apply to DNA, but not to individuals. They denote a change in sequence without any connotation with respect to the function or fitness of that change.

The frequency of different variants can vary widely in different populations, as we will explore in Chapter 10. If a locus in a population has two or more relatively common alleles (typically defined by convention as having an allele frequency >1%), the locus is said to exhibit polymorphism (literally "many forms") in that population; thus such a locus is polymorphic. Most variant alleles, however, are rare; some are so rare as to be found in only a single family and are known as private alleles. Common jargon in genetics came to use polymorphism in reference to a variant rather than a locus, but following expert guidance, for clarity, we suggest use of common variant (rather than polymorphism) or rare variant (rather than mutation). An exception is for the use of single nucleotide polymorphism (SNP) in the context of microarrays, where it is strongly entrenched in the lexicon.

The Concept of Variation

In this chapter we begin by exploring the nature of genomic variation, ranging from the change of a single nucleotide to alterations of an entire chromosome. To recognize a change means that there has to be a gold standard, compared to which the variant shows a difference. As we saw in Chapter 2, there is no single individual whose genome sequence could serve as such a definitive standard for the human species, and thus one arbitrarily designates the most common sequence or arrangement in a population at any one position in the genome as the so-called reference sequence (see Fig. 2.6). As more and more genomes from individuals around the globe are sampled (and thus as more and more variation is detected among the currently 7.9 billion genomes that make up our species), this reference genome is subject to constant evaluation and change. Indeed, a number of international collaborations share and update data on the nature and frequency of DNA variation in different populations in the context of the reference human genome sequence and make the data available through publicly accessible databases that serve as essential resources for scientists, physicians, and other health care professionals (Table 4.1). As we learn more about variation and, in particular, as long-read sequencing allows us to fill holes in the reference genome, updated genome

builds are released by the human genome reference committee; the current reference is hGRC38. Because errors are corrected and new sequences added, it is very important to always specify the build used to annotate a genomic variant.

Variants are sometimes classified by the size of the altered DNA sequence and, at other times, by the functional effect of the change on gene expression. Although classification by size is somewhat arbitrary, it can be helpful conceptually to recognize the spectrum of changes at three different levels:

- Variation in chromosome number that leaves chromosomes intact but changes the number of chromosomes in a cell (**aneuploidy**)
- Alterations that change only a portion of a chromosome and might involve an unbalanced change of a subchromosomal segment or a structural **rearrangement** involving parts of one or more chromosomes (regional variation or **copy number variation [CNV]**)
- Alterations of the sequence of DNA, involving the substitution, **deletion**, or **insertion** of DNA, range from an SNV through small repetitive units (such as trinucleotide repeats) and insertion-deletion variants (**indels**) up to an arbitrarily set (and evolving) limit of approximately 1 kb where such a change becomes a CNV. The basis for and consequences of this third type of variation are the principal focus of this chapter, whereas both chromosome and regional variation will be presented at length in Chapters 5 and 6.

The functional consequences of DNA mutations, even those that change a single **base pair**, run the gamut from being completely innocuous to causing serious

TABLE 4.1 Useful Databases of Information on Human Genetic Diversity

Description	URL
The **Human Genome Project**, completed in 2003, was an international collaboration to map and sequence the genome of our species. The draft sequence of the genome was released in 2001, and the "essentially complete" reference genome assembly was published in 2004.	https://www.genome.gov/human-genome-project http://genome.ucsc.edu/cgi-bin/hgGateway http://www.ensembl.org/Homo_sapiens/Info/Index
The **Single Nucleotide Polymorphism Database (dbSNP)** and the **Structural Variation Database (dbVar)** are databases of small-scale and large-scale variations, including single nucleotide variants, microsatellites, indels, and CNVs.	ncbi.nlm.nih.gov/snp/ ncbi.nlm.nih.gov/dbvar/
The **1000 Genomes Project** created a catalogue of common human genetic variation, using openly consented samples from people who declared themselves to be healthy. All data are publicly available. The International Genome Sample Resource (IGSR) maintains and shares the human genetic variation resource.	www.internationalgenome.org
The **Genome Aggregation Database (gnomAD)** reports variants from 125,748 exomes and 15,708 genomes (141,456 unrelated individuals) aligned on GRCh37 in v2.1 and 76,156 genomes from unrelated individuals aligned on GRCh38 in v3.0.	gnomad.broadinstitute.org
ClinVar is a freely accessible, public archive of reports of the relationships among human variants and phenotypes, with supporting evidence.	www.ncbi.nlm.nih.gov/clinvar
The **Human Gene Mutation Database** is a comprehensive collection of published germline variants associated with or causing human inherited disease (currently including over >210,000 mutations in 8519 genes).	www.hgmd.cf.ac.uk/ac/index.php
The **Database of Genomic Variants** is a curated catalogue of structural variation in the human genome. As of 2023, the database contains over 8 million entries.	dgv.tcag.ca

CNV, Copy number variant; *SNV*, single nucleotide variant.
Updated from Willard HF: The human genome: a window on human genetics, biology and medicine. In Ginsburg GS, Willard HF, editors: *Genomic and personalized medicine*, ed 3, New York, 2016, Elsevier.

illness, all depending on the location, nature, and size of the resulting variant. For example, even a change within a coding **exon** of a gene may have no effect on how a gene is expressed if the change does not alter the primary amino acid sequence of the polypeptide product; even if it does, the resulting change in the encoded amino acid sequence may not alter the functional properties of the protein. Not all variants, therefore, manifest in a clinical phenotype, though they will be reflected as DNA sequence variants.

The Concept of Common Variants

The DNA sequence of a given region of the genome is remarkably similar among chromosomes carried by many different individuals from around the world. In fact, any randomly chosen segment of human DNA of ~1000 bp in length, on average, will differ by only one base pair between the **homologous** segments inherited from that individual's parents (assuming the parents are unrelated). However, across all human populations, hundreds of millions of single nucleotide differences and over a million more complex variants have been identified and catalogued. Because of limited sampling, these figures are likely to underestimate the true extent of genetic diversity in our species. Many populations have yet to be adequately studied. Even in those that have been well studied, the number of individuals examined is too small to reveal most variants with minor allele frequencies below 1% to 2%. Thus, as more people are included in variant discovery projects, additional (and rarer) variants will certainly continue to be uncovered.

Whether a variant is formally considered common or not depends entirely on whether its frequency in a population exceeds a certain threshold, such as 1% of the alleles in that population. It does not depend on what kind of mutation caused it, how large a segment of the genome is involved, or whether it has a demonstrable effect on the individual. Although most common sequence variants are located between genes or within **introns** and are most often inconsequential to the functioning of any gene, others may be located in the coding sequence of genes themselves and result in different protein variants that may lead in turn to distinctive differences in human populations. Still, others are in regulatory regions and may have important effects on **transcription** or **RNA** stability.

One might expect that deleterious variants that cause rare monogenic diseases are unlikely to become considered common variants. Although it is true that the alleles responsible for most clearly inherited clinical conditions are rare, some alleles that have a profound effect on health—such as alleles of genes encoding enzymes that metabolize drugs (e.g., **sensitivity** to abacavir in some individuals infected with human immunodeficiency virus) (Case 1), the sickle cell allele in African populations and others of African and Mediterranean ancestry

(see Chapter 12) (Case 42), or the p.Phe508del variant in *CFTR* that causes cystic fibrosis (see Chapter 13) (Case 12)—are relatively common. Nonetheless, these are exceptions. As more and more genetic variation is discovered and catalogued, it is clear that the vast majority of variants in the genome—whether common or rare—reflect differences in DNA sequence that have no overt significance to health.

Common variants are key elements for the study of human and medical genetics. The ability to distinguish different inherited forms of a gene or different segments of the genome provides critical tools for a wide array of applications, both in research and in clinical practice (see Box 4.1).

BOX 4.1   INHERITED VARIATION IN HUMAN AND MEDICAL GENETICS

Allelic variants can be used as markers for tracking the inheritance of the corresponding segment of the genome in families and in populations. Such variants can be used as follows:
- As powerful research tools for mapping a gene to a particular region of a chromosome by **linkage analysis** or by allelic **association** (see Chapter 11)
- For prenatal diagnosis of genetic disease and for detection of carriers of deleterious alleles (see Chapter 18)
- In blood banking and tissue typing for transfusions and organ transplantation
- In forensic applications such as identity testing for determining paternity, identifying remains of crime victims, or matching DNA from a crime investigation to that of a perpetrator
- To provide genomic-based precision medicine (see Chapter 19), medical care is tailored, for example, to whether an individual carries variants that increase or decrease the **risk** for common adult disorders (such as coronary heart disease, cancer, and diabetes; see Chapter 9) or that influence the efficacy or safety of particular medications (see Chapter 19)

INHERITED COMMON VARIATION IN DNA

The original **Human Genome Project** and the subsequent study of many millions of individuals worldwide have provided vast DNA sequence information. With this information in hand, one can begin to characterize the types and frequencies of common variation found in the human genome and to generate catalogues of the world's human DNA sequence diversity. Such variants can be classified according to how the DNA sequence differs among the different alleles (Table 4.2 and Figs. 4.1 and 4.2).

Single Nucleotide Variants

The simplest and most common of all variants are SNVs. Those that occur at a high population frequency (typically defined as >1% or >5%) have been called SNPs, but more recently, common SNVs. A polymorphic locus characterized by a common SNV usually has

TABLE 4.2 Common Variation in the Human Genome

Type of Variation	Size Range (Approx.)	Basis for the Variant	Number of Alleles
Single nucleotide variant	1 bp	Substitution of one or another base pair at a particular location in the genome	Usually 2
Insertion/deletions (indels)	1 bp–1 kb	*Simple*: Presence or absence of a short segment of DNA 1–1000 bp in length *Microsatellites*: Generally, a 2-, 3-, or 4-nucleotide unit repeated in tandem 5–25 times	*Simple*: 2 *Microsatellites*: typically ≥5
Copy number variant	1 kb–> ≅ 3 Mb	Typically the presence or absence of 1-kb to 1.5-Mb segments of DNA, although tandem duplication of 2, 3, 4, or more copies can also occur	≥2
Inversions	Few bp–>1 Mb	A DNA segment present in either of two orientations with respect to the surrounding DNA	2

bp, Base pair; *kb*, kilobase pair; *Mb*, megabase pair.

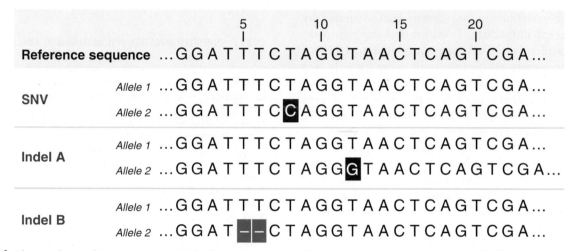

Figure 4.1 Three polymorphisms in genomic DNA from the segment of the human genome reference assembly shown at the top (see also Figure 2.6). The single nucleotide variation *(SNV)* at position 8 has two alleles, one with a T (corresponding to the reference sequence) and one with a C. There are two indels in this region. At indel A, allele 2 has an insertion of a G between positions 11 and 12 in the reference sequence (allele 1). At indel B, allele 2 has a 2 bp deletion of positions 5 and 6 in the reference sequence.

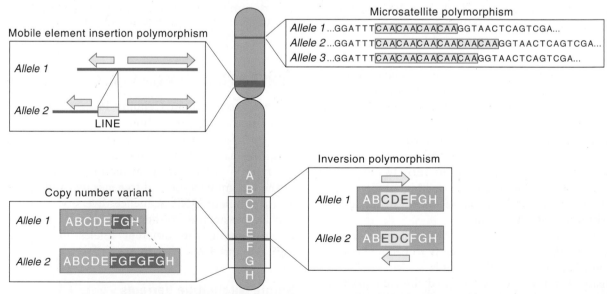

Figure 4.2 Examples of variation in the human genome larger than single nucleotide variants. *Clockwise from upper right*: The microsatellite locus has three alleles, with four, five, or six copies of a CAA trinucleotide repeat. The inversion variant has two alleles corresponding to the two orientations (indicated by the *arrows*) of the genomic segment shown in *green*; such inversions can involve regions up to many megabases of DNA. Copy number variants involve deletion or duplication of hundreds of kilobase pairs to over a megabase of genomic DNA. In the example shown, allele 1 contains a single copy, whereas allele 2 contains three copies of the chromosomal segment containing the F and G genes; other possible alleles with zero, two, four, or more copies of F and G are not shown. The mobile element insertion variant has two alleles, one with and one without insertion of a ~6-kb LINE repeated retroelement; the insertion of the mobile element changes the spacing between the two genes and may alter gene expression in the region.

only two alleles, corresponding to two different bases at that particular location (see Fig. 4.1). Common SNVs are observed, on average, once every 1000 bp. However, their distribution is uneven around the genome; many more are found in noncoding parts of the genome, in introns and in sequences that are some distance from protein-coding genes. Nonetheless, a significant number of SNVs, both common and rare, occur in genes and other known functional elements in the genome. Approximately half of these do not alter the predicted amino acid sequence of the encoded protein and thus are termed **synonymous**, whereas those that do alter the amino acid sequence are called **nonsynonymous**. Other SNVs are candidates to have significant functional consequences, as they introduce or change a **stop codon** (see Table 3.1), or alter a known splice site.

The significance for health of the vast majority of common SNVs is unknown and is the subject of ongoing research. The fact that these variants are common does not mean that they are without detrimental or protective effect on health or longevity. What it does mean is that any effect of common SNVs is likely to involve a relatively subtle altering of disease susceptibility rather than be a direct cause of serious illness.

Insertion-Deletion Variants

A second class of variants result from **insertion** or **deletion** (**indels**) of segments that range from a single base pair up to ~1 kb. Over a million indels have been described among human genomes, numbering in the hundreds of thousands for any one individual. Approximately half of all indels are referred to as simple because they have only two alleles—that is, the presence or absence of the inserted or deleted segment (see Fig. 4.1).

Microsatellite Variants

Other indels, however, are multiallelic due to variable numbers of a segment of DNA in tandem at a particular location. The term satellite comes from the early

observation that this fraction of DNA has a different density, causing separation during centrifugation. Sometimes called **variable number of tandem repeats**, these microsatellites are highly vulnerable to mutation. They consist of DNA cassettes composed of units of several nucleotides—such as TG, CAA, or AAAT—repeated in tandem between one and a few dozen times (see Fig. 4.2). The numbers of repeated units determine the different alleles, sometimes also referred to as **short tandem repeats** (**STRs**). A **microsatellite** locus often has many alleles (repeat lengths) that can be rapidly evaluated by standard laboratory procedures to distinguish different individuals and to infer **familial** relationships (Fig. 4.3). Many tens of thousands of microsatellite loci are known throughout the human genome.

Microsatellites are particularly useful for genetic mapping. Determining the alleles at multiple microsatellite loci is currently the method of choice for **DNA fingerprinting** used for identity testing. For example, the US Federal Bureau of Investigation (FBI) currently uses 20 STRs for its DNA fingerprinting panel. Two individuals (other than **monozygotic twins**) are so unlikely to have exactly the same alleles at all 20 loci that the panel will allow effectively definitive **determination** of whether samples came from the same individual. The information is stored in the FBI's Combined DNA Index System (CODIS).

Mobile Element Insertion Variants

Nearly half of the human genome consists of dispersed families of repetitive elements (see Chapter 2). Although most of the copies of these repeats are stationary, some of them are mobile and contribute to human genetic diversity through the process of **retrotransposition**. As introduced in Chapter 3 in the context of processed pseudogenes, this involves transcription into an RNA, reverse transcription into a DNA sequence, and insertion (i.e., transposition) into another site in the genome. The two most common mobile element families are the *Alu* and long interspersed nuclear elements (LINE) families of repeats, and nearly 10,000 mobile element insertion variants have been

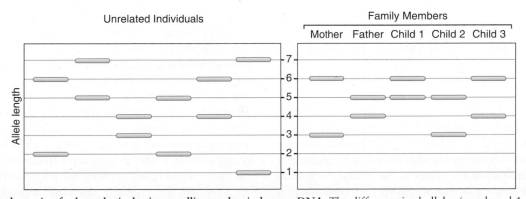

Figure 4.3 **A schematic of a hypothetical microsatellite marker in human DNA.** The different-sized alleles (numbered 1–7) correspond to fragments of genomic DNA containing different numbers of copies of a microsatellite repeat, and their relative lengths are determined by separating them by gel electrophoresis. The shortest allele (allele 1) migrates toward the bottom of the gel, whereas the longest allele (allele 7) remains closest to the top. *Left*, For this multiallelic microsatellite, each of the six unrelated individuals has two different alleles. *Right*, Within a family, the inheritance of alleles can be followed from each parent to each of the three children.

described in different populations. Each polymorphic locus consists of two alleles, one with and one without the inserted mobile element (see Fig. 4.2). Mobile element variants are found on all human chromosomes; although most are found in nongenic regions, a small proportion of them are found within genes. For many of these loci the insertion allele has a frequency of greater than 10% in various populations.

Copy Number Variants

Another important type of human polymorphism includes CNVs, which are conceptually related to indels and microsatellites but involve larger segments of the genome, operationally defined as from 1000 bp to ~3 million bp (i.e., the span between limits of sequencing detection and cytogenetic analysis, respectively). In the general population, variants larger than 500 kb are found in 5% to 10% of individuals, and those encompassing more than 1 Mb in 1% to 2%. The largest CNVs are sometimes in regions of the genome characterized by repeated blocks of homologous sequences called **segmental duplications** (or segdups). The importance of these regions in mediating duplication and deletion of the corresponding segments is discussed further in Chapter 6 in the context of various chromosomal syndromes.

As with indels, smaller CNVs may have only two alleles (i.e., the presence or absence of a segment). Some large CNVs have multiple alleles due to the presence of different numbers of tandem copies of a DNA segment (see Fig. 4.2). In terms of genome diversity, the amount of DNA involved in CNVs vastly exceeds the amount that differs because of SNVs. Compared to the reference genome, the content of any given individual's genome can differ by as much as 30 Mb because of copy number and indel differences.

Notably, since their variable segments can include from one to several dozen genes, CNV loci are frequently implicated in traits that involve altered **gene dosage**. When a CNV is frequent enough, it represents a background of common variation that must be understood to properly interpret alterations in copy number for medical purposes. As with all DNA variation, the significance of different CNV alleles in health and disease susceptibility is the subject of intensive investigation.

Inversions

A final group of structural variants is **inversions**. These regions of the genome, from a few base pairs up to several Mb, are found in either of two orientations (see Fig. 4.2). Most inversions are characterized by regions of sequence homology at the edges of the inverted segment, implicating a process of homologous recombination in their origin. Regardless of orientation, an inversion that does not involve a gain or loss of DNA is balanced. Some can achieve substantial frequencies in the general population. However, anomalous recombination can result in the duplication or deletion of DNA located between the regions of homology—a process associated with clinical disorders that we will explore further in Chapters 5 and 6.

THE ORIGIN AND FREQUENCY OF DIFFERENT TYPES OF MUTATION

Along the spectrum of diversity from rare to common variants, the different kinds of mutation occur in the context of such fundamental processes of cell division as DNA replication, DNA repair, DNA recombination, and **chromosome segregation** in **mitosis** or **meiosis**. The frequency of mutation per locus per cell division is a basic measure of how error prone these processes are, which is of fundamental importance for genome biology and evolution. However, of greatest importance to medical geneticists is the frequency of mutation per disease locus per generation, rather than the overall **mutation rate** across the genome per cell division. Measuring disease-causing mutation rates can be difficult, however, because many mutations cause early embryonic lethality before the result can be recognized in a fetus or newborn. Further, some people with a disease-causing variant may manifest the condition only late in life or may never show signs of the disease. Despite these limitations, we have made great progress in determining the overall frequency—sometimes referred to as the **genetic load**—of all mutations affecting the human species.

These major types of mutation occur at appreciable frequencies in many different cells in the body. In the practice of genetics, we are principally concerned with inherited genome variation; however, all such variation had to originate as a new (*de novo* or spontaneous) change in a germ cell. From this unique start in the population, the ultimate frequency of each variant over time depends on chance and on the principles of inheritance and **population genetics** (see Chapter 10). Although the original mutation would have occurred only in the DNA of a cell in the **germline**, any progeny derived from that cell would then carry it as a constitutional variant in essentially all the cells of the body.

In contrast, **somatic mutations**, depending on when they arise, occur in different proportions of cells throughout the body, but they cannot be transmitted to the next generation of individuals (unless they involved a germline cell). Given the rate of mutation (see later in this section), one would predict that every cell in an individual has a slightly different version of the genome, depending on the number of cell divisions that have occurred since conception. Such genomic **heterogeneity** is particularly likely to be apparent in highly proliferative tissues, such as intestinal epithelia or hematopoietic cells. However, most such variants are not typically detected because, in clinical testing, one usually sequences DNA from many millions of cells, among which the base sequence present at conception will predominate, and rare somatic mutations will be largely invisible and unascertained. Such variants, however, can be of clinical importance in disorders associated with somatic **mosaicism**, caused by mutation in only a subset of cells in certain tissues (see Chapter 7).

While somatic mutations will typically remain undetected within any multicell DNA sample, cancer provides the major exception. The mutational basis for the origins of cancer and the clonal nature of tumor evolution drive certain somatic changes to be present in essentially all the cells of a tumor. Indeed, 1000 to 10,000 somatic variants (and sometimes many more) are readily found in the genomes of most adult tumors, with mutation frequencies and patterns specific to different cancer types (see Chapter 16).

Chromosome Alterations

Events that produce a change in chromosome number because of chromosome missegregation are among the most common sources of variation seen in humans, with a rate of one event per 25 to 50 meiotic cell divisions. This estimate is clearly minimal because the developmental consequences of many such events are likely so severe that the resulting embryos are aborted spontaneously shortly after conception without being detected (see Chapters 5 and 6).

Structural Variation

Alterations affecting the structure or regional organization of chromosomes can arise in a number of different ways. Duplications, deletions, and inversions of a segment of a single chromosome are predominantly the result of homologous recombination between DNA segments with high sequence homology at more than one chromosomal site. Not all structural mutations are the result of homologous recombination, however. Others, such as chromosome translocations and some inversions, can occur at the sites of spontaneous double-stranded DNA breaks. Once breakage occurs at two places anywhere in the genome, the two broken ends can be joined together, even without any obvious sequence homology between the two ends (a process termed nonhomologous end-joining repair). Examples of such mutations will be discussed in Chapter 6.

Mutation in Genes

Gene or DNA variants, including base pair substitutions, insertions, and deletions (Fig. 4.4), can originate by either of two basic mutational mechanisms: errors introduced during DNA replication or arising from a

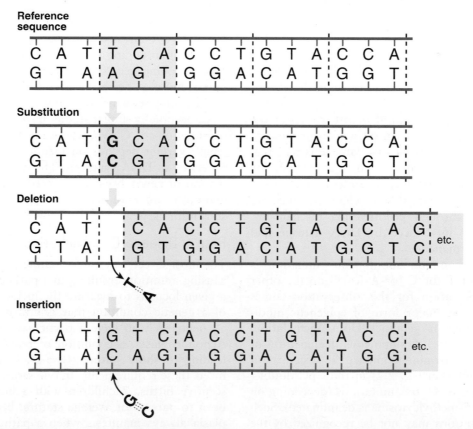

Figure 4.4 **Examples of mutations in a portion of a hypothetical gene with five codons shown (delimited by the *dotted lines*).** The first base pair of the second codon in the reference sequence (shaded in *blue*) is mutated by a base substitution, deletion, or insertion. The base substitution of a G for the T at this position leads to a codon change (shaded in *green*) and, assuming that the upper strand is the sense or coding strand, a predicted nonsynonymous change from a serine to an alanine in the encoded protein (see genetic code in Table 3.1); all other codons remain unchanged. Both the single base pair deletion and insertion lead to a frameshift mutation in which the translational reading frame is altered for all subsequent codons (shaded in *green*), until a termination codon is reached.

failure to properly repair DNA after damage. Many such mutation events are spontaneous, arising during the normal (but imperfect) processes of DNA replication and repair, whereas others are induced by physical or chemical agents called **mutagens**.

DNA Replication Errors

Typically, the process of DNA replication (see Fig. 2.4) is highly accurate. Most replication errors (i.e., bases other than the complementary bases inserted into the double helix) are rapidly removed from the DNA and corrected by a series of DNA repair enzymes. A process termed **DNA proofreading** first recognizes which strand in the newly synthesized double helix contains the incorrect base and then replaces it with the proper complementary base. DNA replication needs to be a remarkably accurate process; otherwise, the burden of mutation on the organism and the species would be intolerable. The enzyme, **DNA polymerase**, faithfully duplicates the two strands of the double helix based on strict base-pairing rules (A pairs with T, C with G) but errs about once in every 10 million bp. Additional proofreading then corrects more than 99.9% of these errors of DNA replication. Thus the overall mutation rate per base as a result of replication errors is a remarkably low 1×10^{-10} per cell division—fewer than one mutation per genome per cell division.

Repair of DNA Damage

In addition to replication errors, about 10,000 to 1,000,000 nucleotides are damaged per human cell per day by (1) spontaneous chemical processes such as depurination, demethylation, or deamination, (2) reaction with chemical mutagens (natural or otherwise) in the environment, or (3) exposure to ultraviolet or ionizing radiation. Some but not all of this damage is repaired. Even if such damage is recognized and excised, the repair machinery may introduce incorrect bases. Thus in contrast to replication-related DNA changes, which are usually corrected through proofreading mechanisms, nucleotide changes introduced by DNA damage and repair are often permanent.

A particularly common spontaneous mutation is the substitution of T for C (or A for G on the other strand). The explanation for this observation comes from considering the major form of **epigenetic** modification in the human genome: **DNA methylation**, introduced in Chapter 3. Spontaneous deamination of 5-methylcytosine to thymine (compare the structures of cytosine and thymine in Fig. 2.2) in the CpG doublet gives rise to C to T or G to A mutations (depending on which strand the 5-methylcytosine is deaminated). Such spontaneous mutations may not be recognized by the DNA repair machinery, thus becoming established in the genome after the next round of DNA replication. More than 30% of all single nucleotide substitutions are of this type, and they occur at a rate 25 times greater than those of other single nucleotide mutations. Thus the CpG doublet represents a true hot spot for mutation in the human genome.

Overall Rate of DNA Mutation

The rate of DNA mutation at specific loci has been estimated using a variety of approaches. The impact of replication and repair errors on the occurrence of new variants throughout the genome can now be determined directly by **whole genome sequencing (WGS)**, using trios consisting of a child and both parents, looking for new sequences in the child that are not present in either parent. The overall rate of new mutations, averaged between maternal and paternal gametes, is $\sim 1.2 \times 10^{-8}$ per base pair per generation. This rate, however, varies from gene to gene and perhaps from population to population, or even individual to individual. This rate of change, combined with considerations of population growth and dynamics, predicts that there must be an enormous number of relatively new (and thus very rare) variants among the current worldwide population of 7.9 billion individuals.

As might be predicted, the vast majority of these will be single nucleotide variants in noncoding portions of the genome and will probably have little or no functional significance. Nonetheless, at the level of populations, the potential collective impact of these new mutation changes on genes of medical importance should not be overlooked. In the United States, for example, with over 4 million live births each year, ~6 million new changes will occur in coding sequences; thus even for a single protein-coding gene of average size, we can anticipate several hundred newborns each year with a new variant in the coding sequence of that gene.

Conceptually similar studies have determined the rate of mutation for CNVs, where the generation of a new length variant depends on recombination, rather than on errors in DNA synthesis. The measured rate of formation of new CNVs ($\approx 1.2 \times 10^{-2}$ per locus per generation) is orders of magnitude higher than that of base substitutions.

Rate of Disease-Causing Variations

The most direct way of estimating the rate of disease-causing mutation, resulting in a **pathogenic variant**, for a given locus is to measure the incidence of new cases of a genetic condition that is clearly recognizable in all neonates who have a particular genetic alteration. Achondroplasia, a condition of reduced bone growth leading to short stature (Case 2), is a condition that meets these requirements. In one series of 242,257 consecutive births, 7 children with achondroplasia were born to parents of average stature; because achondroplasia always manifests when a pathogenic variant is present, all were considered to represent new mutations. Thus the new mutation rate at this locus can be calculated to be 7 new mutations in a total of $2 \times 242,257$ copies of the relevant gene, or $\sim 1.4 \times 10^{-5}$ pathogenic variants per locus per generation. This high mutation rate is particularly striking because virtually all cases of achondroplasia are due to the identical variant: a G to A transition that changes a glycine **codon** to an arginine in the encoded protein.

The rate of pathogenic mutation has been estimated for a number of other disorders in which the occurrence of a new variant was identified by the appearance of a detectable disease (Table 4.3). The measured rates for these and other disorders vary over a 1000-fold range, from 10^{-4} to 10^{-7} mutations per locus per generation. The basis for these differences may be related to some or all of the following: the size of different genes, the fraction of all variants in that gene that will lead to the disease, the age and sex of the parent in whom the mutation occurred, the mutational mechanism, and the presence or absence of mutational hot spots in the gene. Indeed, the high rate of the particular site-specific mutation event in achondroplasia may be partially explained by it being at a hot spot for mutation by deamination, as discussed earlier.

Notwithstanding this range of rates among different genes, the median **gene mutation** rate is $\sim 1 \times 10^{-6}$. Given that there are at least 5000 genes in the human genome in which variants are currently known to cause a discernible disease or other trait (see Chapter 7), ~1 in 200 persons is likely to receive a new pathogenic variant in a known disease-associated gene due to mutation in one or the other parent.

Sex Differences and Age Effects on Mutation Rates

Because the DNA undergoes far more replication cycles in sperm than in ova (see Chapter 2), there is greater opportunity for errors to occur in sperm, suggesting that new variants will be more often paternal than maternal in origin. Indeed, where this has been explored, new variants responsible for certain conditions (e.g., achondroplasia, as just discussed) are usually missense variants that arose nearly always in the paternal germline. Furthermore, the older a man is, the more rounds of replication have preceded the meiotic divisions, thus the frequency of new paternal variants might be expected to increase with the age of the father. Indeed, increased paternal age is correlated with increased incidence of SNVs for a number of disorders (including achondroplasia) and with the incidence of CNVs in autism spectrum disorders (Case 5) and intellectual disability. For other diseases, however, the parent-of-origin and age effects on mutational spectra are, for unknown reasons, not as striking.

TYPES OF MUTATION AND THEIR CONSEQUENCES

In this section we consider the nature of different types of mutation and their effect on the genes involved. Each type of mutation discussed here is illustrated by one or more disease examples. Notably, the **specificity** of the pathogenic variant found in almost all cases of achondroplasia is the exception rather than the rule, and the variants that underlie a single genetic disease are typically heterogeneous among a group of affected individuals. Different cases of a particular disorder will therefore usually be caused by different underlying pathogenic variants in one gene (**allelic heterogeneity**), sometimes in different genes (**locus heterogeneity**). In Chapters 11 and 12 we will turn to the ways in which variants in specific disease-associated genes cause these disorders.

TABLE 4.3 Estimates of Mutation Rates for Selected Human Disease Genes

Disease	Locus (Protein)	Mutation Rate[a]
Achondroplasia (Case 2)	FGFR3 (fibroblast growth factor receptor 3)	1.4×10^{-5}
Aniridia	PAX6 (Pax6)	$2.9–5 \times 10^{-6}$
Duchenne muscular dystrophy (Case 14)	DMD (dystrophin)	$3.5–10.5 \times 10^{-5}$
Hemophilia A (Case 21)	F8 (factor VIII)	$3.2–5.7 \times 10^{-5}$
Hemophilia B (Case 21)	F9 (factor IX)	$2–3 \times 10^{-6}$
Neurofibromatosis, type 1 (Case 34)	NF1 (neurofibromin)	$4–10 \times 10^{-5}$
Polycystic kidney disease, type 1 (Case 37)	PKD1 (polycystin)	$6.5–12 \times 10^{-5}$
Retinoblastoma (Case 39)	RB1 (Rb1)	$5–12 \times 10^{-6}$

[a]Expressed as mutations per locus per generation.
Based on data in Vogel F, Motulsky AG: *Human genetics*, ed 4, Berlin, 1997, Springer-Verlag.

TABLE 4.4 Types of Variation in Human Genetic Disease

Type of Variation	Percentage of Disease-Causing Variants
Nucleotide Substitutions	
• Missense variants (amino acid substitutions)	40%
• Nonsense variants (premature stop codons)	10%
• RNA processing variants (destroy consensus splice sites, cap sites, and polyadenylation sites or create cryptic sites)	10%
• Splice-site variants leading to frameshift mutations and premature stop codons	10%
• Long-range regulatory variants	Rare
Deletions and Insertions	
• Addition or deletions of a small number of bases	25%
• Larger gene deletions, inversions, fusions, and duplications (may be mediated by DNA sequence homology either within or between DNA strands)	5%
• Insertion of a LINE or *Alu* element (disrupting transcription or interrupting the coding sequence)	Rare
• Dynamic variants (expansion of trinucleotide or tetranucleotide repeat sequences)	Rare

Nucleotide Substitutions

Missense Variants

A single nucleotide substitution (or **point mutation** or SNV) in a gene sequence, such as that in the example of achondroplasia, can alter the code in a triplet of bases and cause the nonsynonymous replacement of one amino acid by another in the gene product (see the **genetic code** in Table 3.1 and the example in Fig. 4.4). Such events are called **missense mutations**, creating **missense variants** because they alter the coding (or sense) strand of the gene to specify a different amino acid. Although not all missense variants lead to an observable change in the function of the protein, the resulting protein may fail to work properly, may be unstable and rapidly degraded, or may fail to localize in its proper intracellular position. In many disorders, such as β-thalassemia, most of the variants detected in different patients are missense variants (see Chapter 12).

Nonsense Variants

Point mutation in a DNA sequence that causes the replacement of the normal codon for an amino acid by one of the three termination (or "stop") codons creates a nonsense variant or premature termination codon (PTC; also called stop gain). Because **translation** of **messenger RNA (mRNA)** ceases when a **termination codon** is reached (see Chapter 3), a variant that converts a coding codon into a termination codon causes translation to stop prematurely. In general, mRNAs harboring a PTC are targeted for rapid degradation through a cellular process known as **nonsense-mediated mRNA decay (NMD)**, and no translation is possible. Rarely, transcripts harboring a PTC escape NMD, most predictably if the premature stop codon occurs in last 50 bp of the penultimate exon or anywhere in the final exon of a gene. In this circumstance, a nonsense mutation can often give rise to a truncated protein with altered function.

Rarely, an SNV can alter the normal termination codon (called a stop loss variant), permitting translation to continue until another termination codon in the mRNA is reached further downstream. Such a variant can lead to an abnormal protein product with additional amino acids at its carboxy-terminus. Alternatively, access of a translating **ribosome** into the 3′ **untranslated region** downstream of the normal stop codon can displace proteins that regulate mRNA stability and/or translation.

Variants Affecting RNA Transcription, Processing, and Translation

The normal mechanism by which initial RNA transcripts are made and then converted into mature mRNAs (or final versions of noncoding RNAs) requires a series of modifications, including transcription factor binding, 5′ capping, **polyadenylation**, and splicing (see Chapter 3). All of these steps in RNA maturation depend on specific sequences within the RNA. In the case of **splicing**, two general classes of splicing variants have been described. For introns to be excised from unprocessed RNA and the exons spliced together to form a mature RNA requires particular nucleotide sequences located at or near the exon-intron (5′ donor site) or the intron-exon (3′ acceptor site) junctions. Variants that substitute the required bases at either the splice donor or acceptor site prevent normal **RNA splicing**. Substitution of less conserved adjacent bases has a variable impact on splicing efficiency. A second class of splicing variants involves base substitutions that do not affect the donor or acceptor site sequences themselves, but instead create alternative donor or acceptor sites that compete with the normal sites during RNA processing. Activation of these so-called cryptic splice sites can lead to inappropriate exclusion or inclusion of exonic or intronic sequences, respectively, in the mature mRNA. Thus at least a proportion of the mature mRNA or **noncoding RNA** in such cases may contain improperly spliced intron sequences. Examples of both types of variation are presented in Chapter 12.

For protein-coding genes, even if the mRNA is made, SNVs in the 5′ and 3′ untranslated regions can contribute to disease by changing mRNA stability or translational efficiency, thereby reducing the amount of protein product.

Deletions, Insertions, and Rearrangements

Mutation can also involve the insertion, deletion, or rearrangement of DNA sequences. Some deletions and insertions involve only a few nucleotides and are generally most easily detected by direct sequencing of that part of the genome. In other cases, a substantial segment of a gene or an entire gene is deleted, duplicated, inverted, or translocated to create a novel arrangement of gene sequences—collectively called structural variants. Depending on the exact nature of the deletion, insertion, or rearrangement, a variety of different laboratory approaches can be used to detect the genomic alteration.

Some deletions and insertions affect only a small number of base pairs. When such a variant occurs in a coding sequence and the number of bases involved is not a multiple of three (i.e., not an integral number of codons), the **reading frame** will be altered beginning at the point of the insertion or deletion. The results are called **frameshift variants** (see Fig. 4.4). From the point of the insertion or deletion, a different sequence of codons is thereby generated that encodes incorrect amino acids followed by a termination codon in the shifted frame. This typically leads to degradation of the altered transcript via activation of NMD or, more rarely, an altered and truncated protein product. In contrast, if the number of base pairs inserted or deleted is a multiple of three, then no frameshift occurs, and there will be a simple insertion or deletion of the corresponding amino acids in the otherwise normally translated gene product. Larger insertions or deletions can affect multiple exons of a gene and cause major disruptions of the coding sequence.

One type of insertion mutation involves insertion of a mobile element, such as those belonging to the LINE family of repetitive DNA (LINE-1 [L1] elements). Any of the 146 putatively active L1 elements currently recognized in the human genome are capable of movement by retrotransposition (introduced earlier). Such movement not only generates genetic diversity in our species (see Fig. 4.2) but can cause disease by insertional mutagenesis. For example, in some patients with the severe bleeding disorder hemophilia A **(Case 21)**, **LINE sequences** several kilobases long are found within an exon in the factor VIII gene, interrupting the coding sequence and inactivating the gene. LINE insertions throughout the genome are also common in colon cancer, reflecting retrotransposition in somatic cells (see Chapter 16).

As we discussed earlier in this chapter, duplications, deletions, and inversions of a larger segment of a single chromosome are predominantly the result of homologous recombination between DNA segments with high sequence homology (Fig. 4.5). Disorders arising as a result of such exchanges can be due to a change in the dosage of otherwise wild-type gene products when the homologous segments lie outside the genes themselves (see Chapter 6). Alternatively, such events can lead to a change in the nature of the encoded protein itself when recombination occurs between different genes within a **gene family** (see Chapter 12) or between genes on different chromosomes (see Chapter 16). Abnormal pairing and recombination between two similar sequences in opposite orientation on a single strand of DNA leads to inversion. For example, nearly half of all cases of hemophilia A are due to recombination that inverts a number of exons, thereby disrupting gene structure and rendering the gene incapable of encoding a normal gene product (see Fig. 4.5).

Repeat Expansion Variants

The pathogenic variant in some disorders involves amplification of a simple nucleotide repeat sequence. For example, simple repeats such as $(CCG)_n$, $(CAG)_n$, or $(CCTG)_n$—located in the coding portion of an exon, in an untranslated region of an exon, or even in an intron—may expand during gametogenesis in repeat expansion or dynamic mutation, and interfere with normal gene expression or protein function. An expanded repeat in a coding region will generate an abnormal protein product; in the untranslated regions or introns of a gene, it may interfere with transcription, mRNA processing, or translation. How repeat expansions occur is not completely understood; they are conceptually similar to microsatellites but expand at a much higher rate.

The involvement of simple nucleotide repeat expansions in disease is discussed further in Chapter 7. In such disorders, marked parent-of-origin effects are

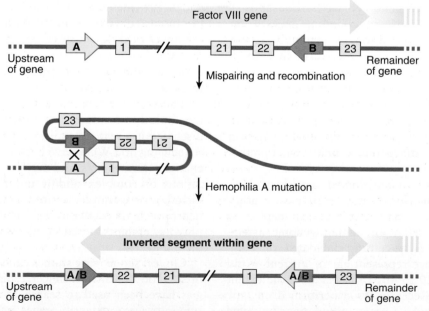

Figure 4.5 Inverted homologous sequences, labeled *A* and *B*, located 500 kb apart on the X chromosome, one upstream of the factor VIII gene, the other in an intron between exons 22 and 23 of the gene. Intrachromosomal mispairing and recombination results in inversion of exons 1 through 22 of the gene, thereby disrupting the gene and causing severe hemophilia.

well known and appear characteristic of the specific disease and/or the particular simple nucleotide repeat involved (see Chapter 13). Such differences may be due to fundamental biologic differences between oogenesis and spermatogenesis but may also result from **selection** against gametes carrying certain repeat expansions.

VARIATION IN INDIVIDUAL GENOMES

The most extensive current inventory of the amount and type of variation in any given genome, relative to the (composite) human reference genome sequence (see Chapter 2), comes from the analysis of individual **diploid** human genome sequences. The first such sequence, that of a male individual, was reported in 2007. Now, hundreds of thousands of individual genomes have been sequenced, some as part of large international research consortia exploring human genetic diversity in health and disease, and others in the context of clinical sequencing to determine the underlying basis of disorders in particular patients.

What degree of genome variation does one detect in such studies? Individual human genomes typically carry ~3.5 million SNVs when compared to the reference genome, of which—depending in part on the population—currently 1% are novel (i.e., not previously documented) (see Box 4.2). This suggests that the number of SNVs described for our species is still incomplete, although presumably the novel fraction will decrease as more genomes from more populations are sequenced.

Within this variation lie variants with clinical impact that are either known, likely, or suspected. Each genome carries 50 to 100 variants that have previously been implicated in known inherited conditions. In addition, each genome carries thousands of nonsynonymous SNVs in protein-coding genes, some of which would be predicted to alter protein function. Each genome also carries ~200 to 500 likely loss-of-function variants, some of which are present at both alleles of a gene in that individual. Within the clinical setting, this realization has important implications for the interpretation of genome sequence data from patients, particularly when trying to predict the impact of variants in genes of currently unknown function (see Chapter 13).

An interesting and unanticipated aspect of individual **genome sequencing** is that each new genome reveals some sequence that is still undocumented or unannotated in the reference human genome assembly. It is estimated that, once fully elucidated, the complete genome sequence representing the current world population will be 20 to 40 Mb larger than the extant reference assembly. Recently WGS performed on only 94 individuals from 44 African populations revealed 33.6 million SNVs, of which 5.7 million (17%) were

novel. This illustrates the extent to which individuals of descent other than European are underrepresented among sequenced cohorts, creating a significant gap in our knowledge of human genetic diversity and our ability to advance **genomic medicine**.

BOX 4.2   VARIATION DETECTED IN A TYPICAL HUMAN GENOME

Individuals vary greatly in a wide range of biologic functions, determined in part by variation among their genomes. Any individual genome will contain (on average) the following:

- ≈3.5 million SNVs compared to the reference genome (varies by population)
- 25,000–50,000 rare variants (private mutations or seen previously in <0.5% of individuals tested)
- ≈65 new (*de novo*) SNVs and indels not detected in parental genomes
- ≈200,000 indels (1–50 bp) (varies by population)
- 500–1000 deletions 1–45 kb, overlapping ≈200 genes
- ≈102 in-frame indels
- ≈132 shifts in reading frame
- 10,000–12,000 synonymous SNVs
- >11,000 nonsynonymous SNVs in 4000–5000 genes
- 175–500 rare nonsynonymous variants
- 1 new nonsynonymous mutation
- ≈474 premature stop codons or splice site disrupting variants
- 250–300 genes with likely loss-of-function variants
- ≈25 genes predicted to be completely inactivated

Clinical Sequencing Studies

In the context of genomic medicine, a key question is the extent to which variation in the sequence and/or expression of one's genome influences the likelihood of disease onset, determines the natural history of disease, and/or provides clues relevant to its management. As just discussed, constitutional genomic variants can have a number of different direct or indirect effects on gene function.

Sequencing of entire genomes (WGS, also referred to as genome sequencing) or of the subset comprising all known coding exons (**exome sequencing**) has been introduced in a number of clinical settings, as will be discussed in greater detail in Chapter 11. Both exome sequencing and WGS have been used to detect *de novo* changes (both SNVs and CNVs) in a variety of conditions of complex and/or unknown etiology. These include, for example, various neurodevelopmental or neuropsychiatric conditions, such as autism, schizophrenia, epilepsy, intellectual disability, and developmental delay.

Clinical sequencing studies can target either germline or somatic variants. In cancer, especially, various strategies have been used to search for somatic variants in tumor tissue to identify genes potentially relevant to cancer progression (see Chapter 16).

Direct-to-Consumer Genomics

Access to laboratory genomic testing has moved into the public realm in recent years, no longer with mainstream medicine as its gatekeeper. Tests are marketed directly to consumers for information ranging from genealogy and ancestry tracing to information about personal health and inherited traits. Targeted screening panels are starting to give way to genome sequencing opportunities. A limited number of specific diagnostic tests have been authorized by the US Food and Drug Administration for marketing. There is considerable public appetite for the sort of individual information being offered commercially, and the massive volume of data being collected and stored has enormous research potential. Notwithstanding or minimizing the significant scientific, ethical, and clinical issues that lie ahead, it is certain that individual genome sequences will be an ongoing active part of medical practice and that some of these will be delivered from patient to practitioner, rather than vice versa.

IMPACT OF GENOMIC VARIATION

Although it will be self-evident to students of human genetics that new pathogenic or rare variants in the population can have clinical consequences, it may appear less obvious that common variants can be clinically relevant. For the proportion of variation that occurs within protein-coding genes, such loci can be studied by examining variation in the proteins encoded by the different alleles. Any one individual is likely to carry two distinct alleles determining structurally differing polypeptides at an estimated 20% of protein-coding loci; when individuals from different ancestral groups are studied, an even greater fraction of proteins has been found to exhibit detectable polymorphism. In addition, even when the gene product is unaltered, the levels of expression of that product may be very different among individuals, determined by a combination of genetic and epigenetic variation, as we saw in Chapter 3.

Thus a striking degree of biochemical individuality exists within the human species in its makeup of enzymes and other gene products. Furthermore, the products of many of the encoded biochemical and regulatory pathways interact in functional and physiologic networks. Each individual, therefore—regardless of state of health—has a unique, genetically determined chemical makeup and responds in a unique manner to environmental, dietary, and pharmacologic influences. This concept of **chemical individuality** first put forward over a century ago by Archibald Garrod, the remarkably prescient British physician introduced in Chapter 1, remains true today. The broad question of what is normal—an essential concept in human biology and in clinical medicine—remains very much

an open and controversial one when it comes to the human genome.

The following chapters will explore this concept of individuality in detail, first in the context of structural genome and chromosome variants (Chapters 5 and 6) and then in terms of intragenic variants that determine the inheritance of genetic disease (Chapter 7) and influence its likelihood in families and populations (Chapter 10).

Assessing the Clinical Significance of a Gene Variant

The American College of Medical Genetics and Genomics and the Association for Molecular Pathology recommend that all variants detected during sequencing of genes for monogenic disease (whether from targeted, exome, or genome sequencing) be classified on a five-level scale, spanning pathogenic, likely pathogenic, of uncertain significance, likely benign, and benign variants. Specialists in molecular diagnostics, human genomics, and **bioinformatics** have developed criteria for assessing where a variant sits among these five categories. None of these criteria are definitive; they must be considered together to provide an overall assessment of the evidence for pathogenicity. These criteria include the following:

- **Population frequency**—If a variant has been seen frequently in a sizable fraction of the general population, beyond what is expected based on the prevalence of the disease, it is considered less likely to be disease causing. Being frequent, however, is no guarantee that a variant is benign. Autosomal **recessive** conditions result from homozygosity for disease-causing variants that may be surprisingly common, largely harbored by asymptomatic **heterozygous** carriers. Conversely, rare variants are not necessarily pathogenic; most variants found in an exome or genome sequence are individually rare.

- **In silico assessment**—Computational algorithms can evaluate how likely a missense variant is to be damaging to the protein, by using information such as whether the amino acid at that position is conserved in **orthologous** proteins (in other species), the structural location of the variant, and machine-learning algorithms. Such tools are limited in their accuracy for predicting functional impact and therefore can never be used alone to definitively determine pathogenicity. They are, however, improving with time, and their contribution to variant assessment may strengthen. Other bioinformatics tools assess the pathogenicity of other types of variants, such as potential splice site variants and other noncoding sequence variants.

- **Functional data**—If a particular variant adversely affects *in vitro* biochemical activity, a function in cultured cells, or the health of a model organism, then it is less likely to be benign. However, it remains possible that a particular variant will appear benign by these criteria and still be disease causing in humans because of a prolonged human life span, environmental triggers, or compensatory genes present in the model organism but not in humans. Conversely, functional effects demonstrated in systems that do not fully represent the human biologic state may falsely implicate a variant as pathogenic. Caution must be exercised to ensure adequate validation of these assays with variants determined to be pathogenic or benign through other types of evidence.

- **Segregation data**—If a particular variant is coinherited with a disease in one or more families or, conversely, does not track with a disease in the family under investigation, then it is more or less likely to be pathogenic. Of course, when only a few individuals are affected, the variant and disease may appear to track by random chance; to be considered strong evidence for pathogenicity, the number of times a variant and disease must be coinherited is generally accepted to be in at least five informative meioses. Finding affected individuals in the family who do not carry the variant would be strong evidence against the variant being pathogenic, but finding unaffected individuals who do carry the variant is less persuasive if the disorder is known to have reduced **penetrance**.

- *De novo* **variant**—The appearance of a severe disorder in a child along with a new variant in a coding exon that neither parent carries (*de novo* variant) is additional evidence for that variant to be pathogenic. However, between one and two new changes occur in the coding regions of genes in every child (see earlier). Only *de novo* variants in genes that are associated with the individual's phenotype are considered evidence for pathogenicity, given a lower prior probability of *de novo* mutation for a small, targeted set of genes.

- **Variant characterization**—A variant may be synonymous, missense, nonsense, a frameshift with a premature termination downstream, or cause a highly conserved splice site change. The impact on the function of the gene can be inferred but, once again, is not definitive. For example, a synonymous change that does not alter an amino acid codon might be thought to be benign but may have deleterious effects on normal splicing and be pathogenic (see examples in Chapter 12). Conversely, one might assume that premature termination or frameshift variants are always deleterious and disease causing; however, such an alteration at the far 3' end of a gene may produce a truncated protein that is still functional and, therefore, be a benign change.

- **Prior occurrence**—Having been seen multiple times among collections of patients with a similar disorder

is important additional evidence that a variant is pathogenic. Even if a missense variant is novel (i.e., never described before) it is more likely to be pathogenic if it occurs at the same position in the protein as other known pathogenic missense variants.

ACKNOWLEDGMENT

We thank Miriam Reuter, Heidi Rehm and Jeff MacDonald for contributing to this chapter.

GENERAL REFERENCES

Olson MV: Human genetic individuality, *Ann Rev Genomics Hum Genet* 13:1–27, 2012.

Strachan T, Read A, editors: *Human molecular genetics* ed 5, New York, 2018, Garland Science.

The 1000 Genomes Project Consortium: An integrated map of genetic variation from 1,092 human genomes, *Nature* 491:56–65, 2012.

Trost B, Loureiro LO, Scherer SW: Discovery of genomic variation across a generation, *Human Molecular Genetics*, Volume 30, Issue R2, 15 October 2021, Pages R174–R186, https://doi.org/10.1093/hmg/ddab209.

Willard HF: The human genome: a window on human genetics, biology and medicine. In Ginsburg GS, Willard HF, editors: *Genomic and personalized medicine* ed 3, New York, 2016, Elsevier.

REFERENCES FOR SPECIFIC TOPICS

Alkan C, Coe BP, Eichler EE: Genome structural variation discovery and genotyping, *Nature Rev Genet* 12:363–376, 2011.

Bagnall RD, Waseem N, Green PM, et al: Recurrent inversion breaking intron 1 of the factor VIII gene is a frequent cause of severe hemophilia A, *Blood* 99:168–174, 2002.

Crow JF: The origins, patterns and implications of human spontaneous mutation, *Nature Rev Genet* 1:40–47, 2000.

Fan S, Kelley DE, Beltrame MH, et al: African evolutionary history inferred from whole genome sequence data of 44 indigenous African populations, *Genome Biol* 20:82, 2019.

Gardner RJ: A new estimate of the achondroplasia mutation rate, *Clin Genet* 11:31–38, 1977.

Karczewski KJ, Francioli LC, Tiao G, et al: The mutational constraint spectrum quantified from variation in 141,456 humans, *Nature* 581:434–443, 2020. https://doi.org/10.1038/s41586-020-2308-7

Kong A, Frigge ML, Masson G, et al: Rate of *de novo* mutations and the importance of father's age to disease risk, *Nature* 488:471–475, 2012.

Lappalainen T, Sammeth M, Friedlander MR, et al: Transcriptome and genome sequencing uncovers functional variation in humans, *Nature* 501:506–511, 2013.

MacArthur DG, Balasubramanian S, Rrankish A, et al: A systematic survey of loss-of-function variants in human protein-coding genes, *Science* 335:823–828, 2012.

McBride CM, Wade CH, Kaphingst KA: Consumers' view of direct-to-consumer genetic information, *Ann Rev Genomics Hum Genet* 11:427–446, 2010.

Richards S, Aziz N, Bale S, et al: Standards and guidelines for the interpretation of sequence variants: a joint consensus recommendation of the American College of Medical Genetics and Genomics and the Association for Molecular Pathology, *Genet Med* 17(5):405–424, 2015. https://doi.org/10.1038/gim.2015.30

Stewart C, Kural D, Stromberg MP, et al: A comprehensive map of mobile element insertion polymorphisms in humans, *PLoS Genet* 7:e1002236, 2011.

Sun JX, Helgason A, Masson G, et al: A direct characterization of human mutation based on microsatellites, *Nature Genet* 44:1161–1165, 2012.

PROBLEMS

1. Variation can arise from a variety of mechanisms, with different consequences. Describe and contrast the types of variation that can have the following effects:
   a. A change in dosage of a gene or genes
   b. A change in the sequence of multiple amino acids in the product of a protein-coding gene
   c. A change in the final structure of an RNA produced from a gene
   d. A change in the order of genes in a region of a chromosome
   e. No obvious effect

2. Aniridia is an eye disorder characterized by the complete or partial absence of the iris and is always present when a pathogenic variant occurs in the responsible gene. In one population, 41 children diagnosed with aniridia were born to parents of normal vision among 4.5 million births during a period of 40 years. Assuming that these cases were due to new mutation events, what is the estimated mutation rate at the aniridia locus? On what assumptions is this estimate based, and why might this estimate be either too high or too low?

3. Which of the following types of variation would be most effective for distinguishing two individuals from the general population: a single nucleotide variant (SNV), a simple indel, or a microsatellite? Explain your reasoning.

4. Compare the likely impact of each of the following on the overall rate of mutation detected in any given genome: age of the parents, hot spots of mutation, intrachromosomal homologous recombination, genetic variation in the parental genomes.

Principles of Clinical Cytogenetics and Genome Analysis

Dimitri J. Stavropoulos

Clinical **cytogenetics** is the study of **chromosomes**, their structure, and their inheritance, as applied to the practice of medicine. It has been apparent for over 50 years that chromosome abnormalities—microscopically visible changes in the number or structure of chromosomes—could account for a number of clinical conditions that are thus referred to as **chromosome disorders**. With their focus on the complete set of **genetic** material, cytogeneticists were the first to bring a genome-wide perspective to the practice of medicine. Today, chromosome analysis—with increasing resolution and precision at both the cytologic and genomic levels—is an important diagnostic procedure in numerous areas of clinical medicine. Current **genome** analyses that use approaches to be explored in this chapter, including chromosomal **microarrays** and **whole genome sequencing (WGS)**, represent impressive improvements in capacity and resolution but ones that are conceptually similar to microscopic methods focusing on chromosomes (Fig. 5.1).

Chromosome disorders form a major category of genetic disease. They account for a large proportion of all spontaneous pregnancy losses, **congenital** malformations, and intellectual disability and play an important role in the pathogenesis of cancer. Specific cytogenetic disorders are responsible for hundreds of distinct **syndromes** that collectively are more common than all the single-gene diseases together. Cytogenetic abnormalities are present in nearly 1% of live births, in ~2% of pregnancies in women older than 35 years who undergo prenatal diagnosis, and in half of all spontaneous, first-trimester pregnancy losses.

The spectrum of analysis from microscopically visible changes in chromosome number and structure to **anomalies** of genome structure and **sequence** detectable at the level of WGS encompasses literally the entire field of medical genetics (see Fig. 5.1). In this chapter we present the general principles of chromosome and genome analysis and focus on the chromosome **variants** and structural variants introduced in the previous chapter. We restrict our discussion to disorders due to genomic imbalance—either for the hundreds to thousands of genes found on individual chromosomes or for smaller numbers of genes located within a particular chromosome region. Application of these principles to some of the most common and best-known chromosomal and genomic disorders will then be presented in Chapter 6.

INTRODUCTION TO CYTOGENETICS AND GENOME ANALYSIS

The general morphology and organization of human chromosomes, as well as their molecular and genomic composition, were introduced in Chapters 2 and 3. Chromosome analysis can be performed for clinical purposes by obtaining peripheral blood and stimulating T lymphocytes to prepare short-term cultures. After a few days, the dividing cells are arrested in **metaphase** with chemicals that inhibit the **mitotic spindle**, and chromosomes are fixed to glass slides and stained by one of several techniques, depending on the particular diagnostic procedure being performed. They are then ready for analysis.

Although ideal for rapid clinical analysis, cell cultures prepared from peripheral blood have the disadvantage of being short lived (3–4 days). Long-term cultures suitable for permanent storage or further studies can be derived from a variety of other tissues. Skin biopsy, a minor surgical procedure, can provide samples of tissue that in culture produce **fibroblasts**, which can be used for a variety of biochemical and molecular studies as well as for chromosome and genome analysis. White blood cells can also be transformed in culture to form **lymphoblastoid** cell lines that are potentially immortal. Bone marrow has the advantage of containing a high proportion of dividing cells so that little if any culturing is required; however, it can be obtained only by the relatively invasive procedure of marrow biopsy. Its main use is in the diagnosis of suspected hematologic malignancies. **Fetal cells** derived from amniotic fluid (amniocytes) or obtained by chorionic villus biopsy can also be cultured successfully for cytogenetic, genomic, biochemical, or molecular analysis. Chorionic villus cells can also be analyzed directly after biopsy, without the need for culturing. Remarkably, small amounts of cell-free fetal DNA are found in the maternal plasma and can be tested by WGS (see Chapter 18 for further discussion).

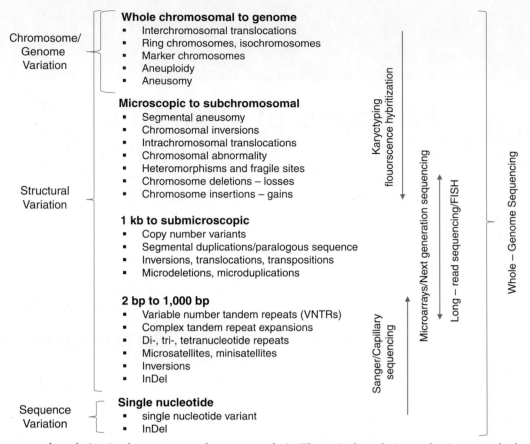

Figure 5.1 Spectrum of resolution in chromosome and genome analysis. The typical resolution and primary methods used to detect them are given for various technologic approaches used routinely in chromosome and genome analysis. See text for details and specific examples. (Redrawn from Trost B, Loureiro LO, Scherer SW: Discovery of genomic variation across a generation. *Hum Mol Genet* 30(2):R174–R186, 2021.)

Molecular analysis of the genome, including WGS, can be carried out on any appropriate clinical material, provided that good-quality DNA can be obtained. Cells need not be dividing for this purpose, and thus it is possible to study DNA from tissue and tumor samples, for example, as well as from peripheral blood. Which approach is most appropriate for a particular diagnostic or research purpose is a rapidly evolving area as the resolution, **sensitivity**, and ease of chromosome and genome analysis increase (see Box 5.1).

Chromosome Identification

The different chromosomes in the genome can be identified cytologically by their characteristic banding patterns after applying specific staining procedures. The most common of these, Giemsa banding (**G-banding**), was developed in the early 1970s and was the first widely used whole genome analytic tool for research and clinical diagnosis that may still apply. It has been the gold standard for the detection and characterization of structural and numerical genomic abnormalities in clinical diagnostic settings for both constitutional (postnatal or prenatal) and acquired (cancer) disorders.

G-banding and other staining procedures can be used to describe individual chromosomes and their variants or abnormalities, using an internationally accepted system of chromosome classification. Fig. 5.2 is an ideogram of the banding pattern of a set of normal human chromosomes at metaphase, illustrating the alternating pattern of light and dark bands used for chromosome identification. The pattern of bands on each chromosome is numbered on each arm from the **centromere** to the **telomere**, as shown in detail in Fig. 5.3 for several chromosomes. The identity of any particular band (and thus the DNA sequences and genes within it) can be described precisely and unambiguously by use of this regionally based and hierarchic numbering system.

Human chromosomes are often classified into three types that can be easily distinguished at metaphase by the position of the centromere, the **primary constriction** visible at metaphase (see Fig. 5.2). **Metacentric** chromosomes have a central centromere and arms of approximately equal length, **submetacentric** chromosomes have an off-center centromere and arms of clearly different lengths, and **acrocentric** chromosomes have the centromere near one end. A potential fourth type of chromosome, **telocentric**, with the centromere at one end and

BOX 5.1 CLINICAL INDICATIONS FOR CHROMOSOME AND GENOME ANALYSIS

Chromosome analysis is indicated as a routine diagnostic procedure for a number of specific conditions encountered in medicine, and some general clinical indications include:

- *Problems of early growth and development.* Failure to thrive, developmental delay, dysmorphic facies, multiple malformations, short stature, ambiguous genitalia, and intellectual disability are frequent findings in children with chromosome abnormalities. Unless there is a definite nonchromosomal diagnosis, genomic analysis should be performed to detect diagnostic genome-wide copy number and sequence variants for patients presenting with any combination of such problems (see Chapter 11).
- *Stillbirth and neonatal death.* The incidence of chromosome abnormalities is much higher among stillbirths (up to ~10%) than among live births (~0.7%). It is also elevated among infants who die in the neonatal period (~10%). For unexplained stillbirths and neonatal deaths, genome-wide copy number and sequence analysis may serve to reveal a genetic etiology. These analyses may provide important information for prenatal or preimplantation genetic diagnosis (see Chapter 18) in future pregnancies.
- *Fertility problems.* Chromosome studies by G-banded **karyotype** are indicated for women with amenorrhea and for couples with a history of infertility or recurrent miscarriage. A chromosome abnormality is seen in one or the other parent in 3–6% of cases in which there is infertility or two or more miscarriages.
- *Structural characterization of genomic imbalances and family follow-up studies.* Copy number variations (CNV) identified by genome-wide copy number analysis may require additional studies by G-banding karyotype or metaphase **fluorescence *in situ* hybridization (FISH)** to characterize the structure of the alteration. A known unbalanced chromosome abnormality may have resulted from a parental balanced **rearrangement**, which will have implications for future pregnancies and potential prenatal diagnosis, as well as potentially for other family members of the **carrier** parent.
- *Neoplasia.* Almost all cancers are associated with one or more chromosome abnormalities (see Chapter 16). Chromosome and genome evaluation in the tumor itself, or in bone marrow for hematologic malignant neoplasms, can offer diagnostic or prognostic information.
- *Pregnancy.* Several prenatal **risk** factors, including advanced maternal age, biochemical markers, and ultrasound findings, are associated with chromosome abnormalities (see Chapter 18). Fetal genome-wide copy number and sequence analysis should be offered as a routine part of prenatal care in such pregnancies. **Noninvasive prenatal screening** using whole genome sequencing of **cell-free DNA** in maternal blood is also available to screen for the most common chromosome disorders.

only a single arm, does not occur in the normal human karyotype, but it is occasionally observed in chromosome rearrangements. The human acrocentric chromosomes (13, 14, 15, 21, and 22) have small, distinctive masses of **chromatin** known as **satellites** attached to their short arms by narrow stalks (called secondary constrictions). The stalks of these five chromosome pairs contain hundreds of copies of genes for ribosomal **RNA** (the major component of ribosomes; see Chapter 3) as well as a variety of repetitive sequences.

The standard G-banded karyotype at a 400- to 550-band stage of resolution, as seen in a typical metaphase preparation, allows detection of deletions and duplications greater than ~5 to 10 Mb (see Fig. 5.1). However, the sensitivity of G-banding at this resolution may be lower in regions of the genome in which the banding patterns are less specific. High-resolution banding (also called **prometaphase** banding) can achieve 850 or more bands in a **haploid** set by staining chromosomes that have been obtained at an early stage of mitosis (**prophase** or prometaphase), when they are still in a relatively uncondensed state (see Chapter 2). Development of high-resolution chromosome analysis in the early 1980s allowed the discovery of a number of new **microdeletion** and microduplication syndrome, caused by smaller genomic rearrangements in the 2-to-3 Mb size range (see Fig. 5.1). However, the time-consuming and technically difficult nature of this cytogenetic method precludes its routine use for whole genome analysis.

In addition to changes in banding pattern, nonstaining gaps, called **fragile sites**, are heritable variants that can be observed at particular chromosome sites that are prone to regional genomic instability induced by stress on DNA replication. Over 100 common and rare (population frequency <5%) fragile sites are documented. Common fragile sites are postulated to drive genomic instability in cancer cells, and a small proportion of rare fragile sites are associated with specific clinical disorders. For example, the rare **fragile site** located at Xq27.3 is caused by an expansion of CGG repeats and is observed in patients with fragile X syndrome (Case 17).

Fluorescence *In Situ* Hybridization (FISH)

Targeted high-resolution chromosome banding was largely replaced in the early 1990s by **FISH**, a method for detecting the presence or absence of a particular DNA sequence or for evaluating the number or structural organization of a chromosome or chromosomal region *in situ* (literally, "in place") in the cell. This convergence of genomic and cytogenetic approaches—variously termed molecular cytogenetics or cytogenomics—dramatically expanded both the scope and precision of chromosome analysis in routine clinical practice.

FISH technology takes advantage of ordered collections of **recombinant** large-insert DNA clones containing DNA from virtually any **locus** in the genome. Clones containing specific human DNA sequences can be labeled with a fluorescent dye and used as probes to detect the corresponding region of the genome in

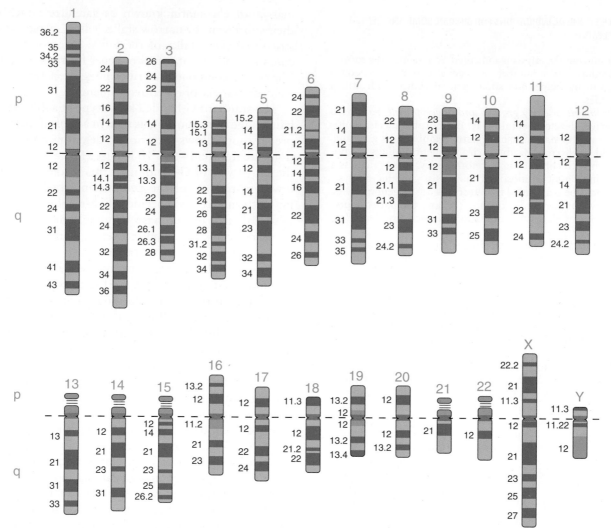

Figure 5.2 **Ideogram showing G-banding patterns for human chromosomes at metaphase, with ~400 bands per haploid karyotype.** As drawn, chromosomes are typically represented with the sister chromatids so closely aligned that they are not recognized as distinct entities. Centromeres are indicated by the primary constriction and narrow *dark gray* regions separating the p and q arms. For convenience and clarity, only the G-dark bands are numbered. For examples of full numbering scheme, see Fig. 5.3. (Redrawn from Shaffer LG, McGowan-Jordan J, Schmid M, editors: ISCN 2013: an international system for human cytogenetic nomenclature, Basel, 2013, Karger.)

chromosome preparations or in **interphase** nuclei for a variety of research and diagnostic purposes (Fig. 5.4).

Although FISH technology provides much higher resolution and **specificity** than G-banded chromosome analysis, it does not allow for efficient analysis of the entire genome. Its use is limited to targeting a specific genomic region based on a clinical diagnosis or suspicion, structural characterization of genomic imbalances and family follow-up studies.

Multiplex Ligation-Dependent Probe Amplification (MLPA)

MLPA is a targeted copy number assay used to detect exon-level deletions and duplications in a gene or targeted chromosome region. This method uses multiplex **polymerase chain reaction (PCR)** to amplify DNA sequences from multiple **exons** simultaneously in one

PCR. The relative quantity of DNA sequence generated from each exon is then compared to amplification of control regions with normal copy number (two copies). Since the total quantity of amplified PCR product is directly proportional to the copy number of each targeted exon in the individual DNA sample, a **heterozygous** deletion (one copy) will produce approximately half as much PCR product when compared to regions with normal copy number (two copies), and a heterozygous duplication (three copies) will generate ~50% more PCR product when compared to regions with normal copy number. This method is limited by the number of targeted regions that can be included in one PCR assay and is not amenable to genome-wide copy number analysis. It is used to investigate a specific gene (e.g., DMD) or known recurrent microdeletion/microduplication syndrome region (e.g., 22q11.2). MLPA can be combined with methylation analysis

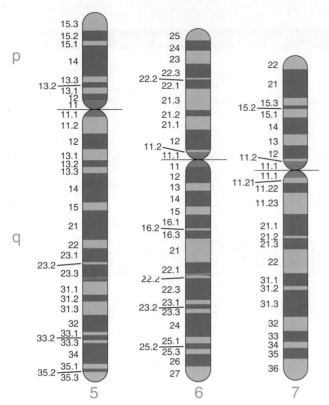

Figure 5.3 Examples of G-banding patterns for chromosomes 5, 6, and 7 at the 550-band stage of condensation. Band numbers permit unambiguous identification of each G-dark or G-light band. The banding nomenclature indicates the chromosome number (1–22,X,Y), the short arm (p) or long arm (q), the region, band, and subband. For example, chromosome 5p15.2 is pronounced as "5-p-one-five-point-2." (Redrawn from Shaffer LG, McGowan-Jordan J, Schmid M, editors: ISCN 2013: an international system for human cytogenetic nomenclature, Basel, 2013, Karger.)

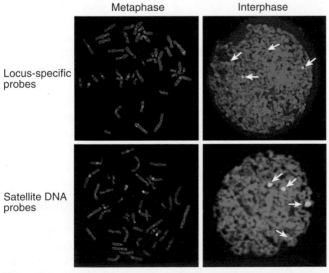

Figure 5.4 Fluorescence *in situ* hybridization to human chromosomes at metaphase and interphase, with different types of DNA probe. *(Top)* Single-copy DNA probes specific for sequences within bands 4q12 (*red* fluorescence) and 4q31.1 (*green* fluorescence). *(Bottom)* Repetitive α-satellite DNA probes specific for the centromeres of chromosomes 18 *(aqua)*, X *(green)*, and Y *(red)* used to count the number of each chromosome in this individual. (Images courtesy M. Katharine Rudd, Emory Genetics Laboratory, Atlanta, Georgia.)

(MS-MLPA) to specifically amplify targeted chromosome regions that are methylated, to determine **imprinting** status. As described in Chapter 8, a subset of the genome is differentially imprinted depending on the parent of origin; and abnormal methylation of these regions can be identified by MS-MPLA to confirm a diagnosis of imprinting disorder (e.g., 15q11.2q13 in Prader-Willi and Angelman syndromes; see [Case 38]).

Genome Analysis Using Microarrays

Chromosome microarray analysis (CMA) has replaced G-banded karyotype as the frontline diagnostic test to detect genome-wide copy number imbalances for most clinical applications. CMA simultaneously queries the whole genome on a glass slide containing regularly spaced DNA probes that represent loci across the entire genome. This technology detects relative copy number gains and losses in a genome-wide manner by hybridizing equal amounts of control and subject DNA to the DNA probes and calculating the ratio of each DNA sample hybridized to each probe. Microarray probes showing equal ratio of subject and control DNA indicate normal copy number at the respective genomic loci. An excess of subject DNA indicates copy number gain, whereas underrepresentation of subject DNA indicates copy number loss at the genomic loci represented by the microarray probes (Fig. 5.5). Microarray platforms may contain copy number probes (see earlier). Alternatively, they may comprise single **nucleotide polymorphism** (SNP) probes that contain versions of sequences corresponding to the variant **alleles** (as introduced in Chapter 4). The data from SNP probes can be plotted on an allele difference plot, which indicates whether a specific SNP locus is **homozygous** for the A allele (AA), homozygous for the B allele (BB), or heterozygous (AB). Normal copy number across a chromosome typically shows the three allele combinations of AA, AB, and BB along its length (see Fig. 5.5). A genomic region of homozygosity (ROH), with AA and BB but no AB track, can be observed when the chromosome region is identical by decent (due to parental **consanguinity**) or when there is **uniparental disomy** (UPD) with both copies of the chromosome inherited from one parent. The identification of several ROHs across the genome of a patient and involving multiple chromosomes suggests parental consanguinity and raises the possibility of a **recessive** disorder. While an ROH affecting only one chromosome raises the possibility of UPD, parental genotype analysis is required to confirm that the ROH is in fact due to UPD.

For routine clinical testing of suspected chromosome disorders, probe spacing on the array provides a resolution as high as 100 kb over the entire unique portion of the human genome. A higher density of probes can be used to achieve even higher resolution (20 kb) over regions of particular clinical interest, such as those

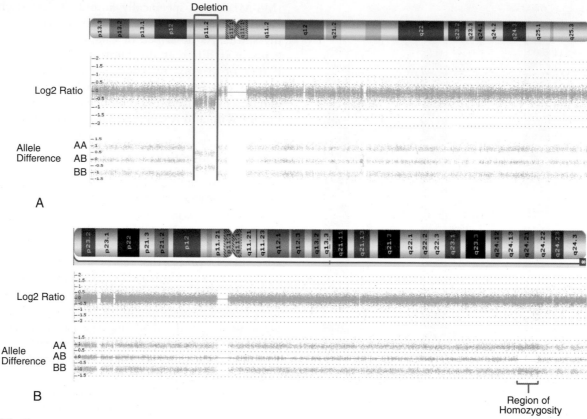

Figure 5.5 **Chromosome microarray analysis to detect copy number variants and regions of homology.** (A) Chromosome 17: G-banding ideogram, followed by an example of copy number and single nucleotide polymorphism (SNP) microarray output, showing the Log2 ratio of fluorescence intensity and allele difference plots. DNA probes *(blue dots)* with a Log2 ratio of 0 indicate diploid copy number. In chromosome region 17p11.2, consecutive probes with a Log2 ratio of −1 indicate a heterozygous deletion of ~3.7 Mb, associated with Smith-Magenis syndrome. (B) Chromosome 18: SNP microarray output plot showing a region of homozygosity of ~6.052 Mb. The total copy number is unaffected, but the allele difference plot shows a stretch of only homozygous genotypes (AA or BB) with no heterozygous genotypes (AB). (Microarray images courtesy of Genome Diagnostics, The Hospital for Sick Children.)

associated with known developmental disorders or congenital anomalies (see Chapter 6). This approach is being used in clinical laboratories to provide high-resolution analysis of targeted clinically significant genes and lower resolution backbone coverage across the rest of the genome. Microarrays have been used successfully to identify chromosome and genome abnormalities in children with unexplained developmental delay, intellectual disability, or birth defects, revealing a number of pathogenic genomic alterations that were not detectable by conventional G-banding. Based on this significantly increased yield (1–3% from karyotype versus 15–20% from microarray), genome-wide arrays have replaced the G-banded karyotype as the routine frontline test for these patient populations.

Two important limitations of this technology bear mentioning, however. First, array-based methods measure only the relative copy number of DNA sequences but not whether they have been translocated or rearranged from their normal position(s) in the genome. Thus further characterization of copy number variants (CNVs) by karyotyping or FISH is important to determine the nature of an abnormality and thus its risk for recurrence

for other family members. Second, high-resolution genome analysis can reveal variants in particular, small differences in copy number, that are of uncertain clinical significance. An increasing number of such variants are being documented and catalogued even from the general population. As we saw in Chapter 4, many are likely to be benign CNVs. Their existence underscores the unique nature of an individual's genome and emphasizes the diagnostic challenge of assessing what is considered normal and what is likely to be pathogenic.

Genome Analysis by Whole Genome Sequencing

On the same spectrum as cytogenetic and microarray analysis, the ultimate resolution for clinical tests to detect chromosomal and genomic disorders would be to sequence genomes in their entirety. Indeed, as the efficiency of WGS has increased and its costs have fallen, it is becoming increasingly practical to sequence samples in a clinical setting (see Fig. 5.1).

The most widely used WGS approach generates millions of short-sequence reads that range between 100 and 500 bp in length, depending on the sequencing platform.

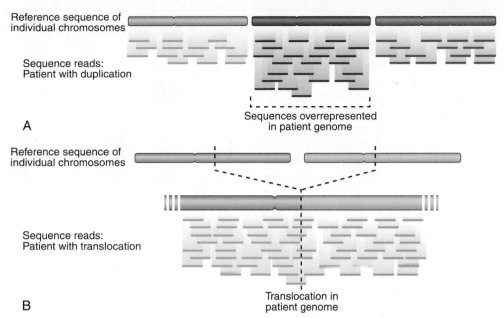

Figure 5.6 **Strategies for detection of numeric and structural chromosome abnormalities by whole genome sequence analysis.** Although only a small number of reads are illustrated schematically here, in practice, many millions of sequence reads are analyzed and aligned to the reference genome to obtain statistically significant support for a diagnosis of aneuploidy or a structural chromosome abnormality. (A) Alignment of sequence reads from a patient's genome to the reference sequence of three individual chromosomes. Overrepresentation of sequences from the *red* chromosome indicates that the patient is aneuploid for this chromosome. (B) Alignment of sequence reads from a patient's genome to the reference sequence of two chromosomes reveals a number of reads that contain contiguous sequences from *both* chromosomes. This indicates a translocation in the patient's genome involving the *blue* and *orange* chromosomes at the positions designated by the *dotted lines*.

An individual's genome is represented by overlapping sequence reads, with typically 30 to 40 reads corresponding to any particular segment of the genome. A genomic region or chromosome with an abnormally low or high representation of those sequence reads is likely to have a numeric or structural abnormality of that genomic region. To detect numeric abnormalities of an entire chromosome it is generally not necessary to sequence a genome to completion; even a limited number of sequences that align to a particular chromosome of interest should reveal whether those sequences are found in the expected number (e.g., equivalent to two copies per **diploid** genome for an **autosome**) or whether they are significantly overrepresented or underrepresented (Fig. 5.6). This concept is now being applied to the prenatal diagnosis of fetal chromosome imbalance (see Chapter 18).

To detect balanced rearrangements of the genome, however, in which DNA in the genome is neither gained nor lost, a more complete genome sequence is required. Here, instead of sequence reads that align perfectly to the reference human genome sequence, one finds rare sequence reads that align to two different and normally noncontiguous regions in the reference sequence (whether on the same chromosome or on different chromosomes) (see Fig. 5.6). This approach has been used to identify the specific genes involved in some cancers, and in children with various congenital defects due to translocations, involving the juxtaposition of sequences that are normally located on different chromosomes. More recently, **bioinformatics** algorithms have been developed to estimate the size of trinucleotide repeat expansions and provide the opportunity to assay known clinically significant loci (such as those involved in fragile X syndrome or Huntington disease) as part of the WGS diagnostic test.

Clinical laboratories are beginning to implement WGS to accurately detect sequence-level variants (single nucleotide variants); insertions/deletions (indels) up to 50 bp and CNVs for genetically heterogeneous disorders; however, CMA and **whole exome sequencing** have so far been the predominant tests used for this purpose due to their lower cost. **Exome** sequencing (ES) generates sequence reads from protein-coding exons, which represent ~1.5% of the genome. This provides accurate detection of exonic sequence–level variants; however, detection of CNVs is less accurate by ES than by WGS because the number of sequence reads generated for each exon can be less consistent, and there is considerable uncertainty of CNV breakpoints due to the large unsequenced chromosome regions between exons. In addition, ES cannot detect balanced rearrangements and noncoding variants. As the cost of WGS continues to decrease, it will replace ES and CMA in genomic diagnostics, providing a much more complete representation of all the variants within an individual's genome.

Although WGS short-read technologies provide a considerable improvement over microarray and ES, the short-read lengths limit the ability to resolve complex structural variation, repetitive regions, and genes with homologous sequence in other regions of the genome (e.g., pseudogenes). The emergence of long-read sequencing technologies that generate sequence reads greater than 10 kb has made it possible to begin to address many of these challenges that can potentially involve clinically relevant genes. Notably, this technology is able to (1) sequence genes without interference of homologous sequence from pseudogenes, (2) provide haplotypes and **phase** variants across large stretches of DNA (>10 kb), (3) sequence large repeat expansions and identify **intervening sequence** that may affect **phenotype** and repeat stability (e.g. involved in *DMPK*, the genes for myotonic dystrophy), and (4) identify balanced and unbalanced translocations, insertions, deletions, duplications, and inversions.

CHROMOSOME ABNORMALITIES

Abnormalities of chromosomes may be either numeric or structural and may involve one or more autosomes, **sex chromosomes,** or both simultaneously. The overall incidence of chromosome abnormalities is ~1 in 154 live births (Fig. 5.7), and their impact is therefore substantial, both in clinical medicine and for society. By far the most common type of clinically significant chromosome abnormality is **aneuploidy,** an abnormal chromosome number due to an extra or missing chromosome. An aneuploid karyotype is typically associated with physical or neurodevelopmental abnormalities, or both. Structural abnormalities (rearrangements involving one or more chromosomes) are also relatively common (see Fig. 5.7). Depending on whether a structural rearrangement leads to an imbalance of genomic content, **disruption** of coding, or regulatory sequence, these may or may not have a phenotypic effect. However, as explained later in this chapter, even individuals with benign balanced chromosome abnormalities may be at an increased risk for abnormal offspring in the subsequent generation.

Chromosome abnormalities are described by a standard set of abbreviations and nomenclature that indicate the nature of the abnormality and (in the case of analyses performed by FISH or microarrays) the technology used. Some of the more common abbreviations and examples of abnormal karyotypes and abnormalities are listed in Table 5.1.

Gene Dosage, Balance, and Imbalance

For chromosome and genomic disorders, it is primarily the quantitative aspects of gene expression that underlie disease, in contrast to single-gene disorders in which pathogenesis often reflects qualitative aspects of a gene's function. The clinical consequences of any particular chromosome alteration will depend on the resulting imbalance of parts of the genome, the specific genes

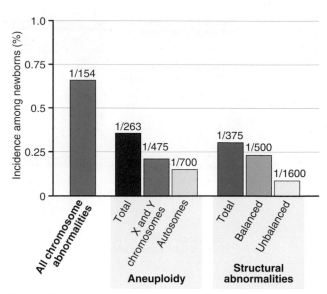

Figure 5.7 Incidence of chromosome abnormalities in newborn surveys, based on chromosome analysis of over 68,000 newborns. (Data summarized from Hsu LYF: Prenatal diagnosis of chromosomal abnormalities through amniocentesis. In Milunsky A, editor: *Genetic disorders and the fetus*, ed 4, Baltimore, 1998, Johns Hopkins University Press, pp 179–248.)

contained in or affected by the alteration, and the likelihood of its transmission to the next generation.

The central concept for thinking about chromosome and genomic disorders is that of **gene dosage** and its balance or imbalance. As we shall see in later chapters, this same concept applies generally to considering some single-gene disorders and their underlying etiology. It takes on uniform importance, however, for chromosome abnormalities, where we are generally more concerned with the dosage of genes within the relevant chromosomal region than with the actual sequence of those genes.

Most genes in the human genome are present in two doses and are expressed from both copies. Some genes, however, are expressed from only a single copy (e.g., imprinted genes and X-linked genes subject to **X inactivation;** see Chapter 3). Extensive analysis of clinical cases has demonstrated that the relative dosage of these genes is critical for normal development. One or three doses instead of two are generally not conducive to normal function for a dosage-sensitive gene or set of genes that is typically expressed from two copies. Similarly, abnormalities of **genomic imprinting** or X inactivation that cause the anomalous expression of two copies or no expression of a gene or set of genes, instead of one, can lead to clinical disorders.

Predicting clinical outcomes for chromosomal and genomic disorders can be an enormous challenge for **genetic counseling,** particularly in the prenatal setting. Many such diagnostic dilemmas will be presented throughout this section and in Chapters 6 and 17, but there are a number of general principles that should be kept in mind as we explore specific types of chromosome abnormality in the sections that follow (see Box 5.2).

TABLE 5.1 Some Abbreviations Used for Description of Chromosomes and Their Abnormalities, With Representative Examples

Abbreviation	Meaning	Example	Example's Condition
		46,XX	Normal female karyotype
		46,XY	Normal male karyotype
arr	Microarray	arr(X,1-22)x2	Normal female
		arr(X,Y)x1,(1-22)x2	Normal male
		arr[GRCh38] 8p23.3(835185_1242591)x1	Deletion in 8p23.3 at genomic position 835185 to 1242591 using Genome Build GRCh38
cen	Centromere		
del	Deletion	46,XX,del(5)(q13)	Female with terminal deletion of one chromosome 5 distal to band 5q13
der	Derivative chromosome	der(1)	Translocation chromosome derived from chromosome 1 and containing the centromere of chromosome 1
dic	Dicentric chromosome	dic(X;Y)	Translocation chromosome containing the centromeres of both the X and Y chromosomes
dup	Duplication		
inv	Inversion	inv(3)(p25q21)	Pericentric inversion of chromosome 3
mar	Marker chromosome	47,XX,+mar	Female with an extra, unidentified chromosome
mat	Maternal origin	arr[GRCh38] 7p22.3(580556_1191665)x3 mat	Maternally inherited duplication in 7p22.3 genomic position 580556 to 1191665 using genome build GRCh38
p	Short arm of chromosome		
pat	Paternal origin		
q	Long arm of chromosome		
r	Ring chromosome	46,X,r(X)	Female with ring X chromosome
rob	Robertsonian translocation	45,XX,rob(14;21)(q10;q10)	Female with balanced Robertsonian translocation in which breakage and reunion have occurred at band 14q10 and band 21q10 in the centromeric regions of chromosomes 14 and 21; however either rob or der may be used.
t	Translocation	46,XX,t(2;8)(q22;p21)	Female with balanced translocation between chromosomes 2 and 8, with breakpoints in bands 2q22 and 8p21
+	Gain of	47,XX,+21	Female with trisomy 21
–	Loss of	45,XY,–22	Male with monosomy 22
/	Mosaicism	mos 47,XX,+21[20]/46,XX[10]	Female with two populations of cells, one with trisomy 21 observed in 20 cells, and one with a normal karyotype observed in 10 cells

Abbreviations from McGowan-Jordan J, Hastings RJ, Adelaide SM editors: *ISCN 2020: an international system for human cytogenetic nomenclature*, Basel, 2020, Karger.

BOX 5.2 UNBALANCED KARYOTYPES AND GENOMES IN LIVEBORNS: GENERAL GUIDELINES FOR COUNSELING

- *Monosomies are more deleterious than trisomies.* Complete monosomies are generally not viable, except for monosomy for the **X chromosome**. Complete trisomies are viable for chromosomes 13, 18, 21, X, and Y.
- *The phenotype in partial (subchromosomal) aneuploidy depends on a number of factors*, including the size of the unbalanced segment, which regions of the genome are affected and which genes are involved, and whether the imbalance is monosomic or trisomic.
- *Risk in cases of inversions depends on the location of the inversion with respect to the centromere and on the size of the inverted segment.* For inversions that do not involve the centromere (paracentric inversions), there is a very low risk for an abnormal phenotype in the next generation. But, for inversions that do involve the centromere (pericentric inversions), the risk for birth defects in offspring may be significant and increases with the size of the inverted segment.
- *For a mosaic karyotype involving any chromosome abnormality, the results from testing one tissue may not accurately represent the extent of mosaicism in other tissues of the body.* Counseling is particularly challenging because the degree of mosaicism in relevant tissues or relevant stages of development is generally unknown. Thus there is uncertainty about the severity of the phenotype.

Abnormalities of Chromosome Number

A human chromosome complement with any number other than 46 is said to be heteroploid. An exact multiple of the haploid chromosome number (n) is called **euploid**, and any other chromosome number is aneuploid.

Triploidy and Tetraploidy

In addition to the diploid (2n) number characteristic of normal somatic cells, two other euploid chromosome complements, **triploid** (3n) and **tetraploid** (4n), are occasionally observed in clinical material. Both triploidy and tetraploidy have been seen in fetuses. Triploidy is observed in 1% to 3% of recognized conceptions; triploid infants can be liveborn, although they do not survive long. Among the few that survive at least to the end of the first trimester of pregnancy, most result from fertilization of an egg by two sperm (**dispermy**). Other cases result from failure of one of the meiotic divisions in either sex, resulting in a diploid egg or sperm. The phenotypic manifestation of a triploid karyotype depends on the source of the extra chromosome set; triploids with an extra set of maternal chromosomes are typically aborted spontaneously early in pregnancy, whereas those with an extra set of paternal chromosomes typically have an abnormal degenerative placenta (resulting in a partial **hydatidiform mole**), with a small fetus. Tetraploids are always 92,XXXX or 92,XXYY and likely result from failure of completion of an early cleavage division of the **zygote**.

Aneuploidy

Aneuploidy is the most common and clinically significant type of human chromosome disorder, occurring in at least 5% of all clinically recognized pregnancies. Most aneuploid individuals have either **trisomy** (three instead of the normal pair of a particular chromosome) or, less often, **monosomy** (only one representative of a particular chromosome). Either trisomy or monosomy can have severe phenotypic consequences.

Trisomy can involve part of a chromosone, but trisomy for a whole chromosome is only occasionally compatible with life. By far the most common type of trisomy in liveborn infants is trisomy 21, the chromosome constitution seen in 95% of patients with Down syndrome (karyotype 47,XX,+21 or 47,XY,+21) (Fig. 5.8). Other trisomies observed in liveborns include trisomy 18 and trisomy 13. It is notable that these autosomes (13, 18, and 21) are the three with the lowest number of genes; presumably, trisomy for autosomes with a greater number of genes is lethal in most instances. Monosomy for an entire chromosome is almost always lethal; an important exception is monosomy for the X chromosome, as seen in Turner syndrome (Case 47). These conditions are considered in greater detail in Chapter 6.

Although the causes of aneuploidy are not fully understood, the most common chromosomal mechanism is meiotic **nondisjunction**. This refers to the failure of a pair of chromosomes to disjoin properly during one of the two meiotic divisions, usually during **meiosis** I. The genomic consequences of nondisjunction during meiosis I and meiosis II are different (Fig. 5.9). If the error occurs during meiosis I, the **gamete** with 24 chromosomes contains both the paternal and the maternal members of the pair. If it occurs during meiosis II, the gamete with the extra chromosome contains both copies of either the paternal or the maternal chromosome. (Strictly speaking, these statements refer only to the paternal or maternal centromere because recombination between homologous chromosomes has usually taken place in the preceding meiosis I, resulting in some genetic differences between the chromatids and thus between the corresponding **daughter chromosomes**; see Chapter 2.)

Proper disjunction of a pair of homologous chromosomes in meiosis I appears relatively straightforward (see Fig. 5.9). In reality, however, it involves a feat of complex engineering that requires precise temporal and spatial control over alignment of the two homologues, their tight connections to each other (**synapsis**), their interactions with the meiotic spindle, and, finally, their release and subsequent movement to opposite poles and to different daughter cells. The propensity for non-disjunction of a chromosome pair has been strongly associated with aberrations in the frequency or placement, (or both), of recombination events in meiosis I, which are critical for maintaining proper synapsis. A chromosome pair with too few (or even no) recombinations, or with recombination too close to the centromere or telomere, may be more susceptible to nondisjunction than a chromosome pair with a more typical number and distribution of recombination events.

In some cases, aneuploidy can result from premature separation of sister chromatids in meiosis I instead of meiosis II. If this happens, the separated chromatids may by chance segregate to the oocyte or to the polar body, leading to an unbalanced gamete.

Nondisjunction can also occur in a mitotic division after formation of the zygote. If this happens at an early cleavage division, clinically significant **mosaicism** may result (see later section). In some malignant cell lines and some cell cultures, mitotic nondisjunction can lead to highly abnormal karyotypes.

Abnormalities of Chromosome Structure

Structural rearrangements result from chromosome breakage, recombination, or exchange, followed by reconstitution into an abnormal combination. Whereas rearrangements can take place in many ways, they are collectively less common than aneuploidy; overall, structural abnormalities are present in ~1 in 375 newborns (see Fig. 5.7). Like numeric abnormalities, structural rearrangements may be present in all cells of a person or in mosaic form.

Structural rearrangements are classified as balanced if the genome has the normal complement of chromosomal material or unbalanced if material is additional or missing. Clearly, these designations depend on the resolution of the method(s) used to analyze a particular rearrangement (see Fig. 5.1); some that appear balanced at the level of high-resolution banding, for example, may be seen as unbalanced when studied with chromosomal microarrays or by DNA sequence analysis. Chromosome rearrangements can be stable, capable of passing through mitotic and meiotic cell divisions unaltered, whereas others are unstable. Some of the more common types of structural rearrangements observed in human chromosomes are illustrated schematically in Fig. 5.10.

Unbalanced Rearrangements

Unbalanced rearrangements are detected in ~1 in 1600 live births (see Fig. 5.7); the phenotype is likely to be abnormal because of **deletion** or duplication of multiple genes, or (in some cases) both. Duplication of part of a chromosome leads to partial trisomy for the genes within that segment; deletion leads to partial monosomy. As a general concept, any change that disturbs normal gene dosage balance can result in abnormal development; a broad range of phenotypes can result, depending on the nature of the specific genes whose dosage is altered in a particular case.

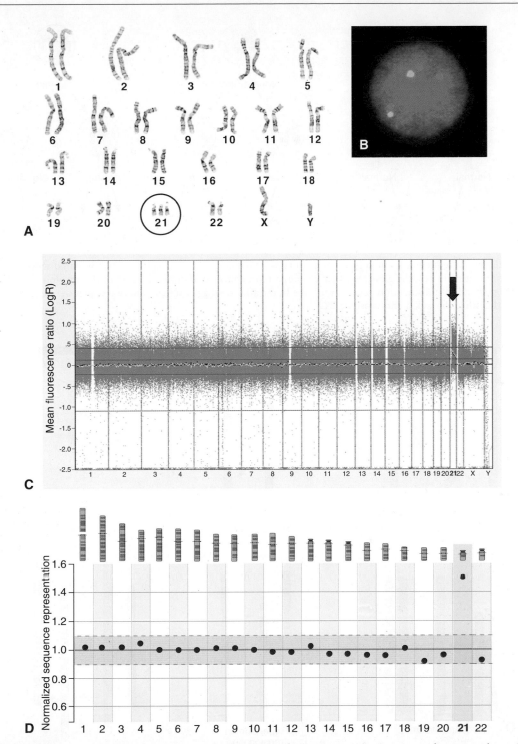

Figure 5.8 Chromosomal and genomic approaches to the diagnosis of trisomy 21. (A) Karyotype from a male patient with Down syndrome, showing three copies of chromosome 21. (B) Interphase fluorescence *in situ* hybridization analysis using locus-specific probes from chromosome 21 (*red*, three spots) and from a control autosome (*green*, two spots). (C) Detection of trisomy 21 in a female patient by whole genome chromosome microarray. Increase in the fluorescence ratio for sequences from chromosome 21 is indicated by the *red arrow*. (D) Detection of trisomy 21 by whole genome sequencing and overrepresentation of sequences from chromosome 21. Normalized sequence representation for individual chromosomes (± SD) in chromosomally normal samples is indicated by the *gray-shaded region*. A normalized ratio of ~1.5 indicates three copies of chromosome 21 sequences instead of two, consistent with trisomy 21. (A, Courtesy Center for Human Genetics Laboratory, University Hospitals of Cleveland; B, courtesy M. Katharine Rudd, Emory Genetics Laboratory; C, courtesy Daynna J. Wolff, Medical University of South Carolina; D, original data from Dan S, Chen F, Choy KW, et al: Prenatal detection of aneuploidy and imbalanced chromosomal arrangements by massively parallel sequencing. *PLoS ONE* 7:e27835, 2012.)

Large structural rearrangements involving imbalance of at least a few megabases can be detected at the level of routine chromosome banding. Detection of smaller changes, however, generally requires higher resolution analysis, involving FISH or chromosomal microarray analysis.

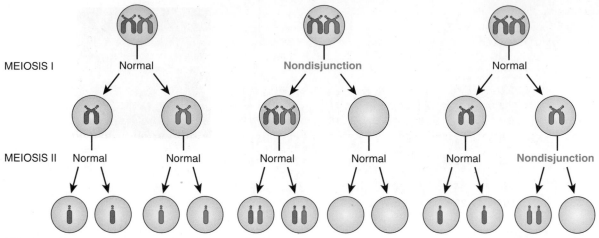

Figure 5.9 The different consequences of nondisjunction at meiosis I *(center)* and meiosis II *(right)*, compared with normal disjunction *(left)*. If the error occurs at meiosis I, the gametes either contain a representative of both members of the chromosome 21 pair or lack a chromosome 21 altogether. If nondisjunction occurs at meiosis II, the abnormal gametes contain two copies of one parental chromosome 21 (and no copy of the other) or lack a chromosome 21.

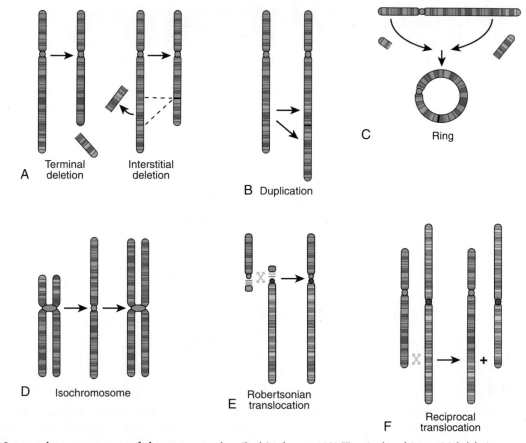

Figure 5.10 **Structural rearrangements of chromosomes, described in the text.** (A) Terminal and interstitial deletions, each generating an acentric fragment that is typically lost. (B) Duplication of a chromosomal segment, leading to partial trisomy. (C) Ring chromosome with two acentric fragments. (D) Generation of an isochromosome for the long arm of a chromosome. (E) Robertsonian translocation between two acrocentric chromosomes, frequently leading to a pseudodicentric chromosome. Robertsonian translocations are nonreciprocal, and the short arms of the acrocentrics are lost. (F) Translocation between two chromosomes, with reciprocal exchange of the translocated segments.

Deletions and Duplications. Deletions involve loss of a chromosome segment, resulting in chromosome imbalance (see Fig. 5.10). A carrier of a chromosomal deletion (with one normal **homologue** and one deleted homologue) is monosomic for the genetic information on the corresponding segment of the normal homologue. The clinical consequences generally reflect **haploinsufficiency** (literally, the inability of a single copy of the genetic material to carry out the functions normally performed by two copies), and, where examined, their severity reflects the size of the deleted segment and the number and function of the specific genes that are deleted. Cytogenetically visible autosomal deletions have an incidence of ~1 in 7000 live births. Smaller, submicroscopic deletions detected by CMA or WGS are much more common, but as mentioned earlier, the clinical significance of many such variants has yet to be determined.

A deletion may occur at the end of a chromosome (terminal) or within a chromosome arm (interstitial). Deletions may originate simply from chromosome breakage and loss of the acentric segment. Numerous deletions have been identified in the course of prenatal diagnosis or in the investigation of dysmorphic patients or those with intellectual disability; specific examples of such cases will be discussed in Chapter 6.

In general, duplication appears to be less harmful than deletion. However, duplication in a gamete results in chromosomal imbalance (i.e., partial trisomy), and the chromosome breaks that generate it may disrupt genes, and can lead to some phenotypic abnormality.

Marker and Ring Chromosomes. Very small, unidentified chromosomes, called **marker chromosomes**, are occasionally seen in chromosome preparations, frequently in a mosaic state. They are usually in addition to the normal chromosome complement and are thus also referred to as supernumerary chromosomes or extra structurally abnormal chromosomes. The prenatal frequency of *de novo* supernumerary marker chromosomes has been estimated to be ~1 in 2500 pregnancies. Because of their small and indistinctive appearance, higher resolution genome analysis (e.g., FISH and/or CMA) is usually required for precise identification.

Larger marker chromosomes contain genomic material from one or both chromosome arms, creating an imbalance for whatever genes are present. Depending on the origin of the marker chromosome, the risk for a fetal abnormality can range from very low to 100%. For reasons not fully understood, a relatively high proportion of such markers derive from chromosome 15 and from the sex chromosomes.

Many marker chromosomes lack telomeres and are **ring chromosomes** that are formed when a chromosome undergoes two breaks, and the broken ends of the chromosome reunite in a ring structure (see Fig. 5.10). Some rings experience difficulties at mitosis, when the two sister chromatids become tangled in their attempt to disjoin at **anaphase**. There may be breakage of the ring followed by fusion, and larger and smaller rings may thus be generated. Because of this mitotic instability it is not uncommon for ring chromosomes to be found in only a proportion of cells.

Isochromosomes. An **isochromosome** is a chromosome in which one arm is missing and the other

duplicated in a mirror-image fashion (see Fig. 5.10). A person with 46 chromosomes carrying an isochromosome therefore has a single copy of the genetic material of one arm (partial monosomy) and three copies of the genetic material of the other arm (partial trisomy). Although isochromosomes for a number of autosomes have been described, the most common isochromosome involves the long arm of the X chromosome—designated i(X)(q10)—in a proportion of individuals with Turner syndrome (see Chapter 6, Case 47). Isochromosomes are also frequently seen in karyotypes of both solid tumors and hematologic malignant neoplasms (see Chapter 16).

Dicentric Chromosomes. A **dicentric** chromosome is a rare type of abnormal chromosome in which two chromosome segments, each with a centromere, fuse end to end. Dicentric chromosomes, despite their two centromeres, can be mitotically stable if one of the two centromeres is inactivated epigenetically or if the two centromeres always coordinate their movement to one or the other pole during anaphase. Such chromosomes are formally called pseudodicentric. The most common pseudodicentrics involve the sex chromosomes or the acrocentric chromosomes (so-called Robertsonian translocations; see later).

Balanced Rearrangements

Balanced chromosomal rearrangements are found in as many as 1 in 500 individuals (see Fig. 5.7) and do not usually lead to a phenotypic effect because all the genomic material is present, even though it is arranged differently (see Fig. 5.10). As noted earlier, it is important to distinguish here between truly balanced rearrangements and those that appear balanced cytogenetically but are really unbalanced at the molecular level. Because of the high frequency of common copy number variants around the genome (see Chapter 4), collectively adding up to differences of many megabases between genomes of unrelated individuals, the concept of what is balanced or unbalanced is subject to ongoing investigation and continual refinement.

Even when structural rearrangements are truly balanced, they can pose a threat to the subsequent generation because carriers are likely to produce unbalanced gametes and therefore have an increased risk for abnormal offspring with unbalanced karyotypes. There is also a possibility that one of the chromosome breaks will disrupt a gene, leading to a **pathogenic variant**. Especially with the use of WGS to examine the nature of apparently balanced rearrangements in patients who present with significant phenotypes, this is an increasingly well-documented cause of disorders in carriers of balanced translocations; such translocations can be a useful clue to the identification of the gene responsible for a particular **genetic disorder**.

Translocations. Translocation involves the movement of chromosome segments between two chromosomes. There are two main types: reciprocal and nonreciprocal.

Reciprocal Translocations. This type of rearrangement results from breakage or recombination involving nonhomologous chromosomes, with reciprocal exchange of the broken-off or recombined segments (see Fig. 5.10). Usually, only two chromosomes are involved, and because the exchange is reciprocal, the total chromosome number and content is unchanged. Such translocations are usually without phenotypic effect; however, like other balanced structural rearrangements, they are associated with a high risk for unbalanced gametes and abnormal progeny. They come to attention either during prenatal diagnosis or when the parents of a clinically abnormal child with an unbalanced translocation are karyotyped. Balanced translocations are more common in couples who have had two or more spontaneous pregnancy losses and in infertile males than in the general population.

Translocations present challenges for the process of chromosome pairing and homologous recombination during meiosis (see Chapter 2). When the chromosomes of a carrier of a balanced **reciprocal translocation** pair at meiosis (Fig. 5.11), they must form a **quadrivalent** to ensure proper alignment of homologous sequences (rather than the typical bivalents seen with normal chromosomes). In typical **segregation**, two of the four chromosomes in the quadrivalent go to each pole at anaphase; however, the chromosomes can segregate from this configuration in several ways, depending on which chromosomes go to which pole. **Alternate segregation,** the usual type of meiotic segregation, produces balanced gametes that have either a normal chromosome complement or contain the two reciprocal chromosomes. Other segregation patterns, however, always yield unbalanced gametes (see Fig. 5.11).

Robertsonian Translocations. Robertsonian translocations are the most common type of chromosome rearrangement observed in our species. They involve two acrocentric chromosomes that fuse near the centromere region with loss of the short arms (see Fig. 5.10). Such translocations are nonreciprocal, and the resulting karyotype has only 45 chromosomes, including the translocation chromosome, which in effect is made up of the long arms of two acrocentric chromosomes. Because, as noted earlier, the short arms of all five pairs of acrocentric chromosomes consist largely of various classes of **satellite DNA**, as well as hundreds of copies of ribosomal RNA genes, loss of the short arms of two

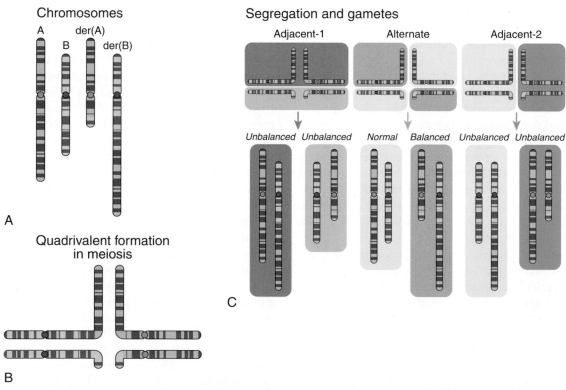

Figure 5.11 (A) Diagram illustrating a balanced translocation between two chromosomes, involving a reciprocal exchange between the distal long arms of chromosomes A and B. (B) Formation of a quadrivalent in meiosis is necessary to align the homologous segments of the two derivative chromosomes and their normal homologues. (C) Patterns of segregation in a carrier of the translocation, leading to either balanced or unbalanced gametes, shown at the bottom. Adjacent-1 segregation (in *red*, top chromosomes to one gamete, bottom chromosomes to the other) leads only to unbalanced gametes. Adjacent-2 segregation (in *green*, left chromosomes to one gamete, right chromosomes to the other) also leads only to unbalanced gametes. Only alternate segregation (in *gray*, upper left/lower right chromosomes to one gamete, lower left/upper right to the other) can lead to balanced gametes.

acrocentric chromosomes is not deleterious; thus the karyotype is considered to be balanced, despite having only 45 chromosomes. Robertsonian translocations are typically, although not always, pseudodicentric (see Fig. 5.10), reflecting the location of the breakpoint on each acrocentric chromosome.

Although **Robertsonian translocations** can involve all combinations of the acrocentric chromosomes, two—designated rob(13;14)(q10;q10) and rob(14;21)(q10;q10)—are relatively common. The translocation involving 13q and 14q is found in ~1 in 1300 persons and is thus by far the most common chromosome rearrangement in our species. Rare individuals with two copies of the same type of Robertsonian translocation have been described; these phenotypically normal individuals have only 44 chromosomes and lack any normal copies of the acrocentrics involved, replaced by two copies of the translocation.

Although a carrier of a Robertsonian translocation does not present with any obvious clinical phenotype, there is a risk for unbalanced gametes and, therefore, for unbalanced offspring. The risk for unbalanced offspring varies according to the particular Robertsonian translocation and the sex of the carrier parent; carrier females in general have a higher risk for transmitting the translocation to an affected child. The chief clinical importance of this type of translocation is that carriers of a Robertsonian translocation involving chromosome 21 are at risk for producing a child with translocation Down syndrome, as will be explored further in Chapter 6.

Insertions. An **insertion** is another type of non-reciprocal translocation that occurs when a segment removed from one chromosome is inserted into a different chromosome or in a different location within the same chromosome, either in its usual orientation with respect to the centromere or inverted. Because they require three chromosome breaks, insertions are relatively rare. Segregation in an insertion carrier can produce offspring with duplication or deletion of the inserted segment, as well as normal offspring and balanced carriers. The average risk for producing an affected child can be up to 50%, and prenatal diagnosis is therefore indicated.

Inversions. An **inversion** occurs when a single chromosome undergoes two breaks and is reconstituted with the segment between the breaks inverted. Inversions are of two types (Fig. 5.12): paracentric, in which both breaks occur in one arm (Greek *para*, beside the centromere); and pericentric, in which there is a break in each arm (Greek *peri*, around the centromere). Pericentric inversions can be easier to identify cytogenetically when they change the proportion of the chromosome arms as well as the banding pattern.

An inversion does not usually cause an abnormal phenotype in carriers because it is a balanced rearrangement.

Its medical significance is for the progeny; a carrier of either type of inversion is at risk for producing unbalanced gametes and offspring. When an inversion is present, a loop needs to form to allow alignment and pairing of homologous segments of the normal and inverted chromosomes in meiosis I (see Fig. 5.12). When recombination occurs within the loop, gametes with balanced chromosome complements (either normal or with the inversion) and gametes with unbalanced complements are formed, depending on the location of recombination events. When the inversion is paracentric, the unbalanced recombinant chromosomes are acentric or dicentric and typically do not lead to viable offspring (see Fig. 5.12); thus the risk that a carrier of a paracentric inversion will have a liveborn child with an abnormal karyotype is very low.

A pericentric inversion, on the other hand, can lead to the production of unbalanced gametes with both duplication and deletion of chromosome segments (see Fig. 5.12). The duplicated and deleted segments are those distal to the inversion. Overall, the risk for the child of a carrier of a pericentric inversion to have an unbalanced karyotype is estimated to be 5% to 10%. Each pericentric inversion, however, is associated with a particular risk, typically reflecting the size and content of the duplicated and deficient segments.

Mosaicism for Chromosome Abnormalities

Sometimes, two or more different chromosome complements are present among the cells in an individual; this situation is called chromosomal mosaicism. Such mosaicism is typically detected by conventional karyotyping, interphase FISH analysis, or chromosomal microarrays.

A common cause of mosaicism is nondisjunction in an early postzygotic mitotic division. For example, a zygote with an additional chromosome 21 might lose the extra chromosome in a mitotic division and continue to develop as a 47,+21/46 mosaic. The effects of mosaicism on development vary with the timing of the nondisjunction event, the nature of the chromosome abnormality, the proportions of the different chromosome complements present, and the tissues affected. It is often believed that individuals who are mosaic for a given trisomy, such as mosaic Down syndrome or mosaic Turner syndrome, are less severely affected than nonmosaic individuals.

When detected in lymphocytes, in cultured cell lines or in prenatal samples, it can be difficult to assess the significance of mosaicism, especially if it is identified prenatally. The proportions of the different chromosome complements seen in the tissue being analyzed (e.g., cultured amniocytes or lymphocytes) may not necessarily reflect the proportions present in other tissues or in the embryo during its early developmental stages. Mosaicism can also arise in cells in culture after they were taken from the individual; thus cytogeneticists

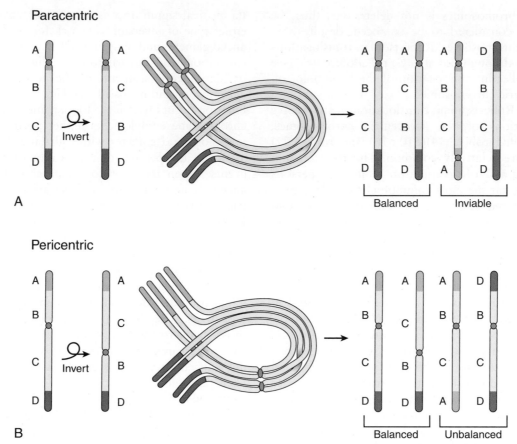

Figure 5.12 Crossing over within inversion loops formed at meiosis I in carriers of a chromosome with segment B-C inverted. (A) Paracentric inversion. Gametes formed after the second meiotic division usually contain either a normal (A-B-C-D) or a balanced (A-C-B-D) copy of the chromosome because the acentric and dicentric products of the crossover are inviable. (B) Pericentric inversion. Gametes formed after the second meiotic division may be balanced (normal or inverted) or unbalanced. Unbalanced gametes contain a copy of the chromosome with a duplication or a deletion of the material flanking the inverted segment (A-B-C-A or D-B-C-D).

attempt to differentiate between true mosaicism, present in the individual, and **pseudomosaicism**, which has occurred in the laboratory. The distinction between these types is not always easy or certain and can lead to major interpretive difficulties in prenatal diagnosis (see Box 2 earlier and Chapter 18).

Incidence of Chromosome Anomalies Visible by Karyotype Analysis

The incidence of different types of chromosomal aberration has been measured in a number of large population surveys and was summarized earlier in Fig. 5.7. The major number disorders of chromosome observed in liveborns are three autosomal trisomies (21, 18, and 13) and four types of sex chromosomal aneuploidy: Turner syndrome (usually 45,X), Klinefelter syndrome (47,XXY), 47,XYY, and 47,XXX (see Chapter 6). Triploidy and tetraploidy account for only a small percentage of cases, typically in spontaneous abortions. The classification and incidence of chromosomal defects measured in these surveys can be used to consider the **fate** of 10,000 conceptuses (Table 5.2).

TABLE 5.2 Outcome of 10,000 Pregnancies[a]

Outcome	Pregnancies	Spontaneous Abortions (%)	Live Births
Total	10,000	1500 (15)	8500
Normal chromosomes	9200	750 (8)	8450
Abnormal chromosomes	800	750 (94)	50
Specific Abnormalities			
Triploid or tetraploid	170	170 (100)	0
45,X	140	139 (99)	1
Trisomy 16	112	112 (100)	0
Trisomy 18	20	19 (95)	1
Trisomy 21	45	35 (78)	10
Trisomy, other	209	208 (99.5)	1
47,XXY, 47,XXX, 47,XYY	19	4 (21)	15
Unbalanced rearrangements	27	23 (85)	4
Balanced rearrangements	19	3 (16)	16
Other	39	37 (95)	2

[a]These estimates are based on observed frequencies of chromosome abnormalities in spontaneous pregnancy losses and in liveborn infants. It is likely that the frequency of chromosome abnormalities in all conceptuses is much higher than this because many undergo spontaneous pregnancy loss before they are recognized clinically.

Live Births

The overall incidence of chromosome abnormalities in newborns is ~1 in 154 births (0.65%) (see Fig. 5.7). Most of the autosomal abnormalities can be diagnosed at birth, but most sex chromosome abnormalities, with the exception of Turner syndrome, are not recognized clinically until puberty (see Chapter 6). Unbalanced rearrangements are likely to come to clinical attention because of abnormal appearance and neurodevelopmental abnormalities in the affected individual. In contrast, balanced rearrangements are rarely identified clinically unless a carrier of a rearrangement has a child with an unbalanced chromosome complement and family studies are undertaken.

Spontaneous Pregnancy Loss

The frequency of chromosome abnormalities in spontaneous pregnancy loss is at least 40% to 50%, and the kinds of abnormalities differ in a number of ways from those seen in liveborns. Somewhat surprisingly, the single most common abnormality in pregnancy loss is 45,X (the same abnormality found in Turner syndrome), which accounts for nearly 20% of chromosomally abnormal spontaneous pregnancy losses but less than 1% of chromosomally abnormal live births (see Table 5.2). Another difference is the distribution of kinds of trisomy; for example, trisomy 16 is not seen at all in live births but accounts for approximately one-third of trisomies in pregnancy losses.

CHROMOSOME AND GENOME ANALYSIS IN CANCER

We have focused in this chapter on constitutional chromosome abnormalities that are seen in most or all of the cells in the body and derive from changes in chromosome structure or number that have been transmitted from a parent (either inherited or occurring *de novo* in the **germline** of a parent) or that have occurred in the zygote in early mitotic divisions.

However, such chromosome abnormalities also occur in somatic cells throughout life and are a hallmark of cancer, both in hematologic **neoplasias** (e.g., leukemias and lymphomas) and in the context of solid tumor progression. An important area in cancer research is the delineation of chromosomal and genomic changes in specific forms of cancer and the relation of the breakpoints of the various structural rearrangements to the process of oncogenesis. The chromosome and genomic changes seen in cancer cells are numerous and diverse. The association of cytogenetic and genome analysis with tumor type and with the effectiveness of therapy is already an important part of the management of patients with cancer; these are discussed further in Chapter 16.

ACKNOWLEDGMENT

We thank Mary Ann George and Mary Shago for contributing to this chapter.

GENERAL REFERENCES

Gardner RJM, Armor D: *Gardner and Sutherland's chromosome abnormalities and genetic counseling,* ed 5, New York, 2018, Oxford University Press.

Feuk L, Carson AR, Scherer SW: Structural variation in the human genome, *Nat Rev Genet* 7(2):85–97, 2006.

McGowan-Jordan J, Hastings RJ, Adelaide SM, editors: *ISCN 2020: an international system for human cytogenetic nomenclature,* Basel, 2020, Karger.

REFERENCES FOR SPECIFIC TOPICS

Baldwin EK, May LF, Justice AN, et al: Mechanisms and consequences of small supernumerary marker chromosomes: from Barbara McClintock to modern genetic-counseling issues, *Am J Hum Genet* 82:398–410, 2008.

Coulter ME, Miller DT, Harris DJ, et al: Chromosomal microarray testing influences medical management, *Genet Med* 13:770–776, 2011.

Dan S, Chen F, Choy KW, et al: Prenatal detection of aneuploidy and imbalanced chromosomal arrangements by massively parallel sequencing, *PLoS ONE* 7:e27835, 2012.

Feng W, Chakraborty A: Fragility extraordinaire: unsolved mysteries of chromosome fragile sites, *Adv Exp Med Biol* 1042:489–526, 2017.

Firth HV, Richards SM, Bevan AP, et al: DECIPHER: database of chromosomal imbalance and phenotype in humans using Ensembl resources, *Am J Hum Genet* 84:524–533, 2009.

Green RC, Rehm IIL, Kohane IS: Clinical genome sequencing. In Ginsburg GS, Willard HF, editors: *Genomic and personalized medicine* ed 2, New York, 2013, Elsevier, pp 102–122.

Higgins AW, Alkuraya FS, Bosco AF, et al: Characterization of apparently balanced chromosomal rearrangements from the Developmental Genome Anatomy Project, *Am J Hum Genet* 82:712–722, 2008.

Ledbetter DH, Riggs ER, Martin CL: Clinical applications of whole-genome chromosomal microarray analysis. In Ginsburg GS, Willard HF, editors: *Genomic and personalized medicine* ed 2, New York, 2013, Elsevier, pp 133–144.

Lee C: Structural genomic variation in the human genome. In Ginsburg GS, Willard HF, editors: *Genomic and personalized medicine* ed 2, New York, 2013, Elsevier, pp 123–132.

Miller DT, Adam MP, Aradhya S, et al: Consensus statement: chromosomal microarray is a first-tier clinical diagnostic test for individuals with developmental disabilities or congenital anomalies, *Am J Hum Genet* 86:749–764, 2010.

Nagaoka SI, Hassold TJ, Hunt PA: Human aneuploidy: mechanisms and new insights into an age-old problem, *Nat Rev Genet* 13:493–504, 2012.

Reddy UM, Page GP, Saade GR, et al: Karyotype versus microarray testing for genetic abnormalities after stillbirth, *N Engl J Med* 367:2185–2193, 2012.

Riggs ER, Andersen EF, Cherry AM, et al: Technical standards for the interpretation and reporting of constitutional copy-number variants: a joint consensus recommendation of the American College of Medical Genetics and Genomics (ACMG) and the Clinical Genome Resource (ClinGen), *Genet Med* 22(2):245–257, 2020.

South ST, Lee C, Lamb AN, et al: ACMG standards and guidelines for constitutional cytogenomic microarray analysis, including postnatal and prenatal applications: revision, *Genet Med* 15:901-909, 2013.

Talkowski ME, Ernst C, Heilbut A, et al: Next-generation sequencing strategies enable routine detection of balanced chromosome rearrangements for clinical diagnostics and genetic research, *Am J Hum Genet* 88:469–481, 2011.

Trost B, Loureiro LO, Scherer SW: Discovery of genomic variation across a generation, *Hum Mol Genet* 30(R2):R174–R186, 2021. https://doi.org/10.1093/hmg/ddab209

PROBLEMS

1. You send a blood sample from an infant with multiple congenital anomalies to the chromosome laboratory for analysis. The laboratory identifies two copy number variants by chromosome microarray, arr[GRCh38] 7q33(136240808_159345973)x3,18q12.3(45466214_80373285)x1. G-banding analysis indicates the child's karyotype is 46,XY,der(18)t(7;18)(q33;q12.3)
   a. What do these results mean?
   b. The laboratory asks for blood samples from the clinically normal parents for analysis. Why?
   c. The laboratory reports the mother's karyotype as 46,XX and the father's karyotype as 46,XY,t(7;18)(q33;q12.3). What does the latter karyotype mean? Referring to the normal chromosome ideograms in Figure 5.2, sketch the translocation chromosome or chromosomes in the father and in his son. Sketch these chromosomes in meiosis in the father. What kinds of gametes can he produce?

2. A spontaneous pregnancy loss is found to have trisomy 18.
   a. What proportion of pregnancies with trisomy 18 are spontaneously lost?
   b. What is the risk that the parents will have a liveborn child with trisomy 18 in a future pregnancy?

3. A newborn child with Down syndrome, when karyotyped, is found to have two cell lines: 70% of her cells have a 47,XX,+21 karyotype, and 30% are normal 46,XX. When did the nondisjunction event likely occur? What is the prognosis for this child?

4. Which of the following persons is or is not expected to be phenotypically normal? For questions 4c and 4d, what are the reproductive risks associated with the chromosome rearrangements assuming the other parent is chromosomally normal?
   a. A female with 47 chromosomes, including a small supernumerary marker chromosome derived from the centromeric region of chromosome 15
   b. A female with the karyotype 47,XX,+13
   c. A person with a balanced reciprocal translocation
   d. A person with a pericentric inversion of chromosome 6

5. For each of the following, state whether chromosome/genome analysis is indicated or not. For which family members, if any? For what kind of chromosome abnormality might the family in each case be at risk?
   a. A pregnant 29-year-old woman and her 41-year-old husband, with no history of genetic defects
   b. A pregnant 41-year-old woman and her 29-year-old husband, with no history of genetic defects
   c. A couple whose only child has Down syndrome
   d. A couple whose only child has cystic fibrosis
   e. A couple who has two boys with global developmental delay and severe intellectual disability

6. Explain the nature of the chromosome abnormality and the method of detection indicated by the following nomenclature.
   a. 46,XX,inv(X)(q21q26)
   b. 46,XX,del(1)(p36.2)
   c. 46,XX.ish del(15)(q11.2q11.2)(SNRPN−,D15S10−)
   d. 46,XX,del(15)(q11.2q13).ish del(15)(SNRPN−,D15S10−)
   e. 46,XX.arr[GRCh38] 1p36.33p36.32(1755688_2633531)x3
   f. 47,XY,+mar.ish der(8)(D8Z1+)
   g. 46,XX,der(13;21)(q10;q10),+21
   h. 45,XY,der(13;21)(q10;q10)

7. A laboratory performs microarray on a 4 year old male with learning disabilities, ventricular septal defect and immune deficiency. This analysis identifies a deletion affecting chromosome 22 at position 18874431 to 20348930 using genome build GRCh38, in chromosome band 22q11.21. Refer to the ISCN microarray nomenclature in Table 5.1 to describe this deletion.

CHAPTER 6

The Chromosomal and Genomic Basis of Disease
Disorders of the Autosomes and Sex Chromosomes

Feyza Yilmaz • Christine R. Beck • Charles Lee

In this chapter we present several of the most common and best understood chromosomal and **genomic disorders** encountered in clinical practice, building on the general principles of clinical **cytogenetics** and **genome** analysis introduced in the previous chapter. Each of the disorders presented here illustrates the principles of dosage balance and imbalance at the level of **chromosomes** and subchromosomal regions of the genome. Because a wide range of phenotypes seen in clinical medicine involves chromosome and subchromosomal **variants**, we include in this chapter the spectrum of disorders that are characterized by intellectual disability or by abnormal or ambiguous sexual development. Although many such disorders can be determined by single **genes**, the clinical approach to evaluation of such phenotypes frequently includes detailed chromosome and genome analysis.

MECHANISMS OF ABNORMALITIES

In this section we consider abnormalities that illustrate the major chromosomal and genomic mechanisms that underlie **genetic** imbalance of entire chromosomes or chromosomal regions. Overall, we distinguish four different categories of such abnormalities, each of which can lead to disorders of clinical significance:

- Disorders due to abnormal **chromosome segregation** (**nondisjunction**)
- Disorders due to recurrent and nonrecurrent chromosomal rearrangements, involving deletions or duplications at genomic hot spots
- Disorders due to unbalanced **familial** chromosomal abnormalities
- Disorders due to chromosomal and genomic events that reveal regions of **genomic imprinting**

The distinguishing features of the underlying mechanisms are summarized in Table 6.1. Although the categories of defects that result from these mechanisms can involve any chromosomes, we introduce them here in the context of autosomal abnormalities.

WHOLE CHROMOSOME ANEUPLOIDY

The most common variant in the human genome involves errors in chromosome segregation, typically leading to production of an abnormal **gamete** that has two copies or no copies of the chromosome involved in the nondisjunction event. Notwithstanding the high frequency of such errors in **meiosis** and, to a lesser extent, in **mitosis**, there are only three well-defined nonmosaic chromosome disorders compatible with postnatal survival in which there is an abnormal dose of an entire **autosome: trisomy** 21 (Down syndrome), trisomy 18, and trisomy 13. It is surely no coincidence that these chromosomes are the ones with the smallest number of genes among all autosomes (see Fig. 2.7). The imbalance for more gene-rich chromosomes is presumably incompatible with long-term survival, and **aneuploidy** for some of these is frequently associated with pregnancy loss (see Table 5.2).

Each of these autosomal trisomies is associated with growth retardation, intellectual disability, and multiple **congenital** anomalies (Table 6.2). Nevertheless, each has a fairly distinctive **phenotype** that is immediately recognizable to an astute clinician in the newborn nursery. Trisomies 18 and 13 are both less common than trisomy 21; survival beyond the first year is rare, in contrast to Down syndrome, in which the average life expectancy is over 50 years of age.

The developmental abnormalities characteristic of any one trisomic state must be determined by the extra dosage of the particular genes on the additional chromosome. Knowledge of the specific relationship between the extra chromosome and the consequent developmental abnormality has been limited to date. Current research, however, is beginning to localize specific genes on the extra chromosome that are responsible for specific aspects of the abnormal phenotype, through direct or indirect modulation of patterning events during early development (see Chapter 15). The principles of **gene dosage** and the likely role of imbalance for individual genes that underlie specific developmental aspects of the phenotype apply to all aneuploid conditions; these are illustrated here in the context of Down syndrome, whereas the other conditions are summarized in Table 6.2.

Down Syndrome

Down syndrome is by far the most common and best known of the chromosome disorders and is the single most common genetic cause of moderate intellectual

TABLE 6.1 Mechanisms of Chromosome Abnormalities and Genomic Imbalance

Category	Underlying Mechanism	Consequences/ Examples
Abnormal chromosome segregation	Nondisjunction	Aneuploidy (Down syndrome, Klinefelter syndrome)
		Uniparental disomy
Recurrent chromosomal syndromes	Recombination at segmental duplications	Duplication/deletion syndromes
		Copy number variation
Nonrecurrent chromosomal abnormalities	Sporadic, variable breakpoints	Deletion syndromes (Cri-du-chat syndrome, 1p36 deletion syndrome)
	De novo balanced translocations	Gene disruption
Unbalanced familial abnormalities	Unbalanced segregation	Offspring of balanced translocations
		Offspring of pericentric inversions
Syndromes involving genomic imprinting	Any event that reveals imprinted gene(s)	Prader-Willi/ Angelman syndromes

disability. The population incidence of Down syndrome (see Table 5.2) in live births is currently estimated to be approximately 1 in 700, reflecting the maternal age distribution for all births and the proportion of older mothers who make use of prenatal diagnosis and selective termination. At ~30 years of age, the **risk** begins to rise sharply, approaching 1 in 10 births in the oldest maternal age group (Fig. 6.1). Even though younger mothers have a much lower risk, their birth rate is much higher, and therefore more than half of the mothers of all newborns with Down syndrome are younger than 35 years.

Down syndrome can usually be diagnosed at birth or shortly thereafter by its characteristic features, which vary among patients but nevertheless produce a distinctive phenotype (Fig. 6.2). Hypotonia may be the first abnormality noticed in the newborn. In addition to characteristic dysmorphic facial features (see Fig. 6.2), the patients are short in stature and have brachycephaly with a flat occiput. The neck is short, with loose skin on the nape. The hands are short and broad, often with a single transverse palmar crease and incurved fifth digits (termed fifth finger clinodactyly).

A major cause for concern in Down syndrome is intellectual disability. Even though in early infancy the child may not seem delayed in development, the delay is usually obvious by the end of the first year. Although the extent of intellectual disability varies among individuals from moderate to mild, many children with Down syndrome develop into interactive and even self-reliant persons, and most attend local schools.

There is a high degree of variability in the phenotype of Down syndrome individuals; specific abnormalities are detected in almost all patients, but others are seen only in a subset of cases. Congenital heart disease is present in about half of all liveborn infants with Down syndrome. Certain malformations, such as duodenal atresia and tracheoesophageal fistula, are much more common in Down syndrome than in other disorders.

TABLE 6.2 Features of Autosomal Trisomies Compatible with Postnatal Survival

Feature	Trisomy 21	Trisomy 18	Trisomy 13
Incidence (live births)	1 in 700	1 in 6000–8000	1 in 5000–15,000
Clinical presentation	Hypotonia, short stature, loose skin on nape, single palmar crease, clinodactyly	Hypertonia, prenatal growth deficiency, characteristic fist clench, rocker-bottom feet	Microcephaly, sloping forehead, characteristic fist clench, rocker-bottom feet, polydactyly
Dysmorphic facial features	Flat occiput, epicanthal folds, upslanting palpebral fissures	Receding jaw, low-set ears	Ocular abnormalities, cleft lip and palate
Intellectual disability	Moderate to mild	Severe	Severe
Other common features	Congenital heart disease	Severe heart malformations	Severe CNS malformations
	Duodenal atresia Risk for leukemia Risk for premature dementia	Feeding difficulties	Congenital heart defects
Life expectancy	60 yr	Typically less than a few months; almost all <1 yr	50% die within first month, >90% within first year

CNS, Central nervous system.

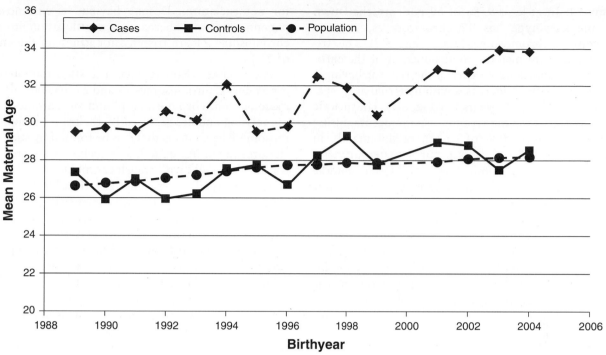

Figure 6.1 Maternal age dependence on the incidence of trisomy 21. Comparison of mean maternal ages at the time of birth. Case *(top)*: maternal age at birth of infant with trisomy 21; control: maternal age at birth of infant without trisomy 21; population: maternal ages at birth of infants in the population from cases and controls. (Data from Allen EG, Freeman SB, Druschel C, et al: Maternal age and risk for trisomy 21 assessed by the origin of chromosome nondisjunction: a report from the Atlanta and National Down Syndrome Projects, *Hum Genet* 125:41–52, 2009; Bull MJ: Down syndrome, *NEJM* 382:2344–2352, 2020.)

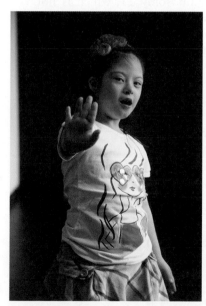

Figure 6.2 **Phenotype of Down syndrome.** Kayla is representing the National Down Syndrome Society (ndss.org). Her hand of greeting shows characteristic short fingers; other typical features include her flattened nasal bridge, small low-set ears, and eyes displaying epicanthal folds and upslanting palpebral fissures. (Photograph by Rick Guidotti, Positive Exposure, www.positiveexposure.org.)

Only ~20% to 25% of trisomy 21 conceptuses survive to birth (see Table 5.2). Among Down syndrome conceptuses, those least likely to survive are those with congenital heart disease; approximately one-fourth of

the liveborn infants with heart defects die before their first birthday. There is a 15-fold increase in the risk for leukemia among individuals with Down syndrome who survive the neonatal period. Premature dementia, associated with the neuropathologic findings characteristic of Alzheimer disease (cortical atrophy, ventricular dilatation, and neurofibrillary tangles), affects nearly all individuals with Down syndrome several decades earlier than the typical age at onset of Alzheimer disease in the general population.

As a general principle it is important to think of this constellation of clinical findings, their variation, and likely outcomes in terms of gene imbalance—the relative overabundance of specific gene products; their impact on various critical pathways in particular tissues and cell types, both early in development and throughout life; and the particular alleles present in an individual's genome, both for genes on the trisomic chromosome and for the many other genes inherited from the parents.

The Chromosomes in Down Syndrome

The clinical diagnosis of Down syndrome usually presents no particular difficulty. Nevertheless, karyotyping is necessary for confirmation and to provide a basis for **genetic counseling**. Although the specific abnormal **karyotype** responsible for Down syndrome usually has little effect on the phenotype of the patient, it is essential for determining the **recurrence risk**.

Trisomy 21. In at least 95% of all patients, the Down syndrome karyotype has 47 chromosomes, with an extra copy of chromosome 21 (see Fig. 5.8). This trisomy results from meiotic nondisjunction of the chromosome 21 pair. As noted earlier, the risk for having a child with trisomy 21 increases with maternal age, especially after the age of 30 years (see Fig. 6.1). The meiotic error responsible for the trisomy usually occurs during maternal meiosis (~90% of cases), predominantly in meiosis I, but ~10% of cases occur in paternal meiosis, often in meiosis II. Typical trisomy 21 is a **sporadic** event, and thus recurrences are infrequent, as will be further discussed later in this chapter.

Approximately 2% of Down syndrome patients are mosaic for two cell populations – one with a normal karyotype and one with a trisomy 21 karyotype. The phenotype may be milder than that of typical trisomy 21, but there is wide variability in phenotypes among mosaic patients, presumably reflecting the variable proportion of trisomy 21 cells in the embryo during early development.

Robertsonian Translocation. Approximately 4% of Down syndrome patients have 46 chromosomes, one of which is a **Robertsonian translocation** between chromosome 21q and the long arm of one of the other **acrocentric** chromosomes (usually chromosome 14 or 22) (see Fig. 5.10). The translocation chromosome replaces one of the normal acrocentric chromosomes, and the karyotype of a Down syndrome patient with a Robertsonian translocation between chromosomes 14 and 21 is therefore 46,XX or XY,rob(14;21)(q10;q10),+21 (see Table 5.1 for nomenclature). Despite having 46 chromosomes, patients with a Robertsonian translocation involving chromosome 21 are trisomic for genes on the entirety of 21q.

A **carrier** of a Robertsonian translocation, involving, for example, chromosomes 14 and 21, has only 45 chromosomes; one chromosome 14 and one chromosome 21 are missing and are replaced by the translocation chromosome. The gametes that can be formed by such a carrier are shown in Fig. 6.3, and such carriers are at risk for having a child with translocation Down syndrome.

Unlike standard trisomy 21, translocation Down syndrome shows no relation to maternal age but has a relatively high recurrence risk in families when a parent, especially a mother, is a carrier of the **translocation**. For this reason, karyotyping of the parents and possibly other relatives is essential before accurate genetic counseling can be provided.

A 21q21q translocation chromosome is seen in a few percent of Down syndrome patients and is thought to originate as an **isochromosome**. It is particularly important to evaluate if a parent is a carrier because all gametes of a carrier of such a chromosome must either contain the 21q21q chromosome, with its double dose of chromosome 21 genetic material, or lack it and have no chromosome 21 representative at all. The potential progeny therefore inevitably have either Down syndrome or **monosomy** 21, which is not viable. Mosaic carriers are at an increased risk (100%) for recurrence, and thus prenatal diagnosis should be considered in any subsequent pregnancy.

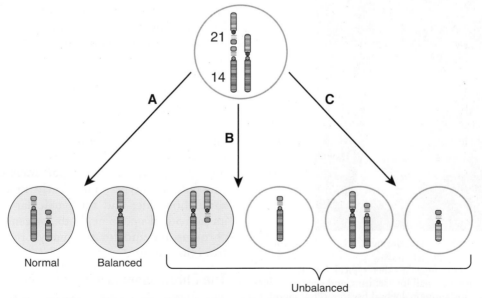

Figure 6.3 Chromosomes of gametes that theoretically can be produced by a carrier of a Robertsonian translocation, rob(14;21). (A) Normal and balanced complements. (B) Unbalanced, with one product containing both the translocation chromosome and the normal chromosome 21, and the reciprocal product containing chromosome 14. (C) Unbalanced, one product with both the translocation chromosome and chromosome 14, and the reciprocal product with chromosome 21 only. Theoretically, there are six possible types of gametes, but three of them appear unable to lead to viable offspring. Only the three shaded gametes *(left)* can lead to viable offspring. Theoretically, the three types of gametes will be produced in equal numbers, and thus, the theoretical risk for a child with Down syndrome should be 1 in 3. However, extensive population studies have shown that unbalanced chromosome complements appear in only ~10% to 15% of the progeny of carrier mothers and in only a few percent of the progeny of carrier fathers who have translocations involving chromosome 21.

Partial Trisomy 21. Very rarely, Down syndrome is diagnosed in a patient in whom only a part of the long arm of chromosome 21 is present in triplicate. These patients are of particular significance because they can show what region of chromosome 21 is likely to be responsible for specific components of the Down syndrome phenotype and what regions can be triplicated without causing that aspect of the phenotype. The most notable success has been the identification of a less than 2-Mb region that is critical for the heart defects seen in ~40% of Down syndrome patients. Sorting out the specific genes crucial to the expression of the Down syndrome phenotype from those that merely happen to be syntenic with them on chromosome 21 is critical for determining the pathogenesis of the various clinical findings.

UNIPARENTAL DISOMY

Chromosome nondisjunction most commonly results in trisomy or monosomy for the particular chromosome involved in the **segregation** error. However, less commonly, it can also lead to a disomic state in which both copies of a chromosome derive from the same parent, rather than one copy being inherited from the mother and the other from the father. This situation, called **uniparental disomy**, is defined as the presence of a disomic cell line containing two chromosomes, or portions thereof, that are inherited from only one parent (see Table 6.1). If the two chromosomes are derived from identical sister **chromatids**, the situation is described as **isodisomy**; if both homologs from one parent are present, the situation is **heterodisomy** (Fig. 6.4).

The most common explanation for uniparental disomy is trisomy rescue due to chromosome nondisjunction in cells of a trisomic conceptus to restore a disomic state. The cause of the originating trisomy is typical meiotic nondisjunction in one of the parental germlines; the rescue results from a second nondisjunction event, this one occurring mitotically at an early postzygotic stage, thus rescuing a fetus that otherwise would most likely be aborted spontaneously (the most common **fate** for any trisomic fetus; see Table 5.2). Depending on the stage and parent of the original nondisjunction event (i.e., maternal or paternal meiosis I or II), the location of meiotic recombination events, and which chromosome is subsequently lost in the postzygotic mitotic nondisjunction event, the resulting fetus or liveborn can have complete or partial isodisomy or heterodisomy for the relevant chromosome.

Although it is not known how common uniparental disomy is overall, it has been documented for most chromosomes in the karyotype by demonstrating uniparental inheritance of polymorphisms in a family. Clinical abnormalities, however, have been demonstrated for only some of these, typically in cases when an imprinted region is present in two copies from one parent (see the section on genomic imprinting later in this chapter) or when a typically **recessive** condition (which would ordinarily imply that both parents are obligate carriers; see Chapter 7) is observed in a patient who has only one documented carrier parent. It is important to stress that, although such conditions frequently come to clinical attention because of variants in individual genes or in imprinted regions, the underlying mechanism in cases of uniparental disomy is abnormal chromosome segregation.

Other Disorders Due to Uniparental Disomy

Although it is unclear how common uniparental disomy is, it may provide an explanation for a disease when an imprinted region (see the section on genomic imprinting later in this chapter) is present in two copies from one parent. Thus physicians and genetic counselors must keep **imprinting** in mind as a possible cause of genetic disorders.

For example, a few patients with cystic fibrosis and short stature have been described with two identical copies of most or the entirety of their maternal chromosome 7. In these cases, the mother happened to be a carrier for cystic fibrosis (Case 12), and because the child received two maternal copies of the **mutant** cystic fibrosis gene and no paternal copy of the normal **allele** at this **locus**, the child developed the disease. The growth failure was unexplained but might be related to loss of unidentified paternally imprinted genes on chromosome 7.

STRUCTURAL VARIANTS AND CLINICAL IMPACT

Structural variants (SVs) are typically defined as changes in DNA that are 50 bp or greater in size. SVs have different types, such as deletions, duplications, insertions, inversions, and translocations, and can potentially impact molecular and cellular processes, regulatory functions, 3D structure, and transcriptional machinery (see Chapter 4).

SVs also include insertions and deletions of mobile elements. Some examples of mobile elements include long interspersed element 1 (LINE-1), *Alu*, short interspersed element (SINE), **variable-number tandem repeat (VNTR)**, and SINE-R/VNTR/*Alu* (SVA) (see Chapter 2). Mobile element insertions into the DNA of gametes or the early embryo can disrupt genes or regulatory elements leading to disease (Table 6.3) (see Chapter 4).

The Impact of Genetic Diversity

The 1000 Genomes Project (1000GP) was initiated to identify genetic variation in the human genome across diverse populations, and it has been instrumental in generating the largest catalog of genomic variants. The 1000GP structural variation analysis group, known as Human Genome Structural Variation Consortium (HGSVC), aims to identify a high-quality map of SVs

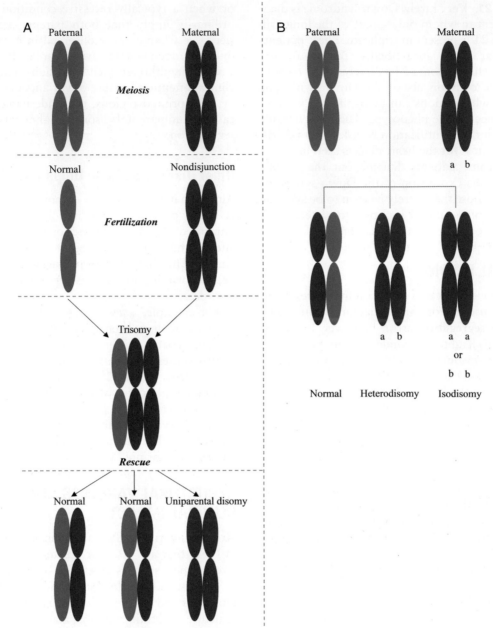

Figure 6.4 Uniparental disomy (UPD), isodisomy, and heterodisomy examples. (A) The formation of UPD. Blue color represents paternal and maroon color represents chromosomes of maternal origin. The nondisjunction could arise in either the maternal or paternal germline. (B) Heterodisomy and isodisomy examples represented. Three offsprings with the following chromosomes are observed: normal biparental inheritance of the example chromosome, maternal heterodisomy with one of each of the mother's chromosomes, and two potential types of uniparental isodisomy with two copies of either of the mother's chromosomes (denoted as *a* and *b*). (Modified from Preece MA, Moore GE: Genomic imprinting, uniparental disomy and foetal growth, *Trends Endocrinol Metabol* 11:270–275, 2000.)

TABLE 6.3 Examples of Mobile Element Insertions and Clinical Phenotypes

Mobile Element	Disease/Disorder
LINE-1	Hemophilia A, Duchenne muscular dystrophy, β-thalassemia trait, hemophilia B, cancer, neurofibromatosis
Alu	Geographic atrophy, familial hypercholesterolemia
SVA	Fukuyama-type congenital muscular dystrophy

and develop new methods to take advantage of both traditional and new genome analysis techniques. Two recent publications from HGSVC not only identify novel variants, including single-nucleotide variants (SNVs), insertions, and deletions, and SVs but also indicated the importance of adopting new technologies, such as long-read sequencing, Strand-Seq, and optical mapping to reveal previously uncharacterized regions of the genome and detect novel variants. The vast majority of genomic variant data derive from individuals of European descent residing in Western countries, which might cause incorrect clinical interpretation of genomic variants. Strikingly, a recent study showed that the African pangenome, built using sequence data from 910 individuals of African descent, contained ~10% more DNA not present in the human reference genome assembly, GRCh38, suggesting that the current reference genome may not fully represent genomic variation in diverse human populations. This is further evidence of the need for *de novo* assemblies of a large number of genomes from underrepresented populations, in order to comprehensively assess the variation in the human genome. A study by Kessler and colleagues suggested that the lack of individuals of African ancestry in variant databases may have resulted in the mischaracterization of variants in the ClinVar and the Human **Gene Mutation** Databases highlighting the fact that additional studies are required to get a better understanding of the human genome diversity and its clinical impact. Several recent large-scale sequencing studies in underrepresented populations, including people of African, Asian, Latinx, and Native American ancestry, have been uploaded to publicly available resources, such as the Genome Aggregation Database (gnomAD).

Segmental Duplications, Copy Number Variants, and Nonallelic Homologous Recombination

Approximately 5% of the human genome consists of low copy repeats called **segmental duplications** (SDs) that are 1000 bp or greater in size, with **paralogous** copies (duplicated copies descended from the same origin) sharing 90% or more sequence identity. Paralogous

copies of SDs either can be in tandem, exist on the same chromosome at some distance (i.e., intrachromosomal SDs), or they can be found on different chromosomes (i.e., interchromosomal SDs). Different SDs can be clustered together into complex regions called SD blocks (Fig. 6.5). High sequence identity between paralogous copies of SDs makes them an excellent substrate for nonallelic **homologous** recombination (NAHR) (Fig. 6.6A). NAHR refers to aberrant recombination resulting from the misalignment of two highly similar paralogous copies of SDs, which further leads to SVs, including deletions, duplications, translocations, and inversions. NAHR is a mechanism that has been shown to cause several genomic disorders, such as Williams-Beuren syndrome (WBS) on chromosome 7q11.23, 15q13.3 **microdeletion**/microduplication syndrome, 16p11.2 microdeletion/microduplication syndrome, and 22q11.2 deletion syndrome (DS) and cat-eye syndrome (CES) (22q11.2 duplication syndrome) on chromosome 22q11.2.

The Impact of Inversions in Genomic Disorders

It is estimated that there are more than 3400 inversions described among humans (based on Database of Genomic Variants 2020-02-05 GRCh38 variant list). An average human genome carries as many as 156 inversions. Inversions can predispose a person to the formation of a new SV that may lead to a genomic disorder. For instance, a study has shown that a ~1.2-Mb **inversion** in the 7q11.23 region is found in 25% of the parent of origin chromosomes of probands with WBS. In other cases, inversions do not seem to have an increased propensity to form a new SV that causes a genomic disorder. For example, a recent study showed that among the

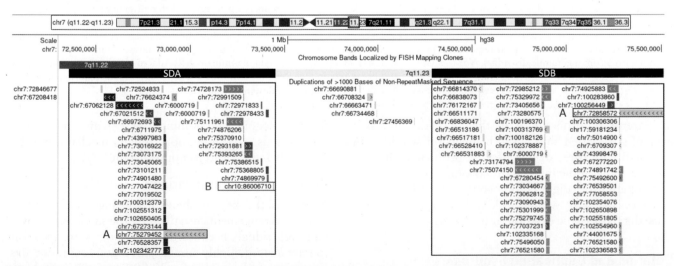

Figure 6.5 Features of segmental duplications (SDs) in the 7q11.2 region of the human genome are represented. Black rectangles, SDA and SDB, represent two SD blocks. Yellow, black, and gray colored rectangles within SD blocks represent individual SDs, and signs embedded to each SD show orientation (>: direct, <: inverted). Text next to each SD shows the genomic position of the other highly similar copy, known as paralogous copy. SDs can be intrachromosomal *(A, red rectangles)*, paralogous copy is present on the same chromosome *(chr7)*, or interchromosomal *(B, blue rectangles)*, paralogous copy is present on a different chromosome (chr10). (Image is obtained from University of California Santa Cruz Genome Browser.)

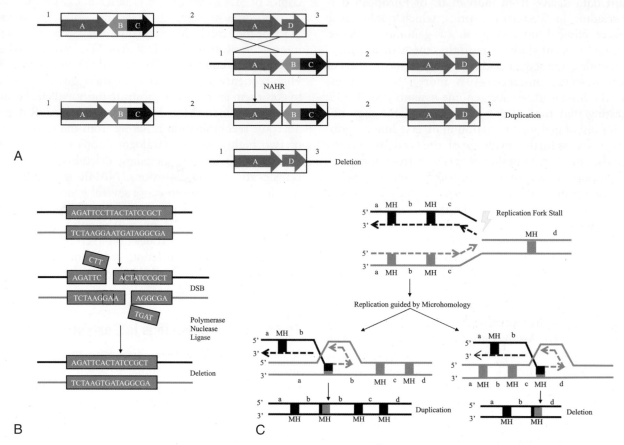

Figure 6.6 **Model of rearrangements underlying genomic disorders.** (A) Nonallelic homologous recombination *(NAHR)*, unequal crossing over between misaligned sister chromatids or homologous chromosomes containing highly homologous copies of segmental duplications can lead to deletion or duplication. (B) Nonhomologous end joining *(NHEJ)*, double-strand breaks (DSBs) occur and NHEJ polymerase, nuclease, and ligase complexes initiate SV formation. Red dashed boxes represent microhomology between the two DNA ends, which is used to guide end joining. The process could result in structural variant formation. (C) Fork stalling or template switching (FoSTeS) and microhomology-mediated break-induced replication (MMBIR) model is represented. When a replication fork encounters a nick (striking arrowhead) in a template strand, one arm of the fork breaks off and results in a collapsed fork. At the single double-strand end, the 5′ end of the lagging strand *(dashed black lines)* is resected, giving a 30 overhang. The 3′ single-strand end of lagging-strand template *(solid red lines)* invades the sister leading-strand DNA *(gray lines)* guided by regions of microhomology *(MH)*, forming a new replication fork. The 3′ end invasion of the lagging-strand template can reform replication forks on different genomic templates before returning to the original sister chromatid and forming a processive replication fork that completes replication. Each line represents a DNA nucleotide strand. New DNA synthesis is shown by dashed lines. For examples of genomic disorders, segmental duplications, and the size of the deleted or duplicated region, see Table 6.4. (Modified from Carvalho CM, Lupski JR: Mechanisms underlying structural variant formation in genomic disorders, *Nat Rev Genet* 17:224–238, 2016; Chang HH, Pannunzio NR, Adachi N, et al: Non-homologous DNA end joining and alternative pathways to double-strand break repair, *Nat Rev Mol Cell Biol* 18:495–506, 2017; Malhotra D, Sebat J: CNVs: harbingers of a rare variant revolution in psychiatric genetics, *Cell* 148:1223–1241, 2012.)

22 parents of probands with the 3q29 deletion syndrome, six carried the ~289-kb inversion within SDA and SDB, and three of the affected probands inherited the inversion on the intact chromosome. However, none of the parent of origin chromosomes carried the larger inversion (~2 Mb) within SDA and SDC, which might caused a pathogenic **deletion** in probands.

Deletion and Duplication Syndromes

Genomic disorders result from gain or loss of hundreds of kilobases of DNA. There are at least two mechanisms whereby SVs can be formed that lead to genomic disorders. NAHR leads to recurrent SVs, whereas nonhomologous end joining (NHEJ) and other non-homologous recombination repair mechanisms (see Fig. 6.6B and C) lead to nonrecurrent SVs.

Recurrent Structural variants

NAHR is the key mechanism causing recurrent SVs. These rearrangements usually have the same size in unrelated individuals because the breakpoints are localized to interspersed, highly similar paralogous copies of SDs. Extensive analysis of over 30,000 patients worldwide has now implicated this general sequence-dependent mechanism in 50 to 100 syndromes involving contiguous gene rearrangements, which collectively are sometimes referred to as genomic disorders. Here we focus on syndromes involving chromosome 22 to illustrate underlying genomic features of this class of disorders.

Deletions and Duplications Involving Chromosome 22q11.2.

A particularly common deletion, 1 in 3400 live births, involves deletions at chromosome region 22q11.2 and is referred to as 22q11.2 deletion syndrome (DS), or DiGeorge syndrome, or velocardiofacial syndrome. This clinical syndrome is caused by a deletion of ~3 Mb within 22q11.2 on one copy of chromosome 22. The deletion and other rearrangements of this region shown in Fig. 6.7 are each mediated by NAHR between SDs in the region.

Patients show characteristic craniofacial **anomalies,** intellectual disability, immunodeficiency, and heart defects, likely reflecting **haploinsufficiency** for one or more of the several dozen genes that are normally found in this region. Because the phenotype is often attributed to deficient copies of multiple, contiguous genes, the term **contiguous gene syndrome** can be applied to this condition. Among the genes deleted, one of the most well studied is the *TBX1* gene, which has been mutated or deleted in as many as 5% of all patients with congenital heart defects, particularly for left-sided outflow tract abnormalities.

The reciprocal duplication of 22q11.2 is much rarer and leads to a series of distinct dysmorphic malformations and birth defects called the 22q11.2 duplication syndrome (see Fig. 6.7).

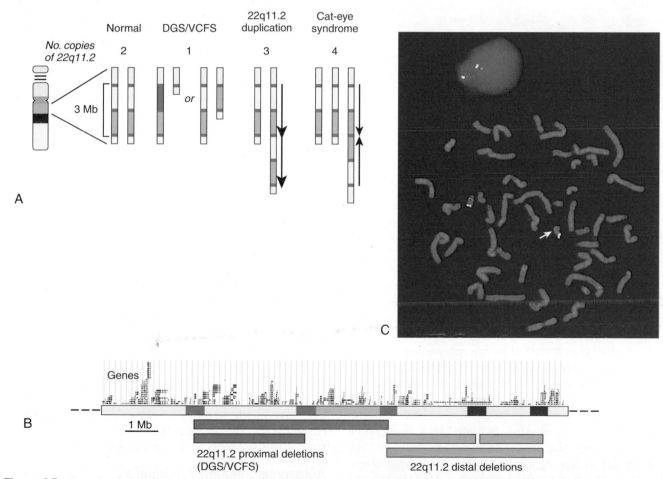

Figure 6.7 **Chromosomal deletions, duplications, and rearrangements in 22q11.2 mediated by homologous recombination between segmental duplications.** (A) Normal karyotypes show two copies of 22q11.2, each containing multiple copies of a family of related segmental duplications within the region *(dark blue).* In DiGeorge syndrome (DGS) or velocardiofacial syndrome (VCFS), a 3-Mb region is deleted from one homologue, removing ~30 genes; in ~10% of patients, a smaller 1.5-Mb deletion (nested within the larger segment) is deleted. The reciprocal duplication is seen in patients with dup(22)(q11.2q11.2). Tetrasomy for 22q11.2 is seen in patients with cat-eye syndrome. Note that the duplicated region in the cat-eye syndrome chromosome is in an inverted orientation relative to the duplication seen in dup(22) patients, indicating a more complex genomic rearrangement involving these segmental duplications. (B) Expanded view of the 22q11.2 genomic region, indicating the common DGS/VCFS deletions *(red)* and more distal deletions (also mediated by recombination involving segmental duplications) that are seen in patients with other phenotypes *(orange).* Genes in the region (from www.genome.ucsc.edu browser) are indicated above the region. (C) Two-color fluorescence *in situ* hybridization analysis of proband with DGS, demonstrating deletion of 22q11.2 on one homologue. Green signal is hybridization to a control region in distal 22q. Red signal shows hybridization to a region in proximal 22q that is present on one copy of the chromosome but deleted from the other *(arrow).* (C, fluorescence *in situ* hybridization image courtesy Kato T, Kosaka K, Kimura M, et al: Thrombocytopenia in patients with 22q11. 2 deletion syndrome and its association with glycoprotein Ib-β, *Genet Med* 5:113–119, 2003.)

TABLE 6.4 Examples of Genomic Disorders Involving Recombination Between Segmental Duplications

Disorder	Location	Genomic Rearrangement Type	Size (Mb)
1q21.1 deletion/ duplication syndrome	1q21.1	Deletion/ duplication	≈0.8
3q29 deletion/ duplication syndrome	3q29	Deletion/ duplication	~1.6
Williams syndrome	7q11.23	Deletion	≈1.6
Prader-Willi/Angelman syndrome	15q11-q13	Deletion	≈3.5
16p11.2 deletion/ duplication syndrome	16p11.2	Deletion/ duplication	≈0.6
Smith-Magenis syndrome	17p11.2	Deletion	≈3.7
dup(17)(p11.2p11.2)		Duplication	
DiGeorge syndrome/ velocardiofacial syndrome	22q11.2	Deletion	≈3.0, 1.5
Cat-eye syndrome/22q11.2 duplication syndrome		Duplication	
Azoospermia (AZFc)	Yq11.2	Deletion	≈3.5

Based on Carvalho CM, Lupski JR: Mechanisms underlying structural variant formation in genomic disorders, *Nat Rev Genet* 17:224–238, 2016; Harel T, Lupski JR: Genomic disorders 20 years on—mechanisms for clinical manifestations, *Clin Genet* 93:439–449, 2018.

The general concepts illustrated for disorders associated with 22q11.2 also apply to many other chromosomal and genomic disorders, some of the most common or more significant of which are summarized in Table 6.4 and Box 6.1.

Nonrecurrent Structural Variants

Nonrecurrent SVs usually do not have the same size in unrelated individuals. The breakpoints of these rearrangements can be localized to anywhere in the genome and are often characterized by microhomologies, small insertions, or blunt ends. At least 70 genomic disorders have now been shown to be caused by nonrecurrent SVs. Although NHEJ is the presumed mechanism for many of these rearrangements, other mechanisms for nonrecurrent SV formation include DNA replication during the aberrant repair and include fork stalling or template switching (FoSTeS) and microhomology-mediated break-induced replication (MMBIR) (see Fig. 6.6B and C). In each of these mechanisms, a stalled replication fork is repaired using microhomology to prime for DNA synthesis.

Nonrecurrent Chromosome Abnormalities

Whereas the abnormalities just described are mediated by the landscape of specific genomic features in particular chromosomal regions, many other chromosome abnormalities are due to deletions or rearrangements that have no definitive mechanistic basis (see Table 6.1). There are

many reports of cytogenetically detectable abnormalities in dysmorphic patients involving events such as deletions, duplications, or translocations of one or more chromosomes in the karyotype (see Fig. 5.10). Overall, cytogenetically visible autosomal deletions occur with an estimated incidence of 1 in 7000 live births. Most of these have been seen in only a few patients and are not associated with recognized clinical syndromes. Others, however, are sufficiently common to allow delineation of clearly recognizable syndromes in which a series of patients have similar abnormalities.

The defining mechanistic feature of this class of abnormalities is that the underlying chromosomal event is nonrecurrent (see Table 6.1); most of them occur *de novo* and have highly variable breakpoints in the particular chromosomal region, thus distinguishing them as a class from those discussed in the previous section.

Autosomal Deletion Syndromes

One long-recognized syndrome is the cri du chat syndrome, in which there is either a terminal or interstitial deletion of part of the short arm of chromosome 5. This deletion syndrome was given its common name because crying infants with this disorder sound like a meowing cat. The facial appearance (Fig. 6.8) is distinctive and includes microcephaly, hypertelorism, epicanthal folds, low-set ears, sometimes with preauricular tags, and micrognathia. The overall incidence of the deletion is estimated to be as high as 1 in 15,000 to 50,000 live births.

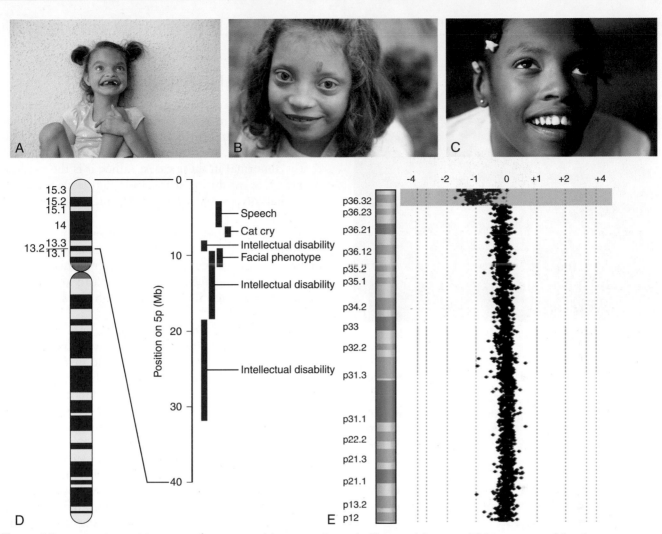

Figure 6.8 Nonrecurrent deletion syndromes. 4p- deletion syndrome is illustrated by two children supported by 4p-supportgroup. org: (A) Kamila's smile reveals missing teeth. (B) Sadie shows what some describe as a Greek warrior helmet facial phenotype. (C) Brielle lives with Cri du chat syndrome (fivepminus.org); here, illustrating characteristic hypertelorism, short philtrum, and epicanthal folds. (D) Phenotype-karyotype map of chromosome 5p, based on chromosomal microarray analysis of a series of del(5p) patients. (E) Chromosomal microarray analysis of ~5-Mb deletion in band 1p36.3 *(red)*, which is undetectable by conventional karyotyping. (A, B and C, Photographs by Rick Guidotti, Positive Exposure, www.positiveexposure.org; D, based on data from Zhang X, Snijders A, Segraves R, et al: High-resolution mapping of genotype-phenotype relationships in cri du chat syndrome using array comparative genome hybridization, *Am J Hum Genet* 76:312–326, 2005; E, courtesy M. Katharine Rudd, Emory Genetics Laboratory, Atlanta, Georgia.)

Most cases of cri du chat syndrome are sporadic; only 10% to 15% of the patients are the offspring of translocation carriers. The breakpoints and extent of the deleted segment of chromosome 5p are highly variable among different individuals, but the critical region missing in all patients with the phenotype has been identified as band 5p15. Many of the clinical findings have been attributed to haploinsufficiency for a gene or genes within specific regions; the degree of intellectual impairment usually correlates with the size of the deletion, although genomic studies suggest that haploinsufficiency for particular regions within 5p14-p15 may contribute disproportionately to severe intellectual disability (see Fig. 6.8).

Although many large deletions can be appreciated by routine karyotyping, detection of other nonrecurrent deletions requires more detailed analysis by microarrays; this is particularly true for abnormalities involving subtelomeric bands of many chromosomes, which can be difficult to visualize well by routine chromosome banding. For example, one of the most common nonrecurrent abnormalities, the chromosome 1p36 deletion syndrome, has a population incidence of 1 in 5000 and involves a wide range of different breakpoints, all within the terminal 10 Mb of chromosome 1p. Approximately 95% of cases are *de novo*, and many (e.g., the case illustrated in Fig. 6.8) are not detectable by routine chromosome analysis.

Typically, and in contrast to the genomic disorders presented in Table 6.4, the breakpoints are highly variable and reflect a range of different mechanisms, including terminal deletion of the **chromosome arm**, as seen

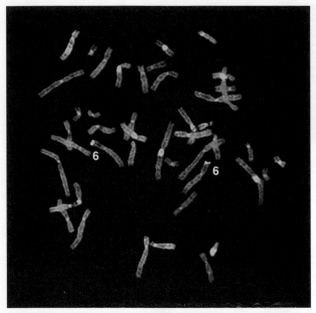

Figure 6.9 A deletion at the long-arm terminus of one chromosome 6 as revealed by subtelomeric fluorescence *in situ* hybridization. Green and red signals reveal intact subtelomeric sequences on the short and long arms of chromosome 6. In this metaphase spread from a patient with congenital abnormalities, we can see the loss of the red signal from one of the chromosome 6s, consistent with a deletion of materials near the long arm terminus of that chromosome. (Courtesy Charles Lee, The Jackson Laboratory for Genomic Medicine, Farmington, Connecticut, United States.)

in 6q deletion (Fig. 6.9), interstitial deletion of a subtelomeric segment, or recombination between copies of repetitive elements, such as *Alu* or LINE-1 (see Chapter 2).

Balanced Translocations With Developmental Phenotypes

Reciprocal translocations are relatively common (see Chapter 5). Most are balanced and involve the precise exchange of chromosomal material between nonhomologous chromosomes; as such, they usually do not have an obvious phenotypic effect. However, among the ~1 in 2000 newborns who have a *de novo* balanced translocation, the risk for a congenital abnormality is empirically elevated several-fold, leading to the suggestion that some balanced translocations involve direct **disruption** of a gene or genes by one or both of the translocation breakpoints.

Detailed analysis of a number of such cases by **fluorescence *in situ* hybridization (FISH)**, microarrays, and targeted or **whole genome sequencing** has identified defects in protein-coding or **noncoding RNA** genes in patients with various phenotypes, ranging from developmental delay to congenital heart defects to autism spectrum disorders. Although the clinical abnormalities in these cases can be ascribed to variants in individual genes located at the site of the translocations, the underlying mechanism

in each case is the chromosomal **rearrangement** itself (see Table 6.1).

Segregation of Familial Abnormalities

The mechanism of pathogenesis here is distinguished from the mechanism of nondisjunction described earlier in this chapter. In contrast to aneuploidy or uniparental disomy, it is not the process of segregation that is abnormal in these cases; rather, it is the random nature of events during segregation that leads to unbalanced karyotypes and thus to offspring with abnormal phenotypes.

In the case of balanced translocations, for example, because the chromosomes involved form a **quadrivalent** in meiosis, the particular combination of chromosomes transmitted to a given gamete can lead to genomic imbalance (see Fig. 5.11), even though the segregation is itself normal.

Another type of familial structural abnormality that illustrates this mechanism involves inversion chromosomes. In this case, segregation of the inverted chromosome and its normal **homologue** during meiosis is typically uneventful; however, unbalanced gametes can be produced as a result of the process of recombination occurring within the inverted segment, in particular for pericentric inversions (see Fig. 5.12). Different inversion chromosomes carry different risks for abnormal offspring, presumably reflecting both the likelihood that a recombination event will occur within the inverted segment and the likelihood that an unbalanced gamete can lead to viable offspring. This overall risk must be determined empirically for use in genetic counseling. Several well-described inversions illustrate this point.

A pericentric inversion of chromosome 3 is one of the few for which sufficient data have been obtained to allow an estimate of the transmission of the inversion chromosome to the offspring of carriers. The inv(3)(p25q21) originated in a couple from Newfoundland in the early 1800s and has since been reported in a number of families whose ancestors can be traced to the Atlantic provinces of Canada. Carriers of the inv(3) chromosome are normal, but some of their offspring have a characteristic abnormal phenotype associated with the presence of a **recombinant chromosome** 3, in which there is duplication of the segment distal to 3q21 and deficiency of the segment distal to 3p25. The other predicted unbalanced gamete, with duplication of distal 3p and deficiency of distal 3q, does not lead to viable offspring. The **empirical risk** for an abnormal pregnancy outcome in inv(3) carriers is greater than 40% and indicates the importance of family chromosome studies to identify carriers and to offer genetic counseling and prenatal diagnosis.

Not all pericentric inversions have a risk for abnormal offspring, however. One of the most common inversions seen in human chromosomes is a small pericentric inversion of chromosome 9, which is present in up to 1% of all individuals. The inv(9)(p11q12) has no known deleterious effect on carriers and does not appear to be associated with a significant risk for miscarriage or unbalanced offspring; the empirical risk is not different from that of the population at large, and it is therefore generally considered a normal variant.

Neurodevelopmental Disorders and Intellectual Disability

Next we consider another class of disorders that frequently require a wide range of chromosomal and genomic approaches for the diagnosis, management, and genetic counseling. Neurodevelopmental disorders are highly heterogeneous, encompassing impairments in cognition, communication, behavior, and motor functioning. Broadly considered, the category of neurodevelopmental disorders includes overlapping diagnoses such as intellectual disability (defined as impairment of cognitive and adaptive functions in childhood), autism spectrum disorder (ASD) (see **Case 5**), and attention-deficit hyperactivity disorder (ADHD). This category can also include various neuropsychiatric conditions such as schizophrenia and bipolar disorder, complex traits of the type that are considered later in Chapter 9.

The overall incidence of intellectual disability and developmental delay is estimated to be at least 2% to 3%, whereas ASD affects as many as 1%. Determining the genetic cause of intellectual disability in most patients is a particular challenge, especially in the absence of other clinical clues or information about the specific gene or region of the genome responsible. Especially in sporadic cases without an obvious family history, a precise diagnosis can be helpful for clinical management and genetic counseling. Thus the full range of screening methods must be considered, including karyotyping and chromosomal microarrays, as well as whole **exome** and whole genome sequencing.

Genomic Imbalance in Neurodevelopmental Disorders

In large studies comparing diagnostic yield in this patient population, chromosomal **microarray** analysis detects pathogenic genomic imbalances in ~12% to 16% of cases, approximately fivefold more than G-banded karyotyping alone; on this basis, chromosomal microarrays are considered the first-tier clinical test to identify genomic imbalance in patients with unexplained intellectual disability or ASD. Although an increase in the presence of multiple rare copy number variants is true both for intellectual disability and for ASD, the copy number variants in patients with intellectual disability tend to be larger and to encompass more genes and are more likely of *de novo* origin than those detected in ASD patients. Several deletion and duplication syndromes,

including 3q29 deletion syndrome, 16p11.2 deletion and duplication syndromes, and 22q11.2 deletion and duplication syndromes, are associated with increased risk of neurodevelopmental and neuropsychiatric disorders. For instance, results from genome-wide analysis of rare copy number variants in 1123 ASD families showed a strong **association** between ASD and *de novo* 7q11.23 duplications. Many hundreds of genes have been implicated to date, with estimates as high as a thousand or more genes in the genome that, when present in too few or too many copies, can lead to neurodevelopmental disorders.

Although screening for the genomic imbalance due to copy number variants is accepted as a diagnostic tool, identifying individual genes and their pathogenic variants remains a significant challenge because of clinical and **genetic heterogeneity**. Some genes appear to be recurrent targets of variation, accounting for up to several percent of cases; exome sequencing can identify *de novo* coding variants with likely or proven pathogenicity in ~15% of patients with severe, sporadic nonsyndromic intellectual disability and in cohorts of patients with the diagnosis of ASD. Whole genome sequencing has also identified likely pathogenic variants, either *de novo* or inherited, in ASD and in intellectual disability.

Clinical Heterogeneity and Diagnostic Overlap

A particular challenge for understanding neurodevelopmental disorders, their etiology, and their clinical course is the extraordinary degree of **clinical heterogeneity**, co-occurrence of symptoms, and diagnostic overlap among them. For cases due either to copy number variants or to single-gene variants, the same defect can lead to different clinical diagnoses in different cases and even in different family members—some with intellectual disability, some with ASD, and some with diagnosed psychiatric conditions. This **heterogeneity** and overlap, even when categorized by genetic/genomic diagnosis rather than clinical diagnosis, suggests the need for further study of **genotype**/phenotype correlations to meaningfully capture the broad range of phenotypes that might emerge among individuals with the same genetic disorder. One important factor is to analyze the effect of the **copy number variant** by comparing affected individuals to their unaffected family members (rather than to unrelated individuals in the general population), thus minimizing confounding effects of the wide range of cognitive and behavioral phenotypes observed even in the general population.

Mechanisms Causing Genomic Disorders
NAHR

This mechanism is also known as unequal **crossing over** that occurs between highly similar copies of SDs (see Fig. 6.6A). Direct copies can result in deletions or duplications, and inverted copies can result in inversions.

NAHR involves crossing over between two paralogous copies and can occur both in meiosis and mitosis at a lower frequency. The positions, homology, and size of the copies impact the rate of NAHR events. Regions of the genome that possess tandemly arranged SDs are more prone to rearrangements. The rate of NAHR varies between SD pairs in the genome, ranging from 2.32×10^{-5} to 8.74×10^{-7}.

NHEJ

This mechanism results in simple, blunt copy number variant endpoints that can have short homologies at the junctions (one to three nucleotides), and unlike NAHR, extensive sequence homology is not required (see Fig. 6.6B). NHEJ can result in an aberrant repair and structural variation of the genome if ligation between double-strand breaks that are not a part of the same lesion occurs. It is possible to observe small deletions or the **insertion** of random nucleotides at the breakpoint junctions. NHEJ is error prone. The breakpoints of SVs formed by NHEJ are frequently observed within mobile elements, such as SINEs and LINEs.

MMBIR

Replication-based repair mechanisms are important when single-strand breaks during the DNA replication process result in collapsed replication forks (see Fig. 6.6C). Variants that occur as a result of this mechanism differ in size and sequence complexity. In addition to microhomology-mediated rearrangements, MMBIR mediated by inverted SDs and coupled with NHEJ can result in complex rearrangements with DUP-TRP/INV-DUP.

DISORDERS ASSOCIATED WITH GENOMIC IMPRINTING

For some disorders the expression of the disease phenotype depends on whether the mutant allele or abnormal chromosome has been inherited from the father or from the mother. As we introduced in Chapter 3, such parent-of-origin effects are the result of **genomic imprinting**.

The effect of genomic imprinting on inheritance patterns in pedigrees will be discussed in Chapter 7. Here, we focus on the relevance of imprinting to clinical cytogenetics, as many imprinting effects come to light because of chromosome abnormalities. Evidence of genomic imprinting has been obtained for a number of chromosomes or chromosomal regions throughout the genome, as revealed by comparing phenotypes of individuals carrying the same cytogenetic abnormality affecting either the maternal or paternal homologue. Although estimates vary, it is likely that as many as several hundred genes in the human genome show imprinting effects. Some regions contain a single imprinted gene; others contain clusters of multiple imprinted genes, spanning in some cases well over 1 Mb along a chromosome.

The hallmark of imprinted genes that distinguishes them from other autosomal loci is that only one allele, either maternal or paternal, is expressed in the relevant tissue. The effect of such mechanisms on the clinical phenotype will necessarily depend on whether a variant (**SNV** and CNV) is present on the maternal or paternal homologue. Among the best-studied examples of the role of genomic imprinting in human disease are Prader-Willi syndrome (Case 38) and Angelman syndrome, and we discuss these next to illustrate the genetic and genomic features of imprinting conditions. An additional example is Beckwith-Wiedemann syndrome.

Prader-Willi and Angelman Syndromes

Prader-Willi syndrome is a relatively common syndrome characterized by neonatal hypotonia followed by obesity, excessive and indiscriminate eating habits, small hands and feet, short stature, hypogonadism, and intellectual disability (Fig. 6.10). Prader-Willi syndrome results from the absence of a paternally expressed imprinted gene or genes. In ~70% of cases of the syndrome there is a cytogenetic deletion of the proximal long arm of chromosome 15 (15q11.2-q13); the deletion is mediated by recombination involving SDs that flank a region of approximately 5 to 6 Mb and in that sense is mechanistically similar to other genomic disorders described earlier (see Table 6.4). However, within this region lies a smaller interval that contains a number of monoallelically expressed genes, some of which are normally expressed only from the paternal copy and others of which are expressed only from the maternal copy. In Prader-Willi syndrome, the deletion is found only on chromosome 15 inherited from the patient's father (Table 6.5). Thus the genomes of these patients have genomic information in 15q11.2-q13 that derives only from their mothers, and the syndrome results from the loss of expression of one or more of the normally paternally expressed genes in the region.

Notably, the low-copy repeats that flank the Prader-Willi and Angelman syndrome regions have also been implicated in other disorders, including duplication or triplication of the region or inverted duplication of chromosome 15. This underscores that although imprinting is responsible for the inheritance and specific clinical findings in Prader-Willi and Angelman syndromes, the underlying mechanism of all these disorders involves unequal recombination of the SDs in the region.

In contrast, in most patients with the rare Angelman syndrome, which is characterized by unusual facial appearance, short stature, severe intellectual disability, spasticity, and seizures, there is a deletion of the same chromosomal region, but now on the chromosome 15

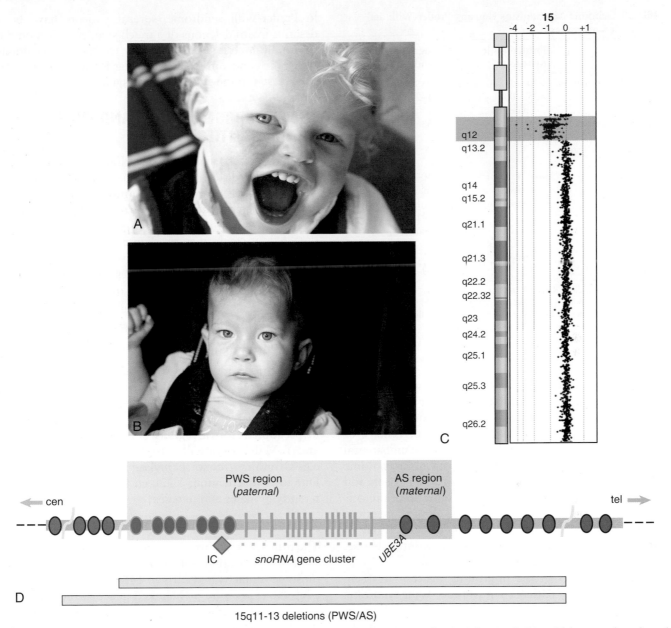

Figure 6.10 (A) Angelman syndrome (AS) (angelman.org) is represented by Jasper, whose smile reveals his widely spaced teeth and large lower jaw. (B) Prader-Willi syndrome (PWS) (pwsausa.org) is represented by Oaklyn, whose face shows almond-shaped eyes and narrow distance between the temple. (C) Chromosomal microarray detection of ~5-Mb deletion in 15q11.2-q13.1 *(red)*. (D) Schematic of the 15q11.2-q13 region. The PWS region (shaded in *blue*) contains a series of imprinted genes *(blue)* that are expressed only from the paternal copy. The AS region (shaded in *pink*) contains two imprinted genes that are expressed only from the maternal copy, including the *UBE3A* gene, which is imprinted in the central nervous system, and variants in which can cause AS. The region is flanked by nonimprinted genes *(purple)* that are expressed from both maternal and paternal copies. Common deletions of the PWS/AS region, caused by recombination between pairs of segmental duplications, are shown in green at the bottom. Smaller deletions of the imprinting center (*IC; orange*) and of a subset of genes in the small nucleolar RNA *(snoRNA)* gene cluster can also lead to PWS. *cen*, Centromere; *tel*, telomere. (Photograph by Rick Guidotti, Positive Exposure, www.positiveexposure.org; C, courtesy M. Katharine Rudd, Emory Genetics Laboratory, Atlanta, Georgia; D, modified from *GeneReviews*. Available from www.ncbi.nlm.nih.gov/books/NBK1116/. Copyright © University of Washington.)

inherited from the mother. Patients with Angelman syndrome therefore have genetic information in 15q11.2-q13 derived only from their fathers. This unusual circumstance demonstrates strikingly that the parental origin of genetic material (in this case, in a segment of

chromosome 15) can have a profound effect on the clinical expression of a defect.

Some patients with Prader-Willi syndrome do not have cytogenetically detectable deletions; instead, they have two cytogenetically normal chromosome 15s, both

TABLE 6.5 Genomic Mechanisms Causing Prader-Willi and Angelman Syndromes

Mechanism	Prader-Willi Syndrome	Angelman Syndrome
15q11.2-q13 deletion	≈70–75% (paternal)	≈75% (maternal)
Uniparental disomy	≈25–30% (maternal)	≈1–2% (paternal)
Imprinting defects (without an imprinting centre deletion)	≈1%	≈3%
Imprinting centre deletion	≈10–15% of patients with an imprinting defect	≈10–15% of patients with an imprinting defect
Gene variants	Rare (small deletions within snoRNA gene cluster)	≈5–10% (*UBE3A* variants)
Unidentified	*<1%*	*≈10–15%*

snoRNA, Small nucleolar RNA.

Data from Beygo J, Buiting K, Ramsden SC, et al: Update of the EMQN/ACGS best practice guidelines for molecular analysis of Prader-Willi and Angelman syndromes, *Eur J Hum Genet* 27:1326–1340, 2019.

of which were inherited from the mother (see Table 6.5). This situation illustrates **uniparental disomy**, introduced previously in this chapter in the section on abnormal chromosome segregation. A smaller percentage of patients with Angelman syndrome also have uniparental disomy, but in their case, with two intact chromosome 15s of paternal origin (see Table 6.5). These patients add further emphasis that, although genomic imprinting is responsible for bringing such cases to clinical attention, the underlying defect in a proportion of cases is one of chromosome segregation, not one of imprinting per se, which is completely normal in these cases.

Primary defects in the imprinting process are seen, however, in a few patients with Prader-Willi syndrome and Angelman syndrome, who have abnormalities in the **imprinting center** itself. As a result, the switch from female to male imprinting during spermatogenesis or from male to female imprinting during oogenesis (see Fig. 3.12) fails to occur. Fertilization by a sperm carrying an abnormally persistent female imprint would produce a child with Prader-Willi syndrome; fertilization of an egg that bears an inappropriately persistent male imprint would result in Angelman syndrome (see Table 6.5).

There is evidence that the major features of the Prader-Willi and Angelman syndrome phenotypes can be accounted for by defects at particular genes within the imprinted region. Variants in the maternal copy of a single gene, the ubiquitin-protein ligase E3A gene (*UBE3A*), have been found to cause Angelman syndrome (see Table 6.5). The *UBE3A* gene is located within the 15q11.2-q13 imprinted region and is normally expressed only from the maternal allele in the central nervous system. Maternally inherited single-gene variants in *UBE3A* account for ~10% of Angelman syndrome cases.

In Prader-Willi syndrome, several patients have been described with deletions of a much smaller region on the paternally inherited chromosome 15, specifically implicating the noncoding small nucleolar **RNA** (snoRNA)116 gene cluster in the etiology of the syndrome.

THE SEX CHROMOSOMES AND THEIR ABNORMALITIES

The X and Y chromosomes have long attracted interest because they differ between the sexes, have their own specific patterns of inheritance, and are involved in primary sex **determination**. They are structurally distinct and subject to different forms of genetic regulation, yet they pair in male meiosis. For all these reasons they require special attention. In this section we review the structure of the **sex chromosomes**, control of the sex determination, and abnormalities of sex development.

The Structure of the Sex Chromosomes

The X Chromosome

One of the chromosomes involved in sex determination is the X chromosome. In 2020, the first telomere-to-telomere assembly of X was finished. There are ~900 genes, many of which are only found on the X. However, genes in **pseudoautosomal regions** are found on both the X and Y. Males are usually affected by X-linked diseases, e.g. Ornithine transcarbamylase deficiency (Fig. 6.11). Due to **X-inactivation**, X-linked traits, may appear differently in males and females.

X Chromosome Inactivation

The principle of X inactivation is that in somatic cells in normal females (but not in normal males), one X chromosome is inactivated early in development, thus equalizing the expression of X-linked genes in the two sexes (see Chapter 3). In normal female development, because the choice of which X chromosome is to be inactivated is a random one that is then maintained clonally, females are mosaic with respect to X-linked gene expression (see Fig. 3.14).

There are many **epigenetic** features, including gene expression, **chromatin** state, noncoding RNA, DNA replication timing, histone variants, and histone modifications, that distinguish the active and inactive X chromosomes in somatic cells (Table 6.6). These features can be useful diagnostically for identifying the inactive X chromosome(s) in clinical material. In patients with extra X chromosomes (whether male or female), any X chromosome in excess of one is inactivated. Thus all **diploid** somatic cells in both males and females have a single active X chromosome, regardless of the total number of X or Y chromosomes present.

The X chromosome contains ~900 genes, but not all of these are subject to inactivation. Notably, the genes that continue to be expressed, at least to some degree,

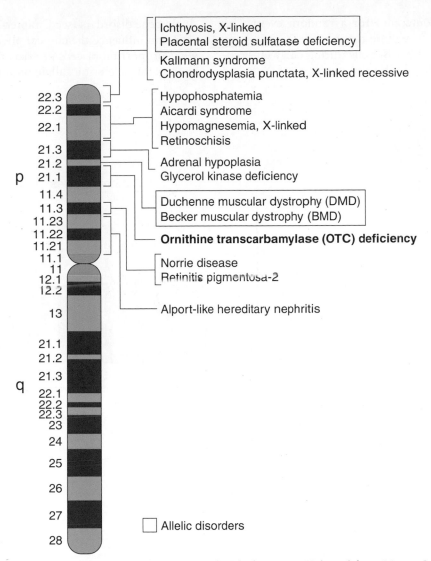

Figure 6.11 The X chromosome structure and disorders associated with the p arm. (Adapted from Morey C, Avner P: Genetics and epigenetics of the X chromosome, *Ann NY Acad Sci 1214*(1), F18–F33, 2010, review is available: Migeon BR: X-linked diseases: susceptible females, *Genet Med* 22.1156–1174, 2020.)

TABLE 6.6 Epigenetic and Chromosomal Features of X Chromosome Inactivation in Somatic Cells

Feature	Active X	Inactive X
Gene expression	Yes; similar to male X	Most genes silenced; ≈15% expressed to some degree
Chromatin state	Euchromatin	Facultative heterochromatin; Barr body
Noncoding RNA	*XIST* gene silenced	*XIST* RNA expressed from Xi only; associates with Barr body
DNA replication timing	Synchronous with autosomes	Late-replicating in S phase
Histone variants	Similar to autosomes and male X	Enriched for macroH2A
Histone modifications	Similar to autosomes and male X	Enriched for heterochromatin marks; deficient in euchromatin marks

Xi, Inactive X.

from the inactive X are not distributed randomly along the X chromosome; many more genes "escape" inactivation on distal Xp (as many as 50%) than on Xq (just a few percent). This finding has important implications for genetic counseling in cases of a partial X chromosome aneuploidy because imbalance for genes on Xp may have greater clinical significance than imbalance for genes on Xq, where the effect is largely mitigated by X inactivation.

Patterns of X Inactivation. X inactivation is normally random in female somatic cells and leads to **mosaicism** for two cell populations expressing alleles from one or the other X. Where examined, most females have approximately equal proportions of cells expressing alleles from the maternal or paternal X (i.e., ~50:50), and ~90% of phenotypically normal females fall within a distribution that extends from ~25:75 to ~75:25 (Fig. 6.12). Such a distribution presumably reflects the expected range of outcomes for a random event (i.e., the choice of which X will be the inactive X) involving a relatively small number of cells during early embryogenesis. For individuals who are carriers for X-linked single-gene disorders (see Chapter 7), this X inactivation ratio can influence the clinical phenotype, depending on what proportion of cells in relevant tissues or cell types express the deleterious allele on the active X.

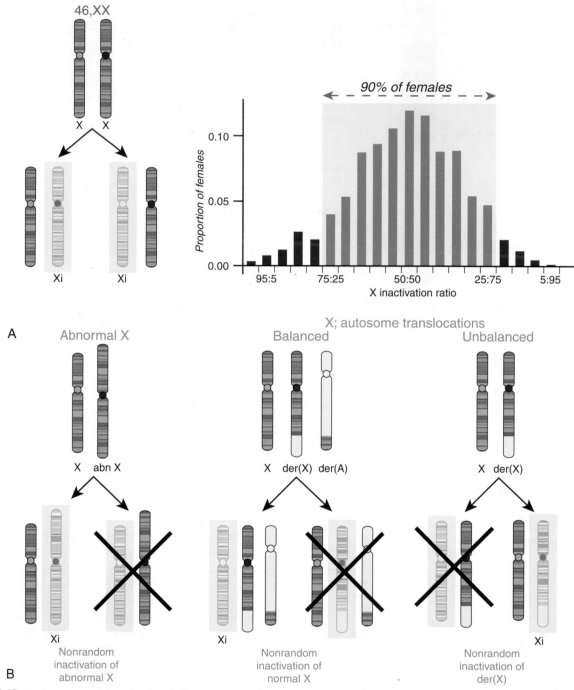

Figure 6.12 X chromosome inactivation in karyotypes with normal or abnormal X chromosomes or X;autosome translocations. (A) Normal female cells (46,XX) undergo random X inactivation, resulting in a mosaic of two cell populations *(left)* in which either the paternal or maternal X is the inactive X (Xi, indicated by *shaded box*). In phenotypically normal females, the ratio of the two cell populations has a mode at 50:50, but with variation observed in the population *(right)*, some with an excess of cells expressing alleles from the paternal X and others with an excess of cells expressing alleles from the maternal X. (B) Individuals carrying a structurally abnormal X (abn X) or X;autosome translocation in a balanced or unbalanced state show nonrandom X inactivation in which virtually all cells have the same X inactive. The other cell population is inviable or at a growth disadvantage because of genetic imbalance and is thus underrepresented or absent. der(X) and der(A) represent the two derivatives of the X;autosome translocation. (B, Data from Amos-Landfraf JM, Cottle A, Plenge RM, et al: X chromosome inactivation patterns of 1005 phenotypically unaffected females, *Am J Hum Genet* 79:493–499, 2006; review is available: Fang H, Disteche CM, Berletch JB: X inactivation and escape: epigenetic and structural features, *Front Cell Dev Biol* 219, 2019.)

However, there are exceptions to the distribution expected for random X inactivation when the karyotype involves a **structurally abnormal X chromosome**. For example, in nearly all patients with unbalanced structural abnormalities of an X chromosome (including deletions, duplications, and isochromosomes), the structurally abnormal chromosome is always the inactive X. Because the initial inactivation event early in embryonic development is likely random, the patterns observed after birth probably reflect secondary **selection** against genetically unbalanced cells that are invisible (see Fig. 6.12). Because of this preferential inactivation of the abnormal X, such X chromosome anomalies have less of an impact on phenotype than unbalanced abnormalities of similar size or gene content involving autosomes.

Nonrandom inactivation is also observed in most cases of X;autosome translocations (see Fig. 6.12). If such a translocation is balanced, the normal X chromosome is preferentially inactivated, and the two parts of the translocated chromosome remain active, again likely reflecting selection against cells in which critical autosomal genes have been inactivated. In the unbalanced offspring of a balanced carrier, however, only the translocation product carrying the **X inactivation center** is present, and this chromosome is invariably inactivated; the normal X is always active. These nonrandom patterns of inactivation have the general effect of minimizing, but not always eliminating, the clinical consequences of the particular chromosomal defect. Because patterns of X inactivation are strongly correlated with clinical outcome, determination of an individual's X inactivation pattern by cytologic or molecular analysis (see Table 6.6) is indicated in all cases involving X;autosome translocations.

The X Inactivation Center. Inactivation of an X chromosome depends on the presence of the X inactivation center region (*XIC*) on that chromosome, whether it is a normal X chromosome or a structurally abnormal X (see Chapter 3). Detailed analysis of structurally abnormal, inactivated X chromosomes led to the identification of the *XIC* within an ~800-kb candidate region in proximal Xq, in band Xq13.2 (Fig. 6.13), which coordinates many, if not all, of the critical steps necessary to initiate and promulgate the silenced chromatin state along the near-entirety of the X chosen to become the inactive X. As introduced in Chapter 3, this complex series of events requires a noncoding RNA gene, *XIST*, that appears to be a key master regulatory locus for the onset of X inactivation. Two additional noncoding RNA genes, *DXZ4* and *FIRRE* are in the interval and have been implicated in various aspects of the development and maintenance of XIC.

X-Linked Intellectual Disability

A long-appreciated aspect of intellectual disability is the excess of males in the affected population, and a large number of variants, microdeletions, or duplications causing X-linked intellectual disability have been documented. The collective incidence of such X-linked defects has been estimated to be as high as 1 in 500 to 1000 live births.

The most common cause of X-linked intellectual disability is a variant in the *FMR1* gene in males with fragile X syndrome (Case 17). However, nearly 100 other X-linked genes have been implicated in X-linked intellectual disability, mostly on the basis of large family studies. Chromosomal microarray analysis has identified presumptive causal copy number variants and insertion-deletions in a further 10% of such families. In addition, exome sequencing efforts summarized in the preceding section to identify *de novo* changes in patients with intellectual disability have revealed an excess of such variants on the X chromosome.

The Y Chromosome

The structure of the Y chromosome and its role in sex development has been determined at both the molecular and genomic levels (Fig. 6.14). In male meiosis, the X and Y chromosomes normally pair by segments at the ends of their short arms (see Chapter 2) and undergo recombination in that region. The pairing segment includes the **pseudoautosomal region** of the X and Y chromosomes, so-called because the X- and Y-linked copies of this region are essentially identical to one another and undergo homologous recombination in meiosis I, like pairs of autosomes. (A second, smaller pseudoautosomal segment is located at the distal ends of Xq and Yq [Fig. 6.15].) By comparison with autosomes and the X chromosome, the Y chromosome is relatively gene poor (see Fig. 2.7) and contains fewer than 100 genes (some of which belong to multigene families), specifying only ~2 dozen distinct proteins. Notably, the functions of a high proportion of these genes are restricted to gonadal and genital development.

Near the pseudoautosomal boundary on the Y chromosome lies the *SRY* gene (*sex-determining region* on the *Y*). It is present in many males with an otherwise normal 46,XX karyotype and is deleted or mutated in a proportion of females with an otherwise normal 46,XY karyotype, thus strongly implicating *SRY* in normal male sex determination. *SRY* is expressed only briefly early in development in cells of the germinal ridge just before **differentiation** of the testis. *SRY* encodes a DNA-binding protein that is likely to be a **transcription factor**, which up-regulates a key autosomal gene, *SOX9*, in the ambipotent gonad, leading ultimately to testes differentiation.

Although there is clear evidence demonstrating the critical role of *SRY* in normal male sexual development, the presence or absence of *SRY* does not explain all cases of abnormal sex determination. Other genes are involved in the sex determination pathway and are discussed later in this chapter.

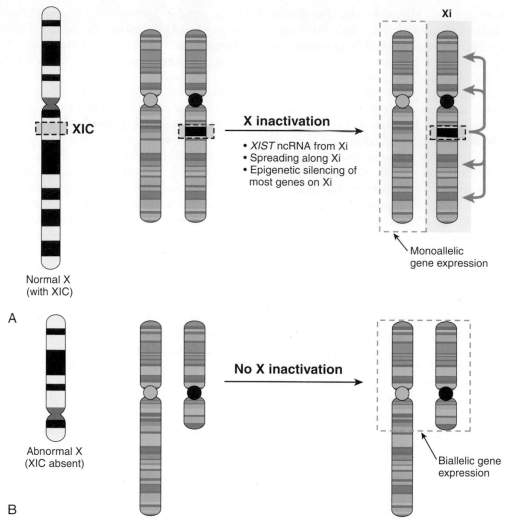

Figure 6.13 X chromosome inactivation and dependence on X inactivation center *(XIC)*. (A) On normal X chromosomes, XIC lies within an ~800-kb candidate region in Xq13.2 that contains a number of noncoding RNA (ncRNA) genes, including *XIST*, the master X inactivation control gene. In early development in XX embryos, the *XIST* RNA spreads along the length of one X, which will become the inactive X (Xi), with epigenetic silencing of most genes on that X chromosome, resulting in monoallelic expression of most, but not all X-linked genes. (B) On structurally abnormal X chromosomes that lack the XIC, X inactivation cannot occur and genes present on the abnormal X are expressed biallelically. Although a fairly large abnormal X is shown here for illustrative purposes, in fact only very small such fragments are observed in female patients, who invariably display significant congenital anomalies, suggesting that biallelic expression of larger numbers of X-linked genes is inconsistent with normal development and is likely inviable.

One or more genes on the long arm of the Y chromosome appear to be important for spermatogenesis because deletions of these regions, AZFa, AZFb, and AZFc, termed azoospermia factors (AZF), lead to low sperm count, ranging from cases of nonobstructive azoospermia (no sperm detectable in semen) to severe oligospermia (<5 million/mL; normal range, 20–40 million/mL). *De novo* deletions of AZFc arise in ~1 in 4000 males and account for ~12% of azoospermic males and ~6% of males with severe oligospermia.

The Control of Sex Determination

The process of sex determination can be thought of as occurring in distinct but interrelated steps:

• Establishment of chromosomal sex (i.e., XY or XX) at the time of fertilization

• Initiation of alternate pathways to differentiation of one or the other gonadal sex, as determined normally by the presence or absence of the testis-determining gene (*SRY*)

• Continuation of sex-specific differentiation of internal and external sexual organs

• Especially after puberty, development of distinctive secondary sexual characteristics to create the corresponding phenotypic sex, as a male or female

Whereas the sex chromosomes play a determining role in specifying chromosomal and gonadal sex, a number of genes located on both the sex chromosomes and the autosomes are involved in sex determination and subsequent sexual differentiation. In most instances, the role of these genes has come to light as a result of patients with various conditions known as **disorders of sex development (DSD)**, and many of these are discussed later in this chapter.

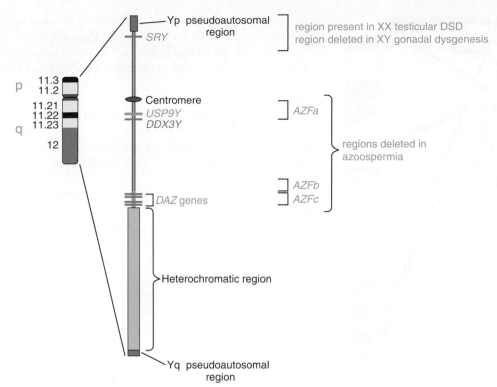

Figure 6.14 The Y chromosome in sex determination and in disorders of sex development (DSDs). Individual genes and regions implicated in sex determination, DSDs, and defects of spermatogenesis are indicated, as discussed in the text.

Embryology of the Reproductive System

By the sixth week of development in both sexes, the primordial germ cells have migrated from their earlier extraembryonic location to the paired genital ridges, where they are surrounded by the sex cords to form a pair of primitive gonads. Up to this time, the developing gonad is ambipotent, regardless of whether it is chromosomally XX or XY (Fig. 6.16).

Development into an ovary or a testis is determined by the coordinated action of a sequence of genes in finely balanced pathways that lead to ovarian development when no Y chromosome is present but tip to the side of testicular development when a Y is present. Under normal circumstances, the ovarian pathway is followed unless the *SRY* gene diverts development into the male pathway.

In the absence of the *SRY* gene, the gonad begins to differentiate to form an ovary, beginning as early as the eighth week of gestation and continuing for several weeks; the cortex develops, the medulla regresses, and **oogonia** begin to develop within follicles (see Fig. 6.16). Beginning at approximately the third month, the oogonia enter meiosis I, but (as described in Chapter 2) this process is arrested at **dictyotene** until ovulation occurs many years later.

In the presence of the *SRY* gene, however, the medullary tissue forms typical testes with seminiferous tubules and Leydig cells that, under the stimulation of chorionic gonadotropin from the placenta, become capable of androgen secretion (see Fig. 6.16). **Spermatogonia,** derived from the primordial germ cells by successive mitoses, line the walls of the seminiferous tubules where they reside together with supporting Sertoli cells, awaiting the onset of puberty to begin spermatogenesis.

In the early embryo, the external genitalia consist of a genital tubercle, paired labioscrotal swellings, and paired urethral folds. From this undifferentiated state, male external genitalia develop under the influence of androgens, beginning at around 12 weeks of gestation. In the absence of a testis (or, more specifically, in the absence of androgens), female external genitalia are formed regardless of whether an ovary is present.

Sex Chromosomal Aneuploidy and Aberration

The most common sex chromosome abnormalities involve aneuploidy for the X and/or Y chromosomes. The phenotypes associated with these chromosomal defects are, in general, less severe than those associated with comparable autosomal disorders because, as discussed earlier, X chromosome inactivation, as well as the low gene content of the Y, minimize the clinical consequences of sex chromosome imbalance. By far the most common sex chromosome defects in liveborn infants and in fetuses are the trisomic types (XXY, XXX, and XYY), but all three are rare in spontaneous abortions. For instance, the incidence of Klinefelter syndrome (XXY) is estimated to be 1 in 650 male births, the incidence of triple X syndrome (XXX) is estimated to be 1 in 1000 females, and the incidence rate of XYY syndrome is

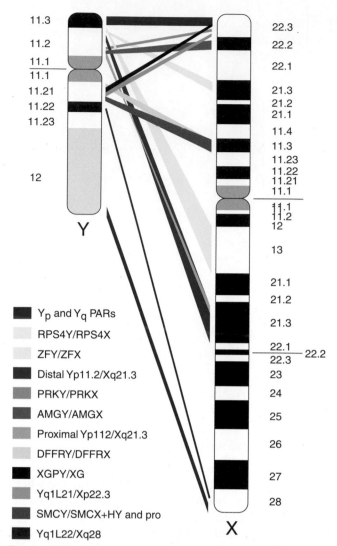

Figure 6.15 legend:

■	Yp and Yq PARs
░	RPS4Y/RPS4X
░	ZFY/ZFX
■	Distal Yp11.2/Xq21.3
▓	PRKY/PRKX
■	AMGY/AMGX
▓	Proximal Yp112/Xq21.3
░	DFFRY/DFFRX
■	XGPY/XG
▓	Yq1L21/Xp22.3
■	SMCY/SMCX+HY and pro
■	Yq1L22/Xq28

Figure 6.15 The human genome X and Y homology chart. (Adapted from Affara N, Bishop C, Brown W, et al: Report of the second international workshop on Y chromosome mapping 1995, *Cytogenet Cell Genet* 73:33–76, 1996.)

1 in 1000 males (Table 6.7). In contrast, monosomy for the X (Turner syndrome Case 47) is less frequent in liveborn infants but is the most common chromosome anomaly reported in spontaneous abortions (see Table 6.7 and Table 5.2).

Klinefelter Syndrome (47,XXY). The incidence of Klinefelter syndrome (Fig. 6.17; Table 6.8) is estimated to be as high as 1 in 650 male births. Approximately half the cases result from nondisjunction in paternal meiosis

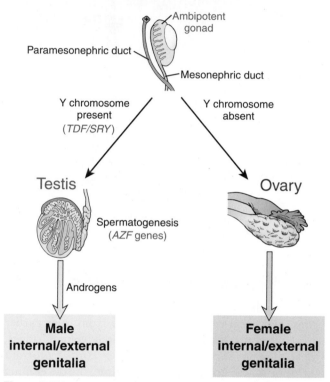

Figure 6.16 Scheme of developmental events in sex determination and differentiation of the male and female gonads from the ambipotent gonad. See text for discussion.

TABLE 6.7 Incidence of Sex Chromosome Abnormalities

Sex	Disorder	Karyotype	Approximate Incidence
Male	Klinefelter syndrome	47,XXY	1/650 males
		48,XXXY	1/25,000 males
		Others (48,XXYY; 49,XXXYY; mosaics)	1/10,000 males
	47,XYY syndrome	47,XYY	1/1000 males
	Other X or Y chromosome abnormalities		1/1500 males
	XX testicular DSD	46,XX	1/20,000 males
		Overall incidence: 1/300 males	
Female	Turner syndrome	45,X	1/4000 females
		46,X,i(Xq)	1/50,000 females
		Others (deletions, mosaics)	1/15,000 females
	Trisomy X	47,XXX	1/1000 females
	Other X chromosome abnormalities		1/3000 females
	XY gonadal dysgenesis	46,XY	1/20,000 females
	Androgen insensitivity syndrome	46,XY	1/20,000 females
		Overall incidence: 1/650 females	

DSD, Disorder of sex development.

Data updated from Robinson A, Linden MG, Bender BG: Prenatal diagnosis of sex chromosome abnormalities. In Milunsky A, ed: *Genetic disorders of the fetus*, ed 4, Baltimore, 1998, Johns Hopkins University Press, pp 249–285; Kanakis GA, Nieschlag E: Klinefelter syndrome: more than hypogonadism, *Metabolism* 86: 135–144, 2018; Cui X, Cui Y, Shi L, Luan J, Zhou X, & Han J: A basic understanding of Turner syndrome: incidence, complications, diagnosis, and treatment, *Intractable Rare Dis Res* 7(4): 223–228, 2018.

I because of a failure of normal Xp/Yp recombination in the pseudoautosomal region. Among cases of maternal origin, most result from errors in maternal meiosis I; maternal age is increased in such cases. Approximately 15% of Klinefelter patients have mosaic karyotypes, most commonly 46,XY/47,XXY. As a group, such mosaic patients have variable phenotypes, and some may have normal testicular development. Patients with Klinefelter syndrome have a several-fold increased risk for learning difficulties, especially in reading, that may require educational intervention. Language difficulties may lead to shyness, unassertiveness, apparent immaturity, and an increased risk for depression. In adulthood, persistent androgen deficiency may result in decreased muscle tone, a loss of libido, and decreased bone mineral density (Box 6.2).

The Mechanism of Sex Reversal

Disorders of sex development (DSD) consists of 46,XY karyotype and 46,XX karyotype. The overall incidence of DSDs associated with a 46,XY karyotype is ~0.6 per million females. Although a number of cytogenetic or single-gene defects have been demonstrated, many

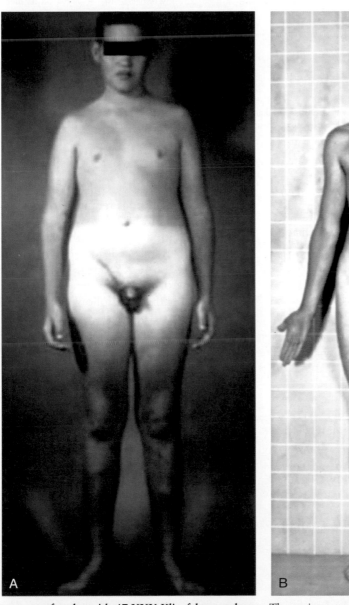
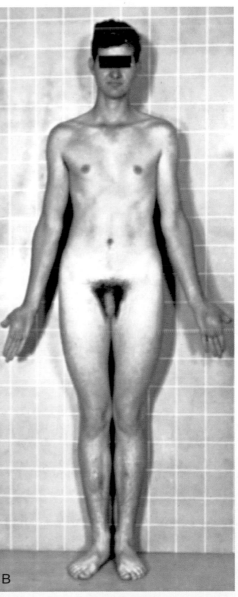

Figure 6.17 **Phenotype of males with 47,XXY Klinefelter syndrome.** The patients are tall and thin and have relatively long legs. They appear physically normal until puberty, when signs of hypogonadism become obvious. Puberty occurs at a normal age, but the testes remain small, and secondary sexual characteristics remain underdeveloped. Note narrow shoulders and chest. Gynecomastia is a feature of some Klinefelter males and is visible in the 16-year-old patient in (A) (A, From Jones KL, Jones MC, del Campo M: *Smith's recognizable patterns of human malformation*, ed 7, Philadelphia, 2013, WB Saunders; B, from Grumbach MM, Hughes IA, Conte FA: Disorders of sex differentiation. In Larsen PR, Kronenberg HM, Melmed S, et al, eds: *Williams textbook of endocrinology*, ed 10, Philadelphia, 2003, WB Saunders.)

TABLE 6.8 Features of Sex Chromosome Aneuploidy Conditions

Feature	47,XXY Klinefelter Syndrome	47,XYY	47,XXX Trisomy X	45,X Turner Syndrome
Prevalence	1 in 650 male births	1 in 1000 male births	1 in 1000 female births	1 in 2500–4000 female births
Clinical phenotype	Tall male (see Fig. 6.17 and text)	Tall, but otherwise typical male appearance	Hypotonia, delayed milestones; language and learning difficulties; tend to be taller than average	Short stature, webbed neck, lymphedema; risk for cardiac abnormalities
Cognition/intelligence	Verbal IQ reduced to low-normal range; educational difficulties	Verbal IQ reduced to low-normal range; language delay; reading difficulties	Normal to low-normal range (both verbal and performance IQ decreased)	Typically normal, but performance IQ lower than verbal IQ
Behavioral phenotype	No major disorders; tendency to poor social adjustments, but normal adult relationships	Subset with specific behavioral problems likely associated with lower IQ	Typically, no behavioral problems; some anxiety and low self-esteem; reduced social skills	Typically normal, but impaired social adjustment
Sex development/fertility	Hypogonadism, azoospermia, infertility	Normal	Reduced fertility in some Premature ovarian failure	Gonadal dysgenesis, delayed maturation, infertility
Variant karyotypes	See Table 6.7		48,XXXX; 49,XXXXX Increased severity with additional Xs	46,Xi(Xq); 45,X/46,XX mosaics; other mosaics

Summarized from Ross JL, Roeltgen DP, Kushner H, et al: Behavioral and social phenotypes in boys with 47,XYY syndrome or 47,XXY Klinefelter syndrome, *Pediatrics* 129:769–778, 2012; Pinsker JE: Turner syndrome: updating the paradigm of clinical care, *J Clin Endocrinol Metab* 97:E994-E1003, 2012; and AXYS, http: www.genetic.org; Skuse D, Printzlau F, Wolstencroft J: Sex chromosome aneuploidies, *Handb Clin Neurol* 147: 355–376, 2018.

BOX 6.2   DISORDERS OF GONADAL DEVELOPMENT

Gonadal dysgenesis refers to a progressive loss of germ cells, typically leading to underdeveloped and dysfunctional (streak) gonads, with consequent failure to develop mature secondary sex characteristics. Complete gonadal dysgenesis (CGD) – as in the case of XX males (now formally designated 46,XX testicular CGD) or XY females (now formally designated 46,XY CGD) – is characterized by normal-appearing external genitalia of the opposite chromosomal sex. Cases with ambiguous external genitalia are said to have partial gonadal dysgenesis. Various types of **gonadal dysgenesis**, their clinical phenotypes, and genetic causes are summarized in Table 6.10.

such cases remain unexplained. Approximately 15% of patients with 46,XY complete gonadal dysgenesis (CGD) have deletions or variants in the *SRY* gene that interfere with the normal male pathway. However, most females with a 46,XY karyotype have an apparently normal *SRY* gene.

The *DAX1* gene in Xp21.3 encodes a transcription factor that plays a dosage-sensitive role in the determination of gonadal sex, implying a tightly regulated interaction between *DAX1* and *SRY*. Although production of *SRY* at a critical point in early development normally leads to testis formation, an excess of *DAX1* resulting from duplication of the gene can apparently suppress the normal male-determining function of *SRY*, leading to ovarian development.

A key master gene in gonadal development and the target of *SRY* signaling is the *SOX9* gene on chromosome 17. *SOX9* is normally expressed early in development in the genital ridge and is required for normal testis formation. Variants in one copy of the *SOX9* gene, typically associated with a skeletal malformation disorder called campomelic dysplasia, lead to complete gonadal dysgenesis in ~75% of 46,XY cases (Table 6.9). In the absence of one copy of the *SOX9* gene, testes fail to form, and the ovarian pathway is followed instead. The phenotype of these patients suggests that the critical step for the male pathway is sufficient *SOX9* expression to drive the formation of testes, normally after up-regulation by the *SRY* gene. In 46,XY CGD, with either a variant in *SRY* or a variant in *SOX9*, the levels of *SOX9* expression remain too low for testis differentiation, allowing ovarian differentiation to ensue.

As many as 10% of patients with a range of 46,XY DSD phenotypes carry variants in the *NR5A1* gene, which encodes a transcriptional regulator of a number of genes, including *SOX9* and *DAX1*. These variants are associated with inadequate androgenization of external genitalia, leading to ambiguous genitalia, partial gonadal dysgenesis, and absent or rudimentary müllerian structures.

The second type of DSDs is a series of phenotypes known as the 46,XX testicular DSDs (previously termed XX sex reversal), which are characterized by the presence of male external genitalia in individuals with an apparently normal 46,XX karyotype. The overall incidence is ~1 in 20,000.

Most patients have a normal male appearance at birth and are not diagnosed until puberty because of small testes, gynecomastia, and infertility, despite otherwise normal-appearing male genitalia and pubic hair

TABLE 6.9 Examples of Genes Involved in Disorders of Sex Development

Gene	Location	Genetic Abnormality	Phenotypic Sex, Disorder
46,XY Karyotype			
SRY	Yp11.3	SRY variant	Female, XY gonadal dysgenesis
DAX1 (NR0B1)	Xp21.3	DAX1 gene duplication	Female, XY gonadal dysgenesis
SOX9	17q24	SOX9 variant	Female, XY gonadal dysgenesis, with campomelic dysplasia
NR5A1	9q33	NRSA1 variant	Ambiguous genitalia, XY partial gonadal dysgenesis
WNT4	1p35	WNT4 gene duplication	Ambiguous genitalia, cryptorchidism
AR	Xq12	AR variant	Female, complete or partial androgen insensitivity syndrome
46,XX Karyotype			
SRY	Yp11.3	SRY gene translocated to X	Male, XX (ovo)testicular DSD
SOX3	Xq27.1	SOX3 gene duplication	Male, XX testicular DSD
SOX9	17q24	SOX9 gene duplication	Male, XX testicular DSD
CYP21A2	6p21.3	CYP21A2 variant	Ambiguous genitalia, virilization, micropenis

DSD, Disorder of sex development.
Updated from Achermann JC, Hughes IA: Disorders of sex development. In Melmed S, Polonsky KS, Larsen PR, et al, eds: *Williams textbook of endocrinology*, ed 12, Philadelphia, 2011, WB Saunders, pp 886–934; and Witchel SF: Disorders of sex development, *Best Pract Res Clin Obstet Gynaecol* 48: 90–102, 2018.

TABLE 6.10 Disorders of Sex Development and Their Characteristics

Disorder	Gonadal Sex	Phenotypic Sex	Characteristics
Sex chromosome DSDs			
Klinefelter syndrome (47,XXY and variants)	Testes (dysgenetic)	Male	Gonadal dysgenesis; hypogonadism; azoospermia
Turner syndrome (45,X)	Ovary (streak gonads)	Female	Gonadal dysgenesis; amenorrhea
46,XX testicular DSD	Testes (bilateral)	Normal male (≈80%) or ambiguous (≈20%)	Most present clinically after puberty with small testes, gynecomastia, azoospermia
46,XX ovotesticular DSD	Testicular and ovarian tissue (ovotestis or one of each)	Ambiguous	Uterus may be present; surgery often required to repair external genitalia; raised as male, female, or intersex
46,XY DSD	Testes (dysgenetic)	Ambiguous	Variable müllerian structures; penoscrotal hypospadias; risk for gonadoblastoma; raised as male or female
46,XY complete gonadal dysgenesis	Undeveloped streak gonads; no sperm production	Female	Normal müllerian structures; risk for gonadoblastoma
46,XY partial gonadal dysgenesis	Regressed testes	Variable (male, female, or ambiguous)	Ambiguous external genitalia with or without müllerian structures; raised as male, female, or intersex
45,X/46,XY mixed gonadal dysgenesis	Asymmetric (dysgenetic testis and streak gonad)	Variable (male, female, or ambiguous)	Variable phenotype, ranging from a typical (short) male to Turner syndrome female; risk for gonadoblastoma

DSD, Disorder of sex development.
Summarized from Achermann JC, Hughes IA: Disorders of sex development. In Melmed S, Polonsky KS, Larsen PR, et al, eds: *Williams textbook of endocrinology*, ed 12, Philadelphia, 2011, WB Saunders, pp 886–934; Pagon RA, Adam MP, Bird TD, et al, eds: GeneReviews [Internet]. Seattle, 1993–2013, University of Washington, Seattle, http://www.ncbi.nlm.nih.gov/books/NBK1116/ and Witchel SF: Disorders of sex development, *Best Pract Res Clin Obstet Gynaecol* 48:90–102, 2018.

(Table 6.10). As described previously in the section on the Y chromosome, most of these individuals are found to have a copy of a normal *SRY* gene translocated to an X chromosome as a result of aberrant recombination.

Those 46,XX males who lack an *SRY* gene, however, are a clinically more heterogeneous group. Approximately 15% to 20% of such patients are identifiable at birth because of ambiguous genitalia, including penoscrotal hypospadias and cryptorchidism (undescended testes); there are no identifiable müllerian structures, and their gender identity is male. A somewhat smaller percentage of patients, however, have both testicular and ovarian tissue, either as an ovotestis or as a separate ovary and testis, a condition known as 46,XX ovotesticular DSD (formerly called true hermaphroditism).

Individuals with either testicular DSD or ovotesticular DSD who lack a translocated *SRY* gene have been the subject of an intense investigation to identify the responsible genetic causes. Duplications of at least two genes have been described, suggesting that increased levels of transcriptional regulators can overcome the absence of *SRY* and initiate the testis-specific pathway (see Table 6.9). Both gene duplications and regulatory variants can increase the level of *SOX9* expression to bypass the requirement for *SRY*. Similarly, duplications of the X-linked *SOX3* gene, which is very closely related in sequence to the *SRY* gene, can stimulate increased *SOX9* expression, replacing the usual need for *SRY* (Box 6.3).

Virilization of 46,XX Infants: Congenital Adrenal Hyperplasia

These patients include those who have 46,XX karyotypes with a normal uterus and ovaries but with

BOX 6.3   OVARIAN DEVELOPMENT AND MAINTENANCE

Ovarian maintenance typically lasts for up to 5 decades in normal females. Loss of normal ovarian function before the age of 40, as seen in ~1% of women, is considered premature ovarian failure (or **premature ovarian insufficiency**). It has long been thought that two X chromosomes are necessary for ovarian maintenance because 45,X females, despite normal initiation of ovarian development *in utero*, are characterized by germ cell loss, oocyte degeneration, and ovarian dysgenesis. Further, patients with 47,XXX or with cytogenetic abnormalities involving Xq, as well as carriers of fragile X syndrome (Case 17), frequently show premature ovarian failure. Because many nonoverlapping deletions on Xq show the same effect, this finding may reflect a need for two structurally normal X chromosomes in oogenesis or simply a requirement for multiple X-linked genes. Nearly a dozen specific genes, such as desert hedgehog gene *(DHH)*, have been implicated in familial cases of premature ovarian failure and in various forms of 46,XX gonadal dysgenesis.

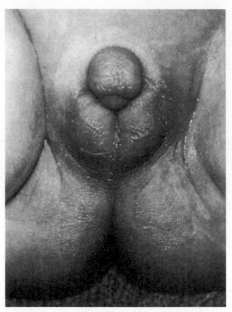

Figure 6.18 Masculinized external genitalia of a 46,XX infant caused by congenital adrenal hyperplasia (virilizing form). See text for discussion. (From Moore KL, Persaud TVN: *The developing human: clinically oriented embryology*, ed 5, Philadelphia, 1993, WB Saunders.)

ambiguous or male external genitalia due to excessive virilization. The majority of such patients have congenital adrenal hyperplasia (CAH), an inherited disorder arising from specific defects in enzymes of the adrenal cortex required for cortisol biosynthesis and resulting in excess androgen production. In addition to being a frequent cause of female virilization, CAH accounts for approximately half of all cases presenting with ambiguous external genitalia. Ovarian development is normal, but excessive production of androgens causes masculinization of the external genitalia, with clitoral enlargement and labial fusion to form a scrotum-like structure (Fig. 6.18).

Androgen Insensitivity Syndrome

There are several forms of androgen insensitivity that result in incomplete masculinization of 46,XY individuals. Here we illustrate the essential principles by considering the X-linked syndrome known as androgen insensitivity syndrome. As the original name indicates, testes are present either within the abdomen or in the inguinal canal, where they are sometimes mistaken for hernias in infants who otherwise appear to be normal females. Although the testes in these patients secrete androgen normally, end-organ unresponsiveness to androgens results from an absence of androgen receptors in the appropriate target cells. The receptor protein, specified by the normal allele at the X-linked androgen receptor (AR) locus, has the role of forming a complex with testosterone and dihydrotestosterone. If the complex fails to form, the hormone fails to stimulate the **transcription** of target genes required for differentiation in the male direction. The molecular defect has been determined in many hundreds of cases and ranges from a complete deletion of the *AR* gene to point variants

in the androgen-binding or DNA-binding domains of the androgen receptor protein. Affected individuals are chromosomal males (karyotype 46,XY) who have apparently normal female external genitalia but have a blind vagina (the female reproductive canal that ends in a sac and does not connect to internal genitalia) and no uterus or fallopian tubes. The incidence of androgen insensitivity is ~1 in 10,000 to 20,000 live births, and both complete and partial forms are known, depending on the severity of the genetic defect. In the complete form (Fig. 6.19), axillary and pubic hair are sparse or absent, and breast development occurs at the appropriate age but without menses; primary amenorrhoea is frequently the presenting clinical finding that leads to a diagnosis.

TECHNOLOGIES USED IN DIAGNOSTIC TESTING

Microarrays, short-read (SR) **whole exome sequencing**, and whole genome sequencing are the most widely utilized cost-effective diagnostic methods (see Chapter 5). But to find novel variations, SV calling methods from *de novo* assembled haplotype-resolved genomes using high-coverage sequencing should be utilized. Accurate detection, genotyping, and annotation of SVs are only a few of the difficulties that must be overcome for accurate SV detection in clinical settings. Determining the frequency of the variants in the population is critical to confirm that they occur at a sufficiently low frequency to call pathogenic variants. While it is possible to evaluate

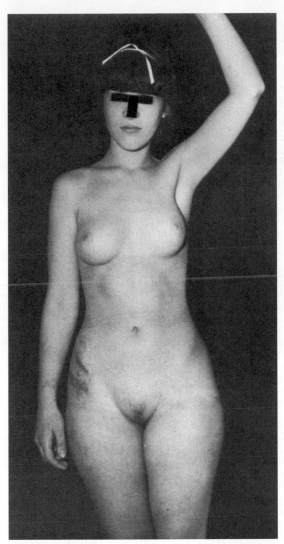

Figure 6.19 Phenotype of a 46,XY individual with complete androgen insensitivity syndrome. Note female body contours, breast development, absence of axillary hair, and sparse pubic hair. (Courtesy L. Pinsky, McGill University, Montreal, Canada.)

that the following algorithms perform better in the deletion or duplication categories: GRIDSS, Lumpy, SVseq2, SoftSV, Manta, and Wham. Numerous SV algorithms are frequently employed to increase the accuracy of SV calling and overlaps across techniques for all types and size ranges of SV are assessed. These findings imply that careful algorithm selection is necessary for each type and size range of SVs to accurately call SVs. Recent research has demonstrated that SV calling based on LR sequencing data should also consider a similar strategy.

An alternate technology is necessary due to the shortcomings of the present cytogenetic techniques, such as chromosomal microarray and SR-based sequencing. Sequencing techniques are quite good at finding SVs, but they struggle to resolve complex regions of the genome precisely, necessitating the use of an orthogonal technique to detect and validate the SVs. Optical mapping is another technique that has been demonstrated to elucidate complex regions in SDs and detect SVs in these regions, some of which are associated with deletion and duplication syndromes. Compared to LR-based sequencing approaches, optical mapping is less expensive and has the capacity to resolve complex SVs, which shows its potential as a diagnostic tool in clinical investigations. Diagnostics depend on the accurate detection of all types of genetic disorders by optical mapping, including deletion and duplication syndromes, aneuploidies, sex chromosomal abnormalities, and disorders involving repeat expansion/contraction.

DATABASES OF GENOMIC VARIANTS

Name	URL	Description
DECIPHER	https://www.deciphergenomics.org/	"The DECIPHER database contains data from 40,078 patients who have given consent for broad data-sharing"
NCBI-ClinVar	https://www.ncbi.nlm.nih.gov/clinvar/	"ClinVar is a public archive with free access to reports on the relationships between human variations and phenotypes, with supporting evidence."
OMIM	https://omim.org/	"Online Mendelian Inheritance in Man, An Online Catalog of Human Genes and Genetic Disorders"
DGV	http://dgv.tcag.ca/dgv/app/home	"Database of genomic variants containing variants identified in individuals without any known diseases or disorders"
gnomAD	https://gnomad.broadinstitute.org/	Genome Aggregation Database

the frequency of SNVs using reference datasets like gnomAD, this is significantly more challenging for SVs, even though several recent population-scale studies provide much-needed SV assessment and annotation. Despite the fact that there are only a few potential SNVs at each site, the number of potential SVs that could affect each site is significantly greater because of the differences in their size and type. The ability to compare SVs to one another is further complicated by this. Because of this, it's essential to use advanced methods like long read (LR) sequencing and genomic data from many diverse populations.

The significance of selecting the proper SV calling algorithm is another facet of SVs. Using simulated and actual whole genome sequencing datasets, Kosugi and colleagues assessed the performance of 69 existing SR sequencing SV detection algorithms. They concluded

GENERAL REFERENCES

Achermann JC, Hughes IA: Disorders of sex development. In Melmed S, Polonsky KS, Larsen PR, editors: *Williams textbook of endocrinology* ed 12, Philadelphia, 2011, WB Saunders, pp 886–934.

Gardner RJM, Sutherland GR, Shaffer LG: *Chromosome abnormalities and genetic counseling*, ed 4, Oxford, England, 2012, Oxford University Press.

Moore KL, Persaud TVN, Torchia MG: *The developing human: clinically oriented embryology*, ed 9, Philadelphia, 2013, WB Saunders.

REFERENCES FOR SPECIFIC TOPICS

100,000 Genomes Project Pilot Investigators, Smedley D, Smith KR, et al: 100,000 genomes pilot on rare-disease diagnosis in health care – preliminary report, *NEJM* 385:1868–1880, 2021.

Allen EG, Freeman SB, Druschel C, et al: Maternal age and risk for trisomy 21 assessed by the origin of chromosome nondisjunction: a report from the Atlanta and National Down Syndrome Projects, *Human Gen* 125:41–52, 2009.

Bartolomei MS, Ferguson-Smith AC: Mammalian genomic imprinting, *Cold Spring Harb Perspect Biol* 3:a002592, 2011.

Baxter R, Vilain R: Translational genetics for diagnosis of human disorders of sex development, *Annu Rev Genomics Hum Genet* 14:371–392, 2013.

Berglund A, Johannsen TH, Stochholm K, et al: Incidence, prevalence, diagnostic delay, and clinical presentation of female 46, XY disorders of sex development, *J Clin Endocrinol Metab* 101:4532–4540, 2016.

Carvalho CM, Lupski JR: Mechanisms underlying structural variant formation in genomic disorders, *Nat Rev Genet* 17:224–238, 2016.

Cassidy SB, Schwartz S, Miller JL, et al: Prader-Willi syndrome, *Genet Med* 14:10–26, 2012.

Chaisson MJ, Sanders AD, Zhao X, et al: Multi-platform discovery of haplotype-resolved structural variation in human genomes, *Nat Comm* 10:1–16, 2019.

Cooper GM, Coe BP, Girirajan S, et al: A copy number variation morbidity map of developmental delay, *Nat Genet* 43:838–846, 2011.

Cui X, Cui Y, Shi L, Luan J, Zhou X, Han J: A basic understanding of Turner syndrome: incidence, complications, diagnosis, and treatment, *Intractable Rare Dis Res* 7(4):223–228, 2018.

de Ligt J, Willemsen H, van Bon BWM, et al: Diagnostic exome sequencing in persons with severe intellectual disability, *NEJM* 367:1921–1929, 2012.

Dittwald P, Gambin T, Szafranski P, et al: NAHR-mediated copy-number variants in a clinical population: mechanistic insights into both genomic disorders and Mendelizing traits, *Genome Res* 23(9):1395–1409, 2013.

Ellison JW, Rosenfeld JA, Shaffer LG: Genetic basis of intellectual disability, *Ann Rev Med* 64:441–450, 2013.

Fang H, Disteche CM, Berletch JB: X inactivation and escape: epigenetic and structural features, *Front Cell Dev Biol*:219, 2019.

Gajecka M, MacKay KL, Shaffer LG: Monosomy 1p36 deletion syndrome, *Am J Med Genet Part C Semin Med Genet* 145C:346–356, 2007.

Gebhardt GS, Devriendt K, Thoelen R, et al: No evidence for a parental inversion polymorphism predisposing to rearrangements at 22q11.2 in the DiGeorge/velocardiofacial syndrome, *Eur J Human Gen* 11:109–111, 2003.

Higgins AW, Alkuraya FS, Bosco AF, et al: Characterization of apparently balanced chromosomal rearrangements from the Developmental Genome Anatomy Project, *Am J Hum Genet* 82:712–722, 2008.

Hughes IA, Davies JD, Bunch TI, et al: Androgen insensitivity syndrome, *Lancet* 380:1419–1428, 2012.

Hughes IA, Houk C, Ahmed SF, et al: Consensus statement on management of intersex disorders, *Arch Dis Child* 91:554–563, 2006.

Huguet G, Ey E, Bourgeron T: The genetic landscapes of autism spectrum disorders, *Ann Rev Genomics Hum Genet* 14:191–213, 2013.

Jiang Y, Yuen RKC, Jin X, et al: Detection of clinically relevant genetic variants in autism spectrum disorder by whole-genome sequencing, *Am J Hum Genet* 93:1–15, 2013.

Kaminsky EB, Kaul V, Paschall J, et al: An evidence-based approach to establish the functional and clinical significance of copy number variants in intellectual and developmental disabilities, *Genet Med* 13:777–784, 2011.

Kanakis GA, Nieschlag E: Klinefelter syndrome: more than hypogonadism, *Metabolism* 86:135–144, 2018.

Kazazian HH Jr, Moran JV: Mobile DNA in health and disease, *NEJM* 377:361–370, 2017.

Kessler MD, Yerges-Armstrong L, Taub MA, et al: Challenges and disparities in the application of personalized genomic medicine to populations with African ancestry, *Nature communications* 7(1):1–8, 2016.

Korbel JO, Tirosh-Wagner T, Urban AE, et al: The genetic architecture of Down syndrome phenotypes revealed by high-resolution analysis of human segmental trisomies, *Proc Natl Acad Sci USA* 106:12031–12036, 2009.

Kosugi S, Momozawa Y, Liu X, et al: Comprehensive evaluation of structural variation detection algorithms for whole genome sequencing, *Genome Biol* 20:1–18, 2019.

Leggett V, Jacobs P, Nation K, et al: Neurocognitive outcomes of individuals with a sex chromosome trisomy: XXX, XYY, or XXY: a systematic review, *Dev Med Child Neurol* 52:119–129, 2010.

Mabb AM, Judson MC, Zylka MJ, et al: Angelman syndrome: insights into genomic imprinting and neurodevelopmental phenotypes, *Trends Neurosci* 34:293–303, 2011.

Malhotra D, Sebat J: CNVs: harbingers of a rare variant revolution in psychiatric genetics, *Cell* 148:1223–1241, 2012.

McDonald-McGinn DM, Sullivan KE, Marino B, et al: 22q11.2 deletion syndrome, *Nat Rev Dis Prim* 1:1–19, 2015.

Miga KH, Koren S, Rhie A, et al: Telomere-to-telomere assembly of a complete human X chromosome, *Nature* 585:79–84, 2020.

Moreno-De-Luca A, Myers SM, Challman TD, et al: Developmental brain dysfunction: revival and expansion of old concepts based on new genetic evidence, *Lancet Neurol* 12:406–414, 2013.

Morris JK, Alberman E, Mutton D, et al: Cytogenetic and epidemiological findings in Down syndrome: England and Wales 1989–2009, *Am J Med Genet A* 158A:1151–1157, 2012.

Mulle JG: The 3q29 deletion confers >40-fold increase in risk for schizophrenia, *Mol Psych* 20:1028–1029, 2015.

Najmabadi H, Hu H, Garshasbi M, et al: Deep sequencing reveals 50 novel genes for recessive cognitive disorders, *Nature* 478:57–63, 2011.

Rodriguez-Martin B, Alvarez EG, Baez-Ortega A, et al: Pan-cancer analysis of whole genomes identifies driver rearrangements promoted by LINE-1 retrotransposition, *Nat Genet* 52:306–319, 2020.

Sanders SJ, Ercan-Sencicek AG, Hus V, et al: Multiple recurrent *de novo* CNVs, including duplications of the 7q11. 23 Williams syndrome region, are strongly associated with autism, *Neuron* 70:863–885, 2011.

Silber SJ: The Y chromosome in the era of intracytoplasmic sperm injection, *Fertil Steril* 95:2439–2448, 2011.

Talkowski ME, Maussion G, Crapper L, et al: Disruption of a large intergenic noncoding RNA in subjects with neurodevelopmental disabilities, *Am J Hum Genet* 91:1128–1134, 2012.

Talkowski ME, Rosenfeld JA, Blumenthal I, et al: Sequencing chromosomal abnormalities reveals neurodevelopmental loci that confer risk across diagnostic boundaries, *Cell* 149:525–537, 2012.

Umehara F, Tate G, Itoh K, et al: A novel variant of desert hedgehog in a patient with 46, XY partial gonadal dysgenesis accompanied by minifascicular neuropathy, *Am J Hum Genet* 67:1302–1305, 2000.

Watson CT, Tomas MB, Sharp AJ, et al: The genetics of microdeletion and microduplication syndromes: an update, *Ann Rev Gen Hum Genet* 15:215–244, 2014.

Weischenfeldt J, Symmns O, Spitz F, et al: Phenotypic impact of genomic structural variation: insights from and for human disease, *Nat Rev Genet* 14:125–138, 2013.

Yilmaz F, Gurusamy U, Mosley T, et al: Multi-modal investigation of the schizophrenia-associated 3q29 genomic interval reveals global genetic diversity with unique haplotypes and segments that increase the risk for non-allelic homologous recombination, *medRxiv*, 2021.

Zarrei M, MacDonald JR, Merico D, Scherer SW. A copy number variation map of the human genome. *Nat Rev Genet.* 2015 Mar; 16(3):172–83. doi:10.1038/nrg3871. Epub 2015 Feb 3. PMID: 25645873.

Zufferey F, Sherr EH, Beckmann ND, et al: A 600 kb deletion syndrome at 16p11.2 leads to energy imbalance and neuropsychiatric disorders, *J Med Genet* 49:660–668, 2013.

PROBLEMS

1. In a woman with a 47,XXX karyotype, what types of gametes would theoretically be formed and in what proportions? What are the theoretical karyotypes and phenotypes of her progeny? What are the actual karyotypes and phenotypes of her progeny?

2. Individuals carrying a copy of the inv(9) described in the text are clinically normal. Provide two possible explanations.

3. The birth incidence rates of 47,XXY and 47,XYY males are approximately equal. Is this what you would expect on the basis of the possible origins of the two abnormal karyotypes? Explain.

4. How can a person with an XX karyotype differentiate as a phenotypically normal male?

5. A small centric ring X chromosome that lacks the X inactivation center is observed in a patient with short stature, gonadal dysgenesis, and intellectual disability. Because intellectual disability is not a typical feature Turner syndrome explain its presence, with or without other associated physical anomalies, in individuals with a 46,X,r(X) karyotype. In a prenatal diagnosis involving a different family, a somewhat larger ring that contains the X inactivation center is detected. What phenotype would you predict for the fetus in this pregnancy?

6. A baby girl with ambiguous genitalia is found to have 21-hydroxylase deficiency of the salt-wasting type. What karyotype would you expect to find? What is the disorder? What genetic counseling would you offer to the parents?

7. What are the expected clinical consequences of the following deletions? If the same amount of DNA is deleted in each case, why might the severity of each be different?
   a. 46,XX,del(13)(pter→p11.1:)
   b. 46,XY,del(Y)(pter→q12:)
   c. 46,XX,del(5)(p15)
   d. 46,XX,del(X)(q23q26)

8. In genetics clinic, five pregnant women inquire about the risk that their fetus has Down syndrome. What are their risks and why?
   a. 23-year-old mother of a previous child with trisomy 21
   b. 41-year-old mother of a previous child with trisomy 21
   c. 27-year-old woman whose niece has Down syndrome
   d. a woman who is a carrier of a 14;21 Robertsonian translocation
   e. a woman whose husband is a carrier of a 14;21 Robertsonian translocation

9. A young girl with Down syndrome is karyotyped and found to carry a 21q21q translocation. With use of standard cytogenetic nomenclature, what is her karyotype?

10. Paracentric inversions generally do not raise the problem of imbalance in offspring. Why not?

Patterns of Single-Gene Inheritance

N e a l   S o n d h e i m e r

In Chapter 1 we introduced and briefly characterized the three main categories of **genetic** disorders – single **gene**, chromosomal, and complex. In this chapter the typical patterns of transmission of single gene disorders are discussed in detail, building on the mechanisms of gene and **genome** transmission presented generally in Chapters 2 and 3; the emphasis here is on the various inheritance patterns of genetic disease in families. Later, in Chapter 9, we will examine more complex patterns of inheritance, including multifactorial disorders that result from the interaction between **variants** at one or more genes, as well as environmental factors.

OVERVIEW AND CONCEPTS

Genotype and Phenotype

For autosomal loci (and X-linked loci in females), the **genotype** of a person at a **locus** is determined by the **alleles** occupying that locus on the two **homologous** chromosomes (Fig. 7.1). Genotype should not be confused with **haplotype**, which refers to the set of alleles at two or more neighboring loci on one of the two homologous chromosomes. More broadly, the term *genotype* can refer to all the allele pairs that collectively make up an individual's genetic constitution across the entire genome. **Phenotype**, as described initially in Chapter 3, is the expression of genotype as a morphologic, clinical, cellular, or biochemical trait, which may be clinically observable or may only be detected by blood or tissue testing. The phenotype can be qualitative – such as the presence or absence of a disease – or can be quantitative, such as measured **body mass index** or a range of blood glucose levels. A phenotype may, of course, be either normal or pathologic in a given individual, but in this book, which emphasizes disorders of medical significance, the focus is on disease phenotypes (i.e., genetic disorders).

When a person has a pair of identical alleles at a locus encoded in nuclear DNA, they are said to be **homozygous**, or a **homozygote**. When the combination of alleles matches to the human reference genome it is referred to as homozygous **wild-type**. It is important to understand that the reference **sequence** is merely one possible combination of alleles and that many allelic variants are not associated with disease.

When two different sets of alleles are present at a locus, a person is **heterozygous**, or a **heterozygote**. The term **compound heterozygote** is used to describe a genotype in which two different variants from a reference sequence are present, rather than one wild-type and one variant allele. These terms (*homozygous*, *heterozygous*, and *compound heterozygous*) can be applied either to a person or to a genotype. In the special case in which an XY male has a variant allele for a gene located on the **X chromosome**, they are referred to as **hemizygous**. **Mitochondrial DNA** is still another special case. In contrast to the two copies of each gene per cell, mitochondrial DNA molecules are typically present in hundreds or thousands of copies per cell (see Chapter 2). For this reason, the terms *homozygous*, *heterozygous*, and *hemizygous* are not used to describe genotypes at mitochondrial loci.

A **single-gene disorder** is one that is determined primarily by the alleles at a single locus. The known single-gene diseases are maintained in *Online Mendelian Inheritance in Man* (OMIM; https://omim.org), an indispensable resource for medical geneticists created by the late Victor A. McKusick. Most of these diseases follow one of the classic inheritance patterns in families (autosomal recessive, autosomal dominant, X linked) and are therefore referred to as **mendelian** because, like the characteristics of the garden peas Gregor Mendel studied, they occur on average in fixed and predictable proportions among the offspring of specific types of matings. OMIM additionally catalogues mitochondrial disorders, defects due to **imprinting**, and disorders where the genetic basis is not yet known, as well as genes of known function.

Pathogenic sequence variants in a single gene may produce diverse phenotypic effects in multiple organ systems, with a variety of signs and symptoms occurring at different points during the life span. To cite just one example, individuals with a **pathogenic variant** in the *VHL* gene can have hemangioblastomas of the brain, spinal cord, and retina; renal cysts; pancreatic cysts; renal cell carcinoma; pheochromocytoma; endolymphatic tumors of the inner ear; as well as tumors of the epididymis in males or of the broad ligament of the uterus in females. All of these disease manifestations stem from the same single variant. Under these

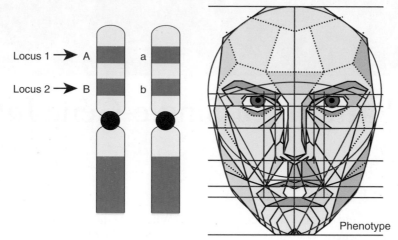

Figure 7.1 **The concepts of genotype and phenotype.** (*Left*) The genotype refers to information encoded in the genome. Diagram of one pair of homologous chromosomes and two loci on that chromosome, Locus 1 and Locus 2, in an individual who is heterozygous at both loci. They have alleles *A* and *a* at locus 1 and alleles *B* and *b* at locus 2. The locus 1 genotype is *Aa*, while the locus 2 genotype is *Bb*. The two haplotypes on these homologous chromosomes are *A-B* and *a-b*. (*Right*) The phenotype is the physical, clinical, cellular, or biochemical manifestation of the genotype, as illustrated here by morphometric aspects of an individual's face.

circumstances, the disorder is said to exhibit **pleiotropy** (from Greek *pleion* and *tropos*, "more turns"), and the expression of the gene defect is said to be **pleiotropic.** Many pleiotropic effects are due to differences in the role of a gene in distinct cell types. With the example of *VHL*, the impact of pathogenic variants in *VHL* is cell type specific because the loss of **cell cycle** regulation gives rise to characteristic problems in specific cell types.

Single-gene disorders affect children disproportionately but not exclusively. Serious single-gene disorders affect 1 in 300 neonates and are responsible for an estimated 16% of pediatric hospitalizations. Although less than 10% of single-gene disorders manifest after puberty, and only 1% occur after the end of the reproductive period, mendelian disorders are nonetheless important to consider in adult medicine. There are hundreds of mendelian disorders whose phenotypes include common adult illnesses such as heart disease, stroke, cancer, and diabetes. Although mendelian disorders are by no means the major contributory factor in causing these common diseases in the population at large, they are important in individual patients because of their significance for the health of other family members and because of the availability of genetic testing and detailed management options for many of them.

Penetrance and Expressivity

For some genetic conditions, a disease-causing genotype is always fully expressed at birth as an abnormal phenotype. Clinical experience, however, teaches that other disorders are not expressed at all or may vary substantially in their signs and symptoms, clinical severity, or age of onset, even among members of a family who all share the same disease-causing genotype. Geneticists use distinct terms to describe such differences in clinical expression.

Penetrance is the probability that an allele or alleles will have *any phenotypic expression at all.* When the frequency of expression of a phenotype is less than 100% – that is, when some of those who have the relevant genotype *completely* fail to express it – the disorder is said to show reduced or incomplete penetrance. Penetrance is all or nothing. It is the percentage of people at any given age with a predisposing genotype who are affected, regardless of the severity.

Penetrance of some disorders is age dependent – that is, it may occur any time, from early in intrauterine development all the way to the postreproductive years. Some disorders are lethal prenatally, whereas others can be recognized prenatally (e.g., by ultrasonography; see Chapter 18) but are consistent with a live born infant; still others may be recognized only at birth (**congenital**). Other disorders have their onset typically or exclusively in childhood or in adulthood. It is even possible that two individuals in the same family with the same disease-causing genotype may develop the disease at very different ages.

In contrast to penetrance, **expressivity** refers not to the presence or absence of a phenotype but to the severity of expression of that phenotype among individuals with the same disease-causing genotype. When the severity of disease differs in people who have the same genotype, the phenotype is said to show variable expressivity. Even in the same family, two individuals carrying the same pathogenic variants may have some signs and symptoms in common, whereas their other disease manifestations may be quite different, depending on which tissues or organs happen to be affected. The challenge to the clinician caring for these families is to not miss very subtle signs of a disorder in a family member and, as a result, either mistake mild expressivity for lack of penetrance or infer that the individual does not have the disease-causing genotype.

PEDIGREES

Single-gene disorders are characterized by their patterns of transmission in families. A usual first step is to obtain information about the patient's family history and to summarize the details in the form of a **pedigree** – a graphical representation of the family tree – with use of standard symbols (Fig. 7.2). Some of these symbols and drawing styles are strongly established, such as the use of a square symbol for a male and a circle for a female. Others vary among users and evolve to accommodate changing needs (e.g., to differentiate sex from gender or

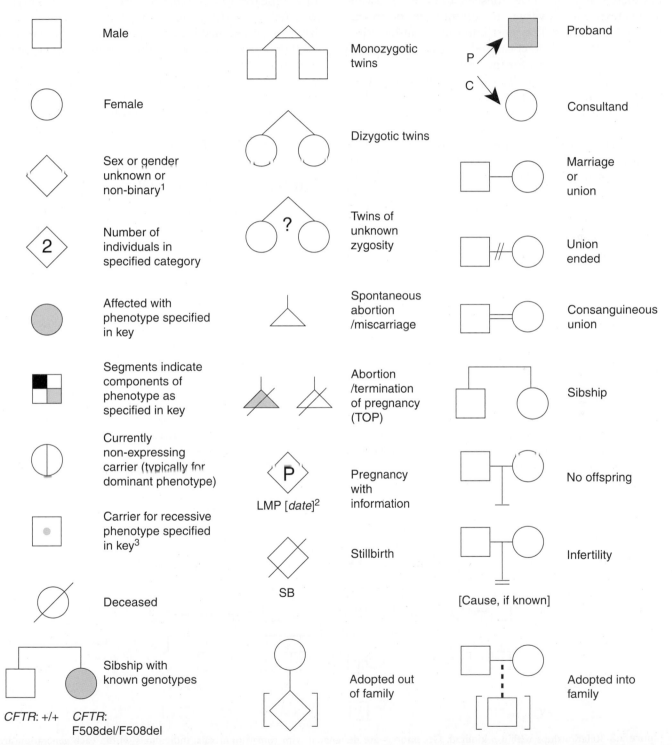

Figure 7.2 Symbols used in pedigree charts. Although there is no uniform system of pedigree notation, the symbols used here are commonly used by professionals in the field of genetic counseling. [1]Modifiers below symbol: AMAB (assigned male at birth), AFAB (assigned female at birth), UAAB (unassigned at birth), no notation = unknown or not specified [2]LMP = last menstrual period (date) [3]Note that this symbol may be inappropriate when multiple genotypes are involved (Practice Resource Focused Revision: Standardized pedigree nomenclature update centered on sex and gender inclusivity: A practice resource of the National Society of Genetic Counselors Robin L. Bennett et al.) *J Genet Couns.* 2022;00:1–11.

to accommodate assisted reproduction options). How to differentiate phenotype and genotype can be a point for consideration, especially as sequence information becomes more prevalent. Many professionals advocate the need for standardization, particularly as computer-generated pedigree drawings become more widespread, but there is not yet one established authority. Drawings in this text reflect a variety of current styles of presenting such pedigrees. The most important considerations are to be clear and practical and to define the symbols and abbreviations used for the drawing.

The extended family depicted in such pedigrees is a **kindred** (Fig. 7.3). An affected individual through whom a family is first brought to medical attention (i.e., is ascertained) is the **proband, propositus,** or **index case.** The person who consults a health professional is referred to as the **consultand** (or perhaps patient or client) who may or may not themselves be affected. Probands and consultands are sometimes differentiated on the pedigree with P or C beside their respective arrows. A family may have more than one proband if they are ascertained through more than one source. Brothers and sisters are called **sibs** or **siblings,** and a family of sibs forms a **sibship.** Relatives are classified as first degree (parents, sibs, and offspring), second degree (grandparents and grandchildren, uncles and aunts, nephews and nieces, and half-sibs), or third degree (e.g., first cousins), and so forth, depending on the number of steps in the pedigree between the two relatives. Couples who have one or more ancestors in common are consanguineous. If the proband is the only affected member in a family, that person is an **isolated** (or sometimes **sporadic**) case. When there is a definitive diagnosis based on comparisons to other patients, well-established patterns of inheritance in other families with the same disorder can often be used as a basis for counseling, even with an **isolated case.**

Examining a pedigree is an essential first step in determining the inheritance pattern of a **genetic disorder** in a family. There are, however, situations that may make this difficult to discern in an individual pedigree. For example, in a family with a lethal disorder affecting a fetus early in pregnancy, one may observe only multiple miscarriages or reduced fertility. For phenotypes with delayed onset, a family may include members who have not yet reached the age at which the disease reveals itself. Nonpenetrance or variable expressivity may make it difficult to obtain accurate information about the existence of relatives carrying a pathogenic genotype. Family relationships may be inaccurately described. Finally, in smaller families, the proband may happen to be the only affected family member, making **determination** of any inheritance pattern very difficult.

PATTERNS OF INHERITANCE

The patterns of inheritance shown by single-gene disorders in families depend chiefly on two factors:

- Whether the chromosomal location of the gene locus is on an **autosome** (chromosomes 1–22), on a **sex chromosome** (X and Y chromosomes), or in the mitochondrial genome
- Whether the phenotype is **dominant** (expressed when only one **chromosome** carries the pathogenic allele) or **recessive** (expressed only when both chromosomes of a pair carry pathogenic alleles at a locus)

The different patterns of transmission of the autosomes, sex chromosomes, and mitochondria during **meiosis** result in distinctive inheritance patterns of pathogenic alleles on these different types of chromosome (see Chapter 2). Because only one of the two copies of each autosome passes into a single **gamete** during meiosis, males and females heterozygous for a

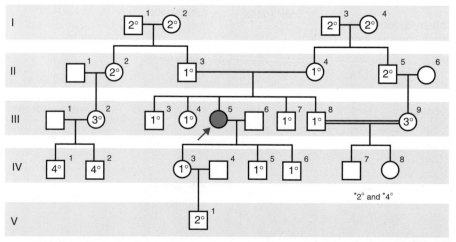

Figure 7.3 Relationships within a kindred. Generations are designated with roman numerals; individuals within each generation are specified by arabic numerals above the symbols. The proband, III-5(*arrow*), represents an isolated case of a genetic disorder. She has four siblings: III-3, III-4, III-7, and III-8. Her partner/spouse is III-6, and they have three children (their F1 progeny). The proband has nine first-degree (1°) relatives (her parents, siblings, and offspring), nine second-degree (2°) relatives (grandparents, uncles and aunts, nieces and nephews, and grandchildren), two third-degree (3°) relatives (first cousins), and four fourth-degree (4°) relatives (first cousins once removed). IV-3, IV-5, and IV-6 are second cousins of IV-1 and IV-2. IV-7 and IV-8, whose parents are consanguineous, are doubly related to the proband: second-degree relatives through their father and fourth-degree relatives through their mother.

pathogenic allele on an autosome have a 50% chance of passing that allele on to any offspring, regardless of the child's sex. Pathogenic alleles on the X chromosome, however, are not distributed equally to sons and daughters. Males pass their **Y chromosome** to their sons and their X to their daughters; they therefore cannot pass an allele on the X chromosome to their sons and always pass the allele to their daughters (unless it is at one of the pseudoautosomal loci; see Chapter 6). Because mitochondria are inherited from the mother only, regardless of the sex of the offspring, variants in the mitochondrial genome are not inherited according to a mendelian pattern. Autosomal, X-linked, and **mitochondrial inheritance** will be discussed in the rest of the chapter that follows.

Dominant and Recessive Traits

Autosomal Loci

As classically defined, a phenotype is recessive if it is expressed only in homozygotes or compound heterozygotes, all of whom lack a wild-type allele, and never in heterozygotes, who do have a wild-type allele. In contrast, a dominant inheritance pattern occurs when a phenotype is expressed in heterozygotes as well as in homozygotes (or compound heterozygotes). For the vast majority of inherited dominant diseases, homozygotes or compound heterozygotes for pathogenic alleles at autosomal loci are more severely affected than are heterozygotes, an inheritance pattern known as **incompletely dominant** (or semidominant). Very few diseases are known in which homozygotes (or compound heterozygotes) show the same phenotype as heterozygotes; such a disorder is referred to as a pure dominant disease. Finally, if phenotypic expression of both alleles at a locus occurs in a compound heterozygote, inheritance is termed **codominant**.

ABO Blood Group. One medically important trait that demonstrates codominant expression is the ABO blood group system important in blood transfusion and tissue transplantation. The *A*, *B*, and *O* alleles at the *ABO* locus form a three-allele system in which two alleles (*A* and *B*) govern expression of either the A or B carbohydrate antigen on the surface of red cells as a codominant trait; a third allele (*O*) results in expression of neither the A nor the B antigen and is recessive. The difference between the A and B antigen is which of two different sugar molecules makes up the terminal sugar on a cell

surface glycoprotein called H. Whether the A or B form of the glycoprotein is made is specified by an enzyme encoded by the *ABO* gene that adds one or the other sugar molecule to the H antigen, depending on which version of the enzyme is encoded by alleles at the *ABO* locus. There are, therefore, four phenotypes possible: O, A, B, and AB (Table 7.1). Type A individuals have antigen A on their red blood cells, type B individuals have antigen B, type AB individuals have both antigens, and type O individuals have neither.

A feature of the ABO groups not shared by other **blood group** systems is the reciprocal relationship, in an individual, between the antigens present on the red blood cells and the antibodies in the serum (see Table 7.1). When the red blood cells lack antigen A, the serum contains anti-A antibodies; when the cells lack antigen B, the serum contains anti-B. Formation of anti-A and anti-B antibodies in the absence of prior blood transfusion is believed to be a response to the natural occurrence of A-like and B-like antigens in the environment (e.g., in bacteria).

X-Linked Loci

For X-linked disorders, a condition expressed only in hemizygotes and never in heterozygotes has traditionally been referred to as an X-linked recessive, whereas a phenotype that is always expressed in heterozygotes as well as in hemizygotes has been called X-linked dominant. Because of **epigenetic** regulation of X-linked gene expression in **carrier** females, due to X chromosome inactivation (introduced in Chapters 3 and 6), it can be difficult to determine phenotypically whether a disease with an X-linked inheritance pattern is dominant or recessive. Some geneticists have, therefore, chosen not to use these terms when describing the inheritance of X-linked disease.

Strictly speaking, the terms *dominant* and *recessive* refer to the inheritance pattern of a phenotype rather than to the alleles responsible for that phenotype. Similarly, a gene is not dominant or recessive; it is the phenotype produced by a particular pathogenic allele in that gene that shows dominant or recessive inheritance.

AUTOSOMAL PATTERNS OF MENDELIAN INHERITANCE

Autosomal Recessive Inheritance

Autosomal recessive disease occurs only in individuals with pathogenic variants on both inherited alleles and no wild-type allele. Such homozygotes or compound heterozygotes

TABLE 7.1 ABO Genotypes and Serum Reactivity

Genotype	Phenotype in RBCs	Reaction With Anti-A	Reaction With Anti-B	Antibodies in Serum
OO	O	−	−	Anti-A, anti-B
AA or AO	A	+	−	Anti-B
BB or BO	B	−	+	Anti-A
AB	AB	+	+	Neither

− Represents no reaction; + represents reaction. *RBC,* Red blood cell.

must have inherited a pathogenic allele from each parent, each of whom is (barring rare exceptions that we will consider later) a heterozygote for that allele.

When a disorder shows recessive inheritance, the pathogenic variant responsible generally reduces or eliminates the function of the gene product: a so-called **loss-of-function** mutation. For example, many recessive diseases are caused by variants that impair or eliminate the function of an enzyme. In a heterozygote, a remaining normal gene copy is able to compensate for the pathogenic allele and prevent the disease from occurring. However, when no wild-type allele is present, as in homozygotes or compound heterozygotes, disease occurs. Disease mechanisms and examples of recessive conditions are discussed in detail in Chapters 12 and 13.

Autosomal recessive disorders may appear whenever two parents are at least **carriers** for the condition, here with the genotype *R/r* (Table 7.2). Carriers are unaffected heterozygotes. In the common case where we consider two carrier parents, the **risk** of transmission of disease is 25%, since each parent passes an allele at random to their offspring. Autosomal recessive disorders may also occur when one parent is a carrier and the other parent has the

disease (genotype *r/r*). In this case the risk of transmission is 50% since the affected parent must transmit a pathogenic allele and the carrier parent transmits the pathogenic allele 50% of the time. Autosomal recessive disorders will always appear in offspring when both parents are affected by the identical condition, since neither parent has a wild-type allele to transmit. Often in autosomal recessive disorders, the proband may be the only affected family member, but if any others are affected, they are usually in the same sibship and not elsewhere in the kindred (Fig. 7.4).

Sex-Influenced Autosomal Recessive Disorders

Because males and females both have the same complement of autosomes, autosomal recessive disorders generally show the same frequency and severity in males and females. There are, however, exceptions. Some autosomal recessive diseases demonstrate a **sex-influenced phenotype** – that is, the disorder is expressed in both sexes but with different frequencies or severity. For example, hereditary hemochromatosis is an autosomal recessive phenotype that is 5 to 10 times more common in males than in females (Case 20). Affected individuals have enhanced absorption of dietary iron that can lead

TABLE 7.2 Autosomal Recessive Inheritance

Two carrier parents			Parent 2 Genotype R/r Gametes		Risk for Disease
			R	r	
Parent 1 genotype R/r	Gametes	R	R/R	R/r	¼ Unaffected (R/R)
		r	R/r	r/r	½ Unaffected carriers (R/r)
					¼ Affected (r/r)
One Carrier and One Affected Parent			Parent 2 genotype r/r gametes		
			r	r	
Parent 1 genotype R/r	Gametes	R	R/r	R/r	½ Unaffected carriers (R/r)
		r	r/r	r/r	½ Affected (r/r)
Two Affected Parents			Parent 2 genotype r/r gametes		
			r	r	
Parent 1 genotype r/r	Gametes	r	r/r	r/r	All affected (r/r)
		r	r/r	r/r	

The wild-type allele is denoted by uppercase R, a pathogenic allele by lowercase r.

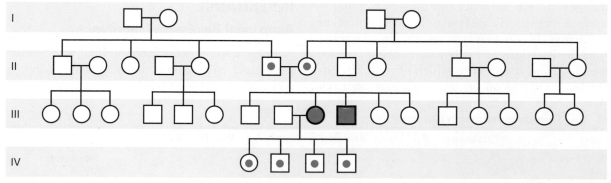

Figure 7.4 Pedigree showing autosomal recessive inheritance. Filled symbols represent individuals affected with the trait. Those with dots represent obligate carriers of the variant allele for the recessive trait but are unaffected. Many others in the pedigree also have significant likelihood to be carriers.

to iron overload and serious damage to the heart, liver, and pancreas. The lower incidence of the clinical disorder in homozygous females is believed to be due to their lower dietary iron intake, lower alcohol usage, and increased iron loss through menstruation.

Gene Frequency and Carrier Frequency

Pathogenic alleles responsible for a recessive disorder are generally rare, so most people will not have even one such copy. Because an autosomal recessive disorder must be inherited from both parents, the risk that any carrier will have an affected child depends partly on the chance that their partner is also a carrier of a pathogenic allele for the condition. Thus, knowledge of the carrier frequency of a disease in the population is clinically important for genetic counseling.

As an example, the most common autosomal recessive disorder in individuals of European ancestry is cystic fibrosis (CF) (Case 12), caused by pathogenic variants in the cystic fibrosis transmembrane conductance regulator (*CFTR*) gene (see Chapter 13). Among this population, ~1 in 2500 individuals has two pathogenic *CFTR* alleles and has the disease, from which we can infer that 1 in 24 individuals is a carrier. (How one calculates heterozygote frequencies in autosomal recessive conditions will be addressed in Chapter 10.) Pathogenic variants may be transmitted from generation to generation without appearing in a homozygous or compound heterozygous state and causing overt disease. The presence of such hidden recessive genes is not revealed unless the carrier has children with someone who also carries a pathogenic allele at the *CFTR* locus and both deleterious alleles are inherited.

Estimates of the number of deleterious alleles in each of our genomes range from 50 to 200, based on examining an individual's complete **exome** or genome sequence for clearly deleterious variants in the coding regions of the genome (see Chapter 4). This estimate is imprecise, however. It may be an underestimate because it does not include variants whose deleterious effect is not obvious from a simple examination of the DNA sequence. Alternatively, it may be an overestimate because it includes variants in many genes that are not known to cause disease.

Consanguinity

Because most pathogenic variants are generally uncommon in the population, people with rare autosomal recessive disorders are often **compound heterozygotes** rather than true homozygotes. One well-recognized exception to this rule occurs when an affected individual inherits the exact same pathogenic allele from both parents because the parents are consanguineous (i.e., they are related and carry the identical allele inherited from a common ancestor). **Consanguinity** in the parents of a patient with a genetic disorder is strong evidence (although not proof) for the autosomal recessive inheritance of that condition. For example, the disorder in the pedigree in Fig. 7.5 is likely to be an autosomal recessive

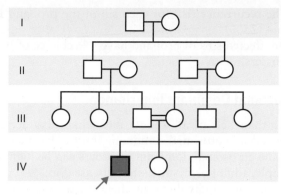

Figure 7.5 Pedigree in which parental consanguinity suggests autosomal recessive inheritance. *Arrow* indicates the proband.

trait, even though other information in the pedigree may seem insufficient to establish this inheritance pattern.

Consanguinity is more frequently found in the background of individuals with very rare conditions than in those with more common recessive conditions. This is because it is less likely that two individuals at random in the population will both be carriers of a very rare disorder by chance alone than it is that they would both be carriers because they inherited the same pathogenic allele from a single common ancestor. For example, in xeroderma pigmentosum (Case 48), a very rare autosomal recessive condition of DNA repair (see Chapter 16), more than 20% of cases occur among the offspring of first cousins. In contrast, in more common recessive conditions, most children are born to ostensibly unrelated persons, each of whom happens by chance to be a carrier. Thus, most affected persons with a relatively common disorder, such as phenylketonuria, do not have consanguineous parents because pathogenic variants are common in the general population. How consanguinity is measured is described in Chapter 10.

The genetic risk to the offspring of related people is not as great as is sometimes imagined. For first cousins, the absolute risk to offspring, including not only known autosomal recessive diseases but also stillbirth, neonatal death, and **congenital** malformation, is 3% to 5%, approximately double the overall background risk of 2% to 3% for offspring born to an unrelated couple (see Chapter 17). Because consanguinity can be seen in any population, it is always important to ascertain in every family.

CHARACTERISTICS OF AUTOSOMAL RECESSIVE INHERITANCE

- An autosomal recessive phenotype, if not isolated, is typically seen only in the sibship of the proband, not in parents, offspring, or other relatives.
- For most autosomal recessive traits, males and females are equally likely to be affected.
- Parents of an affected child are asymptomatic carriers of pathogenic alleles (obligate carriers).
- The parents of the affected person may in some cases be consanguineous. This is especially likely if the gene responsible for the condition is rare in the population.

- The **recurrence risk** for each sib of the proband is 1 in 4 (25%).
- Unaffected sibs of proband have a ⅔ chance of being carriers.

Autosomal Dominant Inheritance

More than half of all known mendelian disorders are inherited as autosomal dominant traits. The incidence of some autosomal dominant disorders can be high. For example, adult polycystic kidney disease (Case 37) occurs in 1 in 1000 individuals in the United States. Other autosomal dominant disorders show a high frequency only in certain populations from specific geographic areas (e.g., the frequency of **familial** hypercholesterolemia [Case 16] affects 1 in 100 for Afrikaner populations in South Africa; myotonic dystrophy affects 1 in 550 in the Charlevoix and Saguenay–Lac Saint Jean regions of northeastern Quebec). The burden of autosomal dominant disorders is further increased because of their hereditary nature; when they are transmitted through families they raise medical and even social problems, not only for individuals but also for whole kindreds, often through many generations.

The risk and severity of dominantly inherited disease in the offspring depend on whether one or both parents are affected and whether the trait is a pure dominant or is incompletely dominant. There are a number of ways that one pathogenic allele can cause a dominantly inherited trait to occur in a heterozygote despite the presence of a normal allele. Disease mechanisms in various dominant conditions are discussed in Chapter 12.

Denoting *D* as the pathogenic variant and *d* as the wild-type allele, the parents of children with an autosomal dominant disease can be two heterozygotes (*D/d*) or, more frequently, a heterozygote (*D/d*) and a homozygote for a normal allele (*d/d*).

As seen in Table 7.3, each child born to a couple where one parent has the *D/d* genotype and the other the *d/d* genotype has a 50% chance of receiving the affected parent's allele *D* and a 50% chance of receiving the normal allele *d*. In the population as a whole, then, the offspring of *D/d* by *d/d* parents are ~50% *D/d* and 50% *d/d*. Of course, each pregnancy is an independent event, not governed by the outcome of previous pregnancies. Thus, within a family, the distribution of affected and unaffected children may be quite different from the theoretic expected ratio of 1:1, especially if the sibship is small. Typical autosomal dominant inheritance can be seen in the pedigree of a family with a dominantly inherited form of hereditary deafness (Fig. 7.6A). In practice, homozygotes for dominant phenotypes are not often seen, but the offspring of two affected individuals with the genotype *D/d* could have a D/D genotype 25% of the time. The potential to observe individuals with the *D/D* genotype may also be limited if the phenotype causes early lethality (see the description of incompletely dominant inheritance later).

Pure Dominant Inheritance

As mentioned earlier, very few human disorders demonstrate a purely dominant pattern of inheritance. Even Huntington disease (Case 24), which is frequently considered to be a pure dominant because the nature and severity of symptoms in heterozygotes and homozygotes is similar, appears to have a somewhat accelerated time course from onset to death in homozygous individuals, compared with that of heterozygotes.

Incompletely Dominant Inheritance

As introduced in Chapter 4, achondroplasia (Case 2) is an incompletely dominant skeletal disorder (short-limbed dwarfism and large head) caused by certain variants in the fibroblast growth factor receptor 3 gene (*FGFR3*). Most individuals with achondroplasia have

TABLE 7.3 Autosomal Dominant Inheritance

One Affected Parent and One Unaffected Parent			Parent 2 Genotype d/d Gametes		Risk for Disease
			d	d	
Parent 1 genotype D/d	Gametes	D	D/d	D/d	½ Affected (D/d) ½ Unaffected (d/d)
		d	d/d	d/d	
Two Affected Parents			Parent 2 genotype D/d gametes		**Risk for Disease**
			D	d	
Parent 1 genotype D/d	Gametes	D	D/D	D/d	Strictly dominant ¾ Affected (D/D and D/d) ¼ Unaffected (d/d) Incompletely dominant ¼ Severely affected (D/D) ½ Affected (D/d) ¼ Unaffected (d/d)
		d	D/d	d/d	

The pathogenic allele causing dominantly inherited disease is denoted by uppercase D; the normal or wild-type allele is denoted by lowercase d.

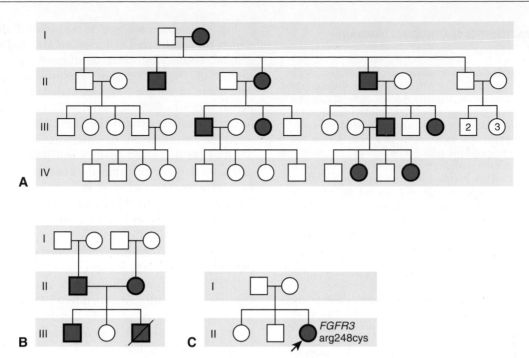

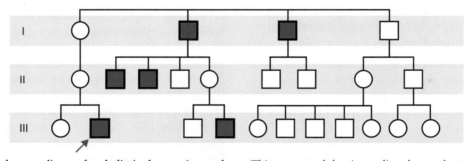

Figure 7.6 (A) Pedigree showing typical inheritance of a form of adult-onset progressive sensorineural hearing loss (DFNA1) inherited as an autosomal dominant trait. (B) Pedigree showing inheritance of achondroplasia, an incompletely dominant (or semidominant) trait. (C) Pedigree showing a sporadic case of thanatophoric dwarfism, a genetic lethal, in the proband (*arrow*).

Figure 7.7 Part of a large pedigree of male-limited precocious puberty. This autosomal dominant disorder can be transmitted by affected males or by unaffected carrier females. Male-to-male transmission shows that inheritance is autosomal, not X linked. Transmission of the trait through carrier females shows that inheritance cannot be Y linked. *Arrow* indicates proband.

normal intelligence and lead normal lives within their physical capabilities. A pedigree with two parents heterozygous for the most common pathogenic variant that causes achondroplasia is shown in Fig. 7.6B. The deceased child, individual III-3, was a homozygote for the condition and had a disorder far more severe than in either parent, resulting in death soon after birth.

Sex-Limited Phenotype in Autosomal Dominant Disease

As discussed earlier for the autosomal recessive condition, hemochromatosis, autosomal dominant phenotypes may also demonstrate a sex ratio that differs significantly from 1:1. Extreme divergence of the sex ratio is seen in **sex-limited phenotypes**, in which the defect is transmitted as an autosomal trait but expressed in only one sex. An example is male-limited precocious puberty, an autosomal dominant disorder in which affected boys develop secondary sexual characteristics and undergo an adolescent growth

spurt at ~4 years of age. In some families, the cause has been traced to variants in the *LCGR* gene, which encodes the receptor for luteinizing hormone; these pathogenic variants constitutively activate the receptor's signaling action, even in the absence of its hormone. The defect shows no effect in heterozygous females. The pedigree in Fig. 7.7 shows that, although the disease can be transmitted by unaffected (nonpenetrant carrier) females, it can also be transmitted directly from father to son, showing that it is autosomal, not X linked.

For disorders in which affected males do not reproduce, however, it is not always easy to distinguish sex-limited autosomal inheritance from X-linked inheritance, because the critical evidence—absence of **male-to-male transmission,** cannot be provided. In that case, other lines of evidence, particularly gene mapping to learn whether the responsible gene maps to the X chromosome or to an autosome (see Chapter 11), can determine the pattern of inheritance and the consequent recurrence risk (Box 7.1).

Effect of Incomplete Penetrance, Variable Expressivity, and New Mutations on Autosomal Dominant Inheritance Patterns

Some of the difficulties raised by incomplete penetrance in fully understanding the inheritance of a disease phenotype are demonstrated by the split-hand/foot malformation, a type of ectrodactyly that can be caused by pathogenic variants in the *DLX5* gene (Fig. 7.8). The split-hand malformation originates in the sixth or seventh week of development, when the hands and feet are forming. Lack of penetrance in pedigrees of split-hand malformation can lead to apparent skipping of generations. This complicates genetic counseling because an at-risk person with normal hands may, nevertheless, carry a pathogenic variant associated with the condition and, thus, be capable of having children who are affected.

Fig. 7.9 is a pedigree of split-hand deformity in which the unaffected sister of an affected man sought genetic counseling. Her mother is a nonpenetrant carrier of the split-hand variant. The literature on split-hand deformity suggests that there is reduced penetrance of ~80% (i.e., only 80% of the people who have the variant exhibit the clinical defect). Using this pedigree information to calculate conditional probabilities (as discussed further in Chapter 17), one can calculate that the risk that the consultant might herself be a nonpenetrant carrier is 17% and her chance of having a child with the abnormality is therefore ~7% (carrier risk × the risk for transmission × penetrance, or 17% × 50% × 80%).

An autosomal dominant inheritance pattern may also be obscured by variable expressivity. Neurofibromatosis 1 (NF1), a common disorder of the nervous system, demonstrates both age-dependent penetrance and variable expressivity in a single family. Some adults may have only multiple flat, irregular pigmented skin lesions, known as café au lait spots, and small benign tumors (hamartomas) called Lisch nodules on the iris of the eye. Other family members can have these signs as well as multiple benign fleshy tumors (neurofibromas) in the skin. Still others may have a much more severe phenotype, with intellectual disability, diffuse plexiform neurofibromas, or malignant tumors of nervous system or muscle in addition to the café au lait spots, Lisch nodules, and neurofibromas. Unless one looks specifically for mild manifestations of the disease in the relatives of the proband, heterozygous carriers may be incorrectly classified as unaffected, noncarriers.

Furthermore, the signs of NF1 may require many years to develop. For example, in the newborn period, less than half of all affected newborns show even the most subtle sign of the disease: an increased incidence of café au lait spots. Eventually, however, multiple café au lait spots and Lisch nodules do appear, so that by adulthood, heterozygotes always demonstrate some sign of the disease. The challenges for diagnosis and genetic counseling in NF1 are presented in (Case 34).

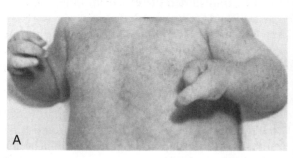
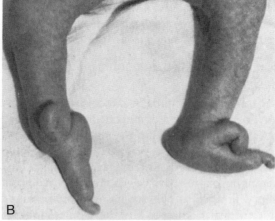

Figure 7.8 Split-hand deformity, an autosomal dominant trait involving the hands and feet, in a 3-month-old boy. (A) Upper part of body. (B) Lower part of body. (From Kelikian H: Congenital deformities of the hand and forearm, Philadelphia, 1974, WB Saunders.)

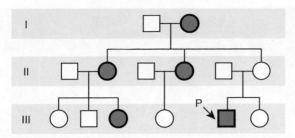

Figure 7.9 Pedigree of split-hand deformity demonstrating of non-penetrance in the mother of the proband (*arrow*) and his sister, the consultand. Reduced penetrance must be taken into account in genetic counseling.

Finally, in classic autosomal dominant inheritance, every affected person in a pedigree has an affected parent, who also has an affected parent, and so on, as far back as the disorder can be traced (see Fig. 7.6A). In fact, however, many dominant conditions of medical importance occur because of a spontaneous, *de novo* mutation in a gamete inherited from a noncarrier parent (see Fig. 7.6C). An individual with an autosomal dominant disorder caused by a new mutation will look like an isolated case, and his or her parents, aunts and uncles, and cousins will all be unaffected noncarriers. This person will still be at risk for passing the altered allele down to his or her own children, however. Once a new mutation has arisen, the variant allele will be transmitted to future generations following standard principles of inheritance; as we discuss in the next section, its survival in the population depends on the fitness of persons carrying it.

Relationship Between New Mutation and Fitness in Autosomal Dominant Disorders

In many disorders, whether a condition demonstrates an obvious pattern of transmission in families depends on whether individuals affected by the disorder can reproduce. Geneticists coined the term **fitness** as a measure of the impact of a condition on reproduction. Fitness is defined as the ratio of the number of offspring of individuals affected with the condition who survive to reproductive age, compared to the number of offspring of individuals who do not carry the pathogenic allele. Fitness ranges from 0 (affected individuals never have children who survive to reproductive age) to 1 (affected individuals have the same number of offspring as unaffected controls). Although we will explore the impact of mutation, **selection**, and fitness on allele frequencies in greater detail in Chapter 10, here we discuss examples that illustrate the major concepts and range of impact of fitness on autosomal dominant conditions.

At one extreme are disorders that have a fitness of 0; patients with such disorders never reproduce, and the disorder is referred to as **genetic lethal**. One example is the severe short-limb dwarfism **syndrome** known as thanatophoric dysplasia that occurs in heterozygotes for certain pathogenic alterations in the *FGFR3* gene (see Fig. 7.6C). Thanatophoric dysplasia is lethal in the neonatal period, and therefore all probands with the

disorder must be due to new mutations because these variants cannot be transmitted to the next generation.

At the other extreme are disorders that have virtually normal reproductive fitness because of a late age of onset or a mild phenotype that does not interfere with reproduction. If the fitness is normal, the disorder will only rarely be the result of new mutation; a patient is much more likely to have inherited the pathogenic variant, and the pedigree is likely to show multiple affected individuals with clear-cut autosomal dominant inheritance. Late-onset progressive hearing loss is a good example of such an autosomal dominant condition, with a fitness of ~1 (see Fig. 7.6A). Thus, there is an inverse relation between the fitness of a given autosomal dominant disorder and the proportion of individuals with the disorder who inherited the defective gene, versus those who received it due to a new mutation. The measurement of mutation frequency and the relation of mutation frequency to fitness will be discussed further in Chapter 10.

It is important to note that fitness is not simply a measure of physical or intellectual disability. Some individuals with an autosomal dominant disorder may appear phenotypically normal but have a fitness of 0; at the other extreme, individuals may have normal or near-normal fitness, despite being affected by an autosomal dominant condition with an obvious and severe phenotype, such as familial Alzheimer disease (**Case 4**).

X-LINKED INHERITANCE

In contrast to genes on the autosomes, genes on the X and Y chromosomes are distributed unequally to males and females in families. The patrilineal inheritance of the Y chromosome is straightforward. However, there are very few strictly Y-linked genes, almost all of which are involved in primary sex determination or the development of secondary male characteristics, as discussed in Chapter 6, and they will not be considered here. Approximately 800 protein-coding and 300 **noncoding RNA** genes have been identified on the X chromosome to date, of which over 300 genes are presently known to be associated with X-linked disease phenotypes. Phenotypes determined by genes on the X have a characteristic sex distribution and a pattern of inheritance that is usually easy to identify and easy to distinguish from the patterns of autosomal inheritance we just explored.

Because males have one X chromosome but females have two, there are only two possible genotypes in males and four in females with respect to pathogenic alleles at an X-linked locus. A male with a pathogenic allele at an X-linked locus is hemizygous for that allele, whereas females may be a homozygote for the wild-type allele, a homozygote for a pathogenic allele, a compound heterozygote for two different pathogenic alleles, or a heterozygous carrier of a pathogenic allele. For example, if X_H is the wild-type allele for an X-linked disease gene and X_h, is the disease allele, the genotypes expected in males and females are as in Table 7.4.

TABLE 7.4 Genotypes and Phenotypes in X-Linked Disease

	Genotypes	Phenotypes
Males	Hemizygous X_H	Unaffected
	Hemizygous X_h	Affected
Females	Homozygous X_H/X_H	Unaffected
	Heterozygous X_H/X_h	Carrier (may or may not be affected)
	Homozygous (or compound heterozygous) X_h/X_h	Affected

X Inactivation, Dosage Compensation, and the Expression of X-Linked Genes

As introduced in Chapters 3 and 6, **X inactivation** is a normal physiologic process in which most of the genes on one of the two X chromosomes in normal females, but not the genes on the single X chromosome in males, are inactivated in **somatic cells**, thus equalizing the expression of most X-linked genes between the two sexes. The clinical relevance of X inactivation in X-linked diseases is profound. It leads to females having two cell populations, which express alleles of X-linked genes from one or the other of the two X chromosomes (see Fig. 3.14 and further discussion in Chapter 6). These two cell populations are thus genetically identical but functionally distinct, and both cell populations in human females can be readily detected for some disorders. For example, in Duchenne muscular dystrophy (Case 14), female carriers exhibit typical mosaic expression of their dystrophin immunostaining (Fig. 7.10). Depending on the pattern of random inactivation of the two X chromosomes, two female heterozygotes for an X-linked disease may have very different clinical presentations because they differ in the proportion of cells that have the pathogenic allele on the active X in a relevant tissue (as seen in **manifesting heterozygotes**, as described later).

Recessive and Dominant Inheritance of X-Linked Disorders

As mentioned earlier in this chapter, the use of the terms *dominant* and *recessive* is different for X-linked conditions than for autosomal disorders. So-called X-linked dominant and recessive patterns of inheritance are typically distinguished on the basis of the phenotype in heterozygous females. Some X-linked phenotypes are consistently apparent clinically in carriers, at least to some degree; these are referred to as dominant. Other X-linked phenotypes are typically not observed in heterozygous females and are considered to be recessive. The difficulty in classifying an X-linked disorder as dominant or recessive arises because females who are heterozygous for the same pathogenic allele in a family may or may not demonstrate the disease, depending on the pattern of random X inactivation and the proportion of the cells in pertinent tissues that have the pathogenic allele on the active or inactive X.

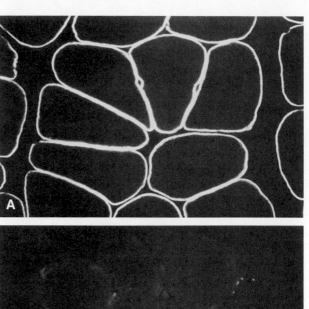
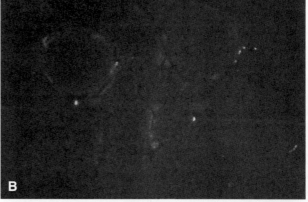
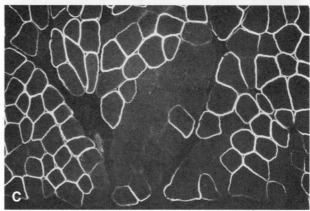

Figure 7.10 **Immunostaining for dystrophin in muscle specimens.** (A) A normal female (×480). (B) A male with Duchenne muscular dystrophy (DMD) (×480). (C) A carrier female (×240). Staining creates the bright signals seen here encircling individual muscle fibers. Muscle from DMD patients lacks dystrophin staining. Muscle from DMD carriers exhibits both positive and negative patches of dystrophin immunostaining, representing fibers with either the normal or pathogenic allele on the active X. Images courtesy K. Arahata, National Institute of Neuroscience, Tokyo.

Nearly a third of X-linked disorders are penetrant in some (but not all) female heterozygotes and cannot be classified as either dominant or recessive. Even for disorders that can be so classified, they show incomplete penetrance that varies as a function of X inactivation patterns, not inheritance patterns. Because clinical expression of an X-linked condition does not depend strictly on the particular gene involved, or even the particular pathogenic variant in the same family, some geneticists have recommended dispensing altogether with the terms *recessive* and *dominant* for X-linked disorders. Be that as it may, the terms are widely applied to X-linked disorders, and we will continue to use them, recognizing that they describe extremes of a continuum of penetrance and expressivity in female carriers of X-linked diseases.

X-Linked Recessive Inheritance

The inheritance of X-linked recessive phenotypes follows a well-defined and easily recognized pattern (Fig. 7.11 and Box 7.2). An X-linked recessive trait is expressed phenotypically in all males who receive the variant allele, and, consequently, X-linked recessive disorders are generally restricted to males.

Hemophilia A is a classic X-linked recessive disorder in which the blood fails to clot normally because of a deficiency of factor VIII, a protein in the clotting cascade (Case 21). The hereditary nature of hemophilia and even its pattern of transmission have been recognized since ancient times, and the condition became known as the "royal hemophilia" because of its occurrence among descendants of Britain's Queen Victoria, who was a carrier.

As in the earlier discussion, suppose X_h represents a pathogenic allele of factor VIII causing hemophilia A, and X_H represents the normal allele. The sons of a male with hemophilia and a noncarrier female receive their father's Y chromosome and a maternal X and are unaffected, but the daughters receive the paternal X chromosome with its hemophilia allele and are obligate carriers. Children of obligate carrier females have four possible genotypes, with equal probabilities (Table 7.5).

The hemophilia of an affected grandfather, which did not appear in any of his own children, has a 50% chance of appearing in each son of his daughters. It will not reappear among the descendants of his sons, however. A daughter of a carrier has a 50% chance of being a carrier herself (see Fig. 7.11). By chance, an X-linked recessive allele may be transmitted undetected through a series of female carriers before it is expressed in a male descendant.

Affected Females in X-Linked Recessive Disease

Although X-linked conditions are classically seen only in males, they can be observed in females under two circumstances. In one, a female can be homozygous for the relevant disease allele. This scenario is unlikely unless her parents are consanguineous; additionally the phenotype can not have a reproductive fitness of 0 in males. However, a few X-linked conditions, such as X-linked color blindness, are sufficiently common and mild that such homozygotes are seen in female offspring of an affected father and a carrier mother.

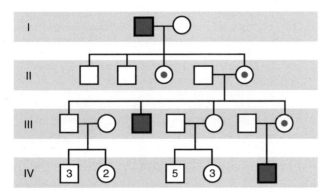

Figure 7.11 Pedigree pattern demonstrating an X-linked recessive disorder such as hemophilia A, transmitted from an affected male through females to an affected grandson and great-grandson.

BOX 7.2 CHARACTERISTICS OF X-LINKED RECESSIVE INHERITANCE

- The incidence of the trait is much higher in males than in females.
- Heterozygous females are usually unaffected, but some may express the condition with variable severity as determined by the pattern of X inactivation.
- The gene responsible for the condition is transmitted from an affected man through all his daughters. Any of his daughters' sons has a 50% chance of inheriting it.
- The pathogenic allele is never transmitted directly from father to son, but it is transmitted by an affected male to all his daughters.
- The pathogenic allele may be transmitted for many generations through a series of carrier females; if so, the affected males in a kindred are related through females.
- A significant proportion of isolated cases are due to new mutation.

TABLE 7.5 X-Linked Recessive Inheritance

Affected Male and Noncarrier Female		Female Genotype X_H/X_H Gametes		Risk for Disease
		X_H	X_H	
Male Genotype X_h/Y	X_h	X_H/X_h	X_H/X_h	All females carriers (X_H/X_h)
Gametes	Y	X_H/Y	X_H/Y	All males unaffected (X_H/Y)
Unaffected Male and Carrier Female		**Female Genotype X_H/X_h Gametes**		**Risk for Disease**
		X_H	X_h	
Male Genotype X_H/Y	X_H	X_H/X_H	X_H/X_h	¼ Noncarrier female (X_H/X_H)
Gametes	Y	X_H/Y	X_h/Y	¼ Carrier female (X_H/X_h)
				¼ Normal male (X_H/Y)
				¼ Affected male (X_h/Y)

The wild-type allele at the X-linked hemophilia locus is denoted as X_H, and the pathogenic allele is denoted as X_h.

More commonly, a female carrier of an X-linked allele who has phenotypic expression of the disease is referred to as a **manifesting heterozygote**. Whether a female carrier will be a manifesting heterozygote depends on a number of features of X inactivation. First, as we saw in Chapter 3, the choice of which X chromosome is to become inactive is random, but it occurs when there is a relatively small number of cells in the developing female embryo. By chance alone, therefore, the fraction of cells in various tissues of carrier females in which the normal or pathogenic allele happens to remain active may deviate substantially from the expected 50%, resulting in **unbalanced** or **skewed X inactivation** (see Fig. 6.12A). A female carrier may have signs and symptoms of an X-linked disorder if the skewed inactivation is unfavorable (i.e., a large majority of the active X chromosomes in pertinent tissues happen to contain the deleterious allele active).

Favorably unbalanced or skewed inactivation also occurs, in which the pathogenic allele is preferentially on the inactive X in some or all tissues of an unaffected heterozygous female. Such skewed inactivation may simply be due to chance alone, as we just saw (albeit in the opposite direction). However, in certain X-linked conditions, there is reduced cell survival (or a proliferative disadvantage) for those cells that originally had the pathogenic allele on the active X early in development. This results in a pattern of highly skewed inactivation that favors cells with the normal allele on the active X in relevant tissues. For example, highly skewed X inactivation is the rule in female carriers of certain X-linked immunodeficiencies, in whom only those early progenitor cells that happen to carry the normal allele on their active X chromosome can populate certain lineages in the immune system.

X-Linked Dominant Inheritance

As discussed earlier, an X-linked phenotype can be described as dominant if it is regularly expressed in heterozygotes. X-linked dominant inheritance (Table 7.6) can readily be distinguished from autosomal dominant inheritance by the lack of **male-to-male transmission**, which is impossible for X-linked inheritance because males transmit the Y chromosome, not the X, to their sons.

Thus the distinguishing feature of a fully penetrant X-linked dominant pedigree (Fig. 7.12) is that all the daughters and none of the sons of affected males are affected; if any daughter is unaffected or any son is affected, the inheritance must be autosomal, not X linked. The pattern of inheritance through females is no different from the autosomal dominant pattern; because females have a pair of X chromosomes just as they have pairs of autosomes, each child of an affected female has a 50% chance of inheriting the trait, regardless of sex. Across multiple families with an X-linked dominant disease, the expression is usually milder in heterozygous females because the pathogenic allele is located on the inactive X chromosome in a proportion of their cells. Thus, most X-linked dominant disorders are incompletely dominant, as is the case with most autosomal dominant disorders (Box 7.3).

> ### BOX 7.3 CHARACTERISTICS OF X-LINKED DOMINANT INHERITANCE
>
> - Affected males with unaffected partners have no affected sons and no unaffected daughters.
> - Both male and female offspring of female carriers have a 50% risk for inheriting the phenotype. The pedigree pattern is similar to that seen with autosomal dominant inheritance.
> - Affected females are approximately twice as common as affected males, but affected females typically have milder (although variable) expression of the phenotype.
> - One example of an X-linked dominant disorder is X-linked hypophosphatemic rickets (also known as vitamin D–resistant rickets), in which the ability of the kidney tubules to reabsorb filtered phosphate is impaired. This disorder fits the criterion of an X-linked dominant disorder in that both sexes are affected, although the serum phosphate level is less depressed and the rickets less severe in heterozygous females than in affected males.

X-Linked Dominant Disorders With Male Lethality

Although most X-linked conditions are typically apparent only in males, a few rare X-linked defects are expressed exclusively, or almost exclusively, in females.

TABLE 7.6 X-Linked Dominant Inheritance

Unaffected Male and Affected Female		Female Genotype X_D/X_d Gametes		Risk for Disease
		X_D	X_d	
Male Genotype X_d/Y	Gametes $\quad X_d$ Y	X_D/X_d X_D/Y	X_d/X_d X_d/Y	¼ Affected females (X_D/X_d) ¼ Unaffected females (X_d/X_d) ¼ Affected males (X_D/Y) ¼ Unaffected males (X_d/Y)
Affected Male and Affected Female		Female Genotype X_d/X_d Gametes		Risk for Disease
		X_d	X_d	
Male Genotype X_D/Y	Gametes $\quad X_D$ Y	X_D/X_d X_d/Y	X_D/X_d X_d/Y	All females affected (X_D/X_d) All males unaffected (X_d/Y)

The wild-type allele at the hypophosphatemic rickets locus is denoted as X_d, and the pathogenic allele is denoted as X_D.

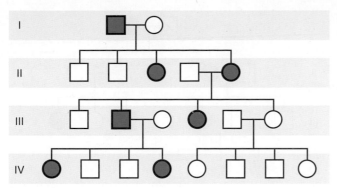

Figure 7.12 Pedigree pattern demonstrating X-linked dominant inheritance.

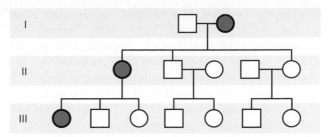

Figure 7.13 Pedigree pattern demonstrating X-linked dominant inheritance of a disorder that is lethal in males during the prenatal period.

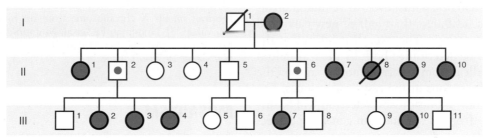

Figure 7.14 Pedigree pattern of familial female epilepsy and cognitive impairment, demonstrating its X-linked dominant inheritance with sparing of males hemizygous for a premature termination variant in the *PCDH19* gene.

These X-linked dominant conditions are lethal in males before birth (Fig. 7.13). Typical pedigrees of these conditions show transmission by affected females, who produce affected daughters, normal daughters, and normal sons in equal proportions (1:1:1); affected liveborn males are not seen.

Rett syndrome (Case 40) is a striking disorder that occurs nearly exclusively in females and meets all criteria for being an X-linked dominant disorder that is usually lethal in hemizygous males. The syndrome is characterized by normal prenatal and neonatal growth and development, followed by the rapid onset of neurologic symptoms in affected girls. The disease mechanism is thought to reflect abnormalities in the regulation of a set of genes in the developing brain; the cause of male lethality is unknown but presumably reflects a requirement during early development for at least one functional copy of the *MECP2* gene on the X chromosome.

X-Linked Dominant Disorders With Male Sparing

Other disorders are manifest only in carrier females because hemizygous males are largely spared the consequences of the variant they carry. One such disorder is female-limited, X-linked epilepsy and cognitive impairment. Affected females are asymptomatic at birth and appear to be developing normally but begin to have seizures, generally in the second year of life, after which development begins to regress. Most affected females go on to be developmentally delayed, which can vary from mild to severe. In contrast, male hemizygotes in

the same families are completely unaffected (Fig. 7.14). The disorder is due to loss-of-function variants in the protocadherin gene 19, an X-linked gene that encodes a cell surface molecule expressed on neurons in the central nervous system.

The explanation for this unusual pattern of inheritance is not clear. It is hypothesized that the epilepsy occurs in females because **mosaicism** for expression of protocadherin 19, resulting from random X inactivation in the brain, disrupts communication between groups of neurons with and without the cell surface protein. Neurons in males uniformly lack the cell surface molecule, but their brains are apparently spared cell-cell miscommunication by a different, compensating protocadherin.

Relationship Between New Mutation and Fitness in X-Linked Disorders

Just as with autosomal dominant disorders, new mutations account for a significant fraction of isolated cases of many X-linked diseases. Males carrying variants causing X-linked disorders are exposed to selection that is complete for some disorders, partial for others, and absent for still others, depending on the fitness of the genotype. Males carrying pathogenic alleles for X-linked disorders such as Duchenne muscular dystrophy (Case 14)—a disease of muscle that affects young boys, do not reproduce. Fitness of affected males is currently 0, although the situation may change as a result of advances in research aimed at therapy for affected boys (see Chapter 14). In contrast, individuals with hemophilia (Case 21) also have reduced fitness, but the condition is not a genetic lethal. Affected males have, on average, ~70% as many offspring as unaffected males do, and fitness of affected males is therefore ~0.70. This fitness may also increase with improvements in the treatment of this disease.

When fitness is reduced, the pathogenic alleles that these males carry are lost from the population. In contrast to autosomal dominant conditions, however, pathogenic alleles for X-linked diseases with reduced fitness may be partially or completely protected from selection when present in females. Thus, even in X-linked disorders with a fitness of 0, less than half of new cases will be due to new mutations. The overall incidence of the disease, then, will be determined both by the transmittal of a pathogenic allele from a carrier mother and by the rate of *de novo* mutations at the responsible locus. The balance between new mutation and selection will be discussed more fully from the **population genetics** perspective in Chapter 10.

PSEUDOAUTOSOMAL INHERITANCE

As we first saw in Chapter 2, meiotic recombination between X-linked loci only occurs between the two homologous X chromosomes and is, therefore, restricted to females. X-linked loci do not participate in meiotic recombination in males, who have a Y chromosome and only one X chromosome. There are, however, a small number of contiguous loci, located at the tips of the p and q arms of the sex chromosomes, that are homologous between X and Y and recombine in male meiosis. As a consequence, during spermatogenesis, a pathogenic allele at one of these loci on the X chromosome can be transferred onto the Y chromosome and passed on to male offspring, thereby demonstrating the male-to-male transmission characteristic of autosomal inheritance. Because these unusual loci on the X and Y mimic autosomal inheritance but are not located on an autosome, they are referred to as pseudoautosomal loci; the segments of the X and Y chromosomes where they are located are referred to as the **pseudoautosomal regions**.

One example of a disease caused by a pathogenic variant at a pseudoautosomal locus is dyschondrosteosis, a dominantly inherited skeletal dysplasia with disproportionate short stature and deformity of the forearms. Although a greater prevalence in females than in males initially suggested an X-linked dominant disorder, the presence of male-to-male transmission clearly ruled out strict X-linked inheritance (Fig. 7.15). Variants in the *SHOX* or *SHOXY* gene, located in the pseudoautosomal region on Xp and Yp, respectively, are responsible for this condition.

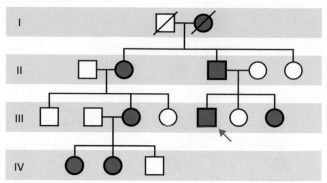

Figure 7.15 Pedigree showing inheritance of dyschondrosteosis due to variants in *SHOX*, a pseudoautosomal gene on the X and Y chromosomes. The *arrow* shows a male who inherited the trait on his Y chromosome from his father. His father, however, inherited the trait on his X chromosome from his mother. From Shears DJ, Vassal HJ, Goodman FR, et al: Mutation and deletion of the pseudoautosomal gene SHOX cause Leri-Weill dyschondrosteosis, *Nat Genet* 19:70–73, 1998.

MOSAICISM

Although we are used to thinking of ourselves as being composed of cells that all carry the same complement of genes and chromosomes, this is in reality an oversimplified view. Mosaicism is the presence in an individual or a tissue of at least two cell lineages that differ genetically but are derived from a single **zygote**. Mutations that occur after conception in a single cell in either prenatal or postnatal life can give rise to clones of cells genetically different from the original zygote because, given the nature of DNA replication, the altered allele will persist in all the clonal descendants of that cell (Fig. 7.16). Mosaicism for numeric or structural abnormalities of chromosomes is a clinically important phenomenon (see Chapters 5 and 17), and **somatic mutation** is recognized as the major contributor to most types of cancer (see Chapter 16).

Mosaicism can affect any cells or tissue within a developing embryo or at any point from after conception to adulthood. It can be a diagnostic dilemma to determine just how widespread the mosaic pattern is. For example, the population of cells that carry a mutation in a mosaic pregnancy might be (a) found only in extraembryonic tissue and not in the embryo proper (**confined placental mosaicism**, see Chapter 18), (b) present in some tissues of the embryo but not in the gametes (pure somatic mosaicism), (c) restricted to the gamete lineage only and nowhere else (pure **germline mosaicism**), or (d) present in both somatic lineages and the **germline**. This all depends on whether the mutation occurred before or after the separation of the **inner cell mass**, the germline cells, and the somatic cells during embryogenesis (see Chapter 18). Because there are ~30 mitotic divisions in the cells of the germline before meiosis in the female and several hundred in the male (see Chapter 2), there is ample opportunity for mutation to occur in germline

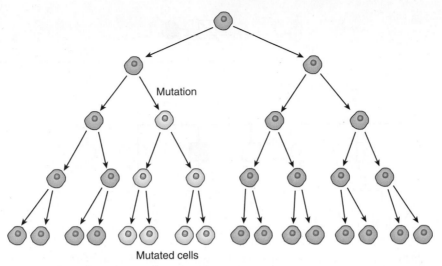

Figure 7.16 Schematic representation of a mutation occurring after conception, during mitotic cell divisions. Such a mutation can lead to a proportion of cells carrying the mutation – that is, to either somatic or germline mosaicism, depending on the stage of embryonic or postnatal development where the mutation occurred.

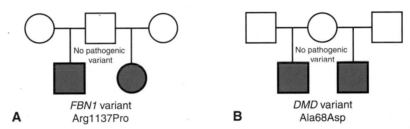

Figure 7.17 Pedigrees demonstrating two affected half-siblings with the autosomal dominant disorder Marfan syndrome (family A) and the X-linked condition Becker muscular dystrophy (family B). In family A, the affected children have the same single nucleotide variant inherited from their father, who is unaffected and does not carry the variant in DNA from examined somatic tissues. He must have been a mosaic for the *FBN1* variant in his germline. In family B, the affected children have the same single nucleotide variant inherited from their mother who is unaffected and does not carry the variant in DNA from examined somatic tissues. She must have been a mosaic for the *DMD* variant in her germline.

cells after the separation from somatic cells, resulting in pure gonadal mosaicism.

Determining whether mosaicism for a mutation is present only in the germline or only in somatic tissues may be difficult. Failure to find evidence in a subset of cells from a readily accessible somatic tissue (e.g., peripheral white blood cells, skin, or buccal cells) does not ensure that the mutation is not present elsewhere in the body, including the germline.

Segmental Mosaicism

A mutation affecting **morphogenesis** and occurring during embryonic development might be manifested as a segmental or patchy abnormality, depending on the stage at which the mutation occurred and the lineage of the somatic cell in which it originated. For example, NF1 (Case 34) is sometimes segmental, affecting only one part of the body. Segmental NF1 is caused by somatic mosaicism for the outcome of a mutation that occurred after conception. Although the parents of such an individual would be unaffected and considered not at risk for transmitting the

mutated allele, a patient with segmental NF1 could be at risk for having an affected child, whose phenotype would be typical for NF1; that is, not segmental. Whether the individual is at risk for transmitting the defect will depend on whether the mutation occurred before separation of germline cells from the somatic cell line.

Germline Mosaicism

In pedigrees with **germline mosaicism**, unaffected individuals with no evidence of a given disease-causing mutation in their genome (as evidenced by the failure to find an altered allele the mutation in DNA extracted from their peripheral white blood cells) may still be at risk for having more than one child who inherited the mutation from them (Fig. 7.17). The existence of germline mosaicism means that geneticists and genetic counselors must be aware that normal examination results and normal gene test results of the parents of a child with an autosomal dominant or X-linked phenotype do not necessarily mean there is no risk of recurrence. The impact of this possibility on risk assessment will be discussed further in Chapter 17.

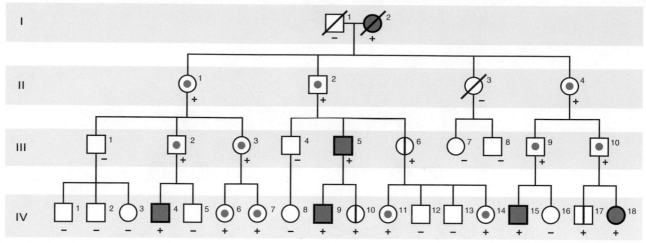

Figure 7.18 Pedigree of a family with paraganglioma syndrome 1 caused by a variant in the *SDHD* gene. Individuals II-1, II-2, II-4, III-2, III-3, III-9, III-10, IV-6, IV-7, IV-11, and IV-14 each inherited the variant from their mothers but are unaffected. However, when the males in this group pass on the variant, those children can be affected. In addition to the imprinting, the family demonstrates the effect of reduced and age-dependent penetrance in the children (III-6, IV-10, IV-17) of heterozygous fathers. The + and − symbols refer to the presence or absence of the *SDHD* variant in this family.

PARENT-OF-ORIGIN EFFECTS ON INHERITANCE PATTERNS

Unusual Inheritance Patterns due to Genomic Imprinting

According to Mendel's laws of heredity, a pathogenic allele of an autosomal gene is equally likely to be transmitted from a parent of either sex to an offspring of either sex; similarly, a female is equally likely to transmit a variant X-linked allele to a child of either sex. Originally, little attention was paid to whether the sex of the parent had any effect on the expression of the genes each parent transmits. As discussed in Chapter 6, we now know that in some genetic disorders, such as Prader-Willi syndrome (Case 38) and Angelman syndrome, expression of the disease phenotype depends on whether the pathogenic allele has been inherited from the father or from the mother. This phenomenon is known as **genomic imprinting**. The hallmark of genomic imprinting is that the sex of the parent who transmits the pathogenic allele determines whether there is expression of the disorder in a child (see Chapter 8). This is very different from sex-limited inheritance (described earlier in this chapter), in which expression of the disease depends on the sex of the child who inherits the pathogenic allele.

Imprinting can cause unusual inheritance patterns: a disorder can appear to be inherited in a dominant manner when transmitted from one parent, but not from the other. For example, the hereditary paragangliomas (PGLs) are a group of autosomal dominant disorders in which multiple tumors develop in sympathetic and parasympathetic ganglia of the autonomic nervous system. Individuals with paraganglioma can also develop a catecholamine-producing tumor known as a pheochromocytoma, either in the adrenal medulla or in sympathetic ganglia along the vertebral column. A pedigree of one type of PGL family, caused by a pathogenic variant in the *SDHD* gene, is shown in Fig. 7.18. The striking observation is that, although both males and females can be affected, this is typically only if they inherited the variant from their father. A male heterozygote who has inherited his variant from his mother will remain unaffected throughout life but is still at a 50% risk for transmitting the variant to each of his children, who are then at high risk for developing the disease.

DYNAMIC MUTATIONS: UNSTABLE REPEAT EXPANSIONS

In all types of inheritance presented thus far in this chapter, the responsible variant allele, once it occurs, is stable when transmitted from one generation to the next; that is, all affected members of a family share the identical inherited variant. In contrast, an entirely different class of genetic disease is has been recognized, diseases due to dynamic mutations that change from generation to generation (see Chapter 4). These conditions are characterized by an unstable expansion within the affected gene of a segment of DNA that consists of tandem repeating units of three or more nucleotides. Many such repeat units consist of three nucleotides, such as CAG or CCG; the repeat being CAGCAGCAGCAG… or CCGCCGCCGCCG, for example. In general, gene loci associated with these diseases are polymorphic; that is, alleles in the normal population have a variable number of repeat units, as we saw in Chapter 4. As the gene is passed from generation to generation, the number of repeats can increase and undergo expansion, far beyond the normal range, leading to abnormalities in gene expression and function.

The discovery of this unusual group of conditions has dispelled the orthodox notions of germline stability and provided a biologic basis for peculiarities of familial transmission (discussed in the next section) that previously had no known mechanistic explanation.

More than 70 diseases are known to result from **unstable repeat expansions** of this type. All of these conditions are primarily neurologic. Here, we will review the inheritance patterns of two different diseases that illustrate the effects that different dynamic mutations can have on patterns of inheritance. A more complete description of the pathogenic mechanisms of unstable repeat disorders is given in Chapter 13.

Polyglutamine Disorders

Several different neurologic diseases share the property that the protein encoded by the implicated gene has a variable-length string of consecutive glutamine residues, which can be encoded by the trinucleotide CAG. These so-called polyglutamine disorders result when an expansion of the CAG repeat leads to a protein with more glutamines than is compatible with normal function. Huntington disease (HD) is a well-known disorder that illustrates many of the common genetic features of such disorders (Case 24). The neuropathology is dominated by degeneration of the striatum and the cortex. Individuals first present clinically in midlife, manifesting a characteristic phenotype of motor abnormalities (chorea, dystonia), personality changes, a gradual loss of cognition, and ultimately death.

For a long time, HD was thought to be a typical autosomal dominant condition with age-dependent penetrance. The disease is transmitted from generation to generation with a 50% risk to each offspring. Heterozygous and homozygous individuals carrying the abnormal allele have very similar phenotypes, although homozygotes may have a more rapid course of their disease. There are, however, obvious peculiarities that cannot be explained by simple autosomal dominant inheritance. First, the disease appears to develop at an earlier and earlier age in successive generations, a phenomenon referred to as **anticipation**. Second, anticipation seems to occur only when the pathogenic allele is transmitted by an affected father and not by an affected mother, a situation known as **parental transmission bias**.

The peculiarities of inheritance of HD are now readily explained by the discovery that the pathogenic allele is composed of an abnormally long CAG expansion in the coding region of the *HTT* gene. Normal individuals carry alleles with between 9 and 35 CAG repeats in their *HTT* gene, with the average being 18 or 19. Individuals affected with HD, however, have 36 or more repeats, with the average being around 46. Repeat numbers of 36 to 50 usually result in disease later in life, which explains the age-dependent penetrance that is a hallmark of this condition. A borderline repeat number of 36 to 39, although usually associated with HD, can be found in a few individuals who show no signs of the disease even at a fairly advanced age. The age of onset varies with how many CAG repeats are present (Fig. 7.19).

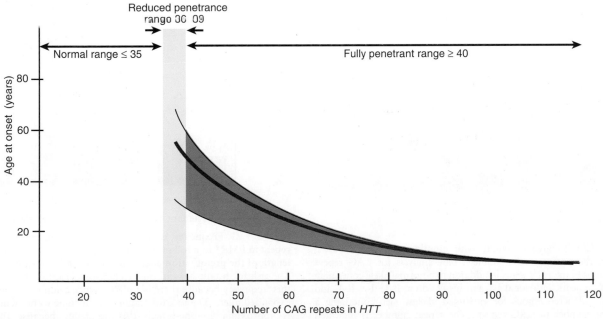

Figure 7.19 Graph correlating approximate age of onset of Huntington disease with the number of CAG repeats found in the *HTT* gene. The *solid line* is the average age of onset, and the *shaded area* shows the range of age of onset for any given number of repeats. (Data courtesy Dr. M. Macdonald, Massachusetts General Hospital, Boston.)

How, then, does an individual come to have an expanded CAG repeat in his or her *HTT* gene? First, the person may have inherited it from a parent who has an allele expanded beyond the normal range but has not yet developed the disease. Second, the person may have inherited an expanded repeat from a parent with repeat length of 36 to 39 which may or may not cause disease in the parent's lifetime but may have expanded on transmission, resulting in earlier-onset disease in later generations (i.e., anticipation). For example, in the pedigree shown in Fig. 7.20, individual I-1, now deceased, was diagnosed with HD at the age of 64 years; he was heterozygous for an expanded allele with 37 CAG repeats and a normal, stable allele with 25 repeats. Four of his children inherited the unstable allele, with CAG repeat lengths ranging from 42 to more than 100 repeats. Finally, unaffected individuals may carry alleles with repeat lengths at the upper limit of the normal range (29–35 CAG repeats) that can expand further during meiosis. CAG repeat alleles at the upper limits of normal that do not cause disease but are capable of expanding into the disease-causing range are known as intermediate alleles (previously **premutations**).

Expansion in *HTT* alleles shows a paternal transmission bias and occurs most frequently during male gametogenesis; thus, the severe early-onset juvenile form of the disease, seen with the largest expansions (70–121 repeats), is always paternally inherited.

Fragile X Syndrome

The fragile X syndrome (Case 17) is the most common heritable form of moderate intellectual disability. The name fragile X refers to a cytogenetic marker on the X chromosome at Xq27.3, a so-called **fragile site** induced in cultured cells in which the **chromatin** fails to condense properly during **mitosis**. The syndrome is inherited as an X-linked disorder with penetrance in females in the 50 to 60% range. The fragile X syndrome has a frequency of 1 in 3000 to 4000 male births; it is so common that it requires consideration in the differential diagnosis of intellectual disability or autism in both males and females.

Like HD, fragile X syndrome is caused by an unstable repeat expansion. However, in this case, a massive expansion of a different triplet repeat, CGG, occurs in the 5′ **untranslated region** of a gene called *FMR1*. The normal number of repeats is up to 55, whereas more than 200 (and even up to several thousand) repeats are found in individuals with the "full" fragile X syndrome allele. The syndrome is due to a lack of expression of the *FMR1* gene and failure to produce the encoded protein. The expanded repeat leads to excessive methylation of cytosines in the **promoter** of *FMR1*. As discussed in Chapter 3, **DNA methylation** at CpG islands prevents normal promoter function and leads to gene silencing.

Triplet repeat numbers between 55 and 200 constitute an intermediate **premutation** stage of the fragile X syndrome. Expansions in this range are unstable when they are transmitted from mother to child and have an increasing tendency to undergo full expansion to more than 200 copies of the repeat during gametogenesis in the female but almost never in the male. The risk for expansion increases dramatically with increasing premutation size (Fig. 7.21). The overall premutation frequency in females in the population is estimated to be greater than 1 in 200.

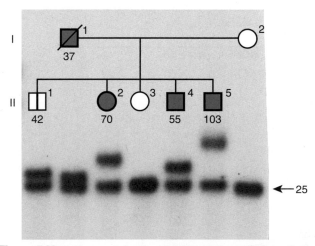

Figure 7.20 Pedigree of family with Huntington disease. Shown beneath the pedigree is a Southern blot analysis for CAG repeat expansions in the *HTT* gene. In addition to a normal allele containing 25 CAG repeats, individual I-1 and his children, II-1, II-2, II-4, and II-5, are all heterozygous for expanded alleles, each containing a different number of CAG repeats. The repeat number is indicated below each individual. II-2, II-4, and II-5 are all affected; individual II-1 is unaffected at the age of 50 years but will develop the disease later in life. (Data courtesy Dr. Ben Roa, Baylor College of Medicine, Houston, Texas.)

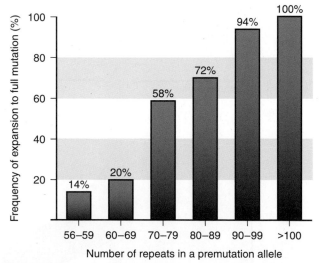

Figure 7.21 Frequency of expansion of a premutation triplet repeat in *FMR1* to a full mutation in oogenesis as a function of the length of the premutation allele carried by a heterozygous female. The risk for fragile X syndrome to her sons is approximately half this frequency because there is a 50% chance a son will inherit the expanded allele. The risk for fragile X syndrome to her daughters is approximately one-fourth this frequency because there is a 50% chance a daughter would inherit the full mutation, and penetrance of the full mutation in a female is ~50%. (From Nolin SL: Familial transmission of the FMR1 CGG repeat, Am J Hum Genet 59:1252-1261, 1996. The University of Chicago Press.)

Similarities and Differences in Huntington Disease and Fragile X Pedigrees

A comparison of HD with the fragile X syndrome reveals some similarities but also many differences, illustrating many of the features of disorders due to dynamic mutations:

- Intermediate/Premutation expansions causing an increased risk for passing on full expansion alleles are the rule in both of these disorders. Anticipation is common in both.
- However, the number of repeats in intermediate alleles for HD is 29 to 35, far smaller than the 55 to 200 repeats in fragile X syndrome premutations.
- Premutation carriers for fragile X syndrome are at risk for adult-onset ataxia (in males) and ovarian failure (in females). Intermediate allele carriers in HD are, by definition, disease-free.
- The expansion of premutation alleles occurs primarily in the female germline in fragile X syndrome; in contrast, the largest expansions causing juvenile-onset HD occur in the male germline.

MATERNAL INHERITANCE OF DISORDERS CAUSED BY VARIANTS IN THE MITOCHONDRIAL GENOME

All the patterns of inheritance described thus far are explained by variants in the nuclear genome, in either autosomal or X-linked genes. However, some inherited diseases that do not show patterns typical of mendelian inheritance are caused by pathogenic variants in the mitochondrial genome (mtDNA), which manifest strictly **maternal inheritance**. Disorders caused by pathogenic variants in mtDNA have several unusual features that result from the unique characteristics of mitochondrial biology and function.

As introduced in Chapter 2, not all the **RNA** and protein synthesized in a cell are encoded in the DNA of the nucleus; a small but important fraction is encoded by genes in mtDNA. The mitochondrial genome consists of 37 genes that encode 13 subunits of enzymes involved in oxidative phosphorylation, as well as ribosomal RNAs and transfer RNAs required for translating the transcripts of the mitochondria-encoded polypeptides. Because mitochondria are essential to the normal functioning of nearly all cells, **disruption** of energy production by pathogenic variants in mtDNA often results in severe disease, affecting many different tissues. Thus, pleiotropy is the rule, not the exception, in mitochondrial disorders.

More than 100 different pathogenic variants have been identified in mtDNA that can cause a range of human diseases—often involving the central nervous and musculoskeletal systems, such as myoclonic epilepsy with ragged-red fibers (Case 33). In this section we will focus on the distinctive pattern of inheritance related to three unusual features of mtDNA: **maternal inheritance**, **replicative segregation**, and **homoplasmy** and **heteroplasmy**. The underlying mechanisms of mitochondrial disorders are discussed in more detail in Chapter 13.

Maternal Inheritance of mtDNA

The first defining characteristic of the genetics of mtDNA is its **maternal inheritance**. Sperm mitochondria are generally not present in the zygote so that only the maternal mtDNA is transmitted to the next generation. Thus, the children of a female who has an mtDNA variant may inherit it, whereas none of the offspring of a male carrying the same variant will. Pedigrees of such disorders are quite distinctive, as shown by the strictly maternal inheritance of an mtDNA variant causing Leber hereditary optic neuropathy (Fig. 7.22). Although maternal inheritance is the general expectation, at least one instance of paternal inheritance of mtDNA has occurred in a patient with a mitochondrial myopathy. Consequently, in individuals with apparently sporadic mtDNA mutations, the rare occurrence of paternal mtDNA inheritance must be considered (Box 7.4).

Replicative Segregation

A second feature of the mitochondrial genome is the stochastic nature of **segregation** during mitosis and meiosis. The number of mtDNA copies per cell is not fixed and is substantially higher than the number of nuclear DNA copies, with cells having as many as hundreds of thousands of mtDNA copies. In addition there is no fixed **phase** of the cell cycle for the replication of mtDNA. At cell division, the copies of mtDNA in each of the

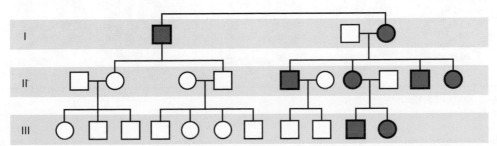

Figure 7.22 Pedigree of Leber hereditary optic neuropathy, a form of adult-onset blindness caused by a defect in mitochondrial DNA. Inheritance is only through the maternal lineage, in agreement with the known maternal inheritance of mitochondrial DNA. Note that no affected male transmits the disease.

mitochondria in each cell sort randomly to the daughter cells, in stark contrast to the highly predictable and programmed segregation of the 46 nuclear chromosomes. This process is known as replicative segregation and can result in significant variability in manifestations of mitochondrial disorders among different tissues and/or individuals.

Homoplasmy and Heteroplasmy

The presence of a high copy number creates an additional distinctive feature in the genetics of mtDNA. The terms *heterozygous* and *homozygous*, used to describe the presence of one or two allelic variants of a nuclear gene, are inexact for mtDNA. Instead, the term for the uniform presence of an identical mitochondrial sequence is homoplasmic. When a variant sequence of mtDNA is also present, within a cell, tissue, or organism, the term used to describe this is heteroplasmic. When a sequence variant first occurs in the mtDNA, it is present in only one of the mtDNA molecules in a mitochondrion. As mtDNA replicates, the mitochondria undergo fission and fusion, and the variant and wild-type DNA are distributed randomly into daughter organelles, which – simply by chance – may contain different proportions of the two allelic variants. The cell, which now contains mitochondria containing different mixtures of mtDNAs, in turn distributes those mitochondria randomly to its daughter cells. Daughter cells may thus have different levels of heteroplasmy (Fig. 7.23). A key feature of the heteroplasmic state is that the ratio of the two allelic variants is not fixed over time and may change with further replication and cell division.

Because the phenotypic expression of a pathogenic variant in mtDNA depends on a quantitative value—the relative proportions of normal- and pathogenic-allele- bearing mtDNA in the cells making up different tissues—reduced penetrance and variable expression are typical features of mitochondrial disorders (Case 33). Most pathogenic variants in mtDNA are only present and transmitted in a state of heteroplasmy, since they would reduce reproductive fitness to 0 if they were homoplasmic. The exceptions (including Leber hereditary optic neuropathy as described earlier) cause disorders that are either incompletely penetrant or are not reproductively lethal.

Maternal inheritance in the presence of heteroplasmy in the mother is associated with additional features of mtDNA genetics that are of medical significance. First, the number of mtDNA molecules within developing oocytes is reduced before being subsequently amplified to the massive number (up to 10^6 copies) seen in mature oocytes. This restriction and subsequent amplification of mtDNA during oogenesis is termed the **mitochondrial genetic bottleneck**. Consequently, variability in the proportion of variant mtDNA molecules seen in the offspring of a mother with heteroplasmy arises, at least in part, from the sampling of a reduced subset of the mtDNAs after the **mitochondrial bottleneck** that occurs in oogenesis. The heteroplasmy of the resulting oocytes is a distribution of values based on the heteroplasmy of the mother herself. As might be expected, mothers with a high heteroplasmy for a pathogenic variant are more likely to have clinically affected offspring than are mothers with a lower proportion. Mothers may also have offspring who, by chance, are homoplasmic for the absence of a pathogenic variant.

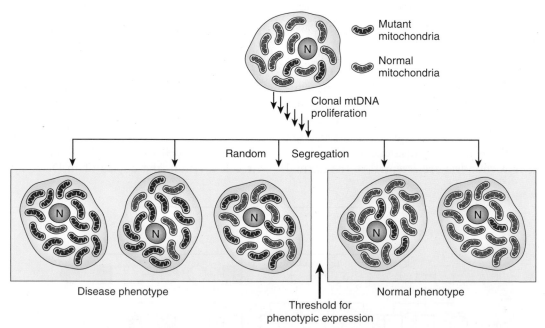

Figure 7.23 Replicative segregation of a heteroplasmic mitochondrial variant. Random partitioning of variant and wild-type mtDNA through multiple rounds of mitosis produces a collection of daughter cells with wide variation in heteroplasmy. Cell and tissue dysfunction results when the fraction of mitochondria that are carrying a variant exceeds a threshold level. *N,* Nucleus.

CORRELATING GENOTYPE AND PHENOTYPE

An important component of medical genetics is identifying and characterizing the genotypes responsible for particular disease phenotypes. In doing so, it is important not to adhere to an overly simplistic view that each disease phenotype is caused uniquely by one particular variant in a specific gene or that pathogenic variants in a particular gene always cause the same phenotype. In fact, there is often substantial **heterogeneity** in the complex relationship(s) among disease phenotypes, the genes that are altered in those diseases, and the nature of the variants found in those genes. Three main types of heterogeneity are distinguished, as will be illustrated in detail in Chapters 12 and 13. Here, we introduce them and outline their distinguishing features.

- **Allelic heterogeneity**, in which different variants in a gene may produce the same phenotype
- **Locus heterogeneity**, in which variants in different genes may cause the same phenotype
- **Clinical** or **phenotypic heterogeneity**, also referred to as a phenotypic diversity at a locus, in which different variants in a gene may result in different phenotypes

Allelic Heterogeneity

There may be more than one pathogenic variant at a locus. Allelic heterogeneity may be responsible for differences in the severity or degree of pleiotropy demonstrated for a particular condition. As one example, more than 2000 different variants have been found worldwide in the cystic fibrosis transmembrane conductance regulator gene (*CFTR*) among patients with CF (Case 12). Sometimes these different variants result in clinically indistinguishable disorders. In other cases, different variants at the same locus produce a similar phenotype but along a continuum of severity. In autosomal recessive disorders, in particular, the fact that many individuals are compound heterozygotes for two different alleles further adds to phenotypic variability of a disorder. For example, homozygotes or compound heterozygotes for many *CFTR* variants have classic CF with pancreatic insufficiency, severe progressive lung disease, and congenital absence of the vas deferens in males, whereas others with combinations of other variants may have lung disease but normal pancreatic function; still others will have only the abnormality of the male reproductive tract.

Allelic heterogeneity may also manifest in the pattern of inheritance demonstrated for a particular condition. For example, in retinitis pigmentosa, a common cause of hereditary visual impairment due to photoreceptor degeneration, some variants in the *ORP1* gene, encoding an oxygen-regulated photoreceptor protein, cause an autosomal recessive form of the disease, whereas others in the same gene result in an autosomal dominant form.

Locus Heterogeneity

Locus heterogeneity describes the situation in which clinically similar and even indistinguishable disorders may arise from variants in different loci in different individuals. For some phenotypes, pedigree analysis alone has been sufficient to demonstrate locus heterogeneity. Taking retinitis pigmentosa again as an example, it was recognized many years ago that the disease occurs in both autosomal and X-linked forms. Now, pedigree analysis combined with gene mapping has demonstrated that this single clinical entity can be caused by variants in at least 96 different genes, of which 89 are autosomal, 6 are X linked, and one is Y linked!

Clinical Heterogeneity

Different variants in the same gene may produce very dissimilar phenotypes in different families: a phenomenon known as clinical or phenotypic heterogeneity. This situation occurs with variants in the *LMNA* gene, which encodes a nuclear membrane protein. Different *LMNA* variants have been associated with at least a half dozen phenotypically distinct disorders, including a form of muscular dystrophy, one form of hereditary dilated cardiomyopathy, one form of the Charcot-Marie-Tooth peripheral neuropathy, a disorder of adipose tissue called lipodystrophy, and the premature aging syndrome known as Hutchinson-Gilford progeria.

IMPORTANCE OF THE FAMILY HISTORY IN MEDICAL PRACTICE

Among medical specialties, medical genetics is distinctive in that it focuses not only on the patient but on the entire family. A comprehensive family history is an important first step in the analysis of any disorder, regardless of whether the disorder is known to be genetic. As the late Barton Childs stated succinctly: "to fail to take a good family history is bad medicine." Despite the sophisticated cytogenetic, molecular, and genome testing now available to geneticists, an accurate family history (including the family pedigree) still remains a fundamental tool for all physicians and genetic counselors. They use it for determining the pattern of inheritance of a disorder in the family, forming a differential diagnosis, determining what genetic testing might be needed, and designing an individualized management and treatment plan for their patients. Furthermore, recognizing a familial component to a medical disorder allows the risk in other family members to be estimated so that proper management, prevention, and counseling can be offered to the patient and the family, as we will discuss in many of the chapters to follow.

ACKNOWLEDGMENT

We thank Carolyn Applegate, Jodie Vento and Cheryl Shuman for contributing to this chapter.

GENERAL REFERENCES

Bennett RL, French KS, Resta RG, et al: Standardized human pedigree nomenclature: update and assessment of the recommendations of the National Society of Genetic Counselors, *J Genet Counsel* 17:424–433, 2008.

Online Mendelian Inheritance in Man (OMIM), Baltimore, 2022, Johns Hopkins University, http://omim.org/

Rimoin DL, Pyeritz RE, Korf BR, editors: *Emery and Rimoin's essential medical genetics*, Oxford, 2013, Academic Press.

Scriver CR, Beaudet AL, Sly WS, et al: *The metabolic and molecular bases of inherited disease*, ed 8, New York, 2000, McGraw Hill. Updated online version available at https://ommbid.mhmedical.com/

PROBLEMS

1. Cathy and Calvin are pregnant for the second time. Their first child, Donald, has cystic fibrosis (CF). Cathy has two brothers, Charles and Colin, and a sister, Cindy. Colin and Cindy are unmarried. Charles is married to an unrelated woman, Carolyn, and has a 2-year-old daughter, Debbie. Cathy's parents are Bob and Betty. Betty's sister Barbara is the mother of Cathy's husband, Calvin. There is no family history of CF except for Donald.
   a. Sketch the pedigree, using standard symbols.
   b. Which people in this pedigree are obligate heterozygotes? Which are likely heterozygotes?

2. George and Grace, who have normal hearing, have eight children; two of their five daughters and two of their three sons have congenital hearing loss. Another couple, Harry and Helen, both with normal hearing, also have eight children; two of their six daughters and one of their two sons are hearing impaired. A third couple, Gilbert and Gisele, each with congenital hearing loss, have four children, who are all affected by hearing loss. Gilbert and Gisele's daughter Hedy marries Horace, a hearing impaired son of George and Grace, and Hedy and Horace in turn have four hearing impaired children. Hedy and Horace's eldest son Isaac marries Ingrid, a daughter of Harry and Helen; although both Isaac and Ingrid are hearing impaired, their six sons all have normal hearing. Sketch the pedigree and answer the following questions. (Hint: How many different types of congenital hearing loss are segregating in this pedigree?)
   a. State the probable genotypes of Isaac and Ingrid's children.
   b. Why are all the children of Gilbert and Gisele and of Hedy and Horace hearing impaired?

3. Consider the following situations:
   a. Retinitis pigmentosa occurs in X-linked and autosomal forms.
   b. Two parents each have a typical case of familial hypercholesterolemia: hypercholesterolemia, arcus corneae, tendinous xanthomas, and deficiency of low-density lipoprotein (LDL) receptors, and family history of the disorder. Their child has very high plasma cholesterol level at birth and within a few years develops xanthomas and generalized atherosclerosis.
   c. A couple with normal vision, from an isolated community, have a child with autosomal recessive gyrate atrophy of the retina. The child grows up, marries another member (with normal vision) of the same community, and has a child with the same eye disorder.
   d. A child has severe neurofibromatosis 1 (NF1). Her father is phenotypically normal; her mother seems clinically normal but has several large café au lait spots and areas of hypopigmentation; slit-lamp examination shows a few Lisch nodules (hamartomatous growths on the iris).
   e. Parents of normal stature have a child with achondroplasia.
   f. An adult male with myotonic dystrophy has cataracts, frontal balding, and hypogonadism, in addition to myotonia.
   g. A man with vitamin D-resistant rickets transmits the condition to all his daughters, who have a milder form of the disease than their father; none of his sons is affected. The daughters have approximately equal numbers of unaffected sons, affected sons, unaffected daughters, and affected daughters, the affected sons being more severely affected than their affected sisters.
   h. A boy has progressive muscular dystrophy with onset in early childhood and is wheelchair-bound by age 12 years. An unrelated man also has progressive muscular dystrophy but is still ambulant at the age of 30 years. Molecular analysis shows that the individuals have a large but different deletion in the dystrophin gene.
   Which of the concepts listed here are illustrated by situations a. to h.?
   - Variable expressivity
   - Consanguinity
   - X-linked dominant inheritance
   - New mutation
   - Allelic heterogeneity
   - Locus heterogeneity
   - Homozygosity for an autosomal dominant trait
   - Pleiotropy

4. Don and his maternal grandfather Barry both have hemophilia A. Don's partner Diane is his maternal first cousin. Don and Diane have one son, Edward, and two daughters,

continued

PROBLEMS—CONT'D

Elise and Emily, all of whom have hemophilia A. They also have an unaffected daughter, Enid.
a. Draw the pedigree.
b. Why are Elise and Emily affected?
c. What is the probability that a son of Elise would have hemophilia? What is the probability that her daughter would have hemophilia?
d. What is the probability that a son of Enid would have hemophilia? A daughter?

5. A couple has a child with NF1. Both parents are clinically normal, and neither of their families shows a positive family history.
a. What is the probable explanation for NF1 in their child?
b. What is the risk for recurrence in other children of this couple?
c. If the husband has another child by a different mother, what would the risk for NF1 be?
d. What is the risk that any offspring of the affected child will also have NF1?

6. Before starting her family, the consultand (arrow) wants to know the risk that a child of hers and her husband's would have a birth defect because they are related (see pedigree). The family history reveals no known recessive disease. What is the chance that such a child could be homozygous for a variant for a recessive disorder carried by the woman who is her great-grandmother and her partner's grandmother?

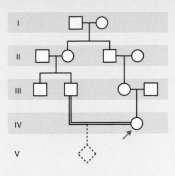

7. Given the following pedigree, what is/are the most likely inheritance pattern(s); possible but less likely inheritance pattern(s); incompatible inheritance pattern(s)? Patterns are autosomal recessive, autosomal dominant, X-linked recessive, X-linked dominant, and mitochondrial. Justify your choices.

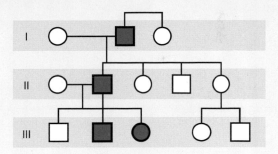

CHAPTER 8

Principles of Clinical Epigenetics

Sarah Goodman • Cheryl Cytrynbaum • Rosanna Weksberg

INTRODUCTION

Epigenetics is a nascent and quickly evolving field. As defined in Chapter 3, epigenetics refers to the study of modifications to DNA or DNA packaging that are transmissible to daughter cells and that do not involve changes to the DNA sequence. A variety of epigenetic marks and phenomena were described earlier, including (1) post-translational modifications of histone proteins, including acetylation, phosphorylation, and methylation; (2) modifications to DNA, such as DNA methylation (also referred to as 5-methylcytosine [5mC]); (3) noncanonical histone variants; (4) noncoding RNAs (e.g., long noncoding RNAs and microRNAs); and (5) X chromosome inactivation. Together, the DNA and histone modifications, as well as molecules that support three-dimensional (3D) DNA structure, constitute the epigenome. To that end, many of these epigenetic marks function in gene regulation by altering the structure of DNA and establishing heterochromatin vs. euchromatin. This modulation of the structural organization of DNA, affecting DNA accessibility and gene expression, orchestrates the cellular and temporal processes that drive normal development, including cell differentiation and steady-state variation in differentiated cells. In this chapter we describe specific topics in the emerging field of clinical epigenetics—that is, the role of epigenetics specifically as it relates to the mechanistic underpinnings of human health and disease.

Our current use of the term epigenetics is quite similar to the original definition described by Conrad Waddington in the 1940s; epigenetics is "the branch of biology which studies the causal interactions between genes and their products, which bring the phenotype into being." Today, the term also encompasses the idea of cellular memory (i.e., molecular changes that are stable and persist long after the original exposure is no longer present), which is especially pertinent to understanding the mechanistic link between environmental exposures, altered gene regulation, and phenotypic outcomes such as increased morbidity and mortality. It is now recognized that there are established pairwise associations between phenotype, genetic variation, epigenetic patterns, and environmental influence that lead us to the central dogma of epigenetics: Epigenetic patterning reflects the relationship between genetic variation and the environment and therefore represents a regulatory stratum above the genome responsible for many types of phenotypic variability. The field has also generated a new vocabulary, often modifying words from the field of genetics, to codify these newly described phenomena (see Box 8.1 for definitions of common epigenetic terms used in this chapter).

BOX 8.1 LIST OF COMMON EPIGENETICS TERMS WITH DEFINITIONS

- **CpG or CpG site:** a cytosine guanine dinucleotide (i.e., a C nucleotide followed by a G nucleotide in the DNA sequence oriented 5′ to 3′). Cytosines in CpG dinucleotides can be methylated, making 5-methylcytosines. CpG methylation is the most abundant form of DNA methylation, although there is non-CpG methylation.
- **DMR (differentially methylated region):** a set of CpGs within a defined locus, which differs between samples; samples used to identify DMRs may differ by tissue type, phenotype, exposure, etc. DMRs are regarded as possible functional regions involved in gene transcriptional regulation, especially when they overlap gene regulatory regions, such as promoters or enhancers.
- **DNA methylation:** the addition of a methyl group, typically to the cytosine in a CpG at position C5, creating 5-methylcytosines. Addition of methyl groups to DNA is carried out by DNA methyltransferases.
- **Epigenome:** the complete set of (described and undescribed) epigenetic marks. Each cell type carries a unique epigenome, which contributes to cellular identity.
- **Epimutation:** a disease-related change in DNA methylation, often occurring at an imprinted locus.
- **EWAS (epigenome-wide association analysis):** a research methodology that takes its name from genome-wide association analysis, in which variation in an epigenetic mark is assessed against a phenotype of interest.
- **Imprinted domain:** a cluster of imprinted genes and associated regulatory elements, including an imprinting center.
- **Imprinting center:** regulatory regions of varying DNA methylation levels established in the germline that act as master cis-regulatory elements to local regions of imprinted genes. Also called imprinting control region.

Recent work in epigenetics has highlighted the role of epigenetics in human health outcomes, specifically the relationship between DNA methylation and genetic variation, including genetic background or population-level variation, **polygenic risk scores**, and single deleterious gene variants. In this context, a risk **allele** can predispose individuals to a certain outcome or phenotype following an exposure, such as an adverse reaction to a medication; the underlying mechanism that drives this reaction may be epigenetic in nature and function via DNA methylation and histone modification changes. As such, if we were to measure DNA methylation in a group of individuals with and without the risk allele, with and without exposure to the medication, the methylation patterns would reflect not just the allele or the exposure, but both. These so-called epialleles represent important biomarkers of the past exposure and may be valuable in a clinical setting. For example, epialleles could provide biologic validation of an exposure to a specific toxin, such as a past exposure to secondhand cigarette smoke in an individual with a respiratory disease and a negative smoking history.

EPIGENETIC MACHINERY

The epigenetic machinery within cells consists of a set of enzymes with specific functions that maintain transcriptional programs and 3D DNA structure, collectively known as epigenetic regulators. Later in the chapter we focus on the epigenetics regulators involved in histone post-translational modifications and DNA methylation. The set of epigenetic regulators involved with histone modifications is much larger than the set targeting DNA methylation due to the large number of epigenetic marks that modify **histones**. As such, histone marks are abbreviated by the histone, the modified amino acid and its position, and the epigenetic mark. For example, H3K9ac denotes acetylation of the ninth amino acid residue (a lysine or K in standard amino acid abbreviation) of the histone H3 protein. Within the two groups of genes (i.e., histone and DNA epigenetic regulators) are so-called writers, erasers, and readers of epigenetic marks. Writers place chemical marks on DNA or histones and often carry the term transferase, which connotes this activity. A few examples include the group DNA methyltransferases, histone-lysine methyltransferases, and histone acetyltransferases. Erasers remove chemical marks and include enzyme groups such as histone deacetylases and histone demethylases. TET enzymes are the erasers of DNA methylation, for which demethylases are not known to exist. Rather TET proteins initiate a stepwise enzymatic process of methyl group removal that results in demethylation. Readers are usually nonenzymatic proteins that bind to specific chemical marks. The fourth and broadest group is remodelers. These enzymes work within large protein complexes to alter **chromatin state/3D structure**, typically at the **nucleosome** level.

This includes changing the conformation of the nucleosome DNA, the position of the nucleosome along the DNA, or exchanging histone variants within a nucleosome. The association between epigenetic regulators and **genetic disorders** will be discussed later in the chapter. Specifically, we will describe a group of **mendelian** neurodevelopmental disorders caused by **pathogenic variants** in genes encoding epigenetic regulators.

Histone and DNA modifications function interdependently, with accumulating evidence for temporal and spatial colocalization of certain groups of epigenetic marks, suggesting the likelihood of combinatorial effects. One example of this interdependency of different modifications is that regions of methylated DNA commonly lack di- and trimethylation of histone H3 at lysine 4 (H3K4me2 and H3K4me3, respectively). While DNA methylation is associated with transcriptional repression, these histone methylation marks (H3K4me2 and H3K4me3) typically occur at transcriptionally active loci. However, there are many known exceptions to these rules. The current hypothesis as to the mutual interdependence of these two marks is that the presence of DNA methylation excludes the histone methyltransferase enzyme from binding and depositing di- and trimethyl groups to H3K4. In fact, many enzymes that act to deposit or remove chemical modification to histone tails have protein domains that are sensitive to DNA methylation. For example, SETDB1 and SETDB2 are two epigenetic writers that function as histone-lysine methyltransferases; both paralogs contain a methyl-CpG-binding domain (MBD), which enables the encoded proteins to localize to methylated DNA in addition to cooperation with other proteins known as binding partners. Inversely, other histone-modifying enzymes can prevent the localization of DNA methylation machineries and protein complexes that lead to chromatin compaction. While we have an incomplete understanding of the crosstalk between DNA and histone modifications, they do not act as **isolated** units. As well, the immense number of possible combinations of various modifications and context **sensitivity** make for an exceptionally complex regulatory mechanism.

EPIGENETICS IN DEVELOPMENT

Now that we have discussed how and where epigenetic marks, particularly DNA methylation, exist in the human genome, we will focus on the critical role of epigenetics in human development. Comprehending how these mechanisms function in development will provide a context for their contributions to pathophysiology of certain diseases and disorders. Arguably, one of the most important roles of DNA methylation occurs during embryonic and fetal development, wherein it participates in regulating cell differentiation, conferring a stable cell/tissue-specific identity. As such, DNA methylation displays tissue- and cell-specific patterns. In fact, tissue of origin is one of the largest determinants of DNA methylation variation in healthy individuals, accounting for greater variation than genetic background.

Epigenetic states are most dynamic during germ cell **specification** and early embryogenesis, two time periods distinguished by epigenetic reprogramming (Fig. 8.1). Our knowledge of these processes comes primarily from studies in mice; however, recent genetic and functional data from human studies have shown that epigenetic reprogramming in the **gametes** and embryo are generally parallel in humans and mouse, although important differences are being identified that require further investigation.

During primordial germ cell specification in a fetus at ~5 weeks of gestation there is global erasure of DNA methylation followed by remethylation and **imprint** acquisition in the differentiating germ cells prior to maturing into oocytes or sperm depending on the sex of the fetus. The resulting highly divergent DNA methylation patterns are associated with distinct differentiated/transcriptional states.

Together, the DNA and histone modifications, as well as molecules that support 3D DNA structure, constitute the epigenome. To that end, after fertilization, the chromatin in the **zygote** is generally open but not transcribed. This is followed by rapid remodeling leading to zygotic genome activation at the eight-cell stage in human embryos. Prior to implantation the embryo undergoes genome-wide DNA methylation reprogramming. This comprises rapid and enzymatically driven/active demethylation of the paternal genome. By comparison, demethylation of the maternal genome occurs mainly through passive demethylation over several cell divisions. The lowest levels of methylation in the maternal genome occur at the **blastocyst** stage, at which time the two parental genomes are comparable.

Importantly, the imprinted loci are excluded from this stage of reprogramming, and gametic imprinting marks are retained (see Fig. 8.1). DNA methylation at these loci is protected from genome-wide demethylation/remethylation in the embryo. The mechanism, although not yet completely understood, involves protein complexes encoded by maternal effect genes. These genes are transcribed from the maternal genome before fertilization, generating transcripts/proteins required by the early embryo before zygotic genome activation occurs at the eight-cell stage. The majority of maternal effect genes have been studied in mice, including their phenotypic outcomes when dysregulated by a targeted **deletion**. Maternal effect genes serve similar functions in humans in that their epigenomic/organizational role is a requirement for normal developmental competence. See **Genomic Imprinting** later for phenotypic outcomes associated with pathogenic variants in these genes.

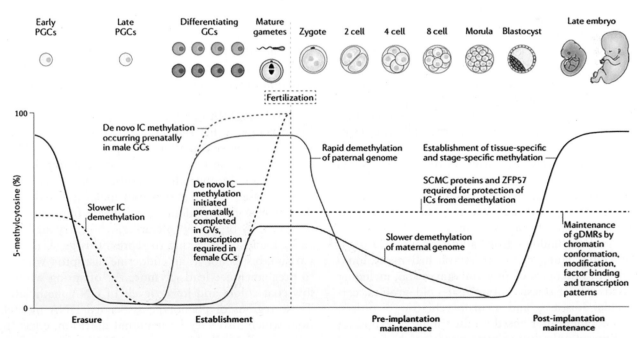

Figure 8.1 **The life cycle of imprints.** DNA methylation reprogramming during human development. Methylation of imprinting centers (ICs) *(dashed black line)* is erased more slowly than that of the rest of the genome *(black line)* in primordial germ cells (PGCs) and reestablished with different kinetics in male (paternal ICs, *dashed blue line*; whole genome, *blue line*) and female (maternal ICs, *dashed red line*; whole genome, *red line*) germ cells. After fertilization, the maternally and paternally derived genomes are widely demethylated, while differential methylation between maternal and paternal IC alleles (50% level) is maintained preimplantation and postimplantation. Factors and events involved in each stage, 5-methylcytosine level and approximate timing of imprint erasure, establishment and preimplantation and postimplantation maintenance are indicated. *gDMRs,* Germline differentially methylated regions; *GVs,* germinal vesicles; *SCMC,* subcortical maternal complex. (From Monk D, Mackay DJG, Eggermann T, et al: Genomic imprinting disorders: lessons on how genome, epigenome and environment interact, *Nat Rev Genet* 20:235–248, 2019. doi:10.1038/s41576-018-0092-0.)

Following implantation, parallel remethylation of the maternal and paternal genomes occurs in a cell-type–dependent and time-dependent manner. Precursor cells (cells that are not yet terminally differentiated) undergo a stepwise differentiation process in which epigenetics plays a critical role. For example, during differentiation, DNA methylation is required to silence pluripotency factors; the promoters of genes associated with pluripotency, such as *Oct4* and *Nanog*, are hypermethylated and silenced. As well, DNA methylation acts to upregulate markers associated with **germ-layer specificity**. In **embryonic stem cells** lacking DNA methylation, differentiation is inhibited. While some epigenetic processes are thought to drive transcriptional programs based on various inputs, spatial and temporal, other epigenetic changes are believed to enforce these changes and create a barrier that prevents dedifferentiation. The results of these tightly orchestrated epigenetic patterns are lineage-specific transcription profiles that confer cellular identity. Moreover, these profiles are maintained across cell divisions, as epigenetic patterns are mitotically heritable.

THE ENVIRONMENT INTERACTS WITH THE EPIGENOME

There is a strong interest in epigenetic mechanisms within the developmental origins of health and disease (DOHaD) field. The DOHaD paradigm posits that environmental factors during fetal development and infancy contribute to chronic disease susceptibility. The seminal research in this field identified geographic links between low birthweight in the United Kingdom associated with increased fetal mortality, as well as adult cardiovascular disease. These findings identified poor *in utero* nutrition and impaired fetal growth as contributing factors to adult cardiovascular disease, initially by observing that regions of England and Wales with the highest rates of coronary heart disease also had increased infant mortality rates in the decades prior. Further work across England and then Europe identified poor prenatal nutrition as an environmental risk for both outcomes, providing strong evidence that prenatal environment contributed to later health outcomes.

Longitudinal findings from adults exposed *in utero* to the Dutch Hunger Winter established many long-term health outcomes of prenatal starvation, including increased risk of obesity, abnormal lipid profiles, cardiovascular disease, and neuropsychiatric disorders. These outcomes differ based on the timing of exposure; those exposed only during early gestations had normal birthweights (but increased risk of obesity), while those exposed at later gestations had reduced birthweights. Importantly, these contrasting phenotypes allow us to define critical periods of development (i.e., during development) for a given biologic system where there exists a window of sensitivity during which certain environmental exposures can cause lasting changes. Here long-term metabolism was altered in response to starvation during early gestation despite the paradoxic healthy birthweights. By contrast, reduced kidney function was observed more prevalently in individuals exposed during midgestation. A continuation of work on this natural experiment also identified corresponding DNA methylation changes, suggesting a role for epigenetics in molecular architecture underlying the physiologic response/changes. Notably, insulin-like growth factor 2 *(IGF2)*, a gene that is critical to prenatal growth and cell proliferation, was found to be hypomethylated (i.e., lower methylation levels that are commonly associated with increased gene activity) in individuals exposed in early gestation, as compared to their unexposed **siblings**. By comparison, this difference in *IGF2* methylation was not observed in pairs of individuals exposed in late gestation and their siblings.

The Agouti mouse model is also a classic example of how epigenetic mechanisms act as a temporal bridge between *in utero* exposures and health outcomes in adulthood. The Agouti gene in mice, which controls fur color via melanin production, is regulated by a cell-type–specific promoter found in the second **exon** of the gene. This promoter results in gene activation during hair follicle cell development. However, the **insertion** of an intracisternal A-particle (IAP) retrotransposon in the Agouti gene results in constitutive expression of this gene (i.e., it is expressed in all cells not just hair follicle cells as the retrotransposon contains a cryptic promoter) (Fig. 8.2). This allele is referred to as A^{vy} or the viable yellow allele. The phenotype of these **mutant** mice includes yellow fur, obesity, type II diabetes, and predisposition to tumors. However, mice with the IAP insertion can have a range of pan-cellular Agouti expression, and the associated phenotypes are dependent on the levels of DNA methylation at the IAP (see Fig. 8.2). Furthermore, a diet rich in methyl donors fed to pregnant Agouti mice can alter the expression of the Agouti gene in the offspring, which will in turn impact long-term health. Mothers **heterozygous** for the A^{vy} allele, when crossed with heterozygous males and fed with a diet high in methyl donors, will more frequently produce healthy brown A^{vy} offspring, who carry high levels DNA methylation acting to repress this gene. By comparison, bisphenol A, an endocrine disruptor, when fed to pregnant mice leads to more A^{vy} offspring with yellow coat colors and lower levels of DNA methylation. These regions of phenotype-associated DNA methylation, which also vary by maternal nutrition, constitute differentially methylated regions (DMRs). The variation in fur color and health outcomes is especially striking when considering that these mice exhibiting a range of fur color and health outcomes are genetically identically individuals. These examples highlight the environmental influence on epigenetic regulation impacting physiologic outcomes, but also how DNA methylation can act as a biosensor of past *in utero* environmental factors.

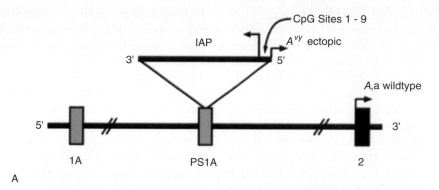

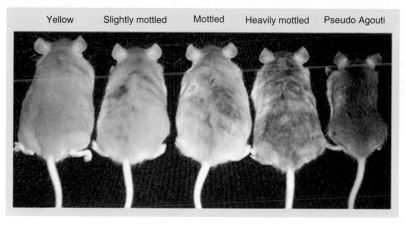

A

B

Figure 8.2 Environmentally induced alterations in the epigenome *in A^{vy} mouse.* (A) The *A^{vy}* allele contains a contraoriented intracisternal A-particle insertion within pseudoexon 1A (PS1A) of the Agouti gene. A cryptic promoter (*short arrowhead* labeled "*A^{vy}* ectopic") drives constitutive ectopic Agouti expression. Transcription of the Agouti gene normally initiates from a developmentally regulated hair cycle–specific promoter in exon 2 (*short arrowhead* labeled "*A,a* wild type"). (B) Genetically identical offspring heterozygous for the viable yellow allele (*A^{vy}/a*) in the Agouti gene representing the five coat color phenotypes, corresponding to different levels of DNA methylation and associated phenotypes, including obesity. Mice shown are the same sex and age. (A, From Dolinoy DC, Huang D, Jirtle RL: Maternal nutrient supplementation counteracts bisphenol A-induced DNA hypomethylation in early development, *Proc Nat Acad Sci* 104(32):13056–13061, 2007. doi:10.1073/pnas.0703739104; B, Jirtle RL: The Agouti mouse: a biosensor for environmental epigenomics studies investigating the developmental origins of health and disease, *Epigenomics* 6(5):447–450, 2014. doi:10.2217/epi.14.58.)

Additional evidence that environmental factors can influence the imprinting process derives from assisted reproductive technologies (ART). Originally developed in the 1970s ART was developed as a treatment for infertility caused by fallopian tube obstruction. Since then, the indications for ART have grown and include couples at increased risk for genetic disorders as well as diverse causes of female and male subfertility or infertility

ART has the potential to disrupt two critical periods of developmental epigenetic reprogramming: oocyte maturation and retention of gametic imprints following fertilization. Ovarian follicular stimulation may activate oocytes that are not yet fully epigenetically reprogramed. In addition, several aspects of ART (*in vitro* fertilization, intracytoplasmic sperm injection, and freezing of embryos) may deregulate preimplantation epigenetic reprogramming. Therefore the reports are not surprising of increased risks of adverse pregnancy outcomes: specifically, low birthweight for gestational age, preterm birth, **congenital** malformations, and increased rate of imprinting disorders, including Beckwith-Wiedemann,

Russell-Silver, Angelman, and Prader-Willi syndromes (see Genomic Imprinting, later). The risk for each of these syndromes in individuals conceived using ART is increased several fold over the general population risk (e.g., for Beckwith-Wiedemann **syndrome** this would raise the risk from 1/13,000 to ~1/2500, although the absolute risk remains low).

In humans, targeted and genome-wide molecular testing in individuals born following ART has identified DNA methylation alterations not only at a specific locus associated with known clinical entities but also variable dysregulation at multiple imprinted loci, a phenomenon known as multilocus imprinting disorder. Studies in humans and model organisms have implicated both ART processes (hormone therapy, *in vitro* culture medium) and primary subfertility issues (oocyte/sperm quality or pathogenic variants in maternal effect genes) as contributors to aberrant epigenetic programming in this complex developmental time period.

We explored earlier the important prenatal environments in relation to epigenetic and phenotypic changes;

however, plasticity does not end at birth. Across the lifespan, DNA methylation patterns continue to change in both predictable and seemingly random ways. These ongoing changes to the epigenome can be illustrated by aging and twin studies, respectively. With regard to the predictable nature of epigenetic patterns across the life span, DNA methylation is the most accurate biologic predictor of chronologic age. For unknown reasons, a small subset of CpGs sites acts as a molecular clock. Furthermore, many health behaviors and disease states are associated with an advanced epigenetic clock (i.e., a predicted age older than one's chronologic age). Significant gaps between the predicted epigenetic age and chronologic age have been associated with increased mortality and morbidity, which may reflect a relationship between DNA methylation and the aging process. However, this phenomenon is not well understood and currently provides little insight into the molecular mechanisms that underlie the aging process, a situation that will likely be clarified by future research.

The second example of DNA methylation patterns across the life span is best observed in **monozygotic twins**, who are born with nonidentical but highly **concordant** DNA methylation patterns. These relatively small DNA methylation differences observed at birth are likely related to differences experienced *in utero* despite sharing an embryonic environment. Following birth, the DNA methylation patterns of monozygotic twins become increasingly divergent with age. This well-described pattern of diverging DNA methylation patterns across the life spans of twins likely occurs in response to ongoing environmental differences as well as stochastic molecular events such as errors in epigenetic machinery. Importantly, DNA methylation differences in monozygotic twins at all ages have been associated with many **discordant** phenotypes, including psychiatric disorders (e.g., schizophrenia and bipolar disorder) and autoimmune diseases (e.g., lupus erythematosus and multiple sclerosis). This work speaks to plasticity that is mediated by DNA methylation beyond the formative years of fetal development and its role as an interface between one's environment and health outcomes.

THE ROLE OF EPIGENETICS IN HUMAN DISEASE

It was the elegant nuclear transfer experiments in mouse embryos that originally led to the discovery that the mammalian maternal and paternal genomic contributions to the fertilized egg, provided by the **haploid** germ cells, have different effects on the developing embryo. Zygotes were created carrying either two nuclei of maternal or paternal origin generating exclusively embryonic or placental tissue, respectively, but no viable embryos. Evidence in humans of the functional difference between the maternal and paternal genomes came from studying human germ cell tumors, specifically **hydatidiform moles** and ovarian teratomas. Hydatidiform moles are androgenetic in origin (two paternal genomes, no maternal genome), while ovarian teratomas are gynogenetic (two maternal genomes, no paternal genome). The histopathologic phenotype of ovarian teratomas reveals well-differentiated fetal structures of all three germ layers (**ectoderm, mesoderm, endoderm**), while the hydatidiform mole contains only extraembryonic trophoblast elements, providing evidence that the maternally and paternally transmitted genomes are not functionally equivalent. We now know that the functional differences between the maternal and paternal genomes are attributed to genomic imprinting.

CATEGORIES OF EPIGENETIC DISORDERS
Genomic Imprinting

As discussed in Chapter 6, imprinted genes are expressed from only one parental allele—that is, although two copies of the gene are present in the cell, only one copy is expressed. Which copy is expressed depends on the parent of origin and is determined by DNA methylation marks. The allele that is expressed is unmethylated, and the allele that is silenced is methylated. Although only a small percentage of human genes undergo genomic imprinting, many of these genes are critical regulators of growth and development, and therefore **disruption** of their normal monoallelic expression results in disorders that often impact both intrauterine and postnatal growth and neurodevelopment. The majority of imprinted genes are found in clusters, called imprinted domains, in specific chromosome regions (i.e., 15q11-13 and 11p15). Each imprinted domain is controlled by one or more independent imprinting control regions that regulate in *cis* the expression of target imprinted genes within the domain. More than 120 imprinted genes have been identified across the human genome (Fig. 8.3). Epigenetic changes that impact imprinting centers (ICs) and result in transcriptional silencing of a gene that is normally active are referred to as epimutations.

The first human disorders recognized to result from genomic imprinting were Prader-Willi syndrome and Angelman syndrome (see Chapter 6). These two neurodevelopmental disorders result from the absence of paternally or maternally expressed genes, respectively, in the chromosome 15q11-13 imprinted region (which contains a cluster of imprinted genes). One of the characteristics of imprinting disorders is molecular **heterogeneity** in that there are several different mechanisms, including epigenetic and/or genetic, that can disrupt gene expression. This is seen with both Prader-Willi and Angelman syndromes, which can occur due to chromosome deletions, **uniparental disomy** (two copies of a single chromosome from one parent) (see Chapter 6; Table 6.5), imprinting defects (i.e., epimutation), and pathogenic sequence variants (*UBE3A* in Angelman syndrome).

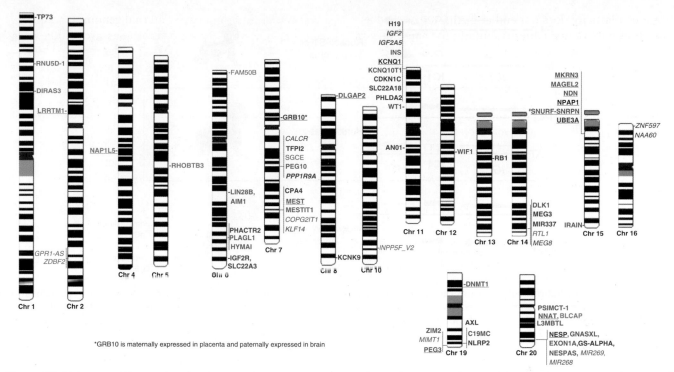

Figure 8.3 **Ideograms of human imprinted genes.** Ideograms were generated using http://www.dna-rainbow.org/ideograms/. An ideogram of each human chromosome known to have an imprinted gene based on the imprinted gene catalogue (http://igc.otago.ac.nz) and GeneImprint portal (http://www.geneimprint.com) is shown. Imprinted genes are listed on each ideogram if they were designated as imprinted in both of the aforementioned human imprinted gene catalogs. *Blue* genes are paternally expressed, red genes are maternally expressed, *black* genes have unknown parent-of-origin expression, *gray* genes have parental expression that is isoform dependent. *Bold* genes are implicated in growth, underlined genes play roles in neurodevelopment. Genes in *italic* have no reported function in growth or neurodevelopment.

Other examples of paired human imprinting disorders are Beckwith-Wiedemann and Russell-Silver syndromes, which are two clinically opposite growth disorders that result from dysregulation of imprinted genes in the chromosome 11p15 region. Beckwith-Wiedemann syndrome is characterized by overgrowth, whereas Russell-Silver syndrome is characterized by intrauterine growth restriction and postnatal growth deficiency. Beckwith-Wiedemann syndrome is also associated with an increased risk for the development of embryonal tumors. The chromosome 11p15 region contains a cluster of imprinted genes that are organized into two distinct imprinted domains, each with its own imprinting control region: the IC1 domain in the telomeric region and the IC2 domain in the centromeric region. The IC1 domain contains the *IGF2* and *H19* genes, and the IC2 domain contains the *CDKN1C*, *KCNQ1*, and *KCNQ1OT1* genes. The genes in these regions undergo parent-of-origin imprinting such that typically IC1 is methylated on the paternally derived chromosome resulting in *IGF2* expression (promotes cell growth and proliferation) and silencing of *H19*. On the maternally derived chromosome IC2 is methylated, resulting in silencing of *KCNQ1OT1* and expression of *KCNQ1* and *CDKN1C* (negative regulator of cell proliferation). Opposite molecular alterations at IC1 and IC2 lead to an imbalance of growth-promoting and/or growth-suppressing genes in this region, either resulting

in overgrowth (Beckwith-Wiedemann) or undergrowth (Russell-Silver). Therefore these conditions are mirror images of each other both clinically and molecularly (Fig. 8.4). Sometimes these two conditions can be seen in the same family when the underlying etiology is a chromosome duplication/deletion that is transmitted through a male versus a female due to parent-of-origin–specific imprinting of the chromosome 11p15 region (Fig. 8.5). The molecular mechanisms that cause these conditions are complex, and similar to the chromosome 15q11-13-related disorders include epigenetic and/or genetic alterations: cytogenetic aberrations, uniparental disomy, loss or gain of methylation at ICs (i.e., epimutation), and pathogenic sequence variants (*CDKN1C* in Beckwith-Wiedemann syndrome [Case 6]).

Whereas imprinting disorders generally result from disturbed methylation in *cis* at one imprinted locus, there are also reports of individuals with multilocus imprinting disorders (MLID) in which there is aberrant methylation of multiple imprinted loci. Individuals with MLID can present with features specific for a single imprinting disorder or overlapping features of multiple imprinting disorders. MLID can be observed in children conceived via ART or caused by pathogenic variants in the patient's genome (e.g., *ZFP57*), or pathogenic variants in maternal effect genes such as *NLRP5* or *PAD16*, which encode proteins that impact imprinted loci in **trans** (see Epigenetics in Development, earlier).

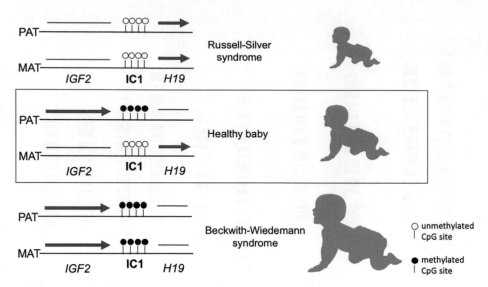

Figure 8.4 Opposite imprinting alterations on 11p15 can cause opposite phenotypes. Schematic representation of imprinting regulation at imprinting center 1 (IC1) in the chromosome 11p15 region. The highlighted box *(middle)* represents normal expression in which IC1 is methylated on the paternally derived chromosome and unmethylated on the maternally derived chromosome, resulting in expression of insulin-like growth factor 2 (IGF2) only from the paternal allele. *(Top)* Loss of methylation at IC1 on the paternal allele results in silencing of IGF2; suppression of IGF2 results in reduced growth and causes Russell-Silver syndrome (RSS). *(Bottom)* Gain of methylation at IC1 on the maternal allele results in activation of IGF2, which promotes growth and causes Beckwith-Wiedemann syndrome (BWS). Loss and gain of methylation at IC2 (not shown here) can also lead to BWS and RSS.

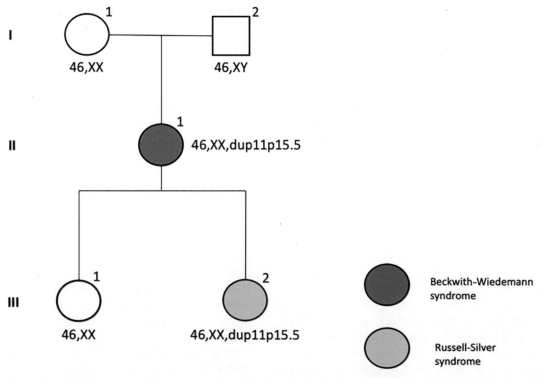

Figure 8.5 Pedigree of a family in which a chromosome 11p15 duplication is segregating; different phenotypes determined by parent-of-origin–specific imprinting. Individual II-1 has a diagnosis of Beckwith-Wiedemann syndrome, which is determined to be due to a *de novo* chromosome duplication of chromosome 11p15 encompassing imprinting center 1 (IC1) on her paternally derived chromosome 11. She therefore has two copies of paternally imprinted genes in this region and one copy of maternally imprinted genes, which leads to relative hypermethylation of IC1. When she passes this chromosome duplication on to her children, the parental imprints will be erased and replaced with maternal imprints. Therefore her daughter (III-2) who inherits the chromosome 11p15 duplication will have two copies of maternally imprinted genes in this region and one copy of paternally imprinted genes, which leads to relative hypomethylation of IC1. This is associated with Russell-Silver syndrome.

Pathogenic variants in maternal effect genes cause variable imprint dysregulation at multiple imprinted loci resulting in a broad range of clinical presentations, including infertility and adverse reproductive outcomes such as hydatidiform moles, recurrent miscarriages, and one or more imprinting disorders. Therefore, when investigating the etiology of MLID where there is a history of infertility and/or adverse pregnancy outcomes, one must consider testing not only the **proband** but also the proband 's mother.

Another consideration in the differential diagnosis of overlapping features of multiple imprinting disorders in the same individual is genome-wide paternal **isodisomy**. While genome-wide uniparental paternal disomy is not associated with a viable pregnancy, **mosaicism** for genome-wide paternal isodisomy has been reported in several individuals with overlapping features of multiple imprinting disorders; specifically, conditions resulting from uniparental disomy of imprinted chromosome regions (6q24, 11p15, 14q32, 15q11, 20q13). Genome-wide paternal uniparental disomy is typically characterized by mosaicism for paternal uniparental and biparental cell lineages. Clinical presentation depends on percentage of mosaic cells and location of the uniparental lineage.

Disorders Involving Unstable Repeat Expansions

Epigenetic mechanisms have been shown to play a critical role in the etiology of disorders due to **unstable repeat expansions** (see Chapter 13). This has been well established for fragile X syndrome, where the expansion of the *FMR1* CGG repeat to a full **mutation** triggers a cascade of epigenetic events, including methylation of the *FMR1* promotor, which leads to reduced or absent production of the fragile X mental retardation protein (FMRP). In males with normal size *FMR1* alleles, the *FMR1* promotor is unmethylated resulting in an open chromatin conformation that allows access of **transcription factors** to the *FMR1* promoter, leading to **transcription** of FMRP. The importance of DNA methylation in mediating the expression of FMRP is illustrated by rare cases of males with full *FMR1* expansion and normal cognition, in whom the *FMR1* promoter has been shown to remain unmethylated.

Many unstable repeat expansion disorders demonstrate **anticipation**, whereby increased disease severity and decreased age of onset are observed in subsequent generations. The basis of anticipation is the tendency for unstable repeats to undergo expansion when transmitted from parent to child. It has been proposed that epigenetic factors are involved in both disease pathogenesis and repeat instability. For example, congenital myotonic dystrophy (CDM1) is the most severe form of myotonic dystrophy type 1, a neuromuscular disease caused by the expansion of a CTG repeat in the *DMPK* gene. CDM1 shows strong genetic anticipation, as well as altered patterns of DNA methylation. Specifically, in individuals with CDM1, *cis*-regulatory elements upstream and downstream of the *DMPK* gene are often aberrantly methylated, thereby altering chromatin structure and gene expression at this locus—that is, impairment of these regulatory elements can lead to increased repeat instability providing early evidence for epigenetic involvement in genetic anticipation.

Disorders of the Epigenetic Machinery

Advances in **genome sequencing** technology have accelerated the discovery of genes involved in mendelian disorders. Over the last decade, an increasing number of mendelian disorders have been recognized to be caused by sequence variants in genes that are important for maintaining normal epigenetic regulation, including writers, erasers, readers, and chromatin remodelers. Although the majority of these syndromes are caused by loss of function of a single allele (haploinsufficiency) suggesting that these proteins function in a dosage-sensitive manner, both autosomal **recessive** and X-linked recessive patterns of inheritance are also described. In contrast to classical imprinting disorders that impact imprinted genes in *cis*, for this group of disorders the epigenetic dysregulation occurs in *trans*, impacting multiple genomic-wide targets. To date, there are over 80 disorders of the epigenetic machinery that have been identified and likely many more yet to be recognized (Fig. 8.6). These disorders are characterized by a wide range of multisystem **anomalies**, with the two most common phenotypic features observed being intellectual disability and growth dysregulation. Several of these disorders will be discussed later.

Disorders of the Epigenetic Machinery: DNA Methylation

There are a small number of genes that regulate DNA methylation marks in contrast to those that regulate histones; these include writers, readers, and erasers. Pathogenic variants in each of these genes are associated with specific phenotypes. Heterozygous germline pathogenic loss-of-function variants in the DNA methyltransferase *DNMT3A* (a writer) cause Tatton-Brown-Rahman syndrome (TBRS), a nonprogressive neurodevelopmental disorder characterized by increased growth, intellectual disability, and dysmorphic facial features. While constitutional pathogenic variants in *DNMT3A* cause TBRS, somatically acquired pathogenic variants in *DNMT3A* are associated with over 20% of acute myeloid leukemia (AML) cases. Notably the same pathogenic variants have been reported in association with both AML and TBRS; however, AML rarely occurs in individuals with TBRS, emphasizing the requirement for multistep

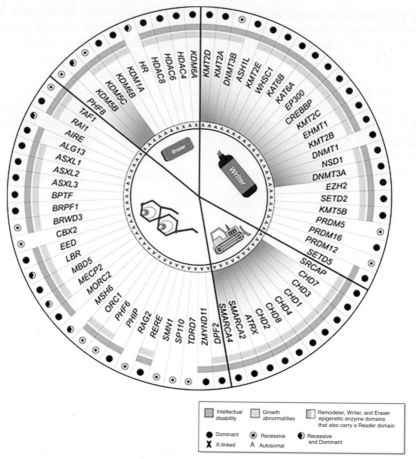

Figure 8.6 Mendelian disorders of the epigenetic machinery. Over 70 genes with defined epigenetic domains (reader, writer, eraser, remodeler, middle icons) have been linked to mendelian phenotypes. The majority of genes cause disease in the heterozygous state *(filled circle)*. Enzyme domains (writer, eraser, remodeler) are mutually exclusive in any given factor but many coexist with a reader domain *(gray shading)*. Intellectual disability is seen in the vast majority *(blue)*, as are growth abnormalities *(orange)*. A = genes on autosomes; X = genes on the X chromosome. (Modified from Fahrner JA, Bjornsson HT: Mendelian disorders of the epigenetic machinery: postnatal malleability and therapeutic prospects, *Human Molecul Genet* 28(2):R254–R264, 2019.)

deregulation in cancer. Although there is an increased cancer (myeloid neoplasms, including AML) risk above the baseline population risk in individuals with TBRS, this does not meet the threshold for clinical surveillance; therefore cancer screening is not recommended for these individuals. There are other epigenetic regulators associated with mendelian disorders for which somatically acquired pathogenic variants are involved in cancers, including *NSD1* and *EZH2*, which encode two histone methyltransferases (writers). Similarly, the phenotypes associated with germline pathogenic variants in these genes (Sotos syndrome and Weaver syndrome, respectively) have an increased cancer risk above the baseline population risk, which does not meet the threshold for clinical surveillance.

Of interest, pathogenic variants in *DNMT1*, the maintenance methyltransferase, are associated with two distinct progressive adult-onset neurologic disorders. These are the only adult-onset conditions associated with pathogenic variants in an epigenetic regulator that we currently recognize and likely result from the ongoing loss of the cell's capacity to maintain critical DNA methylation marks. The specific phenotype is determined by the position of the pathogenic variants in the gene. Hereditary sensory and autonomic neuropathy type 1 with dementia and hearing loss *(HSAN1E)*, associated with variants in exon 20, is a disorder that presents in early adulthood with sensory neuropathy and hearing loss and progresses to dementia. The second syndrome, associated with variants in exon 21 of *DNMT1*, is called autosomal dominant cerebellar ataxia, deafness and narcolepsy and is characterized by adult-onset of narcolepsy followed by the onset of sensorineural deafness, cerebellar ataxia, and ultimately dementia.

Methyl-CpG-binding protein 2 *(MeCP2)*, which functions as a reader of DNA methylation marks, has been studied extensively in part because pathogenic variants in this gene cause a well-recognized neurodevelopmental disorder, Rett syndrome (Case 40), which is characterized by acquired microcephaly, progressive intellectual disability, and loss of motor skills beginning in the first year of life. The majority (90%) of classic Rett syndrome cases are caused by loss-of-function variants in *MeCP2*, located at Xq28. Those with classic Rett syndrome are generally girls who are heterozygous for the loss-of-function variants. When boys with a pathogenic *MeCP2* **variant** or deletion survive until birth they exhibit a severe infantile encephalopathy with seizures.

As described earlier, the TET family of enzymes acts as erasers of DNA methylation marks. Whereas disorders involving writers and readers of DNA methylation have been known for some time, only recently was the first neurodevelopmental disorder impacting the DNA methylation eraser system described. TET3 deficiency, or Beck-Fahrner syndrome (BEFAHRS), is caused by either mono- and biallelic pathogenic variants in *TET3*, which encodes methylcytosine dioxygenase and is characterized by highly variable and nonspecific clinical features, including intellectual disability, features of autism, hypotonia, and dysmorphic facial features. This syndrome can be transmitted in an autosomal recessive or autosomal dominant manner.

Disorders of the Epigenetic Machinery: Histones

The number of genes involved in regulating histone modifications is much larger than for DNA methylation and include writers, erasers, readers, and chromatin remodelers. This group of disorders often presents with overlapping phenotypes, which can make them difficult to differentiate clinically. This phenotypic overlap can be attributed to the fact that the downstream targets of the various epigenetic regulators, which include different genes, are all involved in the regulation of a common pathway to brain and organ development. This means that distinguishing individual disorders is clinically very challenging. For example, Sotos and Weaver syndromes are two overgrowth conditions with overlapping features caused by different genes that function as epigenetic writers, *NSD1* and *EZH2*, respectively. In spite of the fact that these two genes have different downstream targets, these conditions can be difficult to differentiate clinically especially in the first year or two of life. An accurate clinical diagnosis is important for anticipating the natural history as well as clarifying **recurrence risk**. Sotos syndrome is associated with significant intellectual and behavioral problems, whereas Weaver syndrome can have relatively mild or no intellectual deficits. There are also differences with respect to the types of cancers and their respective risks in these two conditions, which is important for anticipatory medical care. With respect to recurrence risks, most cases of Sotos syndrome have a *de novo* etiology, whereas Weaver syndrome is often **familial**, with a milder presentation in a parent only recognized after an affected child is born.

Phenotypic overlap can also be seen when pathogenic variants occur in genes that function as part of multiprotein complexes. In this instance the phenotypic overlap results from the fact that regulation of common downstream targets is disrupted. This can be seen in Kabuki syndrome, a neurodevelopmental disorder characterized by growth deficiency, which can be caused by loss of function variants in one of two genes with opposite functions, *KMT2D* and *KDM6A*. *KMT2D* encodes a histone methyltransferase (writer) and *KDM6A* encodes a histone demethylase (eraser), two proteins that form a complex and have complementary roles in regulating chromatin state and transcriptional activity at a specific set of target genes. *KMT2D* adds a methylation mark associated with open chromatin (H3K4me3), whereas *KDM6A* removes a mark associated with closed chromatin (H3K27me3). Both genes facilitate the opening of chromatin and promote gene expression. Disruption of either gene/protein function will disrupt the balance of open versus closed chromatin at overlapping target genes resulting in the same clinical outcome (i.e., Kabuki syndrome). Identification of the specific genetic etiology is important because pathogenic variants in *KMT2D* are inherited in an autosomal dominant manner and usually occur *de novo*, whereas *KDM6A* is an X-linked recessive gene that can have a high risk of recurrence if inherited from a phenotypically normal **carrier** mother.

There are also distinct clinical conditions with overlapping phenotypes that are caused by pathogenic variants in different genes within the same multiprotein complex. This can be seen with Coffin-Siris syndrome (CSS) and Nicolaides-Baraitser syndrome (NCBRS), two neurodevelopmental disorders that are caused by pathogenic variants in the *ARID1B*, *SMARCB1*, and *SMARCA4* genes (CSS) and *SMARCA2* gene (NCBRS). These genes are all part of the BAF **chromatin remodeling** complex. Although these two conditions have overlapping clinical features, attributable to the common downstream targets of the multiprotein complex that includes the respective causative genes, they also have important differences in natural history that require gene-based diagnosis for optimal management.

DIAGNOSTIC TESTING FOR EPIGENETIC DISORDERS

In light of the fact that the molecular mechanisms that cause imprinting disorders are heterogeneous, one must often utilize more than a single testing methodology to identify the underlying etiology. The hallmark of imprinting disorders is abnormal DNA methylation patterns. The most effective first line of investigation for imprinting disorders is methylation-sensitive **multiplex ligation-dependent probe amplification (MS-MLPA)**. See Chapter 5 for a description of the methodology. The benefit of using MS-MLPA is that it can assess both methylation levels and **copy number variants** across the relevant chromosome region; that is, it can distinguish between methylation abnormalities due to a deletion, uniparental disomy, or imprinting defect. In the case where a methylation abnormality is detected, additional testing may be required to determine the specific underlying molecular etiology. This could involve chromosome **microarray** analysis to look for a chromosome **rearrangement** (e.g., deletion not detectable by the targeted probes utilized in MS-MLPA) or additional molecular testing with parental samples to test for uniparental disomy. If MS-MLPA testing is negative, given the underlying molecular heterogeneity in imprinting disorders, additional testing should be considered: specifically, sequence analysis of relevant imprinted genes (i.e., *CDKN1C* for Beckwith-Wiedemann syndrome or *UBE3A* for Angelman syndrome) and cytogenetic analysis for chromosome rearrangements that can impact imprinting without a change in methylation detectable by MS-MLPA. Identification of the etiology is critical to determining recurrence risk. For instance, a *de novo* methylation abnormality, without a concomitant genetic alteration, would confer a very low recurrence risk, whereas a methylation abnormality due to a deletion at an imprinting control region could confer a 50% risk of recurrence if inherited, depending on parent of origin.

Another consideration in diagnostic testing for imprinting disorders is the fact that the underlying molecular changes may be present in a mosaic state; that is, some cells will have imprinting aberrations and some cells will have appropriate allelic methylation. This is commonly seen with chromosome 11p15 molecular alterations that cause Beckwith-Wiedemann syndrome, and accounts for some of the 20% of patients with a clinical diagnosis who have negative results following comprehensive molecular testing. Therefore one must be aware that a negative test result does not exclude a diagnosis because of the significant rate of somatic mosaicism.

Mendelian disorders of the epigenetic machinery have traditionally been diagnosed via genome sequencing, including targeted single gene or panel testing (if a specific diagnosis is suspected) or genome-wide sequencing. However, sequencing technologies have several limitations, including coverage of noncoding regions, detection of complex sequence variants, and identification of variants of uncertain significance. A promising approach to improving the diagnostic yield of genetic disorders resulting from pathogenic sequence variants in epigenetic regulators involves analysis of genome-wide DNA methylation patterns. In the last few years, unique patterns of DNA methylation alterations, called DNA methylation signatures, have been defined for over 50 different genes. These signatures are developed by comparing peripheral blood–derived DNA for groups of cases with pathogenic variants in a specific gene to controls. The utility of these gene-specific signatures as functional biomarkers for diagnostic testing is increasingly being recognized as a novel tool. These signatures can be used to classify sequence variants of uncertain significance, as either pathogenic or benign, by comparing a DNA methylation profile generated for a specific case to the genome-wide DNA methylation signature

for the gene in question and to controls. Given that the DNA methylation signatures to date have been derived in DNA from whole blood and that DNA methylation marks have cell-type specificity, the current signatures are limited to testing in blood-derived DNA samples. In the future as DNA methylation signatures are identified in other cell types, this technology can be more broadly applied.

DNA METHYLATION AND CANCER DIAGNOSTICS

Cancer, although conventionally considered a genetic disorder, often involves genome-wide epigenetic dysregulation, including alterations to DNA methylation, histone modifications, chromatin remodeling, and microRNA. Given that one important function of eukaryotic DNA methylation is to maintain genomic stability by regulating the expression of **oncogenes** and tumor suppressor genes, it is not surprising that epigenetic dysregulation often contributes to tumor development and progression. Some of this epigenetic dysregulation is driven by somatically acquired pathogenic variants in specific chromatin **modifier genes**. Such variants are frequently observed in malignant cells and can result in aberrant genome-wide methylation changes leading to inappropriately expressed or repressed genes. Pathogenic variants in certain epigenetic regulators are often a hallmark of specific tumor types.

DNA methylation patterns are becoming increasingly recognized as valuable diagnostic and prognostic tools in the cancer realm, particularly with respect to their utility in defining specific tumor types. This is especially important in tumors that escape definition by other molecular and pathologic methods. One particularly difficult challenge that can be addressed by DNA methylation is a cancer of unknown origin (i.e., metastatic disease for which the primary tumor is unknown) because the DNA methylation state of cell type at the time of tumor initiation remains identifiable during tumor development and progression. Therefore the DNA methylation profile of a tumor provides not only data about the current state of the cancer epigenome but also defines the tumor's cell type of origin. As a result, DNA methylation-based clinical diagnosis and prognosis across many different types of primary cancers are now utilized to predict the primary site of metastatic cancers of unknown primaries.

In addition to aiding in the diagnosis of tumor origin, DNA methylation-based diagnostics have been shown to play a valuable role in classifying different tumor subtypes, which can be critical in optimizing treatment/management. One example is the ability to classify tissue samples into one of over 80 central nervous system tumors, and (even more valuable) the ability to identify subgroups within a particular tumor type. This can be seen in the case of medulloblastomas, where DNA methylation signatures have enabled the subclassification so that four different subtypes are now recognized; these subtypes are associated with dramatic prognostic and therapeutic differences. We expect that ongoing advances in DNA methylation-based diagnostics in cancer will be integrated to improve the broader landscape of cancer diagnostics and treatment for patients.

TREATMENT FOR NEURODEVELOPMENTAL DISORDERS CAUSED BY PATHOGENIC VARIANTS IN EPIGENETIC REGULATORS

Historically postnatal treatment of neurodevelopmental disorders was not considered feasible because prior to our understanding of neuroplasticity the brain was considered to be a fully developed organ early in life. Early evidence for possible postnatal treatment of neurodevelopmental disorders came from studies of a mouse model of Rett syndrome, in which the restoration of Mecp2 function led to reversal of advanced neurologic symptoms in adult mice. Given that a large group of neurodevelopmental disorders result from epigenetic dysregulation and that epigenetic changes are considered reversible, epigenetic mechanisms represent an attractive target for therapeutic intervention. Evidence of the efficacy of drugs that target epigenetic dysregulation was initially noted in clinical trials for cancer. Building on this approach, epigenetic therapeutics were trialed in mouse models of two neurodevelopmental disorders, specifically Rubinstein-Taybi syndrome (RTS) and Kabuki syndrome (KS), resulting from pathogenic variants in the epigenetic regulators CREB-binding protein *(CREBBP)* and *KMT2D*, respectively. In the mouse model of RTS, haploinsufficiency of *CREBBP* results in deficit chromatin acetylation as well as intellectual and memory deficits. Treatment using inhibition of histone deacetylase (HDAC) activity ameliorates both the chromatin acetylation and the memory deficit. In the case of KS, pathogenic variants in *KMT2D* cause a closed chromatin state impeding the transcription of genes critical for normal neurodevelopment. Treatment of KS mice with HDAC inhibitors restores the normal open chromatin state at these targets, resulting in improvement of long-term memory deficits. In addition, in a mouse model of KS, treatment with a ketogenic diet (which increases β-hydroxybutyrate levels) was noted to have a similar therapeutic effect. This positive outcome was attributed primarily to the HDAC inhibitor properties of β-hydroxybutyrate. These two models provide further evidence of the potential utility of epigenetic drugs or epigenetic-based therapies in treating neurodevelopment disorders postnatally.

As of the writing of this chapter, some human clinical trials are being developed to evaluate the impact of epigenetic treatment approaches in neurodevelopmental disorders. There is a broad range of potential treatment options for neurodevelopmental disorders (see Chapter 14), including approaches that show promise other than epigenetic drugs. For example, the use of trofinetide, an IGF analog initially studied in mouse models, has now been shown to reduce repetitive behaviors and seizures in females with Rett syndrome (Case 40). Clinical trials are ongoing.

Although these data are very promising, there remain many potential challenges that need to be addressed. One of particular importance is to define the critical brain regions that harbor cells that can be modulated postnatally. In this regard, studies in mouse models of both KS and RTS suggest that hippocampal cells in the dentate gyrus have self-renewal properties that could be channeled into partially rescuing memory and learning deficits in neurodevelopmental disorders. Other questions to be addressed include navigating the blood-brain barrier and windows of opportunity for successful treatment. Furthermore, current epigenetic agents do not target loci with aberrant epigenetic patterns but alter the epigenetic status at many sites across the genome, which may be associated with a number of adverse effects in unrelated cell types and pathways. Future progress in addressing these challenges is required to enable effective treatments of neurodevelopmental disorders.

FUTURE DIRECTIONS

In this chapter we have introduced many different facets of epigenetics and their relative applications, and a number of important themes clearly arise. Foremost, there is mounting evidence pointing to a role for epigenetic changes in health risk and disease in response to both genetic variation and environmental or lifestyle influences. Such epigenetic patterns have been shown to play a role not only in mendelian disorders but also in complex diseases and health outcomes that arise from certain environmental exposures. The dynamic and reversible nature of epigenetic changes permits a level of adaptability or plasticity that greatly exceeds the capacity of DNA sequence alone and thus is relevant both to the origins and the potential treatment of disease. Current obstacles to fully understanding the role of epigenetic aberrations in disease pathophysiology include (1) the sheer complexity of the epigenome, which consists of many interrelated and context-dependent chemical marks; (2) a unique epigenome that exists for each cell type and changes across the life span, especially during development; and (3) baseline levels of stochastic and nonstochastic variation among individuals, similar to that in the human genome. A number of large-scale epigenomics projects (akin to the original **Human Genome Project**) have been initiated to catalogue DNA methylation sites genome-wide (the so-called methylome), to evaluate CpG landscapes across the genome, to discover new histone variants and modification patterns in various tissues, and to document positioning of nucleosomes around the genome in different cell types and in samples from both healthy individuals and those with cancer or other diseases. These analyses are part of a broad effort (called the **ENCODE Project** [*Enc*yclopedia of *DNA Elements*]) to explore epigenetic patterns in chromatin genome-wide in order to better understand control of gene expression in different tissues or disease states. The data from such efforts can then be channeled into refining our understanding of the role of epigenetics in human health and disease and as a platform for improving personalized medicine approaches to diagnostics and therapeutics.

GENERAL REFERENCES

Bird A: Perceptions of epigenetics, *Nature* 447(7143):396–398, 2007. https://doi.org/10.1038/nature05913

Greally JM: A user's guide to the ambiguous word "epigenetics", *Nat Rev Mol Cell Biol* 19(4):207–208, 2018. https://doi.org/10.1038/nrm.2017.135

Smith ZD, Meissner A: DNA methylation: roles in mammalian development, *Nat Rev Genet* 14(3):204–220, 2013. https://doi.org/10.1038/nrg3354

Tucci V, Isles AR, Kelsey G, et al: Genomic imprinting and physiological processes in mammals, *Cell* 176(5):952–965, 2019. https://doi.org/10.1016/j.cell.2019.01.043

Ziller MJ, Gu H, Muller F, et al: Charting a dynamic DNA methylation landscape of the human genome, *Nature* 500(7463):477–481, 2013. https://doi.org/10.1038/nature12433

SPECIFIC REFERENCES

Aref-Eshghi E, Rodenhiser DI, Schenkel LC, et al: Genomic DNA methylation signatures enable concurrent diagnosis and clinical genetic variant classification in neurodevelopmental syndromes, *Am J Hum Genet* 102(1):156–174, 2018. https://doi.org/10.1016/j.ajhg.2017.12.008

Azzi S, Abi Habib W, Netchine I: Beckwith-Wiedemann and Russell-Silver syndromes: from new molecular insights to the comprehension of imprinting regulation, *Curr Opin Endocrinol Diabetes Obes* 21(1):30–38, 2014. https://doi.org/10.1097/MED.0000000000000037

Barker DJ: The origins of the developmental origins theory, *J Intern Med* 261(5):412–417, 2007. https://doi.org/10.1111/j.1365-2796.2007.01809.x

Capper D, Jones DTW, Sill M, et al: DNA methylation-based classification of central nervous system tumours, *Nature* 555(7697):469–474, 2018. https://doi.org/10.1038/nature26000

Chater-Diehl E, Goodman SJ, Cytrynbaum C, et al: Anatomy of DNA methylation signatures: emerging insights and applications, *Am J Hum Genet* 108(8):1359–1366, 2021. https://doi.org/10.1016/j.ajhg.2021.06.015

Cortessis VK, Azadian M, Buxbaum J: Comprehensive meta-analysis reveals association between multiple imprinting disorders and conception by assisted reproductive technology, *J Assist Reprod Genet* 35(6):943–952, 2018. https://doi.org/10.1007/s10815-018-1173-x

Dolinoy DC, Huang D, Jirtle RL: Maternal nutrient supplementation counteracts bisphenol A-induced DNA hypomethylation in early development, *Proc Natl Acad Sci U S A* 104(32):13056–13061, 2007. https://doi.org/10.1073/pnas.0703739104

Fahrner JA, Bjornsson HT: Mendelian disorders of the epigenetic machinery: postnatal malleability and therapeutic prospects, *Hum Mol Genet* 28(2):R254–R264, 2019. https://doi.org/10.1093/hmg/ddz174

Fraga MF, Ballestar E, Paz MF: Epigenetic differences arise during the lifetime of monozygotic twins, *Proc Natl Acad Sci U S A* 102(30):10604–10609, 2005. https://doi.org/10.1073/pnas.0500398102

Guo F, Yan L, Guo H, et al: The transcriptome and DNA methylome landscapes of human primordial germ cells, *Cell* 161(6):1437–1452, 2015. https://doi.org/10.1016/j.cell.2015.05.015

Heijmans BT, Tobi EW, Stein AD, et al: Persistent epigenetic differences associated with prenatal exposure to famine in humans, *Proc Natl Acad Sci U S A* 105(44):17046–17049, 2008. https://doi.org/10.1073/pnas.0806560105

Horvath S, Raj K: DNA methylation-based biomarkers and the epigenetic clock theory of ageing, *Nat Rev Genet* 19(6):371–384, 2018. https://doi.org/10.1038/s41576-018-0004-3

Kalish JM, Conlin LK, Bhatti TR, et al: Clinical features of three girls with mosaic genome-wide paternal uniparental isodisomy, *Am J Med Genet A* 161A(8):1929–1939, 2013. https://doi.org/10.1002/ajmg.a.36045

Kraan CM, Godler DE, Amor DJ: Epigenetics of fragile X syndrome and fragile X-related disorders, *Dev Med Child Neurol* 61(2):121–127, 2019. https://doi.org/10.1111/dmcn.13985

Lanni S, Pearson CE: Molecular genetics of congenital myotonic dystrophy, *Neurobiol Dis* 132:104533, 2019. https://doi.org/10.1016/j.nbd.2019.104533

Moran S, Martinez-Cardus A, Sayols S, et al: Epigenetic profiling to classify cancer of unknown primary: a multicentre, retrospective analysis, *Lancet Oncol* 17(10):1386–1395, 2016. https://doi.org/10.1016/S1470-2045(16)30297-2

PROBLEMS

1. a. When in human fetal development does genome-wide epigenetic reprogramming occur?
   b. How does this type of reprogramming differ by parent of origin?

2. Genetically identical Agouti mice heterozygous for the Avy or the viable yellow allele can display a range of phenotypes, including obesity and coat color differences. Describe the underlying epigenetic changes associated with expression of the Agouti gene and nutritional manipulations that can alter phenotypic presentation.

3. Assisted reproductive technologies (ART) increase the risk of a specific group of epigenetic disorders. Name this group of disorders, as well as two specific disorders within this category.

4. Mendelian disorders of the epigenetic machinery are characterized by a wide range of multisystem anomalies; however, these diverse disorders share some phenotypic features.
   a. List two common clinical features that are often observed.
   b. Describe two epigenetic functions of the proteins encoded by genes that cause such disorders when they carry pathogenic variants.

5. What is a DNA methylation signature? What is its application in clinical diagnostics for constitutional disorders of the epigenetic machinery and in the field of oncology?

6. Name a drug with an epigenetic mode of action.

CHAPTER 9

Complex Inheritance of Common Multifactorial Disorders

Cristen J. Willer • Gonçalo R. Abecasis

Common diseases such as heart disease, cancer, diabetes, neuropsychiatric disease, and asthma cause morbidity and premature mortality in nearly two of every three individuals (Table 9.1). Many of these diseases "run in families" – cases seem to cluster among the relatives of affected individuals more frequently than in similarly situated unrelated individuals. The inheritance of these diseases generally does not follow one of the **mendelian** patterns seen in the **single-gene disorders** described in Chapter 7. This is because these common diseases rarely result simply from inheriting a specific **genetic** defect at a single **gene** (or locus), as is the case for classical **dominant** and **recessive** mendelian disorders. Instead, they result from the combined effects of multiple genetic **variants** and environmental risk factors. Together, these genetic and environmental **risk** factors alter susceptibility to disease. For this reason, these disorders are considered to be **multifactorial** in origin, and the **familial** clustering generates a pattern of inheritance that is referred to as **complex**.

The familial clustering seen with multifactorial disorders can be explained by recognizing that family members share a greater proportion of their genetic information and environmental exposures than individuals chosen at random in the population. Thus the relatives of an affected individual are more likely to experience the same genes, as well as gene-gene and gene-environment interactions that led to disease susceptibility than are individuals who are unrelated to the **proband**. The pattern is complex because the contribution of chance events and because the combined effects of multiple environmental and genetic risk factors are not easy to predict and can result in a wide variety of patterns of disease **segregation** across families.

In this chapter we first address the question of how we infer that genetic variants predispose to common diseases. We then describe how studies of familial aggregation and twin studies are used by geneticists to quantify the relative contributions of genetic variation and environment and show how these tools have been applied to **multifactorial diseases**. We describe a few examples of complex disorders where information

has emerged about the specific nature of the genetic and environmental contributions to disease. Finally, we discuss how understanding of the genetic basis of common diseases enables **polygenic risk scores (PRS)** and predictions of individual disease risk that may soon impact clinical care in prevention, diagnosis, and individualized therapeutics.

For most common diseases a number of genetic variants contributing to disease susceptibility have now been identified, mainly through large-scale genetic association studies (https://www.ebi.ac.uk/gwas/). Still, the specific genes, variants, and environmental factors that contribute to disease risk have not yet been fully identified for the vast majority of common multifactorial diseases. Completing the task and identifying all genetic and environmental factors that contribute to each disease is challenging work to which you, dear reader, might contribute – it is our hope that this chapter will give you a helpful introduction to the process.

A more detailed understanding of the approaches that geneticists use to identify the genetic factors underlying complex disease first requires a full appreciation of the distribution of genetic variation in different populations. This topic is presented in Chapter 10, after which we will turn, in Chapter 11, to discussion of the specific population-based epidemiological approaches that geneticists are using to identify the particular genes and variants contributing to conditions with **complex inheritance**.

Ultimately, finding the genes and variants that interact with the environment to contribute to disease susceptibility will give us a better understanding of the underlying processes leading to common multifactorial diseases and, perhaps, better tools for prevention or treatment.

QUALITATIVE AND QUANTITATIVE TRAITS

The first step in a genetic analysis of disease is often to summarize the disease state for each individual. For convenience, disease states for multifactorial diseases with complex inheritance are most often summarized as discrete or binary traits (classifying individuals as

TABLE 9.1 Frequency of Different Types of Genetic Disease

Type	Incidence at Birth (per 1000)	Prevalence at Age 25 (per 1000)	Population Prevalence (per 1000)
Disorders due to genome and chromosome alterations	6	1.8	3.8
Disorders due to single-gene variants	10	3.6	20
Disorders with multifactorial inheritance	≈50	≈50	≈600

Data from Rimoin DL, Connor JM, Pyeritz RE: *Emery and Rimoin's principles and practice of medical genetics*, ed 3, Edinburgh, 1997, Churchill Livingstone.

affected cases or unaffected controls) but can also be summarized using continuous **quantitative traits** or even discrete ordinal scales. At first glance, a binary classification strategy is the simpler approach; a disease, such as asthma, obesity, or hearing loss, is classified as present or absent in each individual being studied. Distinguishing between individuals who have a disease and those who do not may not always be straightforward and may require detailed examination, specialized testing, or even arbitrary distinctions and cutoff points. As an alternative to detailed examination of each study participant, many contemporary studies use automated algorithms for assigning disease states to individuals based on electronically encoded information in their medical records. A popular set of strategies in this class is the use of PheCodes, a disease state definition based on presence or absence of one or more billing, diagnostic, or procedure codes in the medical record. It's worth noting that while these strategies can be extremely practical and have enabled many successful gene-mapping experiments, they can also result in arbitrary or inconsistent classification of individual individuals (e.g., depending on the choices their health care provider might have made in diagnosis, testing, billing, or treatment). In some cases, multiple instances of a code in the electronic health record are required for a more confident diagnosis, and individuals with unclear **phenotypes** are excluded from both the case and control groups.

Quantitative traits can often avoid arbitrary boundaries between cases and controls. Instead of classifying individuals as asthmatic cases and nonasthmatic controls, we might measure their lung capacity or the number of emergency room visits per year. Instead of classifying individuals as hard-of-hearing cases or normal-hearing controls, we might use a quantitative measure to quantify the loudness or pitch of sounds each individual can hear. Instead of classifying individuals as obese or nonobese, we might measure their weight or **body mass index**. Quantitative traits are also commonly used to summarize disease-related measurable physiologic or biochemical quantities such as blood pressure, serum cholesterol concentration, or activity levels that vary among individuals within a population.

The Normal Distribution

As is often the case with physiologic quantities, such as systolic blood pressure, a graph of the number (or the fraction) of individuals in the population (y-axis) having a particular quantitative value (x-axis) approximates the familiar, bell-shaped curve known as the **normal** (or **gaussian**) **distribution** (Fig. 9.1A). The position of the peak and the width of the curve of the **normal distribution** are governed by two quantities, the mean (μ) and the variance (σ^2), respectively. The mean is the arithmetic average of the values, and because – for many traits – more people have values for the trait near the average, the curve ordinarily has its peak at the mean value. The variance (or its square root, σ, the standard deviation [SD]) is a measure of how much spread there is in the values to either side of the mean and therefore determines the breadth of the curve.

Any physiologic quantity that can be measured in a sample of a population is a quantitative phenotype, and the mean and variance for that sample can be calculated and used to approximate the underlying mean and variance of the population from which the sample was drawn. For example, the systolic blood pressure of thousands of men in two different age groups is shown in Fig. 9.1B. The systolic blood pressure of the younger cohort is nearly symmetric; in the older age group, however, the curve becomes more skewed (asymmetric), with more individuals with systolic blood pressures above the mean than below.

The normal distribution provides guidelines for setting the limits of the normal range. A normal range is often defined as the values of a quantitative trait that are seen in ~95% of the population. Statistical theory states that when the values of a quantitative trait in a population follow the bell-shaped normal curve (i.e., are normally distributed), ~5% of the population will have measurements more than 2 SD above or below the population mean. It is important to note that an individual may be perfectly healthy (i.e., "normal") despite having a trait value outside the normal range. Furthermore, since 5% of the population will, by definition, be outside the normal range, when many traits are measured and thus classified, each individual will typically be extreme in several traits. It's important to note that this concept of normal range should not be confused with health and disease. For example, because body mass is typically high in industrialized societies, many individuals within the normal range (e.g., within 2 SD of the mean) might be considered clinically obese. As another example, because the human body can physiologically tolerate variation in platelet levels, the extreme platelet levels used to diagnose clinical conditions like thrombocytosis

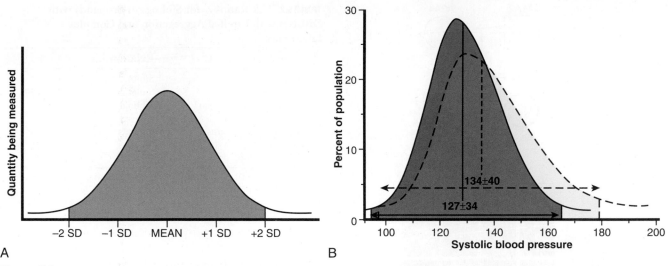

Figure 9.1 (A) The normal gaussian distribution, with mean (average) and standard deviation (SD) indicated. For many traits, the "normal" range is considered the mean ±2 SD, as indicated by the shaded region. (B) Distribution of systolic blood pressure in ~3300 men aged 40–45 *(solid line)* and ~2200 men aged 50–55 *(dotted line)*. The mean and ±2 SD are shown above double-headed arrows. (B, Data from Sive PH, Medalie JH, Kahn HA, et al: Distribution and multiple regression analysis of blood pressure in 10,000 Israeli men, *Am J Epidemiol* 93:317–327, 1971.)

or thrombocytopenia are far outside the normal range. In general the normal distribution and the normal range are a statistical convenience but cannot be used directly to diagnose health and disease.

For convenience, many genetic analyses assume that traits follow this bell-shaped normal distribution in the population. Although this is approximately true for many traits (such as height, weight, total cholesterol, and blood pressure in younger individuals), it is clearly not the case in other cases (such as triglyceride levels, number of moles in skin, or number of children in a family). For convenience, many genetic studies map the original measurements, which may not be normally distributed, to a new measurement scale that is normally distributed. This can provide much more flexibility in the choice of analysis strategy. The process typically works by rank-ordering the quantitative measurements (first highest among 100, second highest among 100, etc.) and then mapping these ranks to corresponding values in a simulated normal distribution (2.58 SD, 2.17 SD, etc.). The inverse normal distribution function is used to tabulate the expected values in the simulated normal distribution. This popular strategy handles outlier values or nonnormality in the original measured values and provides genetic results in SD units allowing for easier comparison between different studies.

FAMILIAL AGGREGATION AND CORRELATION

Allele Sharing Among Relatives

The more closely related two individuals are, the more **alleles** they share in common, on average (see Chapter 7). The most extreme example of allele sharing is identical (**monozygotic [MZ]**) **twins** (see later in this chapter),

who have the same alleles at every **locus**, with possibly a few small exceptions arising from somatic variants. The next most closely related individuals are typically first-degree relatives, such as a parent offspring or **sibling** pairs, including fraternal (**dizygotic [DZ]**) **twins**. In a parent-child pair, the child shares at least one allele out of two (50% of alleles) in common with the parent at every genetic location. This shared allele is on the **chromosome** the child inherited from that parent; sharing on the chromosome inherited from the other parent can result from **consanguinity**, very distant relatedness, or chance. Siblings (including DZ twins) also share 50% or more of their alleles on average, but this can vary along the **genome**. This is because, at a given locus, a pair of siblings inherits the same two chromosomes from their parents ¼ of the time, inherits one chromosome in common ½ the time, and inherits no chromosomes in common the remaining ¼ of the time (Fig. 9.2). At any one locus, in the absence of consanguinity, the average number of chromosomes that a sibling pair is expected to share identical by descent (i.e., alleles that are identical because they are copies of the same ancestral chromosome) is:

$$\tfrac{1}{4}(2\,\text{alleles}) + \tfrac{1}{4}(0\,\text{allele}) + \tfrac{1}{2}(1\,\text{allele}) = 0.5 + 0.5 + 0 = 1\,\text{allele}$$

The more distantly related two members of a family are, the fewer alleles they are expected to inherit from a common ancestor.

Familial Aggregation in Binary Traits

If genetic variants modify disease risk, relatives of an affected individual will have a greater-than-expected rate of the disease than unrelated individuals with similar nongenetic risk profiles (familial aggregation of

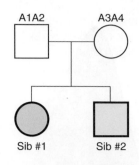

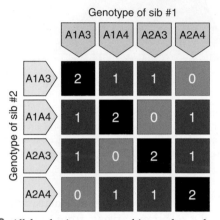

Figure 9.2 Allele sharing at an arbitrary locus between sibs concordant for a disease. The parents' genotypes are shown as *A1A2* for the father and *A3A4* for the mother. All four possible genotypes for sib #1 are given across the top of the table, and all four possible genotypes for sib #2 are given along the left side of the table. The numbers inside the boxes represent the number of alleles both sibs have in common for all 16 different combinations of genotypes for both sibs. For example, the upper left-hand corner has the number 2 because sib #1 and sib #2 both have the genotype *A1A3* and so have both *A1* and *A3* alleles in common. The bottom left-hand corner contains the number 0 because sib #1 has genotype *A1A3*, whereas sib #2 has genotype *A2A4*, so there are no alleles in common.

disease). This is because closely related family members are expected to share, on average, some disease predisposing alleles. Next, we will discuss two approaches to measuring familial aggregation: **relative risk ratios** and family history case-control studies.

Relative Risk Ratio

One way to measure familial aggregation of a disease is by comparing the frequency of the disease in the relatives of an affected proband with its disease frequency (prevalence) in the general population. The **relative risk ratio** λ_r (where the subscript r refers to relatives) is defined as:

$$\lambda_r = \frac{\text{Prevalence of the disease in the relatives of an affected person}}{\text{Prevalence of the disease in the general population}}$$

The value of λ_r as a measure of familial aggregation depends both on how frequently a disease occurs in

TABLE 9.2 Risk Ratios λ_s for Siblings of Probands with Diseases with Familial Aggregation and Complex Inheritance

Disease	Relationship	λ_s
Schizophrenia	Siblings	12
Autism	Siblings	150
Manic-depressive (bipolar) disorder	Siblings	7
Type 1 diabetes mellitus	Siblings	35
Crohn disease	Siblings	25
Multiple sclerosis	Siblings	24

Data from Rimoin DL, Connor JM, Pyeritz RE: *Emery and Rimoin's principles and practice of medical genetics*, ed 3, Edinburgh, 1997, Churchill Livingstone; King RA, Rotter JI, Motulsky AG: *The genetic basis of common diseases*, ed 2, Oxford, England, 2002, Oxford University Press.

relatives of an affected individual (the numerator) and on the population prevalence (the denominator); the larger λ_r is, the greater the familial aggregation. This estimate is typically performed within a specific type of close relative (e.g., siblings, offspring, identical twins). The population prevalence enters into the calculation because the more common a disease is, the greater the likelihood that apparent aggregation may be a coincidence. A value of $\lambda_r = 1$ indicates that a relative is no more likely to develop the disease than is any individual in the population, whereas a value greater than 1 indicates that a relative is more likely to develop the disease. Examples of relative risk ratios determined for various diseases in samples of siblings (λ_s where s is for siblings) are shown in Table 9.2. Since many diseases have sex- and/or age-specific prevalences, it is important to ensure relatives and reference populations are appropriately matched with respect to these factors.

Family History Case-Control Studies

Another approach to estimating familial aggregation is the **case-control study**, in which individuals with a disease (the cases) are compared with suitably chosen individuals without the disease (the controls), with respect to family history of disease (as well as other factors, such as environmental exposures, occupation, geographic location, parity, and previous illnesses). To assess a possible genetic contribution to familial aggregation of a disease, the frequency with which the disease is found in the extended families of the cases (positive family history) is compared with the frequency of positive family history among suitable controls, matched for age and ancestry. Spouses can be used as controls in this situation because they usually match the cases in age and ancestry and share the same household environment (provided the disease is of similar prevalence in males and females). Other frequently used controls are individuals with unrelated diseases matched for age, sex, and ancestry. Thus, for example, in a study of multiple sclerosis (MS), ~3.5% of first-degree relatives of patients with MS also had MS, a prevalence that was much higher than among first-degree relatives of matched controls without

MS (0.2%). That is, the **odds** of having a first-degree relative with MS were 18 times higher among, people with MS than among controls. (In Chapter 11, we will discuss how one calculates **odds ratios** in case-control studies.) One can conclude therefore that substantial familial aggregation is occurring in MS, thereby providing evidence of a genetic predisposition to this disease. These types of studies are somewhat vulnerable to recall bias, since diseased individuals are more likely to be aware of the disease status of similarly affected relatives.

Measuring the Genetic Contribution to Quantitative Traits

Sharing of alleles that govern a particular quantitative trait affects the distribution of values of that trait in family members. The more sharing of alleles that govern a quantitative trait there is among relatives, the more similar values of the trait are expected to be. The effect of genetic variation on quantitative traits is often measured and reported in two related ways: **correlation** between relatives and **heritability**.

Familial Correlation

Just like the relative risk ratios are used to summarize aggregation of disease within families, there are analogous strategies to summarize whether quantitative traits aggregate within families. Checking for these patterns of familial aggregation provides important clues about the role of genetic variation in each trait. Prior to studying the genetic factors underlying a trait, it is important to first establish that the trait has a genetic component. Geneticists answer this question in a few different ways. The tendency for the values of a physiologic measurement to be more similar among relatives is summarized through the correlation of these physiologic quantities among relatives. The coefficient of correlation (symbolized by the letter r) is a statistical measure of correlation applied to a pair of measurements, such as a child's serum cholesterol level and that of a parent. A positive correlation between the cholesterol measurements in two groups of relatives exists if it is found that a higher level in the first individual (e.g., the child) predicts a proportionately higher level in the relative (e.g., the parent). When a correlation exists, a graph of values in the proband and his or her relatives, in which each point represents a proband-relative pair of values, will tend to cluster around a straight line. The value of r can range from 0 when there is no correlation to +1 for perfect positive correlation. In the example of serum cholesterol, Fig. 9.3 shows a modest positive correlation ($r = 0.294$) between serum cholesterol level of mothers

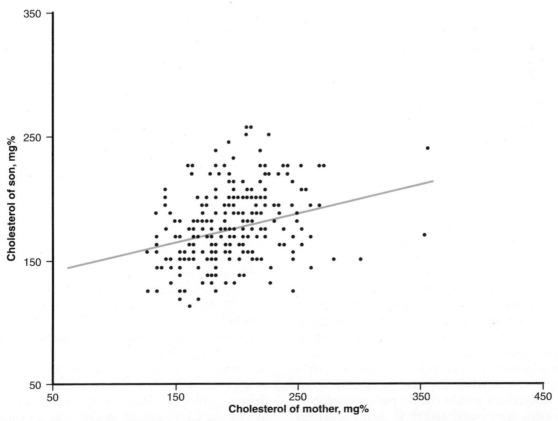

Figure 9.3 Plot of serum cholesterol levels in a group of mothers aged 30–39 and in their male children aged 4–9 years. Each dot represents a mother-son pair of measurements. The straight line is a "best fit" through the data points. (Data from Johnson BC, Epstein FH, Kjelsberg MO: Distributions and familial studies of blood pressure and serum cholesterol levels in a total community – Tecumseh, Michigan. *J Chronic Dis* 18:147–160, 1965.)

aged 30 to 39 and those of their male children aged 4 to 9. A negative correlation exists when an increase in the first individual's measurement predicts a lower measurement in relatives. The measurements are still correlated but in the opposite direction. In such a case, the value of r can range from 0 to −1 for a perfect negative correlation. This is relatively rare in genetic studies of relatives, but it can occur in other settings where correlations are used to summarize relationships between measurements (e.g., an individual's activity levels might be negatively correlated with body mass).

Heritability

The concept of heritability of a quantitative trait (symbolized as H^2) was developed to describe how much the genetic differences between individuals in a population contribute to variability of that trait in the population. H^2 is defined as the fraction of the variation in a quantitative trait that is due to genetic variation in the broadest sense, regardless of the mechanism by which the various alleles affect the phenotype. The higher the heritability, the greater the contribution of genetic differences among people to the variability of the trait in the population. The value of H^2 varies from 0, if **genotype** contributes nothing to the total phenotypic variance in a population, to 1, if genotype is totally responsible for the phenotypic variance in that population.

Heritability of a human trait is a theoretical quantity that is usually estimated from the correlation between measurements of that trait among relatives of known degrees of relatedness, such as parents and children, siblings, or, as we shall see later in this chapter, twins.

DETERMINING THE RELATIVE CONTRIBUTIONS OF GENES AND ENVIRONMENT TO COMPLEX DISEASE

Distinguishing Between Genetic and Environmental Influences Using Family Studies

For both qualitative and quantitative traits, similarities among family members are most likely the result of shared genetics and shared environment, such as socioeconomic status, local environment, dietary habits, or cultural behaviors, all of which are frequently shared among family members but are generally considered to be of nongenetic origin. Given evidence of familial aggregation of a disease or correlation of a quantitative trait, geneticists attempt to separate the relative contributions of genotype and environment to the phenotype using a variety of approaches. Historically, when sample sizes were smaller and genetic data were less available, researchers would collect **pedigree** information from cases (probands) and their family members. This would enable estimates of disease risk in different relatives, grouped by their shared genetics (e.g., 50% genetic sharing in parent-offspring pairs or full siblings, 25% genetic sharing in grandparent-grandchild

pairs, avuncular or half-sibling pairs) and an evaluation of whether the degree of similarity between individuals attenuates in proportion to their genetic relatedness. Another common attempt to control for shared environment is to compare the concordance of disease status in MZ or identical twins with that in same-sex DZ or fraternal twins. Since twins share much of their environment *in utero* and early childhood whether identical or fraternal, it is convenient to hypothesize that any difference in concordance is due to the difference in genetic sharing (100% sharing for identical twins and ~50% sharing for fraternal twins). More recently, with the development of biobanks (i.e., very large-scale collections of research participants, coupled with genetic data and large-scale electronic health records), heritability of many phenotypes and diseases can be efficiently examined using very distant relative pairs identified by comparing their genetic data directly. For example, we might hypothesize that for a genetic trait, concordance of disease status or correlation between quantitative measurements will be higher between individuals who share 4% of their genetic material than between individuals who share 2% of their genetic material. We next discuss some possibilities in more detail.

Attenuation of Risk for Progressively More Distant Relatives

One approach is to compare λ_r measurements or quantitative trait correlations between relatives of varying degrees of relatedness to the proband. For example, if genes predispose to a disease, one would expect λ_r to be greatest for MZ twins, to be somewhat smaller for first-degree relatives such as sibs or parent-child pairs, and to continue to decrease as allele-sharing decreases among the more distant relatives in a family (see Fig. 7.3).

To illustrate this approach, consider cleft lip with or without cleft palate, or CL(P), one of the most common **congenital** malformations, affecting 1.4 per 1000 newborns worldwide. CL(P) originates as a failure of fusion of embryonic tissues that will go to make up the upper lip and the hard palate at approximately day 35 of gestation. It is a multifactorial disorder with complex inheritance; for reasons that are not well understood, ~60% to 80% of those affected with CL(P) are males. Despite the similarity in names, CL(P) is usually etiologically distinct from **isolated** cleft palate (i.e., without cleft lip).

CL(P) is heterogeneous and includes forms in which the clefting is only one feature of a **syndrome** that includes other features, known as syndromic CL(P), as well as forms that are not associated with other birth defects, which are known as nonsyndromic CL(P). Syndromic CL(P) can be inherited as a mendelian single-gene disorder or can be caused by **chromosome disorders** (especially trisomy 13 and 4p⁻ deletion syndrome) (see Chapter 6) or **teratogenic** exposure (rubella embryopathy, thalidomide, or anticonvulsants) (see

TABLE 9.3 Risk for Cleft Lip with or without Cleft Palate in a Child Depending on the Number of Affected Parents and Other Relatives

| | Risk for CL(P) (%) | | |
| | No. of Affected Parents | | |
Affected Relatives	0	1	2
None	0.1	3	34
One sibling	3	11	40
Two siblings	8	19	45
One sibling and one second-degree relative	6	16	43
One sibling and one third-degree relative	4	14	44

CL(P), Cleft lip with or without cleft palate.

Chapter 15). Nonsyndromic CL(P) can also be inherited as a single-gene disorder but more commonly is a **sporadic** occurrence and demonstrates some degree of familial aggregation without an obvious mendelian inheritance pattern.

The risk for CL(P) in a child increases as a function of the number of relatives the child has who are affected with CL(P) and the more closely related they are to the child (Table 9.3). The simplest explanation for this is that the more closely related one is to the proband and, the more probands there are in the family, the more likely one is to inherit disease-susceptibility alleles, thus increasing risk for the disorder.

Another approach is to compare the disease relative risk ratio in biological relatives of the proband with that in biologically unrelated family members (e.g., adoptees or spouses), all living in the same household environment. Returning to MS, for example, λ_r is 190 for MZ twins and 20 to 40 for first-degree biological relatives (parents, children, and sibs). In contrast, λ_r is 1 for the adopted siblings of an affected individual, suggesting that most of the familial aggregation in MS is genetic rather than the result of a shared environment. A similar analysis can be carried out for quantitative traits such as blood pressure: No correlation exists between a child's blood pressure and that of the child's adopted siblings, in contrast to the positive correlation for blood pressure of biological siblings, all living in the same household.

Distinguishing Between Genetic and Environmental Influences Using Twin Studies

Of all methods used to separate genetic and environmental influences, geneticists have historically relied most heavily on twin studies.

Twinning

MZ and DZ twins are "experiments of nature" that provide an excellent opportunity to separate environmental

and genetic influences on phenotypes in humans. MZ twins arise from the cleavage of a single fertilized **zygote** into two separate zygotes early in embryogenesis (see Chapter 14). They occur in ~0.3% of all births, without large differences among different populations. At the time the zygote cleaves in two, MZ twins start out with identical genotypes at every locus and are therefore often thought of as having identical genomes.

In contrast, DZ twins arise from the simultaneous fertilization of two eggs by two sperm; genetically, DZ twins are siblings who share a womb and, like all siblings, share, on average, 50% of the alleles at all loci. DZ twins are of the same sex half the time and of opposite sex the other half. In contrast to MZ twins, DZ twins occur with a frequency that varies as much as fivefold in individuals with different ancestries - e.g., 0.2% among individuals with Asian ancestry and 1% of births in parts of Africa.

Disease Concordance in MZ and DZ Twins

When twins have the same disease, they are said to be **concordant** for that disorder. Conversely, when only one member of the pair of twins is affected and the other is not, the relatives are **discordant** for the disease. An examination of how frequently MZ twins are concordant for a disease is a powerful method for determining whether genotype alone is sufficient to produce a particular disease. The differences between a disease that is mendelian from one that shows complex inheritance are immediately evident. Using sickle cell disease (Case 42) as an example of a mendelian disorder, if one MZ twin has sickle cell disease, the other twin will always have the disease as well. In contrast, as an example of a multifactorial disorder, when one MZ twin has type 1 diabetes mellitus (previously known as insulin-dependent or juvenile diabetes) the other twin will also have type 1 diabetes only ~40% of such twin pairs. *Disease concordance of less than 100% in MZ twins is strong evidence that nongenetic factors play a role in the disease.* Such factors could include environmental influences, such as exposure to infection or diet, as well as other effects, such as somatic variation, effects of aging, or **epigenetic** changes in gene expression in one twin compared with the other.

MZ and same-sex DZ twins share a common intrauterine environment and biological sex and are usually reared together in the same household by the same parents. Thus a comparison of concordance for a disease between MZ and same-sex DZ twins shows how frequently disease occurs when relatives who experience the same prenatal and often the same postnatal environment have the same alleles at every locus (MZ twins) and how often it occurs when they share 50% of alleles in common (DZ twins). *Greater concordance in MZ versus DZ twins is strong evidence of a genetic component to the disease*, as shown in Table 9.4 for a number of disorders.

Estimating Heritability from Twin Studies

Just as twins are be used to separate the roles of genes and environment in qualitative disease traits, twins are also used to estimate the heritability of a quantitative trait using the correlation in the values of a physiologic measurement in MZ and DZ twins. If one assumes that the alleles affecting the trait exert their effect additively (which is certainly overly simplistic and probably incorrect in many cases), MZ twins, who share 100% of their alleles, have twice the amount of allele sharing compared to DZ twins, who share 50% of their alleles on average. H^2, introduced earlier in this chapter, can therefore be approximated by taking twice the difference in the correlation coefficient r for a quantitative trait between MZ twins (r_{MZ}) and r between same-sex DZ twins (r_{DZ}) (as given by Falconer's formula):

$$H^2 = 2 \times (r_{MZ} - r_{DZ})$$

If the variability of the trait is determined chiefly by environment, the correlation within pairs of DZ twins will be similar to that seen between pairs of MZ twins; there will be little difference in the value of r for MZ and DZ twins. Thus, $r_{MZ} - r_{DZ} = \approx 0$, and H^2 will approach 0. At the other extreme, however, if the variability is determined exclusively by genetic makeup, the correlation coefficient r between MZ pairs will approach 1, whereas r between DZ twins will be half of that. Now, $r_{MZ} - r_{DZ} = \approx \frac{1}{2}$, and therefore H^2 will be approximately $2 \times (\frac{1}{2}) = 1$.

Twins Reared Apart

Although a rare occurrence, twins are sometimes separated at birth for social reasons and placed in different homes, thus providing an opportunity to observe individuals of identical or half-identical genotypes reared in different environments. Such studies have been used primarily in research on psychiatric disorders, substance use, and eating disorders, in which strong environmental influences within the family are believed to play a role in the development of disease. For example, in one study of obesity, the **body mass index** (**BMI**; weight/height², expressed in kg/m²) was measured in MZ and DZ twins reared in the same household versus those reared apart (Table 9.5). Although the average BMI among MZ or DZ twins was similar, regardless of whether they were reared together or apart, the pairwise correlation for BMI between a pair of twins was much higher for MZ than for DZ twins. Also interesting is that the higher correlation between MZ and DZ twins was independent of whether the twins were reared together or apart, which suggests that genetics has a highly significant impact on adult weight and consequently on the risk for obesity and its complications.

Limitations of Familial Aggregation and Heritability Estimates From Family and Twin Studies

Potential Sources of Bias

There are a number of difficulties in measuring and interpreting λ_s. One is that studies of familial aggregation of disease are subject to various forms of bias. There is **ascertainment bias**, which arises when families with more than one affected sibling are more likely to come to a researcher's attention, thereby inflating the sibling recurrence risk λ_s. Ascertainment bias is

TABLE 9.4 Concordance Rates in MZ and DZ Twins for Various Multifactorial Disorders

Disorder	Concordance (%)* MZ	Concordance (%)* DZ
Nontraumatic epilepsy	70	6
Multiple sclerosis	18	2
Type 1 diabetes	40	5
Schizophrenia	46	15
Bipolar disease	62	8
Osteoarthritis	32	16
Rheumatoid arthritis	12	3
Psoriasis	72	15
Cleft lip with or without cleft palate	30	2
Systemic lupus erythematosus	22	0

*Rounded to the nearest percent.
DZ, Dizygotic; *MZ*, monozygotic.
Data from Rimoin DL, Connor JM, Pyeritz RE: *Emery and Rimoin's principles and practice of medical genetics*, ed 3, Edinburgh, 1997, Churchill Livingstone; King RA, Rotter JI, Motulsky AG: *The genetic basis of common diseases*, Oxford, England, 1992, Oxford University Press; Tsuang MT: Recent advances in genetic research on schizophrenia, *J Biomed Sci* 5:28–30, 1998.

TABLE 9.5 Pairwise Correlation of BMI Between MZ and DZ Twins Reared Together and Apart

Twin Type	Rearing	Men No. of Pairs	Men BMI*	Men Pairwise Correlation	Women No. of Pairs	Women BMI*	Women Pairwise Correlation
Monozygotic	Apart	49	24.8 ± 2.4	0.70	44	24.2 ± 3.4	0.66
	Together	66	24.2 ± 2.9	0.74	88	23.7 ± 3.5	0.66
Dizygotic	Apart	75	25.1 ± 3.0	0.15	143	24.9 ± 4.1	0.25
	Together	89	24.6 ± 2.7	0.33	119	23.9 ± 3.5	0.27

*Mean ± 1 SD.
BMI, Body mass index; *DZ*, dizygotic; *MZ*, monozygotic.
Data from Stunkard AJ, Harris JR, Pedersen NL, et al: The body-mass index of twins who have been reared apart, *NEJM* 322:1483–1487, 1990.

also a problem for twin studies. Many studies rely on asking one twin with a particular disease to recruit the other twin to participate in a study (volunteer-based ascertainment), rather than ascertaining them first as twins through a twin registry and only then examining their health status (population-based ascertainment). Volunteer-based **ascertainment** can give biased results because twins, particularly MZ twins who may be emotionally close, are more likely to volunteer if they are concordant than if they are not, which inflates the concordance rate.

Similarly, because case-control studies of family history often rely, for practical reasons, on taking a history from the proband rather than examining all the relatives directly, there may be recall bias, in which a proband may be more likely to know of family members with the same or similar disease. Such biases will inflate the level of familial aggregation.

Other difficulties arise in measuring and interpreting heritability. The same trait may yield different measurements of heritability in different populations because of different allele frequencies or diverse environmental conditions. For example, heritability measurements of height would be lower when measured in a population with widespread famine that stunts growth in childhood as compared to the same population after food becomes plentiful. Heritability of a trait should therefore not be thought of as an intrinsic, universally applicable measure of "how genetic" the trait is, because it depends on the population and environment in which the estimate is being made. Although heritability estimates are still made in genetic research, most geneticists consider them to be only preliminary but convenient estimates of the role of genetic variation in phenotypic variation.

Potential Genetic or Epigenetic Differences

Despite the evident power of twin studies, one must caution against thinking of such studies as perfectly controlled experiments that compare individuals who share either half or all of their genetic variation and are exposed either to the same or to different environments. Studies of MZ twins assume the twins are genetically identical. Although this is mostly true, genotype and gene expression patterns may come to differ between MZ twins because of genetic or epigenetic changes that occur after the cleavage event that produced the MZ twin embryos. For example, genotype may differ due to somatic **rearrangements** and/or rare **somatic mutations** that occur after the cleavage event (see Chapter 3). Epigenetic changes may occur in response to environmental or stochastic factors, thus leading to differences in gene expression between MZ twins. (Female MZ twins have an additional source of variability because of the stochastic nature of **X inactivation** patterns in various tissues, as presented in Chapter 6.)

Other Limitations

Another problem may arise when assuming that the environmental exposure of MZ and DZ twins has been held constant when they are reared together but not when twins are reared apart. Environmental exposures, including even intrauterine environment, may vary for twins reared in the same family. For example, MZ twins frequently share a placenta, and there may be a disparity between the twins in blood supply, intrauterine development, and birthweight. For late-onset diseases, such as neurodegenerative disease of late adulthood, the assumption that MZ and DZ twins are exposed to similar environments throughout their adult lives becomes less and less valid, and thus a difference in concordance provides less strong evidence for genetic factors in disease causation. Conversely, one assumes that by determining disease concordance in MZ twins reared apart, one is measuring the effect of different environments on the same genotype. However, the environment of twins reared apart may actually not be as different as one might suppose. *Thus no twin study is a perfectly controlled assessment of genetic versus environmental influence.*

Finally, caution is necessary when generalizing from twin studies. The most extreme situation would be when the phenotype being studied is only sometimes genetic in origin; that is, nongenetic phenocopies may exist. If genotype alone causes the disease in half the pairs of twins (MZ twin concordance of 100%) in your sample and a nongenetic phenocopy affects only one twin of the other half of twin pairs in your sample (MZ twin concordance of 0%), twin studies will show an intermediate level of 50% concordance that really applies to neither form of the disease.

Genome-wide Association Studies

Lei Sun and Wei Deng

Complex diseases and traits are influenced by a combination of genetic and environmental risk factors. In the last decade, genome-wide association studies (GWAS) have been particularly fruitful in identifying disease susceptibility loci and biologic pathways, elucidating the genetic architecture of many complex diseases. The concept of **GWAS** is elegantly simple: examining each individual genetic variant – usually a biallelic locus (which is typically either a single nucleotide polymorphism [SNP] or an **insertion** deletion variant or indel) – for evidence of **association** with a disease phenotype or quantitative trait. Individual variant results can point to specific regions of the genome that are associated with a disease or trait. Sometimes the association signal implicates a protein-altering variant, which has a simple interpretation in terms of biologic and functional consequences, but most of the time the association signal falls among the noncoding regions of the genome. Many approaches have been developed to map associated genetic variants to their effector genes, but for complex disease the most sophisticated approaches only guess the correct gene a little over half of the time.

These individual association results, over the entire genome, reveal the landscape of phenotype-genotype associations, where the association evidence is often summarized pictorially by the famous **Manhattan plot** of $-\log 10$ p-values (Fig. 9.4). More recently, some have proposed a Brisbane plot enumerating the number of independently associated variants within a specified window size (useful for GWAS with many findings), or a Miami plot showing results from two similar GWASs above and below the horizontal axis (i.e., a reflection) (Figs. 9.5 and 9.6).

Polygenic Risk Scores

Lei Sun and Wei Deng

In addition to discovery of novel association signals, GWAS have enabled the estimation of genetic effects associated with millions of individual SNPs across a range of complex diseases. The magnitude of these effects for each genetic variant is typically small compared to established clinical risk factors. As the higher risk allele at each SNP locus only moderately increases the risk of disease, it is natural to construct a composite score that can potentially capture the overall genetic burden across the genome. This is indeed the idea behind the PRS: a weighted sum of the numbers of the risk alleles of all associated SNPs, where the weights are derived from effect size estimates from GWAS.

The earlier **polygenic** risk research focused on association, and one of the most prominent early examples of PRS was in schizophrenia. There, a large number of SNPs individually below the genome-wide detection threshold (of p-value $< 5 \times 10^{-8}$, which is the threshold typically used to allow for millions of tests for common variants distributed throughout the genome) was used to construct a PRS highly associated with schizophrenia status.

More recent PRS research has focused on the utility of PRS for prediction of individuals at risk of disease, on the ability of PRS to help refine diagnoses by separating different types of cases, and on the ability of PRS to aid in the **selection** of optimal treatment regimes. For example, a higher PRS is capable of identifying individuals with a higher disease risk: Individuals with PRS values in the top 1% of the distribution have at least a threefold increase in risk of developing coronary artery disease, atrial fibrillation, type 2 diabetes, inflammatory bowel disease, or breast cancer. Indeed, PRS of this magnitude could have many clinical utilities: They might inform screening strategies, motivate health-related behavior changes, and potentially help identify treatment targets for precision medicine. PRS for breast cancer was the first to be implemented in the CanRisk/BOADICEA risk algorithm, which was used clinically to predict individuals at higher risk of breast cancer, and became available for prediction of coronary artery disease by at least one

private company in 2022 (Color). In the case of diagnostic refinement, PRS was found to distinguish between type 1 and type 2 diabetes, which had previously been assigned primarily based on age of onset.

The construction of a good PRS, predictive of the risk of a disease, requires a systematic approach to (1) powerfully identify associated SNPs, (2) accurately estimate their genetic effects on the disease, and (3) ensure the PRS is applied to the appropriate people (e.g., whose age, ancestry, and clinical risk profiles are similar to those in whom the genetic effects were originally estimated). The ideal PRS construction should include all disease-associated SNPs and no others; a realistic PRS typically not only misses some of the truly associated SNPs but includes false positives due to limited power of GWAS. The low power of GWAS is a direct result of moderate-to-weak effects of individual SNPs on a complex disease with polygenic inheritance. The estimation of effect can be challenging, as it is often biased toward discovery – otherwise known as the winner's curse – where the estimated genetic effect of an SNP is inflated relative to the true value. Finally, to avoid data dredging (also known as p-hacking), for both (1) and (2) above, a (discovery) sample of individuals is used, which is independent of the (target) sample of individuals where the PRS is evaluated for prediction accuracy.

While statistical methodology in capturing the polygenic risk associated with diseases has progressed significantly, for many complex diseases and quantitative traits the amount of phenotypic variance explained by PRS derived from GWASs is modest. Thus for most common diseases we are still evaluating the value of PRS in the clinic and in other settings where they might influence the health and wellbeing of individuals. With the availability of biobank-scale studies and more sophisticated PRS methods, we expect incremental improvement in the predictiveness of PRS, particularly for diseases with few clinical predictors.

A major methodologic issue in the construction of a PRS is population **heterogeneity**, also known as the transportability issue. Because genetic effect sizes may vary according to the ancestral background of the study population, the PRS weights derived in one population might not translate well into another. Another major gap is the lack of methods to include SNPs from the **X chromosome**, thus missing 5% of the **haploid** genome. Finally, the genetic risk for a disease, predicted using PRS, has a theoretical upper bound that depends on the population-specific heritability of the disease. This is not to say, however, that heritability limits the absolute disease risk for an individual. Consider the well-known example of familial breast cancer, whereby individuals with **pathogenic variants** in the *BRCA1* gene can have a substantially increased risk of early-onset cancer, even though these relatively highly penetrant variants only account for a small number of breast cancer cases overall and only explain a small proportion of cancer heritability in the populations where they occur.

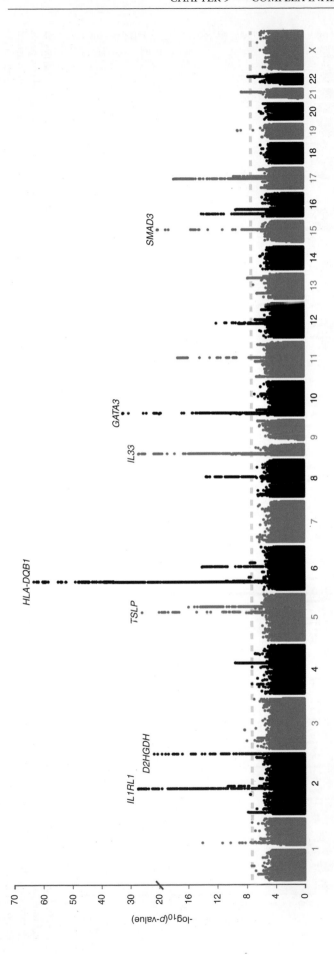

Figure 9.4 Manhattan plot example for a genome-wide association analysis of asthma in UK Biobank. The association analysis compares genotypes at millions of genetic variants between asthma cases, defined on the basis of diagnosis codes in their individual medical records, and controls. The results of each comparison are summarized in a *p*-value which is plotted in the graph. The top few association signals have been labeled with the name of the nearest gene. (The figure is based on the UK Biobank association analyses reported in Taliun D, Harris DN, Kessler MD, et al: Sequencing of 53,831 diverse genomes from the NHLBI TOPMed Program, *Nature* 590: 290–299, 2021. https://doi.org/10.1038/s41586-021-03205-y.)

Meanwhile, the clinical use of PRS is not without caveats. A main controversy is the potential health disparity resulting from the fact that most large GWAS and PRS have been conducted and tested only in large samples of European ancestry. Second, the interpretation of a PRS score (e.g., relative vs. absolute risk) can sometimes be a barrier in clinical settings, requiring continued education of clinicians to help them to better disclose results to families. Third, it remains an open question how best to combine PRS and modifiable clinical risk factors to inform disease prevention. Finally, standardized reporting of PRS results will facilitate knowledge **translation**.

EXAMPLES OF COMMON MULTIFACTORIAL DISEASES WITH A GENETIC CONTRIBUTION

In this section and the next, we turn to considering examples of several common conditions that illustrate general concepts of multifactorial disorders and their complex inheritance, as summarized in the accompanying box (see Box 9.1).

BOX 9.1 CHARACTERISTICS OF INHERITANCE OF COMPLEX DISEASES

- Genetic variation contributes to diseases with complex inheritance, but these diseases are not single-gene disorders and do not demonstrate a simple mendelian pattern of inheritance.
- Diseases with complex inheritance often demonstrate familial aggregation because close relatives of an affected individual are likely to also share disease-predisposing alleles.
- Diseases with complex inheritance are more common among the close relatives of a proband and become less common in relatives who are less closely related and therefore share fewer predisposing alleles. Greater concordance for disease is expected among monozygotic versus **dizygotic twins**.
- However, pairs of relatives who share disease-predisposing genotypes at relevant loci may still be discordant for phenotype (show lack of penetrance) because of the crucial role of nongenetic factors in disease causation. The most extreme examples of lack of **penetrance** despite identical genotypes are discordant **monozygotic twins**.

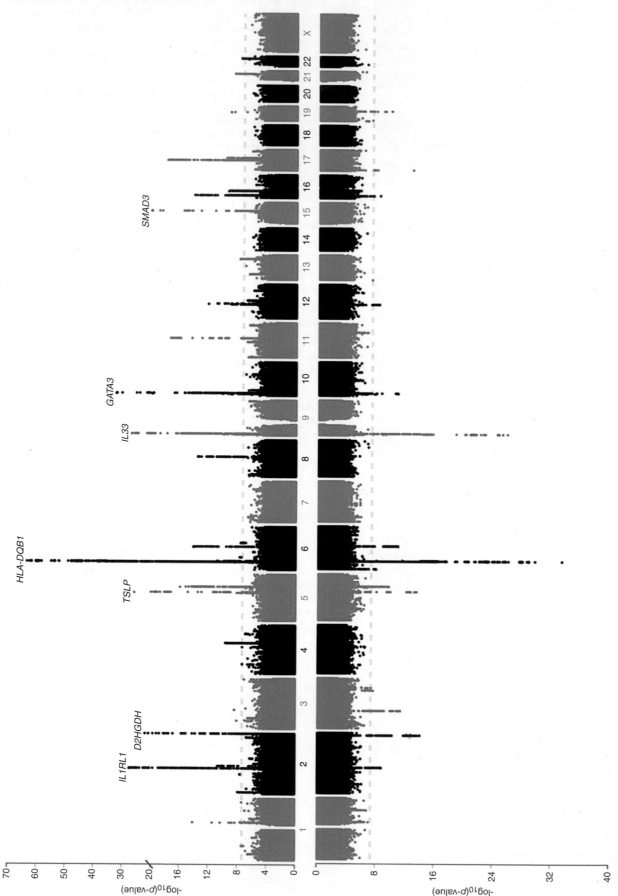

Figure 9.5 Miami plot example for a genome-wide association analysis of asthma and nasal polyps in UK Biobank. The association analysis on the top panel compares genotypes at millions of genetic variants between asthma cases, defined on the basis of diagnosis codes in their individual medical records, and controls. The analysis on the bottom panel compares genotypes at the same variants between individuals with nasal polyps and controls. Note the many shared signals between the two analyses. The results of each comparison are summarized in a *p*-value, which is plotted in the graph. The top few association signals have been labeled with the name of the nearest gene in the asthma portion of the plot. (The figure is based on the UK biobank association analyses reported in Taliun D, Harris DN, Kessler MD, et al: Sequencing of 53,831 diverse genomes from the NHLBI TOPMed Program, *Nature* 590: 290–299, 2021. https://doi.org/10.1038/s41586-021-03205-y.)

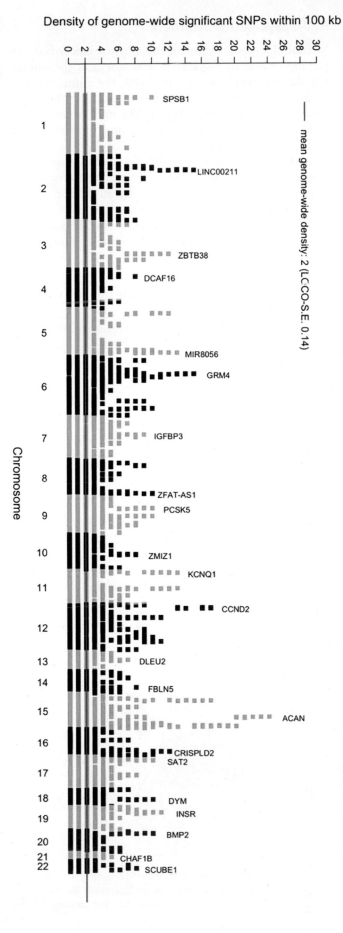

Figure 9.6 Brisbane plot example for a genome-wide association analysis of height in 5.3-m individuals. Each dot shows one of the 12,111 independent genome-wide significant variants associated with height. Density was calculated as the number of other independent associated variants within 100 kb. (Figure from height GWAS in Yengo L, Vedantam S, Marouli E, et al: A saturated map of common genetic variants associated with human height, *Nature* 610(7933):704–712, 2022. https:doi.org/10.1038/s41586-022-05275-y.)

Multifactorial Congenital Malformations

Many common congenital malformations, occurring as isolated defects and not as part of a syndrome, are multifactorial and demonstrate complex inheritance (Table 9.6). Among these, **congenital heart malformations** are some of the most common and serve to illustrate the current state of understanding of other categories of congenital malformation.

Congenital heart defects (CHDs) occur at a frequency of ~4 to 8 per 1000 births. They are a heterogeneous group, caused in some cases by single-gene or chromosomal mechanisms and in others by exposure to teratogens, such as rubella infection or maternal diabetes. The cause is usually unknown, however, and the majority of cases are believed to be multifactorial in origin.

There are many types of CHDs, with different population incidences and **empirical risks**. It is known that when heart defects recur in a family, however, the affected children do not necessarily have exactly the same anatomic defect but instead show recurrence of lesions that are similar with regard to developmental mechanisms (see Chapter 14). By using developmental mechanisms as a classification scheme, five main groups of CHDs can be distinguished:

- Flow lesions
- Defects in cell migration

TABLE 9.6 Some Common Congenital Malformations With Multifactorial Inheritance

Malformation	Approximate Population Incidence (per 1000)
Cleft lip with or without cleft palate	0.4–1.7
Cleft palate	0.4
Congenital dislocation of hip	2*
Congenital heart defects	4–8
Ventricular septal defect	1.7
Patent ductus arteriosus	0.5
Atrial septal defect	1.0
Aortic stenosis	0.5
Neural tube defects	2–10
Spina bifida and anencephaly	Variable
Pyloric stenosis	1,[†] 5*

*Per 1000 males.
[†]Per 1000 females.

Data from Carter CO; Genetics of common single malformations, *Br Med Bull* 32:21–26, 1976; Nora JJ: Multifactorial inheritance hypothesis for the etiology of congenital heart diseases: The genetic environmental interaction, *Circulation* 38:604–617, 1968; Lin AE, Garver KL: Genetic counseling for congenital heart defects, *J Pediatr* 113:1105–1109, 1988.

- Defects in cell death
- Abnormalities in extracellular matrix
- Defects in targeted growth

The subtype of congenital heart malformations known as flow lesions illustrates the familial aggregation and elevated risk for recurrence in relatives of an affected individual, all characteristic of a complex trait (Table 9.7). Flow lesions, which constitute ~50% of all CHDs, include hypoplastic left heart syndrome, coarctation of the aorta, atrial septal defect of the secundum type, pulmonary valve stenosis, a common type of ventricular septal defect, and other forms (Fig. 9.7). Up to 25% of individuals with flow lesions, particularly tetralogy of Fallot, may have the **deletion** of chromosome region 22q11 seen in the velocardiofacial syndrome (see Chapter 6).

Certain isolated CHDs are inherited as multifactorial traits. Until more is known, the figures shown in Table 9.7 can be used as estimates of the **recurrence risk** for flow lesions in first-degree relatives. There is, however, a rapid falloff in risk (to levels not much higher than the population risk) in second- and third-degree relatives of index patients with flow lesions. Similarly, relatives of index patients with types of CHDs other than flow lesions can be offered reassurance that their risk is not much greater than that of the general population. For further reassurance, many CHDs can now be assessed prenatally by ultrasonography (see Chapter 18).

Neuropsychiatric Disorders

Mental illnesses are some of the most common and perplexing of human diseases, affecting 4% of the human population worldwide. As of 2020, the annual cost in medical care and social services exceeds $200 billion in the United States alone. Among the most severe of the mental illnesses are schizophrenia and bipolar disease (manic-depressive illness).

Schizophrenia affects 1% of the world's population. It is a devastating psychiatric illness, with onset commonly in late adolescence or young adulthood, and is characterized by abnormalities in thought, emotion, and social relationships, often associated with delusional thinking and disordered mood. A genetic contribution

TABLE 9.7 Population Incidence and Recurrence Risks for Various Flow Lesions

Defect	Population Incidence (%)	Frequency in Sibs (%)	λ_s
Ventricular septal defect	0.17	4.3	25
Patent ductus arteriosus	0.083	3.2	38
Atrial septal defect	0.066	3.2	48
Aortic stenosis	0.044	2.6	59

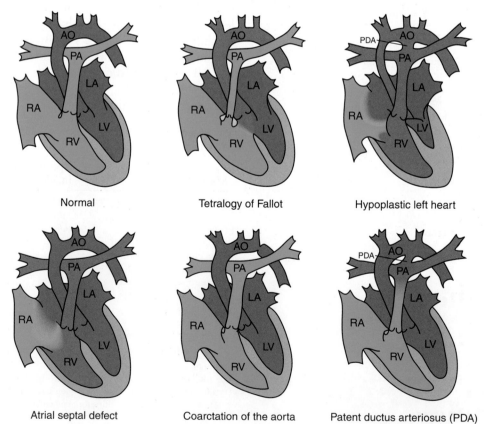

Normal   Tetralogy of Fallot   Hypoplastic left heart

Atrial septal defect   Coarctation of the aorta   Patent ductus arteriosus (PDA)

Figure 9.7 Diagram of various flow lesions seen in congenital heart disease. Blood on the left side of the circulation is shown in red, on the right side in blue. Abnormal admixture of oxygenated and deoxygenated blood is purple. *AO*, Aorta; *LA*, left atrium; *LV*, left ventricle; *PA*, pulmonary artery; *RA*, right atrium; *RV*, right ventricle.

TABLE 9.8 Recurrence Risks and Relative Risk Ratios in Schizophrenia Families

Relation to Individual Affected by Schizophrenia	Recurrence Risk (%)	λ_r
Child of two schizophrenic parents	46	23
Child	9–16	11.5
Sibling	8–14	11
Nephew or niece	1–4	2.5
Uncle or aunt	2	2
First cousin	2–6	4
Grandchild	2–8	5

TABLE 9.9 Recurrence Risks and Relative Risk Ratios in Bipolar Disorder Families

Relation to Individual Affected With Bipolar Disease	Recurrence Risk (%)*	λ_r
Child of two parents with bipolar disease	50–70	75
Child	27	34
Sibling	20–30	31
Second-degree relative	5	6

*Recurrence of bipolar, unipolar, or schizoaffective disorder.

to schizophrenia is supported by both twin and family aggregation studies. MZ concordance in schizophrenia is estimated to be 40% to 60%; DZ concordance is 10% to 16%. The recurrence risk ratio is elevated in first- and second-degree relatives of individuals with schizophrenia (Table 9.8).

Although there is considerable evidence of a genetic contribution to schizophrenia, only a subset of the genes and alleles that predispose to the disease has been identified to date. A major exception is the small percentage (<2%) of all schizophrenia that is found in individuals with interstitial deletions of particular chromosomes, such as the 22q11 deletion responsible for the velocardiofacial syndrome. It is estimated that 25% of individuals with 22q11 deletions develop schizophrenia, even in the absence of many or most of the other physical signs of the syndrome. The mechanism by which a deletion of 3 Mb of DNA on 22q11 (see Fig. 6.7) causes mental illness in individuals with this syndrome is unknown. Chromosomal **microarrays** have been used to scan the entire genome for other deletions and duplications, many too small to be detectable by standard cytogenetic approaches, as introduced in Chapter 5. These studies have revealed numerous deletions and duplications (copy number variants) throughout the genome in both normal individuals and individuals with a variety of psychiatric and neurodevelopmental disorders (see Chapter 6). In particular, small (1–1.5 Mb) interstitial deletions at 1q21.1, 15q11.2, and 15q13.3 have been implicated repeatedly in a small fraction of individuals with schizophrenia. For the vast majority of people with schizophrenia, however, genetic lesions are not known, and counseling therefore relies on empirical risk figures (see Table 9.8).

Bipolar disease is predominantly a mood disorder in which episodes of mood elevation, grandiosity, high-risk dangerous behavior, and inflated self-esteem (mania) alternate with periods of depression, decreased interest in what are normally pleasurable activities, feelings of worthlessness, and suicidal thinking. The prevalence of bipolar disease is 0.8%, approximately equal to that of schizophrenia, with a similar age at onset. The seriousness of this condition is underscored by the high rate of suicide in affected individuals.

A genetic contribution to bipolar disease is strongly supported by twin and family aggregation studies. MZ twin concordance is 40% to 60%; DZ twin concordance is 4% to 8%. Disease risk is also elevated in relatives of affected individuals (Table 9.9). One striking aspect of bipolar disease in families is that the condition has variable **expressivity**; some members of the same family demonstrate classic bipolar illness, others have depression alone (unipolar disorder), and others carry a diagnosis of a psychiatric syndrome that involves both thought and mood (schizoaffective disorder). Even less is known about genes and alleles that predispose to bipolar disease than is known for schizophrenia; in particular, although an increase in *de novo* deletions or duplications has been identified in bipolar psychosis, recurrent **copy number variants** involving particular regions of the genome have not been identified. Counseling therefore typically relies on empirical risk figures (see Table 9.9).

Coronary Artery Disease

Coronary artery disease (CAD) kills ~500,000 individuals in the United States yearly and is one of the most frequent causes of morbidity and mortality in the developed world. CAD due to atherosclerosis is the major cause of the nearly 1.5 million cases of myocardial infarction (MI) and the more than 200,000 deaths from acute MI occurring annually. In the aggregate, CAD costs more than $143 billion in health care expenses alone each year in the United States, not including lost productivity. For unknown reasons, males are at higher risk for CAD both in the general population and within affected families.

Family studies have repeatedly supported a role for heredity in CAD, particularly when it occurs in relatively young individuals. The pattern of increased risk suggests that when the proband is female or young there is likely to be a greater genetic contribution to MI in the family, thereby increasing the risk for disease in the proband's relatives. For example, the recurrence risk (Table 9.10) in male first-degree relatives of a female proband is sevenfold greater than that in the general population, compared with the 2.5-fold increased risk in female relatives of a male proband.

When the proband is young (<55 years) and female, the risk for CAD is more than 11 times greater than that of the general population. Having multiple relatives affected at a young age increases risk substantially as well. Twin studies also support a role for genetic variants in CAD (Table 9.11).

TABLE 9.10 Risk for Coronary Artery Disease in Relatives of a Proband

Proband	Increased Risk for CAD in a Family Member*
Male	3-fold in male first-degree relatives
	2.5-fold in female first-degree relatives
Female	7-fold in male first-degree relatives
Female <55 yr	11.4-fold in male first-degree relatives
Two male relatives <55 yr	13-fold in first-degree relatives

*Relative to the risk in the general population.
CAD, Coronary artery disease.
Data from Silberberg JS: Risk associated with various definitions of family history of coronary heart disease, *Am J Epidemiol* 147:1133–1139, 1998.

A few mendelian disorders leading to CAD are known. Familial hypercholesterolemia (Case 16), an autosomal dominant defect of the low-density lipoprotein (LDL) receptor discussed in Chapter 13, is one of the most common of these but accounts for only ~5% of survivors of MI. Most cases of CAD show multifactorial inheritance, with both nongenetic and genetic predisposing factors. There are many stages in the evolution of atherosclerotic lesions in the coronary artery. What begins as a fatty streak in the intima of the artery evolves into a fibrous plaque containing smooth muscle, lipid, and fibrous tissue. These intimal plaques become vascular and may bleed, ulcerate, and calcify, thereby causing severe vessel narrowing as well as providing fertile ground for thrombosis, resulting in sudden, complete occlusion and MI. Given the many stages in the evolution of atherosclerotic lesions in the coronary artery, it is not surprising that many genetic differences affecting the various pathologic processes involved could predispose to or protect from CAD (Fig. 9.8; also see box). Additional risk factors for CAD include other disorders that are themselves multifactorial with genetic components, such as hypertension,

TABLE 9.11 Twin Concordance Rates and Relative Risks for Fatal Myocardial Infarction When Proband Had Early Fatal Myocardial Infarction*

Sex of the Twins	Concordance MZ Twins	Increased Risk† in an MZ Twin	Concordance DZ Twins	Increased Risk† in a DZ Twin
Male	0.39	6–8-fold	0.26	3-fold
Female	0.44	15-fold	0.14	2.6-fold

*Early myocardial infarction defined as age <55 years in males, age <65 years in females.
†Relative to the risk in the general population.
DZ, Dizygotic; MZ, monozygotic.
Data from Marenberg ME: Genetic susceptibility to death from coronary heart disease in a study of twins, *NEJM* 330:1041–1046, 1994.

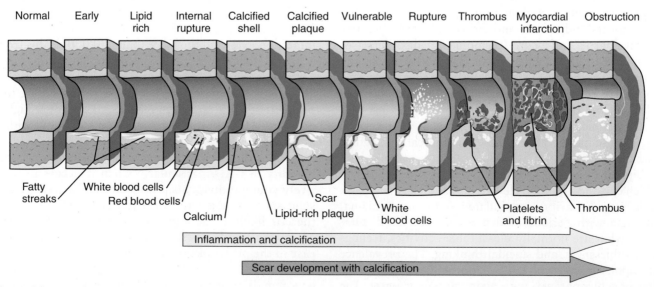

Figure 9.8 Sections of coronary artery demonstrating the steps leading to coronary artery disease. Genetic and environmental factors operating at any or all of the steps in this pathway can contribute to the development of this complex, common disease. (Modified from an original figure courtesy Larry Almonte, with permission.)

obesity, and diabetes mellitus. The metabolic and physiologic derangements represented by these disorders also contribute to enhancing the risk for CAD. Finally, diet, physical activity, systemic inflammation, and smoking are environmental factors that also play a major role in influencing the risk for CAD. Given all the different processes, metabolic derangements, and environmental factors that contribute to the development of CAD, it is easy to imagine that genetic susceptibility to CAD could be a complex multifactorial condition (see Box 9.2).

BOX 9.2 GENES AND GENE PRODUCTS INVOLVED IN THE STEPWISE PROCESS OF CORONARY ARTERY DISEASE

A large number of genes and gene products have been suggested and, in some cases, implicated in promoting one or more of the developmental stages of coronary artery disease. These include genes involved in the following:
- Serum lipid transport and metabolism – cholesterol, apolipoprotein E, apolipoprotein C-III, the low-density lipoprotein (LDL) receptor, and lipoprotein(a) – as well as total cholesterol level. Elevated LDL cholesterol level and triglyceride levels, both of which elevate the risk for coronary artery disease, are themselves quantitative traits with significant heritabilities.
- Vasoactivity, such as angiotensin-converting enzyme.
- Blood coagulation, platelet adhesion, and fibrinolysis, such as plasminogen activator inhibitor 1, and the platelet surface glycoproteins Ib and IIIa.
- Inflammatory and immune pathways.
- Arterial wall components.

CAD is often an incidental finding in family histories of individuals with other genetic diseases. In view of the high recurrence risk, physicians and genetic counselors may need to consider whether first-degree relatives of people with CAD should be evaluated further and offered counseling and therapy, even when CAD is not the primary genetic problem for which the patient or relative has been referred. Such an evaluation is clearly indicated when the proband is young, particularly if the proband is female.

EXAMPLES OF MULTIFACTORIAL TRAITS FOR WHICH SPECIFIC GENETIC AND ENVIRONMENTAL FACTORS ARE KNOWN

Up to this point we have described some of the epidemiologic approaches involving family and twin studies that are used to assess the extent to which there may be a genetic contribution to a complex trait. It is important to realize, however, that studies of familial aggregation, disease concordance, or heritability do not specify how many loci there are, which loci and alleles are involved,

or how a particular genotype and set of environmental influences interact to cause a disease or to determine the value of a particular physiologic measurement. In most cases, all we can show is that there is some genetic contribution and estimate its magnitude. These genetic contributions reflect the aggregate effects of many variants that might number in hundreds or thousands. There are, however, a few multifactorial diseases with complex inheritance for which we have begun to identify the genetic and, in some cases, environmental factors responsible for increasing disease susceptibility. We give a few examples in the next part of this chapter, illustrating increasing levels of complexity.

Modifier Genes in Mendelian Disorders

As discussed in Chapter 7, allelic variation at a single locus can explain variation in the phenotype in many single-gene disorders. However, even for well-characterized mendelian disorders known to be due to defects in a single gene, variation at other gene loci may impact some aspect of the phenotype, illustrating features of complex inheritance.

In cystic fibrosis (CF) **(Case 12)**, for example, whether an individual has pancreatic insufficiency requiring enzyme replacement can be explained largely by which genetic changes are present in the *CFTR* gene (see Chapter 13). The correlation is imperfect, however, for other phenotypes. For example, the variation in the degree of pulmonary disease seen in CF patients remains unexplained by **allelic heterogeneity**. It has been proposed that the genotype at other genetic loci could act as genetic modifiers, that is, genes whose alleles have an effect on the severity of pulmonary disease seen in CF. For example, reduction in forced expiratory volume after 1 second (FEV_1), calculated as a percentage of the value expected for CF patients (a CF-specific FEV_1 percent), is a quantitative trait commonly used to measure deterioration in pulmonary function in CF. A comparison of CF-specific FEV_1 percent in affected MZ versus affected DZ twins provides an estimate of the heritability of the severity of lung disease in CF patients of ~50%. This value is independent of the specific *CFTR* allele(s) (because both kinds of twins will have the same pathogenic CF variants).

Two loci harboring alleles responsible for modifying the severity of pulmonary disease in CF are known: *MBL2*, a gene that encodes a serum protein called mannose-binding lectin; and the *TGFB1* locus encoding the cytokine transforming growth factor β (TGFβ). Mannose-binding lectin is a plasma protein in the innate immune system that binds to many pathogenic organisms and aids in their destruction by phagocytosis and complement activation. A number of common alleles that result in reduced blood levels of the lectin exist at the *MBL2* locus in European populations. Lower levels of mannose-binding lectin appear associated with worse outcomes for CF lung disease, perhaps because low levels of lectin result in difficulties with containing respiratory pathogens, particularly *Pseudomonas*. Alleles at the *TGFB1* locus that result in higher TGFβ production are also associated with worse outcome, perhaps because TGFβ promotes lung scarring and fibrosis after inflammation. Thus both *MBL2* and *TGFB1* are **modifier genes**, variants at which – while they do not cause CF – can modify the clinical phenotype associated with disease-causing alleles at the *CFTR* locus.

Digenic Inheritance

The next level of complexity is a disorder determined by the additive effect of the genotypes at two or more loci. One clear example of such a disease phenotype has been found in a few families of patients with a form of retinal degeneration called retinitis pigmentosa (RP) (Fig. 9.9). Affected individuals in these families are heterozygous for pathogenic alleles at two different loci (**double heterozygotes**). One locus encodes the photoreceptor membrane protein peripherin and the other encodes a related photoreceptor membrane protein called Rom1. **Heterozygotes** for only one or the other of these **mutations** are unaffected. Thus the RP in this family is caused by the simplest form of multigenic inheritance, inheritance due to the effect of variant alleles at two loci, without any known environmental factors that greatly influence disease occurrence or severity. The proteins encoded by these two genes are likely to have overlapping physiologic function because they are both located in the stacks of membranous disks found in retinal photoreceptors. It is the additive effect of having an abnormality in two proteins with overlapping function that produces disease.

A multigenic model has also been proposed in a few families with Bardet-Biedl syndrome, a rare **birth defect** characterized by obesity, variable degrees of intellectual disability, retinal degeneration, polydactyly, and genitourinary malformations. Fourteen different genes have been found in which pathogenic variants cause the syndrome. Although inheritance is clearly autosomal recessive in most families, a few families appear to demonstrate **digenic inheritance**, in which the disease occurs only when an individual is homozygous or compound heterozygous for mutations at one of these 14 loci and is heterozygous for a variant at another of the loci.

Gene-Environment Interactions in Venous Thrombosis

Another example of gene-gene interaction predisposing to disease is found in the group of conditions referred to as hypercoagulability states, in which venous or arterial clots form inappropriately and cause life-threatening complications of thrombophilia (Case 46). With hypercoagulability, however, there is a third factor, an environmental influence that in the presence of the predisposing genetic factors increases the risk for disease even more.

One such disorder is idiopathic cerebral vein thrombosis, a disease in which clots form in the venous system of the brain, causing catastrophic occlusion of cerebral veins in the absence of an inciting event such as infection or tumor. It affects young adults, and although quite rare (<1 per 100,000 in the population), it carries a high mortality rate (5–30%). Three relatively common factors – two genetic and one environmental – that lead to abnormal coagulability of the clotting system are each known to individually increase the risk for cerebral vein thrombosis (Fig. 9.10):

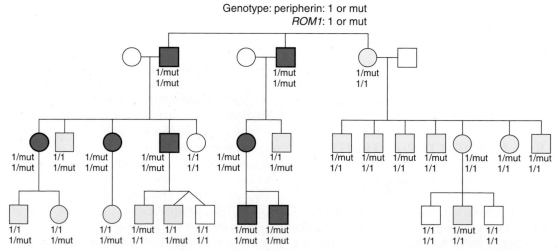

Figure 9.9 Pedigree of a family with retinitis pigmentosa due to digenic inheritance. Dark blue symbols are affected individuals. Each individual's genotypes at the peripherin locus *(first line)* and *ROM1* locus *(second line)* are written below each symbol. The normal allele is 1; the allele carrying a mutation is mut. Light blue symbols are unaffected, despite carrying a pathogenic variant in one or the other gene. (Redrawn from Kajiwara K, Berson EL, Dryja TP: Digenic retinitis pigmentosa due to pathogenic variants at the unlinked peripherin/RDS and ROM1 loci, *Science* 264:1604–1608, 1994.)

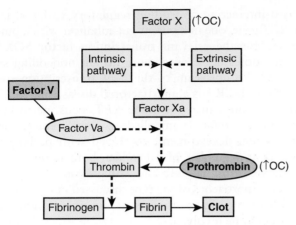

Figure 9.10 The clotting cascade relevant to factor V Leiden and prothrombin variants. Once factor X is activated, through either the intrinsic or extrinsic pathway, activated factor V promotes the production of the coagulant protein thrombin from prothrombin, which in turn cleaves fibrinogen to generate fibrin required for clot formation. Oral contraceptives *(OC)* increase blood levels of prothrombin and factor X as well as a number of other coagulation factors. The hypercoagulable state can be explained as a synergistic interaction of genetic and environmental factors that increase the levels of factor V, prothrombin, factor X, and others to promote clotting. Activated forms of coagulation proteins are indicated by the letter *a*. *Solid arrows* are pathways; *dashed arrows* are stimulators.

- A **missense variant** in the gene for the clotting factor, factor V
- A variant in the 3′ **untranslated region (UTR)** of the gene for the clotting factor prothrombin
- The use of oral contraceptives

A common allele of factor V, factor V Leiden (FVL) **(Case 46)**, in which arginine is replaced by glutamine at position 506 (Arg506Gln), has a frequency of ~2.5% in populations of European origin but is rarer in other population groups. This alteration affects a cleavage site used to degrade factor V, thereby making the protein more stable and able to exert its procoagulant effect for a longer duration. Heterozygous **carriers** of FVL, ~5% of the European population, have a risk for cerebral vein thrombosis that, although still quite low, is 7-fold higher than that in the general population; **homozygotes** have a risk that is 80-fold higher.

The second genetic risk factor, a pathogenic variant in the **prothrombin** gene, changes a G to an A at position 20210 in the 3′ UTR of the gene (prothrombin g.20210 G>A). Approximately 2.4% of individuals of European ancestry are heterozygotes, but it is rare in other groups. This change appears to increase the level of prothrombin **mRNA**, resulting in increased translation and elevated levels of the protein. Being heterozygous for the prothrombin 20210 G>A allele raises the risk for cerebral vein thrombosis three- to sixfold.

The use of oral contraceptives containing synthetic estrogen increases the risk for thrombosis 14- to 22-fold, independent of genotype at the factor V and prothrombin loci, probably by increasing the levels of many clotting factors in the blood. Although using oral contraceptives and being heterozygous for FVL cause only a modest increase in risk compared with either factor alone, oral contraceptive use in a heterozygote for prothrombin 20210 G>A raises the **relative risk** for cerebral vein thrombosis 30- to 150-fold!

There is also interest in the role of FVL and prothrombin 20210 G>A alleles in deep venous thrombosis (DVT) of the lower extremities, a condition that occurs in ~1 in 1000 individuals per year, far more common than idiopathic cerebral venous thrombosis. Mortality due to DVT (primarily due to pulmonary embolus) can be up to 10%, depending on age and the presence of other medical conditions. Many environmental factors are known to increase the risk for DVT and include trauma, surgery (particularly orthopedic surgery), malignant disease, prolonged periods of immobility, oral contraceptive use, and advanced age.

The FVL allele increases the relative risk for a first episode of DVT 7-fold in heterozygotes; heterozygotes who use oral contraceptives see their risk increased 30-fold compared with controls. Heterozygotes for prothrombin 20210 G>A also have an increase in their relative risk for DVT of two- to threefold. Notably, **double heterozygotes** for FVL and prothrombin 20210 G>A have a relative increased risk of 20-fold – a risk approaching a few percent of the population.

Thus each of these three factors, two genetic and one environmental, on its own increases the risk for an abnormal hypercoagulable state; having two or all three of these factors at the same time raises the risk even more, to the point that thrombophilia screening programs for selected populations may be indicated in the future.

Multiple Coding and Noncoding Elements in Hirschsprung Disease

A more complicated set of interacting genetic factors has been described in the pathogenesis of a developmental abnormality of the enteric nervous system in the gut known as Hirschsprung disease (HSCR). In HSCR, there is complete absence of some or all of the intrinsic ganglion cells in the myenteric and submucosal plexuses of the colon. An aganglionic colon is incapable of peristalsis, resulting in severe constipation, symptoms of intestinal obstruction, and massive dilatation of the colon (megacolon) proximal to the aganglionic segment. The disorder affects ~1 in 5000 newborns of European ancestry but is twice as common among Asian infants. HSCR occurs as an isolated birth defect 70% of the time, as part of a chromosomal syndrome 12% of the time, and as one element of a broad constellation of congenital abnormalities in the remainder of cases. Among individuals with HSCR as an isolated birth defect, 80% have only a single, short aganglionic segment of colon at the level of the rectum (hence, HSCR-S), whereas 20%

have aganglionosis of a long segment of colon, the entire colon or, occasionally, the entire colon plus the ileum (hence, HSCR-L).

Familial HSCR-L is often characterized by patterns of inheritance that suggest dominant or recessive inheritance, but consistently with reduced penetrance. HSCR-L is most commonly caused by loss-of-function missense or nonsense mutations in the *RET* gene, which encodes RET, a receptor tyrosine kinase. A small minority of families have pathogenic variants in genes encoding ligands that bind to RET, but with even lower penetrance than those families with *RET* variants.

HSCR-S is the more common type of HSCR and has many of the characteristics of a disorder with complex genetics. The relative risk ratio for sibs, λ_s, is very high (~200), but MZ twins do not show perfect concordance, and families do not show any obvious mendelian inheritance pattern for the disorder. When pairs of siblings concordant for HSCR-S were analyzed genome wide to see which loci and which sets of alleles at these loci each sib had in common with an affected brother or sister, alleles at three loci (including *RET*) were found to be significantly shared, suggesting gene-gene interactions and/or multigenic inheritance; indeed, most of the concordant sibpairs were found to share alleles at all three loci. Although the non-*RET* loci have yet to be identified, Fig. 9.11 illustrates the range of interactions necessary to account for much of the penetrance of HSCR in even this small cohort of patients.

Pathogenic variants of HSCR mutations have now been described at over a dozen loci, with *RET* mutations being by far the most common. The current data suggest that the *RET* gene is implicated in nearly all individuals with HSCR and, in particular, have pointed to two interacting noncoding regulatory variants near the *RET* gene, one in a potent gut **enhancer** with a binding site for the relevant **transcription factor** SOX10 and the other at an even more distant noncoding site some 125 kb upstream of the *RET* **transcription** start site. Thus HSCR-S is a multifactorial disease that results from mutations in or near the *RET* locus, perturbing the normally tightly controlled process of enteric nervous system development, combined with pathogenic variants at a number of other loci, both known, such as EDNRB and GDNF, and still unknown. Current genomic approaches of the type discussed in Chapter 11 suggest the possibility that many dozens of additional genes could be involved.

The identification of common, low-penetrant variants in noncoding elements serves to illustrate that the gene variants responsible for modifying expression of a multifactorial trait may be subtle in how they exert their effects on gene expression and, as a consequence, on disease penetrance and expressivity. It is also sobering to realize that the underlying genetic mechanisms for this relatively well-defined congenital malformation have turned out to be so surprisingly complex; still, they are likely to be far simpler than are the mechanisms involved in the more common complex diseases, such as diabetes.

Type 1 Diabetes Mellitus

A common complex disease for which some of the underlying genetic architecture is being delineated is diabetes mellitus. Diabetes occurs in two major forms: type 1 (T1D) (sometimes referred to as insulin dependent [IDDM]) and type 2 (T2D) (sometimes referred to as non–insulin dependent [NIDDM]), representing ~10%

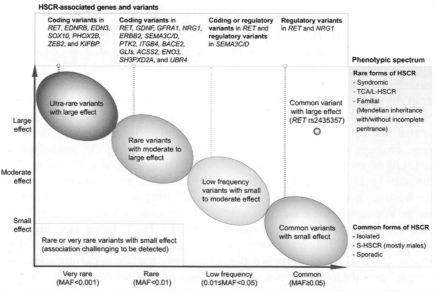

Figure 9.11 Current understanding of the genetic factors underlying inheritance of HSCR. As with most complex traits, genetic susceptibility can be explained by common variants with relatively small impacts on individual risk, and a spectrum towards very rare alleles with a substantial impact on risk. HSCR shows phenotypic severity differences - whereas syndromic HSCR and TCA/L-HSCR are more rare and severe, whereas sporadic S-HSCR is more common. (From Karim A, Tang CS, Tam PK. The Emerging Genetic Landscape of Hirschsprung Disease and Its Potential Clinical Applications. Front Pediatr 2021;9:638093.)

and 88% of all cases, respectively. Familial aggregation is seen in both types of diabetes, but in any given family usually only T1D or T2D is present. They differ in typical onset age, MZ twin concordance, and association with particular genetic variants at particular loci. Here, we focus on T1D to illustrate the major features of complex inheritance in diabetes.

T1D has an incidence in the population of European ancestry of ~2 per 1000 (0.2%), but this is lower in African and Asian ancestry populations. It usually manifests in childhood or adolescence. It results from autoimmune destruction of the β cells of the pancreas, which normally produce insulin. A large majority of children who will go on to have T1D develop multiple autoantibodies early in childhood against a variety of endogenous proteins, including insulin, well before they develop overt disease.

There is strong evidence for genetic factors in T1D: concordance among MZ twins is ~40%, which far exceeds the 5% concordance in DZ twins. The lifetime risk for T1D in siblings of an affected proband is ~7%, resulting in an estimated λ_s of ≈ 35. However, the earlier the age of onset of the T1D in the proband, the greater is λ_s.

The Major Histocompatibility Complex

The major genetic factor in T1D is the **major histocompatibility complex (MHC)** locus, which spans some 3 Mb on chromosome 6 and is the most highly polymorphic locus in the human genome, with over 200 known genes (many involved in immune functions) and well over 2000 alleles known in populations around the globe (Fig. 9.12). On the basis of structural and functional differences, two major subclasses, the class I and class II genes, correspond to the **human leukocyte antigen (HLA)** genes, originally discovered by virtue of their importance in tissue transplantation between unrelated individuals. The HLA class I (HLA-A, HLA-B, HLA-C) and class II (HLA-DR, HLA-DQ, HLA-DP) genes encode cell surface proteins that play a critical role in the presentation of antigen to lymphocytes, which cannot recognize and respond to an antigen unless it is complexed with an HLA molecule on the surface of an antigen-presenting cell. Within the MHC, the HLA class I and class II genes are by far the most highly polymorphic loci (see Fig. 9.12).

The original studies showing an association between T1D and alleles designated as *HLA-DR3* and *HLA-DR4* relied on a serologic method in use at that time for distinguishing between different HLA alleles, one that was based on immunologic reactions in a test tube. This method has long been superseded by direct **determination** of the DNA **sequence** of different alleles, and sequencing of the MHC in a large number of individuals has revealed that the serologically determined "alleles" associated with T1D are not single alleles at all (see Box 9.3). Both *DR3* and *DR4* can be subdivided into a dozen or more alleles located at a locus now termed *HLA-DRB1*.

BOX 9.3 HUMAN ANTIGEN ALLELES AND HAPLOTYPES

The human leukocyte antigen (HLA) system can be confusing at first because the nomenclature used to define and describe different HLA alleles has undergone a fundamental change with the advent of widespread DNA sequencing of the major histocompatibility complex (MHC). According to the older system of HLA nomenclature, the different alleles were distinguished from one another serologically. However, as the genes responsible for encoding the class I and class II MHC chains were identified and sequenced (see Fig. 9.12), single HLA alleles initially defined serologically were shown to consist of multiple alleles defined by different DNA sequence variants even within the same serological allele. The 100 serologic specificities at *HLA-A, B, C, DR, DQ,* and *DP* loci now comprise more than 1300 alleles defined at the DNA sequence level! For example, what used to be a single *B27* allele defined serologically is now referred to as *HLA-B*2701, HLA-B*2702,* and so on, based on DNA-based genotyping.

The set of HLA alleles at the different class I and class II loci on a given chromosome together form a **haplotype**. Within any one ancestral group, some HLA alleles and haplotypes are found commonly; others are rare or never seen. The differences in the distribution and frequency of the alleles and haplotypes within the MHC are the result of complex genetic, environmental, and historical factors at play in each of the different populations. The extreme levels of genetic variation at HLA loci and their resulting haplotypes have been extraordinarily useful for identifying associations of particular variants with specific diseases (see Chapter 11), many of which (as one might predict) are autoimmune disorders, associated with an abnormal immune response apparently directed against one or more self antigens resulting from **polymorphism** in immune response genes.

Furthermore, it is now clear that the association between certain *DRB1* alleles and T1D is due, in part, to alleles at two other class II loci, *DQA1* and *DQB1*, located ~80 kb away from *DRB1*, that form a particular combination of alleles with each other (i.e., a haplotype) that is typically inherited as a unit (due to linkage disequilibrium; see Chapter 11). *DQA1* and *DQB1* encode the α and β chains of the class II DQ protein. Certain combinations of alleles at these three loci form a haplotype that increases the risk for T1D more than 11-fold over that for the general population, whereas other combinations of alleles reduce the risk 50-fold. The DQB1*0303 allele contained in this protective haplotype results in the amino acid aspartic acid at position 57 of the DQB1 product, whereas other amino acids at this position (alanine, valine, or serine) confer susceptibility. In fact, ~90% of individuals with T1D are homozygous for *DQB1* alleles that do not encode aspartic acid at position 57. It is likely that differences in antigen binding, determined by which amino acid is at position

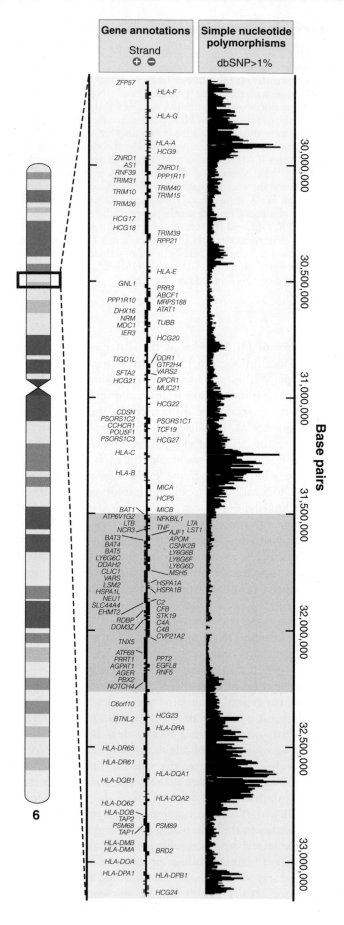

Figure 9.12 Genomic landscape of the major histocompatibility complex (MHC). The classic MHC is shown on the short arm of chromosome 6, comprising the class I region *(yellow)* and class II region *(blue)*, both enriched in human leukocyte antigen (HLA) genes. Sequence-level variation is shown for single nucleotide polymorphisms (SNPs) found with at least 1% frequency. Remarkably high levels of genetic variation are seen in regions containing the classic HLA genes where variation is enriched in coding exons involved in defining the antigen-binding cleft. Other genes *(pink)* in the MHC region show lower levels of genetic variation. *dbSNP*, Minor allele frequency in the SNP database. (Modified from Trowsdale J, Knight JC: Major histocompatibility complex genomics and human disease, *Annu Rev Genom Hum Genet* 14:301–323, 2013.)

57, contribute directly to the autoimmune response that destroys the insulin-producing cells of the pancreas. Other loci and alleles in the MHC, however, are also important, as can be seen from the fact that some individuals with T1D have an aspartic acid at this position.

Genes Other Than Class II Major Histocompatibility Complex Loci in Type 1 Diabetes

The MHC haplotype alone accounts for only a portion of the genetic contribution to the risk for T1D in siblings of a proband. Family studies in T1D (Table 9.12) suggest that even when siblings share the same MHC class II haplotypes, the risk for disease is only ~17%, still well below the MZ twin concordance rate of ~40%. Thus there must be other genes elsewhere in the genome that contribute to the development of T1D (assuming that MZ twins and sibs have similar environmental exposures). Indeed, genetic association studies (to be described in Chapter 11) indicate that variation at more than 50 different loci around the genome can increase susceptibility to T1D, although most have very small effects on increasing disease susceptibility.

TABLE 9.12 Empirical Risks for Counseling in Type 1 Diabetes

Relationship to Affected Individual	Risk for Development of Type 1 Diabetes (%)
None	0.2
MZ twin	40
Sibling	7
Sibling with no DR haplotypes in common	1
Sibling with 1 DR haplotype in common	5
Sibling with 2 DR haplotypes in common	17*
Child	4
Child of affected mother	3
Child of affected father	5

*20–25% for particular shared haplotypes.
MZ, Monozygotic.

It is important to stress, however, that genetic factors alone do not cause T1D because the MZ twin concordance rate is only ~40%, not 100%. Until a more complete picture develops of the genetic and nongenetic factors that cause T1D, risk counseling using HLA haplotyping must remain empirical (see Table 9.12).

Alzheimer Disease

Alzheimer disease (AD) (Case 4) is a fatal neurodegenerative disease that affects 1% to 2% of the US population. It is the most common cause of dementia in older adults and is responsible for more than half of all cases of dementia. As with other dementias, patients experience a chronic, progressive loss of memory and other cognitive functions, associated with loss of certain types of cortical neurons. Age, sex, and family history are the most significant risk factors for AD. Once a person reaches 65 years of age, the risk for any dementia, and AD in particular, increases substantially with age and female sex (Table 9.13).

AD can be diagnosed definitively only postmortem, on the basis of neuropathologic findings of characteristic protein aggregates (β-amyloid plaques and neurofibrillary tangles; see Chapter 13). The most important constituent of the plaques is a small (39–42 amino acid) peptide, Aβ, derived from cleavage of a normal neuronal protein, the amyloid protein precursor. The secondary structure of Aβ gives the plaques the staining characteristics of amyloid proteins.

In addition to three rare autosomal dominant forms of the disease (see Chapter 13), in which disease onset is in the third to fifth decade, there is a common form of AD with onset after the age of 60 years (late onset). This form has no obvious mendelian inheritance pattern but shows familial aggregation and an elevated relative risk ratio ($\lambda_s = \approx 4$) typical of disorders with complex inheritance. Twin studies have been inconsistent but suggest MZ concordance of ~50% and DZ concordance of ~18%.

The ε4 Allele of Apolipoprotein E

The major locus with alleles found to be significantly associated with common late-onset AD is *APOE*, which encodes apolipoprotein E. Apolipoprotein E is a protein component of the LDL particle and is involved in clearing LDL through an interaction with high-affinity receptors in the liver. Apolipoprotein E is also a constituent of amyloid plaques in AD and is known to bind the Aβ peptide. The *APOE* gene has three alleles, ε2, ε3, and ε4, due to substitutions of arginine for two different cysteine residues in the protein (see Chapter 13).

When the genotypes at the *APOE* locus were analyzed in individuals with AD and controls, a genotype with at least one ε4 allele was found two to three times more frequently among patients compared with controls in both the general US and Japanese populations (Table 9.14), with much less of an association in Hispanic and African populations. Even more striking is that the risk for AD appears to increase further if both *APOE* alleles are ε4, through an effect on the age at onset of AD; individuals with two ε4 alleles have an earlier onset of disease than those with only one. In a study of people with AD and unaffected controls, the age at which AD developed in the affected individuals was earliest for ε4/ε4 homozygotes, next for ε4/ε3 heterozygotes, and significantly less for the other genotypes (Fig. 9.13).

In the population in general, the risk for developing AD by age 80 is approaching 10%. The ε4 allele is clearly a predisposing factor that increases the risk for development of AD by shifting the age at onset to an earlier age, such that ε3/ε4 heterozygotes have a 40% risk for developing the disease, and ε4/ε4 have a 60% risk by age 85. Despite this increased risk, other genetic and environmental factors must be important because a significant proportion of ε3/ε4 and ε4/ε4 individuals live to extreme old age with no evidence of AD. There are also reports of association between the presence of the ε4 allele and neurodegenerative disease after traumatic head injury (as seen in professional boxers, football players, and soldiers who have suffered blast injuries), indicating that at least one environmental factor, brain trauma, can interact with the ε4 allele in the pathogenesis of AD.

TABLE 9.13 Cumulative Age- and Sex-Specific Risks for Alzheimer Disease and Dementia

Time Interval Past Age 65 Yr	Risk for Development of AD (%)	Risk for Development of Any Dementia (%)
65–80 yr		
Male	6.3	10.9
Female	12	19
65–100 yr		
Male	25	32.8
Female	28.1	45

AD, Alzheimer disease.
Data from Seshadri S, Wolf PA, Beiser A, et al: Lifetime risk of dementia and Alzheimer's disease. The impact of mortality on risk estimates in the Framingham Study, *Neurology* 49:1498–1504, 1997.

TABLE 9.14 Association of Apolipoprotein E ε4 Allele With Alzheimer Disease*

	Frequency			
	United States		**Japan**	
Genotype	AD	Control	AD	Control
ε4/ε4; ε4/ε3; or ε4/ε2	0.64	0.31	0.47	0.17
ε3/ε3; ε2/ε3; or ε2/ε2	0.36	0.69	0.53	0.83

*Frequency of genotypes with and without the ε4 allele among Alzheimer disease (AD) patients and controls from the United States and Japan.

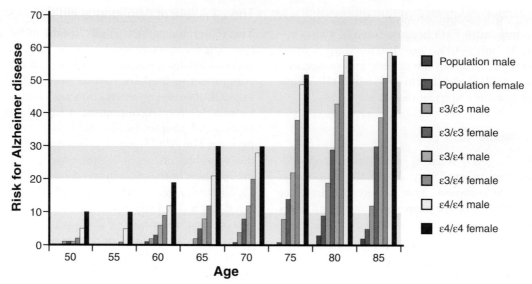

Figure 9.13 Chance of developing Alzheimer disease as a function of age for different APOE genotypes for each sex. At one extreme is the ε4/ε4 homozygote, who has a ≈40% chance of remaining free of the disease by the age of 85 years, whereas an ε3/ε3 homozygote has ≈70% to ≈90% chance of remaining disease free at the age of 85 years, depending on the sex. General population risk is also shown for comparison. (Modified from Roberts JS, Cupples LA, Relkin NR, et al: Genetic risk assessment for adult children of people with Alzheimer's disease: the Risk Evaluation and Education for Alzheimer's Disease (REVEAL) study, *J Geriatr Psychiatry Neurol* 18:250–255, 2005.)

The ε4 variant of APOE represents a prime example of a predisposing allele: It predisposes to a complex trait in a powerful way but does not predestine any individual carrying the allele to the disease. Additional genes as well as environmental effects are also clearly involved; although several of these appear to have a significant effect, most remain to be identified. In general, testing of asymptomatic people for the APOE ε4 allele remains controversial because knowing that one is a heterozygote or homozygote for the ε4 allele does not mean one will develop AD, and there are no preventative interventions to reduce disease risk in more susceptible individuals (see Chapter 19).

THE CHALLENGE OF MULTIFACTORIAL DISEASE WITH COMPLEX INHERITANCE

The greatest challenge facing medical genetics and **genomic medicine** going forward is unraveling the complex interactions between the variants at multiple loci and the relevant environmental factors that underlie the susceptibility to common multifactorial disease. This area of research is the central focus of the field of population-based **genetic epidemiology** (to be discussed more fully in Chapter 10). The field is developing rapidly, and it is clear that the genetic contribution to many more complex diseases in humans will be elucidated in the coming years. Such understanding will, in time, allow the development of novel preventive and therapeutic measures for the common disorders that cause such significant morbidity and mortality in the population.

GENERAL REFERENCES

Chakravarti A, Clark AG, Mootha VK: Distilling pathophysiology from complex disease genetics, *Cell* 155:21–26, 2013.
Rimoin DL, Pyeritz RE, Korf BR: *Emery and Rimoin's essential medical genetics*, Waltham, MA, 2020, Academic Press (Elsevier).
Scott W, Ritchie M: *Genetic analysis of complex disease*, ed 3, Hoboken, NJ, 2022, John Wiley and Sons.

REFERENCES FOR SPECIFIC TOPICS

Baylis RA, Smith NL, Klarin D, et al: Epidemiology and genetics of venous thromboembolism and chronic venous disease, *Circ Res* 128:1988–2002, 2021.
Bellenguez C, Küçükali F, Jansen IE, et al: New insights into the genetic etiology of Alzheimer's disease and related dementias, *Nat Genet* 54:412–436, 2022.
Bigdeli TB, Fanous AH, Li Y, et al: Genome-wide association studies of schizophrenia and bipolar disorder in a diverse cohort of US veterans, *Schizophr Bull* 47(2):517–529, 2021.
Grant SFA, Wells AD, Rich SS: Next steps in the identification of gene targets for type 1 diabetes, *Diabetologia* 63:2260–2269, 2020.
Karim A, Tang CS, Tam PK: The emerging genetic landscape of Hirschsprung disease and its potential clinical applications, *Front Pediatr* 9:638093, 2021. https://doi.org/10.3389/fped.2021.638093
Khera AV, Chaffin M, Aragam KG, et al: Genome-wide polygenic scores for common diseases identify individuals with risk equivalent to monogenic mutations, *Nat Genet* 50:1219–1224, 2018. https://www.nature.com/articles/s41588-018-0183-z
Matzaraki M, Kumar V, Wijmenga C, et al: The MHC locus and genetic susceptibility to autoimmune and infectious diseases, *Genome Bio* 18:76, 2017.
Shoaib M, Ye Q, IglayReger H, et al: Evaluation of polygenic risk scores to differentiate between type 1 and type 2 diabetes, *Genet Epidemiol.* 2023. https://doi.org/10.1002/gepi.22521
Uffelmann E, Huang QQ, Munung NS, et al: Genome-wide association studies, *Nat Rev Methods Primers* 1:59, 2021.
Wu P, Gifford A, Meng X, et al: Mapping ICD-10 and ICD-10-CM codes to phecodes: Workflow development and initial evaluation, *JMIR Med Inform* 7(4):e14325, 2019. https://doi.org/10.2196/14325

PROBLEMS

1. For a specific disease, the concordance rate in monozygotic (MZ) twins is 80% and the concordance rate in dizygotic (DZ) twins is 20%. What does this tell us about whether there are genetic or environmental contributions to susceptibility for this disease?

2. Match the genetic mapping technique that would be most cost-effective to find genetic predictors in each scenario:

a. Searching for the disease-causing variant in a large pedigree with 4-5 related individuals who have a rare disease	i. Genome-wide association study using array-based genotyping and imputation
b. Searching for common variants that increase susceptibility to a disease in a large case-control sample with well-studied ancestry	ii. Exome sequencing with linkage analysis
c. Searching for specific effector genes for a large number of diseases in a biobank sample	iii. Exome or genome sequencing with gene-based burden testing

3. One of the most important challenges in human genetics is keeping up with the rapidly evolving literature about each trait. Pick a complex disease of your choice and find the largest genome wide association study published in the last 5 years and compare it to one published 5 years before that. If you don't have a favorite complex disease, consider atrial fibrillation as a potential example.

   a. How many disease loci were identified in each of the two studies?

   b. What was the strongest signal in each of the studies, defined by p-value? Summarize disease allele frequency, odds ratio and nearest gene of all genome-wide hits.

   c. What was the strongest signal in each of the studies, defined by odds ratio? Summarize disease allele frequency, odds ratio and nearest gene.

   d. Did the two studies focus on similar questions? What new questions did the new study consider?

CHAPTER 10

Population Genetics for Genomic Medicine

Alice B. Popejoy

INTRODUCTION TO POPULATION GENETICS FOR GENOMIC MEDICINE

We have explored in previous chapters the nature of genetic and genomic variation, mechanisms and types of **mutation**, and the inheritance of **alleles** (genetic variants) in families. Throughout, we have alluded to observed differences in allele frequencies across the globe, whether assessed by examining **single nucleotide variants (SNVs)**, **insertions** and **deletions** (indels), or copy number variants (CNVs) in the **genomes** of many thousands of individuals. We have also discussed how the incidence and prevalence of some **genetic disorders** may differ among populations, and how discoveries have been made by selectively sampling individuals with specific **phenotypes**. Here we take a deeper look into the assumptions and limitations of how populations are defined in **genomics** research and medicine, considering in greater detail the underlying forces that shift or maintain allele frequencies over time.

Identifying genetic susceptibilities to diseases is a key objective of medical genetics, with a critical role in clinical diagnosis and **genetic counseling**. Concepts and observations from **population genetics** inform our understanding of the genetic architecture of health and disease by observing how **variants** may differ in frequency, effect size, and phenotypic expression in human populations. When we refer to a population frequency, we consider a hypothetical **gene pool** as a collection of all the alleles at a particular **locus** for the entire population. The frequency of an allele is thus its proportion among all alleles at the same locus in a population.

In this chapter, we describe a central organizing concept of population genetics, Hardy-Weinberg equilibrium (HWE), and its utility for genomics and clinical genetics in understanding the relationship between allele and **genotype** frequencies. Assumptions of the Hardy-Weinberg principle are considered in the context of factors that cause true or apparent **deviation** from equilibrium in real, as opposed to idealized, populations.

Clinical genetics is primarily concerned with rare, often *de novo* mutations that cause genetic conditions and may severely impact function, with similar incidences across populations. Genetic variants that impact function and reproduction are rare in nearly *all* human populations because they are eliminated from the gene pool through **natural selection**. These variants are most often *de novo* – not inherited – so there is typically no link between genetic ancestral origins and the incidence of these pathogenic mutations. Most human genomic variation is shared among all groups, so there are exceedingly rare cases of clinically relevant variants that are found exclusively in one category or group of patients. The exception to this rule is when a defined ancestral group has experienced a bottleneck that reduces and then regrows the population with a subset of its original genetic variants. This increases the chance of maintaining a **pathogenic variant** in the population, as selective pressure is weaker than in a more genetically diverse population.

Population genetics is the quantitative study of the distribution of genetic variation in populations, including trends in the frequencies of genes and genotypes over time. Differences in the frequencies of alleles that cause genetic disease are of particular interest to the medical geneticist and genetic counselor because they contribute to differences in disease **risk** among populations. Nevertheless, it is important to consider what we do not know and examine our baseline assumptions about genetic etiologies of health and disease. We present clinical examples to illustrate how the creation of genomic knowledge, as in all fields, depends on who is included in the underlying research, how their attributes are represented, and what categories are used to classify or stratify people into groups.

The distributions of genetic variants and attributes in families, communities, and geographic regions are driven by a combination of social, environmental, and biological factors. Social scientists, anthropologists, and evolutionary biologists employ mathematical descriptions of shifting allele frequencies across geographic regions and time to reconstruct our evolutionary histories. Knowing about differences in allele frequencies across populations may be important for physicians to predict an increased likelihood of certain conditions in patients with *specific* ancestral origins linked to a pathogenic variant. However, it is important to keep in mind that most genetic variation that is used to describe ancestral origins is selectively neutral or has an unknown biological function.

With today's access to genome sequencing technology, considering all types of variation, we know that all humans share an average of 99% of our **DNA** sequences across the genome. The relatively small proportion of our genomes that do vary (**polymorphism**) do not differentiate us into discrete social categories; on the contrary, greater genomic variation has been observed *within* broad groupings (e.g., based on "race" or "ethnicity") than between them. Nevertheless, humans tend to make meaning out of anecdotal observations, attributing physical or health-related differences we observe to underlying attributes of broad semantic categories that reinforce social stereotypes. This is one mechanism by which biological or scientific racism is enacted in genetics. Data subjects are often stratified into groups to make statistical comparisons, which (with sufficient sample sizes) may yield average differences that offer a biased confirmation of natural classes. Some have used these findings to argue for the inevitability of systemic inequities. This chapter touches on the history and impact of classifying humans into nominal groupings, making the case for genetics researchers and clinicians to understand the origins and assumptions underlying conceptual and functional models used to create and apply knowledge.

Statistical methods have been used to identify variants that can differentiate many individuals into broad "continental ancestry" groupings based on allele frequencies observed across geographic regions. Such **ancestry informative markers (AIMs)** often lack functional relevance, but they have been used as a proxy for genomic background, which may inflate estimated genetic distances between groups. When such variants are associated with complex, multifactorial traits (with both genetic and environmental influences) such as obesity, diabetes, heart disease, and asthma, it is difficult to determine the true causal factors driving statistically significant **associations**, because social determinants of health influence the environment differently across sociocultural groups. A central challenge for human genomics research is thus teasing apart causal factors that drive phenotypic variation from confounders that are associated with patterns of both genotype and phenotype variation.

Stratification is not inherently problematic as a statistical strategy to reduce the complexity of genomic and environmental backgrounds, but there are deep scientific and ethical flaws in approaches that collapse these nuanced dimensions of variation into static population descriptors such as race, ethnicity, and ancestry. European colonization, slavery, and **eugenics** have institutionalized conceptual frameworks tied to categories of difference, preserving hierarchies of power. These frameworks have persisted in colonized societies and science, with implications for analytic approaches still used today in biomedical research.

Racial categories are constructed using poorly defined criteria that subdivide humankind using physical appearance (i.e., skin color, hair texture, and facial features) combined with characteristic identities that have their origins in the geographical, historical, cultural, religious, and linguistic backgrounds of the communities in which an individual was born and raised. Physical traits linked to racial and ethnic stereotypes may be influenced by genetics. However, genetic variation and diverse phenotypes exist across all populations, so attempts to equate continental origins with race are misguided. DNA alone cannot be used to assign someone to a social identity group, and it is primarily nongenetic, social and systemic factors that create the conditions for observed group-level differences in health outcomes.

Concept of race and racism are important in discussions of social and health policy, tracking disparities in outcomes and social determinants of health. Longstanding systemic and structural factors create differences in health outcomes among racial groups, which can contribute to confounding and disparities in the quality of care, such as timely screening and test referrals. Thus, race may be used as a proxy for the effects of racism, but not as a proxy for genetic background or to calculate genetic disease risk.

Building on themes from previous chapters, we paint a detailed picture of global genomic diversity that is largely shared among all human populations, and the factors that influence shifts in relative frequencies of genetic variants over time. We demonstrate the importance of African genomic diversity for all populations, highlighting the need for clinically relevant data on **genetic heterogeneity**, structural variation, and **haplotype** diversity across the globe. These data will inform our understanding of genetic etiologies of health and disease in everyone and must be included in public databases. Finally, we seek to clarify common misconceptions about human populations and diversity that could exacerbate health disparities in genomics and medicine.

HUMAN ORIGINS AND FOUNDER EFFECTS OF SERIAL MIGRATION

Our species (*Homo sapiens*) is comprised of more than 7 billion members, all of whom share a common ancestral lineage on the African continent dating back ~200,000 years ago. Fig. 10.1 illustrates the origin of modern humans in Southern Africa and suggests a series of migrations north through the continent beginning ~100,000 years ago. Subsequent dispersals of subsets of these migratory modern human ancestors led our species out of Africa to populate the other continents, such that we are thought to have reached South America ~15,000 years ago.

Migration can change allele frequencies through the process of **gene flow**, defined as the slow diffusion

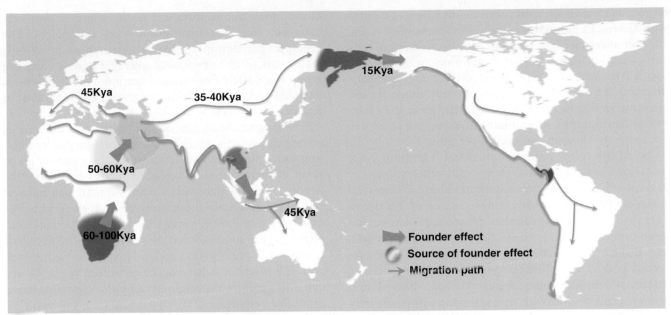

Figure 10.1 Ancient dispersal patterns of modern humans during the past 100,000 years. This map highlights demic events that began with a source population in southern Africa 60 to 100 kya and concluded with the settlement of South America approximately 12 to 14 kya. *Wide arrows* indicate major founder events during the demographic expansion into different continental regions. *Colored arcs* indicate the putative source for each of these founder events. *Thin arrows* indicate potential migration paths. Many additional migrations occurred during the Holocene. From Henn BM, Cavalli-Sforza LL, Feldman MW. The great human expansion. *Proceedings of the National Academy of Sciences of the United States of America.* 109:17758–64. PMID 23077256. https://doi.org/10.1007/S12045-019-0830-4

of variants, or alleles, across a barrier. Gene flow usually involves a large population and a gradual change in allele frequencies. The allele frequencies of migrant populations gradually merge into the gene pool of the population into which they have migrated, a process referred to as **genetic admixture**. The term *migration* is used here in the broad sense of crossing a reproductive barrier, which may be social or cultural (not necessarily geographic) and does not require physical movement from one region to another.

During serial migration events a subset of the genomic variation from the original population travels with the migratory group into the new population. These events create **founder effects**, which are marked by a reduction in genomic diversity from the original, ancestral population to the new subpopulation. Founder events such as bottlenecks, the reduction in size and subsequent regrowth of a population whereby it loses a large portion of its original diversity, create so-called founder populations. In populations that have experienced a bottleneck (e.g., European ancestry groups), we observe greater genetic homogeneity (lower heterozygosity) than would be expected, based on the overall estimated population size. Founder populations thus have lower effective population sizes (N_e) relative to their census populations, and various estimators for genetic diversity use this concept to model human population history.

Founder populations with small N_e are relevant for clinical genetics, because individuals with these ancestries are generally at a greater risk of accumulating genetic diseases that are rare in other populations.

Dominant deleterious mutations can rise to high frequency more easily when there are fewer potential reproductive partners, as this reduces competition in the form of alternative alleles. For example, the high incidence of Huntington disease (Case 24) among inhabitants around Lake Maracaibo, Venezuela, resulted from genetic isolation following the introduction of a (likely European) genetic variant that causes Huntington disease.

Similarly, French-Canadians in the Saguenay-Lac-Saint-Jean region of Quebec are at greater risk for the autosomal **recessive** condition hereditary type I tyrosinemia. If untreated, this condition causes hepatic failure and renal tubular dysfunction due to deficiency of fumarylacetoacetase, an enzyme in the degradative pathway of tyrosine. The disease incidence was estimated (in 1994) at 1 in 1846, with the pathogenic allele **carrier** frequency estimated at 1 in 22. Nearly all pathogenic alleles observed in Saguenay-Lac-Saint-Jean patients are due to the same variant inherited through a shared lineage of recent common ancestor(s). This observation is consistent with the history of this population, which is a known founder population or genetic isolate, meaning there was reduced genetic variation among individuals who originally founded the population, followed by population growth and a paucity of new alleles flowing into it.

As a result of serial founder events throughout our history, nearly all human genomic variation in modern populations is only a subset of the variation that exists in Africa, the ancestral homeland of our species, and the current home of modern human populations with more genetic diversity compared to anywhere else in the world. African populations and individuals with recent African ancestries have the largest effective population sizes, with genomic evidence pointing to Indigenous South Africans having the most diverse and anciently diverged genomes. It is a common error to think of these ancestral genomes as an artifact of the past; they have in fact continued to accumulate variation and to experience effects of natural selection over time.

In addition to standing ancestral variation, new mutations arise – albeit slowly – and other sources of variation have been introduced in different ancestral lineages. Evidence (mostly from studies of European ancestry populations) suggests *Homo sapiens* encountered other early hominid species such as Neanderthals and Denisovans – whose genetic fragments were preserved in cold, dry climates. Segments of these archaic hominids' **chromosomes** appear to have flowed into human genomes through introgression approximately ~50 to 90k years ago. By comparing human genomes to DNA extracted from excavated bone fragments, ancient DNA researchers estimate that 1% to 4% of the DNA of modern humans may be derived from these species.

While there is little evidence of archaic hominid introgression into human populations in regions of the world marked by hot and humid climates, (which are not conducive to the preservation of DNA in ancient remains), it is likely that such introgression events occurred wherever other hominid species met and mingled with ancient *Homo sapiens*.

DEFINING HUMAN POPULATIONS TO CHARACTERIZE DIVERSITY

There are many ways to define a population – whether criteria are based on geography, societal and cultural factors, geopolitical or national borders, or any other features that may be considered characteristic of individuals within a group. Whether an individual or group is designated as belonging to a "population" depends on the classification framework, and how it is implemented in practice. Many designated "populations" have nothing to do with genetics – such as the census population of a large, urban metropolis. The specific criteria that are used to define a population often flow from certain research or clinical objectives and may also be influenced by social, cultural, and political factors that privilege certain approaches. Who has the authority to determine such classification criteria also plays an important role in defining human populations.

Decisions made by researchers and clinicians about how to classify participants or patients into groups strongly influence population-level estimates such as allele frequencies and disease prevalence. Methods used to detect and interpret combinations and mixtures of these alleles, and to investigate how they impact our health, play an important role in what is generally accepted about average group-level differences. For example, population-level statistics such as point estimates that serve to represent averages across an entire group (e.g., allele frequencies) are influenced by who is included and excluded from the group, and their level of genetic relatedness.

The magnitude of genetic similarities and differences among individuals defined by some category or population descriptor thus impacts the accuracy of any given point estimate for that category. It also influences the precision with which such a point estimate can be used to make predictions about individuals in the group. For example, population categories such as "Asian" and "African" are so broad that they describe more than half of the world population and land mass. The vast genetic and environmental **heterogeneity** within such groups call into question the reliability of point estimates based on such groupings.

In contrast, populations with less total variability are more likely to yield group-level estimates that reflect a greater number of individuals in the category. For example, populations that have experienced bottlenecks have less overall diversity in the underlying gene pool and population mean and median values may be more informative. This is important because it means that research methods or approaches to estimating disease risk based on point estimates have differential validity and utility across population groups, benefiting those with less variability (i.e., European ancestries).

Many clinical case studies present population allele frequencies as point estimates corresponding to different race, ethnicity, or ancestry categories. Unfortunately, these terms are conceptualized and used in vastly different ways among clinical genetics professionals and researchers, so summary statistics that are based on such poorly or broadly defined groupings may be unreliable and inconsistent, depending on the underlying characteristics of the groups.

Genetic ancestry and ethnicity represent different kinds of information, so direct comparisons cannot be made between them (despite misguided attempts to 'valide' self-identified race or ethnicity using estimated proportions of DNA shared with 'known' population reference datasets). Most people are not limited to one ancestry or ethnic identity, and these identity concepts can change over time. As such, ontological frameworks and methodologies in population genetics that force a single-group assignment are conceptually inconsistent, insufficient for characterizing the spectrum of human cultural and genomic diversity, and are becoming increasingly obsolete.

For example, while "Ashkenazi Jewish" represents a cultural or ethnic designation without specific geographic constraints, its related definition of having "ancestry from Africa, the Middle East, or the Mediterranean" is geographically diverse and includes a vast array of social and cultural identities. For many years, carrier screening for autosomal recessive diseases such as for Tay-Sachs disease used a risk-based strategy that relied on self-described ethnicity; this approach is now known to introduce inaccuracy into the screening process. Thus, recent recommendations from the American College of Medical Genetics and Genomics (ACMG) note that carrier screening paradigms should be agnostic to race, ethnicity, and ancestry.

Carrier screening, referrals for genetic testing, and reporting risk predictions to patients or other care providers have relied on patient self-reported information about race, ethnicity, or ancestry. Certain populations may be at higher risk for conditions that are not routinely screened for, but only individuals who have self-identified with (or for whom a provider has determined their membership in) these populations would have access to those screenings. In some circumstances, physicians may not think to refer patients for genetic testing unless they fit the stereotype of the population known to be at high risk, and insurance companies may not cover genetic testing for certain conditions unless a patient has disclosed information about their background that is consistent with population-specific elevated risk of disease. Thus, whether and how patients are classified into population groups or categories is of great importance here.

Expanded carrier screening has received much attention and has the potential to alleviate some of the pitfalls of relying on proxy measures and poorly defined population groups to guide clinical decision-making. However, once the results of genetic tests are received, there are additional uses for population-level information about patients that inform the interpretation and curation of findings.

A survey of clinical genetics professionals and researchers, conducted mainly in the United States, revealed that patient self-reported race and ethnicity information may be used to make decisions about ordering tests, interpreting results, and reporting findings to patients. At least 18% of respondents reported that this information may have been entered into a patient's medical record without asking them directly. Fewer than 5% of clinical genetics professionals who responded to the survey reported that they conduct ancestry analyses or have access to ancestry estimates based on patients' DNA for the purpose of clinical variant interpretation and **gene** curation. This means that social categories are used as a proxy for genomic background in clinical genetics.

Cultural and political contexts shape the way we collect and use information about patients' social/cultural identities and ancestral backgrounds – and asking for a person's race or ethnicity is illegal in some parts of the world. It is important for clinical genetics professionals to know about the risks of relying too heavily on this information to make predictions or decisions in the clinical setting. Box 10.1 offers descriptions of "race," "ethnicity," and "ancestry" that have been useful for genomics researchers.

BOX 10.1 DESCRIPTIONS OF RACE, ETHNICITY, AND ANCESTRY

"Race," "ethnicity," and "ancestry" are often used interchangeably, yet they have no universal definitions. We provide brief descriptions of our usage below. For extensive discussion in context of genomics, including recommendations from professional organizations, see Banda et al. (2015); Mersha and Abebe (2015); Race, Ethnicity, and Genetics Working Group (2005).

Race: A culturally and politically charge term, for which definitions and meaning are context-specific. Race is related to individual and/or group identity and is often linked to stereotypes of visible physical attributes such as skin and hair pigmentation. The concept of race is tightly linked to social power dynamics and has historically been used to justify hierarchies of power, discrimination, and oppression in an unequal society. Social and cultural conditions may differ among racial groups, on average, and these differences may lead to environmental effects such as chronic stress and unequal access to goods and services, including healthcare and nutrition. These inequities can affect environmental risk for complex diseases and/or potentially interact with genetics to affect risk.

Ethnicity: Describes people as belonging to cultural groups, usually on the basis of shared language, traditions, foods, etc. Ethnicity has often been used interchangeably with race and is similarly ambiguous. To the extent that traits are affected by social and environmental differences, ethnicity has previously served as a proxy for health and disease risk at the population level as a result of social, cultural and community effects described above. There is no universal agreement on a system of "ethnic" groupings worldwide. Some ethnic groups may share genetic factors due to similar ancestral origins; other groups may be more social and cultural in nature.

Ancestry: Meaning varies by context. Here, we use the term to denote genetic ancestry, a description of the population(s) from which an individual's recent biological ancestors originated, as reflected in the DNA inherited from those ancestors. Genetic ancestry can be estimated via comparison of participant's genotypes to global reference populations, so incomplete availability of these references can create biased estimates. We note that different methods of calculating genetic ancestry can yield different results. Thus, discreet labeling of ancestral populations oversimplifies the complexity of human genetic variation and demography. Nevertheless, accounting for systemic differences in allele frequencies and **linkage disequilibrium** is necessary for genetic analyses. In this paper, diversity in genomics is described primarily in terms of ancestry.

From Peterson RE, Kuchenbaecker K, Walters RK, et al: Genome-wide association studies in ancestrally diverse populations: Opportunities, methods, pitfalls, and recommendations, *Cell* 179(3):589-603, 2019. https://doi.org/10.1016/j.cell.2019.08.051

History and Influence of Eugenics on Population Genetics

Countless atrocities have been committed in the name of perceived differences among human beings, from oppression, discrimination, and displacement to slavery and genocide. In the United States, Jim Crow laws were enacted upon the abolition of slavery and persisted overtly through the 1960s, which forced **segregation** of "Black" and "white" people to preserve exploitative power dynamics and justify economic and social injustice. The ideological underpinning of segregating hospitals and clinical care was that white and Black people needed different *medical care* due to perceived differences in biology. However, there are no unique, fundamental genetic differences between groups of people who identify as "white" or "Black," and the persistence of this racial binary in genomics research has contributed to misconceptions and harm.

Many in human genomics may not realize how the field's history is rooted in the American Eugenics Movement, which provided a false sense of scientific legitimacy to Nazi propaganda during WWII. Indeed, the *Annals of Human Genetics* was originally called the *Annals of Eugenics*, founded in 1925 by an English eugenics thought leader, Francis Galton. Mentees of Galton's became the journal's editors, including Karl Pearson and R.A. Fisher, who developed statistical methods we still use today. They include the chi-square test, p-values, analysis of variance (ANOVA), and principal component analysis (PCA). Another of Galton's mentees, Charles Davenport, used taxonomic frameworks classify humans, the scientific endeavor of biological racism. The idea that racial groups were genetically distinct predates eugenics, back to early European slave traders who devized categories that dehumanized people with darker skin to justify their enslavement and exploitation. While it may feel uncomfortable to engage the history of these ideologies researchers and physicians must understand how they persist in our scientific and clinical methodologies so that we can heal the wounds of the past, moving forward with greater care and precision.

Aristotle's *Scala Naturae* laid the foundation for Carl Linnaeus's 1737 *Systema Naturae*, a taxonomy of humans subdivided into four continental groups based on skin color: "whitish European," "reddish American," "tawny Asian," and "blackish African"; a fifth category described "wild and monstrous humans, unknown groups, and more or less abnormal people." Such taxonomic classes strike a shuddering resemblance to continent- or race-based categories that persist in human genomics. It is everyone's responsibility to reflect on this to ensure our studies are robust to the conceptual and mathematical influence of constructed social hierarchies rooted in biological racism.

It is a powerful and pervasive myth that genetics are *primarily* responsible for differences we observe across geographic regions, cultural contexts, and social or political identities. Eugenic scientists invoked natural class theory, but also relied on genetic essentialism–the notion that genetics are necessary and sufficient for all phenotypes. Early in the field's history, statistical geneticist R.A. Fisher was commissioned by Leonard Darwin to develop mathematical models that could provide a biological explanation for trait differences between groups of individuals. It is widely accepted today that the social and culture-bound traits that eugenicists focused on (e.g., imbecility and promiscuity) are not caused by genetics. However, concepts and statistical methods that Fisher developed to explain how such traits occurred more frequently within families are still used today. Twin studies of inherited contributions to disease – using Fisher's *Heritability* – were conducted on children imprisoned in concentration camps during WWII. **Heritability** estimates from twin studies have motivated **GWAS** of social phenomena (e.g., educational attainment) despite their problematic assumptions and historical abuses.

Heritability estimates have curiously remained central to certain branches of human genetics and social science. Causal relationships between exposures and outcomes can rarely be proven, because there is no way to disentangle the impact of shared family or cultural environment (twins reared apart are often raised by relatives or other community members) and the impact of shared genetic variation within those extended family communities. In particular, for complex, or multifactorial, traits (in which the environment plays a role), it is important to acknowledge the limitations of this heuristic. Heritability estimates cannot truly distinguish between genetic and nongenetic effects, and there must be a proposed mechanism justify claims that genetics could influence purely social outcomes.

There is no scientific basis for using broad social categories or sweeping statistical assumptions to infer anyone's precise genomic variation, so we need to develop better methods and conceptual frameworks to bolster our interpretation of genomics. Researchers, clinicians, professional societies, and funding agencies are dealing with problems introduced by the legacy of using race, ethnicity, and ancestry in biomedical research and medicine. Eliminating race-based clinical algorithms may reduce health disparities, but in the absence of robust data from diverse populations, the standard of care is biased toward white people of European descent. Collecting this information is illegal in some countries; thus rendering invisible the influence of social stigma and discrimination on health outcomes. We must be able to track health and healthcare disparities, while avoiding unscientific and unethical applications of broad social categories.

Complex Disease and Confounding

It is important to recognize the role of confounding in the causal pathway from exposures to health outcomes.

Confounding can create spurious associations (e.g., between continental ancestry and disease risk), even if there is no genetic basis for the condition. Statistical associations observed between outcomes and exposures are confounded when there is another, unmeasured or hidden factor that is both causally linked to the outcome of interest and associated with the exposure. This generates statistical **correlations** between measured exposure(s) and outcome(s) despite the absence of a causal relationship. Fig. 10.2 (B) illustrates confounding by social determinants of health (SDOH) and group categories (race, ethnicity, and ancestry) in a causal pathway for complex traits.

The true cause(s) of these traits could be nongenetic, environmental factors at a higher prevalence in the population, and/or genetic factors that are difficult to identify due to small effect sizes across multiple loci. **Linkage disequilibrium (LD)**, or the non-independence of allele frequencies along segments of chromosomes that are inherited together, creates additional statistical challenges. In an association study, the true causal variant cannot be distinguished from other variants that are in LD with it. If there is confounding by SDOH associated with genetic ancestry and an outcome of interest, ancestral patterns of LD may create group-specific genetic signals that are not causal.

One example of uncontrolled confounding leading to harmful and false conceptions is the belief that genetics primarily drives racial or ethnic differences in health outcomes, or other complex traits with environmental components. Because some racial and ethnic groupings are associated with genetic ancestry at the global, or continental, level (i.e., African, Asian, European, Latin American, etc.), genetic variation that happens to be more prevalent in some groups than others (by chance) may be mistaken for causal genetic factors contributing to

intergroup differences in traits. Instead, these are caused by environmental factors that also differ among groups. In these cases, nongenetic factors confound the relationship between ancestry-associated traits or outcomes and genetic variation shared in ancestry-associated cultural groups.

Identity by Descent Versus Allele Sharing in Unrelated Individuals

Throughout recorded history and still today, humans have migrated around the world and exchanged DNA with one another such that our ancestral roots live in our genomes as mixtures of chromosomal segments (haplotypes) that have been inherited through our maternal and paternal lineages. When these lineages are related, segments of maternal and paternal chromosomes in an individual will be shared in the manner of being identical by descent (IBD), meaning they descend from a recent common ancestor. In contrast, genomic loci that have shared variation in a large population with multiple ancestries, or between ancestral groups, are considered identical by state (IBS) and do not necessarily share a *recent* common ancestral origin.

IBD sharing between maternal and paternal chromosomes is a result of **consanguinity**, or reproduction between genetically related individuals. This, like founder effects, leads to an increase in the frequency of autosomal recessive traits because carriers of the same recessive allele are more likely to meet and reproduce. The kinds of recessive disorders seen in the offspring of related parents may be very rare and unusual in the general population. This is because consanguineous mating allows an uncommon allele inherited from a heterozygous common ancestor to become homozygous.

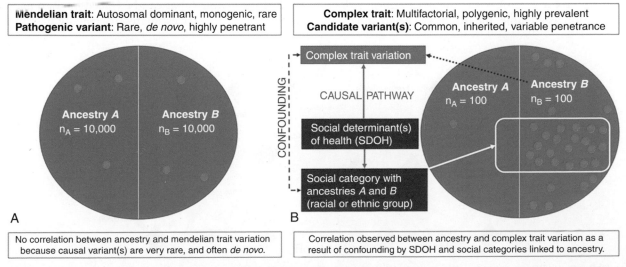

Figure 10.2 (A) Mendelian traits are typically rare, due to deleterious effects of *de novo* variants that are unlikely to be inherited by subsequent generations so individuals with different ancestries have a similar risk profile. (B) Complex traits are common, caused by combined genetic, social, and other environmental factors. Ancestry may appear to influence disease risk if it is associated with the trait of interest and social determinants of health.

IBD sharing is more prevalent in genetic isolates, small populations derived from a limited number of common ancestors who tended to mate only among themselves. Reproduction between two apparently "unrelated" individuals in a genetic isolate may have the same risk for certain recessive conditions as that observed in consanguineous reproduction because the individuals are both carriers via inheritance from common ancestors within the isolate. Fig. 10.3A illustrates a simplified path of alleles shared IBD, inherited from parents who are related or have recent, closely shared ancestry (cryptic relatedness); in contrast, Fig. 10.3B shows alleles IBS that are *de novo* mutations and/or inherited independently.

The concept of a coalescent describes the joining together of distinct lineages or alleles backward in time (t) to a most recent common ancestor (MRCA). Coalescent theory is used to estimate t for two copies of an allele or haplotype (collection of linked alleles) that are shared IBD (Fig. 10.3A). In contrast, identical alleles are IBS (Fig. 10.3B) when they arise through independent processes such as mutation or inheritance through different ancestral lineages. The relative number of alleles (or average lengths of stretches of chromosomes) shared IBD among individuals in a population is proportional to the effective population size. Smaller N_e leads to greater IBD sharing, on average, because there are fewer haplotypes circulating in the population. This leads to a greater prior probability that two recessive deleterious alleles will be inherited by chance through closely or distantly related ancestral lineages.

Assortative mating describes a phenomenon in which certain groups of individuals have – for a variety of historical, cultural, or religious reasons – remained relatively genetically separate during modern times. When mate **selection** in a population is restricted for any reason to members of a particular group, and that group happens to have a variant with a higher frequency than the population as a whole, the result will be an apparent excess of **homozygotes** in the overall population beyond what one would predict.

A clinically important aspect of assortative mating is the tendency to choose partners with similar traits, such as **congenital** deafness or blindness. In such cases, the genotypes of two reproductive partners at loci influencing the trait are not predicted from population allele frequencies. For example, consider achondroplasia (Case 2), an autosomal dominant form of skeletal dysplasia with a population incidence of 1 per 15,000 to 1 per 40,000 live births. Offspring homozygous for the achondroplasia variant have a severe, lethal form of skeletal dysplasia that is almost never seen unless both parents have achondroplasia and are thus heterozygous for the variant. This would be highly unlikely to occur by chance, except for assortative mating among those with achondroplasia.

When reproductive partners have autosomal recessive disorders caused by the same pathogenic variant or by allelic variants in the same gene, all their offspring will also have the disease. Even if there is **locus heterogeneity** with assortative mating, the chance that two individuals carry pathogenic variants in the same locus is increased over what it would be under true **random mating**, and therefore likelihood of the trait in their offspring is also increased.

Genetic Ancestry and Population Structure

The concept of genetic ancestry may seem more scientifically valid and concrete than self-reported measures like race and ethnicity because it is based on genetic information; however, it also lacks a firm "ground truth." Genetic ancestry is a dynamic and relative measure; estimates can change over time depending on the reference data and methods used, all of which have inherent assumptions and limitations. Often reported as percentages of the genome that can be traced back to ancestral populations, ancestry estimates are usually based on the

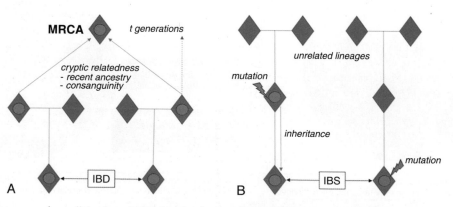

Figure 10.3 (A) Coalescence of an allele shared identical by descent (IBD) between two individuals traced back to their most recent common ancestor (MRCA) *t* generations ago; and (B) *de novo* or recently inherited alleles identical by state (IBS) in unrelated individuals. *Blue diamonds* are individuals and the *edges* connecting them indicate their relations in a pedigree; *orange circles* and *arrows* represent pathogenic variants, their origins traced forward being inheritance and backward being coalescence in lineages.

average proportion of an individual's DNA that most closely matches a given reference dataset with assigned population labels (compared to all other reference data available for the analysis). This means that the more robust and geographically specific reference datasets are, the higher the resolution achieved for reported proportions of population-specific ancestry.

For example, most direct-to-consumer (DTC) genetic ancestry companies can predict specific geographic origins for individuals' European ancestry components (e.g., a small village in Northern Ireland) but often report ancestry components at the continental level for regions that are underrepresented among reference datasets, such as "Sub-Saharan Africa." Representation in genomic reference datasets disproportionately excludes the most genetically diverse ancestries while including mostly Europeans. Since genetic ancestry is estimated using reference data, individuals with ancestries from regions of the world that have yet to be broadly included in genomics research may not receive accurate, detailed, or informative ancestry proportion results. Similarly, imputation (the process of filling in of alleles that are missing from genotype data using some reference dataset), is less accurate in groups with greater genetic diversity that is missing from reference resources.

Alleles that differ in their frequencies among preconstructed ancestry groupings are referred to as **ancestry informative markers** (AIMs). AIMs have been identified to differentiate among broad geographical groupings (e.g., African, East Asian, South Asian, European, Middle Eastern, Native American, and Pacific Islanders). Such markers have been used for charting human migration patterns, for documenting historical admixture between or among populations, and for determining the degree of genetic diversity among ancestral population groups. Studies of hundreds of thousands of AIMs from across the genome have been used to distinguish and determine the genome-wide relationships among many different populations.

Since AIMs are selected to maximize differences between predefined groups, they should not be considered representative of genome-wide variation among those groups. **Polymorphisms** that happen to occur at higher frequencies in certain groups of individuals may be identified as AIMs by chance, even if the grouping scheme is not otherwise biologically meaningful. Predefined groups are often based on sociocultural categories or their respective broad, continental groupings; they influence the loci that are selected, then those AIMS may be treated as a proxy for genomic background. This has downstream implications for research and quality control measures that rely on AIMs (e.g., to identify population-specific reference panels, impute missing genomic information, or test the accuracy of various analytic methods).

In 2008, population geneticist John Novembre and colleagues famously published results of a principal component analysis (PCA) that appear to reconstruct the geography of Europe using genotype data sampled from countries across the continent (Fig. 10.4). Subsequently, many genomics researchers have used PCA and other statistical clustering methods like admixture analysis that reduce the complexity of data to visualize population structure. While these approaches may provide some insight, they also have limitations and may be misleading.

Novembre and colleagues have published concerns about the potential for confusion about global genetic population structure because of these methods. For example, geographic clusters that appear distinct in the PCA plot of Europe are genetically very similar, but the figure may mislead people into thinking they have large overall genetic differences. In the case of Europe, clines or gradients in allele frequencies are roughly aligned with latitude and longitude, as humans migrated East-West and South-North across the continent. This pattern of allele frequencies mirroring geography is unique to Europe, and the structure shown only emerges after >100k loci are included in the analysis because allele frequency differences are so small. Genetic variation among populations may be falsely perceived as divided among regional groups, though few alleles are restricted to just one region of the world.

Data from the US Population Architecture using Genomics and Epidemiology (PAGE) study were used to visualize population structure with PCA (Fig. 10.5). Each colored dot in the plot of principal components (PCs) 1 and 2 represents an individual research participant, and its color corresponds to the self-reported race or ethnicity category selected by the participant. The dots are positioned relative to one another according to similarities and differences in genotypes across the genome. We can see from the spread of these individuals across PCs that there is a complex spectrum of shared variation that cannot be adequately represented by categorical data structures. This illustrates why sociocultural categories used in the US Census cannot be considered genetically differentiated; there is a continuous distribution of genomic variation within and among groups such that most variants are shared and their frequency distributions overlap.

Misclassification results from individuals being assigned to the wrong analytic group in a study (e.g., case being classified incorrectly as a control, or vice versa). In clinical algorithms that rely on racial and ethnic classification, misclassification could be considered the incorrect attribution of a category-based mean value to an individual patient. Furthermore, classification error is almost certain due to genetic heterogeneity within racial and ethnic groups that violate baseline assumptions and motivations for applying population- or group-level adjustments. If genetic ancestry were used instead of self-reported measures of racial or ethnic identity, the preselected nature of

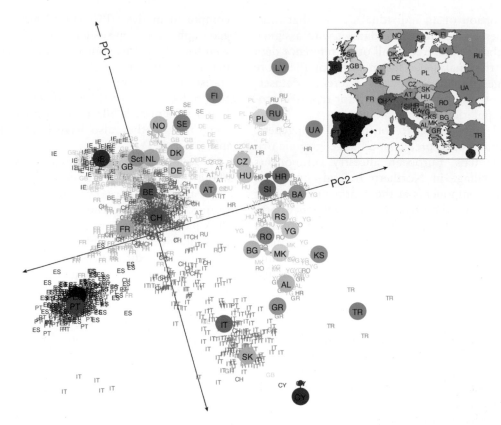

Figure 10.4 A statistical summary of genetic data from 1387 Europeans based on principal component axis one (PC1) and axis two (PC2). *Small colored labels* represent individuals and *large colored points* represent median PC1 and PC2 values for each country. The inset map provides a key to the labels. The PC axes are rotated to emphasize the similarity to the geographic map of Europe. AL, Albania; AT, Austria; BA, Bosnia-Herzegovina; BE, Belgium; BG, Bulgaria; CH, Switzerland; CY, Cyprus; CZ, Czech Republic; DE, Germany; DK, Denmark; ES, Spain; FI, Finland; FR, France; GB, Great Britain; GR, Greece; HR, Croatia; HU, Hungary; IE, Ireland; IT, Italy; KS, Kosovo; LV, Latvia; MK, Macedonia; NO, Norway; NL, Netherlands; PL, Poland; PT, Portugal; RO, Romania; RS, Serbia and Montenegro; RU, Russia; Sct, Scotland; SE, Sweden; SI, Slovenia; SK, Slovakia; TR, Turkey; UA, Ukraine; YG, Yugoslavia. From Novembre J, Johnson T, Bryc K. et al. Genes mirror geography within Europe. *Nature* 456:98–101, 2008. https://doi.org/10.1038/nature07331

AIMs and then using those to classify individuals into discrete groupings may create the exact same problems as race and ethnicity categories. That is, ancestry categories that are semantic variations of racial and ethnic groupings do no better at describing genomic variation because human genetic diversity is a narrow spectrum of [mostly] shared alleles at gradually changing, relative frequencies.

Humans from different regions of the world have genetic similarities and differences that may have nothing to do with geography. Whereas there may be geographic trends in aggregate, an allele frequency cannot be used to determine an individual's genotype. Even Duffy **blood group** alleles, which are classically known for differences in frequencies by geography, can be seen on every continent, with clines or gradients showing clear variation *within* those regions. Earlier versions of this very textbook have described blood group variation according to geographic, racial, and ethnic categories (which change over time and across cultural contexts) but today, we have enough genetic data to establish that neither is genomic variation restricted to such

categories nor is it easily characterized by any categorical framework.

To illustrate this point, Fig. 10.6 showcases continuous global frequencies of the three common Duffy blood group alleles (*FY*A*, *FY*B*, and *FY*B^ES*), which have historically been used as the canonical example of geographic **differentiation**. We highlight here that not all parts of Africa have a high frequency of the *FY*B^ES* allele that confers protection against malarial infection via the *Plasmodium* parasites, and some other parts of the world (not in Africa) have elevated frequencies as well. In geographic locations where *Plasmodium* species causing malaria in humans are endemic, the protective allele is highly prevalent. All three common Duffy alleles are present at a range of frequencies across the Americas, and none are restricted to a single continent or large geographic region that corresponds to continental ancestry groupings.

There are many different factors that can explain how differences in disease incidence, prevalence, and allele frequencies arise among biogeographic populations. In cases where genetic variants are contributing

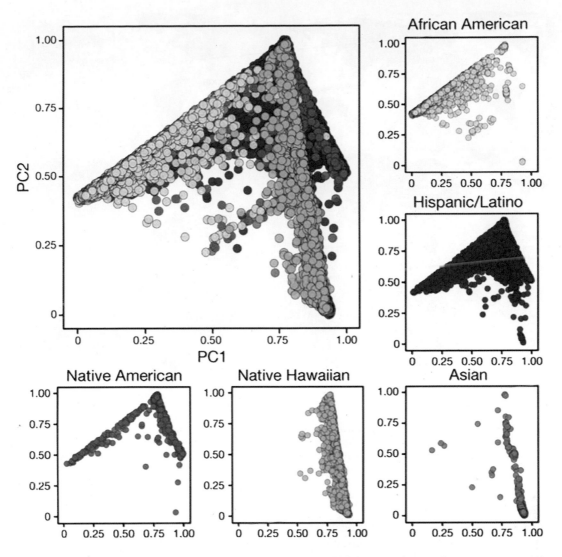

Figure 10.5 Inclusion of multiethnic samples enables discovery and replication in GWAS. The population substructure that is present in the multiethnic sample of PAGE (n = 49,839) reveals complex patterns preventing meaningful stratification. PC1 and PC2 show major patterns of variation, stratified by self-identified race/ethnicity. Individuals denoted by *orange* self-identified as "Other." From Wojcik GL, Graff M, Nishimura KK, et al. Genetic analyses of diverse populations improves discovery for complex traits, *Nature* 570:514–518, 2019. https://doi.org/10.1038/s41586-019-1310-4

to disease etiology, it is possible that inheritance of an ancestral haplotype containing a pathogenic variant is more likely, given reported or estimated ancestry of an individual patient. However, disease-causing alleles that reduce the **fitness** of an individual tend to be rare in populations that are sufficiently large (such that other haplotypes are frequent enough to outcompete one that is pathogenic). In smaller populations that have been genetically isolated from others, or in situations where environmental conditions enhance the fitness of carriers of pathogenic variants and create a **heterozygote advantage**, it is possible to see disease-causing alleles at frequencies higher than would be expected given disease prevalence. Other factors include **genetic drift**, which applies to benign variants that rise to high frequency due to physical proximity

to fitness-enhancing alleles, without having direct impact on the phenotype.

If the overall population is sufficiently large, the frequency of an allele in a small subset of the population will not change the total population allele frequency. However, the larger the subset of carriers relative to the total population, the greater the chance that it will alter the population allele frequency. Therefore, classification of individuals into population categories important because the relationship between the numerator (number of observations) and the denominator (total population under investigation) determines the allele frequency. In practice, estimates of allele frequencies are used in combination with disease prevalence and incidence to determine genotype frequencies, given their modes of inheritance.

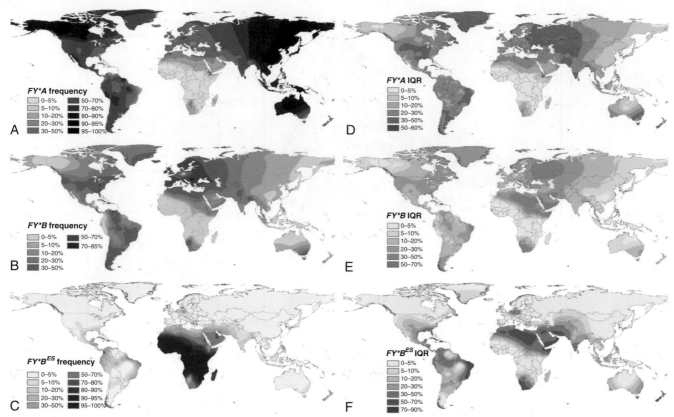

Figure 10.6 Global Duffy blood group allele frequencies and uncertainty maps. A, B, and C correspond to $FY*A$, $FY*B$, and $FY*B^{ES}$ allele frequency maps, respectively (median values of the prediction posterior distributions); D–F show the respective interquartile ranges (IQR) of each allele frequency map (25–75% interval). Predictions are made on a 5×5 km grid in Africa and a 10×10 km grid elsewhere. From Howes R, Patil A, Piel F. et al. The global distribution of the Duffy blood group. *Nat Commun* 2:266, 2011. https://doi.org/10.1038/ncomms1265

Most sections in this chapter have thus far dealt with the complexity of defining human populations, characterizing ancestry and genetic population structure, and accounting for nongenetic factors associated with systemic inequities that may create erroneous correlations among group-level phenotypic differences, ancestry estimates, and sociocultural categories. While it is important to recognize limitations of point estimates and other discrete measures to characterize continuous variables (e.g., genomic variant distributions in human populations), there is utility in calculating allele and genotype frequencies to inform genomic research and medicine. In the next section, we describe how to calculate these frequencies and offer clinically relevant examples.

ALLELE AND GENOTYPE FREQUENCIES

For autosomal loci, the size of the gene pool at one locus is twice the number of individuals (2 N) in the population because each autosomal genotype consists of two alleles. Consider a population that is structured by recent ancestry or migration from another population, such that 10% of the total population contains a group in which the **minor allele frequency**

(MAF) for a biallelic, autosomal recessive disease is 5% ($q = 0.05$). Since the trait has two alleles whose frequencies sum to 1 in the population ($p + q = 1$), we can infer the other allele's frequency to be $p = 0.95$ in this group by subtracting the frequency of q from 1. In the remaining 90% of the total population, the frequency of this pathogenic variant is so small that it is not observed and presumed to be absent such that $q \approx 0$ and $p \approx 1$.

Let us continue with the Duffy blood group example to illustrate the relationship between allele and genotype frequencies in populations. Consider the gene *ACKR1* (atypical chemokine receptor 1) on chromosome 1 (1q23.2), which encodes the major subunit of the Duffy blood group system and serves as an entry point for *Plasmodium vivax*, an important parasite causing malaria. Hundreds of variants have been observed in this gene with varying functional consequences. We will focus on a single nucleotide variant (SNV) in the **promoter** region of *ACKR1* (rs2814778 in Ensembl), which confers protection against malarial infection and exhibits allele frequency differences across global populations. We draw on data from the 1000 Genomes (1KG) Project to calculate allele frequencies from observed genotype

TABLE 10.1 Genotype Frequencies and Derived Allele Frequencies for *ACKR1* Duffy Blood Group Allele rs2814778 in the 5′ UTR From the 1000 Genomes (1KG) Project

Genotype for *ACKR1* rs2814778	Number of Individuals	Observed Genotype Frequency	Allele	Derived Allele Frequencies
T|T	1793	0.716		
C|T	88	0.035	T	0.734
C|C	623	0.249	C	0.266
Total	2504	1.000		

From The 1000 Genomes Project Consortium: A global reference for human genetic variation, *Nature* 526:68–74, 2015. doi:10.1038/nature15393. Genotype frequencies were obtained online from Ensembl (https://www.Ensembl.org) in October 2022.

TABLE 10.2 Allele Frequencies for *ACKR1* Duffy Blood Group Allele rs2814778 in the 5′ UTR From Three Populations in the 1000 Genomes (1KG) Project

1KG Population Label	Alleles for *ACKR1* rs2814778	Allele Counts per Population	Allele Frequencies
African Caribbean in Barbados (ACB)	T	22	0.115
	C	170	0.885
African Ancestry in Southwest US (ASW)	T	25	0.205
	C	97	0.795
Esan in Nigeria (ESN)	T	0	0.0
	C	198	1.0
Total (2N = 512)	T	47	0.092
	C	465	0.908

From The 1000 Genomes Project Consortium: A global reference for human genetic variation, *Nature* 526:68–74, 2015. doi:10.1038/nature15393. Allele counts and frequencies were obtained online from Ensembl (https://www.Ensembl.org) in October 2022.

frequencies. Table 10.1 reports the genotype frequencies for homozygous (T|T and C|C) and heterozygous (C|T) individuals.

Because each homozygous individual has two copies of the same allele, and heterozygous individuals have one copy of each allele, the frequency of each allele is twice the number of individuals in the population homozygous for the allele, plus the number of **heterozygotes**, divided by the total number of alleles in the population or 2N:

$$T: \frac{(2 \times 1793) + (1 \times 88)}{2504 \times 2} = 0.734$$

$$C: \frac{(2 \times 623) + (1 \times 88)}{2504 \times 2} = 0.266$$

Rather than calculating the frequency of each allele independently, the calculated frequency of one allele can simply be subtracted from one (e.g., 1 − 0.734 = 0.266) because the frequencies of the two alleles must add up to 1 (recall $p + q = 1$). Now consider that genotype and allele frequencies differ across geographic regions due to the protective nature of this allele in regions with malarial parasites. Table 10.2 provides more granular frequency data that we hope will contribute to developing an intuition about diversity among African ancestry populations.

Data from the 1KG Project can be used to assess global allele and genotype frequencies for discrete geographic regions that have been sampled for large-scale genome sequencing, but it is important to keep in mind that this sampling scheme does not account for all the global genomic variation that exists (most of which has been unsampled to date); it simply tells us about the subset of variation among project participants. Fig. 10.7 illustrates genomic diversity across the 1KG dataset, showing the greatest number of variants in samples from Africa

and reinforcing the fact that most variants (gray-shaded pieces of the pie charts) are shared across continents.

Hardy-Weinberg Equilibrium

As we have shown, a sample of individuals with known genotypes in a population can be used to derive estimates of allele frequencies by simply counting the alleles in individuals with each genotype. How about the converse? Can we calculate the proportion of the population with various genotypes once we know the allele frequencies?

Deriving genotype frequencies from allele frequencies is not as straightforward as counting because we do not know in advance how the alleles are distributed among homozygotes and heterozygotes. If a population meets certain assumptions, however, there is a simple mathematical equation for calculating genotype frequencies from allele frequencies. This equation is known as Hardy-Weinberg equilibrium (HWE), named after Godfrey Hardy, an English mathematician, and Wilhelm Weinberg, a German physician, who formulated it in 1908.

The Hardy-Weinberg principle has two critical components. The first is that under certain ideal conditions (see Box 10.2), a simple relationship exists between allele frequencies and genotype frequencies in a population. To illustrate the utility of Hardy-Weinberg for understanding the relationship between allele and genotype frequencies, we offer here a step-by-step visual mathematical proof that under the right conditions, allele and genotype frequencies remain constant in each generation for a population in HWE.

First, we start with genotypes that are observed in a population and simulate all possible reproductive pairings between individuals of each possible genotype. In this example, we consider a biallelic locus with alleles A and a, such that there are three possible genotypes: two are homozygous (AA or aa) and one is heterozygous (Aa).

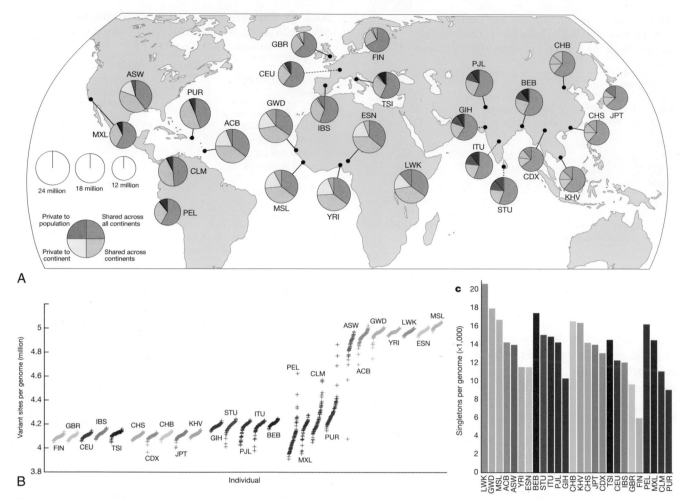

Figure 10.7 Population sampling in the 1000 Genomes (1KG) Project. (A) Polymorphic variants within sampled populations. The area of each pie is proportional to the number of polymorphisms within a population. Pies are divided into four slices, representing variants private to a population (*darker color* unique to population), private to a continental area (*lighter color* shared across continental group), shared across continental areas (*light gray*), and shared across all continents (*dark gray*). *Dashed lines* indicate populations sampled outside of their ancestral continental region. (B) The number of variant sites per genome. (C) The average number of singletons per genome. From The 1000 Genomes Project Consortium. A global reference for human genetic variation. *Nature* 526:68–74, 2015. https://doi.org/10.1038/nature15393

Predicted offspring (F₁) genotypes, given genotypes of possible parent mating pairs (P₁,₂) in a population

Parent Generation (P₁,₂) Possible Mating Pairs		P₁ Genotype: AA		P₁ Genotype: Aa		P₁ Genotype: aa	
		A	**A**	**A**	**a**	**a**	**a**
P₂ Genotype: AA	A	AA	AA	AA	Aa	Aa	Aa
	A	AA	AA	AA	Aa	Aa	Aa
P₂ Genotype: Aa	A	AA	AA	AA	Aa	Aa	Aa
	a	Aa	Aa	Aa	aa	aa	aa
P₂ Genotype: aa	a	Aa	Aa	Aa	aa	aa	aa
	a	Aa	Aa	Aa	aa	aa	aa

The table above uses Punnett squares to illustrate all possible genotypes present in a generation of offspring (F1) resulting from all possible combinations of genotypes in the parent generation (P), given two alleles A and a: AA, Aa, and aa. Assuming that there is no mutation or other violations of HWE conditions, the proportions of genotypes in F1 can be calculated by plugging in the P1 genotype pairings as such:

Offspring genotype frequencies given parental genotypes, assuming Hardy-Weinberg conditions (no mutation)

Parent (p) Genotypes	AA	Aa		aa
AA	AA_{F1} $(AA \times AA)_p(1.0)$	AA_{F1} $(Aa \times AA)_p(0.5)$	Aa_{F1} $(Aa \times AA)_p(0.5)$	Aa_{F1} $(aa \times AA)_p(1.0)$
Aa	AA_{F1} $(AA \times Aa)_p(0.5)$	AA_{F1} $(Aa \times Aa)_p(0.25)$	Aa_{F1} $(Aa \times Aa)_p(0.25)$	Aa_{F1} $(aa \times Aa)_p(0.5)$
	Aa_{F1} $(AA \times Aa)_p(0.5)$	Aa_{F1} $(Aa \times Aa)_p(0.25)$	aa_{F1} $(Aa \times Aa)_p(0.25)$	aa_{F1} $(aa \times Aa)_p(0.5)$
aa	Aa_{F1} $(AA \times aa)_p(1.0)$	Aa_{F1} $(Aa \times aa)_p(0.5)$	aa_{F1} $(Aa \times aa)_p(0.5)$	aa_{F1} $(aa \times aa)_p(1.0)$

Suppose p is the frequency of allele A, and q is the frequency of allele a in the gene pool, such that $p + q = 1$ for a hypothetical biallelic trait. Substituting in the frequency variables p and q (below) for their respective alleles in F1 genotype proportion equations (above), the table below expresses offspring genotype proportions for all possible mating pairs in P in terms of p and q.

Genotype frequencies in offspring generation (F1), given parental genotype frequencies; assuming two alleles (A and a) are in HWE with population allele frequencies Freq[A] = p and Freq[a] = q; such that p + q = 1.

Parent (P) Genotype Frequencies	$AA = p^2$	$Aa = 2pq$		$aa = q^2$
$AA = p^2$	AA_{F1} $(p^2 \times p^2)(1.0) = p^4$	AA_{F1} $(2pq \times p^2)(0.5) = p^3q$	Aa_{F1} $(2pq \times p^2)(0.5) = p^3q$	Aa_{F1} $(q^2 \times p^2)(1.0) = p^2q^2$
$Aa = 2pq$	AA_{F1} $(p^2 \times 2pq)(0.5) = p^3q$	AA_{F1} $(2pq \times 2pq)(0.25) = p^2q^2$	Aa_{F1} $(2pq \times 2pq)(0.25) = p^2q^2$	Aa_{F1} $(q^2 \times 2pq)(0.5) = pq^3$
	Aa_{F1} $(p^2 \times 2pq)(0.5) = p^3q$	Aa_{F1} $(2pq \times 2pq)(0.25) = p^2q^2$	aa_{F1} $(2pq \times 2pq)(0.25) = p^2q^2$	aa_{F1} $(q^2 \times 2pq)(0.5) = pq^3$
$aa = q^2$	Aa_{F1} $(p^2 \times q^2)(1.0) = p^2q^2$	Aa_{F1} $(2pq \times q^2)(0.5) = pq^3$	aa_{F1} $(2pq \times q^2)(0.5) = pq^3$	aa_{F1} $(q^2 \times q^2)(1.0) = q^4$

Now let us assume alleles combine into genotypes randomly; that is, mating in the population is completely random with respect to the genotypes at this locus. The chance that two A alleles will pair up to give the AA genotype is then p^2; the chance that two a alleles will come together to give the aa genotype is q^2; and the chance of having one A and one a pair, resulting in the Aa genotype, is $2pq$ (the factor 2 comes from the fact that the A allele could be inherited from one parent and the a allele from the other, or vice versa). This applies to all autosomal loci and to the X chromosome in females, but not to X-linked loci in males who have just one X chromosome.

The Hardy-Weinberg principle states that the frequency of the three genotypes AA, Aa, and aa is given by the terms of the binomial expansion of $(p + q)^2 = p^2 + 2pq + q^2 = 1$.

If allele frequencies do not change from generation to generation, the proportion of genotypes will not change either; that is, the *genotype frequencies from generation to generation will remain constant (at equilibrium) in the population if the allele frequencies (p and q) remain constant*. When there is random mating in a population at HWE equilibrium, and genotypes AA, Aa, and aa are present in the proportions $p^2:2pq:q^2$, then genotype frequencies in the next generation will remain in the same relative proportions, $p^2:2pq:q^2$. This is proven as follows:

Constant Genotype frequency Proportions for a Population in Hardy-Weinberg Equilibrium (HWE)

P — Genotype frequencies in the parent generation (P) can be used to predict genotype frequencies in the first generation of offspring (F1) by adding up the resulting genotype frequencies from all possible mating pairs ($P_{1,2}$).

	AA p^2	:	Aa $2pq$	:	aa q^2
AA x AA:	$p^2p^2 = \mathbf{p^4}$	:	0	:	0
AA x Aa:	$p^2q + p^3q = \mathbf{2p^3q}$	:	$p^3q + p^3q = \mathbf{2p^3q}$	:	0
AA x aa:	0	:	$p^2q^2 + p^2q^2 = \mathbf{2p^2q^2}$	:	0
Aa x Aa:	$\mathbf{p^2q^2}$	:	$p^2q^2 + p^2q^2 = \mathbf{2p^2q^2}$	:	$\mathbf{p^2q^2}$
Aa x aa:	0	:	$pq^3 + pq^3 = \mathbf{2pq^3}$	:	$pq^3 + pq^3 = \mathbf{2pq^3}$
aa x aa:	0	:	0	:	$\mathbf{q^4}$

F1

AA	Aa	aa
$\mathbf{p^4 + 2p^3p + p^2p^2}$	$\mathbf{2p^3q + 2p^2q^2 + 2p^2q^2 + 2pq^3}$	$\mathbf{p^2p^2 + 2pq^3 + q^4}$
$= p^2(p^2 + 2pq + q2)$	$= 2pq(p^2 + 2pq + q^2)$	$= q^2(p^2 + 2pq + q^2)$
$= p^2(p + q)^2$	$= 2pq(p + q)^2$	$= q^2(p + q)^2$
$= p^2(1)^2$	$= 2pq(1)^2$	$= q^2(1)^2$

AA	$\mathbf{= p^2}$	:	Aa	$\mathbf{= 2pq}$	:	aa	$\mathbf{= q^2}$

F2 — Genotype frequency Proportions remain constant in a population under Hardy-Weinberg conditions.

AA p^2	+	Aa $2pq$	+	aa q^2	$= 1$

It is important to note that HWE does not require any particular values for p and q; whatever allele frequencies happen to be present in the population will result in genotype frequencies of $p^2:2pq:q^2$, and these relative genotype frequencies will remain constant from generation to generation as long as the allele frequencies remain constant and the other conditions introduced in Box 10.2 are met.

This principle can be adapted for genes with more than two alleles. For example, if a locus has three alleles, with frequencies p, q, and r, the genotypic distribution can be determined from $(p + q + r)^2 = 1$. In general terms, the genotype frequencies for any known number of alleles a_n with allele frequencies $p_1, p_2, \ldots p_n$ can be derived from the terms of the expansion of $(p_1 + p_2 + \ldots p_n)^2$.

Applying HWE to the *ACKR1* (Duffy blood group) example given earlier, with relative frequencies of the two alleles in the 1KG Project dataset 0.734 (for the T allele) and 0.266 (for the C allele), the relative proportions of the three combinations of alleles (genotypes) are $\Pr[T|T] = p^2 = 0.734 \times 0.734 = 0.539$ (for an individual having two T alleles), $\Pr[C|C] = q^2 = 0.266 \times 0.266 = 0.071$ (for two C alleles), and $\Pr[C|T] = 2pq = (0.734 \times 0.266) + (0.734 \times 0.266) = 0.39$ (for individuals with one T and one C allele).

These genotype frequencies were calculated assuming HWE; so, when applied to a population of 2504 individuals, the derived numbers of people with the three different genotypes (TT:CT:CC) should be equivalent

BOX 10.2 HARDY-WEINBERG EQUILIBRIUM ASSUMPTIONS

The principle of Hardy-Weinberg equilibrium rests on the assumption that genotype frequency proportions remain constant over time because of the following:

- **Random mating.** Reproductive pairings are random with respect to the locus in question.
- **No genetic drift.** The population under study is sufficiently large such that alleles are not likely to dramatically rise or drop in frequency by random chance.
- **No mutation.** Rate of mutation is low such that allele frequencies are not impacted.
- **No selection.** Individuals are equally capable of passing on their genes, regardless of genotype, preserving equality between each allele frequency and its chance of being inherited.
- **No gene flow.** There has been no significant migration of individuals between populations with significantly different allele frequencies.

A population that appears to meet these assumptions is in Hardy-Weinberg equilibrium.

to the observed genotype frequencies from the 1KG dataset. However, when we do this calculation (total population size × genotype frequency), the proportions of individuals with each genotype are 1350:977:177. This is very different from the actual *observed* proportions in Table 10.1 (1793:88:623), which indicates that the assumptions of HWE do not hold for the "population" defined as all individuals in the 1KG dataset. This makes sense, because the sampling scheme of the project was meant to identify individuals from different parts of the world to enable comparisons of average frequencies across the globe and cannot be considered a single population in HWE. Two key HWE assumptions that are violated in this scenario are: (1) Random mating, because we would not expect individuals to meet and reproduce with people from across the globe with equal chance compared to those close by; and (2) selection, since we know this allele is under positive selective pressure in locations that have a high incidence of malaria.

Now, let us try this exercise again with a different variant in the same gene (e.g., *ACKR1* rs36007769; Ensembl) that is **synonymous** and therefore not predicted to change the protein, such that its frequency is not under the influence of natural selection (unless it is in strong LD with a functionally relevant variant that is under selection and carries it along). We can again use HWE to calculate *predicted* genotype frequencies from *observed* allele frequencies in 1KG and compare those results to the *observed* genotype frequencies reported for this dataset in Ensembl.

Table 10.3 reports observed allele counts and frequencies for the synonymous SNV rs36007769 in the *ACKR1* (Duffy blood group) gene, as reported in Ensembl for the 1KG Project (Phase 3) dataset. Recall that the HWE equation $p^2 + 2pq + q^2 = 1$ can be used to calculate expected genotype frequencies, given observed allele frequencies such that the first and third terms (p^2 and q^2) are the expected frequencies of homozygous genotypes for alleles p and q, respectively, and the second term ($2pq$) is the expected frequency of heterozygotes. Table 10.4 reports the results of these calculations as *derived* genotype frequencies.

TABLE 10.3 Allele Counts and Frequencies for the *ACKR1* Duffy Blood Group Allele rs36007769 observed and reported by the 1000 Genomes (1KG) Project

Allele in *ACKR1* rs36007769	Observed Allele Counts	Observed Allele Frequencies
G	4990	0.996
A	18	0.004
Total	5008	1.0

From The 1000 Genomes Project Consortium: A global reference for human genetic variation, *Nature* 526:68–74, 2015. doi:10.1038/nature15393. Accessed online via Ensembl.

TABLE 10.4 Genotype Counts and Frequencies for the *ACKR1* Duffy Blood Group Allele rs36007769 Observed in the 1000 Genomes (1KG) Project and Derived Using HWE

rs36007769 Genotypes	Observed Genotype Counts	Observed Genotype Frequencies	Derived Genotype Frequencies (HWE)
G|G	2486	0.993	$p^2 = (0.996)^2$ = 0.992
A|G	18	0.007	$2pq = 2(0.996)$ (0.004) = 0.008
A|A	0	0	$q^2 = (0)^2 = 0$

Comparing these derived frequencies (0.992:0.008: 0.0) to *observed* genotype frequencies in the 1KG dataset (0.993:0.007:0.0), we can see that they are roughly equivalent. Given that the assumptions of HWE hold, we would expect these genotype frequencies to remain constant generation after generation. Although the 1KG dataset is not a genetically homogeneous population and it includes samples from many different parts of the world, the absence of selection acting on this variant and the fact that it is rare in a relatively large population (defined as the dataset) mean that genotype frequency calculations based on HWE are still useful.

Upon further inspection of the incidence of this variant, 5 occurrences are in Central and South American ancestry (AMR) populations and 13 occurrences are in European ancestry (EUR) populations. Using the reported allele frequencies in those populations from 1KG, AMR (G: 0.993, A: 0.007), and EUR (G: 0.987, A: 0.013) to calculate expected genotype frequencies with HWE, they are equivalent to reported frequency proportions in AMR (0.986:0.014:0) and EUR (0.974:0.026:0). This suggests that HWE holds for each of these populations for this specific variant, and thus their frequency proportions should persist in subsequent generations.

Applying Hardy-Weinberg Equilibrium to Autosomal Recessive Traits

The major practical application of the Hardy-Weinberg principle in medical genetics is in genetic counseling for autosomal recessive conditions. For a disease such as phenylketonuria (PKU), there are hundreds of different pathogenic alleles with frequencies that vary among different population groups defined by geography and/ or ethnicity (see Chapter 13). Affected individuals can be homozygoues for the same pathogenic allele, but they are often **compound heterozygotes** for different pathogenic variants (see Chapter 7). For many conditions, it is convenient to consider all disease-causing alleles together and treat them as a single pathogenic allele, with frequency q, even when there is significant **allelic heterogeneity** among pathogenic alleles. Similarly, the combined frequency of all benign or nonpathogenic alleles, p, is given by $1 - q$.

Suppose we would like to know the frequency of all disease-causing PKU alleles in a population for use in genetic counseling, for example, to inform couples of their risk for having a child with PKU. If we were to attempt to determine the frequency of disease-causing PKU alleles directly from genotype frequencies, we would need to know the frequency of heterozygotes in the population, a frequency that cannot be measured directly because of the recessive nature of PKU. This is because heterozygotes are asymptomatic silent carriers (see Chapter 7), and their frequency in the population (i.e., $2pq$) cannot be reliably determined directly from phenotype observation.

However, the frequency of affected homozygotes/compound heterozygotes for disease-causing alleles in the population (i.e., q^2) could be determined directly, by counting the number of babies with PKU born over a given time period and identified through newborn screening (see Chapter 19), divided by the total number of babies screened during that same time period. Now, using HWE, we can calculate the pathogenic allele frequency (q) from the observed frequency of homozygotes/compound heterozygotes alone (q^2), thereby providing an estimate ($2pq$) of the frequency of heterozygotes for use in genetic counseling.

To illustrate this example further, consider a population in which the frequency of PKU is approximately 1 per 4500. If we group all disease-causing alleles together and treat them as a single allele with frequency q, then the frequency of affected individuals $q^2 = 1/4500$. From this, we calculate $q = 0.015$, and thus $2pq = 0.029$. The carrier frequency for all disease-causing alleles lumped together in this population is therefore approximately 3%. For an individual known to be a carrier of PKU through the birth of an affected child in the family, there would then be an approximately 3% chance that he or she would find a new mate from the same population who would also be a carrier, and this estimate could be used to provide genetic counseling. Note, however, that this estimate applies only to the population in question; if the new mate was from a different genetic ancestral population where the frequency of PKU is much lower (e.g., 1 per 200,000), their chance of being a carrier would be only 0.6%.

In this example, all PKU-causing alleles are collapsed for the purpose of estimating q. For other conditions, however, such as hemoglobin disorders that we will consider in Chapter 12, different pathogenic alleles can lead to very different conditions, and therefore it would make no sense to group all pathogenic alleles together, even when the same locus is involved. Instead, the frequencies of alleles leading to different phenotypes (e.g., sickle cell disease and β-thalassemia in the case of different pathogenic alleles at the β-globin locus) are calculated separately.

Allele and Genotype Frequencies in X-Linked Conditions

Recall from Chapter 7 that, for X-linked genes, there are three female genotypes but only two possible male genotypes. To illustrate the relationship between allele and genotype frequencies when a gene of interest is X linked, we use the trait known as X-linked red-green color blindness, which is caused by structural variants in genes encoding cell receptors that respond to photons of light at wavelengths we perceive as red and green (*OPN1LW* and *OPNMW*, respectively) that are adjacent to one another on the X chromosome. We use color blindness as an example because, as far as we know, it is not a deleterious trait (except for possible difficulties with traffic lights), and persons with color blindness are not subject to selection.

In this example, we use the symbol *cb* to represent variants conferring some variation of color blindness and the symbol + for variants without color blindness, with frequencies q and p, respectively (Table 10.5). Because females have two X chromosomes, their genotypes are distributed like autosomal genotypes, but because color blindness variants are recessive, their homozygous and heterozygous genotypes are typically not distinguishable. In contrast, males with only one X chromosome will exhibit the trait with a single copy of a *cb* variant. As such, the frequency of color blindness in females is much lower than that in males (<1%).

Frequencies of the two types of variants (*cb* and +) can be determined directly from the prevalence of the corresponding phenotypes in *males*. So, if the prevalence of colorblindness in a population of biologically male individuals (with an X and a Y chromosome) is roughly 8%, the frequency of *cb* variants in the population is likewise 0.08. Genotypes of unaffected females (homozygous or heterozygous) cannot be determined by looking at phenotypes; frequencies of variants for the trait that were ascertained by looking at phenotype frequencies in male individuals can be used to determine approximate variant frequencies for females using HWE. As shown in Table 10.5, ~15% of females are unaffected carriers. Among these heterozygous unaffected individuals, those who are pregnant with a male fetus have a 50% chance of giving birth to a male child with colorblindness (because they have a 50% chance of passing on the X^{cb} variant and this is the only X chromosome a male will receive from either parent). In contrast, a female fetus receives two copies of the X chromosome, so the 50% probability of an unaffected carrier transmitting the *cb* variant is instead the chance that a female fetus will also be a silent carrier.

TABLE 10.5 X-Linked Genotype Frequencies and Prevalence of Color Blindness

Biological Sex	Phenotypes	Prevalence	Genotypes	Genotype Frequencies	Variant Frequencies
Male (X/Y)	*Colorblindness*	*cb* 8%+ 92%	[Y] X^{cb}	0.08	$q = 0.08$
	Unaffected		[Y] X^+	0.92	$p = 0.92$
Female (X/X)	*Colorblindness*	*cb* <1%	$X^{cb}X^{cb}$	$q^2 = (0.08)^2 = 0.0064$	
	Unaffected		$X^{cb}X^+$	$2pq = 2(0.08)(0.92) = 0.1472$	
			X^+X^+	$p^2 = (0.92)^2 = 0.8464$	

Violating Assumptions of Hardy-Weinberg Equilibrium

Underlying the principle of Hardy-Weinberg equilibrium and its use are several assumptions (see Box 10.2), not all of which can be met (or reasonably inferred to be met) by all populations. In this section, we provide a high-level overview of the conditions and factors that contribute to violations of HWE assumptions: (1) nonrandom mating, (2) genetic drift, (3) mutation, (4) selection, and (5) gene flow. We have seen examples of these throughout the chapter, as population genetics is concerned with modeling and measuring shifts in allele frequencies.

First, we have seen nonrandom mating at work in small genetic isolates, or founder populations, which (by definition) are isolated from reproduction events outside the group. In human populations, assortative mating, underlying population structure, or cryptic relatedness due to shared recent ancestry, and consanguinity can all lead to nonrandom mate choices. Assortative mating is a type of nonrandom mating in which individuals in a population engage in preferential reproductive choices. This may increase the frequency of variants contributing to traits that influence individuals in these reproductive choices and other variants in LD with them.

Genetic drift refers to changes in allele frequencies over time due to random chance, which occur more quickly in smaller populations. When a new mutation occurs in a small population, its frequency is represented by only one copy among all the copies of that gene in the population. Random effects of the environment or other chance occurrences that are *independent* of the genotype (i.e., events that occur for reasons unrelated to whether an individual is carrying a pathogenic variant) can produce significant changes in the frequency of the disease allele when the population is small. Such chance occurrences disrupt Hardy-Weinberg equilibrium and cause the allele frequency to change from one generation to the next. During the next few generations, although the population size of the new group remains small, there may be considerable fluctuation until allele frequencies come to a new equilibrium as the population increases in size.

HWE assumes no genetic drift – which requires an absence of migration in and out of the population by groups whose allele frequencies at loci of interest differ drastically from those of the population under HWE assumptions. This is a phenomenon called **gene flow**, whereby alleles are exchanged into and out of populations via migration and reproduction among individuals from different populations. Gene flow disrupts HWE because allele frequencies can change when new alleles are introduced into a population. Similarly, **mutation** (see Chapter 4) introduces new allelic variants into a population at random, which can influence stability of allele frequencies. When these newly introduced alleles (either through gene flow or mutation) confer some

evolutionary advantage over existing alleles in the population, they will naturally rise in frequency due to pressures of natural selection, thereby disrupting HWE.

Changes in allele frequencies due to selection or mutation usually occur slowly, in small increments, and cause much less deviation from HWE, at least for recessive diseases. This is because rates of new mutations are generally well below the frequency of heterozygotes for autosomal recessive diseases. The addition of new pathogenic alleles to the gene pool thus has little effect (in the short term) on allele frequencies for such diseases. In addition, most deleterious recessive alleles are hidden in asymptomatic heterozygotes and thus are not subject to selection. Consequently, selection is not likely to have major short-term effects on allele frequencies of these recessive alleles. Therefore, to a first approximation, HWE may apply even for alleles that cause severe autosomal recessive disease. Importantly, however, for dominant or X-linked conditions, mutation and selection *do* perturb allele frequencies from what would be expected under HWE, by substantially reducing or increasing certain genotypes in just a few generations.

In practice, some violations of HWE we have discussed are more disruptive than others when applying the principle to human populations. For example, violating the assumption of random mating can cause large deviations from the expected frequency of individuals homozygous for an autosomal recessive condition. In contrast, changes in allele frequency due to mutation, selection, or migration usually cause more minor and gradual deviations from HWE. When HWE assumptions do not hold for a particular disease allele at a particular locus, it may be instructive to investigate *why* the allele and its associated genotypes are not in equilibrium as this may provide clues about the pathogenesis of the condition or point to historical events that have affected the frequency of alleles in different population groups over time.

Mutation and Selection Balance in Traits With Different Modes of Inheritance

In this section, we examine the concepts of mutation and selection through the lens of fitness, a heuristic device that indicates the likelihood of a mutation at a particular locus being eliminated, becoming stable, or becoming (over time) the predominant allele (or fixed) in a population. The frequency of an allele in a population at any given time represents a balance between the rate at which new alleles appear through mutation and the influence of selection on these alleles. If the **mutation rate** or the effectiveness of selection is altered, the allele frequency is expected to change.

More formally, whether an allele is transmitted to the succeeding generation depends on its fitness, ω, which is a quantitative measure for the expected (average) number of offspring of affected persons who survive to reproductive age. This measure is called relative fitness when compared with that of an appropriate control group. If a pathogenic allele is just as likely to be represented in the next generation compared to functionally neutral alleles, $\omega = 1$. If an allele causes death or sterility, purifying, or negative, **selection** acts against it completely, and $\omega = 0$. Values between 0 and 1 indicate transmission of the variant, and values of $\omega > 1$ indicate positive selection increasing the variant's frequency in a population.

A related parameter is the coefficient of selection, s, which is a measure of the *loss* of fitness and is defined as $1 - \omega$, that is, the proportion of pathogenic alleles that are *not* passed on and are therefore lost due to negative selection. When a genetic condition limits reproduction such that $\omega = 0$ and $s = 1$, the variant conferring this trait is referred to as a **genetic lethal**. In the genetic sense, a variant that prevents reproduction by an adult is just as "lethal" as one that causes a very early miscarriage of an embryo, because in neither case is the variant transmitted to the next generation. Fitness is thus the outcome of the joint effects of survival and fertility. In the biological sense, relative fitness has no connotation of superior endowment but is simply a measure of comparative ability to contribute alleles to the next generation, on *average*.

The frequency of pathogenic alleles in a population represents a balance between loss of pathogenic alleles through the effects of selection and gain of pathogenic alleles through recurrent mutation. A stable allele frequency will then be reached at whatever level balances the two opposing forces: one (selection) that removes pathogenic alleles from the gene pool and one (*de novo* mutation) that adds new ones back. The **mutation rate** per generation, μ, at a locus with pathogenic variants must be sufficient to account for the fraction of all pathogenic alleles that are lost by selection from each generation. That is,

$$\mu = sq$$

where μ is the mutation rate, s is the coefficient of selection, and q is the allele frequency.

If a pathogenic allele for a condition has a dominant mode of inheritance and is deleterious but not lethal, affected persons may reproduce but will nevertheless contribute fewer than the average number of offspring to the next generation; that is, $0 < \omega < 1$. Such a variant will be lost through selection at a rate proportional to the reduced fitness of heterozygotes. For example, consider a phenotypic trait that reduces the fitness of affected persons to an average of one-fifth the number of children compared to unaffected persons in a population. The relative fitness is thus $\omega = 0.20$, and the coefficient of selection, $s = 1 - \omega = 0.80$. This means that in the next generation of offspring, only 20% of pathogenic alleles are passed on.

When the frequency of such conditions appears stable from one generation to the next, new mutations are most likely responsible for replacing 80% of the pathogenic alleles predicted to be lost through selection. If the fitness of affected persons suddenly improves (e.g., because of medical advances or removal of other barriers to reproduction for individuals with the condition), the observed incidence in the population is predicted to increase and reach a new equilibrium. Retinoblastoma (Case 39) and other dominant embryonic tumors with childhood onset are examples of conditions that now have a greatly improved prognosis compared to when they were first described, which may have increased the frequency of such conditions in the population.

Selection against pathogenic alleles with a recessive mode of inheritance has less of an effect on population frequencies than selection against dominant variants, because only a small proportion of these alleles cooccur in homozygotes, with phenotypic presentation that exposes them selective pressure. Even if there were complete selection against homozygotes ($\omega = 0$), as in many lethal autosomal recessive conditions, it would take many generations to reduce the allele frequency appreciably because most pathogenic alleles are carried by unaffected carriers (heterozygotes).

For example, the frequency of pathogenic alleles causing Tay-Sachs disease, q, can be as high as 1.5% in Ashkenazi Jewish populations. Given this value $q = 0.015$; $p = 1 - 0.015 = 0.95$; thus the proportion of heterozygous individuals is expected to be $2pq = 2(0.015)(0.95) = 0.029$. This means approximately 3% of individuals in such a population are expected to carry one copy of the pathogenic variant. In contrast, only 1 individual per 4500 ($q^2 = 0.015 \beta 0.015 = 0.0002$) is homozygous for the pathogenic allele, such that selection can act on the recessive phenotype. The proportion of all pathogenic variants among homozygotes in such a population is thus:

$$\frac{2 \times 0.0002}{(2 \times 0.0002) + (1 \times 0.03)} \approx 0.0132$$

such that <2% of all pathogenic variants in the population are in affected individuals, whose condition would be exposed to negative selection in the absence of effective treatment.

We hope this example offers mathematical intuition as to why recessive variants are slow to influence allele frequencies in a population, due to the relatively small number of pathogenic variants that are subjected to selection at any given time. Reduction or removal of selection against an autosomal recessive disorder by successful treatment (e.g., as in the case of PKU) would have just as slow an effect on increasing the allele frequency over many generations. Thus, *if mating is random, genotypes in autosomal recessive diseases are considered to be in Hardy-Weinberg equilibrium, despite selection against homozygotes for the recessive allele*. It follows that the mathematical relationship between genotype and allele frequencies described by HWE holds for most practical purposes in the case of an autosomal recessive disease.

In contrast to recessive pathogenic alleles, dominant pathogenic alleles are exposed *directly* to selection. Consequently, the effects of selection and mutation are more obvious and can be more readily measured for dominant traits. A genetic lethal dominant allele, if fully penetrant, will be exposed to selection in heterozygotes, thus removing all alleles responsible for the disorder in a single generation. Several human diseases are thought to be autosomal dominant traits with zero or near-zero fitness and thus always result from *de novo*, rather than inherited, autosomal dominant variants. This is a point of great significance for genetic counseling, and examples of these conditions are listed in Table 10.6.

In some of these conditions, the specific pathogenic alleles are known, and family studies have revealed *de novo* mutations in affected individuals that were not inherited from the parents. In other conditions, the responsible genes are not known, but paternal age effects (Chapter 4) have been observed, which suggests a possible mechanism of *de novo* mutations in the paternal **germline**. The implication for genetic counseling is that parents of a child with an autosomal dominant (but genetically lethal) condition will typically have a very low risk of recurrence in subsequent pregnancies because the condition would require another independent *de novo* mutation. A caveat to keep in mind is the possibility of **germline mosaicism** (See Fig. 7.17) and the possibility of abundant *de novo* mutations in a germline heavily exposed to **mutagens**.

In clinically relevant conditions that have an X-linked recessive mode of inheritance, selection acts on **hemizygous** males but not in heterozygous females, except for the small proportion of females who are **manifesting heterozygotes** with reduced fitness (see Chapter 7).

In this brief discussion, we assume that heterozygous females do not have reduced fitness. Because males have one X chromosome and females have two, the pool of X-linked alleles in the entire population's gene pool is partitioned, such that one-third of pathogenic alleles are in males and two-thirds are in females.

As we saw in the case of autosomal dominant variants, pathogenic alleles lost through selection must be replaced by recurrent new mutations to maintain the observed disease incidence. If the incidence of an X-linked condition is not changing, and selection is operating (only) against hemizygous males, the mutation rate, μ, must equal the coefficient of selection, s (i.e., the proportion of pathogenic alleles that are *not* passed on), times q (the pathogenic allele frequency), adjusted by a factor of 3, since *selection is operating only on the third of pathogenic alleles in the population that are present in males*. The equation is thus:

$$\mu = sq/3$$

For an X-linked genetic lethal condition, $s = 1$, and one-third of all copies of the pathogenic allele are lost from each generation; so, at equilibrium, these must be replaced by *de novo* mutations. Thus, roughly one-third of all persons who have X-linked lethal disorders are predicted to carry a *de novo* mutation, and their unaffected mothers have a low risk of future pregnancies harboring the same disorder (in the absence of germline mosaicism). The remaining two-thirds of mothers of individuals with an X-linked lethal disorder are predicted to be carriers, each with a 50% *future* risk of conceiving an affected child, given that it is male. However, the prediction that two-thirds of mothers of individuals with an X-linked lethal disorder are carriers of a disease-causing variant assumes that mutation rates in males and in females are equal.

Given that the germline mutation rate is higher in males with advanced paternal age than in females, the chance of a *de novo* mutation occurring in the egg is very low. (Note: the impact on genetic counseling related to these sex-dependent considerations of mutation rates will be discussed in Chapter 17). Most mothers of affected children are carriers, having most likely inherited novel variants from unaffected fathers, which they then have a 50% chance of passing on to their children. Taking advantage of the statistical property that the *probability of two independent events occurring is equal to the product of probabilities of each separate event*,

$$\Pr[A \text{ and } B] = \Pr[A] \times \Pr[B]$$

where A and B are independent events, we can therefore calculate the total risk of an unaffected carrier of an X-linked condition having a child with the condition as:

$$\Pr[\text{male child}] \times \Pr[\text{passing on the pathogenic allele}]$$
$$= (0.5)(0.5) = 0.25$$

TABLE 10.6 Genetic Conditions Occurring via *De Novo* Mutations With Zero Fitness

Condition/ Phenotype	Description
Atelosteogenesis	Early lethal form of short-limbed skeletal dysplasia
Cornelia de Lange syndrome	Intellectual disability, micromelia, synophrys, and other abnormalities; can be caused by pathogenic variants in the *NIPBL* and other genes
Developmental and epileptic encephalopathy	Intellectually disability and early-onset seizures; can be caused by *de novo* variants in >50 different genes
Osteogenesis imperfecta, type II	Perinatal lethal type, with a defect in type I collagen (*COL1A1*, *COL1A2*) (see Chapter 13)
Thanatophoric dysplasia	Early lethal form of skeletal dysplasia due to specific *de novo* pathogenic variants in the *FGFR3* gene (see Fig. 7.6 C)

such that the probability that an unaffected carrier will give birth to a child with an X-linked genetic lethal condition is 25% or one-fourth, given that the other parent is not affected.

In less severe disorders, such as hemophilia A (Case 21), the proportion of affected individuals representing new mutations is less than one-third (~15%). Because the treatment of hemophilia has improved significantly, the total frequency of pathogenic alleles can be expected to rise rapidly and to reach a new equilibrium. Assuming that the mutation rate at this locus stays the same over time, the *proportion* of those with hemophilia whose pathogenic variant arises *de novo* will decrease, but the overall *incidence* of the disease will increase. Such a change would have significant implications for genetic counseling for this condition (see Chapter 17).

Although certain pathogenic alleles may be deleterious in homozygotes, there may be environmental conditions in which heterozygotes for some conditions have *increased* fitness relative to homozygotes for both the pathogenic allele and the reference allele. This is called **heterozygote advantage** because even a slightly greater relative fitness of heterozygotes can lead to an increase in frequency of an allele that is severely detrimental in homozygotes. This is because heterozygotes greatly outnumber homozygotes in the population. A situation in which selective forces operate to both *maintain* a deleterious allele and *remove* it from the gene pool is often referred to as balancing selection.

A well-known example of heterozygote advantage is resistance to malaria in individuals who are heterozygous for the pathogenic allele that causes sickle cell disease (Case 42). This pathogenic variant in the β-globin gene *HBB* has reached its highest frequency in certain regions of Africa and Southeast Asia, where malaria is endemic and heterozygotes have greater relative fitness than either type of homozygote, due to their resistance to malarial infection. In the presence of (mosquito) **vectors** that carry malaria-inducing parasites, homozygotes without the trait allele are highly susceptible; they may become infected and are severely (even fatally) affected. Homozygotes for the pathogenic allele are even more disadvantaged, with a relative fitness that approaches zero due to severely debilitating hematological disease (see Chapter 12).

Heterozygotes, on the other hand, have red blood cells that are inhospitable to the malarial parasite but do not typically undergo the characteristic sickling that leads to pain crises in active sickle cell disease. As such, these heterozygotes have a much greater relative fitness than homozygotes for the typical β-globin allele. Over time, the pathogenic allele for sickle cell disease has reached a frequency as high as 0.15 in some areas of the world that are endemic for malaria, far higher than could be accounted for by recurrent mutation alone.

Heterozygote advantage in sickle cell disease offers a clear example of how assumptions of HWE are violated when the mathematical relationship between allele and genotype frequencies diverges from expected values, (in this case) due to the effects of balancing selection. To firmly ground this example, let us consider the sickle cell allele in the β-globin gene *HBB*, rs334 (c.20 A>T [p.Glu7Val]), in which the pathogenic allele β^S is under balancing selection due to heterozygote advantage. Let us define the benign (nonpathogenic) allele β^+ such that the two alleles β^S and β^+ give rise to three genotypes: $\beta^+|\beta^+$ (unaffected; homozygous), $\beta^+|\beta^S$ (unaffected carriers; heterozygous), and $\beta^S|\beta^S$ (affected).

In a study of whole-genome sequence data from 2932 individuals aggregated across the 1000 Genomes Project, the African Genome Variation Project, and Qatar, balancing selection on the sickle cell variant β^S is estimated to have conferred strong heterozygote advantage, having reached its equilibrium frequency of 12% after 87 generations (while the initial mutation is dated back 259 generations, or ~7300 years ago). Using the β^S allele's reported equilibrium frequency of 0.12 (q), we can calculate the expected ratio of genotypes under HWE ($p^2:2pq:q^2$) and compare this to observed genotype frequencies in the 1KG dataset for populations that have the β^S allele at or near its equilibrium frequency.

Given that $q = 0.12$ and $p = 1 - q$, the frequency of $p = 1 - 0.12 = 0.88$. From this, we can use HWE to calculate expected genotype frequencies as follows: Pr[affected homozygotes ($\beta^S|\beta^S$)] = q^2 = (0.12) * (0.12) = 0.014; Pr[unaffected homozygotes ($\beta^+|\beta^+$)] = p^2 = (0.88) * (0.88) = 0.774; and Pr[heterozygotes ($\beta^S|\beta^+$)] = $2pq$ = 2*(0.88) * (0.12) = 0.211. Thus the expected genotype proportions of $p^2:2pq:q^2$ are 0.774:0.211:0.014.

Investigating rs334 allele frequencies in the 1KG dataset through Ensembl, two populations sampled from Africa appear to have the β^S allele at or near its equilibrium frequency (0.12): the Esan in Nigeria (ESN) with β^S at 12.1% and the Mende in Sierra Leone (MSL) with β^S at 12.4% in the population. Observed genotype frequencies for these populations are as follows: 0.758:0.242:0 (for ESN) and 0.753:0.247:0 (for MSL). In both these populations, the observed proportions of heterozygous ($\beta^S|\beta^+$) individuals exceed what was predicted assuming HWE, whereas the observed number of unaffected homozygotes ($\beta^+|\beta^+$) and affected homozygotes ($\beta^S|\beta^S$) are below what was predicted. This trend reflects balancing selection at this locus, illustrating how forces of selection, operating both negatively on the relatively rare $\beta^S|\beta^S$ genotype and positively on the more common $\beta^S|\beta^+$ genotype, cause deviation from HWE.

The effects of balancing selection on malaria resistance are also apparent in other infectious diseases. For example, many people with the severe renal disease known as focal segmental glomerulosclerosis are homozygotes for certain alleles in the coding region of the *APOL1* gene that encodes the apolipoprotein L1. Apolipoprotein L1 is a serum factor that kills the trypanosome parasite

Trypanosoma brucei, which causes trypanosomiasis (sleeping sickness). The same variants that increase one's risk of severe kidney disease in homozygotes tenfold over the rest of the population protect heterozygotes carrying these variants against trypanosomes (e.g., *T. brucei rhodesiense*) that have developed resistance to **wild-type** apolipoprotein L1. As a result, the frequency of heterozygous carriers for these alleles can be as high as ~45% in parts of the world in which the rhodesiense trypanosomiasis is endemic.

GENOMIC VARIATION AND BIASES IN POPULATION DATASETS

The type and amount of information available to researchers and clinicians for our work is the foundation for discoveries, diagnostics, treatment regimens, and approaches to measuring outcomes. Missing data is inevitable – but uncertainty arises in the interpretation and portability of findings when the amount and type of data available is missing or of differential quality in a nonrandom ways, that is, if certain groups or patient populations are better represented in databases than others, for example.

Ascertainment bias refers to systemic biases in observations that steer our research or interpretations in a direction based on what is observed – without having any knowledge of that which remains unobserved (and could potentially change the result or interpretation if revealed). For example, >80% of genomics research to date has been conducted on people of mostly European ancestries, so population reference data and genomic databases are heavily biased toward a European genomic background. Fig. 10.8 shows broad ancestry groups of GWAS participants from 2003 to 2018, compared with the world's population, showing Europeans are vastly overrepresented among GWAS participants relative to their global census representation.

The impact of this European bias is far-reaching, such that genetic tests are designed primarily to capture variation that commonly contributes to disease on a European genomic background (or is associated with the causal variant via Linkage Disequilibrium; see Chapter 11). **Genetic** or **locus heterogeneity** in a trait means that variation in different regions of the genome can be pathogenic for the same trait. The ascertainment bias toward prevalence in European ancestries contributes to higher rates of variants of unknown or uncertain significance (VUS) in non-Europeans, as well as higher rates of false negative diagnoses, due to missing genetic heterogeneity.

Higher false positive rates have also been documented, as in the case of a variant associated with hypertrophic cardiomyopathy (and curated as pathogenic based on information from European ancestry individuals), which was later shown to be benign in African American patients – after many had already undergone an invasive prophylactic intervention. Exclusion of individuals with recent African ancestries is a mistake for any study of the genetic underpinnings of health and disease, due to the wealth of genetic variation that exists in African populations. Fig. 10.9 illustrates this point by showcasing not only how much ancestral variation is present across the African continent (relative to reference data) but also how biased representations of global genomic diversity can be when restricted to continental ancestry groupings that seek to "balance" representation across the canonical discrete categories, as in Fig. 10.9B.

Information disparity in the genomic knowledgebase between individuals with primarily European ancestries and everyone else is responsible for differences in the utility and accuracy of clinical genetic testing. This further exacerbates health and health care disparities at

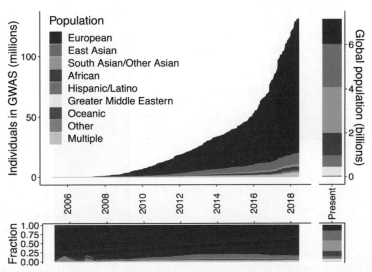

Figure 10.8 Ancestry of GWAS participants over time, as compared with the global population. Cumulative data, as reported by the GWAS catalog. Individuals whose ancestry is "not reported" are not shown. From Martin et al. Clinical use of current polygenic risk scores may exacerbate health disparities, *Nat Genet* 51:584–591, 2019. https://doi.org/10.1038/s41588-019-0379-x

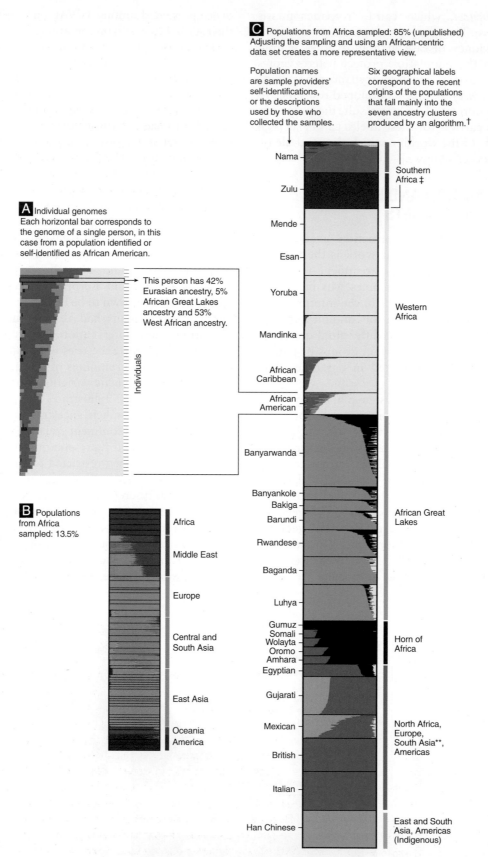

C Populations from Africa sampled: 85% (unpublished)
Adjusting the sampling and using an African-centric data set creates a more representative view.

Population names are sample providers' self-identifications, or the descriptions used by those who collected the samples.

Six geographical labels correspond to the recent origins of the populations that fall mainly into the seven ancestry clusters produced by an algorithm.[†]

A Individual genomes
Each horizontal bar corresponds to the genome of a single person, in this case from a population identified or self-identified as African American.

This person has 42% Eurasian ancestry, 5% African Great Lakes ancestry and 53% West African ancestry.

B Populations from Africa sampled: 13.5%

Figure 10.9 Compiling genotype data from individuals can show the genetic diversity of populations. (A) An analysis from 2008* suggested significant genetic differences between seven continental populations (B) But only 13.5% of the populations represented were from Africa. Boosting representation to 85% and sampling more broadly across the continent (C) underlines that the level of genetic variation within Africa is equivalent to that seen between continents. Figure adapted from Carlson J, Henn BM, Al-Hindi DR, Ramachandran S. Counter: the weaponization of genetics research by extremists, *Nature* 610: 2022.
**South Asia appears twice because Gujarati people in India have intermediate allele frequencies.

the population level due to structural racism that disproportionately impacts Black patients of all ancestries (e.g., the well-documented undertreatment of pain in African Americans). We will ground this discussion in the practical context of clinical variant interpretation.

Guidelines for clinical variant interpretation protocols published by Association for Molecular Pathology (AMP) and the American College of Medical Genetics and Genomics (ACMG) include population-level information (e.g., allele frequency in population databases), among other data (e.g., functional evidence) to guide decisions about whether to designate a variant as benign, likely benign, likely pathogenic, pathogenic, or uncertain significance. For variants detected in European populations, the genomic knowledgebase is robust and reliable enough such that the absence of a variant from population databases can be considered evidence for pathogenicity. This is because these populations are well represented among reference datasets, so the absence of a variant can be reasonably interpreted as evidence that it is not tolerated in the population.

In contrast, most global populations have not been included in genomic datasets at a comparable rate or magnitude, so this interpretation may be subject to limited certainty. Instead, it may be that absence or very low frequency of a variant in population databases reflects insufficient representation, and more rigorous sampling would reveal higher population-allele frequencies than would be consistent with predicted pathogenicity of the variant. Several efforts are underway to improve diversity and inclusion in genomic databases; Box 10.3 details two of these examples.

As biomedical researchers and clinicians, we must acknowledge that the ways in which we collect,

BOX 10.3 "A TALE OF TWO INITIATIVES" (BY LAURA ARBOUR)

The Genome Aggregation Database (gnomAD) is an international collaborative effort of researchers utilizing available data sources of genomic variation compiled through the Broad Institute (https://gnomad.broadinstitute.org). It is used frequently as a clinical tool in the diagnosis of rare, severe, genetic disease. The frequency of variants present in the dataset and reported geographical ancestry of origin are openly available to clinicians and researchers, which aids in the first steps of consideration for pathogenicity of variants (common variants are unlikely to cause severe, early onset disease). The combination of whole genomes and exomes of more than 140,000 unrelated individuals contributes to the genomic reference database. Although there are ongoing efforts to increase diversity in public genomic databases including gnomAD, the problem is that not all populations are represented in available datasets for a multitude of reasons, therefore not all children or families with rare genetic conditions will have the same opportunity for a precise diagnosis in a timely manner. The lack of genomic reference data increases the "genomic divide," where those with the greatest health disparities benefit least from genomic advances.

The impact of lack of Indigenous genomic data is staggering when it is considered that there are more than 370 million Indigenous people spanning 90 countries worldwide (https://www.un.org/esa/socdev/unpfii/documents/5session_factsheet1.pdf.).

Two initiatives aim to address this issue for Indigenous patients with genetic conditions. In parallel, the Silent Genomes Project (Canada) and the Aotearoa Variome (New Zealand) are developing genomic data reference databases that are prioritized for genomic health care (https://www.frontiersin.org/articles/10.3389/fpubh.2020.00111/full) and may also be used for health research. These initiates are led or co-led by Indigenous scholars, and variant use and release mechanisms are being developed and are informed by long-standing ethical frameworks from within their respective countries ("DNA on Loan" and the Te Mata Ira guidelines for medical genomics with Māori) and are consistent with the recent International Indigenous Data

Sovereignty Interest Group "CARE" principles, CARE being the acronym for "Collective Benefit, Authority to Control, Responsibility and Ethics" (https://datascience.codata.org/articles/10.5334/dsj-2020-043/). The CARE principles are Indigenous focused but are meant to complement the "FAIR principles (Findable, Accessible, Interopcrable, Reusable) which are Guiding Principles for scientific data management and stewardship" (https://www.nature.com/articles/sdata201618). The CARE principles support the notion of benefit for, and self-determination of, Indigenous people, consistent with the United Nations Declaration of the Rights of Indigenous Peoples (adopted by the UN General Assembly in 2007 and endorsed by law in Canada [Bill C-15] in 2021).

Both the Silent Genomes Project and Aotearoa Variome will start with sequencing the samples of consented individuals within their countries. Storage, use, and release of variants for clinical and possibly research purposes is being informed by local Indigenous perspectives and governance mechanisms. The Silent Genomes Project will also assess the efficacy of the Indigenous Background Variant Library (IBVL) in a cohort of Indigenous children who have gone through diagnosis without the IBVL. The primary goal of both initiatives is to reduce, and not increase, health disparities with genomic advances.

References (also integrated above):

https://www.un.org/esa/socdev/unpfii/documents/5session_factsheet1.pdf

https://www.genomics-aotearoa.org.nz/projects/aotearoa-nz-genomic-variome

https://www.bcchr.ca/silent-genomes-project

Indigenous genomic databases: Pragmatic considerations and cultural contexts

NR Caron, M Chongo, M Hudson, L Arbour, WW Wasserman, S Robertson, S Correard, P Wilcox: *Front Public Health* 8:111, 2020. doi:10.3389/fpubh.2020.00111; https://www.nature.com/articles/sdata201618

https://datascience.codata.org/articles/10.5334/dsj-2020-043/

https://www.un.org/development/desa/indigenous-peoples/declaration-on-the-rights-of-indigenous-peoples.html

https://www.mltaikins.com/indigenous/senate-passes-undrip-bill-c-15/

analyze, visualize, and report or publish our data on human population genetics are crucially important. Our analytic approaches are heavily influenced by the historical, cultural, social, and political contexts in which we conduct our research and clinical practices. How we think about and represent categories of difference and similarity within and among populations matters – both for science and medicine, but also for society. Members of the public with harmful political agendas have weaponized figures illustrating admixture mapping that are published in peer-reviewed journals (e.g., Fig. 10.9B), claiming such clustering methods support their ideologies that are steeped in biological racism. We must counter these efforts and work to prevent further misconceptions from spreading, through responsible and trustworthy research and reporting.

Until we have a more robust and complete picture of global genomic variation and how it contributes to complex disease etiology, it is imperative that we exercise caution when implementing existing (and new) methodologies to analyze genome-wide data. For example, **polygenic risk scores**, or polygenic scores (PRS), have the potential to exacerbate both conceptual and practical issues related to equity in human population genetics and medicine. Figs. 10.10 and 10.11 provide a high-level overview of how PRS are constructed, and the

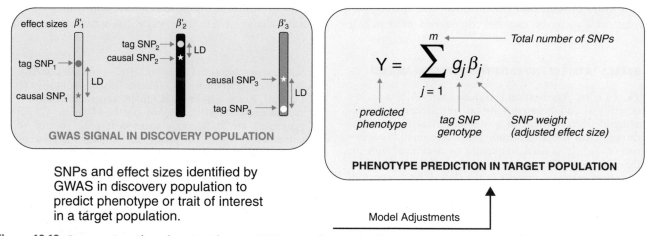

Figure 10.10 Construction of a polygenic risk score (PRS) to predict a trait of interest (Y) in a target population using SNPs associated with the trait (g_j) and their effect sizes (βj) in a genome-wide association study (GWAS) in a discovery population. Variants identified by GWAS in the discovery population are not necessarily causing or contributing to variation of the trait in the discovery population, but these "tag SNPs" are linked to causal SNP(s) such that they signal a candidate region to be further investigated.

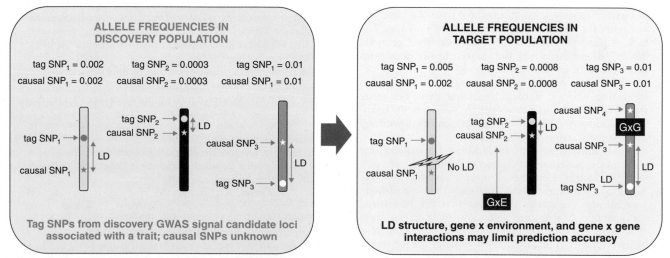

Figure 10.11 Allele frequencies of tag SNPs and causal SNPs are equal in the discovery population because these variants are in linkage disequilibrium (LD). When LD structure differs between discovery and target populations, associations between tag SNPs and causal SNPs in the discovery GWAS may not be replicated in the target population, limiting the predictive power of this model. Differences in environmental factors and gene-by-environment interactions (GxE) between discovery and target populations may impact the accuracy of prediction in the target population, particularly for multifactorial traits. The presence of other variants in the causal pathway with gene-by-gene interactions (GxG, or epistatic effects) in one population, but not the other, may also limit the portability of PRS between populations.

conceptual as well as technical pitfalls of trying to predict phenotypic variation in one (target) population using GWAS results from another (discovery) population.

In this simplified model, PRS construction involves several assumptions about homogeneity in genetic contributions to disease, allele frequencies, LD structure, GxG, and GxE between a discovery population and the target (prediction) population. Allele frequencies and LD structure may differ substantively between populations (depending on how they are defined and their underlying characteristics). Similarly, differential GxE and GxG between populations can dramatically affect the results of genomic investigations and obscure the role of genetic variants in disease etiology. Clinical professionals must be aware that PRS still have a long way to go before one could argue that they offer enhanced utility beyond the current standards of care and could make matters worse in the meantime.

What is true of PRS is the same for all approaches we use in genomic research and medicine. We must critically examine our underlying assumptions about what factors contribute most to health and disease, consider the impact of those assumptions, investigate the history and biases of approaches we seek to use, and question the foundations of what we think we know – to make room for more curiosity and innovation that will lead to novel discoveries and more precise **genomic medicine**.

ACKNOWLEDGMENT

Some language and sections included in this chapter were inherited from previous (published) versions of the textbook. Laura Arbour contributed "A Tale of Two Initiatives". Conversations with clinical genetics professionals and other interdisciplinary collaborations through the NIH-funded Clinical Genome Resource (ClinGen) Ancestry & Diversity Working Group helped motivate the development of new content for this revision.

We thank Sonja Rasmussen for contributing to this chapter.

GENERAL REFERENCES

Li CC: *First course in population genetics*, Pacific Grove, 1975, Boxwood Press.

Nielsen R, Slatkin M: *An introduction to population genetics*, Sunderland, 2013, Sinauer Associates, Inc.

Dorothy R: *Fatal invention: How Science, Politics, and Big Business Re-Create Race in the Twenty-First Century*, New York, 2011, New Press.

Popejoy AB, Crooks KR, Fullerton SM, et al: Clinical Genome Resource (ClinGen) Ancestry and Diversity Working Group: Clinical genetics lacks standard definitions and protocols for the collection and use of diversity measures, *Am J Hum Genet* 107(1):72–82, 2020. https://doi.org/10.1016/j.ajhg.2020.05.005

Royal CD, Novembre J, Fullerton SM, et al: Inferring genetic ancestry: opportunities, challenges and implications, *Am J Hum Genet* 86:661–673, 2010.

REFERENCES FOR SPECIFIC TOPICS

American Society of Human Genetics: ASHG denounces attempts to link genetics and racial supremacy, *Am J Hum Genet* 103:636, 2018.

Behar DM, Yunusbayev B, Metspalu M, et al: The genome-wide structure of the Jewish people, *Nature* 466:238–242, 2010.

Borrell LN, Elhawary JR, Fuentes-Afflick E, et al: Race and genetic ancestry in medicine – A time for reckoning with racism, *N Engl J Med* 384:474–480, 2021. https://doi.org/10.1056/NEJMms2029562

Corona E, Chen R, Sikora M, et al: Analysis of the genetic basis of disease in the context of worldwide human relationships and migration, *PLoS Genet* 9:e1003447, 2013.

Gregg AR, Aarabi M, Klugman S, et al: ACMG Professional Practice and Guidelines Committee: Screening for autosomal recessive and X-linked conditions during pregnancy and preconception: a practice resource of the American College of Medical Genetics and Genomics (ACMG, *Genet Med* 23(10):1793–1806, 2021. https://doi.org/10.1038/s41436-021-01203-z

Henn BM, Cavalli-Sforza LL, Feldman MW: The great human expansion. *Proceedings of the National Academy of Sciences of the United States of America* 109:17758–64. PMID 23077256. https://doi.org/10.1007/S12045-019-0830-4

Howes R, Patil A, Piel F, et al: The global distribution of the Duffy blood group. *Nat Commun* 2:266, 2011. https://doi.org/10.1038/ncomms1265

Kaseniit KE, Haque IS, Goldberg JD, Shulman LP, Muzzey D: Genetic ancestry analysis on >93,000 individuals undergoing expanded carrier screening reveals limitations of ethnicity-based medical guidelines, *Genet Med* 22(10):1694–1702, 2020. https://doi.org/10.1038/s41436-020-0869-3

Kumar R, Seibold MA, Aldrich MC, et al: Genetic ancestry in lung-function predictions, *N Engl J Med* 363:321–330, 2010.

Lewontin RC: The apportionment of human diversity. In: Dobzhansky T, Hecht MK, Steere WC, editors: *Evolutionary biology: volume*, 6, New York, 1972, Springer.

Martin A, Kanai M, Kamatani Y, Okada Y, Neale BM, Daly MJ: Clinical use of current polygenic risk scores may exacerbate health disparities, *Nat Genet* 51:584–591, 2019. https://doi.org/10.1038/s41588-019-0379-x

Novembre J, Johnson T, Bryc K, et al: Genes mirror geography within Europe. *Nature* 456:98–101, 2008. https://doi.org/10.1038/nature07331

Novembre J, Peter BM: Recent advances in the study of fine-scale population structure in humans. *Curr Opin Genet Dev* 41:98–105, 2016. https://doi.org/10.1016/j.gde.2016.08.007

Peterson RE, Kuchenbaecker K, Walters RK, et al: Genome-wide association studies in ancestrally diverse populations: Opportunities, methods, pitfalls, and recommendations, *Cell* 179(3):589–603, 2019. https://doi.org/10.1016/j.cell.2019.08.051

Richards S, Aziz N, Bale S, et al: Standards and guidelines for the interpretation of sequence variants: a joint consensus recommendation of the American College of Medical Genetics and Genomics and the Association for Molecular Pathology, *Genet Med* 17:405–423, 2015. https://doi.org/10.1038/gim.2015.30

Sankararaman S, Mallick S, Dannemann M, et al: The genomic landscape of Neanderthal ancestry in present-day humans, *Nature* 507:354–357, 2014.

Shriner D, Rotimi CN: Whole-genome-sequence-based haplotypes reveal single origin of the sickle allele during the Holocene Wet Phase, *Am J Hum Genet* 102(4):547–556, 2018. https://doi.org/10.1016/j.ajhg.2018.02.003. Epub 2018 Mar 8. PMID: 29526279; PMCID: PMC5985360.

Wastnedge E, Waters D, Patel S, et al: The global burden of sickle cell disease in children under five years of age: a systematic review and meta-analysis, *J Global Health* 8(2):021103, 2018. https://www.ncbi.nlm.nih.gov/pmc/articles/PMC6286674/

Wexler (Need REF for Venezuela finding)

Wojcik GL, Graff M, Nishimura KK, et al: Genetic analyses of diverse populations improves discovery for complex traits, *Nature* 570:514–318, 2019. https://doi.org/10.1038/s41586-019-1310-4

PROBLEMS

1. A short tandem repeat (STR) variant consists of 5 different alleles, each with a frequency of 0.20 in a population.
   a. What proportion of individuals in this population would you expect to be homozygous at this locus?
   b. What proportion of the population is likely to be heterozygous at this locus?
   c. What proportion of individuals would be homozygous, and what proportion would be heterozygous if the 5 alleles had different frequencies of 0.40, 0.30, 0.15, 0.10, and 0.05?

2. In a population with allele frequencies in Hardy-Weinberg equilibrium, three genotypes are present in the following proportions: A/A, 0.81; A/a, 0.18; a/a, 0.01.
   a. What are the allele frequencies of A and a?
   b. What will their frequencies be in the next generation, assuming the conditions of Hardy-Weinberg equilibrium hold?

3. In a screening program designed to detect carriers of an autosomal recessive condition, the carrier frequency in a specific founder population was approximately 4%.
   a. Calculate the frequency of the pathogenic allele in this population (assuming only one).
   b. If the genetic fitness of affected individuals is zero, what proportion of possible reproductive pairings in this population could produce an affected child?
   c. What is the prevalence of unaffected carriers among offspring of couples in which both partners are heterozygous for the trait?
   d. If the pathogenic allele for this condition had the same frequency but were instead inherited through an autosomal dominant mode of inheritance (fully penetrant), what would be the frequency of unaffected adult carriers? What if it were X-linked dominant? X-linked recessive?

4. Which of the following populations is in Hardy-Weinberg equilibrium, based on the information provided?
   a. A/A, 0.70; A/a, 0.21; a/a, 0.09.
   b. A/A, 0.32; A/a, 0.64; a/a, 0.04.
   c. A/A, 0.64; A/a, 0.32; a/a, 0.04.
   What explanations could you offer to explain the frequencies in those populations that are not in equilibrium?

5. You are consulted by a couple, Meera and Arjun, who tell you that Meera's sister has Hurler syndrome (a mucopolysaccharidosis) and that they are concerned that they might have a child with the same syndrome. Hurler syndrome is inherited as an autosomal recessive trait with an estimated prevalence of 1 in 90,000 individuals in a large population.
   a. What is the chance that Arjun is heterozygous for the pathogenic allele?
   b. What is the chance that Meera is a carrier of the pathogenic allele for Hurler syndrome?
   c. If Meera and Arjun are not genetically related through their parents (no consanguinity), what is the risk that Meera and Arjun's first child will have Hurler syndrome?
   d. If Meera and Arjun share the same population ancestry, or received similar continental-level ancestry results from a direct-to-consumer genetic testing company, what is the risk that their first child will have the syndrome?

6. In a certain population, each of 3 serious neuromuscular conditions—autosomal dominant facioscapulohumeral muscular dystrophy, autosomal recessive Friedreich ataxia, and X-linked recessive Duchenne muscular dystrophy—has an incidence of approximately 1 in 25,000 individuals.
   a. What are the frequencies of pathogenic alleles for each of these conditions?
   b. Suppose that each condition could be treated such that affected individuals could have children. What would be the resulting effect on the incidence of each condition? Why?

7. As discussed in this chapter, the autosomal recessive condition tyrosinemia type I has an incidence of 1 in 685 individuals in one population in the province of Quebec, but approximately 1 in 100,000 elsewhere. What is the frequency of the variant associated with tyrosinemia in these two groups? Suggest possible explanations for the difference in allele frequencies between the population in Quebec and populations elsewhere.

Identifying the Genetic Basis for Human Disease

Christian R. Marshall

This chapter provides an overview of how geneticists study families and populations to identify **genetic** contributions to disease. Whether a disease is inherited in a recognizable **mendelian** pattern, as illustrated in Chapter 7, or occurs at a higher frequency in relatives of affected individuals, as explored in Chapter 9, it is specific genomic **variants** that either cause disease directly or influence the susceptibility to disease. **Genome** research has provided geneticists with a catalogue of all known human genes, knowledge of their location and structure, and an ever growing list of tens of millions of variants in DNA sequence found among individuals in different populations. As we saw in previous chapters, some of these variants are common, others are rare, and still others are ultrarare or even private to families or individuals. Whereas some variants clearly have functional consequences associated with disease **risk**, others are certainly neutral. For most, their significance for human health and disease is unknown.

In Chapter 4, we dealt with the effect of **mutation**, which alters one or more genes or loci to generate variant **alleles** and **polymorphism**. In Chapters 7 and 9, we examined the role of genetic factors in the pathogenesis of various mendelian or complex disorders. In this chapter, we discuss how geneticists go about discovering the particular genes implicated in disease and the variants they contain that underlie or contribute to human diseases, focusing on three approaches:

- The first approach, **linkage analysis**, is family based. Linkage analysis takes explicit advantage of family **pedigrees** to follow the inheritance of a disease among family members and to test for consistent, repeated coinheritance of the disease with a particular genomic region or even with a specific variant(s), whenever the disease is passed on in a family.
- The second approach, genome-wide **association** analysis, is population based. Association analysis takes advantage of the entire history of a population to look for increased or decreased frequency of a particular allele or set of alleles in a cohort of affected individuals compared with a control set of unaffected individuals from that same population. It is particularly

useful for complex and **multifactorial diseases** that do not show a mendelian inheritance pattern.

- The third approach involves direct genome-wide sequencing of affected individuals and their parents and/or other individuals in the family or population. Genome-wide sequencing refers to sequencing the entire **genome** or sequencing the coding portion of the genome, the **exome**. This approach has been broadly adopted by geneticists, mainly due to the advancement of next-generation sequencing technologies that have reduced the cost of DNA sequencing a millionfold from the original reference genome sequenced for the **Human Genome Project**. Genome-wide sequencing is particularly useful for rare mendelian disorders in which linkage analysis is not possible because there are not enough families to do such analysis, or because the disorder is a **genetic lethal** that always results from new mutations and is never inherited. Although this approach allows an unbiased analysis of genes, examination of the resulting billions (or in the case of the exome, tens of millions) of bases of DNA requires a robust filtering strategy for identification of disease alleles. Using a strategy to pare down variants coupled with the emergence of matchmaking programs has been extremely successful in **gene** discovery for hundreds of rare **genetic disorders**.

Use of linkage, association, and genome-wide sequencing to identify disease-associated genes has had an enormous impact on our understanding of the pathogenesis and pathophysiology of many diseases. In time, knowledge of the genetic contributions to disease will also suggest new methods of prevention, management, and treatment.

GENETIC BASIS FOR LINKAGE ANALYSIS AND ASSOCIATION

A fundamental feature of human biology is that each generation reproduces by combining **haploid gametes** containing 23 **chromosomes** that resulted from independent **assortment** and recombination of homologous chromosomes (see Chapter 2). To understand fully the concepts underlying genetic linkage analysis and tests for association, it is necessary to review briefly the behavior of chromosomes and genes during **meiosis**, as they are passed from one generation to the next. Some of this information repeats the classic material on gametogenesis presented in Chapter 2, illustrating it with new information that has become available as a result of the Human Genome Project and its applications to the study of human variation.

Independent Assortment and Homologous Recombination in Meiosis

During meiosis I, homologous chromosomes line up in pairs along the meiotic spindle. The paternal and maternal **homologues** exchange **homologous** segments by crossing over and creating new chromosomes that are a patchwork-like effect consisting of alternating portions of the grandparental chromosomes (see Fig. 2.15). In the family illustrated in Fig. 11.1, examples of recombined chromosomes are shown in the offspring of each generation, with the individual in generation III shown to inherit a maternal chromosome that contains segments derived from all four of his maternal grandparents' chromosomes (generation I). The creation of such patchwork chromosomes emphasizes the notion of human genetic individuality: each chromosome inherited by a child from a parent is never exactly the same as either of the two copies of that chromosome in the parent.

Homologous chromosomes differ substantially at the DNA sequence level. As discussed in Chapter 4, these differences at the same position (locus) on a pair of homologous chromosomes are **alleles**. Alleles that are common (generally considered to be those carried by 1% or more of the population) constitute a polymorphic locus. Allelic variants on homologous chromosomes allow geneticists to trace each segment of a chromosome inherited by a particular child to determine if and where recombination events have occurred along the homologous chromosomes. There are now hundreds of millions of **genetic markers** across diverse populations available to serve as genetic markers for this purpose.

Alleles at Loci on Different Chromosomes Assort Independently

Assume there are two polymorphic loci, 1 and 2, on different chromosomes, with alleles A and a at **locus 1** and alleles B and b at locus 2 (Fig. 11.2). Suppose an

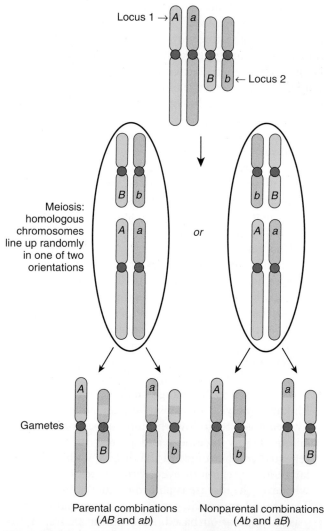

Figure 11.2 **Independent assortment of alleles at two loci, 1 and 2, when they are located on different chromosomes.** Assume that alleles A and B were inherited from one parent, a and b from the other. The two chromosomes can line up on the metaphase plate in meiosis I in one of two equally likely combinations, resulting in independent assortment of the alleles on these two chromosomes.

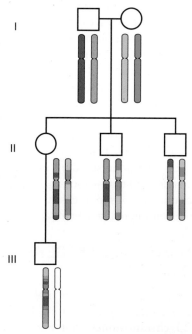

Figure 11.1 **The effect of recombination on the origin of various portions of a chromosome.** Because of crossing over in meiosis, the copy of the chromosome the boy (generation III) inherited from his mother is a mosaic of segments of all four of his grandparents' copies of that chromosome. The blank chromosome represents the chromosome inherited from the boy's father.

individual's **genotype** at these loci is *Aa* and *Bb*; that is, she is heterozygous at both loci, with alleles *A* and *B* inherited from her father and alleles *a* and *b* inherited from her mother. The two different chromosomes will line up on the **metaphase** plate at meiosis I in one of two combinations with equal likelihood. After recombination and chromosomal **segregation** are complete, there will be four possible combinations of alleles in a gamete: *AB, ab, Ab,* and *aB*. Each combination is as likely to occur as any other, a phenomenon known as independent assortment. Because *AB* gametes contain only her paternally derived alleles, and *ab* gametes only her maternally derived alleles, these gametes are designated parental. In contrast, *Ab* or *aB* gametes, each containing one paternally derived allele and one maternally derived allele, are termed nonparental gametes. On average, half (50%) of gametes will be parental (*AB* or *ab*) and 50% nonparental (*Ab* or *aB*).

Alleles at Loci on the Same Chromosome Assort Independently If At Least One Crossover Between Them Always Occurs

Now suppose that an individual is heterozygous at two loci, 1 and 2, with alleles *A* and *B* paternally derived and *a* and *b* maternally derived, but the loci are on the same chromosome (Fig. 11.3). Genes that reside on the same chromosome are said to be syntenic (literally, "on the same thread"), regardless of how close together or how far apart they lie on that chromosome.

How will these alleles behave during meiosis? We know that between one and four **crossovers** occur between homologous chromosomes during meiosis I when there are two **chromatids** per homologous chromosome. If no crossing over occurs within the segment of the chromatids between the loci 1 and 2 (and ignoring whatever happens in segments outside the interval between these loci), then the chromosomes we see in the gametes will be *AB* and *ab*, which are the same as the original parental chromosomes; a parental chromosome is therefore a nonrecombinant chromosome. If crossing over occurs at least once in the segment between the loci, the resulting chromatids may be either nonrecombinant or *Ab* and *aB*, which are not the same as the parental chromosomes; such a nonparental chromosome is therefore a **recombinant chromosome** (shown in Fig. 11.3). One, two, or more recombinations occurring between two loci at the four-chromatid stage result in gametes that are 50% nonrecombinant (parental) and 50% **recombinant** (nonparental), which is precisely the same proportions one sees with independent assortment of alleles at loci on different chromosomes. Thus if two syntenic loci are sufficiently far apart on the same chromosome to ensure at least one crossover between them in every meiosis, then the ratio of recombinant to

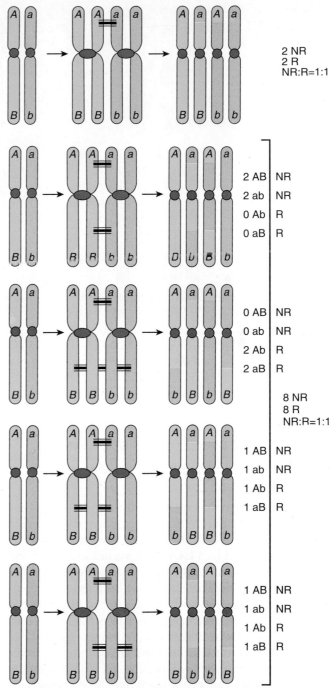

Figure 11.3 Crossing over between homologous chromosomes *(black horizontal lines)* in meiosis is shown between chromatids of two homologous chromosomes on the left. Crossovers result in new combinations of maternally and paternally derived alleles on the recombinant chromosomes present in gametes, shown on the right. If no crossing over occurs in the interval between loci 1 and 2, only parental (nonrecombinant) allele combinations, *AB* and *ab*, occur in the offspring. If one or two crossovers occur in the interval between the loci, half the gametes will contain a nonrecombinant combination of alleles and half the recombinant combination. The same is true if more than two crossovers occur between the loci (not illustrated here). *NR,* Nonrecombinant; *R,* recombinant.

nonrecombinant genotypes will be, on average, 1:1— just as if the loci were on separate chromosomes and assorting independently.

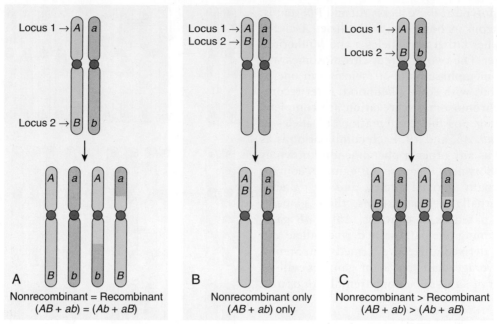

Figure 11.4 **Assortment of alleles at two loci, 1 and 2, when they are located on the same chromosome.** (A) The loci are far apart and at least one crossover between them is likely to occur in every meiosis. (B) The loci are so close together that crossing over between them is not observed, regardless of the presence of crossovers elsewhere on the chromosome. (C) The loci are close together on the same chromosome but far enough apart that crossing over occurs in the interval between the two loci only in some meioses but not in most others.

Recombination Frequency and Map Distance

Frequency of Recombination as a Measure of Distance Between Loci

Suppose now that two loci are on the same chromosome but are either far apart, very close together, or somewhere in between (Fig. 11.4). As we just saw, when the loci are far apart (see Fig. 11.4A), at least one crossover will occur in the segment of the chromosome between loci 1 and 2, and there will be gametes of both the nonrecombinant genotypes (*AB* and *ab*) and recombinant genotypes (*Ab* and *aB*), in equal proportions (on average) in the offspring. On the other hand, if two loci are so close together on the same chromosome that crossovers never occur between them, there will be no recombination; the nonrecombinant genotypes (parental chromosomes *AB* and *ab* in Fig. 11.4B) are transmitted together all of the time, and the frequency of the recombinant genotypes *Ab* and *aB* will be 0. In between these two extremes is the situation in which two loci are far enough apart that one recombination between the loci occurs in some meioses but not in others (see Fig. 11.4C). In this situation we observe nonrecombinant combinations of alleles in the offspring when no crossover occurred and recombinant combinations when a recombination has occurred. The frequency of recombinant chromosomes at the two loci will fall between 0 and 50%. The crucial point is that the closer together two loci are, the smaller the recombination frequency and the fewer recombinant genotypes in the offspring.

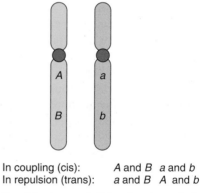

| In coupling (cis): | *A* and *B* | *a* and *b* |
| In repulsion (trans): | *a* and *B* | *A* and *b* |

Figure 11.5 Possible phases of alleles *A* and *a* and alleles *B* and *b*.

Detecting Recombination Events Requires Heterozygosity and Knowledge of Phase

Detecting the recombination events between loci requires that (1) a parent be heterozygous (informative) at both loci and (2) we know which allele at locus 1 is on the same chromosome as which allele at locus 2. In an individual who is heterozygous at two syntenic loci, one with alleles *A* and *a*, the other *B* and *b*, **phase** refers to which allele at the first locus is on the same chromosome with which allele at the second locus (Fig. 11.5). The set of alleles on the same homologue (*A* and *B*, or *a* and *b*) are said to be in *cis* (or in coupling) and form what is referred to as a **haplotype**. In contrast, alleles on the different homologues (*A* and *b*, or *a* and *B*) are in *trans* (or in repulsion) (see Fig. 11.5).

Fig. 11.6 shows a pedigree of a family with multiple individuals affected by autosomal **dominant** retinitis pigmentosa (RP), a degenerative disease of the retina that causes progressive blindness in association with abnormal retinal pigmentation. As shown, individual I-1 is heterozygous at both marker locus 1 (with alleles *A* and *a*) and marker locus 2 (with alleles *B* and *b*), as well as heterozygous for the disorder (*D* is the disease allele, *d* is the normal allele). The alleles *A-D-B* form one haplotype, and *a-d-b* the other. Because we know her spouse is homozygous at all three loci and can only pass on the *a*, *b*, and *d* alleles, we can easily determine which alleles the children received from their mother and thus trace the inheritance of her RP-causing allele or her normal allele at that locus, as well as the alleles at both marker loci in her children. Close inspection of Fig. 11.6 allows one to determine whether each child has inherited a recombinant or a nonrecombinant haplotype from the mother.

However, if the mother (I-1) had been homozygous *bb* at locus 2, then all children would have inherited a maternal *b* allele, regardless of whether they received a **mutant** *D* or normal *d* allele at the *RP9* locus. Because she is not informative at locus 2 in this scenario, it would be impossible to determine whether recombination had

occurred. Similarly, if the information provided for the family in Fig. 11.6 was simply that individual I-1 was heterozygous, *Bb*, at locus 2 and heterozygous for an autosomal dominant form of RP, but the phase was not known, one could not determine which of her children were nonrecombinant between the *RP9* locus and locus 2 and which were recombinant. Thus, **determination** of who is or is not a recombinant requires that we know whether the *B* or *b* allele at locus 2 was on the same chromosome as the mutant *D* allele for RP in individual I-1 (see Fig. 11.6).

Linkage and Recombination Frequency

Linkage is the term used to describe a departure from the independent assortment of two loci, or, in other words, the tendency for alleles at loci that are close together on the same chromosome to be transmitted together, as an intact unit, through meiosis. Analysis of linkage depends on determining the frequency of recombination as a measure of how close two loci are to each other on a chromosome. A common notation for recombination frequency (as a proportion, not a percentage) is the Greek letter theta, θ, where θ varies from 0 (no recombination at all) to 0.5 (independent assortment). If two loci are so close together that $\theta = 0$ between them (as in Fig. 11.4B), they are said to be completely linked; if they are so far apart that $\theta = 0.5$ (as in Fig. 11.4A), they are assorting independently and are unlinked. In between these two extremes are various degrees of linkage.

Genetic Maps and Physical Maps

The **map distance** between two loci is a theoretical concept that is based on actual data—the extent of observed recombination, θ, between the loci. Map distance is measured in units called **centimorgans (cM)**, defined as the genetic length over which, on average, one crossover occurs in 1% of meioses. (The centimorgan is $\frac{1}{100}$ of a "morgan," named after Thomas Hunt Morgan, who first observed genetic recombination in the fruit fly, *Drosophila*.) Therefore a **recombination fraction** of 1% (i.e., $\theta = 0.01$) translates approximately into a map distance of 1 cM. As we discussed before in this chapter, the recombination frequency between two loci increases proportionately with the distance between two loci only up to a point, because once markers are far enough apart that at least one recombination will always occur, the observed recombination frequency will equal 50% ($\theta = 0.5$), no matter how physically far apart the two loci are.

To accurately measure true genetic map distance between two widely spaced loci, therefore, one has to use markers spaced at short genetic distances (≤ 1 cM) in the interval between these two loci, and then add up the values of θ between the intervening markers; the values of θ between pairs of closely neighboring markers will be good approximations of the genetic distances between them. Using this approach, the genetic length of an entire human genome has been measured and,

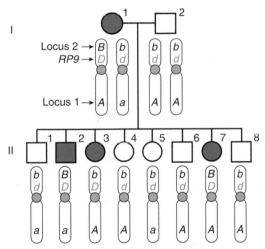

Figure 11.6 Coinheritance of the gene for an autosomal dominant form of retinitis pigmentosa (RP), with marker locus 2 and not with marker locus 1. Only the mother's contribution to the children's genotypes is shown. The mother (I-1) is affected with this dominant disease and is heterozygous at the *RP9* locus (*Dd*) as well as at loci 1 and 2. She carries the *A* and *B* alleles on the same chromosome as the mutant *RP9* allele (*D*). The unaffected father is homozygous normal (*dd*) at the *RP9* locus as well as at the two marker loci (*AA* and *bb*); his contributions to his offspring are not considered further. Two of the three affected offspring have inherited the *B* allele at locus 2 from their mother, whereas individual II-3 inherited the *b* allele. The five unaffected offspring have also inherited the *b* allele. Thus, seven of eight offspring are nonrecombinant between the *RP9* locus and locus 2. However, individuals II-2, II-4, II-6, and II-8 are recombinant for *RP9* and locus 1, indicating that meiotic crossover has occurred between these two loci.

interestingly, found to differ between the sexes. When measured in female meiosis, genetic length of the human genome is ~60% greater ($\approx$4596 cM) than when it is measured in male meiosis (2868 cM), and this sex difference is consistent and uniform across each **autosome**. The sex-averaged genetic length of the entire haploid human genome, which is estimated to contain ~3.3 billion **base pairs** of **DNA**, or $\approx$3300 Mb (see Chapter 2), is 3790 cM, for an average of ~1.15 cM/Mb.

Pairwise measurements of recombination between genetic markers separated by 1 Mb or more gives a fairly constant ratio of genetic distance to physical distance of ~1 cM/Mb. However, when recombination is measured at much higher resolution, such as between markers spaced less than 100 **kb** apart, recombination per unit length becomes nonuniform and can range over four orders of magnitude (0.01–100 cM/Mb). When viewed on the scale of a few tens of kilobase pairs of DNA, the apparent linear relationship between physical distance in base pairs and recombination between polymorphic markers located millions of base pairs of DNA apart is, in fact, the result of an averaging of so-called hot spots of recombination interspersed among regions of little or no recombination. Hot spots occupy only ~6% of **sequence** in the genome and yet account for ~60% of all the meiotic recombination in the human genome. The impact of this nonuniformity of recombination at high resolution is discussed next, as we address the phenomenon of linkage disequilibrium.

Linkage Disequilibrium

It is generally the case that the alleles at two loci will not show any preferred phase in the population if the loci are linked, but at a distance of 0.1 to 1 cM or more. For example, suppose loci 1 and 2 are 1 cM apart. Suppose further that allele *A* is present on 50% of the chromosomes in a population and allele *a* on the other 50%, whereas at locus 2, a disease susceptibility allele *S* is present on 10% of chromosomes and the protective allele *s* is on 90% (Fig. 11.7). Because the frequency of the *A-S* haplotype (freq(*A-S*)) is simply the product of the frequencies of the two alleles—freq(*A*) × freq(*S*) = 0.5 × 0.1 = 0.05—the alleles are said to be in linkage equilibrium (see Fig. 11.7A). That is, the frequencies of the four possible haplotypes, *A-S*, *A-s*, *a-S*, and *a-s* follow directly from the allele frequencies of *A*, *a*, *S*, and *s*.

However, as we examine haplotypes involving loci that are very close together, we find that knowing the allele frequencies for these loci individually does not allow us to predict the four haplotype frequencies. The frequency of any one of the haplotypes, freq(*A-S*) for example, may not be equal to the product of the frequencies of the individual alleles that make up that haplotype; in this situation, freq(*A-S*) ≠ freq(*A*) × freq(*S*), and

Linkage equilibrium: Haplotype frequencies are as expected from allele frequencies

		Allele frequencies at locus 2	
		freq(S) = 0.1	freq(s) = 0.9
Allele frequencies at locus 1	freq(A) = 0.5	Haplotype A-S freq(A-S) = 0.05	Haplotype A-s freq(A-s) = 0.45
	freq(a) = 0.5	Haplotype a-S freq(a-S) = 0.05	Haplotype a-s freq(a-s) = 0.45

A

Linkage disequilibrium: Haplotype frequencies diverge from what is expected from allele frequencies

		Allele frequencies at locus 2	
		freq(S) = 0.1	freq(s) = 0.9
Allele frequencies at locus 1	freq(A) = 0.5	Haplotype A-S freq(A-S) = 0	Haplotype A-s freq(A-s) = 0.5
	freq(a) = 0.5	Haplotype a-S freq(a-S) = 0.1	Haplotype a-s freq(a-s) = 0.4

B

Partial linkage disequilibrium: Haplotype frequencies are rarer than expected from allele frequencies

		Allele frequencies at locus 2	
		freq(S) = 0.1	freq(s) = 0.9
Allele frequencies at locus 1	freq(A) = 0.5	Haplotype A-S freq(A-S) = 0.01	Haplotype A-s freq(A-s) = 0.49
	freq(a) = 0.5	Haplotype a-S freq(a-S) = 0.09	Haplotype a-s freq(a-s) = 0.41

C

Figure 11.7 Tables demonstrating how the same allele frequencies can result in different haplotype frequencies indicative of linkage equilibrium, strong linkage disequilibrium, or partial linkage disequilibrium. (A) Under linkage equilibrium, haplotype frequencies are as expected from the product of the relevant allele frequencies. (B) Loci 1 and 2 are located very close to one another, and alleles at these loci show strong **linkage disequilibrium**. Haplotype *A-S* is absent and *a-s* is less frequent (0.4 instead of 0.45) compared to what is expected from allele frequencies. (C) Alleles at loci 1 and 2 show partial linkage disequilibrium. Haplotypes, *A-S* and *a-s* are underrepresented compared to what is expected from allele frequencies. Note that the allele frequencies for *A* and *a* at locus 1 and for *S* and *s* at locus 2 are the same in all three tables; it is the way the alleles are distributed in haplotypes, shown in the central four cells of the table, that differs.

the alleles are thus said to be in **linkage disequilibrium** (**LD**). The **deviation** ("delta") between the expected and actual haplotype frequencies is called D and is given by:

$$D = \text{freq}(A\text{-}S) \times \text{freq}(a\text{-}s) - \text{freq}(A\text{-}s) \times \text{freq}(a\text{-}s)$$

D ≠ 0 is equivalent to saying the alleles are in LD, whereas D = 0 means the alleles are in linkage equilibrium.

Examples of LD are illustrated in Fig. 11.7B and C. Suppose one discovers that *all* chromosomes carrying allele *S* also have allele *a*, whereas none has allele *A* (see Fig. 11.7B). Then allele *S* and allele *a* are said to be in complete LD. As a second example, suppose the *A-S* haplotype is present on only 1% of chromosomes in the population (see Fig. 11.7C). The *A-S* haplotype has a frequency much below what one would expect on the basis of the frequencies of alleles *A* and *S* in the population as a whole, and D < 0, whereas the haplotype *a-S* has a frequency much greater than expected and D > 0. In other words, chromosomes carrying the susceptibility allele *S* are enriched for allele *a* at the expense of allele *A*, compared with chromosomes that carry the protective allele *s*. Note, however, that the individual allele frequencies are unchanged; it is only how they are distributed into haplotypes that differ, and this is what determines if there is LD.

Linkage Disequilibrium Has Both Biologic and Historical Causes

What causes LD? When a pathogenic allele first enters the population (by mutation or by immigration of a founder who carries the altered allele), the particular set of alleles at polymorphic loci linked to the disease locus constitutes a disease-associated **haplotype** (Fig. 11.8). The degree to which this original disease-associated haplotype will persist over time depends in part on the probability that recombination removes the disease-associated allele from the original haplotype and onto chromosomes with different sets of alleles at these linked loci. The speed with which recombination will move the

pathogenic allele onto a new haplotype depends on a number of factors:

- The number of generations (and therefore the number of opportunities for recombination) since the mutation first appeared.
- The frequency of recombination per generation between the loci. The smaller the value of θ, the greater is the chance that the disease-associated haplotype will persist intact.
- Processes of **natural selection** for or against particular haplotypes. If a haplotype combination undergoes either positive **selection** (and is preferentially passed on) or experiences negative selection (and is less readily passed on), it will be either over- or under-represented in that population.

Measuring Linkage Disequilibrium

Although conceptually valuable, the discrepancy, D, between the expected and observed frequencies of haplotypes is not a good way to quantify LD because it varies not only with degree of LD but also with the allele frequencies themselves. To quantify varying degrees of LD, therefore, geneticists often use a measure derived from D, referred to as D′ (see Box 11.1). D′ is designed to vary from 0, indicating linkage equilibrium, to a maximum of ±1, indicating very strong LD. LD is a result, not only of genetic distance, but of the amount of time

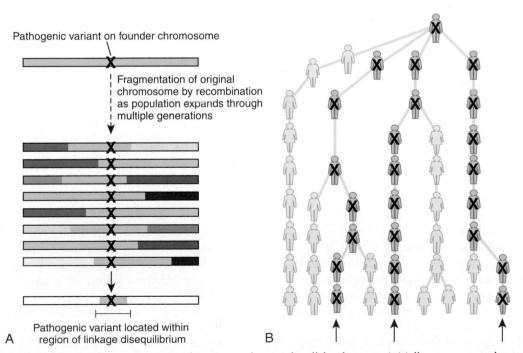

Figure 11.8 (A) With each generation, meiotic recombination exchanges the alleles that were initially present at polymorphic loci on a chromosome on which a disease-associated (pathogenic) variant arose (▬) for other alleles present on the homologous chromosome. Over many generations, the only alleles that remain in coupling phase with the variant are those at loci so close to the disease associated locus that recombination between the loci is very rare. These alleles are in linkage disequilibrium with the pathogenic variant and constitute a disease-associated haplotype. (B) Affected individuals in the current generation *(arrows)* carry the pathogenic variant (**X**) in linkage disequilibrium with the disease-associated haplotype (individuals in *blue*). Depending on the age of the pathogenic variant and other population genetic factors, a disease-associated haplotype ordinarily spans a region of DNA of a few kb to a few hundred kb. (Modified from original figures of Thomas Hudson, McGill University, Canada.)

during which recombination had a chance to occur and the possible effects of selection for or against particular haplotypes. Different populations, therefore, living in different environments and with different histories can have different values of D′ between the same two alleles at the same locus in the genome.

BOX 11.1 MEASURING LINKAGE DISEQUILIBRIUM

$$D' = D/F$$

where $D = \text{freq}(A\text{-}S) \times \text{freq}(a\text{-}s) - \text{freq}(A\text{-}s) \times \text{freq}(a\text{-}S)$

and F is a correction factor that helps account for the allele frequencies.
The value of F depends on whether D itself is a positive or negative number.

F = the smaller of $\text{freq}(A) \times \text{freq}(s)$ or $\text{freq}(a) \times \text{freq}(S)$ if D > 0
F = the smaller of $\text{freq}(A) \times \text{freq}(S)$ or $\text{freq}(a) \times \text{freq}(s)$ if D < 0

Clusters of Alleles Form Blocks Defined by Linkage Disequilibrium

Analysis of pairwise measurements of D′ for neighboring variants, particularly common **single nucleotide variants (SNVs)**, across the genome reveals a complex genetic architecture for LD. Contiguous SNVs can be grouped into clusters of varying size, in which the SNVs in any one cluster show high levels of LD with each other but not with SNPs outside that cluster (Fig. 11.9). For example, the nine polymorphic loci in cluster 1 (see Fig. 11.9A), each consisting of two alleles, have the potential to generate $2^9 = 512$ different haplotypes; yet, only five haplotypes constitute 98% of all haplotypes seen. The absolute values of |D′| between SNVs within the cluster are well above 0.8. Clusters of loci with alleles in high LD across segments of only a few kilobase pairs to a few dozen kilobase pairs are termed LD blocks.

The size of an LD block encompassing alleles at a particular set of polymorphic loci is not identical in all populations. African populations have smaller blocks, averaging 7.3 kb per block across the genome, compared with 16.3 kb in Europeans; Chinese and Japanese block sizes are comparable to each other and are intermediate, averaging 13.2 kb. This difference in block size is almost certainly the result of the smaller number of generations since the founding of the non-African populations compared with populations in Africa, thereby limiting the time in which there has been opportunity for recombination to break up regions of LD.

Is there a biologic basis for LD blocks, or are they simply genetic phenomena reflecting human (and genome) history? It appears that biology contributes to LD block structure in that the boundaries between LD blocks often coincide with meiotic recombination hot spots, discussed earlier (see Fig. 11.9C). Such recombination hot spots would break up any haplotypes spanning them into two

shorter haplotypes more rapidly than average, resulting in linkage equilibrium between SNPs on one side and the other side of the hot spot. The **correlation** is by no means exact, and many apparent boundaries between LD blocks are not located over evident recombination hot spots. This lack of perfect correlation should not be surprising, given what we have already surmised about LD: it is affected not only by how likely a recombination event is (i.e., where the hot spots are) but also by the age of the population, the frequency of the haplotypes originally present in the founding members of that population, and whether there has been either positive or negative selection for particular haplotypes.

STRATEGIES FOR DISCOVERY OF DISEASE-ASSOCIATED GENES

In clinical medicine, a disease state is defined by a collection of phenotypic findings seen in a patient or group of patients. Designating such a disease as "genetic"—inferring the existence of a gene whose alteration is responsible for or contributes to the disease—comes from detailed genetic analysis, applying the principles outlined in Chapters 7 and 9. However, surmising the existence of a gene or genes in such a way does not tell us which of the ~20,000 coding and ~18,000 **noncoding genes** in the genome is involved, what its function might be, or how it causes or contributes to the disease.

Strategies for discovery of genes associated with human disease have evolved over the years, from gene mapping to genome-wide sequencing. Combining these two approaches has provided an effective strategy. Mapping of such genes has historically been a critical and necessary first step in identifying the gene(s) in which certain variants are responsible for causing or increasing susceptibility to disease. Mapping the gene focuses attention on a region of the genome in which to carry out a systematic analysis of all the genes in that region, to identify variation that contributes to the disease. The marked fall in cost of DNA sequencing over the last decade has made it feasible to take a genome-wide sequencing approach to gene discovery. Sequencing the genomes (or just the coding portion of the genome, the exome) of cohorts with similar **phenotypes**, followed by systematic filtering, has proven a powerful approach for gene discovery. This is especially true for disorders with a new (*de novo*) dominant mechanism that may be intractable to gene mapping. Incorporation of gene mapping information into the filtering strategy of genome-wide sequencing has also proven an effective approach to narrow in on loci that are associated with disease.

Regardless of strategy, identification of the gene that harbors the DNA variants responsible for either causing a mendelian disorder or increasing susceptibility to a genetically complex disease, allows the full spectrum of variation in that gene to be studied. We can determine the degree of **allelic heterogeneity**, the **penetrance** of

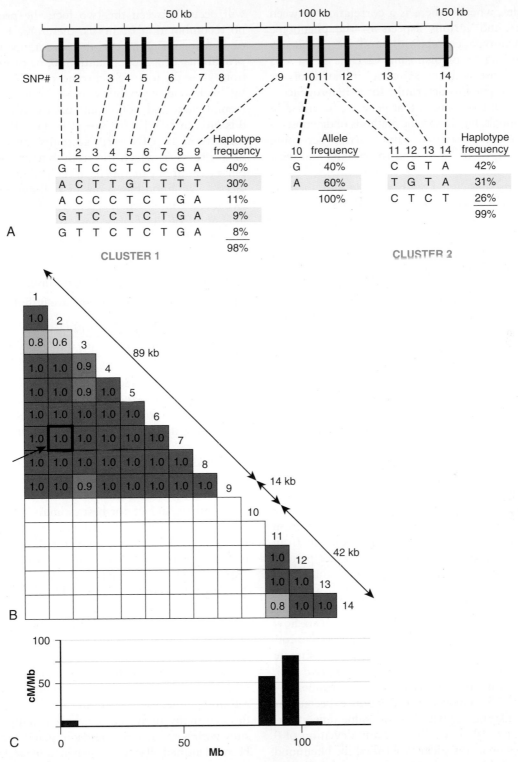

Figure 11.9 (A) A 145-kb region of chromosome 4 containing 14 single nucleotide polymorphic loci (SNPs). In cluster 1, containing SNPs 1 through 9, five of the $2^9 = 512$ theoretically possible haplotypes are responsible for 98% of all the haplotypes in the population, reflecting substantial linkage disequilibrium (LD) among these SNP loci. Similarly, in cluster 2, only three of the $2^4 = 16$ theoretically possible haplotypes involving SNPs 11 to 14 represent 99% of all the haplotypes found. In contrast, alleles at SNP 10 are found in linkage equilibrium with the SNPs in cluster 1 and cluster 2. (B) A schematic diagram in which each red box contains the pairwise measurement of the degree of LD between two SNPs (e.g., the *arrow* points to the box, *outlined in black*, containing the value of D' for SNPs 2 and 7). The higher the degree of LD, the darker the color in the box, with maximum D' values of 1.0 occurring when there is complete LD. Two LD blocks are detectable, the first containing SNPs 1 through 9, and the second SNPs 11 through 14. Between blocks, the 14-kb region containing SNP 10 shows no LD with neighboring SNPs 9 or 11 or with any of the other SNP loci. (C) A graph of the ratio of map distance to physical distance (cM/Mb), showing that a recombination hot spot is present in the region between SNP 10 and cluster 2, with values of recombination that are 50- to 60-fold above the average of ~1.15 cM/Mb for the genome. (Based on data and diagrams provided by Thomas Hudson, Quebec Genome Center, Montreal, Canada.)

different alleles, whether there is a correlation between certain alleles and various aspects of the phenotype (genotype-phenotype correlation), and the frequency of disease-causing or predisposing variants in various populations. Those with the same or similar disorders can also be examined to determine **locus heterogeneity**. Once the gene and variants in that gene are identified in affected individuals, highly specific methods of diagnosis—including prenatal diagnosis and **carrier** screening (see Chapter 18)—can be offered to patients and their families.

The variants associated with disease can then be modeled in other organisms, which allows us to use powerful genetic, biochemical, and physiologic tools to better understand the disease pathogenesis. Finally, armed with an understanding of gene function and how disease-alleles affect that function, we can begin to develop specific therapies to prevent or ameliorate the disorder (see Chapter 14). Indeed, much of the material in the next few chapters about the etiology, pathogenesis, mechanism, and treatment of various diseases begins with identification of the genes involved. Here, we examine the major approaches used to discover these genes, as outlined at the beginning of this chapter.

MAPPING HUMAN DISEASE GENES BY LINKAGE ANALYSIS

Determining Whether Two Loci Are Linked

Linkage analysis is a method of mapping genes that uses studies of recombination in families to determine whether two genes show linkage when passed from one generation to the next. We use information from the known or suspected mendelian inheritance pattern (dominant, recessive, X-linked) to determine which family members have inherited a recombinant or a nonrecombinant chromosome.

To decide whether two loci are linked and, if so, how close or far apart they are, we rely on two pieces of information. First, using the family data in hand, we estimate θ, the recombination frequency between the two loci. Next, we ascertain whether θ is statistically significantly different from 0.5, which is the fraction expected for unlinked loci. Estimating θ and, at the same time, determining the statistical significance of any deviation of θ from 0.5, relies on a statistical tool called the likelihood ratio (as discussed later in the chapter).

Linkage analysis begins with a set of actual family data with N individuals. Based on a mendelian inheritance model, count the number of chromosomes, r, that show recombination between the allele causing the disease and informative alleles at various polymorphic loci around the genome (so-called markers). The number of chromosomes that do not show recombination is therefore N − r. With each meiosis, the recombination fraction, θ, is the unknown probability that a recombination

will occur between the two loci; the probability that no recombination occurs is, therefore, 1 − θ. Because each meiosis is an independent event, one multiplies the probability of a recombination, θ, or of no recombination, (1 − θ), for each chromosome. The formula for the likelihood (probability) of observing this number of recombinant and nonrecombinant chromosomes when θ is unknown is $\{N!/r!(N-r)!\}\theta^r(1-\theta)^{(N-r)}$. (The factorial term, $N!/r!(N-r)!$, accounts for all the possible birth orders in which the recombinant and nonrecombinant children can appear in the pedigree.) Calculate a second likelihood based on the null hypothesis that the two loci are unlinked, i.e., that $\theta = 0.50$. The ratio of the likelihood of the family data supporting linkage with unknown θ to the likelihood that the loci are unlinked is the **odds** in favor of linkage and is given by:

$$\frac{\text{Likelihood of the data if loci are linked at distance }\theta}{\text{Likelihood of the data if loci are unlinked}(\theta = 0.5)} =$$

$$\frac{\{N!/r!(N-r)!\}\theta^r(1-\theta)^{(N-r)}}{\{N!/r!(N-r)!\}\left(\frac{1}{2}\right)^r\left(\frac{1}{2}\right)^{(N-r)}}$$

Fortunately, the factorial terms are always the same in the numerator and denominator of the likelihood ratio, and therefore they cancel each other out and can be ignored. If $\theta = 0.5$, the numerator and denominator are the same and the odds equal 1.

Statistical theory tells us that when the value of the likelihood ratio for all values of θ between 0 and 0.5 are calculated, the value of θ with the greatest likelihood ratio is, in fact, the best estimate of the recombination fraction and is referred to as θ_{max}. By convention, the computed likelihood ratio for different values of θ is usually expressed as the $\log_{10}$ and is called the **LOD score** (Z), where LOD stands for *l*ogarithm of the *od*ds. The use of logarithms allows likelihood ratios calculated from different families to be combined by simple addition instead of having to multiply them together.

How is LOD score analysis actually carried out in families with mendelian disorders? (See the accompanying box.) Return to the family shown in Fig. 11.6, in which the mother has an autosomal dominant form of retinitis pigmentosa. There are dozens of forms of this disease, many of which have been mapped to specific sites within the genome and the genes for which have been identified. Typically, when a new family comes to clinical attention, one does not know which form of RP a patient has. In this family, the mother is also heterozygous for two marker loci on chromosome 7: locus 1 in distal 7q and locus 2 in 7p14. Suppose we know (from other family data) that the disease allele *D* is in **coupling** with allele *A* at locus 1 and allele *B* at locus 2. Given this phase, one can see that there has been recombination between RP and locus 2 in only one of her eight children: her daughter II-3. The alleles at the disease locus, however, show no tendency to follow the alleles at locus 1 or alleles at any of the other hundreds of marker loci tested on the other autosomes. Thus, although the RP locus involved in this family could, in principle, have mapped anywhere in the human genome, the linkage data suggest that the responsible RP locus lies in the region of chromosome 7 near marker locus 2.

To provide a quantitative assessment of this suspicion, suppose we let θ be the "true" recombination fraction between RP and locus 2—the fraction we would see if we had unlimited offspring to test. The likelihood ratio for this family is

$$\frac{(\theta)^1(1-\theta)^7}{\left(\frac{1}{2}\right)^1\left(\frac{1}{2}\right)^7}$$

and reaches a maximum LOD score of $Z_{max} = 1.1$ at $\theta_{max} = 0.125$.

The value of θ that maximizes the likelihood ratio, θ_{max}, may be the best estimate for θ given the data, but how good an estimate is it? This is reflected in the magnitude of the LOD score. By convention, a LOD score of +3 or greater (equivalent to greater than $1000:1$ odds in favor of linkage) is considered firm evidence that two loci are linked; that is, that θ_{max} is statistically significantly different from 0.5. In our RP example, $\frac{7}{8}$ of the offspring are nonrecombinant and $\frac{1}{8}$ are recombinant. The $\theta_{max} = 0.125$, but the LOD score is only 1.1: enough to raise a suspicion of linkage but insufficient to prove linkage because Z_{max} falls far short of 3.

Combining LOD Score Information Across Families

Just as each meiosis in a family that produces a non-recombinant or recombinant offspring is an independent event, so too are the meioses that occur in different families. We can, therefore, combine the likelihoods in the numerators and denominators of each family's likelihood **odds ratio**. Suppose two additional families with RP were studied; one showed no recombination between locus 2 and RP in four children and the other showed no recombination in five children. The individual LOD scores can be generated for each family and added together (Table 11.1). Because the maximum LOD score, Z_{max}, exceeds 3 at $\theta_{max} = \approx 0.06$, the RP gene in this group of families is linked to locus 2 at a recombination distance of ≈ 0.06. Because the genomic location of marker locus 2 is known to be at 7p14, the RP in this family can be mapped to the 7p14 region. The *RP9*

gene is a likely candidate – one of the identified loci for a form of autosomal dominant RP.

If, however, some of the families being used for the study were to have RP due to **pathogenic variants** at a different locus, the LOD scores between families would diverge, with some showing a trend to being positive at small values of θ and others showing strongly negative LOD scores at these values. Thus, in linkage analysis involving more than one family, unsuspected locus heterogeneity can obscure what may be real evidence for linkage in a subset of families.

Phase-Known and Phase-Unknown Pedigrees

In the RP example just discussed, we assumed that we knew the phase of marker alleles on chromosome 7 in the affected mother in that family. Let us now look at the implications of knowing phase in more detail.

Consider the three-generation family with autosomal dominant neurofibromatosis, type 1 (NF1) (Case 34) in Fig. 11.10. The affected mother, II-2, is heterozygous at both the NF1 locus *(D/d)* and a marker locus *(A/a)*, but (as shown in Fig. 11.10A) we have no genotype information on her parents. The two affected children received the *A* alleles along with the *D* disease allele, and the one unaffected child received the *a* allele along with the normal *d* allele. Without knowing the phase of these alleles in the mother, either all three offspring are recombinants or all three are nonrecombinants. Because both possibilities are equally likely in the absence of any other information, we consider the phase on her two chromosomes to be *D-a* and *d-A* half of the time and

BOX 11.2 LINKAGE ANALYSIS OF MENDELIAN DISEASES

Linkage analysis is used when there is a particular mode of inheritance (autosomal dominant, autosomal recessive, or X-linked) that explains the inheritance pattern. LOD score analysis allows mapping of genes with variants for phenotypes that follow mendelian inheritance.
The LOD score gives both:
- a best estimate of the recombination frequency, θ_{max}, between a marker locus and the disease locus; and
- an assessment of the strength of evidence for linkage at that value of θ_{max}. For the LOD score, Z, values above 3 are considered strong evidence.

Linkage at a particular θ_{max} of a given gene locus to a marker with known physical location implies proximity between the two. The smaller the θ_{max} the closer the locus-of-interest is to the linked marker locus.

TABLE 11.1 LOD Score for Three Families With Retinitis Pigmentosa

	0.00	0.01	0.05	0.06	0.07	0.10	0.125	0.20	0.30	0.40
Family 1	—	0.38	0.95	1.00	1.03	1.09	**1.1**	1.03	0.80	0.46
Family 2	**1.2**	1.19	1.11	1.10	1.08	1.02	0.97	0.82	0.58	0.32
Family 3	**1.5**	1.48	1.39	1.37	1.35	1.28	1.22	1.02	0.73	0.39
Total	—	3.05	3.45	**3.47**	3.46	3.39	3.29	2.87	2.11	1.17

Individual Z_{max} for each family is shown in **bold**. The overall $Z_{max} = 3.47$ at $\theta_{max} = 0.06$.

D-A and d-a the other half (which assumes the alleles in these haplotypes are in linkage equilibrium). To calculate the overall likelihood of this pedigree, we then add the likelihood calculated assuming one phase in the mother to that assuming the other phase. The overall likelihood $= \frac{1}{2}\theta^0(1-\theta)^3 + \frac{1}{2}(\theta^3)(1-\theta)^0$; the likelihood ratio for this pedigree, then, is:

$$\frac{\frac{1}{2}(1-\theta)^3(\theta^0) + \frac{1}{2}(\theta^3)(1-\theta)^0}{\frac{1}{8}}$$

giving a maximum LOD score of $Z_{max} = 0.602$ at $\theta_{max} = 0$.

If, however, additional genotype information in the maternal grandfather, I-1, becomes available (as in Fig. 11.10B), the phase can now be determined to be D-A (i.e., the NF1 allele D was in coupling with the A in individual II-2). In light of this new information, the three children can now be scored definitively as non-recombinants, and we no longer have to consider the possibility of the opposite phase. The numerator of the likelihood ratio now becomes $(1 - \theta)^3(\theta^0)$ and the maximum LOD score, $Z_{max} = 0.903$ at $\theta_{max} = 0$. Thus knowing the phase increases the power of the data available to test for linkage.

Gene Finding in a Common Mendelian Disorder by Linkage Mapping: Cystic Fibrosis

The application of **linkage mapping** to medical genetics using the approaches outlined has met with many successes. Here we describe one such historical example, using linkage analysis and LD to narrow down the location of the gene responsible for the common autosomal **recessive** disease, cystic fibrosis (CF) (Case 12).

Because of its relatively high frequency, particularly in populations of European descent, and (at the time) the little understanding of its pathogenesis, CF represented a prime candidate for identifying the gene responsible by first using linkage to find the gene's location. DNA samples from nearly 50 multiplex CF families were analyzed for linkage between CF and hundreds of DNA markers throughout the genome. Eventually, linkage of CF to markers on the long arm of chromosome 7 was identified. Linkage to additional DNA markers in 7q31-q32 narrowed the location of the CF gene to a ~500 kb region of chromosome 7.

At this point, however, an important feature of CF genetics emerged: although the closest linked markers were still some distance from the CF gene, it became clear that there was significant LD between the disease locus and a particular haplotype of nearby markers. Regions with the greatest degree of LD were analyzed for gene sequences, leading to the isolation of the gene responsible in 1989. As described in detail in Chapter 13, this gene, which was named the CF transmembrane conductance regulator (*CFTR*), showed an interesting spectrum of variants. A 3 bp **deletion** (then called ΔF508) that removed a phenylalanine at position 508 in the protein was found in ~70% of all variant CF alleles in northern European populations, but never among normal alleles at this locus. Although subsequent studies have demonstrated many hundreds of variant *CFTR* alleles worldwide, it was the high frequency of the ΔF508 variant in the families used to map the CF locus and the LD between it and alleles at polymorphic marker loci nearby, that proved so helpful in the ultimate identification of the *CFTR* gene.

Mapping of the CF locus and cloning of the *CFTR* gene made possible a wide range of research advances and clinical applications, from basic pathophysiology to molecular diagnosis for **genetic counseling**, prenatal diagnosis, animal models, and finally effective treatments for the disorder (see Chapters 13 and 14).

Mapping Human Disease Genes by Association

Designing an Association Study

An entirely different approach to identification of the genetic contribution to disease relies on finding particular alleles that are associated with the disease in a sample from the population. In contrast to linkage analysis, this approach does not depend upon there being a mendelian inheritance pattern and is, therefore, better

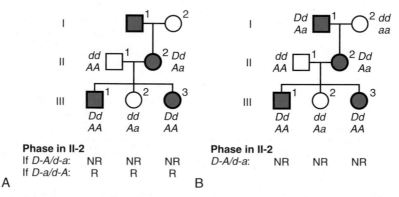

Figure 11.10 Linkage autosomal dominant neurofibromatosis, type 1 (NF1). (A) Phase of the disease allele *D* and marker alleles *A* and *a* in individual II-2 is unknown. (B) Availability of genotype information for generation I allows a determination that the disease allele *D* and marker allele *A* are in coupling in individual II-2. *NR*, Nonrecombinant; *R*, recombinant.

suited for discovering the genetic contributions to disorders with **complex inheritance** (see Chapter 9). It is important to note that here, alleles can harbor either SNVs or CNVs associated with disease. The increased or decreased frequency of a particular allele in affected individuals, compared to that in unaffected individuals, is known as a disease association. There are two designs commonly used for association studies:

- **Case-control studies.** Individuals with the disease (cases) are selected in a population, along with a matching group without disease (controls). Genotypes of individuals in the two groups are determined and used to populate a two-by-two table (see table below).
- **Cross-sectional or cohort studies.** A random sample of the population is chosen and analyzed with respect to the disease phenotype in question and individually genotyped for selected markers. A cross-sectional study involves a single time point, whereas a cohort study takes place over time. The numbers of individuals with and without disease and with and without an allele (or genotype or haplotype) of interest are used to fill out the cells of a two-by-two table.

Odds Ratios and Relative Risks

The two different types of association studies report the strength of association, using either the odds ratio (OR) or relative risk (RR).

In a case-control study, the frequency of a particular marker (e.g., a **human leukocyte antigen [HLA]** haplotype or a particular SNV allele or haplotype) is compared between the selected affected and unaffected individuals. Association between disease and genotype is then calculated by an **odds ratio** (OR).

	Cases	Controls	Totals
With genetic marker*	a	b	a + b
Without genetic marker	c	d	c + d
Totals	a + c	b + d	

*A genetic marker can be an allele, a genotype, or a haplotype.

Using the two-by-two table, the odds of a marker carrier developing the disease is the ratio (a/b) of the number of marker carriers who develop the disease (a) to the number of marker carriers who do not develop the disease (b). Similarly, the odds of a noncarrier developing the disease is the ratio (c/d) of noncarriers who develop the disease (c) to the number of noncarriers who do not develop the disease (d). The disease OR is then the ratio of these odds.

$$OR = \frac{a/b}{c/d} = \frac{ad}{bc}$$

An OR that differs from 1 means there is an association of the disease with the genetic marker, whereas OR = 1 means there is no association.

Alternatively, if the association study was designed as a cross-sectional or **cohort study**, the strength of an association can be measured by the **relative risk (RR)**. The RR is the ratio of the proportion of those with the disease who carry a particular marker allele ([a/(a + b)]) to the proportion of those without the disease who carry that marker ([c/(c + d)]).

$$RR = \frac{a/(a + b)}{c/(c + d)}$$

Again, an RR that differs from 1 means there is an association of disease with the genetic marker, whereas RR = 1 means there is no association. (The RR introduced here should not be confused with Relative Risk Ratio (λ_r), (i.e., risk ratio in relatives) discussed in Chapter 9. λ_r is the prevalence of a particular disease phenotype in an affected individual's relatives versus that in the general population.)

For diseases that are rare (i.e., a << b and c << d), a case-control design with calculation of the OR is best because any random sample of a population is unlikely to contain sufficient numbers of affected individuals to be suitable for a cross-sectional or cohort study design. Note, however, that when a disease is rare, and calculating an OR in a **case-control study** is the only practical approach, OR is a good approximation for RR. (Examine the formula for RR and convince yourself that, when a << b and c << d, (a + b) ≈ b and (c + d) ≈ d; thus, RR ≈ OR.)

The information obtained in an association study comes in two parts. The first is the magnitude of the association itself. The further the RR or OR diverges from 1, the greater is the effect of the genetic variant on the association. However, an OR or RR for an association is a statistical measure and requires a test of statistical significance. The significance of any association can be assessed with a chi-square test, asking whether if the frequencies of the marker classifications (a, b, c, and d in the two-by-two table) differ significantly from what would be expected if there were no association (i.e., if the OR or RR were equal to 1.0). A common way of expressing whether there is statistical significance to an estimate of OR or RR is to provide a 95% (or 99%) confidence interval. The confidence interval is the range within which one would expect the OR or RR to fall 95% (or 99%) of the time by chance alone in a sample taken from the population. If a confidence interval excludes the value 1.0, then the OR or RR deviates significantly from what would be expected if there were no association with the marker locus being tested; thus, the null hypothesis (of no association) can be rejected at the corresponding significance level. (Later in this chapter we will explain why a level of 0.05 or 0.01 is inadequate for assessing statistical significance when multiple genomic marker loci are tested simultaneously for association.)

To illustrate these approaches we first consider a case-control study of cerebral vein thrombosis (CVT), which we introduced in Chapter 9. In this study, suppose a group of 120 individuals with CVT and 120 matched controls were genotyped for the 20210 G>A allele in the prothrombin gene (see Chapter 9).

	Cases With CVT	Controls Without CVT	Totals
20210 G>A allele present	23	4	27
20210 G>A allele absent	97	116	213
Total	120	120	240

CVT, Cerebral vein thrombosis.

Because this is a case-control study, we will calculate an odds ratio: OR = (23/4)/(97/116) = ≈6.9 with 95% confidence limits of 2.3 to 20.6. The effect size of 6.9 is substantial, and 95% confidence limits exclude 1.0, thereby demonstrating a strong and statistically significant association between the 20210 G>A allele and CVT. Stated simply, individuals carrying the prothrombin 20210 G>A allele have nearly seven times greater odds of having the disease than do those who do not carry this allele.

To illustrate a longitudinal cohort study, calculating RR instead of OR—consider statin-induced myopathy, a rare but well-recognized adverse drug reaction that can develop in some individuals during statin therapy to lower cholesterol. In one study, subjects enrolled in a cardiac protection study were randomized to receive 40 mg of the statin drug, simvastatin, or placebo. Over 16,600 participants exposed to the statin were genotyped for a variant (Val174Ala) in the *SLCO1B1* gene—which encodes a hepatic drug transporter, and were watched for development of the adverse drug response. Out of the entire genotyped group exposed to the statin, 21 developed myopathy. Examination of their genotypes showed that the RR for developing myopathy associated with the presence of the Val174Ala allele was ~2.6, with 95% confidence limits of 1.3 to 5.1. Thus, there is a statistically significant association between the Val174Ala allele and statin-induced myopathy. Those carrying this allele are at moderately increased risk for developing this adverse drug reaction, relative to those who do not carry this allele.

One common misconception concerning an association study is that the more significant the *p*-value, the stronger is the association. In fact, a significant *p*-value for an association does not provide information concerning the magnitude of the effect of an associated allele on disease susceptibility. Significance is a statistical measure that describes how likely it is that the population sample used for the association study could have yielded an observed OR or RR that differs from 1.0, simply by chance. In contrast, the actual magnitude of the OR or RR—how far it diverges from 1.0—is a measure of the

impact a particular variant (or genotype or haplotype) on increasing or decreasing disease likelihood.

Genome-Wide Association Studies

The Haplotype Map (HapMap)

Association studies for human disease genes were once limited to particular sets of variants in restricted sets of genes. These were chosen, either for convenience or because they were thought to be involved in a pathophysiologic pathway relevant to a disease, making them logical candidate genes for the disease under investigation. Many such association studies were undertaken before the Human Genome Project era, using HLA or **blood group** loci, for example, because these were highly polymorphic and easily genotyped in case-control studies. Ideally, however, one would like to test systematically for an association between any disease of interest and every one of the tens of millions of rare and common alleles in the genome, in an unbiased fashion without preconception of what genes and genetic variants might be contributing to the disease.

Association analyses on a genome scale are referred to as **genome-wide association studies (GWAS)**. Such an undertaking for all known variants is impractical for many reasons. It can, however, be approximated by genotyping cases and controls for a mere 300,000 to 1 million individual variants located throughout the genome, to search for association with the disease or trait in question. The success of this approach depends on exploiting LD: as long as a variant responsible for altering disease susceptibility is in LD with one or more of the genotyped variants within an LD block, a positive association should be detectable between that disease and the alleles in the LD block.

Developing such a set of markers led to the launch of the Haplotype Mapping (HapMap) Project, one of the biggest human **genomics** efforts to follow completion of the Human Genome Project. The HapMap Project began in four geographically distinct groups—a primarily European population, a West African population, a Han Chinese population, and a population from Japan—and included collecting and characterizing millions of SNP loci and developing methods to genotype them rapidly and inexpensively. HapMap version 3 expanded coverage and diversity to include genotyping of 1.6 million common SNP loci as well as common CNVs in more than 1000 reference individuals from 11 global populations. Subsequently, **whole genome sequencing** has been applied to many populations in what is referred to as the 1000 Genomes Project, resulting in a massive expansion in the database of DNA variants available for GWAS among different populations around the globe.

Gene Mapping by Genome-Wide Association Studies

The purpose of the HapMap was not just to gather basic information about the distribution of LD across the human genome. Its primary purpose was to provide a powerful new tool for finding the genetic variants that contribute to human disease and other traits, by making possible an approximation to an idealized, full-scale, genome-wide association. The driving principle behind this approach is straightforward: detecting an association with alleles within an LD block pinpoints the genomic region within the block as likely to contain the disease-associated allele. Consequently, although the approach does not typically pinpoint the actual variant responsible functionally for the disease association, this region will be the place to focus additional studies to find the allelic variant(s) directly involved in the disease process.

Historically, detailed analysis of conditions associated with high-density variants in the class I and class II HLA regions has exemplified this approach (see Box 11.3). However, with the tens of millions of variants now available in different populations, this approach can be broadened to examine the genetic basis of virtually any complex disease or trait. Indeed, to date, thousands of GWAS have uncovered an enormous number of naturally occurring variants associated with a variety of genetically common and complex multifactorial diseases. These range from diabetes and inflammatory bowel disease to rheumatoid arthritis and neuropsychiatric disease, and include traits such as stature and pigmentation. Research to uncover the underlying biologic basis for these associations will be ongoing for years to come.

Finding the Genes Contributing to a Complex Disease by Genome-Wide Association: Age-Related Macular Degeneration

Genome-wide association has proven effective in identifying hundreds of genes and alleles associated with genetically complex disorders. The power of these approaches has increased enormously with the introduction of highly efficient and less expensive technologies for genome analysis. Here we describe an example of using GWAS to find multiple allelic variants in genes that increase susceptibility to age-related macular degeneration (AMD) (Case 3), a devastating disorder that robs older adults of their vision.

AMD is a progressive degenerative disease of the portion of the retina responsible for central vision. It causes blindness in 1.75 million Americans older than 50 years. The disease is characterized by the presence of drusen, which are clinically visible, discrete extracellular deposits of protein and lipids behind the retina in the region of the macula (Case 3). Although there is ample evidence for a genetic contribution to the disease, most individuals with AMD are not in families with a likely mendelian pattern of inheritance. Environmental contributions are also important, as shown by the increased risk for AMD in cigarette smokers compared with nonsmokers.

BOX 11.3 HUMAN LEUKOCYTE ANTIGEN AND DISEASE ASSOCIATION

Among more than 1000 genome-trait or genome-disease associations from around the genome, the region with the highest concentration of associations to different phenotypes is the human leukocyte antigen (HLA) region. In addition to the association of specific alleles and haplotypes to type 1 diabetes discussed in Chapter 9, association of various HLA polymorphisms has been demonstrated for a wide range of conditions. Most, but not all of these are autoimmune; that is, associated with an abnormal immune response apparently directed against one or more self-antigens. These associations are thought to be related to variation in the immune response resulting from polymorphism in immune response genes.

The functional basis of most HLA-disease associations is unknown. HLA molecules are integral to T-cell recognition of antigens. Different HLA alleles are thought to result in structural variation in these cell surface molecules, leading to differences in capacity of the proteins to interact with antigen and the T-cell receptor in the initiation of an immune response. This affects such critical processes as immunity against infections and self-tolerance to prevent autoimmunity.

Ankylosing spondylitis, a chronic inflammatory disease of the spine and sacroiliac joints, is one example. More than 95% of those with ankylosing spondylitis are *HLA-B27* positive; the risk for developing ankylosing spondylitis is at least 150 times higher for people who have certain *HLA-B27* alleles than for those who do not. These alleles lead to HLA-B27 heavy chain misfolding and inefficient antigen presentation.

In other disorders, the association between a particular HLA allele or haplotype and a disease is not due to functional differences in immune response genes themselves. Instead, the association is due to a particular allele being present at a very high frequency on chromosomes that also happen to contain disease-causing variants in another gene within the **major histocompatibility complex** region. One example is hemochromatosis (Case 20), a common disorder of iron overload. More than 80% of individuals with hemochromatosis are homozygous for a common variant, Cys282Tyr, in the hemochromatosis gene *(HFE)* and have *HLA-A*0301* alleles at their *HLA-A* locus. The association is not the result of *HLA-A*0301*, however. *HFE* is involved with iron transport or metabolism in the intestine; *HLA-A*, as a class I immune response gene, has no effect on iron transport. The association is due to proximity of the two loci and LD between the Cys282Tyr *HFE* mutation and the *A*0301* allele at *HLA-A*.

Initial case-control GWAS of AMD revealed association of two common SNP loci near the complement factor H *(CFH)* gene. The most frequent at-risk haplotype containing these alleles was seen in 50% of cases versus only 29% of controls (OR = 2.46; 95% confidence interval [CI], 1.9–53.11). Homozygosity for this haplotype was found in 24.2% of cases, compared to only 8.3% of the controls (OR = 3.51; 95% CI, 2.13–5.78). A search through the SNPs within the LD block containing the AMD-associated haplotype revealed a **nonsynonymous** SNP in the *CFH* gene that substituted a histidine for tyrosine at position 402 of the CFH protein (Tyr402His). The Tyr402His alteration, which has an allele frequency of 26 to 29% in European and African populations, showed an even stronger association with AMD than did the two SNPs that showed an association in the original GWAS.

Given that drusen contain complement factors and that CFH is found in retinal tissues around drusen, it is believed that the Tyr402His variant is less protective against the inflammation that is thought to be responsible for drusen formation and retinal damage. Thus, Tyr402His is likely to be the variant at the *CFH* locus responsible for increasing the risk for AMD.

More recent GWAS of AMD, using more than 7600 cases and more than 50,000 controls and millions of variants genome wide, have revealed that alleles at a minimum of 19 loci are associated with AMD, with genome-wide significance of $P < 5 \times 10^{-8}$. A popular way to summarize GWAS in graphic form is to plot the $-\log_{10}$ significance levels for each associated variant in a **Manhattan plot** (so named because it is thought to bear a somewhat fanciful similarity to the skyline of New York City) (Fig. 11.11). The ORs for AMD of these variants range from a high of 2.76 for a gene of unknown function, *ARMS2*, and 2.48 for *CFH* to 1.1 for many other genes involved in multiple pathways, including the complement system, atherosclerosis, blood vessel formation, and others.

In this example of AMD, a complex disease, GWAS led to the identification of strongly associated common SNPs that in turn were in LD with a common coding SNP in the gene that appears to be the functional variant involved in the disease. This discovery in turn led to the identification of other SNPs in the complement cascade and elsewhere that can also predispose to or protect against the disease. Taken together, these results give important clues to the pathogenesis of AMD and suggest that the complement pathway might be a fruitful target for novel therapies. Equally interesting is that GWAS revealed that a novel gene of unknown function, *ARMS2*, is also involved, thereby opening up an entirely new line of research into the pathogenesis of AMD.

Gene Mapping by Analysis of Copy Number Variation

Association studies have been successful in uncovering both common and rare risk alleles for common neuropsychiatric disorders. The Psychiatric Genomics Consortium (PGC) is a large international consortium that promotes global collaboration for the study of 11 psychiatric disorders: ADHD, Alzheimer disease, autism, bipolar disorder, eating disorders, major depressive disorder, obsessive-compulsive disorder/Tourette syndrome, posttraumatic stress disorder, schizophrenia, substance use disorders, and all other anxiety disorders. For complex brain disorders such as these, it has become clear that extremely large numbers of cases and controls (i.e., >10,000 samples) are necessary for markers to reach statistical significance; these numbers are well beyond what single study analysis can achieve. The PGC GWAS group aims to conduct rigorous large-scale-analysis for

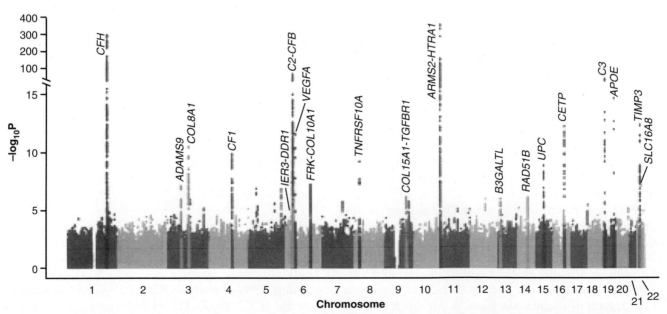

Figure 11.11 Manhattan plot of genome-wide association studies (GWAS) of age-related macular degeneration using ~1 million genome-wide single nucleotide polymorphism (SNP) alleles located along all 22 autosomes on the x-axis. Each blue dot represents the statistical significance [expressed as $-\log_{10}(P)$ plotted on the y-axis], confirming a previously known association; green dots are the statistical significance for novel associations. The discontinuity in the y-axis is needed because some of the associations have extremely small P values $< 1 \times 10^{-16}$. (From Fritsche LG, Chen W, Schu M, et al: Seven new loci associated with age-related macular degeneration. *Nature Genet* 17:1783–1786, 2013.)

psychiatric disorders (i.e., to gather data from multiple studies and platforms into one large dataset and perform GWAS). This approach has proven effective in increasing the number of associated loci recognized for disorders (e.g., for schizophrenia, the number of associated loci increased from 22 using 20,000 subjects to 108 using 150,000 subjects).

One of the beneficial by-products of genotyping so many individuals, typically performed with SNP **microarray**, is the ability to interrogate the data for copy number variation (CNV). Rare CNVs are known to cause several neuropsychiatric conditions, some with high penetrance. Since highly penetrant CNVs are individually rare and tend to have nonrecurrent breakpoints, large cohorts are needed to show statistical association and precisely map regions and genes. For example, in Fig. 11.12 we can see a CNV map overlapping the *NRXN1* gene on chromosome 2 in 20,000 cases and controls. This method has been used to find dozens of genomic loci or specific genes associated with neuropsychiatric disorders.

Pitfalls in Design and Analysis of GWAS

Association methods are powerful tools for pinpointing precisely the genes that contribute to genetic disease, by demonstrating not only the genes, but also the particular alleles responsible. These methods are relatively easy to perform because one needs samples only from

a set of unrelated affected individuals and controls, not laborious collection of samples from many members of a pedigree.

Association studies must be interpreted with caution, however. One serious limitation of association studies is the problem of totally artifactual association caused by population stratification (see Chapter 10). If a population is stratified into separate subpopulations (e.g., by ethnicity or religion) and members of one subpopulation rarely mate with members of other subpopulations, then a disease that happens to be more common in one subpopulation can appear (incorrectly) to be associated with any alleles that also happen to be more common in that subpopulation than in the population as a whole. Factitious association due to population stratification can be minimized, however, by careful selection of matched controls. In particular, one form of quality control is to make sure the cases and controls have similar frequencies of alleles whose frequencies differ markedly between populations (**ancestry informative markers** as we discussed in Chapter 10). If the frequencies seen in cases and controls are similar, then unsuspected or cryptic stratification is unlikely.

In addition to the problem of stratification producing false-positive associations, false-positive results in GWAS can arise if an inappropriately lax test for statistical significance is applied. This is because, as the number of alleles being tested for a disease association

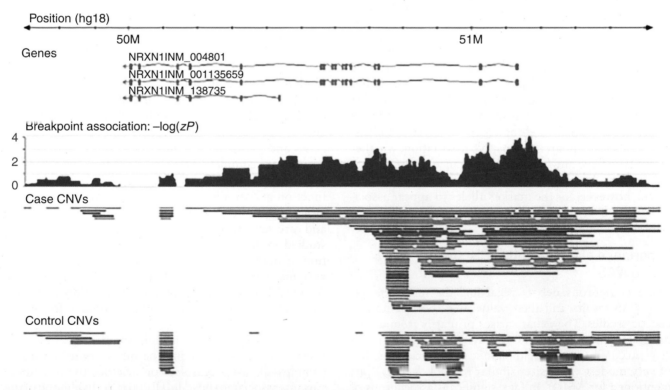

Figure 11.12 Copy number breakpoint mapping at the *NRXN1* gene locus in cases diagnosed with schizophrenia. Manhattan plot of copy number variation breakpoint associations at the *NRXN1* locus in cases with schizophrenia versus controls. The three isoforms of *NRXN1* are shown in pink. Rare copy number deletions *(red bars)* and duplications *(blue)* are mapped in schizophrenia cases (n = 21,094) and population controls (n = 20,227).

increases, the risk of finding associations by chance alone also increases—a concept in statistics known as the problem of **multiple hypothesis testing**. To understand why the cutoff for statistical significance must be much more stringent when multiple hypotheses are being tested, imagine flipping a coin 50 times and having it come up heads 40 times. Such a result has a probability of occurring only once in ~100,000 times. However, if the same experiment were repeated a million times, chances are greater than 99.999% that at least one coin flip experiment out of the million performed will result in 40 or more heads! Thus, even rare events that occur by chance alone in an experiment become frequent when the experiment is repeated over and over again. This is why, when testing for an association with hundreds of thousands to millions of variants across the genome, tens of thousands of variants could appear associated with $P < 0.05$ by chance alone. This makes a typical cutoff for statistical significance of $P < 0.05$ far too low to point to a true association. Instead, a significance level of $P < 5 \times 10^{-8}$ is considered to be more appropriate for GWAS that tests hundreds of thousands to millions of variants. Even with appropriately stringent cutoffs for genome-wide significance, however, false-positive results due to chance alone will still occur. To take this into account, a properly performed GWAS usually includes a replication study in a different, completely independent group of individuals to show that alleles near the same locus are associated. A caveat, however, is that alleles that show association may be different in different ancestral groups.

Finally, it is important to emphasize that if an association is found between a disease and a marker allele that is part of a dense haplotype map, one cannot infer a functional role for that marker allele in increasing disease susceptibility. Because of the nature of LD, all alleles in LD with an allele at a locus involved in the disease will show apparently positive association, whether or not they have any functional relevance in disease predisposition. An association based on LD is still quite useful, however; for the marker alleles to appear associated, they likely sit within an LD block that also harbors the actual disease locus.

Importance of Associations Discovered with GWAS

There is vigorous debate regarding the interpretation of GWAS results and their value as a tool for human genetic studies. The debate arises primarily from a misunderstanding of what an OR or RR means. Many properly executed GWAS yield significant associations, but of very modest effect size (similar to the OR of 1.1 just mentioned for AMD). In fact, significant associations of smaller and smaller effect size have become more common as larger and larger sample sizes are used. This has led to the suggestion that GWAS are of little value

because the effect size of the association, as measured by OR or RR, is too small to implicate the gene and pathway identified by that variant in the pathogenesis of the disease. This is faulty reasoning on two accounts.

First, ORs are a measure of the impact of a specific allele (e.g., the *CFH* Tyr402His allele for AMD) on complex pathogenetic pathways, such as the alternative complement pathway, of which CFH is a component. The subtlety of that impact is determined by how that allele perturbs the biologic function of the gene in which it is located, not by whether the gene harboring that allele might be important in disease pathogenesis. Studies, for example, of individuals with different autoimmune disorders, such as rheumatoid arthritis, systemic lupus erythematosus, and Crohn disease, reveal modest associations, but with some of the same variants. This suggests common pathways leading to these distinct but related diseases, an observation that may illuminate their pathogenesis.

Second, even if the effect size of any one variant is small, GWAS demonstrate that many of these disorders are indeed extremely **polygenic**, even more so than previously suspected. Thousands of variants, most of which individually contribute little to disease likelihood (ORs between 1.01 and 1.1) in aggregate, account for a substantial fraction of clustering of these diseases within certain families (see Chapter 9). Indeed genotypes from all of the variants can be combined into a number called a **polygenic risk score** (PRS) (see Chapter 9). The PRS reflects a person's inherited susceptibility to a disease, and the effect size can be as high as with some rare penetrant variants.

Most alleles found by GWAS may indeed have modest effect size, but there is a critical and perhaps most fundamental finding of GWAS: the genetic architecture of some of the most common complex diseases may involve hundreds to thousands of loci harboring variants of small effect in many genes and pathways. These genes and pathways are important to our understanding of how complex diseases occur, even if each allele exerts but subtle effects on gene regulation or protein function and on disease susceptibility. It is also important to note the potential interplay between common and rare variants in disease susceptibility. This has been studied in depth in schizophrenia, with the identification of both rare variants with high OR and common variants of low OR contributing to risk (Fig. 11.13). An overall risk profile that combines a PRS with rare variants will perhaps be come available for many disorders.

Thus, GWAS remains an important human genetics research tool for dissecting the many contributions to complex disease, regardless of whether the individual variants associated substantially raise the likelihood of the disease in individuals who carry them (see Chapter 17). There are more than 300,000 mapped associations in the genome (https://www.ebi.ac.uk/gwas/home). We

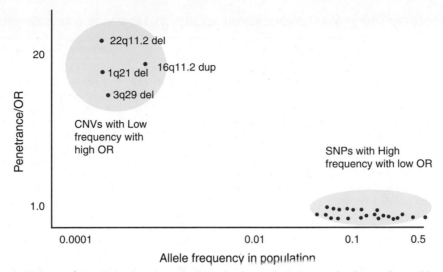

Figure 11.13 Common and rare variant allele spectrum of schizophrenia. Penetrance in the form of an odds ratio (OR) is shown on the y-axis with allele frequency on the y-axis. Both rare and common variation contribute to schizophrenia risk with rare CNVs acting with OR of 10 to 20. Common SNPs associated with schizophrenia have OR of ~1 to 1.5. (From Sullivan PF, Daly MJ, O'Donovan M. Genetic architectures of psychiatric disorders: the emerging picture and its implications. *Nat Rev Genet* 13(8):537-551, 2012. https://doi.org/10.1038/nrg3240.)

anticipate many more genetic variants responsible for complex diseases to be identified by genome-wide association and that deep sequencing of such regions will uncover the variants or collections of variants functionally responsible for the disease. Such findings should provide powerful insights and potential therapeutic targets for many of the common diseases that cause so much morbidity and mortality.

FINDING GENES RESPONSIBLE FOR DISEASE BY GENOME-WIDE SEQUENCING

Thus far in this chapter we have focused on two approaches to map and then identify genes involved in disease: linkage analysis and GWAS. Now we turn to a third approach, involving direct genome-wide sequencing of affected individuals, along with their parents and/or other family members, or a population cohort with the same clinical diagnosis. Characteristics, strengths, and weaknesses of linkage, association, and genome-wide sequencing methods for disease gene identification are summarized in Box 11.4.

The development of vastly improved and high-throughput methods of DNA sequencing has cut the cost of sequencing by six orders of magnitude from that spent for the Human Genome Project's reference sequence. This has opened new possibilities for discovering the genes and variants responsible for diseases, particularly for rare mendelian disorders. As introduced in Chapter 4, these new technologies make it possible to generate a **whole genome sequence (GS)** or, in what is a cost-effective compromise, sequence for the less than 2% of the genome containing the exons of genes, referred to as a **whole exome sequence** or **exome sequencing (ES)**.

Comparison of Exome and Whole Genome Sequencing

Both exome and **genome sequencing** fall into the category of genome-wide sequencing (i.e., taking an unbiased approach to interrogating a genome). ES involves sequencing of the coding portion of the genome, where, during the library preparation step, gene exons are targeted or captured. There are several commercially available kits available for ES and all involve either a **hybridization** or PCR step to enrich for the exonic portion of the genome. Further customization is often possible to boost and thus provide better coverage for certain variant types (e.g., mitochondrial variants) or clinically relevant regions (e.g., known pathogenic variants). The application of ES has been instrumental in the discovery of genes responsible for rare mendelian disorders, given its cost effectiveness, allowing the sequencing of more samples compared to more costly GS. However, there are both design and technical limitations in using ES, including the inability to analyze noncoding changes (e.g., deep intronic or regulatory regions) unless specifically targeted, the dropout of some coding sequence due to capture inefficiencies (high GC content exons), and limited ability to resolve more complex genetic mechanisms (e.g., structural rearrangements, repeat expansions). With the cost of sequencing continuing to drop it is becoming more feasible to use GS for gene discovery.

The application of GS can address many of the technical limitations of ES (see Box 11.5). First, since there is no capture process, GS is not prone to dropout of more complex or high GC regions and, thus, provides better coverage of the coding regions of the genomes. Second, noncoding regions of the genome are

BOX 11.4 METHODS OF DISCOVERY: COMPARISON OF LINKAGE, ASSOCIATION METHODS, AND GENOME-WIDE SEQUENCING

Linkage	Association	Genome-Wide Sequencing
• Follows inheritance of a disease trait and regions of the genome from individual to individual in family pedigrees • Looks for regions of the genome harboring disease alleles; uses polymorphic loci to mark which region an individual has inherited from which parent • Uses hundreds to thousands of informative markers across the genome • Not designed to find the specific variant responsible for or predisposing to the disease; can only demarcate where the variant can be found within (usually) one or a few megabases • Relies on recombination events occurring in families during only a few generations to allow measurement of the genetic distance between a disease gene and markers on chromosomes • Requires sampling of families, not just people affected by the disease • Loses power when disease has complex inheritance with substantial lack of penetrance • Most often used to map disease-causing variants with strong enough effects to cause a mendelian inheritance pattern	• Tests for altered frequency of particular alleles or haplotypes in individuals with a disease, compared with population controls • Examines particular alleles or haplotypes for their contribution to the disease • Uses anywhere from a few markers in targeted genes to hundreds of thousands of markers for genome-wide analyses • Can occasionally pinpoint the variant functionally responsible for the disease; more often, defines a disease-containing haplotype over a 1- to 10-kb interval • Relies on finding a set of alleles, including the disease gene, that remained together for many generations due to lack of recombination among the markers • Can be carried out on case-control or cohort samples from populations • Is sensitive to population stratification artifact, although this can be controlled by proper case-control designs or the use of family-based approaches • Is the best approach for finding variants with small effect that contribute to complex traits	• Determines variation in the whole genome or coding sequence (exome) in unbiased approach in families or cohorts • Requires robust filtering strategy to narrow down rare variants based on segregation and expected disease mode • Filtering can be within a family or across individuals with the same clinical diagnosis • Can be used in conjunction with linkage data to aid in narrowing down region of the genome with causative variant • Designed to precisely identify causative variant that is functionally responsible for the disease • Does not rely on linked variants and is particularly useful for finding *de novo* dominant variants that are intractable to linkage or association studies • Can use either family- or cohort-based analysis • Designed to identify rare disease-causing variants but can perform genome-wide association studies • Confirmation of gene disease association greatly enhanced with submission to GeneMatcher

sequenced, including deep **intronic**, regulatory regions and **noncoding RNA**, which may harbor pathogenic variation. Third, GS has the potential to detect nearly all classes of genetic variation, including those that are intractable to ES, such as complex structural variation, repeat expansions, and medically important genes with high homology (e.g., *SMN1*). A comparison of variant classes detectable by ES and GS is shown in Box 11.5. There are still many challenges in interpretation of the large amount of rare variation sequenced in a GS; however, advancements in algorithms and annotation allow us to take better advantage of GS and have led to finding causative variants in many cases whose ES results had been uninformative.

BOX 11.5 COMPARISON OF VARIANT CLASSES DETECTED FROM WHOLE EXOME AND WHOLE GENOME SEQUENCING

Category	ES	GS
Small Variants	Yes	Yes
Copy Number Variants	Yes, limited sensitivity	Yes
Balanced Structural Variants	No	Yes
Mitochondrial Variants	Yes, requires boosting	Yes
Repeat Expansions	No	Yes, but limited
Homologous Regions	Some	Some

Filtering Genome-Wide Sequence Data to Find Potential Causative Variants

It is now possible, given our current knowledge of the genome, to systematically filter sequence data from millions of variants to yield a handful of rare variants that are potentially functional. For example, consider a family trio consisting of a child affected with a rare disorder and his parents. GS is performed for all three, yielding, typically, over 4 to 5 million differences relative to the human genome reference sequence (see Chapter 4). Which of these variants is responsible for the disease? Extracting useful information from this massive amount of data relies on creating a variant filtering strategy, based on a variety of reasonable assumptions about which variants are more likely to be causative.

There are many possible filtering strategies that will arrive at the same causative variant. Outcome can be influenced by the type of data generated (GS or ES), the potential inheritance pattern in the family, previous genetic testing, and whether you are looking for a known cause (e.g., diagnostic testing) versus gene discovery. Regardless, it is important to create a robust and systematic filtering scheme that can be used consistently to produce repeatable results in subsequent cases. Most filtering strategies will rely on location of the variant, its predicted functional effect on the gene product, population frequency, and inheritance pattern. Once these basic filters have been applied to narrow the number of variants, they can be further interrogated for clinical correlation, plausible biologic function, known expression, prior observation in other cases, and previous classifications. One example of a filtering scheme that can be used to sort through these variants is shown in Fig. 11.14; the order of filtering can be altered to produce similar results.

1. *Location with respect to protein-coding genes.* Keep variants that are within or near exons of protein-coding genes, and discard variants deep within introns or intergenic regions. It is possible, of course, that the variant responsible might lie in a noncoding RNA

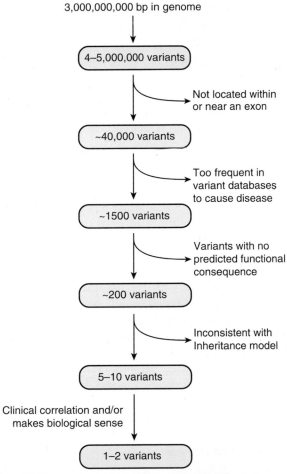

gene or in regulatory sequence located some distance from a gene, as introduced in Chapter 3. However, these are currently more difficult to assess; as a simplifying assumption, it is reasonable to focus initially on protein coding genes. If the filtering scheme does not yield interesting candidates, one can always go back and assess noncoding variants. **Splicing** assessment algorithms are becoming better at predicting splice variants in deep intronic regions.

2. *Population frequency.* Keep rare variants from step 1 by discarding common variants with allele frequencies greater than expected for a rare disorder. For filtering, one would typically pick an allele frequency cutoff of between 0.03 and 0.05. Common variants are highly unlikely to be responsible for a rare disease whose population prevalence is much less than the q^2 predicted by Hardy-Weinberg equilibrium (see Chapter 10).

3. *Deleterious nature of the variant.* Keep variants from step 2 that cause loss of function changes, including nonsense, frameshift, or those that alter highly conserved (canonical) splice sites. Keep nonsynomous variants that are predicted to be damaging. Discard synonymous or intronic changes that have no predicted effect on gene function.

4. *Consistency with likely inheritance pattern.* If the disorder is considered most likely to be autosomal recessive, keep any variants from step 3 that are found in both copies of a gene in an affected child. The child need not be homozygous for the same deleterious variant but could be a **compound heterozygote** for two different deleterious changes in the same gene (see Chapter 7). If this hypothesized mode of inheritance is correct, then the parents should both be heterozygous for the variant(s). If the parents are consanguineous, the candidate genes and variants may be further filtered by requiring that the child be a true **homozygote** for the same variant derived from a single common ancestor (see Chapter 10). If the disorder is severe and seems more likely to be due to a new mutation for a dominant trait, keep variants from step 3 that are *de novo* changes in the child and are not present in either parent. Finally, if there is suspicion of an X-linked disorder and the child is male, one can focus on **hemizygous** variants that are inherited from a heterozygous mother.

In the end, millions of variants can be filtered down to a handful occurring in a small number of genes. Once the filtering reduces the number of genes and alleles to a manageable number, they can be further assessed for other characteristics. Do any of the genes have a known function or tissue expression pattern that would be expected of a potential disease gene? Is the gene involved in other disease phenotypes, or does it have a role in pathways with other genes in which variation can cause similar or different phenotypes? Is the gene under constraint such that loss of function variants are

Figure 11.14 Representative filtering scheme for whole-genome sequencing of a family consisting of two unaffected parents and an affected child, reducing the millions of variants detected down to a small number that can be assessed for biologic and disease relevance. The initial enormous collection of variants is reduced into smaller and smaller bins by applying filters that remove variants unlikely to be causative, based on assuming that variants of interest are likely to be located near a gene, will disrupt its function, and are rare. Each remaining candidate gene is then assessed for whether the variants are inherited in a manner that fits the most likely inheritance pattern of the disease, whether a variant occurs in a candidate gene that makes biologic sense given the phenotype in the affected child, and whether other affected individuals also have causative variants in that gene.

rarely observed? Finally, has the variant been observed and classified in others, or has pathogenic variation in the gene been observed in others with the disease? Finding causative variation in one of these genes in other affected individuals would lend evidence that this was the responsible gene and variant in the original trio.

In some cases, one gene from the list in step 4 may rise to the top as a candidate because its involvement makes biologic or genetic sense, or it is known to be causative in other affected individuals. In other cases, however, the gene responsible may turn out to be entirely unanticipated on biologic grounds, or may not be causative in other affected individuals because of locus heterogeneity (i.e., pathogenic variants in other as yet undiscovered genes can cause a similar disease).

Such variant assessments require extensive use of public genomic databases and software tools. These include the human genome reference sequence, databases of allele frequencies (e.g., 1000 genomes and gnomAD), software that assesses how deleterious an amino acid substitution might be to gene function, collections of known disease-causing variants (e.g., ClinVar or disease specific), and databases of functional networks and biologic pathways. The enormous expansion of this information over the past few years, fueled by genome-wide sequencing of millions of cases and controls, has played a crucial role in facilitating gene discovery and molecular diagnosis of rare mendelian disorders, as we discuss in the next section.

FILTERING STRATEGIES FOR IDENTIFICATION OF DISEASE-CAUSING GENES

In the previous section we discussed filtering schemes for a single family to identify variants causing disease. But what if nothing is identified or there are interesting candidates that are lacking enough evidence to definitively link to disease? For rare mendelian disorders, analysis of a single affected individual is often inadequate for gene discovery, making other study designs and strategies necessary. This involves traditional mapping

approaches as well as other common genetic strategies that have been adapted for genome-wide sequencing. Generally, sequencing of multiple affected individuals within a family or sequencing of unrelated individuals with the same clinical diagnosis is necessary. Deciding which cases are the most informative to sequence is highly influenced by the suspected mode of inheritance and whether the variants are expected to be inherited or due to new (*de novo*) mutations. Fig. 11.15 shows some examples of strategies employed for gene identification using genome-wide sequencing. This is not an exhaustive list but includes strategies for finding disease-causing genes based on variant inheritance and sharing across affected individuals.

For families demonstrating autosomal recessive inheritance, genome-wide sequencing and filtering strategies are relatively straightforward. In those families with no known **consanguinity** or not belonging to a founder population, compound heterozygous is the most likely disease model. Sequencing of affected sibling pairs is highly effective since there are very few shared compound heterozygous variants. In smaller families, sequencing of parents is useful to filter out variants that are both coming from one parent (in *cis*). In those families with expected or known consanguinity, causative variants are expected to be homozygous. Sequencing of sibling pairs or other affected relatives and prioritizing homozygous variants is an extremely effective strategy that has led to many new gene discoveries. If possible, sequencing of more distantly related individuals will aid in further reducing the number of shared homozygous variants. Homozygosity mapping with SNP microarrays to predetermine chromosomal loci with overlapping stretches of homozygosity in affected individuals can be used to narrow regions. However, with the cost of sequencing decreasing, current strategies typically only use the genome-wide data for homozygosity mapping, or to sequence more individuals and look for shared homozygous variants. Finally, for those families showing X-linked recessive inheritance, one can look for shared variants on chromosome X in males and filter out autosome variants. However, one must

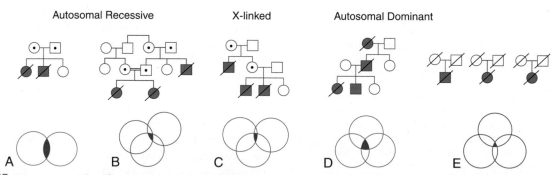

Figure 11.15 **Disease gene identification strategies using genome-wide sequencing for different suspected modes of inheritance. Strategies (A–E) are detailed in the text.** Filled symbols indicate affected individuals, and empty symbols are unaffected. Obligate carriers are denoted with a dot. Cross lines depict individuals undergoing genome-wide sequencing, with circles below indicating variant sets and overlapping strategies for detection of causative variants.

be cautious in this approach that there is unequivocal evidence that the transmission is X-linked and not potentially autosomal recessive.

The use of genome-wide sequencing for identifying genes causing inherited dominant disorders can be more challenging. This strategy involves looking for shared variants in affected individuals and excluding variants present in unaffected individuals. In principle, finding the causative variant can be difficult owing to the number of rare variants that are private to a family. To effectively filter variants down to a manageable number to interpret, sequencing of many affected and unaffected individuals is necessary, which can be costly especially if using GS. This can be partially mitigated in large families by using the principles of linkage that we discussed earlier in the chapter. Performing linkage to define a disease locus, then strategically sequencing a few distantly related individuals, can be a cost-effective approach to gene identification. If there are no candidates in the linked region, it raises the possibility of variant classes that may not be detectable due to technical limitations of genome-wide sequencing or that the causative variant is noncoding and difficult to interpret without functional assays.

Genome-wide sequencing has been particularly successful for discovery of disorders caused by *de novo* dominant variants—a disease mode that is intractable to linkage studies. These disorders tend to be severe genetic lethals, with variants not passed on to subsequent generations. There are relatively few *de novo* events per exome

(1–2) and genome (50–70); overlapping *de novo* events in two unrelated individuals with a similar phenotype can be sufficient to show disease causation, although overlap by chance is possible. The *de novo* overlap strategy has been particularly useful in finding causes for disorders with high genetic and phenotypic **heterogeneity**, such as syndromic forms of autism spectrum disorder and intellectual disability. Pooling of large case cohorts is often necessary to find *de novo* variants in the same gene, given their individually rare participation in a genotypically heterogeneous pool. Genes identified using this strategy are more likely to overlap by chance as the number of family trios sequenced increases. Thorough investigation of genotype and phenotype correlation is imperative to establish disease gene associations.

Each of the strategies above can be hindered by genetic and phenotypic heterogeneity and the rarity of the disorders that remain unsolved. Indeed, much of the low-hanging fruit for rare disease associations has been discovered, and the majority of cases that undergo genome-wide sequencing are unsolved. It is clear that for study of exceedingly rare disorders or new disease mechanisms, international collaboration is necessary, as no one cohort will likely have the numbers to make robust disease associations. One such effort is the Matchmaker Exchange (MME), which uses a federated network of data sharing to solve undiagnosed cases and facilitates publication of case series describing new disease genes (Fig. 11.16). The MME provides a genetic

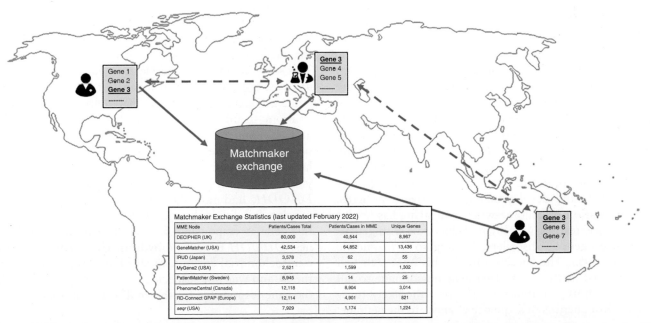

Matchmaker Exchange Statistics (last updated February 2022)			
MME Node	Patients/Cases Total	Patients/Cases in MME	Unique Genes
DECIPHER (UK)	80,000	40,544	8,967
GeneMatcher (USA)	42,534	64,852	13,436
IRUD (Japan)	3,578	62	55
MyGene2 (USA)	2,521	1,599	1,302
PatientMatcher (Sweden)	8,945	14	25
PhenomeCentral (Canada)	12,118	8,904	3,014
RD-Connect GPAP (Europe)	12,114	4,901	821
seqr (USA)	7,929	1,174	1,224

Figure 11.16 International collaboration through matchmaker exchange (MME). For rare mendelian disorders, federated networks of data sharing can facilitate solutions for undiagnosed cases and establish genotype-phenotype correlations. Candidate genes without established disease associations, sequenced as either part of research or clinical service, can be submitted to MME via several projects. Matching genes can be linked between submitters for more detailed phenotype-genotype correlation. In the example here, researchers and clinicians from three centers have submitted candidate genes *(solid lines)* for affected individuals to MME, with gene 3 in common. Direct connections between submitters *(dotted bidirectional arrows)* can then be established to further study potential causal relationships. The insert includes a snapshot of federated databases that link into MME with the number of cases and genes submitted.

Growth of Gene-phenotype Relationships
31 Dec 2021

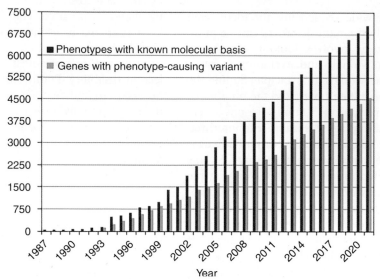

Figure 11.17 Growth of phenotype and disease gene associations. Growth of gene association with disease phenotype has steadily increased due to the advent of genome-wide sequencing combined with data sharing.

matchmaking service that connects multiple researchers or clinicians who have patients with similar phenotypes and variants in the same candidate gene. Multiple nodes feed into MME, with a growing collective dataset of more than 150,000 cases submitted from 99 countries. As sequencing becomes less expensive, these datasets will continue to grow.

The increased application of genome-wide sequencing coupled with sharing of data has played a pivotal role in our understanding of gene-disease associations, leading to a rapid increase in gene discovery over the last 10+ years. Since the application of GS or ES to rare mendelian disorders was first described in 2009, many hundreds of such disorders have been studied, and the causative variants found among hundreds of previously unrecognized disease genes (Fig. 11.17). These discoveries feed back into diagnostic testing where they not only provide information useful for genetic counseling in the families involved, but may inform clinical management and the potential development of effective treatments. The application of genome-wide sequencing has grown in diagnostic testing, notably in individuals with genetically heterogenous disorders, leading to a diagnostic yield of ~30%. The success rate of this approach will only increase as the costs of sequencing continue to fall and with improved ability to interpret the likely functional consequences of sequence changes in the genome.

Example: Identification of the Gene Causing Postaxial Acrofacial Dysostosis

The genome-wide sequencing approach just outlined was used in the study of a family in which two siblings affected with a rare **congenital** malformation, known as postaxial acrofacial dysostosis (POAD), were born to two unaffected, unrelated parents. Individuals with this disorder have small jaws, missing or poorly developed digits on the ulnar sides of their hands, underdevelopment of the ulna, cleft lip, and clefts (colobomas) of the eyelids. The disorder was thought to be autosomal recessive, because some parents of an affected child are consanguineous, and because a few families are like the one here, with multiple affected siblings born to unaffected parents—both findings that are hallmarks of recessive inheritance (see Chapter 7). This small family alone was clearly inadequate for linkage analysis. Instead, all four members of the family had their entire genomes sequenced and analyzed.

From an initial list of more than 4 million variants and assuming autosomal recessive inheritance of the disorder in both affected children, a filtering scheme similar to that described earlier (see Figs. 11.14 and 11.15) yielded only four possible candidate genes. One of these, *DHODH*, had rare damaging variants in two other unrelated individuals with POAD, thereby identifying this gene as responsible for the disorder in these families. *DHODH* encodes dihydroorotate dehydrogenase, a mitochondrial enzyme involved in **pyrimidine** biosynthesis, and was not suspected on biologic grounds to be the gene responsible for this **malformation syndrome**.

Limitations of Genome-Wide Sequencing and Future Outlook

Although the genome-wide sequencing approach has proved powerful for both gene discovery and diagnosis of rare mendelian disease, it still has limitations. Most groups report diagnostic yields in the 20 to 40% range, depending on clinical indication, which leaves the majority of cases without an identified causative variant and answer. There are several reasons for this observation. First, some disorders are intractable to standard genome-wide sequencing, including methylation disorders (e.g., Prader-Willi and Angelman syndromes) or those involving certain types of **Uniparental disomy (UPD)** if parents are not sequenced (i.e., heterodisomy). Second (and related), genome-wide sequencing may miss certain classes of variation that are difficult to detect by routine short-read sequencing alone (e.g., balanced changes, repeat expansions). As discussed earlier, whole genome sequencing has technological advantages over exome sequencing, with the ability to detect a broader range of variation; however, there are still limitations in accurately detecting or resolving complex regions of the genome. Third, variation is detected that is difficult to interpret with our current understanding of the genome. This is particularly true of genome sequencing and the rare variation detected in noncoding and regulatory genomic regions. Finally, at present, whole genome sequencing cannot actually sequence the entire genome in any one individual. Cost limits most of the sequencing to short-reads and aligning back to a reference genome (termed resequencing) to detect variation. Some sequence is too complex and/or highly homologous or repetitive to be technically sequenced or mapped back to the reference genome. Additionally, sequence novel to one's genome, i.e., not in the reference assembly, will be filtered out even though it may be pathogenic.

Such limitations are starting to be addressed in several ways. Improvements in both sequencing technology and informatics algorithms for variant detection allow a more accurate catalogue of genomic variation. The increasing number of genomes sequenced and the subsequent aggregation of data allow more accurate interpretation of variation. In addition, the advancement of other -omic technologies, such as **RNA** sequencing or methylation experiments, are proving to be valuable tests ancillary to genome-wide sequencing for the interpretation of noncoding variation. The emergence of long-read sequencing technology (reads up to 10–100 kb in length) has provided insight into regions of the genome that have been intractable to short-read sequencing, including highly homologous or repetitive regions, with detection of variation previously unseen. Long-read technology can also be used to advance *de novo* assembly of genomes, rather than reference-based assembly, to get a more complete picture of the genome. These advances will lead to a better understanding of our genome, its variation, and its relation to disease.

ACKNOWLEDGMENT

We wish to thank Ada Hamosh and Gregory Costain for contributing to this chapter.

GENERAL REFERENCES

Altshuler D, Daly MJ, Lander ES: Genetic mapping in human disease, *Science* 322:881–888, 2008.

Boycott KM, Azzariti DR, Hamosh A, et al: Seven years since the launch of the Matchmaker Exchange: The evolution of genomic matchmaking, *Hum Mutat*, 2022. https://doi.org/10.1002/humu.24373. Online ahead of print. PMID: 35537081.

Boycott KM, Vanstone MR, Bulman DE, et al: Rare-disease genetics in the era of next-generation sequencing: Discovery to translation, *Nat Rev Genet* 14:681–691, 2013.

Gilissen C, Hoischen A, Brunner HG, et al: Disease gene identification strategies for exome sequencing, *Eur J Hum Genet* 20:490–497, 2012.

Manolio TA: Genomewide association studies and assessment of the risk of disease, *NEJM* 363:166–176, 2010.

Risch N, Merikangas K: The future of genetic studies of complex human diseases, *Science* 273:1516–1517, 1996.

Sullivan PF, Daly MJ, O'Donovan M: Genetic architectures of psychiatric disorders: The emerging picture and its implications, *Nat Rev Genet* 13:537–551, 2012.

Terwilliger JD, Ott J: *Handbook of human genetic linkage*, Baltimore, 1994, Johns Hopkins University Press.

REFERENCES FOR SPECIFIC TOPICS

Abecasis GR, Auton A, Brooks LD, et al: An integrated map of genetic variation from 1,092 human genomes, *Nature* 491:56–65, 2012.

Bainbridge MN, Wiszniewski W, Murdock DR, et al: Whole-genome sequencing for optimized patient management, *Science Transl Med* 3:87re3, 2011.

Bush WS, Moore JH: Genome-wide association studies, *PLoS Computational Biol* 8:e1002822, 2012.

Denny JC, Bastarache L, Ritchie MD, et al: Systematic comparison of phenome-wide association study of electronic medical record data and genome-wide association data, *Nat Biotechnol* 31:1102–1110, 2013.

Fritsche LG, Chen W, Schu M, et al: Seven new loci associated with age-related macular degeneration, *Nat Genet* 17:1783–1786, 2013.

Gonzaga-Jauregui C, Lupski JR, Gibbs RA: Human genome sequencing in health and disease, *Ann Rev Med* 63:35–61, 2012.

Hindorff LA, MacArthur J, Morales J, et al: A catalog of published genome-wide association studies, 2015. www.genome.gov/gwastudies

International HapMap Consortium: A second generation human haplotype map of over 3.1 million SNPs, *Nature* 449:851–861, 2007.

Kircher M, Witten DM, Jain P, et al: A general framework for estimating the relative pathogenicity of human genetic variants, *Nat Genet* 46:310–315, 2014.

Koboldt DC, Steinberg KM, Larson DE, et al: The next-generation sequencing revolution and its impact on genomics, *Cell* 155:27–38, 2013.

Lionel AC, Costain G, Monfared N, et al: Improved diagnostic yield compared with targeted gene sequencing panels suggests a role for whole-genome sequencing as a first-tier genetic test, *Genet Med* 20:435–443, 2018.

Manolio TA: Bringing genome-wide association findings into clinical use, *Nat Rev Genet* 14:549–558, 2014.

Marshall CR, Howrigan DP, Merico D, et al: Contribution of copy number variants to schizophrenia from a genome-wide study of 41,321 subjects, *Nat Genet* 49:27–35, 2016.

Matise TC, Chen F, Chen W, et al: A second-generation combined linkage-physical map of the human genome, *Genome Res* 17:1783–1786, 2007.

Roach JC, Glusman G, Smit AF, et al: Analysis of genetic inheritance in a family quartet by whole-genome sequencing, *Science* 328:636–639, 2010.

Robinson PC, Brown MA: Genetics of ankylosing spondylitis, *Mol Immunol* 57:2–11, 2014.

SEARCH Collaborative Group: *SLCO1B1* variants and statin-induced myopathy—A genomewide study, *NEJM* 359:789–799, 2008.

Stahl EA, Wegmann D, Trynka G, et al: Bayesian inference analyses of the polygenic architecture of rheumatoid arthritis, *Nat Genet* 44:4383–4391, 2012.

Yang Y, Muzny DM, Reid JG, et al: Clinical whole-exome sequencing for the diagnosis of mendelian disorders, *NEJM* 369:1502–1511, 2013.

Yuen RK, Merico D, Bookman M, et al: Whole genome sequencing resource identifies 18 new candidate genes for autism spectrum disorder, *Nat Neurosci* 20:602–611, 2017.

PROBLEMS

1. In the early days of gene mapping the Huntington disease (HD) locus was found to be tightly linked to a DNA common variant on chromosome 4. In the same study, however, linkage was ruled out between HD and the locus for the polymorphic MNSs blood group, which also maps to chromosome 4. What is the explanation?

2. LOD scores *(Z)* between a common variant in the α-globin locus on the short arm of chromosome 16 and an autosomal dominant disease (e.g., polycystic kidney disease) was analyzed in a series of British and Dutch families, with the following data:

θ	0.00	0.01	0.10	0.20	0.30	0.40
Z	−∞	23.4	24.6	19.5	12.85	5.5

$Z_{max} = 25.85$ at $\theta_{max} = 0.05$

How would you interpret these data?

In a subsequent study, a large family from Sicily with what looks like the same disease was also investigated for linkage to α-globin, with the following results:

θ	0.00	0.10	0.20	0.30	0.40
LOD scores (Z)	−∞	−8.34	−3.34	−1.05	−0.02

How would you interpret the data in this second study?

3. This pedigree was obtained in a study designed to determine whether a pathogenic variant in one of the genes coding for a γ-crystallin protein, *CRYGD*, may be responsible for an autosomal dominant form of cataract. The filled-in symbols in the pedigree indicate family members with cataracts. The letters indicate three alleles at the *CRYGD* locus on chromosome 2. If you examine each affected person who has passed on the cataract to his or her children, how many of these represent a meiosis that is informative for linkage between the cataract and *CRYGD*? In which individuals is the phase known between the cataract pathogenic variant and the *CRYGD* alleles? Are there any meioses in which a crossover must have occurred to explain the data? What would you conclude about linkage between the cataract and the *CRYGD* gene from this study? What additional studies might be performed to confirm or reject the hypothesis?

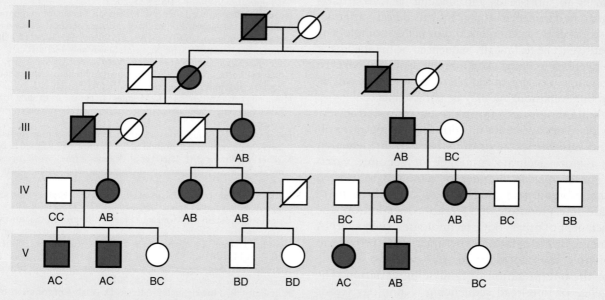

Pedigree for question 3

4. Genome-wide sequencing has become an effective strategy for the discovery of genes causing rare mendelian disorders and refers to either whole exome (ES) or whole genome sequencing (GS).
   a. Define whole exome sequencing and describe conceptually how it is performed?
   b. What are the advantages and disadvantages of GS compared to ES?

5. Review the pedigree in Fig. 11.10B. If the unaffected grandmother, I-2, had been an *A/a* heterozygote, would it be possible to determine the phase in the affected parent, individual II-2?

6. In the pedigree below, showing a family with X-linked hemophilia A, can you determine the phase of the variant factor VIII allele *(h)* and the normal allele *(H)* with respect to variant alleles *M* and *m* in the mother of the two affected boys?

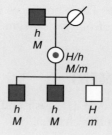

continued

PROBLEMS—CONT'D

Pedigree of X-linked hemophilia. The affected grand-father in the first generation has the disease (allele *h*) and allele *M* at a polymorphic locus on the X chromosome.

7. Relative risk calculations are used for cohort studies and not case-control studies. To demonstrate why, imagine a case-control study for the effect of a genetic variant on disease susceptibility. The investigator has ascertained as many affected individuals (a + c) as possible and then arbitrarily chooses a set of (b + d) controls. They are genotyped as to whether a variant is present: a/(a + c) of the affected have the variant, whereas b/(b + d) of the controls have the variant.

	Disease Present	Disease Absent
Variant present	a	b
Variant absent	c	d
	a + c	b + d

Calculate the odds ratio (OR) and relative risk (RR) for the association between the variant being present and the disease being present.

Now, imagine the investigator arbitrarily decided to use three times as many unaffected individuals, $3 \times (b + d)$, as controls. The investigator has every right to do so because it is a case-control study and the numbers of affected and unaffected are not determined by the prevalence of the disease in the population being studied, as they would be in a cohort study. Assume the distribution of the variant remains the same in this control group as with the smaller control group—that is, $3b/[3 \times (b + d)] = b/(b + d)$ carrying the allele.

	Disease Present	Disease Absent
Variant present	a	3b
Variant absent	c	3d
	a + c	$3 \times (b + d)$

Recalculate the OR and RR with this new control group. Do the same when an arbitrary control group is an n-tuple of the original control group—that is, the size of the control group is $n \times (b + d)$.

The Molecular Basis of Genetic Disease

Gregory Costain

GENERAL PRINCIPLES AND LESSONS FROM THE HEMOGLOBINOPATHIES

The term molecular disease, introduced in 1949, refers to disorders in which the primary disease-causing event is an alteration, either inherited or acquired, affecting a **gene(s)**, its structure, and/or its expression. In this chapter we first outline the basic **DNA variant** types and associated mechanisms underlying monogenic (**single-gene**) **disorders**. We then illustrate their molecular and clinical consequences using inherited diseases of hemoglobin—the hemoglobinopathies—as examples. This overview of mechanisms is expanded on in Chapter 13 to include other **genetic** diseases that illustrate key principles of genetics in medicine.

A genetic disease occurs when an alteration in the DNA of an essential gene changes the amount or function, or both, of the gene products—typically **messenger RNA (mRNA)** and protein, but occasionally specific noncoding RNAs (ncRNAs) with structural or regulatory functions. Although almost all known single-gene disorders result from variants that affect the function of a protein, a few exceptions to this generalization are now known. These exceptions are diseases due to variants in ncRNA genes, including microRNA (miRNA) genes that regulate specific target genes, and mitochondrial genes that encode **transfer RNAs (tRNAs**; see Chapter 13) . In this chapter we restrict our attention to diseases caused by defects in protein-coding genes.

It is essential to understand genetic disease at the molecular level because this knowledge is the foundation of rational therapy. By 2022, the online version of *Mendelian Inheritance in Man* listed over 7000 **phenotypes** for which the molecular basis is known. Although it is impressive that the basic molecular defect has been found in so many disorders, it is sobering to realize that the pathophysiology is not entirely understood for any genetic disease. Sickle cell disease (Case 42), discussed later in this chapter, was the first disease to be characterized at the molecular level and remains among the best characterized of all inherited disorders; even here, knowledge is incomplete. Genetically informed therapies for hemoglobinopathies are now emerging as a realistic prospect in the clinic, thanks in part to an increasingly sophisticated understanding of the genetic pathomechanisms.

EFFECT OF PATHOGENIC VARIANTS ON PROTEIN FUNCTION

DNA variants within protein-coding genes have been primarily found to cause disease through one of four different effects on protein function (Fig. 12.1). The most common effect by far is a loss of function of the protein. Many important conditions arise, however, from other mechanisms: a gain of function, the acquisition of a novel property by the affected protein, or the expression of a gene at the wrong time (heterochronic expression) and/or in the wrong place (**ectopic expression**).

Loss-of-Function Variants

The loss of function of a gene may result from alteration of its coding, regulatory, or other critical sequences due to **nucleotide** substitutions, **deletions, insertions**, or **rearrangements**. A loss of function due to deletion, leading to a reduction in **gene dosage**, is exemplified by the α-thalassemias (Case 44), which are most commonly due to deletion of α-globin genes (see later discussion); by **chromosome**-loss diseases (Case 27), such as monosomies like Turner **syndrome** (see Chapter 6) (Case 47); and by acquired somatic variants that occur in **tumor-suppressor genes** in many cancers, such as retinoblastoma (Case 39) (see Chapter 16). Many other types of variants can also lead to a complete loss of function, and all are illustrated by the β-thalassemias (see later discussion), a group of hemoglobinopathies that result from a reduction in the abundance of β-globin, one of the major adult hemoglobin proteins in red blood cells.

The severity of a disease due to loss-of-function variants generally correlates with the amount of function lost. In many instances, the retention of even a small percent of residual function by the abnormal protein greatly reduces the severity of the disease.

Gain-of-Function Variants

Variants may also enhance one or more of the normal functions of a protein; in a biologic system, however, more is not necessarily better, and disease may result. It

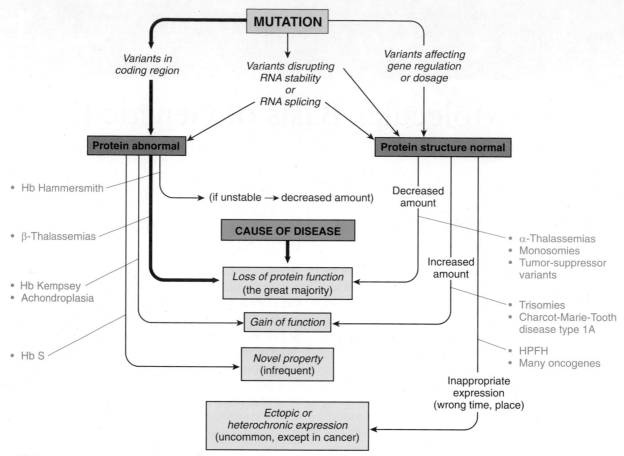

Figure 12.1 A general outline of the mechanisms by which disease-causing variants produce disease. Variants in the coding region result in structurally abnormal proteins that have a loss or gain of function or a novel property that causes disease. Variants in noncoding sequences are of two general types: those that alter the stability or splicing of the messenger RNA (mRNA) and those that disrupt regulatory elements or change gene dosage. Variants in regulatory elements alter the abundance of the mRNA or the time or cell type in which the gene is expressed. Variants in either the coding region or regulatory domains can decrease the amount of the protein produced. *HPFH,* Hereditary persistence of fetal hemoglobin.

is critical to recognize when a disease is due to a gain-of-function variant because the treatment must necessarily differ from disorders due to other mechanisms, such as loss-of-function variants. Gain-of-function variants fall into two broad classes:

- Variants that increase the production of a normal protein. Some variants cause disease by increasing the synthesis of a normal protein in cells in which the protein is normally present. The most common variants of this type are due to increased gene dosage, which generally results from duplication of part or all of a chromosome. As discussed in Chapter 6, the classic example is **trisomy** 21 (Down syndrome), which is due to the presence of three copies of chromosome 21. Other important diseases arise from the increased dosage of single genes, including one form of **familial** Alzheimer disease due to a duplication of the amyloid precursor protein (βAPP) gene (see Chapter 13), and the peripheral nerve degeneration Charcot-Marie-Tooth disease type 1A (Case 8), which generally results from duplication of the gene for peripheral myelin protein 22 (*PMP22*).

- Variants that enhance one normal function of a protein. Rarely, a variant in the coding region may increase the ability of each protein molecule to perform one or more of its normal functions, even though this increase is detrimental to the overall physiologic role of the protein. For example, the missense variant that creates hemoglobin Kempsey locks hemoglobin into its high oxygen affinity state, thereby reducing oxygen delivery to tissues. Another example of this mechanism is the missense variation in the *FGFR3* gene that causes achondroplasia (Case 2), the most common skeletal dysplasia.

Novel Property Variants

In a few diseases, a change in the amino acid sequence confers a novel property on the protein, without necessarily altering its normal functions. The classic example of this mechanism is sickle cell disease (Case 42), which, as we will see later in this chapter, is due to an amino acid substitution that has no effect on the ability of sickle hemoglobin to transport oxygen. Rather, unlike normal hemoglobin, sickle hemoglobin chains aggregate when they are deoxygenated and form abnormal polymeric fibers that deform red blood cells. That novel property variants are infrequent is not surprising because most amino acid substitutions are either neutral or detrimental to the function or stability of a protein that has been finely tuned by evolution.

Variants Associated With Heterochronic or Ectopic Gene Expression

An important class of variants includes those that lead to inappropriate expression of the gene at an abnormal time or place. These variants occur in the regulatory regions of the gene. Cancer can be driven by expression of a gene that normally promotes cell proliferation—a proto-**oncogene**—in cells in which the gene is not normally expressed (see Chapter 16). Some variants in hemoglobin **regulatory elements** lead to the continued expression in adults of the γ-globin gene, which is normally expressed at high levels only in fetal life. Such γ-globin gene variants cause a benign phenotype called hereditary persistence of fetal hemoglobin (Hb F), as we explore later in this chapter.

HOW VARIANTS DISRUPT THE FORMATION OF BIOLOGICALLY NORMAL PROTEINS

Disruptions of the normal functions of a protein that result from the different types of variants outlined earlier can be well exemplified by the broad range of diseases due to variants in the globin genes, as we will discuss in the second part of this chapter. To form a biologically active protein (such as the hemoglobin molecule), information must be transcribed from the nucleotide sequence of the gene to the mRNA and then translated into the polypeptide, which then undergoes progressive stages of maturation (see Chapter 3). Variants can disrupt any of these steps (Table 12.1). As we shall see next, abnormalities in five of these stages are illustrated by various hemoglobinopathies; the others are exemplified by diseases to be presented in Chapter 13.

THE RELATIONSHIP BETWEEN GENOTYPE AND PHENOTYPE IN GENETIC DISEASE

Key molecular concepts that can account for differences in the observed clinical phenotype associated with a genetic disease are:
- **Allelic heterogeneity**
- **Locus heterogeneity**
- Effect of **modifier genes**

Each of these concepts is illustrated by variants in the α-globin and/or β-globin genes (Table 12.2).

Allelic Heterogeneity

Genetic **heterogeneity** is most commonly due to the presence of multiple **alleles** at a single **locus**, a situation referred to as allelic **heterogeneity** (see Chapter 7 and Table 12.1). In some instances there may be a clear **genotype**-phenotype correlation between a specific allele and a specific phenotype. The most common explanation for the effect of allelic heterogeneity on the clinical

TABLE 12.1 Eight Steps at Which DNA Variants Can Disrupt the Production of a Normal Protein

Step	Phenotype Example
Transcription	Thalassemias due to reduced or absent production of a globin mRNA because of deletions or variants in regulatory or splice sites of a globin gene
	Hereditary persistence of fetal hemoglobin, which results from increased postnatal transcription of one or more γ-globin genes
Translation	Thalassemias due to nonfunctional or rapidly degraded mRNAs with nonsense or frameshift variants
Polypeptide folding	More than 70 hemoglobinopathies are due to abnormal hemoglobins with amino acid substitutions or deletions that lead to unstable globins that are prematurely degraded (e.g., Hb Hammersmith)
Posttranslational modification	I-cell disease, a lysosomal storage disease that is due to a failure to add a phosphate group to mannose residues of lysosomal enzymes. The mannose 6-phosphate residues are required to target the enzymes to lysosomes (see Chapter 13)
Assembly of monomers into a holomeric protein	Types of osteogenesis imperfecta in which an amino acid substitution in a procollagen chain impairs the assembly of a normal collagen triple helix (see Chapter 13)
Subcellular localization of the polypeptide or the holomer	Familial hypercholesterolemia variants (class 4), in the carboxyl terminus of the LDL receptor, that impair the localization of the receptor to clathrin-coated pits, preventing the internalization of the receptor and its subsequent recycling to the cell surface (see Chapter 13)
Cofactor or prosthetic group binding to the polypeptide	Types of homocystinuria due to poor or absent binding of the cofactor (pyridoxal phosphate) to the cystathionine synthase **apoenzyme** (see Chapter 13)
Function of a correctly folded, assembled, and localized protein produced in normal amounts	Diseases in which the altered protein is mostly normal but one of its critical biologic activities is altered by an amino acid substitution (e.g., in Hb Kempsey, impaired subunit interaction locks hemoglobin into its high oxygen affinity state)

LDL, Low-density lipoprotein; *mRNA,* messenger RNA.

TABLE 12.2 Types of Heterogeneity Associated With Genetic Disease

Type of Heterogeneity	Definition	Example From the Hemoglobinopathies
Genetic		
Allelic heterogeneity	The occurrence of more than one allele at a locus	β-Thalassemia
Locus heterogeneity	The **association** of more than one locus with a clinical phenotype	Thalassemia can result from variants in either the α-globin or β-globin genes
Clinical or phenotypic	The association of more than one phenotype with variants at a single locus	Sickle cell disease and β-thalassemia each result from distinct β-globin gene variants

phenotype is that alleles that confer more residual function on the altered protein are often associated with a milder form of the principal phenotype associated with the disease. In some instances, however, alleles that confer some residual protein functions are associated with only one or a subset of the phenotypes seen with a missing or completely nonfunctional allele (frequently termed a **null allele**). As we will explore more fully in Chapter 13, this situation prevails with certain variants of the cystic fibrosis gene, *CFTR*, that lead to a phenotypically different condition—**congenital** absence of the vas deferens, but not to the other manifestations of cystic fibrosis. An important exception to this rule relates to variants that act in a **dominant-negative** fashion, as exemplified by select missense variants in the genes encoding components of type I collagen that result in a more severe form of osteogenesis imperfecta than with a null allele (see Chapter 13).

A second explanation for allele-based differences in phenotype is that a specific property of the protein may be more perturbed by a particular variant. This situation is well illustrated by Hb Kempsey, a β-globin allele that maintains the hemoglobin in a high oxygen affinity structure. This causes polycythemia because the reduced peripheral delivery of oxygen is misinterpreted by the hematopoietic system as being due to an inadequate production of red blood cells.

The consequences of a specific variant on the function of a protein can be unpredictable. No one would have foreseen that the β-globin allele associated with sickle cell disease would lead to the formation of globin polymers that deform erythrocytes to a sickle cell shape (see later in this chapter). However, sickle cell disease is also unusual in that it results only from a single specific variant—the p.Glu6Val substitution in the β-globin chain—whereas most genetic diseases can arise from any of a number of different DNA-level variants in the corresponding gene.

Locus Heterogeneity

Genetic heterogeneity also arises when variants at more than one locus can result in a specific clinical condition—a situation termed locus heterogeneity (see Chapter 7). This phenomenon is illustrated by the finding that thalassemia can result from variants in either the α-globin or β-globin chain genes (see Table 12.2). Once locus heterogeneity has been documented, careful comparison of the phenotype associated with each gene sometimes reveals that the phenotype is not as homogeneous as initially believed.

Modifier Genes

Sometimes even the most robust genotype-phenotype relationships are found not to hold for a specific individual. Such phenotypic variation can, in principle, be ascribed to nongenetic (e.g., environmental, stochastic) factors or to the action of other genes, termed modifier genes (see Chapter 9). Identified modifier genes for specific human monogenic disorders are growing in number; however, there remain relatively few examples with clinically relevant effect sizes or therapeutic significance. As described later in this chapter, individuals with β-thalassemia who also have a deletion at the α-globin locus can have a less severe phenotype.

HUMAN HEMOGLOBIN AND ASSOCIATED DISEASES

To illustrate in greater detail the concepts introduced in the first section of this chapter, we now turn to disorders of hemoglobin. These hemoglobinopathies are collectively the most common monogenic diseases in humans, and major contributors to global morbidity. The World Health Organization estimates that more than 5% of the world's population are **heterozygous carriers** of genetic variants associated with clinically important disorders of hemoglobin. Hemoglobinopathies are also important because their molecular and biochemical pathology is better understood than perhaps that of any other group of genetic diseases. Indeed, our understanding of the basic anatomy of a gene (Chapter 3) arose in large part from studying these prototypical monogenic disorders of hemoglobin. Before the hemoglobinopathies are discussed in depth, it is important to briefly introduce the normal aspects of the globin genes and hemoglobin biology.

Structure and Function of Hemoglobin

Hemoglobin is the oxygen carrier in vertebrate red blood cells. Each hemoglobin molecule consists of four subunits: two α- (or α-like) globin chains and two β- (or β-like) globin chains. Each subunit is composed of a polypeptide chain, globin, and a prosthetic group, heme. The latter is an iron-containing pigment that combines with

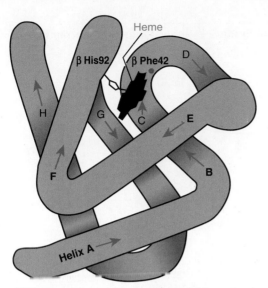

Figure 12.2 The structure of a hemoglobin subunit. Each subunit has eight helical regions, designated A to H. The two most conserved amino acids are shown: p.His92, the histidine to which the iron of heme is covalently linked; and p.Phe42, the phenylalanine that wedges the porphyrin ring of heme into the heme "pocket" of the folded protein. See discussion of Hb Hammersmith and Hb Hyde Park, which have substitutions for p.Phe42 and p.His92, respectively, in the β-globin molecule.

oxygen to give the molecule its oxygen-transporting ability (Fig. 12.2). The predominant adult human hemoglobin, Hb A, has an $\alpha_2\beta_2$ structure in which the four chains are folded and fit together to form a globular tetramer.

As with all proteins that have been strongly conserved throughout evolution, the **tertiary structure** of globins is constant; virtually all globins have seven or eight helical regions (depending on the chain) (see Fig. 12.2). Variants that disrupt this tertiary structure invariably have pathologic consequences. In addition, variants that substitute a highly conserved amino acid or that replace one of the nonpolar residues—which form the hydrophobic shell that excludes water from the interior of the molecule, are likely to cause a hemoglobinopathy (see Fig. 12.2). Like all proteins, globin has sensitive areas, in which variants cannot occur without affecting function, and insensitive areas, in which variations are more freely tolerated.

The Globin Genes

In addition to Hb A, with its $\alpha_2\beta_2$ structure, there are five other normal human hemoglobins, each of which has a tetrameric structure like that of Hb A, consisting of two α or α-like chains and two non-α chains (Fig. 12.3A). The genes for the α and α-like chains are clustered in a tandem arrangement on chromosome 16. Note that there are two identical α-globin genes, designated α1 and α2, on each **homologue**. The β- and β-like globin genes, located on chromosome 11, are close family members that, as described in Chapter 3, undoubtedly arose from a common ancestral gene (see Fig. 12.3A). Illustrating this close evolutionary relationship, the β- and δ-globins differ in only 10 of their 146 amino acids.

Developmental Expression of Globin Genes and Globin Switching

The expression of the various globin genes changes during development, a process referred to as globin switching (see Fig. 12.3B). Note that the genes in the α- and β-globin clusters are arranged in the same **transcriptional** orientation and, remarkably, the genes in each cluster are situated in the same order in which they are expressed during development. The temporal switches of globin synthesis are accompanied by changes in the principal site of erythropoiesis (see Fig. 12.3B). The three embryonic globins are made in the yolk sac from the third to eighth weeks of gestation, but at approximately the fifth week, hematopoiesis begins to move from the yolk sac to the fetal liver. Hb F $(\alpha_2\gamma_2)$, the predominant hemoglobin throughout fetal life, constitutes ~70% of total hemoglobin at birth. In adults, however, Hb F represents only a few percent of the total hemoglobin, although this can vary from less than 1% to ~5% in different individuals.

β-chain synthesis becomes significant near the time of birth, and by 3 months of age almost all hemoglobin is of the adult form: Hb A $(\alpha_2\beta_2)$ (see Fig. 12.3B). In diseases due to variants that decrease the abundance of β-globin, such as β-thalassemia (see later section), strategies to increase the normally small amount of γ-globin (and therefore of Hb F $[\alpha_2\gamma_2]$) produced in adults are proving to be successful in ameliorating the disorder (see Chapter 14).

The Developmental Regulation of β-Globin Gene Expression: The Locus Control Region

Elucidation of the mechanisms that control expression of the globin genes has provided generalizable insights into both normal and pathologic biologic processes. The expression of the β-globin gene is only partly controlled by the **promoter** and two **enhancers** in the immediate flanking DNA (see Chapter 3). A requirement for additional regulatory elements was first suggested by the identification of individuals who had no gene expression from any of the genes in the β-globin cluster, even though the genes themselves (including their individual regulatory elements) were intact. These informative patients were found to have large deletions upstream of the β-globin complex that removed an ~20 **kb** domain—now called the **locus control region** (LCR), located ~6 kb upstream of the ε-globin gene (Fig. 12.4). The resulting disease, εγδβ-thalassemia, is described later in this chapter. These cases show us that the LCR is required for the expression of all genes in the β-globin cluster.

The LCR is defined by five DNase I hypersensitive sites (see Fig. 12.4): genomic regions that are unusually open to certain proteins (including the enzyme DNase I) used experimentally to reveal potential regulatory sites. Within the context of the **epigenetic** packaging of **chromatin** (see Chapter 3), these sites maintain an open chromatin

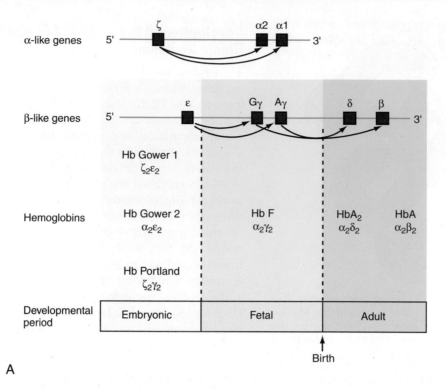

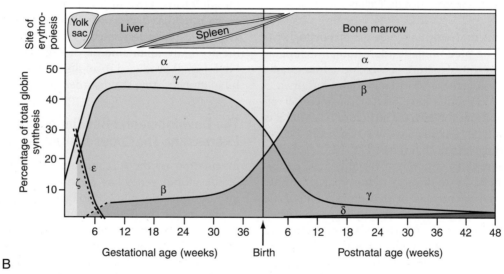

Figure 12.3 **Organization of the human globin genes and hemoglobins produced in each stage of human development.** (A) The α-like genes are on chromosome 16, the β-like genes on chromosome 11. The *curved arrows* refer to the switches in gene expression during development. (B) Development of erythropoiesis in the human fetus and infant. Types of cells responsible for hemoglobin synthesis, organs involved, and types of globin chain synthesized at successive stages are shown. (A, Redrawn from Stamatoyannopoulos G, Nienhuis AW: Hemoglobin switching. In Stamatoyannopoulos G, Nienhuis AW, Leder P, et al, editors: *The molecular basis of blood diseases*, Philadelphia, 1987, WB Saunders; B, redrawn from Wood WG: Haemoglobin synthesis during fetal development, *Br Med Bull* 32:282–287, 1976.)

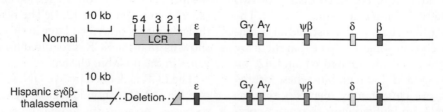

Figure 12.4 **The β-globin locus control region (LCR).** Each of the five regions of open chromatin *(arrows)* contains several consensus binding sites for both erythroid-specific and ubiquitous transcription factors. The precise mechanism by which the LCR regulates gene expression is unknown. Also shown is a deletion of the LCR that has led to εγδβ-thalassemia, which is discussed in the text. (Redrawn from Kazazian Jr HH, Antonarakis S: Molecular genetics of the globin genes. In Singer M, Berg P, editors: *Exploring genetic mechanisms*, Sausalito, 1997, University Science Books.)

configuration that gives **transcription factors** access to the regulatory elements that mediate the expression of each of the β-globin genes in erythroid cells (see Chapter 3). The LCR, along with its associated DNA-binding proteins, interacts with the genes of the β-globin locus to form a nuclear domain called the **active chromatin hub**, where β-globin gene expression takes place. The sequential switching of gene expression that occurs among the five members of the β-globin gene complex during development results from the sequential association of the active chromatin hub with the different genes in the cluster, as the hub moves from the most proximal gene in the complex (the ε-globin gene in embryos) to the most distal (the δ- and β-globin genes in adults).

The clinical significance of the LCR could extend beyond those individuals with deletions of the LCR who fail to express the genes of the β-globin cluster. Components of the LCR may prove relevant to gene therapy (see Chapter 14) for disorders of the β-globin cluster, wherein a goal is for the therapeutic normal copy of the gene in question to be expressed at the correct time in life and in the appropriate tissue. Knowledge of the molecular mechanisms that underlie globin switching may also make it feasible to up-regulate the expression of the γ-globin gene in those with β-thalassemia (who have variants only in the β-globin gene) because Hb F ($\alpha_2\gamma_2$) is an effective oxygen carrier in adults who lack Hb A ($\alpha_2\beta_2$) (see Chapter 14).

Gene Dosage, Developmental Expression of the Globins, and Clinical Disease

The differences, both in the gene dosage of the α- and β-globins (four α-globin and two β-globin genes per **diploid genome**) and in their patterns of expression during development, are important to an understanding of the pathogenesis of many hemoglobinopathies. A variant in a β-globin gene affects 50% of the β chains, whereas a single α-chain variant affects only 25% of the α chains. β-globin variants have no prenatal consequences because γ-globin is the major β-like globin before birth, with Hb F constituting 75% of the total hemoglobin at term (see

Fig. 12.3B). In contrast, because α chains are the only α-like components of hemoglobin 6 weeks after conception, α-globin variants cause severe disease in both fetal and postnatal life.

THE HEMOGLOBINOPATHIES

Hereditary disorders of hemoglobin can be divided into the following three broad groups, which, in some rare instances, overlap:

- Structural alterations of the amino acid sequence of the globin polypeptide, altering properties such as its ability to transport oxygen, or reducing its stability. An example is sickle cell disease (Case 42) due to a missense variant that makes deoxygenated β-globin relatively insoluble, changing the shape of the red cell (Fig. 12.5).
- Thalassemias, which are diseases that result from the decreased abundance of one or more of the globin chains (Case 44). The decrease can result from reduced production of a globin chain or, less commonly, from a variant that destabilizes the chain. The resulting imbalance in the ratio of the α:β chains underlies the pathophysiology of these conditions. Examples include promoter variants that decrease expression of the β-globin mRNA to cause β-thalassemia.
- Hereditary persistence of fetal hemoglobin, a group of clinically benign conditions that impair the perinatal switch from γ-globin to β-globin synthesis. An example of a causal variant is a deletion that removes both the δ- and β-globin genes but leads to continued postnatal expression of the γ-globin genes, to produce Hb F, which is an effective oxygen transporter (see Fig. 12.3).

Hemoglobin Structural Alterations

Most variant hemoglobins result from **single nucleotide variants** in one of the globin genes. More than 500 abnormal hemoglobins have been described, and approximately half of these are clinically significant. The hemoglobin structural alterations can be separated

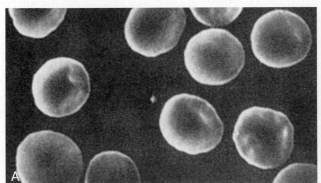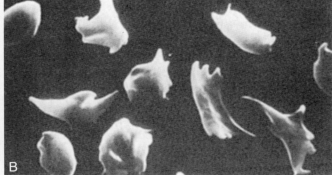

Figure 12.5 Scanning electron micrographs of red cells from a patient with sickle cell disease. (A) Oxygenated cells are round and full. (B) The classic sickle cell shape is produced only when the cells are in the deoxygenated state. (From Kaul DK, Fabry ME, Windisch P, et al: Erythrocytes in sickle cell anemia are heterogeneous in their rheological and hemodynamic characteristics, *J Clin Invest* 72:22, 1983.)

TABLE 12.3 Major Classes of Hemoglobin Structural Alterations

Class Example[a]	Amino Acid Substitution	Pathophysiological Effect of Variant	Inheritance
Hb S	β chain: p.Glu6Val	Deoxygenated Hb S polymerizes → sickle cells → vascular occlusion and hemolysis	AR
Hb Hammersmith	β chain: p.Phe42Ser	An unstable Hb → Hb precipitation → hemolysis; also low oxygen affinity	AD
Hb M-Hyde Park	β chain: p.His92Tyr	The substitution makes oxidized heme iron resistant to methemoglobin reductase → Hb M, which cannot carry oxygen → cyanosis (asymptomatic)	AD
Hb Kempsey	β chain: p.Asp99Asn	The substitution keeps the Hb in its high oxygen affinity structure → less oxygen to tissues → polycythemia	AD
Hb E	β chain: p.Glu26Lys	The variant → an abnormal Hb *and* decreased synthesis (abnormal RNA splicing) → mild thalassemia[b] (see Fig. 12.11)	AR

[a]Hemoglobin variants are often named after a location related to the first described patient(s).
[b]Additional β-chain gene variants that cause β-thalassemia are depicted in Table 12.5.
AD, Autosomal dominant; *AR*, autosomal recessive; *Hb M*, methemoglobin (See text.)

into the following three classes, depending on the clinical phenotype (Table 12.3):

- Alterations that cause hemolytic anemia, most commonly because they make the hemoglobin tetramer unstable.
- Alterations with modified oxygen transport, due to increased or decreased oxygen affinity or to the formation of **methemoglobin**—a form of globin incapable of reversible oxygenation.
- Alterations due to variants in the coding region that cause thalassemia because they reduce the abundance of a globin polypeptide. Most of these variants impair the rate of synthesis of the mRNA or otherwise affect the level of the encoded protein.

Hemolytic Anemias

Hemoglobins With Novel Physical Properties: Sickle Cell Disease. Sickle cell hemoglobin is of great clinical importance in many parts of the world, affecting millions. The causal variant is a single nucleotide substitution that changes the **codon** of the sixth amino acid of β-globin from glutamic acid to valine (GAG → GTG: p.Glu6Val) (see Table 12.3). Homozygosity for this variant is the cause of sickle cell disease (Case 42). The disease has a characteristic geographic distribution: occurring most frequently in equatorial Africa and less commonly in the Mediterranean area, India, Spanish-speaking regions in the Western Hemisphere, or in countries to which people from these regions have migrated. Approximately 1 in 400 Black persons in the United States is born with sickle cell disease.

Clinical Features. Sickle cell disease is a severe autosomal **recessive** hemolytic condition characterized by a tendency of the red blood cells to become grossly abnormal in shape (i.e., take on a sickle shape) under conditions of low oxygen tension (see Fig. 12.5). **Heterozygotes**—who are said to have sickle cell trait, are, generally, clinically unaffected, but their red cells can sickle when subjected to very low oxygen pressure. Occasions when this occurs are uncommon, although heterozygotes appear to be at **risk** for splenic infarction, especially at high altitude (e.g., in airplanes with reduced cabin pressure) or when exerting themselves to extreme levels in athletic competition. The heterozygous state is present in ~8% of Black individuals in the United States, but in areas where the sickle cell allele (β^S) frequency is high (e.g., West Central Africa), up to 25% of the newborn population is heterozygous for the allele.

The Molecular Pathology of Hb S. In the 1950s, Vernon Ingram discovered that the abnormality in sickle cell hemoglobin was a replacement of one of the 146 amino acids in the β chain of the hemoglobin molecule. All the clinical manifestations of sickle cell hemoglobin are consequences of this single change in the β-globin gene. Ingram's discovery was the first demonstration in any organism that a variant in a **structural gene** could cause an amino acid substitution in the corresponding protein. Because the substitution is in the β-globin chain, the formula for sickle cell hemoglobin is written as $\alpha_2\beta_2^S$ or, more precisely, $\alpha_2 A\beta_2^S$. A heterozygote has a mixture of the two types of hemoglobin, A and S, summarized as $\alpha_2 A\beta_2 A/\alpha_2 A\beta_2^S$, as well as a hybrid hemoglobin tetramer, written as $\alpha_2 A\beta A\beta^S$. Strong evidence indicates that the sickle cell variant arose in West Africa, but that it occurred independently elsewhere. The β^S allele has attained high frequency in malaria endemic areas of the world because it confers protection against malaria in heterozygotes (see Chapter 10).

Sickling and Its Consequences. The molecular and cellular pathology of sickle cell disease is summarized in Fig. 12.6. Hemoglobin molecules containing the altered β-globin subunits are normal in their ability to perform their principal function of binding oxygen (provided they have not polymerized, as described next), but in deoxygenated blood they are only one-fifth as soluble as normal hemoglobin. Under conditions of low oxygen tension, this relative insolubility of deoxyhemoglobin S causes the sickle hemoglobin molecules to aggregate in the form of rod-shaped polymers or fibers (see Fig. 12.6). These molecular rods distort the $\alpha_2\beta_2^S$ erythrocytes to a sickle shape that prevents them from squeezing single file through capillaries—as do normal red cells, thereby blocking blood flow and causing local ischemia. They may also cause disruption of the red cell membrane

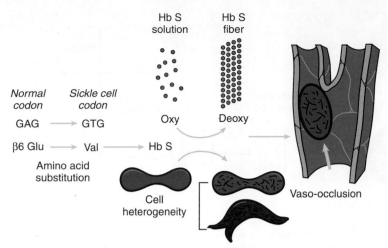

Figure 12.6 **The pathogenesis of sickle cell disease.** (Redrawn from Ingram V: Sickle cell disease: molecular and cellular pathogenesis. In Bunn HF, Forget BG, editors: *Hemoglobin: Molecular, genetic, and clinical aspects,* Philadelphia, 1986, WB Saunders.)

(hemolysis) and release of free hemoglobin, which can have deleterious effects on the availability of vasodilators, such as nitric oxide, thereby exacerbating the ischemia.

Modifier Genes Determine the Clinical Severity of Sickle Cell Disease. It has long been known that a strong modifier of the clinical severity of sickle cell disease is the patient's level of Hb F ($\alpha_2\gamma_2$), higher levels being associated with less morbidity and lower mortality. The physiologic basis of the ameliorating effect of Hb F is clear: Hb F is a perfectly adequate oxygen carrier in postnatal life and inhibits the polymerization of deoxyhemoglobin S.

Until recently, however, it was not certain whether the variation in Hb F expression was heritable. Genome-wide association studies (GWAS) (see Chapter 11) have demonstrated that single nucleotide variants (SNPs) at three polymorphic loci (SNPs)—the γ-globin gene and two genes that encode transcription factors, BCL11A and MYB—account for 40 to 50% of the variation in the levels of Hb F in individuals with sickle cell disease. Moreover, the Hb F–associated SNPs are associated with the painful clinical episodes thought to be due to capillary occlusion caused by sickled red cells (see Fig. 12.6). Individuals with heterozygous loss-of-function variants in *BCL11A* (gene) have a rare neurogenetic disorder but also hereditary persistence of fetal hemoglobin.

The genetically driven variations in the level of Hb F are also associated with variation in the clinical severity of β-thalassemia (discussed later) because the reduced abundance of β-globin (and thus of Hb A [$\alpha_2\beta_2$]) in that disease is partly alleviated by higher levels of γ-globin and, thus, of Hb F ($\alpha_2\gamma_2$). The discovery of these genetic modifiers of Hb F abundance not only explains much of the variation in the clinical severity of sickle cell disease and β-thalassemia, but highlights a general principle introduced in Chapter 9: modifier genes can play a major role in determining the clinical and physiologic severity of a single-gene disorder.

BCL11A, a Silencer of γ-Globin Gene Expression in Adult Erythroid Cells. The identification of genetic modifiers of Hb F levels, particularly BCL11A, has opened great therapeutic potential. The product of the *BCL11A* gene is a transcription factor that normally silences γ-globin expression, thus shutting down Hb F production postnatally. Accordingly, drugs that suppress BCL11A activity postnatally, thereby increasing the expression of Hb F, might be of great benefit to those with sickle cell disease and β-thalassemia (see Chapter 14). In addition, preliminary clinical trial data suggest that post-transcriptional genetic silencing of *BCL11A* may be an effective treatment for sickle cell disease.

Trisomy 13, MicroRNAs, and MYB—Another Silencer of γ-Globin Gene Expression. The indication from GWAS that MYB is an important regulator of γ-globin expression has received further support from an unexpected direction: studies investigating the basis for the persistent increased postnatal expression of Hb F that is observed in individuals with trisomy 13 (see Chapter 6). Two miRNAs, miR-15a and miR-16-1, directly target the 3′ **untranslated region (UTR)** of the *MYB* mRNA, thereby reducing *MYB* expression. The genes for these two miRNAs are located on chromosome 13; their extra dosage in trisomy 13 is predicted to reduce *MYB* expression to below normal levels, thereby partly relaxing the postnatal suppression of γ-globin gene expression normally mediated by the MYB protein. This leads to increased expression of Hb F (Fig. 12.7).

Unstable Hemoglobins. The unstable hemoglobins are due largely to single nucleotide variants that cause denaturation of the hemoglobin tetramer in mature red blood cells. The denatured globin tetramers are insoluble and precipitate to form inclusions (Heinz bodies) that damage the red cell membrane and cause hemolysis of mature red blood cells in the vascular tree (Fig. 12.8, showing a Heinz body due to β-thalassemia).

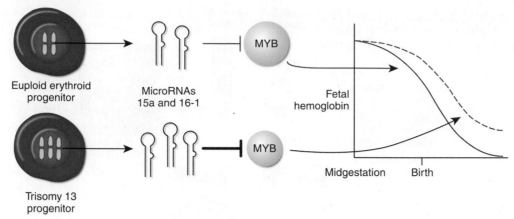

Figure 12.7 **A model demonstrating how elevations of microRNAs 15a and 16-1 in trisomy 13 can result in elevated fetal hemoglobin expression.** The basal level of these microRNAs moderates expression of targets such as the *MYB* gene during erythropoiesis. In the case of trisomy 13, elevated levels of these microRNAs result in additional down-regulation of MYB expression, which in turn results in a delayed switch from fetal to adult hemoglobin and persistent expression of fetal hemoglobin. (Redrawn from Orkin SH: Disorders of hemoglobin synthesis: The thalassemias. In Stamatoyannopoulos G, Nienhuis AW, Leder P, et al, editors: *The molecular basis of blood diseases*, Philadelphia, 1987, WB Saunders, pp. 106–126.)

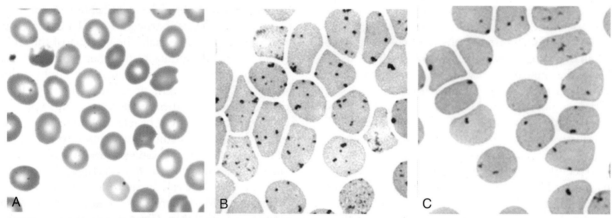

Figure 12.8 **Visualization of one pathologic effect of the deficiency of β chains in β-thalassemia: the precipitation of the excess normal α chains to form a Heinz body in the red blood cell.** Peripheral blood smear and Heinz body preparation. The peripheral smear (A) shows "bite" cells with pitted-out semicircular areas of the red blood cell membrane as a result of removal of Heinz bodies by macrophages in the spleen, causing premature destruction of the red cell. The Heinz body preparation (B) shows increased Heinz bodies in the same specimen when compared to a control (C). (From Hoffman R, Furie B, McGlave P, et al: *Hematology: Basic principles and practice*, ed 5, 2008, Elsevier.)

The amino acid substitution in the unstable hemoglobin, Hb Hammersmith (β-chain p.Phe42Ser; see Table 12.3), leads to denaturation of the tetramer and consequent hemolysis. This variant is notable because the substituted phenylalanine residue is one of the two amino acids that are conserved in all globins in nature (see Fig. 12.2). It is, therefore, not surprising that substitutions of this phenylalanine produce serious alterations in hemoglobin function. In normal β-globin, the bulky phenylalanine wedges the heme into a "pocket" in the folded β-globin monomer. Its replacement by serine, a smaller residue, creates a gap that allows the heme to slip out of its pocket. In addition to its instability, Hb Hammersmith has a low oxygen affinity, which can cause cyanosis in heterozygotes carriers.

In contrast to variants that destabilize the tetramer, other variants destabilize the globin monomer and never

form the tetramer, causing chain imbalance and thalassemia (see following section).

Variants With Altered Oxygen Transport

Variants that alter the ability of hemoglobin to transport oxygen, although rare, are of general interest because they illustrate how a variant can impair one function of a protein (in this case, oxygen binding and release) and yet leave the other properties of the protein relatively intact. For example, the variants that affect oxygen transport generally have little or no effect on hemoglobin stability.

Methemoglobins. Oxyhemoglobin is the form of hemoglobin that is capable of reversible oxygenation; its heme iron is in the reduced (or ferrous) state. The heme iron tends to oxidize spontaneously to the ferric form and the resulting molecule—referred to as methemoglobin, is incapable of reversible oxygenation. If significant amounts of methemoglobin accumulate in the blood, cyanosis results. Maintenance of the heme iron in the reduced state is the role of the enzyme, methemoglobin reductase. In several altered globins (either α or β), substitutions in the region of the heme pocket affect the heme-globin bond in a way that makes the iron resistant to the reductase. Although heterozygotes for these abnormal hemoglobins are cyanotic (a sign), they are asymptomatic. The homozygous state is presumably lethal. One example of a β-chain methemoglobin is Hb Hyde Park (see Table 12.3), in which the conserved histidine (p.His92 in Fig. 12.2) to which heme is covalently bound has been replaced by tyrosine (p.His92Tyr).

Hemoglobins With Altered Oxygen Affinity. Variants that alter oxygen affinity demonstrate the importance of subunit interaction for the normal function of a multimeric protein such as hemoglobin. In the Hb A tetramer, the α:β interface has been highly conserved throughout evolution. It is subject to significant movement between the chains when the hemoglobin shifts from the oxygenated (relaxed) to the deoxygenated (tense) form of the molecule. Substitutions in residues at this interface, exemplified by the β-globin **mutant** Hb Kempsey (see Table 12.3), prevent the normal oxygen-related movement between the chains; the variant "locks" the hemoglobin into the high oxygen affinity state, reducing oxygen delivery to tissues and causing polycythemia.

Thalassemia: An Imbalance of Globin-Chain Synthesis

The thalassemias are collectively the most common human single-gene disorders in the world (Case 44). They are a heterogeneous group of diseases of hemoglobin synthesis in which variants reduce the synthesis or stability of either the α-globin or β-globin chain to cause α-thalassemia or β-thalassemia, respectively. The resulting imbalance in the ratio of the α:β chains underlies the pathophysiology. The chain that is produced at the normal rate is in relative excess; in the absence of a complementary chain with which to form a tetramer, the excess normal chains eventually precipitate in the cell, damaging the membrane and leading to premature red blood cell destruction. The excess β or β-like chains are insoluble and precipitate in both red cell precursors (causing ineffective erythropoiesis) and in mature red cells (causing hemolysis) because they damage the cell membrane. The result is anemia (lack of red blood cells) in which the red cells are both hypochromic (i.e., pale red cells) and microcytic (i.e., small red cells).

The name thalassemia (from the Greek *thalassa*, sea) was first used to signify that the disease was discovered in persons of Mediterranean origin. Both α-thalassemia and β-thalassemia, however, have a high frequency in many populations; α-thalassemia is more prevalent and more widely distributed. The high frequency of thalassemia is due to the protective advantage against malaria that it confers on carriers, analogous to the **heterozygote advantage** of sickle cell hemoglobin carriers (see Chapter 10). There is a characteristic distribution of the thalassemias in a band around the Old World—in the Mediterranean, the Middle East, and parts of Africa, India, and Asia.

An important clinical consideration is that alleles for both types of thalassemia, as well as for structural alterations in hemoglobin, do often coexist in an individual. As a result, interactions may occur among different alleles of the same globin gene, or among variant alleles of different globin genes.

The α-Thalassemias

Genetic disorders of α-globin production disrupt the formation of both fetal and adult hemoglobins (see Fig. 12.3), causing intrauterine as well as postnatal disease. In the absence of α-globin chains with which to associate, the chains from the β-globin cluster are free to form a homotetrameric hemoglobin. Hemoglobin with a γ_4 composition is known as Hb Barts, and the β_4 tetramer is called Hb H. Because neither of these hemoglobins is capable of releasing oxygen to tissues under normal conditions, they are completely ineffective oxygen carriers. Consequently, fetuses with severe α-thalassemia and high levels of Hb Barts suffer severe intrauterine hypoxia and develop massive generalized fluid accumulation: a condition called hydrops fetalis. In milder α-thalassemias, an anemia develops because of the gradual precipitation of the Hb H in the erythrocyte. The formation of Hb H inclusions in mature red cells and the removal of these inclusions by the spleen damages the cells, leading to their premature destruction.

Deletions of the α-Globin Genes. The most common molecular causes of α-thalassemia are gene deletions. The high frequency of deletions in the α-chain genes, compared with, for example, the β-chain genes, is a consequence of having two identical α-globin genes on each chromosome 16 (see Fig. 12.3A). This arrangement of tandem **homologous** α-globin genes facilitates misalignment, due to homologous pairing and subsequent recombination between the α1 gene domain on one chromosome and the corresponding α2 gene region on the other (Fig. 12.9). Evidence supporting this pathogenic mechanism of nonallelic homologous recombination is provided by reports of individuals with a triplicated α-globin gene complex. Deletions or other alterations of one, two, three, or all four copies of the α-globin gene cause a proportionately severe hematologic abnormality (Table 12.4).

Individuals with two normal and two abnormal α-globin genes are said to have α-thalassemia trait.

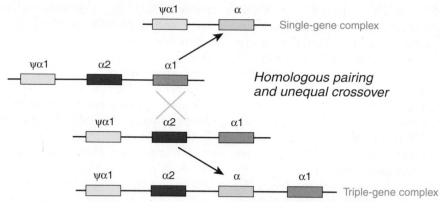

Figure 12.9 The probable mechanism underlying the most common form of α-thalassemia, which is due to deletions of one of the two α-globin genes on a chromosome 16. Misalignment, homologous pairing, and recombination between the α1 gene on one chromosome and the α2 gene on the homologous chromosome result in the deletion of one α-globin gene. (Redrawn from Kazazian HH: The thalassemia syndromes: Molecular basis and prenatal diagnosis in 1990, *Semin Hematol* 27:209–228, 1990.)

TABLE 12.4 Clinical States Associated With α-Thalassemia Genotypes

Clinical Condition	Number of Functional α Genes	α-Globin Gene Genotype	α-Chain Production
"Normal"	4	αα/αα	100%
Silent carrier	3	αα/α−	75%
α-Thalassemia trait (mild anemia, microcytosis)	2	α−/α− or αα/−−	50%
Hb H (β₄) disease (moderately severe hemolytic anemia)	1	α−/−−	25%
Hydrops fetalis or homozygous α-thalassemia (Hb Barts: γ₄)	0	−−/−−	0%

This can result from either of two genotypes (−−/αα or −α/−α), differing in whether the deletions are in *cis* or in **trans**. The α-thalassemia trait is distributed throughout the world. However, heterozygosity for deletion of both copies of the α-globin gene in *cis* (−−/αα genotype) is largely restricted to Southeast Asians. Offspring of two carriers of this deletion allele may receive two −−/−− chromosomes, leading to Hb Barts (γ₄) and hydrops fetalis. In other populations, however, α-thalassemia trait is usually the result of the *trans* −α/−α genotype, which cannot give rise to −−/−− offspring.

In addition to α-thalassemia variants that result in deletion of the α-globin genes, variants that delete only the LCR of the α-globin complex can cause α-thalassemia. In fact, similar to the observations with respect to the β-globin LCR, such deletions were critical for demonstrating the existence of this regulatory element at the α-globin locus.

Other Forms of α-Thalassemia. In all the classes of α-thalassemia described earlier, deletions in the α-globin genes or variants in their *cis*-acting **sequences** account for the reduction of α-globin synthesis. Other types of α-thalassemia occur much less commonly. One important rare form of α-thalassemia is ATR-X syndrome, which is associated with both α-thalassemia and intellectual disability. It illustrates the importance of epigenetic packaging of the genome in the regulation of gene expression (see Chapters 3 and 8). The **X chromosome**

ATRX gene encodes a **chromatin remodeling** protein that functions, in *trans*, to activate the expression of the α-globin genes. The ATRX protein belongs to a family of proteins that function within large multiprotein complexes to change DNA topology. ATR-X syndrome is one of several monogenic diseases that result from variants in chromatin remodeling proteins (chromatinopathies; see Chapter 8).

ATR-X syndrome was initially recognized as unusual because the first families in which it was identified were northern Europeans, a population in which the deletion forms of α-thalassemia are uncommon. All affected individuals were males with severe intellectual disability, together with a wide range of other abnormalities, including characteristic facial features, skeletal defects, and urogenital malformations. This diversity of phenotypes suggests that ATRX regulates the expression of numerous other genes besides the α-globins.

In those with ATR-X syndrome, the reduction in α-globin synthesis is due to accumulation at the α-globin gene cluster of a histone variant (see Chapter 3) called macroH2A. This accumulation reduces α-globin gene expression and causes α-thalassemia. To date, all variants in the *ATRX* gene associated with ATR-X syndrome involve partial loss of function, leading to hematologic defects that are mild, compared with those seen in the classic forms of α-thalassemia.

Individuals with ATR-X syndrome have abnormalities in **DNA methylation** patterns to indicate that the

ATRX protein is also required to establish or maintain the methylation pattern in certain domains of the genome. This may be by modulating access of the DNA methyltransferase enzyme to its binding sites. This finding is noteworthy because variants in *MECP2*, which encodes a protein that binds to methylated DNA, cause Rett syndrome (Case 40) by disrupting the epigenetic regulation of genes in regions of methylated DNA, leading to neurodevelopmental regression. Normally, ATRX and the MeCP2 protein interact; impairment of this interaction due to ATRX variants may contribute to the intellectual disability seen in ATR-X syndrome.

The β-Thalassemias

The β-thalassemias share many features with α-thalassemia. In β-thalassemia, the decrease in β-globin production causes a hypochromic, microcytic anemia. An imbalance in globin synthesis is due to the excess of α chains. The latter are insoluble and precipitate (see Fig. 12.8) in both red cell precursors (causing ineffective erythropoiesis) and mature red cells (causing hemolysis) because they damage the cell membrane. In contrast to α-globin, however, the β chain is important only in the postnatal period. Consequently, the onset of β-thalassemia is not apparent until a few months after birth, when β-globin normally replaces γ-globin as the major non–α chain (see Fig. 12.3B). Only the synthesis of the major adult hemoglobin, Hb A, is reduced. The level of Hb F is increased in β-thalassemia, not because of a reactivation of the γ-globin gene expression that was switched off at birth, but because of selective survival and perhaps increased production of the minor population of adult red blood cells that contain Hb F.

In contrast to α-thalassemia, the β-thalassemias are usually due to single nucleotide variants rather than to deletions (Table 12.5). In many regions of the world where β-thalassemia is common, there are so many different β-thalassemia variants that individuals with this condition are more likely to be **compound heterozygotes** (i.e., carrying two different β-thalassemia alleles) than to be **homozygotes** for one allele. Most individuals with two β-thalassemia alleles have thalassemia major: a condition characterized by severe anemia and the need for lifelong medical management. When the β-thalassemia alleles allow so little production of β-globin that no Hb A is present, the condition is designated β^0-thalassemia. Clinically, affected individuals are dependent on red blood cell transfusions. If some Hb A is detectable, the affected individual has β^+-thalassemia. Although the severity of the clinical disease depends on the combined effect of the two alleles present, until recently, survival into adult life was unusual.

Infants with homozygous β-thalassemia present with anemia once the postnatal production of Hb F decreases—generally before 2 years of age. At present, in most countries, treatment of the thalassemias is based on correction of the anemia and the increased marrow expansion by blood transfusion; the consequent excess iron accumulation is controlled by administration of chelating agents. Bone marrow transplantation is effective, but this is an option only if an HLA-matched family member can be found. Gene therapy options are now emerging in clinical practice (see Chapter 14).

Carriers of one β-thalassemia allele are clinically well and are said to have thalassemia minor. Such individuals have hypochromic, microcytic red blood cells

TABLE 12.5 The Molecular Basis of Some Causes of Simple β-Thalassemia

Type	Example								Phenotype
RNA splicing defects (see Fig. 12.11C)	Abnormal acceptor site of intron 1: AG → GG								β^0
Promoter variants	Variant in the ATA box								β^+
	−31	−30	−29	−28		−31	−30	−29	−28
	A	T	A	A	→	G	T	A	A
Abnormal RNA cap site	A → C transversion at the mRNA cap site								β^+
Polyadenylation signal defects	AATAAA → AACAAA								β^+
Nonsense variants	Codon 39								β^0
	gln → stop								
	CAG → UAG								
Frameshift variants	Codon 16 (1 bp deletion)								β^0
	Normal	trp	gly	lys	val	asn			
		15	16	17	18	19			
		UGG	GGC	AAG	GUG	AAC			
		UGG	GCA	AGG	UGA				
	Variant	trp	ala	arg	stop				
Synonymous variants	Codon 24								β^+
	gly → gly								
	GGU → GGA								

Derived in part from Weatherall DJ, Clegg JB, Higgs DR, et al: The hemoglobinopathies. In Scriver CR, Beaudet AL, Sly WS, et al, editors: *The metabolic and molecular bases of inherited disease*, ed 7, New York, 1995, McGraw-Hill, pp. 3417–3484; Orkin SH: Disorders of hemoglobin synthesis: the thalassemias. In Stamatoyannopoulos G, Nienhuis AW, Leder P, et al, editors: *The molecular basis of blood diseases*, Philadelphia, 1987, WB Saunders, pp. 106–126.
[a]One other hemoglobin structural variant that causes β-thalassemia is shown in Table 12.3.
mRNA, Messenger RNA.

and may have a slight anemia that can be misdiagnosed initially as iron deficiency. The diagnosis of thalassemia minor can be supported by hemoglobin electrophoresis, which generally reveals an increase in the level of Hb A_2 ($\alpha_2\delta_2$). In many countries, thalassemia minor is sufficiently common to require diagnostic distinction from iron deficiency anemia and to be a frequent source of referral for prenatal diagnosis of affected homozygous fetuses (see Chapter 18).

α-Thalassemia Alleles as Modifier Genes of β-Thalassemia. In human genetics, one of the best examples of a modifier gene comes from co-existence of β-thalassemia and α-thalassemia alleles in a population. In such populations, β-thalassemia homozygotes may also inherit an α-thalassemia allele. The clinical severity of the β-thalassemia is sometimes ameliorated by the presence of the α-thalassemia allele, which acts as a modifier. The imbalance of globin chain synthesis that occurs in β-thalassemia (due to the relative excess of α chains) is reduced by the decrease in α-chain production that results from the α-thalassemia gene deletion.

β-Thalassemia, Complex Thalassemias, and Hereditary Persistence of Fetal Hemoglobin. Almost every type of DNA variant known to reduce the synthesis of an mRNA or protein has been identified as a cause of β-thalassemia. The following overview of these genetic defects is, therefore, instructive about variant mechanisms in general, by describing the molecular basis of one of the most common and severe genetic diseases in the world. Variants of

the β-globin gene complex are separated into two broad groups with different clinical phenotypes. One group, which accounts for the great majority of patients, impairs the production of β-globin alone and causes simple β-thalassemia. The second group consists of large deletions that cause the complex thalassemias, in which the β-globin gene is removed, as well as one or more of the other genes—or the LCR—in the β-globin cluster. Finally, we are informed about the regulation of globin gene expression through some deletions within the β-globin cluster that do not cause thalassemia, but rather, a benign phenotype termed the hereditary persistence of fetal hemoglobin (i.e., the persistence of γ-globin gene expression throughout adult life).

Molecular Basis of Simple β-Thalassemia. Simple β-thalassemia results from a remarkable diversity of molecular defects, predominantly single nucleotide variants, in the β-globin gene (Fig. 12.10; see Table 12.5). Most variants causing simple β-thalassemia lead to a decrease in the abundance of the β-globin mRNA. These include promoter variants, **RNA splicing** variants (the most common), mRNA capping or tailing variants, and frameshift or nonsense variants that introduce premature **termination codons** within the coding region of the gene. A few hemoglobin structural alterations also impair processing of the β-globin mRNA, as exemplified by Hb E (described later).

RNA Splicing Variants. Most β-thalassemia cases with a decreased abundance of β-globin mRNA have abnormalities in RNA splicing. Dozens of defects of

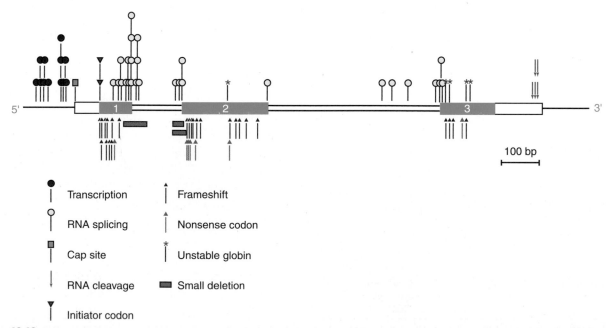

Figure 12.10 Representative point variants and small deletions that cause β-thalassemia. Note the distribution of variants throughout the gene and that the variants affect virtually every process required for the production of normal β-globin. More than 100 different β-globin point variants are associated with simple β-thalassemia.

this type have been described, and their combined clinical burden is substantial. These variants have acquired high visibility because their effects on **splicing** are often unexpectedly complex, and analysis of the altered mRNAs has contributed extensively to knowledge of the sequences critical to normal RNA processing (introduced in Chapter 3). The splice defects are separated into three groups (Fig. 12.11) depending on the region of the unprocessed RNA in which the variant is located.

- Splice junction variants include those at the canonical 5′ donor or 3′ acceptor splice junctions of the **introns** or in the **consensus sequences** surrounding the junctions. The critical nature of the conserved GT dinucleotide at the 5′ intron donor site and of the AG at the 3′ intron acceptor site (see Chapter 3) is demonstrated by the complete loss of normal splicing that results from variants in these dinucleotides (see Fig. 12.11B). Inactivation of the normal acceptor site elicits the use of other acceptor-like sequences elsewhere in the RNA precursor molecule. These alternative sites are termed **cryptic splice sites** because they are not used by the splicing apparatus if the correct site is available. Cryptic donor or **acceptor splice sites** can be found in either exons or introns.

- Intronic variants enhance the use of a cryptic splice site by making it more similar or identical to the normal splice site. The activated cryptic site then competes with the normal site, with variable effectiveness. This reduces the abundance of the normal mRNA by decreasing splicing from the correct site, which remains perfectly intact (see Fig. 12.11C). Cryptic splice site variants are often leaky, which means that some use of the normal site occurs, producing a β+-thalassemia phenotype.

- Coding sequence changes that affect splicing result from variants in the **open reading frame** that activate a cryptic splice site in an exon, whether or not they also change the amino acid sequence (see Fig. 12.11D). For example, a mild form of β+-thalassemia results from a variant in codon 24 (see Table 12.5) that activates a cryptic splice site but does not change the encoded amino acid (both GGT and GGA code for glycine [see Table 3.1]); this is an example of a **synonymous** variant that is not neutral in its effect.

Nonfunctional mRNAs. Some mRNAs are nonfunctional and cannot direct the synthesis of a complete polypeptide, because the variant generates a premature **stop codon**, which prematurely terminates **translation**. Two β-thalassemia variants near the amino terminus exemplify this effect (see Table 12.5). In one (p. Gln39Ter), the failure in translation is due to a single nucleotide substitution that creates a nonsense variant. In the other, a frameshift variant results from a single **base pair** deletion early in the open **reading frame**, removing the first nucleotide from codon 16, which normally encodes glycine. In the reading frame that results, a premature stop codon is quickly encountered downstream, well before the normal termination signal. Because no β-globin is made from these alleles, both types of nonfunctional mRNA variants cause β0-thalassemia in the homozygous state. In some instances, frameshifts near the carboxyl terminus of the protein allow most of the mRNA to be translated normally or to produce elongated globin chains, resulting in a variant hemoglobin rather than null alleles.

In addition to ablating the production of the β-globin polypeptide, premature stop variants, including the two described earlier, often lead to reduced abundance of the abnormal mRNA; indeed, the mRNA may be undetectable. The mechanism underlying this phenomenon—called **nonsense-mediated mRNA decay**, appears to be restricted to nonsense codons located more than 50 bp upstream of the final exon-exon junction.

Defects in Capping and Tailing of β-Globin mRNA. Several β+-thalassemia variants highlight the critical nature of post-transcriptional modifications of mRNAs. For example, the 3′ UTR of almost all mRNAs ends with a polyA sequence, and if this sequence is not added, the mRNA is unstable. As introduced in Chapter 3, **polyadenylation** of mRNA first requires enzymatic cleavage of the mRNA, which occurs in response to a signal for the cleavage site, AAUAAA, that is found near the 3′ end of most eukaryotic mRNAs. Individuals with a substitution that changes the signal sequence to AACAAA produce only a minor fraction of correctly polyadenylated β-globin mRNA.

Hemoglobin E: A Structurally Altered Hemoglobin With Thalassemia Phenotypes

Hb E is probably the most common structurally abnormal hemoglobin in the world, occurring at high frequency in Southeast Asia, where there are at least 1 million homozygotes and 30 million heterozygotes. Hb E is a β-globin variant (p.Glu26Lys) that reduces the rate of synthesis of the abnormal β chain. It is another example of a coding sequence variant that impairs normal splicing by activating a cryptic splice site (see Fig. 12.11D). Although Hb E homozygotes are asymptomatic and only mildly anemic, individuals who are genetic compounds of Hb E and another β-thalassemia allele have clinically relevant phenotypes that are largely determined by the severity of the other allele.

Complex Thalassemias and the Hereditary Persistence of Fetal Hemoglobin

As mentioned earlier, large deletions that cause the complex thalassemias remove the β-globin gene plus one or more other genes—or the LCR—from the β-globin cluster. Thus, affected individuals have reduced expression

Normal splicing pattern

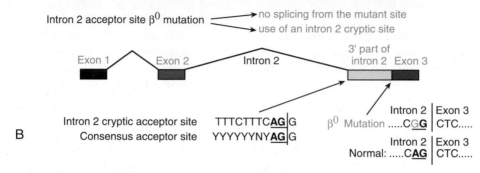

Mutation destroying a normal splice acceptor site and activating a cryptic site

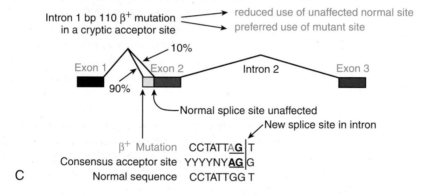

Mutation creating a new splice acceptor site in an intron

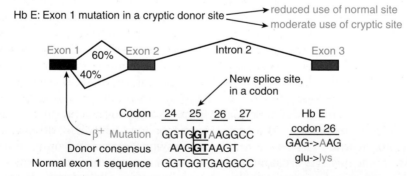

Mutation enhancing a cryptic splice donor site in an exon

Figure 12.11 **Examples of variants that disrupt normal splicing of the β-globin gene to cause β-thalassemia.** (A) Normal splicing pattern. (B) An intron 2 variant (IVS2-2A>G) in the normal splice acceptor site aborts normal splicing. This variant results in the use of a cryptic acceptor site in intron 2. The cryptic site conforms perfectly to the consensus acceptor splice sequence (where Y is either pyrimidine, T or C). Because exon 3 has been enlarged at its 5′ end by inclusion of intron 2 sequences, the abnormal alternatively spliced messenger RNA (mRNA) made from this mutant gene has lost the correct open reading frame and cannot encode β-globin. (C) An intron 1 variant (G > A in nucleotide 110 of intron 1) activates a cryptic acceptor site by creating an AG dinucleotide and increasing the resemblance of the site to the consensus acceptor sequence. The globin mRNA thus formed is elongated (19 extra nucleotides) at the 5′ side of exon 2; a premature stop codon is introduced into the transcript. A β+ thalassemia phenotype results because the correct acceptor site is still used, although at only 10% of the wild-type level. (D) In the Hb E defect, the missense variant (p.Glu26Lys) in codon 26 in exon 1 activates a cryptic donor splice site in codon 25 that competes effectively with the normal donor site. Moderate use is made of this alternative splicing pathway, but the majority of RNA is still processed from the correct site, and mild β+ thalassemia results. (Modified from Stamatoyannopoulos G, Grosveld F: Hemoglobin switching. In Stamatoyannopoulos G, Majerus PW, Perlmutter RM, et al, editors: *The molecular basis of blood diseases*, ed 3, Philadelphia, 2001, WB Saunders.)

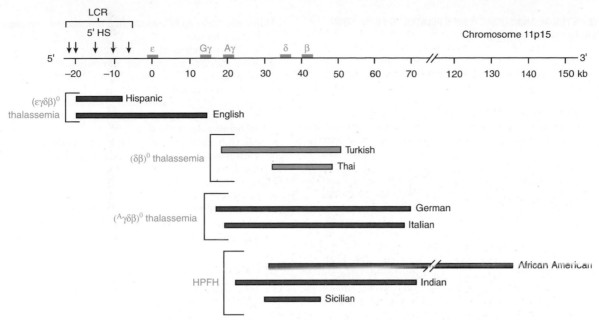

Figure 12.12 Location and size of deletions of various $(\varepsilon\gamma\delta\beta)^0$-thalassemia, $(\delta\beta)^0$-thalassemia, $(^A\gamma\delta\beta)^0$-thalassemia, and HPFH mutants. Note that deletions of the locus control region (LCR) abrogate the expression of all genes in the β-globin cluster. The deletions responsible for δβ-thalassemia, $^A\gamma\delta\beta$-thalassemia, and HPFH overlap (see text). *HPFH*, Hereditary persistence of fetal hemoglobin; *HS*, hypersensitive sites.

of β-globin and one or more of the other β-like chains. These disorders are named according to the genes deleted (e.g., $[\delta\beta]^0$-thalasscmia or $[A\gamma\delta\beta]^0$-thalassemia) (Fig. 12.12). Deletions that remove the β-globin LCR start ~50 to 100 kb upstream of the β-globin gene cluster and extend 3′ to varying degrees. Although some of these deletions (such as the Hispanic deletion shown in Fig. 12.12) leave all or some of the genes at the β-globin locus completely intact, they ablate expression from the entire cluster to cause $(\varepsilon\gamma\delta\beta)^0$-thalassemia. Such variants demonstrate the total dependence of gene expression from the β-globin gene cluster on the integrity of the LCR (see Fig. 12.4).

A second group of large β-globin gene cluster deletions of medical significance are those that leave at least one of the γ genes intact (such as the English deletion in Fig. 12.12). Individuals carrying such variants have one of two clinical manifestations, depending on the deletion: either $\delta\beta^0$-thalassemia, or a benign condition called hereditary persistence of fetal hemoglobin (HPFH) that is due to disruption of the perinatal switch from γ-globin to β-globin synthesis. Homozygotes with either of these conditions are viable because the remaining γ gene(s) are still active after birth, instead of switching off as would normally occur. As a result, Hb F ($\alpha_2\gamma_2$) synthesis continues postnatally at a high level and compensates for the absence of Hb A.

The clinically innocuous nature of HPFH that results from the substantial production of γ chains is due to a higher level of Hb F in heterozygotes (17–35% Hb F) than is generally seen in $\delta\beta^0$-thalassemia heterozygotes

(5–18% Hb F). Because the deletions that cause $\delta\beta^0$-thalassemia overlap with those that cause HPFH (see Fig. 12.12), it is not clear why patients with HPFH have higher levels of γ gene expression. One possibility is that some HPFH deletions bring enhancers closer to the γ-globin genes. Insight into the role of regulators of Hb F expression, such as BCL11A and MYB (see earlier discussion), has been partly derived from the study of individuals with complex deletions of the β-globin gene cluster. For example, the study of several individuals with HPFH due to rare deletions of the β-globin gene cluster identified a 3.5 kb region, near the 5′ end of the δ-globin gene, that contains binding sites for BCL11A, the critical **silencer** of Hb F expression in the adult.

Public Health Approaches to Preventing Thalassemia

Large-Scale Population Screening. The clinical severity of many forms of thalassemia, combined with their high frequency, imposes a tremendous health burden on many societies. To reduce the high incidence of the disease in some parts of the world, governments have introduced successful thalassemia control programs based on offering or requiring thalassemia carrier screening of individuals of childbearing age in the population (see Box 12.1). As a result of such programs, in many parts of the Mediterranean, the birth rate of affected newborns has been reduced by as much as 90%, through programs of education directed both to the general population and to health care providers.

Worldwide, approximately 70,000 infants are born each year with β-thalassemia, at high economic cost to health care systems and at great emotional cost to affected families.

To identify individuals and families at increased risk for the disease, screening is done in many countries. National and international guidelines recommend that screening not be compulsory and that education and **genetic counseling** should inform decision making.

Widely differing cultural, religious, economic, and social factors significantly influence the adherence to guidelines. For example:

In Sardinia, a program initiated in 1975 involves voluntary screening, followed by testing of the extended family once a carrier is identified.

In Greece, screening is voluntary, is available both premaritally and prenatally, requires informed consent, is widely advertised by the mass media and in military and school programs, and is accompanied by genetic counseling for carrier couples.

In Iran and Turkey, these practices differ only in that screening is mandatory premaritally (but in all countries with mandatory screening, carrier couples have the right to marry if they wish).

Major obstacles to more effective population screening for β-thalassemia.

The principal obstacles include the facts that pregnant individuals may feel overwhelmed by the array of tests offered to them, many health professionals have insufficient knowledge of genetic disorders, appropriate education and counseling are costly and time consuming, it is commonly misunderstood that informing an individual about a test is equivalent to obtaining consent, and the effectiveness of mass education varies greatly, depending on the community or country.

The effectiveness of well-executed β-thalassemia screening programs.

In populations where β-thalassemia screening has been effectively implemented, the reduction in the incidence of the disease has been striking. For example, in Sardinia, screening between 1975 and 1995 reduced the incidence from 1 per 250 to 1 per 4000 individuals. Similarly, in Cyprus, the incidence of affected births fell from 51 in 1974 to none up to 2007.

[a]Based on Cousens NE, Gaff CL, Metcalfe SA, et al: Carrier screening for β-thalassaemia: A review of international practice, *Eur J Hum Genet* 18:1077–1083, 2010.

Screening Restricted to Extended Families. The initiation of screening programs for thalassemia can be a major economic and logistical challenge. However, work in Pakistan and Saudi Arabia has demonstrated the effectiveness of a screening strategy that may be broadly applicable in countries where consanguineous marriages are common. In the Rawalpindi region of Pakistan, β-thalassemia was found to be largely restricted to a specific group of families that came to attention because there was an identifiable index case (see Chapter 7). In 10 extended families with such an **index case,** testing of almost 600 persons established that ~8% of the married couples examined consisted of two carriers; outside of these 10 families, no couple at risk was identified among 350 randomly selected pregnant people and their partners. All carriers reported that the information provided was used to avoid further pregnancy if they already had two or more healthy children or, for couples with only one or no healthy children, for prenatal diagnosis. Although the long-term impact of this program must be established, extended family screening of this type may contribute importantly to the control of recessive diseases in parts of the world where a cultural preference for consanguineous marriage is present. In other words, because of **consanguinity,** disease gene variants are trapped within extended families, so that an affected child indicates an extended family at high risk for the disease.

The initiation of carrier testing and prenatal diagnosis programs for thalassemia requires not only the education of the public and of physicians but the establishment of skilled central laboratories and the consensus of the population to be screened (see Box). Whereas population-wide programs to control thalassemia are inarguably less expensive than the cost of lifetime care for a large population of affected individuals, the temptation for governments or physicians to pressure individuals into accepting such programs must be avoided. The autonomy of the individual in reproductive decision making—a bedrock of modern bioethics, and the cultural and religious views of their communities must be respected.

GENERAL REFERENCES

Higgs DR, Engel JD, Stamatoyannopoulos G: Thalassaemia, *Lancet* 379:373–383, 2012.

Higgs DR, Gibbons RJ: The molecular basis of α-thalassemia: a model for understanding human molecular genetics, *Hematol Oncol Clin North Am* 24:1033–1054, 2010.

McCavit TL: Sickle cell disease, *Pediatr Rev* 33:195–204, 2012.

Roseff SD: Sickle cell disease: a review, *Immunohematol* 25:67–74, 2009.

Taher AT, Musallam KM, Cappellini MD: β-thalassemias, *N Engl J Med* 384:727–743, 2021.

Weatherall DJ: The role of the inherited disorders of hemoglobin, the first "molecular diseases," in the future of human genetics, *Annu Rev Genomics Hum Genet* 14:1–24, 2013.

REFERENCES FOR SPECIFIC TOPICS

Bauer DE, Orkin SH: Update on fetal hemoglobin gene regulation in hemoglobinopathies, *Curr Opin Pediatr* 23:1–8, 2011.

Ingram VM: Gene mutations in human haemoglobin: the chemical difference between normal and sickle cell haemoglobin, *Nature* 180:326–328, 1957.

Ingram VM: Specific chemical difference between the globins of normal human and sickle-cell anaemia haemoglobin, *Nature* 178:792–794, 1956.

Kervestin S, Jacobson A: NMD, a multifaceted response to premature translational termination, *Nat Rev Mol Cell Biol* 13:700–712, 2012.

Pauling L, Itano HA, Singer SJ, et al: Sickle cell anemia, a molecular disease, *Science* 110:543–548, 1949.

Sankaran VG, Lettre G, Orkin SH, et al: Modifier genes in mendelian disorders: the example of hemoglobin disorders, *Ann N Y Acad Sci* 1214:47–56, 2010.

Steinberg MH, Sebastiani P: Genetic modifiers of sickle cell disease, *Am J Hematol* 87:795–803, 2012.

Weatherall DJ: The inherited diseases of hemoglobin are an emerging global health burden, *Blood* 115:4331–4336, 2010.

PROBLEMS

1. A newborn female dies of hydrops fetalis attributable to α-thalassemia. Draw a pedigree with genotypes illustrating to the biological parents the genetic basis of this disease. Explain why a Melanesian couple, whom they met in the hematology clinic and who both also have α-thalassemia trait, are unlikely to have a similarly affected child.

2. Why are most individuals with β-thalassemia compound heterozygotes for causal DNA variants in the β-globin gene? In what situation(s) might you anticipate that an individual with β-thalassemia would likely have two identical β-globin alleles (i.e., to be homozygous for the causal DNA variant)?

3. Tony, a young male of self-identified Italian ancestry, is found to havehas non-transfusion-dependent β-thalassemia, with a hemoglobin concentration of 7 g/dL (normal, amounts are 10 to 13 g/dL). When you perform a Northern blot of his reticulocyte RNA, you unexpectedly find three β-globin mRNA bands, one of normal size, one larger than normal, and one smaller than normal. What variant mechanism(s) could account for the presence of three bands like this observation in an individual with β-thalassemia? In this patient, the fact that the anemia is mild suggests that a significant fraction of normal β-globin mRNA is being made. What type(s) of variants would allow this to occur?

4. A man is heterozygous for Hb M Saskatoon, a hemoglobin missense structural alteration in which the normal amino acid His is replaced by Tyr at position 63 of the β chain. His mate is heterozygous for Hb M Boston, in which His is replaced by Tyr at position 58 of the α chain. Heterozygosity for either of these mutant variant alleles produces methemoglobinemia. Outline the possible genotypes and phenotypes of their offspring.

5. A child has a paternal uncle and a maternal aunt with sickle cell disease; both of her parents do not have sickle cell disease. What is the probability that the child has sickle cell disease?

6. A woman has sickle cell trait, and her mate is heterozygous for Hb C. What is the probability that their child has no abnormal hemoglobin?

7. Match the following:

_____ complex β-thalassemia	1. detectable Hb A
_____ β+-thalassemia	2. three
_____ number of α-globin genes missing in Hb H disease	3. β-thalassemia
_____ two different variant alleles at a locu	4. α-thalassemia
_____ ATR-X syndrome	5. high-level β-chain expression
_____ insoluble β chains	6. α-thalassemia trait
_____ number of α-globin genes missing in hydrops fetalis with Hb Barts	7. compound heterozygote
_____ locus control region	8. δβ genes deleted
_____ α–/α– genotype	9. four
_____ increased Hb A2	10. intellectual disability

8. Exome sequencing is organized for a child with unexplained intellectual disability, who also has non-transfusion-dependent β-thalassemia. Although this reveals a genetic cause for the intellectual disability, the molecular basis of the β-thalassemia phenotype is not elucidated, as only a single heterozygous pathogenic variant in the β-globin gene is identified. List possible explanations.

9. What are some possible explanations for the fact that thalassemia control programs, such as the successful one in Sardinia, have not reduced the birth rate of newborns with severe thalassemia to zero? For example, in Sardinia from 1999 to 2002, approximately two to five such infants were born each year.

The Molecular, Biochemical, and Cellular Basis of Genetic Disease

Ada Hamosh

In this chapter we extend our examination of the molecular and biochemical basis of **genetic** disease beyond the hemoglobinopathies to include other diseases and the abnormalities in **gene** and protein function that cause them. In Chapter 12, we presented an outline of the general mechanisms by which **pathogenic variants** cause disease (see Fig. 12.1) and reviewed the steps at which they can disrupt the synthesis or function of a protein (see Table 12.1). Those outlines provide a framework for understanding the pathogenesis of all genetic disease. However, pathogenic **variants** in other classes of proteins often disrupt cell and organ function by processes that differ from those illustrated by the hemoglobinopathies, and we explore them in this chapter.

To illustrate these other types of disease mechanisms, we now examine well-known disorders such as phenylketonuria (PKU), cystic fibrosis (CF), **familial** hypercholesterolemia, Duchenne muscular dystrophy (DMD), and Alzheimer disease (AD). Some less common disorders are included because they best demonstrate a specific principle. The importance of selecting representative disorders becomes apparent now that pathogenic variants in over 4500 genes have been associated with a clinical **phenotype**. One anticipates that many more of the ~20,000 protein coding genes in the human **genome** will be associated with both monogenic and genetically complex diseases.

DISEASES DUE TO PATHOGENIC VARIANTS IN DIFFERENT CLASSES OF PROTEINS

Proteins carry out an astounding number of functions, some of which are presented in Fig. 13.1. Pathogenic variants in virtually every functional class of protein can lead to genetic disorders. In this chapter we describe important genetic diseases that affect representative proteins selected from the groups shown in Fig. 13.1; other proteins listed, as well as the conditions associated with them, are described in the Cases section.

Housekeeping Proteins and Specialty Proteins in Genetic Disease

Proteins can be separated into two general classes on the basis of their pattern of expression. Housekeeping proteins are present in virtually every cell and have fundamental roles in the maintenance of cell structure and function; tissue-specific **specialty proteins** are produced in one or few cell types and have unique functions that contribute to the individuality of the cells in which they are expressed. Most cell types in humans express 10,000 to 15,000 protein-coding genes. Knowledge of the tissues in which a protein is expressed, particularly at high levels, may help in understanding the pathogenesis of a disease.

Two broad generalizations can be made about the relationship between the site of a protein's expression and the site of disease.

- First (and somewhat intuitively), pathogenic variants in a tissue-specific protein most often produce a disease restricted to that tissue. However, there may be secondary effects on other tissues. Pathogenic variants in tissue-specific proteins may cause abnormalities primarily in organs that do not express the protein at all; ironically, the tissue expressing the abnormal protein may be unaffected by the pathologic process. This situation is exemplified by PKU, discussed in depth in the next section. PKU is due to the absence of phenylalanine hydroxylase (PAH) activity in the liver, but it is the brain (which expresses very little of this enzyme), not the liver, that is damaged by the high blood levels of phenylalanine resulting from the lack of hepatic PAH.

- Second, although housekeeping proteins are expressed in most or all tissues, the clinical effects of pathogenic variants in such proteins are frequently limited to one or few tissues, for at least two reasons. Most often, the housekeeping protein in question is normally expressed abundantly in one or few tissues where it serves a specialty function. This situation is illustrated by Tay-Sachs disease, as discussed later

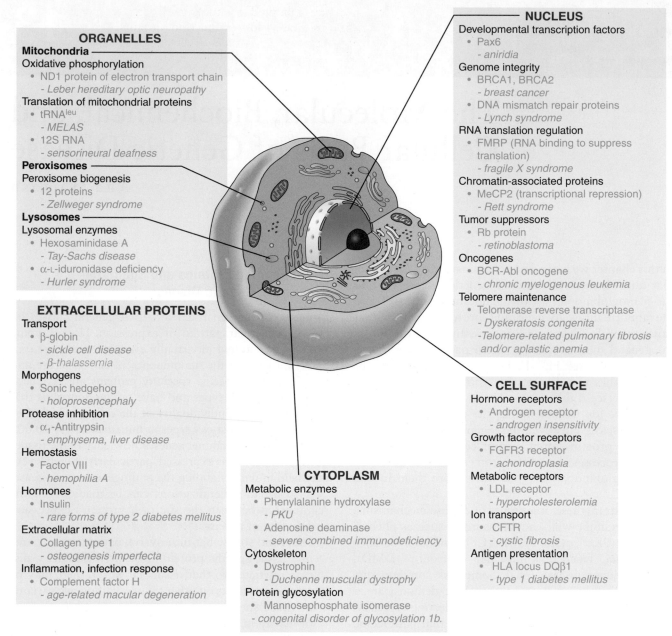

ORGANELLES

Mitochondria
Oxidative phosphorylation
- ND1 protein of electron transport chain
  - *Leber hereditary optic neuropathy*
Translation of mitochondrial proteins
- tRNA^{leu}
  - *MELAS*
- 12S RNA
  - *sensorineural deafness*

Peroxisomes
Peroxisome biogenesis
- 12 proteins
  - *Zellweger syndrome*

Lysosomes
Lysosomal enzymes
- Hexosaminidase A
  - *Tay-Sachs disease*
- α-L-iduronidase deficiency
  - *Hurler syndrome*

EXTRACELLULAR PROTEINS

Transport
- β-globin
  - *sickle cell disease*
  - *β-thalassemia*
Morphogens
- Sonic hedgehog
  - *holoprosencephaly*
Protease inhibition
- α$_1$-Antitrypsin
  - *emphysema, liver disease*
Hemostasis
- Factor VIII
  - *hemophilia A*
Hormones
- Insulin
  - *rare forms of type 2 diabetes mellitus*
Extracellular matrix
- Collagen type 1
  - *osteogenesis imperfecta*
Inflammation, infection response
- Complement factor H
  - *age-related macular degeneration*

NUCLEUS
Developmental transcription factors
- Pax6
  - *aniridia*
Genome integrity
- BRCA1, BRCA2
  - *breast cancer*
- DNA mismatch repair proteins
  - *Lynch syndrome*
RNA translation regulation
- FMRP (RNA binding to suppress translation)
  - *fragile X syndrome*
Chromatin-associated proteins
- MeCP2 (transcriptional repression)
  - *Rett syndrome*
Tumor suppressors
- Rb protein
  - *retinoblastoma*
Oncogenes
- BCR-Abl oncogene
  - *chronic myelogenous leukemia*
Telomere maintenance
- Telomerase reverse transcriptase
  - *Dyskeratosis congenita*
  - *Telomere-related pulmonary fibrosis and/or aplastic anemia*

CELL SURFACE
Hormone receptors
- Androgen receptor
  - *androgen insensitivity*
Growth factor receptors
- FGFR3 receptor
  - *achondroplasia*
Metabolic receptors
- LDL receptor
  - *hypercholesterolemia*
Ion transport
- CFTR
  - *cystic fibrosis*
Antigen presentation
- HLA locus DQβ1
  - *type 1 diabetes mellitus*

CYTOPLASM
Metabolic enzymes
- Phenylalanine hydroxylase
  - *PKU*
- Adenosine deaminase
  - *severe combined immunodeficiency*
Cytoskeleton
- Dystrophin
  - *Duchenne muscular dystrophy*
Protein glycosylation
- Mannosephosphate isomerase
  - *congenital disorder of glycosylation 1b.*

Figure 13.1 Examples of the classes of proteins associated with diseases with a strong genetic component (most are monogenic), and the part of the cell in which those proteins normally function. *CDG1b (MPI-CDG)*, Congenital disorder of glycosylaton type 1b (mannosephosphate isomerase, congenital disorder of glycosylation); *CFTR*, cystic fibrosis transmembrane regulator; *FMRP*, fragile X messenger ribonucleoprotein; *HLA*, human leukocyte antigen; *LDL*, low-density lipoprotein; *MELAS*, mitochondrial encephalomyopathy with lactic acidosis and strokelike episodes; *PKU*, phenylketonuria.

(and in (Case 43). The enzyme affected in this disorder is hexosaminidase A, which is expressed in virtually all cells, but its absence leads to a fatal neurodegeneration while leaving nonneuronal cell types unscathed. In other instances, another protein with overlapping biologic activity may be expressed in the unaffected tissue, thereby lessening the impact of the loss of function by the variant **allele** – a situation known as genetic **redundancy**. Unexpectedly, even pathogenic variants in genes seeming as essential to every cell, such as actin, can result in viable offspring.

DISEASES INVOLVING ENZYMES

Enzymes are the catalysts that mediate the efficient conversion of a substrate to a product. The diversity of substrates on which enzymes act is huge. Accordingly, the human genome contains more than 3700 genes that encode enzymes, and there are hundreds of human diseases – the **enzymopathies** – that involve enzyme defects. We first discuss one of the best-known groups of inborn errors of metabolism, the hyperphenylalaninemias.

Aminoacidopathies

The Hyperphenylalaninemias

The abnormalities that lead to an increase in the blood level of phenylalanine, most notably PAH deficiency or PKU, illustrate almost every principle of **biochemical genetics** related to enzyme defects. The biochemical causes of hyperphenylalaninemia are illustrated in Fig. 13.2, and the principal features of the diseases associated with the biochemical defect at the six known hyperphenylalaninemia loci are presented in Table 13.1. All the genetic disorders of phenylalanine metabolism are inherited as autosomal **recessive** conditions and are due to loss-of-function variants, either in the gene encoding PAH or in genes required for the synthesis or reutilization of the PAH cofactor, tetrahydrobiopterin (BH$_4$), or (rarely) in *DNAJC12*, which encodes a chaperone for PAH.

Phenylketonuria. Classic PKU is the epitome of the enzymopathies. It results from pathogenic variants in the gene encoding PAH, which converts phenylalanine to tyrosine (see Fig. 13.2 and Table 13.1). The discovery of PKU in 1934 marked the first demonstration of a

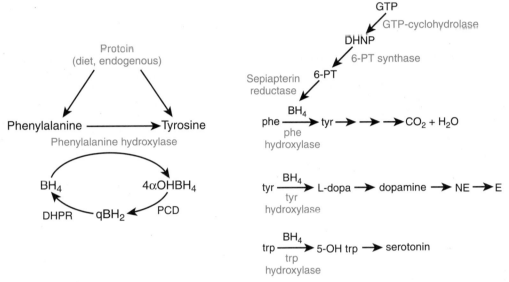

Figure 13.2 The biochemical pathways affected in the hyperphenylalaninemias. *BH$_4$*, tetrahydrobiopterin; *4αOHBH$_4$*, 4α-hydroxytetrahydrobiopterin; *qBH$_2$*, quinonoid dihydrobiopterin, the oxidized product of the hydroxylation reactions, which is reduced to BH$_4$ by dihydropteridine reductase (DHPR); *PCD*, pterin 4α-carbinolamine dehydratase; *phe*, phenylalanine; *tyr*, tyrosine; *trp*, tryptophan; *GTP*, guanosine triphosphate; *DHNP*, dihydroneopterin triphosphate; *6-PT*, 6-pyruvoyltetrahydropterin; *L-dopa*, L-dihydroxyphenylalanine; *NE*, norepinephrine; *E*, epinephrine; *5-OH trp*, 5-hydroxytryptophan.

TABLE 13.1 Locus Heterogeneity in the Hyperphenylalaninemias

Biochemical Defect	Incidence/10⁶ Births	Enzyme Affected	Treatment
Variants in the Gene Encoding Phenylalanine Hydroxylase			
Classic PKU	5–350 (depending on the population)	PAH	Low-phenylalanine diet*
Variant PKU	Less than classic PKU	PAH	Low-phenylalanine diet (less restrictive than that required to treat PKU); BH$_4$
Non-PKU hyperphenylalaninemia	15–75	PAH	None, or a much less restrictive low-phenylalanine diet; BH$_4$ in untreated individuals with phenylalanine levels >300
Variants in Genes Encoding Enzymes of Tetrahydrobiopterin Metabolism			
Impaired BH$_4$ recycling	<1	PCD DHPR	Low-phenylalanine diet + L-dopa, 5-HT, carbidopa (+ folinic acid for DHPR patients)
Impaired BH$_4$ synthesis	<1	GTP-CH 6-PTS	Low-phenylalanine diet + L-dopa, 5-HT, carbidopa and pharmacological doses of BH$_4$
Variants in the Gene Encoding the PAH chaperone			
Impaired chaperone and stabilization of PAH	<1	DNAJC12	Low-phenylalanine diet + L-dopa, 5-HT, carbidopa and pharmacological doses of BH$_4$

BH$_4$, Tetrahydrobiopterin; *DHPR*, dihydropteridine reductase; *GTP-CH*, guanosine triphosphate cyclohydrolase; *5-HT*, 5-hydroxytryptophan; *PAH*, phenylalanine hydroxylase; *PCD*, pterin 4α-carbinolamine dehydratase; *PKU*, phenylketonuria; *6-PTS*, 6-pyruvoyltetrahydropterin synthase.
*BH$_4$ supplementation may increase the PAH activity of some patients in this group.

genetic defect as a cause of intellectual disability. Because patients with PKU cannot degrade phenylalanine, it accumulates in body fluids and damages the developing central nervous system. A small fraction of phenylalanine is metabolized to produce increased amounts of phenylpyruvic acid, the keto acid responsible for the name of the disease. Ironically, although the enzymatic defect has been known for many decades, the precise pathogenetic mechanism(s) by which increased phenylalanine damages the brain is still uncertain. Importantly, the neurologic damage is largely avoided by reducing the dietary intake of phenylalanine. The management of PKU is a paradigm of the treatment of the many metabolic diseases whose outcome can be improved by preventing accumulation of an enzyme substrate and its derivatives; this therapeutic principle is described further in Chapter 14.

Variant Phenylketonuria and Nonphenylketonuria Hyperphenylalaninemia. Classical PKU results from a virtual absence of PAH activity (<1% of that in controls) and is defined by untreated phenylalanine (phe) levels of more than 1200 µmol/L. Less severe phenotypes – designated mild or variant PKU (phe levels 400–1200 µmol/L), and non-PKU (or benign) hyperphenylalaninemia (phe levels <400 µmol/L) (see Table 13.1) – result when the **mutant** PAH enzyme has some residual activity. The fact that a very small amount of residual enzyme activity can have a large impact on phenotype is another general principle of the enzymopathies (see Box 13.1).

BOX 13.1 MUTANT ENZYMES AND DISEASE: GENERAL CONCEPTS

The following concepts are fundamental to the understanding and treatment of enzymopathies.

- **Inheritance patterns**
  Enzymopathies are almost always recessive or X-linked (see Chapter 7). Most enzymes are produced in quantities significantly in excess of minimal biochemical requirements so that heterozygotes (typically with ~50% of residual activity) are clinically normal. In fact, many enzymes may maintain normal substrate and product levels with less than 10% of full activity, a point relevant to the design of therapeutic strategies (e.g., for homocystinuria due to cystathionine synthase deficiency—see Chapter 14). The enzymes of porphyrin synthesis are exceptions (see discussion of acute intermittent porphyria in main text, later).

- **Substrate accumulation or product deficiency**
  Because the function of an enzyme is to convert a substrate to a product, all of the pathophysiologic consequences of enzymopathies can be attributed either to the accumulation of the substrate (as in PKU), to the deficiency of the product (as in glucose-6-phosphate dehydrogenase deficiency (**Case 19**), or to some combination of the two (Fig. 13.3).

- **Diffusible vs macromolecular substrates**
  An important distinction can be made between enzyme defects in which the substrate is a small molecule (such as phenylalanine, which can be readily distributed throughout body fluids by diffusion or transport) and defects in which the substrate is a macromolecule (such as a mucopolysaccharide or glycosaminoglycan, which remains trapped within its organelle or cell). The pathologic change of the macromolecular diseases, such as Tay-Sachs disease, is confined to the tissues in which the substrate accumulates. In contrast, the site of the disease in the small molecule disorders is often unpredictable because the free-moving unmetabolized substrate or its derivatives can damage cells remote from the affected enzyme, as in PKU.

- **Loss of multiple enzyme activities**
  An individual with a single-gene defect may have loss of function in more than one enzyme. There are several possible mechanisms: the enzymes may use the same cofactor (e.g., BH_4 deficiency); the enzymes may share a common subunit or an activating, processing, or stabilizing protein (e.g., the GM_2 gangliosidoses); the enzymes may all be processed by a common modifying enzyme, and in its absence, they may be inactive, or their uptake into an organelle may be impaired (e.g., I-cell disease, in which failure to add mannose 6-phosphate to many lysosomal enzymes abrogates the ability of cells to recognize and import the enzymes); or a group of enzymes may be absent or ineffective if the organelle in which they are normally found is not formed or is abnormal (e.g., Zellweger **syndrome**, a disorder of peroxisome biogenesis).

- **Phenotypic homology**
  The pathologic and clinical features resulting from an enzyme defect are often shared by diseases involving other enzymes that function in the same area of metabolism (e.g., the mucopolysaccharidoses) as well as by the different phenotypes that can result from partial versus complete defects of one enzyme. Partial defects often present with clinical abnormalities that are a subset of those found with the complete deficiency, although the etiologic relationship between the phenotypes may not be immediately obvious. For example, partial deficiency of the **purine** enzyme, hypoxanthine-guanine phosphoribosyltransferase, causes only hyperuricemia, whereas complete deficiency causes hyperuricemia with a profound neurologic disease, Lesch-Nyhan syndrome, which resembles cerebral palsy and is characterized by severe self-injurious behavior.

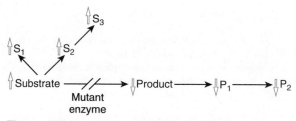

Figure 13.3 A model metabolic pathway showing that the potential effects of an enzyme deficiency include accumulation of the substrate *(S)* or derivatives of it *(S₁, S₂, S₃)* and deficiency of the product *(P)* or compounds made from it *(P₁, P₂)*. In some cases, the substrate derivatives are normally only minor metabolites that may be formed at increased rates when the substrate accumulates (e.g., phenylpyruvate in phenylketonuria).

Variant PKU includes individuals who require only some dietary phenylalanine limitations, less restrictive than for classic PKU, because their blood phenylalanine levels are more moderate and less damaging to the brain. With classic PKU, the plasma phenylalanine levels are more than 1200 µmol/L on a normal diet, whereas non-PKU hyperphenylalaninemia is defined by plasma phenylalanine concentrations above the upper limit of normal (120 µmol/L) but below those seen in classic PKU. If the increase in non-PKU hyperphenylalaninemia is small (<400 µmol/L, termed benign hyperphenylalaninemia), no treatment is required; these individuals come to clinical attention only through newborn screening (see Chapter 19). They are followed to ensure that levels do not rise into the treatment range. Their normal phenotype has been the best indication of the safe target level of plasma phenylalanine in treating classic PKU. The association of these three clinical phenotypes with variants in the *PAH* gene is a clear example of **allelic heterogeneity** leading to **clinical heterogeneity** (see Table 13.1).

Allelic and Locus Heterogeneity in the Hyperphenylalaninemias

Allelic Heterogeneity in the PAH Gene. A striking degree of allelic heterogeneity at the *PAH* locus – more than 1200 different variants worldwide – has been identified among individuals with hyperphenylalaninemia associated with classic PKU, variant PKU, or benign hyperphenylalaninemia (see Table 13.1). Seven variants account for a majority of known pathogenic alleles in populations of European descent, whereas six others represent the majority of *PAH* pathogenic variants in Asian populations. The remaining disease-causing variants are individually rare. To record and make this information publicly available, a *PAH* variant database has been developed by an international consortium.

The allelic heterogeneity at the *PAH* locus has major clinical consequences. Most important is that most individuals with hyperphenylalaninemia are **compound heterozygotes** (i.e., they have two different disease-causing alleles) (see Chapter 7). This allelic heterogeneity accounts for much of the enzymatic and phenotypic heterogeneity among affected individuals. Thus pathogenic variants that eliminate or dramatically reduce PAH activity generally cause classic PKU, whereas greater residual enzyme activity is associated with milder phenotypes. However, **homozygous** patients with certain PAH variants have phenotypes ranging all the way from classic PKU to non-PKU hyperphenylalaninemia. Accordingly, other unidentified biologic variables – undoubtedly including modifier genes – generate variation in the phenotype for a given **genotype**. This lack of a strict genotype-phenotype **correlation**, initially somewhat surprising, is now recognized as a feature of most single-gene diseases, highlighting that even monogenic traits like PKU are not genetically simple disorders.

Defects in Tetrahydrobiopterin Metabolism. In 1% to 3% of individuals with elevated phenylalanine, the *PAH* gene is normal, and the hyperphenylalaninemia results from a defect in one of the steps in the biosynthesis or regeneration of BH_4 – the cofactor for PAH (see Table 13.1 and Fig. 13.2). The association of a single biochemical phenotype, such as hyperphenylalaninemia, with variants in different genes, is an example of **locus heterogeneity** (see Table 13.1). The proteins encoded by genes that manifest locus heterogeneity generally act at different steps in a single biochemical pathway: another principle of genetic disease illustrated by hyperphenylalaninemia (see Fig. 13.2). BH_4-deficient patients were first recognized because they developed profound neurologic problems in early life, despite the successful administration of a low-phenylalanine diet. This poor outcome is due in part to the requirement for the BH_4 cofactor by two other enzymes: tyrosine hydroxylase and tryptophan hydroxylase. These hydroxylases are critical for the synthesis of the monoamine neurotransmitters, dopamine, norepinephrine, epinephrine, and serotonin (see Fig. 13.2).

The locus heterogeneity of hyperphenylalaninemia is significant because the treatment of patients with a defect in BH_4 metabolism differs markedly from that for subjects with pathogenic variants in *PAH*, in two ways. First, because the PAH enzyme is itself normal in individuals with BH_4 defects, its activity can be restored by large doses of oral BH_4, leading to reduction in plasma phenylalanine levels. This practice highlights the principle of product replacement in the treatment of some genetic disorders (see Chapter 14). Consequently, phenylalanine restriction can be significantly relaxed for those with defects in BH_4 metabolism, and some actually tolerate an unrestricted diet. Second, one must try to normalize the neurotransmitters in the brains of these patients by administering the products of tyrosine hydroxylase and tryptophan hydroxylase: L-dopa and 5-hydroxytryptophan, respectively (see Fig. 13.2 and Table 13.1).

A novel form of hyperphenylalaninemia with movement disorder and sometimes with cognitive impairment is caused by biallelic pathogenic variants in *DNAJC12*, which codes for a member of the HSP40 family of proteins. It functions as a cochaperone (with members of the HSP70 family of proteins) of the aromatic hydroxylases, including PAH, tyrosine hydroxylase, and tryptophan hydroxylases 1 and 2. So far, more than 20 patients have been described. This condition will be identified by elevated phenylalanine on newborn screening and requires sequencing of the gene for diagnosis.

Remarkably, pathogenic variants in sepiapterin reductase, an enzyme in the BH_4 synthesis pathway, do not cause hyperphenylalaninemia. Only dopa-responsive dystonia is seen, due to impaired synthesis of dopamine and serotonin (see Fig. 13.2). Alternative pathways may exist for the final step in BH_4 synthesis, bypassing the sepiapterin reductase deficiency in peripheral tissues, an example of genetic redundancy.

For these reasons, all hyperphenylalaninemic infants must be evaluated to determine whether their hyperphenylalaninemia is the result of an abnormality in PAH, in BH_4 metabolism, or in the chaperone. The hyperphenylalaninemias thus illustrate the critical importance of obtaining a specific molecular diagnosis in all patients with a genetic disease phenotype. The underlying genetic defect may not be what one first suspects, and the treatment can vary accordingly.

Tetrahydrobiopterin Responsiveness With PAH Variants. Many individuals with variants in the *PAH* gene (rather than in BH_4 metabolism) will also respond to large oral doses of BH_4 cofactor, with a substantial decrease in plasma phenylalanine. BH_4 supplementation is therefore an important adjunct therapy for PKU patients of this type, allowing a less restricted dietary intake of phenylalanine. The affected individuals most likely to respond are those with significant residual PAH activity (i.e., those with variant PKU and non-PKU hyperphenylalaninemia), but a minority of individuals with classic PKU are also responsive. The presence of residual PAH activity does not, however, guarantee an effect of BH_4 administration on plasma phenylalanine levels. Rather, the degree of BH_4 responsiveness will depend on the specific properties of each altered PAH protein, reflecting the allelic heterogeneity underlying *PAH* variants.

The provision of increased amounts of a cofactor is a strategy that has been used for the treatment of many inborn errors of enzyme metabolism, as discussed further in Chapter 14. In general, a cofactor comes into contact with the protein component of an enzyme (termed an **apoenzyme**) to form the active **holoenzyme**, which consists of both the cofactor and the otherwise inactive apoenzyme. Illustrating this strategy, BH_4 supplementation exerts its beneficial effect through one or more mechanisms, all of which result from increased cofactor in contact with the altered PAH apoenzyme. These mechanisms include stabilization of the enzyme, protection of the enzyme from degradation by the cell, and increase in cofactor supply for an altered enzyme with low affinity for BH_4.

Newborn Screening. PKU is the prototype of genetic diseases for which mass newborn screening is justified (see Chapter 19) because (1) it is relatively common in some populations (up to ~1 in 2900 live births), (2) mass screening is feasible, (3) failure to treat has severe consequences (profound intellectual disability), and (4) treatment is effective if begun early in life. To allow time for the postnatal increase in blood phenylalanine levels, the test is performed after 24 hours of age. Central laboratories assay blood from a heel prick for blood phenylalanine levels and phenylalanine-to-tyrosine ratio. Positive test results must be confirmed quickly because delays in treatment beyond 4 weeks postnatally have profound effects on intellectual outcome. The current recommendation is to initiate treatment within the first week of life.

Maternal Hyperphenylalaninemia. Originally, the low-phenylalanine diet was discontinued in mid-childhood for most individuals with PKU. It was later found, however, that almost all offspring of women with PKU not on treatment are clinically abnormal; most are severely delayed developmentally, and many have microcephaly, growth impairment, and malformations, particularly of the heart. As predicted by principles of **mendelian** inheritance, these children are heterozygotes; their neurodevelopmental delay is not due to their own genetic constitution but to the highly teratogenic effect of elevated phenylalanine in the maternal circulation. Accordingly, women with PKU who are planning pregnancies must achieve tight metabolic control with a low-phenylalanine diet and BH_4 supplementation (if responsive) prior to conception.

Lysosomal Storage Diseases: A Unique Class of Enzymopathies

Lysosomes are membrane-bound organelles containing an array of hydrolytic enzymes involved in the degradation of a variety of biologic macromolecules. Pathogenic variants in these hydrolases are unique because they lead to the accumulation of their substrates inside the lysosome, where the substrates remain trapped because their large size prevents their egress from the organelle. Their accumulation and sometimes toxicity interferes with normal cell function, eventually causing cell death. Moreover, the substrate accumulation underlies one uniform clinical feature of these diseases – their unrelenting progression. In most of these conditions, substrate storage increases the mass of the affected tissues and organs. When the brain is affected, the picture is one of neurodegeneration. The clinical phenotypes are very distinct and often make the diagnosis of a storage disease straightforward. More than 50 lysosomal hydrolase or lysosomal membrane transport deficiencies, almost all inherited as autosomal recessive conditions, have been described. Historically these diseases were untreatable. However, bone marrow transplantation and enzyme replacement therapy have dramatically improved the prognosis of these conditions (see Chapter 14).

Tay-Sachs Disease

Tay-Sachs disease (Case 43) is one of a group of heterogeneous lysosomal storage diseases, the GM_2 gangliosidoses, that result from the inability to degrade a sphingolipid, GM_2 ganglioside (Fig. 13.4). The biochemical lesion is a marked deficiency of hexosaminidase A (hex A). Although the enzyme is ubiquitous, the disease has its clinical impact almost solely on the brain, the predominant site of GM_2 ganglioside synthesis. Catalytically active hex A is the product of a three-gene system (see Fig. 13.4). These genes encode the α and β subunits of the enzyme (the *HEXA* and *HEXB* genes,

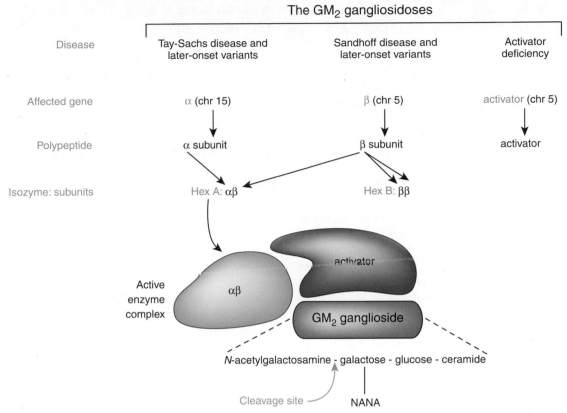

Figure 13.4 **The three-gene system required for hexosaminidase A activity and the diseases that result from defects in each of the genes.** The function of the activator protein is to bind the ganglioside substrate and present it to the enzyme. *Hex A*, Hexosaminidase A; *Hex B*, hexosaminidase B; *NANA*, N-acetyl neuraminic acid. (Modified from Sandhoff K, Conzelmann E, Neufeld EF, et al: The GM$_2$ gangliosidoses. In Scriver CR, Beaudet AL, Sly WS, et al, editors: *The metabolic bases of inherited disease*, ed 6, New York, 1989, McGraw-Hill, pp 1807–1839.)

respectively) and an activator protein that must associate with the substrate and the enzyme before the enzyme can cleave the terminal N-acetyl-β-galactosamine residue from the ganglioside.

The clinical manifestations of defects in the three genes are indistinguishable, but they can be differentiated by enzymatic analysis. Pathogenic variants in the *HEXA* gene affect the α subunit and disrupt hex A activity to cause Tay-Sachs disease (or less severe variants of hex A deficiency). Defects in the *HEXB* gene or in the gene encoding the activator protein impair the activity of both hex A and hex B (see Fig. 13.4) to produce Sandhoff disease or activator protein deficiency (which is very rare), respectively.

The clinical course of Tay-Sachs disease is tragic. Affected infants appear normal until ~3 to 6 months of age but then gradually undergo progressive neurologic deterioration until death at 2 to 4 years. The effects of neuronal death can be seen directly in the form of the cherry-red spot in the retina (Case 43). In contrast, *HEXA* alleles associated with some residual activity lead to later-onset forms of neurologic disease, with manifestations including lower motor neuron dysfunction and ataxia due to spinocerebellar degeneration. In contrast to the infantile disease, vision and intelligence usually remain normal, although psychosis develops in one-third of these patients. Finally, **pseudodeficiency alleles** (discussed next) cause no disease.

Hex A Pseudodeficiency Alleles and Their Clinical Significance. An unexpected consequence of screening for Tay-Sachs **carriers** in the Ashkenazi Jewish population was the discovery of a unique class of hex A alleles, the pseudodeficiency alleles. Although the two pseudodeficiency alleles are clinically benign, individuals identified as pseudodeficient in screening tests are genetic compounds with a **pseudodeficiency allele** on one **chromosome** and a common Tay-Sachs variant on the other chromosome. These individuals have a low level of hex A activity (~20% of controls) that is adequate to prevent GM$_2$ ganglioside accumulation in the brain. The importance of hex A pseudodeficiency alleles is twofold. First, they complicate prenatal diagnosis because a pseudodeficient fetus could be incorrectly diagnosed as affected. More generally, the recognition of the hex A pseudodeficiency alleles indicates that screening programs for other genetic diseases must recognize that comparable alleles may exist at other loci and may confound the correct characterization of individuals in screening or diagnostic tests.

Population Genetics. In many monogenic diseases, some alleles are found at higher frequency in some populations than in others (see Chapter 10). This situation is illustrated by Tay-Sachs disease, in which three alleles account for 99% of the variants found in Ashkenazi

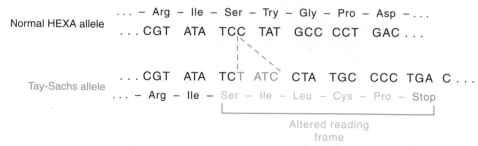

Figure 13.5 Four-base insertion (TATC) in the hexosaminidase A (hex A) gene in Tay-Sachs disease, leading to a frameshift. This variant is the major cause of Tay-Sachs disease in Ashkenazi Jews. No detectable hex A protein is made, accounting for the complete enzyme deficiency observed in these infantile-onset patients.

Jewish patients, the most common of which accounts for 80% of cases (Fig. 13.5). Approximately 1 in 27 Ashkenazi Jews is a carrier of a Tay-Sachs allele, and the incidence of affected infants was 100 times higher than in other populations, prior to screening. A **founder effect** or **heterozygote advantage** is the most likely explanation for this high frequency (see Chapter 10). Because most Ashkenazi Jewish carriers will have one of the three common alleles, a practical benefit of the molecular characterization of the disease in this population is the degree to which carrier screening has been simplified.

ALTERED PROTEIN FUNCTION DUE TO ABNORMAL POSTTRANSLATIONAL MODIFICATION

Congenital Disorders of Glycosylation

Approximately 50% of all proteins and 80% of those in blood are glycosylated and need appropriate sugar moieties added to function properly. A broad class of monogenic disease is the **congenital** disorders of glycosylation (CDGs), involving over 160 different genes (Fig. 13.6): most are autosomal recessive and a few are X-linked. They usually present in infancy with multisystem problems, including failure to thrive, liver disease, hypotonia, intestinal disease (often protein-losing enteropathy), developmental delay, eye and skeletal **anomalies**, immunologic abnormalities, and may or may not include brain and/or neurodevelopmental abnormalities. CDGs are divided into two main groups: type I CDGs comprise defects in the assembly of the dolichol lipid-linked oligosaccharide (LLO) chain and its transfer to the nascent protein; type II CDGs are due to defects in the processing of the protein-bound glycans either late in the endoplasmic reticulum or in the Golgi apparatus. Screening for N-linked glycosylation disorders can be achieved by isoelectric focusing of transferrin, a heavily glycosylated plasma protein. Decrease in the proportion of tetrasialo-transferrin with increases of asialo- or di- or trisialotransferrin, suggest the diagnosis, which then needs molecular confirmation. Because the multipathway, or type II, CDGs require sequencing and the

manifestations are so variable, increasingly the diagnosis is established by direct genome-wide investigation through either **exome** or **genome sequencing**.

One example is CDG due to pathogenic variants in *MPI*, called MPI-CDG or CDG1b. This condition spares cognitive development but manifests in infancy with severe failure to thrive, protein-losing enteropathy, hypoglycemia, and coagulation defects. Treatment with high-dose mannose (1 g/kg body weight) results in elimination of hypoglycemia, protein-losing enteropathy, and coagulation defects. Despite treatment, some patients have manifested liver fibrosis in adulthood, so long-term follow-up is essential.

A Loss of Glycosylation: Mucolipidosis II or I-Cell Disease

Some proteins have information contained in their primary amino acid **sequence** that directs them to their subcellular residence, whereas others are localized on the basis of posttranslational modifications. This latter mechanism is true of the acid hydrolases found in lysosomes, but this form of cellular trafficking was unrecognized until the discovery of I-cell disease, a severe autosomal recessive lysosomal storage disease. The disorder has a range of phenotypic effects involving facial features, skeletal changes, growth retardation, and intellectual disability and survival of less than 10 years. The cytoplasm of cultured skin **fibroblasts** from individuals with I-cell disease contains numerous abnormal lysosomes, or inclusions (hence the term inclusion [I] cells).

In I-cell disease, the cellular levels of many lysosomal acid hydrolases are greatly diminished, and instead they are found in excess in body fluids, including blood. This unusual situation arises because the hydrolases in these patients have not been properly modified posttranslationally. A typical hydrolase is a glycoprotein, the sugar moiety containing mannose residues, some of which are phosphorylated. The mannose-6-phosphate residues are essential for recognition of the hydrolases by receptors on the cell and lysosomal membrane surface. In I-cell disease there is a defect in the enzyme that transfers a phosphate group to the mannose residues. The fact that many enzymes are affected is consistent with the diversity of clinical abnormalities seen in these patients.

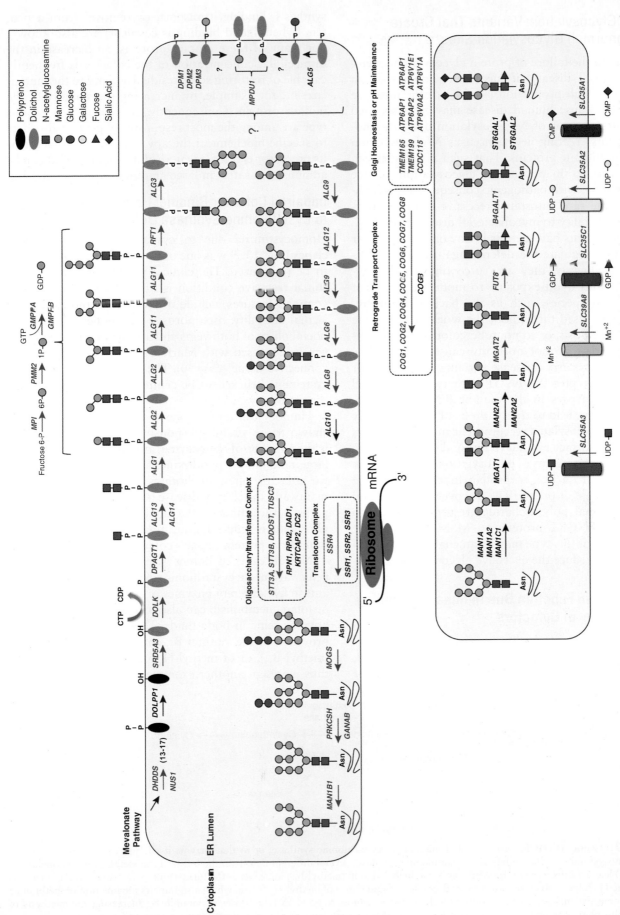

Figure 13.6 A schematic of the *N*-linked pathway highlighting those genes required for both the initial steps of lipid-linked oligosaccharide synthesis and several key components for glycan processing within the Golgi. These genes highlighted in red represent known loci for glycosylation disorders. The *blue arrow* indicates MPI. Supplementation with pharmacologic doses of mannose can drive this reaction to create extra mannose-6-phosphate. (Adapted from Ng BG, Freeze HH: Perspectives on glycosylation and its congenital disorders, *Trends Genet* 34(6):466–476, 2018. https://doi.org/10.1016/j.tig.2018.03.002.)

Gains of Glycosylation: Variants That Create New (Abnormal) Glycosylation Sites

In contrast to the failure of protein glycosylation exemplified by I-cell disease, it has been shown that an unexpectedly high proportion (~1.5%) of the missense variants that cause human disease may be associated with abnormal gains of N-glycosylation due to pathogenic variants creating new consensus N-glycosylation sites in the mutant proteins. That such novel sites can actually lead to inappropriate glycosylation of the mutant protein, with pathogenic consequences, is highlighted by the rare autosomal recessive disorder, mendelian susceptibility to mycobacterial disease (MSMD).

MSMD patients have defects in any one of a number of genes that regulate the defense against some infections. Consequently, they are susceptible to disseminated infections upon exposure to moderately virulent mycobacterial species, such as the bacillus Calmette-Guérin (BCG) used throughout the world as a vaccine against tuberculosis, or to nontuberculous environmental bacteria that do not normally cause illness. Some MSMD patients carry missense variants in the gene for interferon-γ receptor 2 *(IFNGR2)* that generate novel N-glycosylation sites in the mutant IFNGR2 protein. These novel sites lead to the synthesis of an abnormally large, overly glycosylated receptor. The mutant receptors reach the cell surface but fail to respond to interferon-γ. Variants leading to gains of glycosylation have also been found to lead to a loss of protein function in several other monogenic disorders. The discovery that removal of the abnormal polysaccharides restores function to the mutant IFNGR2 proteins in MSMD offers hope that disorders of this type may be amenable to chemical therapies that reduce the excessive glycosylation.

Loss of Protein Function Due to Impaired Binding or Metabolism of Cofactors

Some proteins acquire biologic activity only after they associate with cofactors, such as BH_4 in the case of PAH, as discussed earlier. Variants that interfere with cofactor synthesis, binding, transport, or removal from a protein (when ligand binding is covalent) are also known. For many of these mutant proteins, an increase in the intracellular concentration of the cofactor is frequently capable of restoring some residual activity to the mutant enzyme, for example, by increasing the stability of the mutant protein. Consequently, enzyme defects of this type are among the most responsive of genetic disorders to specific biochemical therapy because the cofactor or its precursor is often a water-soluble vitamin that can be administered safely in large amounts (see Chapter 14).

Impaired Cofactor Binding: Homocystinuria Due to Cystathionine Synthase Deficiency

Homocystinuria due to cystathionine synthase deficiency (Fig. 13.7) was one of the first aminoacidopathies to be recognized. The clinical phenotype of this autosomal recessive condition is often dramatic. The most common features include dislocation of the lens, intellectual disability, osteoporosis, long bones, and thromboembolism of both veins and arteries, a phenotype that can be confused with Marfan syndrome, a disorder of connective tissue (**Case 30**). The accumulation of homocysteine is believed to be central to most, if not all, of the pathology.

Homocystinuria was one of the first genetic diseases shown to be vitamin responsive; pyridoxal phosphate is the cofactor of the enzyme, and the administration of large amounts of pyridoxine, the vitamin precursor of the cofactor, often ameliorates the biochemical abnormality and the clinical disease (see Chapter 14). In many patients, the affinity of the mutant enzyme for pyridoxal phosphate is reduced, indicating that altered conformation of the protein impairs cofactor binding.

Not all cases of homocystinuria result from pathogenic variants in cystathionine synthase. Pathogenic variants in five different enzymes of cobalamin (vitamin B_{12}) or folate metabolism can also lead to increased levels of homocysteine in body fluids. These variants impair the provision of the vitamin B_{12} cofactor, methylcobalamin (methyl-B_{12}), or of methyl-H_4-folate (see Fig. 13.7) and thus represent another example (like the defects in BH_4

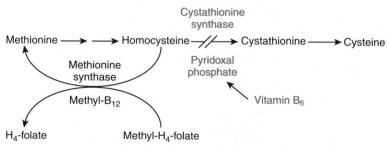

Figure 13.7 Genetic defects in pathways that impinge on cystathionine synthase, or in that enzyme itself, and cause homocystinuria. Classic homocystinuria is due to defective cystathionine synthase. Several different defects in the intracellular metabolism of cobalamins (not shown) lead to a decrease in the synthesis of methylcobalamin (methyl-B_{12}) and thus in the function of methionine synthase. Defects in methylene-H_4-folate reductase *(not shown)* decrease the abundance of methyl-H_4-folate, which also impairs the function of methionine synthase. Some patients with cystathionine synthase abnormalities respond to large doses of vitamin B_6, increasing the synthesis of pyridoxal phosphate, thereby increasing cystathionine synthase activity and treating the disease (see Chapter 14).

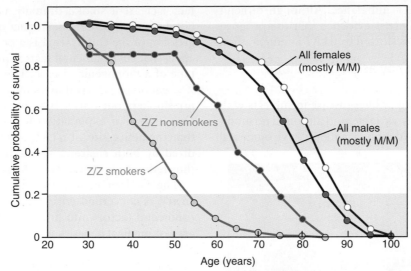

Figure 13.8 The effect of smoking on the survival of patients with α_1-antitrypsin deficiency. The curves show the cumulative probability of survival to specified ages of smokers, with or without α_1-antitrypsin deficiency. (Redrawn from Larson C: Natural history and life expectancy in severe α_1-antitrypsin deficiency, Pi Z, *Acta Med Scand* 204:345–351, 1978.)

synthesis that lead to hyperphenylalaninemia) of genetic diseases due to defects in the biogenesis of enzyme cofactors. The clinical manifestation of these disorders is variable but includes megaloblastic anemia, developmental delay, and failure to thrive. These conditions, all of which are autosomal recessive, are often partially or completely treatable with high doses of vitamin B_{12}.

Pathogenic Variants of an Enzyme Inhibitor: α_1-Antitrypsin Deficiency

α_1-Antitrypsin (α1AT) deficiency is an important autosomal recessive condition associated with a substantial **risk** for chronic obstructive lung disease (emphysema) (Fig. 13.8) and cirrhosis of the liver. The α1AT protein belongs to a major family of protease inhibitors, the *ser*ine *pro*tease *in*hibitors or serpins; *SERPINA1* is the formal gene name. Notwithstanding the **specificity** suggested by its name, α1AT actually inhibits a wide spectrum of proteases, particularly elastase released from neutrophils in the lower respiratory tract.

In populations of European descent, α1AT deficiency affects ~1 in 6700 persons, and ~4% are carriers. A dozen or so α1AT alleles are associated with an increased risk for lung or liver disease, but only the Z allele (p.Glu342Lys) is relatively common. The reason for the relatively high frequency of the Z allele in European populations is unknown, but analysis of DNA haplotypes suggests a single origin with subsequent spread throughout northern Europe. Given the increased risk for emphysema, α1AT deficiency is an important public health problem, affecting an estimated 60,000 persons in the United States alone.

The α1AT gene is expressed principally in the liver, which normally secretes α1AT into plasma. Approximately 17% of Z/Z homozygotes present with

neonatal jaundice, and ~20% of this group subsequently develop cirrhosis. The liver disease associated with the Z allele is thought to result from a novel property of the mutant protein – its tendency to aggregate, trapping it within the rough endoplasmic reticulum (ER) of hepatocytes. The molecular basis of the Z protein aggregation is a consequence of structural changes in the protein that predispose to the formation of long beadlike necklaces of mutant α1AT polymers. Thus, like the sickle cell disease variant in β-globin (see Chapter 12), the Z allele of α1AT is a clear example of a variant that confers a novel property on the protein (in both of these examples, a tendency to aggregate) (see Fig. 12.1).

Both sickle cell disease and the α1AT deficiency associated with homozygosity for the Z allele are examples of inherited conformational diseases. These disorders occur when a variant causes the shape or size of a protein to change in a way that predisposes it to self-association and tissue deposition. Notably, some fraction of the mutant protein is invariably correctly folded in these disorders, including α1AT deficiency. Note that not all conformational diseases are single-gene disorders, as illustrated, for example, by nonfamilial AD (discussed later) and prion diseases.

The lung disease associated with the Z allele of α1AT deficiency is due to the alteration of the normal balance between elastase and α1AT, which allows progressive degradation of the elastin of alveolar walls (Fig. 13.9). Two mechanisms contribute to the elastase α1AT imbalance. First, the block in the hepatic secretion of the Z protein, although not complete, is severe, and Z/Z patients have only ~15% of the normal plasma concentration of α1AT. Second, the Z protein has only ~20% of the ability of the normal α1AT protein to inhibit neutrophil elastase. The infusion of normal α1AT is used in some patients to augment the level of α1AT in the plasma, to rectify the elastase:α1AT imbalance. Although difficult to prove definitively, there is evidence that the progression of the lung disease is slowed by α1AT augmentation.

α₁-Antitrypsin Deficiency as an Ecogenetic Disease

The development of lung or liver disease in subjects with α1AT deficiency is highly variable, and although no modifier genes have yet been identified, a major environmental

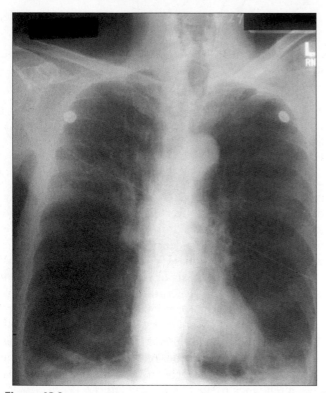

Figure 13.9 A posteroanterior chest radiograph of an individual carrying two Z alleles of the α1AT gene, showing the hyperinflation and basal hyperlucency characteristic of emphysema. (From Stoller JK, Aboussouan LS: α₁-Antitrypsin deficiency, *Lancet* 365: 2225–2236, 2005.)

factor, cigarette smoke, dramatically influences the likelihood of emphysema. The impact of smoking on the progression of the emphysema is a powerful example of the effect that environmental factors may have on the phenotype of a monogenic disease. Thus, for persons with the Z/Z genotype, survival after 60 years of age is ~60% in nonsmokers but only ~10% in smokers (see Fig. 13.8). One molecular explanation for the effect of smoking is that the active site of α1AT, at methionine 358, is oxidized by both cigarette smoke and inflammatory cells, thus reducing its affinity for elastase by 2000-fold.

The field of ecogenetics, illustrated by α1AT deficiency, is concerned with the interaction between environmental factors and different human genotypes. This area of medical genetics is one of increasing importance as genotypes are identified that entail an increased risk for disease on exposure to certain environmental agents (e.g., drugs, foods, industrial chemicals, and viruses). At present, the most highly developed area of ecogenetics is that of **pharmacogenetics**, presented in Chapter 19.

Dysregulation of a Biosynthetic Pathway: Acute Intermittent Porphyria

Acute intermittent porphyria (AIP) is an autosomal **dominant** disease associated with intermittent neurologic dysfunction. The primary defect is a deficiency of porphobilinogen (PBG) deaminase, an enzyme in the biosynthetic pathway of heme, required for the synthesis of both hemoglobin and hepatic cytochrome p450 drug-metabolizing enzymes (Fig. 13.10). All individuals with AIP have a ~50% reduction in PBG deaminase enzymatic activity, whether their disease is clinically latent (90% of patients throughout their lifetime) or clinically expressed (~10%). This reduction is consistent with the autosomal dominant inheritance pattern (see Chapter 7). Homozygous deficiency of PBG deaminase, a critical enzyme in heme biosynthesis, would presumably be

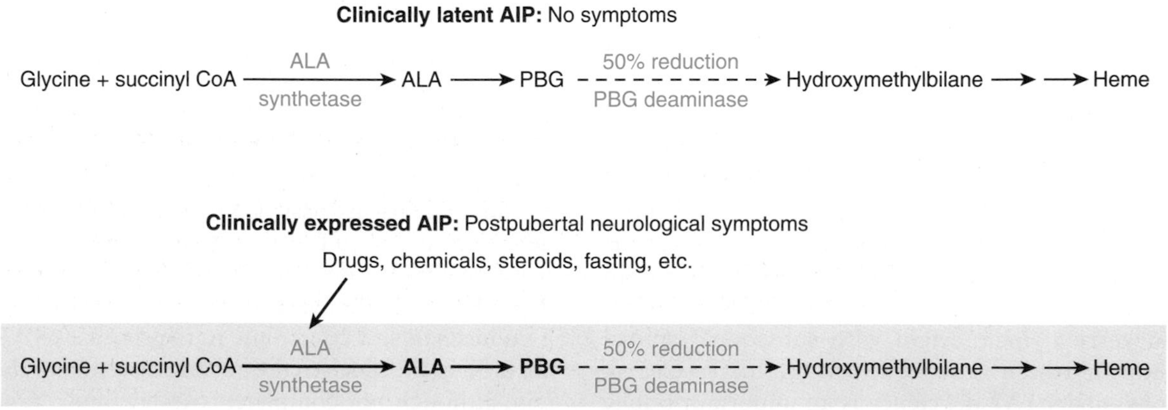

Clinically latent AIP: No symptoms

Glycine + succinyl CoA $\xrightarrow{\text{ALA synthetase}}$ ALA $\longrightarrow$ PBG $\dashrightarrow[\text{PBG deaminase}]{50\% \text{ reduction}}$ Hydroxymethylbilane $\longrightarrow$ $\longrightarrow$ Heme

Clinically expressed AIP: Postpubertal neurological symptoms

Drugs, chemicals, steroids, fasting, etc.

Glycine + succinyl CoA $\xrightarrow{\text{ALA synthetase}}$ **ALA** $\longrightarrow$ **PBG** $\dashrightarrow[\text{PBG deaminase}]{50\% \text{ reduction}}$ Hydroxymethylbilane $\longrightarrow$ $\longrightarrow$ Heme

Figure 13.10 The pathogenesis of acute intermittent porphyria *(AIP)*. Patients with AIP who are either clinically latent or clinically affected have approximately half the control levels of porphobilinogen *(PBG)* deaminase. When the activity of hepatic δ-aminolevulinic acid *(ALA)* synthase is increased in carriers by exposure to inducing agents (e.g., drugs, chemicals), the synthesis of ALA and PBG is increased to a level that the PBG deaminase can't handle. The residual PBG deaminase activity (~50% of controls) is overloaded, and the accumulation of ALA and PBG causes clinical disease. *CoA*, Coenzyme A. (Redrawn from Kappas A, Sassa S, Galbraith RA, et al: The porphyrias. In Scriver CR, Beaudet AL, Sly WS, et al, editors: *The metabolic bases of inherited disease*, ed 6, New York, 1989, McGraw-Hill, pp 1305–1365.)

incompatible with life. AIP illustrates one molecular mechanism by which an autosomal dominant disease may manifest only episodically.

The pathogenesis of the nervous system disease is uncertain but may be mediated directly by the increased levels of δ-aminolevulinic acid (ALA) and PBG that accumulate due to the 50% reduction in PBG deaminase (see Fig. 13.10). The peripheral, autonomic, and central nervous systems are all affected, and the clinical manifestations are diverse. Indeed, this disorder is one of the great mimics in clinical medicine, with manifestations ranging from acute abdominal pain to psychosis.

Clinical crises in AIP are elicited by a variety of precipitating factors: drugs (most prominently the barbiturates, and to this extent, AIP is a pharmacogenetic disease; see Chapter 19); some steroid hormones (clinical disease is rare before puberty or after menopause); and catabolic states, including reducing diets, intercurrent illnesses, and surgery. The drugs provoke the clinical manifestations by interacting with drug-sensing nuclear receptors in hepatocytes, which then bind to transcriptional regulatory elements of the ALA synthetase gene, increasing the production of both ALA and PBG. In normal individuals the drug-related increase in ALA synthetase is beneficial because it increases heme synthesis, allowing greater formation of hepatic cytochrome P450 enzymes that metabolize many drugs. In patients with AIP, however, the increase in ALA synthetase causes the accumulation of ALA and PBG because of the 50% reduction in PBG deaminase activity (see Fig. 13.10). The fact that half of the normal activity of PBG deaminase is inadequate to cope with the increased requirement for heme synthesis in some situations accounts for both the dominant inheritance of the condition and the episodic nature of the clinical illness.

DEFECTS IN RECEPTOR PROTEINS

The recognition of a class of diseases due to defects in receptor molecules began with the identification by Goldstein and Brown of the low-density lipoprotein (LDL) receptor as the polypeptide affected in the most common form of familial hypercholesterolemia. This disorder, which leads to a greatly increased risk for myocardial infarction, is characterized by elevation of plasma cholesterol carried by LDL, the principal cholesterol transport protein in plasma. Goldstein and Brown's discovery has cast much light on normal cholesterol metabolism and on the biology of cell surface receptors in general. LDL receptor deficiency is representative of a number of disorders now recognized to result from receptor defects.

Familial Hypercholesterolemia: A Genetic Hyperlipidemia

Familial hypercholesterolemia is one of a group of metabolic disorders called the hyperlipoproteinemias. These

TABLE 13.2 Four Genes Associated With Familial Hypercholesterolemia

Mutant Gene Product	Pattern of Inheritance	Effect of Disease-Causing Variants	Typical LDL Cholesterol Level (Normal Adults: ~120 mg/dL)
LDL receptor	Autosomal dominant	Loss of function	Heterozygotes: 350 mg/dL Homozygotes: 700 mg/dL
Apoprotein B-100	Autosomal dominant*	Loss of function	Heterozygotes: 270 mg/dL Homozygotes: 320 mg/dL
ARH adaptor protein	Autosomal recessive†	Loss of function	Homozygotes: 470 mg/dL
PCSK9 protease	Autosomal dominant	Gain of function	Heterozygotes: 225 mg/dL

*Principally in individuals of European descent.
†Principally in individuals of Italian and Middle Eastern descent.
LDL, Low-density lipoprotein.
Partly modified from Goldstein JL, Brown MS: The cholesterol quartet, *Science* 292:1310–1312, 2001.

diseases are characterized by elevated levels of plasma lipids (cholesterol, triglycerides, or both) carried by apolipoprotein B (apoB)–containing lipoproteins. Other monogenic hyperlipoproteinemias, each with distinct biochemical and clinical phenotypes, have also been recognized.

In addition to variants in the LDL receptor gene (Table 13.2), abnormalities in three other genes can lead to familial hypercholesterolemia (Fig. 13.11). Remarkably, all four of the genes associated with familial hypercholesterolemia disrupt the function or abundance either of the LDL receptor at the cell surface or of apoB, the major protein component of LDL and a ligand for the LDL receptor. Because of its importance, we first review familial hypercholesterolemia due to pathogenic variants in the LDL receptor. We also discuss variants in the *PCSK9* protease gene; although gain-of-function variants in this gene cause hypercholesterolemia, the greater importance of *PCSK9* lies in the fact that several common loss-of-function sequence variants lower plasma LDL cholesterol levels, conferring substantial protection from coronary heart disease.

Familial Hypercholesterolemia Due to Pathogenic Variants in the LDL Receptor

Pathogenic variants in the LDL receptor gene *(LDLR)* are the most common cause of familial hypercholesterolemia (Case 16). The receptor is a cell surface protein responsible for binding LDL and delivering it to the cell interior. Elevated plasma concentrations of LDL cholesterol lead to premature atherosclerosis (accumulation of cholesterol by macrophages in the subendothelial space of major arteries) and increased risk for heart attack and stroke in both untreated **heterozygote** and **homozygote**

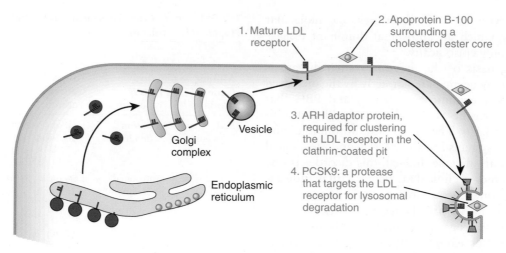

Figure 13.11 The four proteins associated with familial hypercholesterolemia. The low-density lipoprotein *(LDL)* receptor binds apoprotein B-100. Pathogenic variants in the LDL receptor-binding domain of apoprotein B-100 impair LDL binding to its receptor, reducing the removal of LDL cholesterol from the circulation. Clustering of the LDL receptor–apoprotein B-100 complex in clathrin-coated pits requires the ARH adaptor protein, which links the receptor to the endocytic machinery of the coated pit. Homozygous variants in the ARH protein impair the internalization of the LDL:LDL receptor complex, thereby impairing LDL clearance. PCSK9 protease activity targets LDL receptors for lysosomal degradation, preventing them from recycling back to the plasma membrane (see text).

carriers of mutant alleles. Physical stigmata of familial hypercholesterolemia include xanthomas (cholesterol deposits in skin and tendons) (Case 16) and premature arcus corneae (deposits of cholesterol around the periphery of the cornea). Few diseases have been as thoroughly characterized; the sequence of pathologic events from the affected locus to its effect on individuals and populations has been meticulously documented.

Genetics. Familial hypercholesterolemia due to pathogenic variants in the *LDLR* gene is inherited as an autosomal semidominant trait. Both homozygous and **heterozygous** phenotypes are known, and a clear **gene dosage** effect is evident; the disease manifests earlier and much more severely in homozygotes than in heterozygotes, reflecting the greater reduction in the number of LDL receptors and the greater elevation in plasma LDL cholesterol (Fig. 13.12). Homozygotes may have clinically significant coronary artery disease in childhood and, if untreated, few live beyond the third decade. The heterozygous form of the disease, with a population frequency of ~2 per 1000, is one of the most common single-gene disorders. Heterozygotes have levels of plasma cholesterol that are approximately twice those of controls (see Fig. 13.12). Because of the inherited nature of familial hypercholesterolemia, it is important to make the diagnosis in the ~5% of survivors of premature (<50 years of age) myocardial infarction who are heterozygotes for an LDL receptor defect. It is important to stress, however, that among those in the general population with plasma cholesterol concentrations above the 95th percentile for age and sex, only ~1 in 20 has familial hypercholesterolemia; most such individuals have an uncharacterized hypercholesterolemia due to multiple common genetic variants, as presented in Chapter 9.

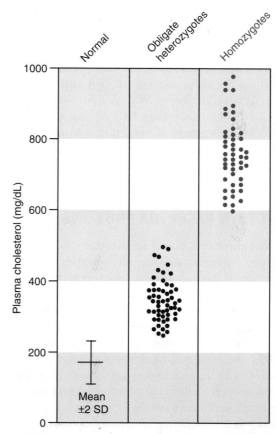

Figure 13.12 Gene dosage in low-density lipoprotein (LDL) deficiency. Shown is the distribution of total plasma cholesterol levels in 49 patients homozygous for deficiency of the LDL receptor, their parents (obligate heterozygotes), and normal controls. (Redrawn from Goldstein JL, Brown MS: Familial hypercholesterolemia. In Scriver CR, Beaudet AL, Sly WS, et al, editors: *The metabolic bases of inherited disease*, ed 6, New York, 1989, McGraw-Hill, pp 1215–1250.)

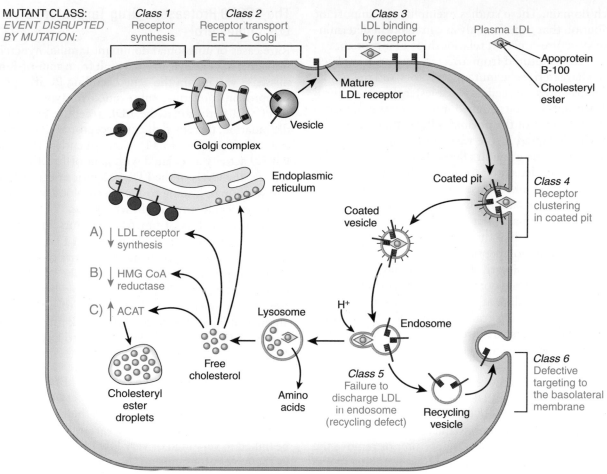

Figure 13.13 The cell biology and biochemical role of the low-density lipoprotein *(LDL)* receptor and the six classes of variants that alter its function. After synthesis in the endoplasmic reticulum (ER), the receptor is transported to the Golgi apparatus and subsequently to the cell surface. Normal receptors are localized to clathrin-coated pits, which invaginate, creating coated vesicles and then endosomes, the precursors of lysosomes. Normally, intracellular accumulation of free cholesterol is prevented because the increase in free cholesterol *(A)* decreases the formation of LDL receptors, *(B)* reduces *de novo* cholesterol synthesis, and *(C)* increases the storage of cholesteryl esters. The biochemical phenotype of each class of mutant is discussed in the text. *ACAT,* Acyl-coenzyme A:cholesterol acyltransferase; *HMG CoA reductase,* 3-hydroxy-3-methylglutaryl coenzyme A reductase. (Modified from Brown MS, Goldstein JL: The LDL receptor and HMG-CoA reductase – Two membrane molecules that regulate cholesterol homeostasis, *Curr Top Cell Regul* 26:3–15, 1985.)

Cholesterol Uptake by the LDL Receptor. Normal cells obtain cholesterol from either *de novo* synthesis or the uptake from plasma of exogenous cholesterol bound to lipoproteins, especially LDL. The majority of LDL uptake is mediated by the LDL receptor, which recognizes apoprotein B-100, the protein moiety of LDL. LDL receptors on the cell surface are localized to invaginations (coated pits) lined by the protein clathrin (Fig. 13.13). Receptor-bound LDL is brought into the cell by endocytosis of the coated pits, which ultimately evolve into lysosomes in which LDL is hydrolyzed to release free cholesterol. The increase in free intracellular cholesterol reduces endogenous cholesterol formation by suppressing the rate-limiting enzyme of the synthetic pathway, 3-hydroxy-3-methylglutaryl coenzyme A (HMG CoA) reductase. Cholesterol not required for cellular metabolism or membrane synthesis may be reesterified for storage as cholesteryl esters, a process stimulated by the activation of acyl-coenzyme

A:cholesterol acyltransferase (ACAT). The increase in intracellular cholesterol also reduces synthesis of the LDL receptor (see Fig. 13.13).

Classes of Variants in the LDL Receptor

More than 1100 different variants have been identified in the *LDLR* gene, and these are distributed throughout the gene and protein sequence. Not all of the reported changes are functionally significant, and some disturb receptor function more severely than others. The great majority of alleles are single **nucleotide** substitutions, small **insertions,** or **deletions**; structural rearrangements account for only 2% to 10% of the *LDLR* alleles in most populations. The mature LDL receptor has five distinct structural domains that for the most part have distinguishable functions that mediate the steps in the life cycle of an LDL receptor, shown in Fig. 13.13. Analysis of the effect on the receptor of variants in each domain has played an important role in defining the function of each domain. These studies exemplify the important contribution that genetic analysis can make in determining the structure-function relationships of a protein.

Fibroblasts cultured from affected patients have been used to characterize the mutant receptors and the resulting disturbances in cellular cholesterol metabolism. *LDLR* variants can be grouped into six classes, depending on which step of the normal cellular itinerary of the receptor is disrupted by the variant (see Fig. 13.13).

- Class 1 variants are null alleles that prevent the synthesis of any detectable receptor; they are the most common type of disease-causing variants at this locus. In the remaining five classes, the receptor is synthesized normally, but its function is impaired.

- Class 2 variants (like those in classes 4 and 6) define features of the polypeptide critical to its subcellular localization. The relatively common class 2 variants are designated transport deficient because the LDL receptors accumulate at the site of their synthesis, the ER, instead of being transported to the Golgi complex. These alleles are predicted to prevent proper folding of the protein, an apparent requisite for exit from the ER.

- Class 3 variant receptors reach the cell surface but are incapable of binding LDL.

- Class 4 variants impair localization of the receptor to the coated pit, and consequently the bound LDL is not internalized. These variants alter or remove the cytoplasmic domain at the carboxyl terminus of the receptor, demonstrating that this region normally targets the receptor to the coated pit.

- Class 5 variants are recycling-defective alleles. Receptor recycling requires the dissociation of the receptor and the bound LDL in the endosome. Variants in the epidermal growth factor precursor homology domain prevent the release of the LDL ligand. This failure leads to degradation of the receptor, presumably because an occupied receptor cannot return to the cell surface.

- Class 6 variants lead to defective targeting of the mutant receptor to the basolateral membrane, a process that depends on a sorting signal in the cytoplasmic domain of the receptor. Variants affecting the signal can mistarget the mutant receptor to the apical surface of hepatic cells, thereby impairing the recycling of the receptor to the basolateral membrane and leading to an overall reduction of endocytosis of the LDL receptor.

The PCSK9 Protease, a Drug Target for Lowering LDL Cholesterol

Rare cases of autosomal dominant familial hypercholesterolemia have been found to result from gain-of-function missense variants in the gene encoding PCSK9 protease (proprotein convertase subtilisin/kexin type 9). The role of PCSK9 is to target the LDL receptor for lysosomal degradation, thereby reducing receptor abundance at the cell surface (see Fig. 13.11). Consequently, the increase in PSCK9 activity associated with gain-of-function variants reduces the levels of the LDL receptor at the cell surface below normal, leading to increased blood levels of LDL cholesterol and coronary heart disease.

Conversely, loss-of-function variants in the *PCSK9* gene result in an increased number of LDL receptors at the cell surface by decreasing the activity of the protease. More receptors increase cellular uptake of LDL cholesterol, lowering cholesterol and providing protection against coronary artery disease. Notably, the complete absence of PCSK9 activity in the few known individuals with two *PCSK9* null alleles appears to have no adverse clinical consequences.

Some PCSK9 Sequence Variants Protect Against Coronary Heart Disease. The link between monogenic familial hypercholesterolemia and the *PCSK9* gene suggested that common sequence variants in *PCSK9* might be linked to very high or very low LDL cholesterol levels in the general population. Importantly, several *PCSK9* sequence variants are strongly linked to low levels of plasma LDL cholesterol (Table 13.3). For example, a study that used US census definitions showed that in the Black population one of two *PCSK9* nonsense variants is found in 2.6% of all subjects; each variant is associated with a mean reduction in LDL cholesterol of ~40%. This reduction in LDL cholesterol has a powerful protective effect against coronary artery disease, reducing the risk by ~90%; only ~1% of Black subjects carrying one of these two *PCSK9* nonsense variants developed coronary artery disease over a 15-year period, compared to almost 10% of individuals without either variant. A missense allele (p.Arg46Leu) is more common in white US census category populations (3.2% of subjects) but appears to confer only a ~50% reduction in coronary heart disease. These findings have major public health implications because they suggest that modest but lifelong reductions in plasma LDL

TABLE 13.3 *PCSK9* Variants Associated With Low LDL Cholesterol Levels

Sequence Variant	Population Frequency	LDL Cholesterol Level (Normal ≤~100 mg/dL)	Impact on Incidence of Coronary Heart Disease
Null or dominant negative alleles	Rare genetic compounds, one dominant negative heterozygote	7–16 mg/dL	Unknown, but likely to greatly reduce risk
Tyr142Stop or Cys679Stop	Black heterozygotes: 2.6%	Mean: 28% (38 mg/dL)	90% reduction
Arg46Leu	white heterozygotes: 3.2%	Mean: 15% (20 mg/dL)	50% reduction

LDL, Low-density lipoprotein.

Derived from Cohen JC, Boerwinkle E, Mosley TH, et al: Sequence variants in *PCSK9*, low LDL, and protection against coronary heart disease, *N Engl J Med* 354: 1264–1272, 2006.

cholesterol levels of 20 to 40 mg/dL would significantly decrease the incidence of coronary heart disease in the population. The strong protective effect of *PCSK9* loss-of-function alleles, together with the apparent absence of any clinical sequelae in subjects with a total absence of PCSK9 activity, made PCSK9 a strong candidate target for drugs that inactivate or diminish the activity of the enzyme (see Chapter 14).

Finally, these discoveries emphasize how the investigation of rare genetic disorders can lead to important new knowledge about the genetic contribution to common genetically complex diseases.

Clinical Implications of the Genetics of Familial Hypercholesterolemia. Early diagnosis of the familial hypercholesterolemias is essential both to permit the prompt application of cholesterol-lowering therapies to prevent coronary artery disease and to initiate genetic screening of first-degree relatives. With appropriate drug therapy, familial hypercholesterolemia heterozygotes have a normal life expectancy. For homozygotes, onset of coronary artery disease can be remarkably delayed by plasma apheresis (which removes the hypercholesterolemic plasma) but will ultimately require liver transplantation.

Finally, the elucidation of the biochemical basis of familial hypercholesterolemia has had a profound impact on the treatment of the vastly more common forms of **sporadic** hypercholesterolemia by leading to the development of the statin class of drugs that inhibit *de novo* cholesterol biosynthesis (see Chapter 14). Newer therapies include monoclonal antibodies that directly target PCSK9 and lower LDL cholesterol by an additional 60% in clinical trials, prompting approval and use around the world.

TRANSPORT DEFECTS

Cystic Fibrosis

Since the 1960s, CF has been one of the most publicly visible of all human monogenic diseases (Case 12). It is the most common autosomal recessive **genetic disorder** of children in populations of European ancestry in the United States, with an incidence of ~1 in 2500 births (and thus a carrier frequency of ~1 in 25), whereas it is much less prevalent in other population groups, such as Blacks (1 in 15,000 births) and Asians (1 in 31,000 births). The isolation of the CF gene (called *CFTR*, for *CF t*ransmembrane *r*egulator) (see Chapter 11) more than 30 years ago was one of the first illustrations of the power of molecular genetic and genomic approaches to identify disease genes. Physiologic analyses have shown that the CFTR protein is a regulated chloride channel located in the apical membrane of the epithelial cells affected by the disease.

The Phenotypic Features of Cystic Fibrosis. The lungs and exocrine pancreas are the principal organs affected by CF (Case 12), but a major diagnostic feature is increased sweat sodium and chloride concentrations

(often first noted when parents kiss their infant). CF is most commonly identified by newborn screening in regions of the world where that is offered. Elsewhere, in most CF patients, the diagnosis is initially based on the clinical pulmonary or pancreatic findings and on an elevated level of sweat chloride. Less than 2% of patients have normal sweat chloride concentration despite an otherwise typical clinical picture; in these cases, molecular analysis can be used to ascertain whether they have pathogenic variants in the *CFTR* gene.

The pancreatic defect in CF is a maldigestion syndrome due to the deficient excretion of pancreatic enzymes (lipase, trypsin, chymotrypsin). Approximately 5% to 15% of patients with CF have enough residual pancreatic exocrine function for normal digestion and are designated "pancreatic sufficient." Moreover, patients with CF who are pancreatic sufficient have better growth and overall prognosis than the majority, who are "pancreatic insufficient." The clinical heterogeneity of the pancreatic disease is at least partly due to allelic heterogeneity, as discussed later.

Many other features are observed in CF patients. For example, neonatal lower intestinal tract obstruction (meconium ileus) occurs in 10% to 15% of CF newborns. The genital tract is also affected; females with CF have some reduction in fertility, but more than 98% of males with CF are infertile because they lack the vas deferens, a phenotype known as congenital bilateral absence of the vas deferens (CBAVD). In a striking example of allelic heterogeneity giving rise to a partial phenotype, it has been found that some infertile males who are otherwise well (i.e., have no pulmonary or pancreatic disease) have CBAVD associated with specific variants in the *CFTR* gene. Similarly, some individuals with idiopathic chronic pancreatitis are carriers of variants in *CFTR* yet lack other clinical signs of CF.

The CFTR Gene and Protein. The *CFTR* gene has 27 **exons** and spans ~190 kb of DNA. The CFTR protein encodes a large integral membrane protein of ~170 kD (Fig. 13.14). The protein belongs to the ABC (*ATP* [adenosine triphosphate]–*b*inding *c*assette) family of transport proteins. At least 27 ABC transporters have been implicated in mendelian disorders and complex trait phenotypes.

The CFTR chloride channel has five domains, shown in Fig. 13.14: two membrane-spanning domains, each with six transmembrane sequences; two nucleotide (ATP)–binding domains; and a regulatory domain with multiple phosphorylation sites. The importance of each domain is demonstrated by the identification of CF-causing missense variants in each of them (see Fig. 13.14). The pore of the chloride channel is formed by the 12 transmembrane segments. ATP is bound and hydrolyzed by the nucleotide-binding domains, and the energy released is used to open and close the channel. Regulation of the channel is mediated, at least in part, by phosphorylation of the regulatory domain.

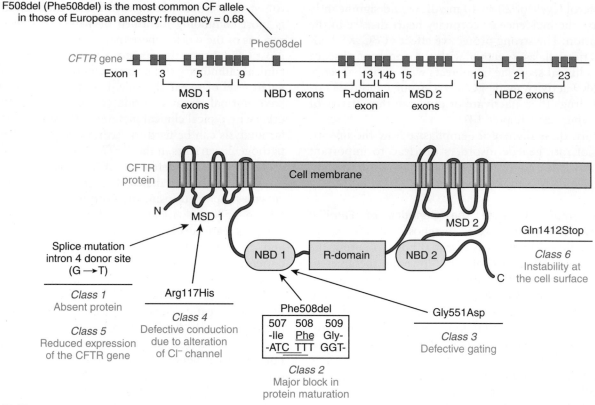

Figure 13.14 **The structure of the *CFTR* gene and a schematic of the CFTR protein.** Selected variants are shown. The exons, introns, and domains of the protein are not drawn to scale. Phe508del results from the deletion of TCT or CTT, replacing the Ile codon with ATT, and deleting the Phe codon. *CF*, Cystic fibrosis; *MSD*, membrane-spanning domain; *NBD*, nucleotide-binding domain; *R-domain*, regulatory domain. (Based on Zielinski J: Genotype and phenotype in cystic fibrosis, *Respiration* 67:117–133, 2000.)

The Pathophysiology of Cystic Fibrosis. CF is due to abnormal fluid and electrolyte transport across epithelial apical membranes. This abnormality leads to disease in the lung, pancreas, intestine, hepatobiliary tree, and male genital tract. The physiologic abnormalities have been most clearly elucidated for the sweat gland. The loss of CFTR function means that chloride in the duct of the sweat gland cannot be reabsorbed, leading to a reduction in the electrochemical gradient that normally drives sodium entry across the apical membrane. This defect leads, in turn, to the increased chloride and sodium concentrations in sweat. The effects on electrolyte transport due to the abnormalities in the CFTR protein have also been carefully studied in airway and pancreatic epithelia. In the lung, the hyperabsorption of sodium and reduced chloride secretion result in a depletion of airway surface liquid. Consequently, the mucous layer of the lung may become adherent to cell surfaces, disrupting the cough and cilia-dependent clearance of mucus and providing a niche favorable to *Pseudomonas aeruginosa*, the major cause of chronic pulmonary infection in CF.

The Genetics of Cystic Fibrosis

Pathogenic Variants in the Cystic Fibrosis Transmembrane Regulator Polypeptide. The most common CF pathogenic variant is a deletion of a phenylalanine residue at position 508 (p.Phe508del, shortened to F508del) in the first ATP-binding fold (NBD1; see Fig. 13.14), accounting for ~70% of all CF alleles in populations of European ancestry. In these populations, only seven other pathogenic variants are more frequent than 0.5%, and the remainder are each quite rare. Variants of all types have been identified, but the largest single group (nearly half) are missense substitutions. The remainder are point variants of other types, and less than 1% are genomic rearrangements. Although nearly 2000 *CFTR* gene sequence variants have been associated with disease, the actual number of missense variants that are disease-causing is uncertain because few have been subjected to functional analysis. However, a project called the Clinical and Functional **Translation** of CFTR (CFTR2 project; cftr2.org) has succeeded in assigning pathogenicity to more than 466 *CFTR* variants (including 174 missense variants and in frame deletions), which together account for at least 96% of all *CFTR* alleles worldwide.

Although the specific biochemical abnormalities associated with most CF alleles are not known, six general classes of dysfunction of the CFTR protein have been identified to date. Alleles representative of each class are shown in Fig. 13.14.

• Class 1 variants are null alleles – no CFTR polypeptide is produced. This class includes alleles with premature stop codons or those that generate highly unstable **RNAs**. Because CFTR is a glycosylated membrane-spanning protein, it must be processed in the endoplasmic reticulum and Golgi apparatus to be glycosylated and secreted.

- Class 2 variants impair the folding of the CFTR protein, thereby arresting its maturation. The F508del variant typifies this class; this misfolded protein cannot exit from the endoplasmic reticulum. However, the biochemical phenotype of the F508del protein is complex because it also exhibits defects in stability and activation in addition to impaired folding.
- Class 3 variants allow normal delivery of the CFTR protein to the cell surface but disrupt its function (see Fig. 13.14). The prime example is the p.Gly551Asp variant that impedes the opening and closing of the CFTR ion channel at the cell surface.
- Class 4 variants are located in the membrane-spanning domains and, consistent with this localization, have defective chloride ion conduction.
- Class 5 variants reduce the number of *CFTR* transcripts.
- Class 6 mutant proteins are synthesized normally but are unstable at the cell surface.

A Cystic Fibrosis Genocopy: Pathogenic Variants in the Epithelial Sodium Channel Gene *SCNN1*.

Although *CFTR* is the only gene that has been associated with classic CF, several families with nonclassic presentations (including CF-like pulmonary infections, less severe intestinal disease, elevated sweat chloride levels) have been found to carry pathogenic variants in the epithelial sodium channel gene *SCNN1*, a **genocopy**, that is, a phenotype that, although genetically distinct, has a very closely related phenotype. This finding is consistent with the functional interaction between the CFTR protein and the epithelial sodium channel. Its main clinical significance, at present, is the demonstration that patients with nonclassic CF display locus heterogeneity and that if *CFTR* pathogenic variants are not identified in a particular case, abnormalities in *SCNN1* must be considered.

Genotype-Phenotype Correlations in Cystic Fibrosis.

Because all patients with the classic form of CF appear to have pathogenic variants in the *CFTR* gene, clinical heterogeneity in CF must arise from allelic heterogeneity, from the effects of other modifying loci, or from nongenetic factors. Independent of the *CFTR* alleles that a particular patient may have, a significant genetic contribution from other (modifier) genes to several CF phenotypes has been recognized, with effects on lung function, neonatal intestinal obstruction, and diabetes.

Two generalizations have emerged from the genetic and clinical analysis of patients with CF. First, the specific *CFTR* genotype is a good predictor of exocrine pancreatic function. For example, patients homozygous for the common F508del variant or for predicted null alleles generally have pancreatic insufficiency. On the other hand, alleles that allow the synthesis of a partially functional CFTR protein, such as Arg117His (see Fig. 13.14), tend to be associated with pancreatic sufficiency.

Second, however, the specific *CFTR* genotype is a poor predictor of the severity of pulmonary disease. For example, among patients homozygous for the F508del variant, the severity of lung disease is variable. One reason for this poor phenotype-genotype correlation is inherited variation in the gene encoding transforming growth factor β1 (TGFβ1), as also discussed in Chapter 9. Overall, the evidence indicates that *TGFB1* alleles that increase TGFβ1 expression lead to more severe CF lung disease, perhaps by modulating tissue remodeling and inflammatory responses. Other genetic modifiers of CF lung disease, including alleles of the interferon-related developmental regulator 1 gene *(IFRD1)* and the interleukin-8 gene *(IL8)*, may act by influencing the ability of the CF lung to tolerate infection. Similarly, a few modifier genes have been identified for other CF-related phenotypes, including diabetes, liver disease, and meconium ileus.

The Cystic Fibrosis Gene in Populations.

At present, it is not possible to account for the high frequency of disease-causing *CFTR* alleles (about 1 in 25) among populations of European descent (see Chapter 9). The disease is much less frequent in others, although it has been reported in those of Indigenous, African, and Asian descent (e.g., ~1 in 90,000 Hawaiians of Asian descent). The F508del allele is the only one found to date that is common in virtually all populations of European ancestry, but its frequency among all pathogenic alleles varies significantly in different European populations, from 88% in Denmark to 45% in southern Italy.

In populations in which the F508del allele frequency is ~70% of all mutant alleles, ~50% of patients are homozygous for the F508del allele; an additional 40% are genetic compounds for F508del and another mutant allele. In addition, ~70% of CF carriers have the F508del variant. As noted earlier, except for F508del, other variants at the *CFTR* locus are rare, although in specific populations some alleles are relatively common.

Population Screening.

Both carrier screening and newborn screening for CF is offered universally in the United States, Canada, Australia, New Zealand, most of western Europe, Russia, Brazil, Argentina, and Chile.

Genetic Analysis of Families of Patients and Prenatal Diagnosis.

The high frequency of the F508del allele is useful when CF patients without a family history present for DNA diagnosis. The identification of the F508del allele, in combination with a panel of 127 common variants suggested by the American College of Medical Genetics and **Genomics**, can be used to predict the status of family members for confirmation of disease (e.g., in a newborn or a sibling with an ambiguous presentation), carrier detection, and prenatal diagnosis. Given the vast knowledge of *CFTR* variants in many populations, direct variant detection is the method of choice for genetic analysis. For couples with a 25% risk, preimplantation genetic testing following *in vitro* fertilization can be offered; alternatively, for fetuses with a 1 in 4 risk, prenatal diagnosis by DNA analysis at 10 to 12 weeks, with tissue obtained by chorionic villus biopsy, is the method of choice (see Chapter 18).

Molecular Genetics and the Treatment of Cystic Fibrosis. Historically, the treatment of CF has been directed toward controlling pulmonary infection and improving nutrition. Increasing knowledge of the molecular pathogenesis has made it possible to design pharmacologic interventions that modulate CFTR function in most patients (see Chapter 14). Alternatively, **gene transfer therapy** may be possible in the future for CF, but there are many difficulties.

DISORDERS OF STRUCTURAL PROTEINS

The Dystrophin Glycoprotein Complex: Duchenne, Becker, and Other Muscular Dystrophies

Like CF, Duchenne muscular dystrophy (DMD) has long received attention from the general and medical communities as a relatively common, severe, and progressive muscle-wasting disease with relentless clinical deterioration (Case 14). The isolation of the gene affected in this X-linked disorder and the characterization of its protein (named dystrophin because of its association with DMD) have given insight into every aspect of the disease, greatly improved the **genetic counseling** of affected families, and suggested strategies for treatment. The study of dystrophin led to the identification of a major complex of other muscular dystrophy–associated muscle membrane proteins, the dystrophin glycoprotein complex (DGC), described later in this section.

The Clinical Phenotype of Duchenne Muscular Dystrophy. Affected boys are normal for the first 1 to 2 years of life but develop muscle weakness by 3 to 5 years of age, when they begin to have difficulty climbing stairs and rising from a sitting position. The child is typically confined to a wheelchair by the age of 12 years. Although DMD is currently incurable, recent advances in the management of pulmonary and cardiac complications (which were leading causes of death in boys with DMD) have changed the disease from a life-limiting to a life-threatening disorder. In the preclinical and early stages of the disease, the serum level of creatine kinase is grossly elevated (50–100 times the upper limit of normal) because of its release from diseased muscle. The brain is also affected; on average, there is a moderate decrease in IQ of ~20 points.

The Clinical Phenotype of Becker Muscular Dystrophy. Becker muscular dystrophy (BMD) is also due to pathogenic variants in the dystrophin gene, but the BMD alleles produce a much milder phenotype and patients often remain ambulant beyond the teenage years. In general, patients with BMD carry variant alleles that maintain the **reading frame** of the protein and thus express some dystrophin, albeit often an altered product at reduced levels. Dystrophin is generally demonstrable in the muscle of patients with BMD (Fig. 13.15). In contrast, patients with DMD have little or no detectable dystrophin.

The Genetics of Duchenne Muscular Dystrophy and Becker Muscular Dystrophy

Inheritance. DMD has an incidence of ~1 in 3300 live male births, with a calculated **mutation rate** of 10^{-4}, an order of magnitude higher than the rate observed in genes involved in most other genetic diseases (see Chapter 4). In fact, given a production of ~8×10^7 sperm per day, a normal male produces a sperm with a new **mutation** in the *DMD* gene every 10 to 11 seconds! In Chapter 7, DMD was presented as a typical X-linked recessive disorder that is lethal in males, so that one-third of cases are predicted to be due to new mutations and two-thirds of patients have carrier mothers (see also Chapter 17). The great majority of carrier females have no clinical manifestations, although ~70% have slightly elevated levels of serum creatine kinase. In accordance with random inactivation of the **X chromosome** (see Chapter 6), however, the X chromosome carrying the normal *DMD* allele appears to be inactivated above a critical threshold of cells in some female heterozygotes. Nearly 20% of adult female carriers have some muscle weakness; whereas in 8%, life-threatening cardiomyopathy and serious proximal muscle disability occur. In rare instances, females have been described with DMD. Some have X;**autosome** translocations (see Chapter 6), whereas others have only one X chromosome (Turner syndrome) with a *DMD* pathogenic variant on that chromosome.

BMD accounts for ~15% of the variants at the locus. An important genetic distinction between these allelic phenotypes is that whereas DMD is a **genetic lethal**, the reproductive **fitness** of males with BMD is high (up to ~70% of normal) so that they can transmit the mutant gene to their daughters. Consequently, and in contrast to DMD, a high proportion of BMD cases are inherited, and relatively few (only ~10%) represent new mutations.

The DMD Gene and Its Product. The most remarkable feature of the *DMD* gene is its size, estimated to be >2000kb, or ~1.5% of the entire X chromosome. This huge gene is among the largest known in any species, by an order of magnitude. The high mutation rate can be at least partly explained by the fact that the locus is a large target for mutation but, as described later, it is also structurally prone to deletion and duplication. The *DMD* gene is complex, with 79 exons and seven tissue-specific promoters. In muscle, the large (14-kb)

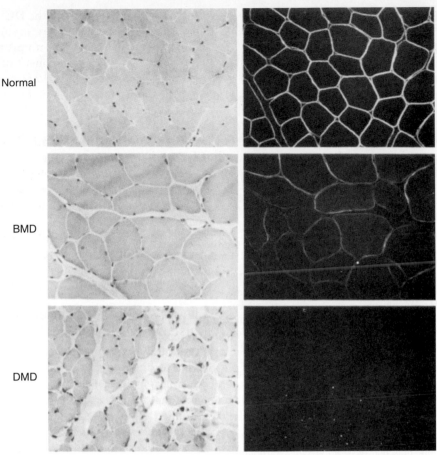

Figure 13.15 Microscopic visualization of the effect of pathogenic variants in the dystrophin gene in a patient with Becker muscular dystrophy *(BMD)* and a patient with Duchenne muscular dystrophy *(DMD)*. *(Left column)* Hematoxylin and eosin staining of muscle. *(Right column)* Immunofluorescence microscopy staining with an antibody specific to dystrophin. Note the localization of dystrophin to the myocyte membrane in normal muscle, the reduced quantity of dystrophin in BMD muscle, and the complete absence of dystrophin from the myocytes of the DMD muscle. The amount of connective tissue between the myocytes in the DMD muscle is increased. (Courtesy K. Arahata, National Institute of Neuroscience, Tokyo.)

dystrophin transcript encodes a huge 427-kD protein. In accordance with the clinical phenotype, the protein is most abundant in skeletal and cardiac muscle, although many tissues express at least one dystrophin isoform.

The Molecular and Physiologic Defects in Becker Muscular Dystrophy and Duchenne Muscular Dystrophy. The most common molecular defects in patients with DMD are deletions (60% of alleles), which are not randomly distributed. Rather, they are clustered in either the 5′ half of the gene or in a central region that encompasses an apparent deletion hot spot. The mechanism of deletion in the central region is unknown, but it appears to involve the **tertiary structure** of the genome and, in some cases, recombination between *Alu* repeat sequences (see Chapter 2) in large central **introns**. Point variants account for approximately one-third of the alleles and are randomly distributed throughout the gene.

The absence of dystrophin in DMD destabilizes the myofiber membrane, increasing its fragility and allowing increased Ca^{++} entry into the cell, with subsequent activation of inflammatory and degenerative pathways.

In addition, the chronic degeneration of myofibers eventually exhausts the pool of myogenic stem cells that are normally activated to regenerate muscle. This reduced regenerative capacity eventually leads to the replacement of muscle with fat and fibrotic tissue.

The Dystrophin Glycoprotein Complex. Dystrophin is a **structural protein** that anchors the DGC at the cell membrane. The DGC is a veritable constellation of polypeptides associated with more than a dozen genetically distinct muscular dystrophies (Fig. 13.16). This complex serves several major functions. First, it is thought to be essential for the maintenance of muscle membrane integrity, by linking the actin cytoskeleton to the extracellular matrix. Second, it is required to position the proteins in the complex at the sarcolemma. Although the function of many of the proteins in the complex is unknown, their association with diseases of muscle indicates that they are essential components of the complex. Pathogenic variants in several of these proteins cause autosomal recessive limb girdle muscular dystrophies and other congenital muscular dystrophies (see Fig. 13.16).

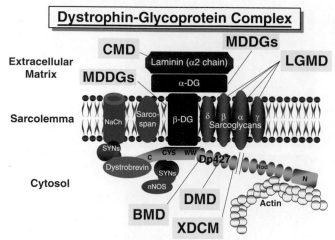

Figure 13.16 In muscle, dystrophin links the extracellular matrix (laminin) to the actin cytoskeleton. Dystrophin interacts with a multimeric complex composed of the dystroglycans (DG), the sarcoglycans, the syntrophins, and dystrobrevin. The α,β-dystroglycan complex is a receptor for laminin and agrin in the extracellular matrix; pathogenic variants in 14 glycosyltransferase genes affecting the complex cause various forms of muscular dystrophy with or without brain and eye involvement (MDDGs, muscular dystrophy-dystroglycanopathies). The function of the sarcoglycan complex is uncertain, but it is integral to muscle function; pathogenic variants in the sarcoglycans have been identified in limb girdle muscular dystrophies *(LGMD)*. Pathogenic variants in laminin type 2 (merosin) cause a congenital muscular dystrophy *(CMD)*. The branched structures represent glycans. The WW domain of dystrophin is a tryptophan-rich, protein-binding motif. *BMD*, Becker muscular dystrophy; *DMD*, Duchenne muscular dystrophy; *Syn*, Syntrophins; *XDCM*, X-linked dilated cardiomyopathy. (Courtesy R. Cohn, The Hospital for Sick Children, Toronto.)

That each component of the DGC is affected by variants that cause other types of muscular dystrophies highlights the principle that no protein functions in isolation but rather is a component of a biologic pathway or a multiprotein complex. Variants in the genes encoding other components of a pathway or a complex often lead to genocopies.

Posttranslational Modification of the Dystrophin Glycoprotein Complex. Five of the muscular dystrophies associated with the DGC result from pathogenic variants in glycosyltransferases, leading to hypoglycosylation of α-dystroglycan. That five proteins are required for the posttranslational modification of one other polypeptide testifies to the critical nature of glycosylation to the function of α-dystroglycan in particular but, more generally, to the importance of posttranslational modifications for the normal function of most proteins.

Clinical Applications of Gene Testing in Muscular Dystrophy

Prenatal Diagnosis and Carrier Detection. With gene-based technologies, accurate carrier detection and prenatal diagnosis are available for most families with a history of DMD. In the 60% to 70% of families in whom the allele results from a deletion or duplication, the presence or absence of the defect can be assessed by examination of fetal DNA using methods that assess the gene's genomic continuity and size (see Fig. 13.17).

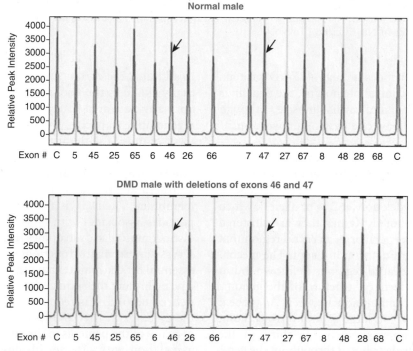

Figure 13.17 Diagnosis of Duchenne muscular dystrophy *(DMD)* involves screening for deletions and duplications by a procedure called multiplex ligation-dependent probe amplification (MLPA). MLPA allows the simultaneous analysis of all 79 exons of the *DMD* gene in a single DNA sample and can detect exon deletions and duplications in males or females. Each amplification peak represents a single *DMD* gene exon, after separation of the amplification products by capillary electrophoresis. *(Top panel)* The amplification profiles of 16 exons of a normal male sample. Control (C) DNAs are included at each end of the scan. The MLPA DNA fragments elute according to size, which is why the exons are not numbered sequentially. *(Bottom panel)* The corresponding amplification profile from a DMD patient with a deletion of exons 46 and 47. (Courtesy P. N. Ray, the Hospital for Sick Children, Toronto.)

In most other families, single nucleotide variants can be identified by sequencing of the coding region and intron-exon boundaries. Because the disease has a very high frequency of new mutations and is not manifested in carrier females, ~80% of Duchenne boys are born into families with no previous history of the disease (see Chapter 7). Thus the incidence of DMD will not decrease substantially until universal prenatal or preconception screening for the disease is possible.

Maternal Mosaicism. If a boy with DMD is the first affected member of his family, and if his mother is not found to carry the variant in her lymphocytes, the usual explanation is that he has a new mutation at the *DMD* locus. However, ~5% to 15% of such cases appear to be due to maternal gonadal **mosaicism**, in which case the **recurrence risk** is significant (see Chapter 7).

Therapy. At present, only symptomatic treatment is available for DMD. The possibilities for rational therapy for DMD have greatly increased with the understanding of the normal role of dystrophin in the myocyte. Some of the therapeutic considerations are discussed in Chapter 14.

Pathogenic Variants in Genes That Encode Collagen or Other Components of Bone Formation: Osteogenesis Imperfecta

Osteogenesis imperfecta (OI) is a group of inherited disorders that predispose to skeletal deformity and easy fracturing of bones, even with little trauma (Fig. 13.18). The combined incidence of all forms of the disease is ~1 per 10,000. Approximately 95% of affected individuals have heterozygous pathogenic variants in one of two genes, *COL1A1* and *COL1A2*, that encode the chains of type I collagen, the major protein in bone. A remarkable degree of clinical variation has been recognized, from lethality in the perinatal period to only a mild increase in fracture frequency. The clinical heterogeneity is explained by both locus and allelic heterogeneity; the phenotypes are influenced by which chain of type I procollagen is affected and according to the type and location of the pathogenic variant at the locus. The major phenotypes and genotypes associated with variants in the type I collagen genes are outlined in Table 13.4.

Normal Collagen Structure and Its Relationship to Osteogenesis Imperfecta

It is important to appreciate the major features of normal type I collagen to understand the pathogenesis of OI. The type I procollagen molecule is formed from two proα1(I) chains (encoded by *COL1A1*) and

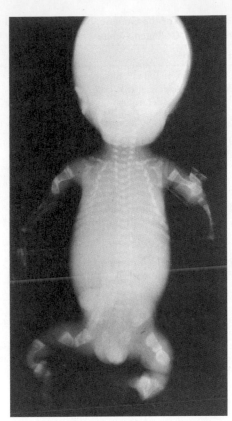

Figure 13.18 Radiograph of a premature (26 weeks of gestation) infant with the perinatal lethal form (type II) of osteogenesis imperfecta. The skull is relatively large and unmineralized and was soft to palpation. The thoracic cavity is small, the long bones of the arms and legs are short and deformed, and the vertebral bodies are flattened. All the bones are undermineralized. (Courtesy T. Costa, The Hospital for Sick Children, Toronto.)

one similar but distinct proα2(I) chain (encoded by *COL1A2*) (Fig. 13.19).

Proteins composed of subunits, like collagen, are often subject to variants that prevent subunit association by altering the subunit interfaces. The triple helical (collagen) section is composed of 338 tandemly arranged Gly-X-Y repeats; proline is often in the X position, and hydroxyproline or hydroxylysine is often in the Y position. Glycine, the smallest amino acid, is the only residue compact enough to occupy the axial position of the helix, and consequently, variants that substitute other residues for those glycines are highly disruptive to the helical structure.

Several features of procollagen maturation are of special significance to the pathophysiology of OI. First, the assembly of the individual proα chains into the trimer begins at the carboxy terminus, and triple helix formation progresses toward the amino terminus. Consequently, variants that alter residues in the carboxy-terminal part of the triple helical domain are more disruptive because they interfere earlier with the propagation of the triple helix (Fig. 13.20). Second, the

TABLE 13.4 Summary of the Genetic, Biochemical, and Molecular Features of the Types of Osteogenesis Imperfecta Due to Variants in Type 1 Collagen Genes

Type	Phenotype	Inheritance	Biochemical Defect	Gene Defect
Defective Production of Type I Collagen*				
I	**Mild:** blue sclerae, brittle bones but no bone deformity	Autosomal dominant	All the collagen made is normal (i.e., solely from the normal allele), but the quantity is reduced by half	Largely null alleles that impair the production of proα1(I) chains, such as defects that interfere with mRNA synthesis
Structural Defects in Type I Collagen				
II	**Perinatal lethal:** severe skeletal abnormalities, dark sclerae, death within 1 mo (see Fig. 13.18)	Autosomal dominant (new mutation)	Production of abnormal collagen molecules due to substitution of the glycine in Gly-X-Y of the triple helical domain located, in general, throughout the protein	Missense variants in the glycine codons of the genes for the α1 and α2 chains
III	**Progressive deforming:** with blue sclerae; fractures, often at birth; progressive bone deformity, limited growth	Autosomal dominant†		
IV	**Normal sclerae, deforming:** mild-moderate bone deformity, short stature, fractures	Autosomal dominant		

mRNA, Messenger RNA.

*A few patients with type I disease have substitutions of glycine in one of the type I collagen chains.

†Rare cases are autosomal recessive.

Modified from Byers PH: Disorders of collagen biosynthesis and structure. In Scriver CR, Beaudet AL, Sly WS, et al, eds: *The metabolic basis of inherited disease,* ed 6, New York, 1989, McGraw-Hill, pp 2805–2842; Byers PH: Brittle bones – Fragile molecules: disorders of collagen structure and expression, *Trends Genet* 6:293–300, 1990.

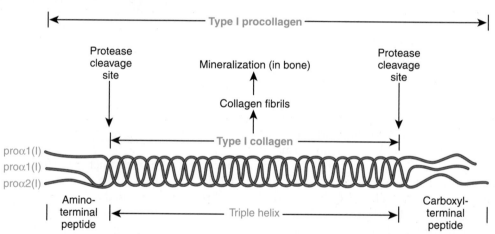

Figure 13.19 The structure of type I procollagen. Each collagen chain is made as a procollagen triple helix that is secreted into the extracellular space. The amino- and carboxyl-terminal domains are cleaved extracellularly to form collagen; mature collagen fibrils are then assembled and, in bone, mineralized. Note that type I procollagen is composed of two proα1(I) chains and one proα2(I) chain. (Redrawn from Byers PH: Disorders of collagen biosynthesis and structure. In Scriver CR, Beaudet AL, Sly WS, et al, editors: *The metabolic bases of inherited disease,* ed 6, New York, 1989, McGraw-Hill, pp 2805–2842.)

posttranslational modification (e.g., proline or lysine hydroxylation; hydroxylysyl glycosylation) of procollagen continues on any part of a chain not assembled into the triple helix. Thus, when triple helix assembly is slowed by a change, the unassembled sections of the chains amino-terminal to the defect are modified excessively, which slows their secretion into the extracellular space. Overmodification may also interfere with the formation of collagen fibrils. As a result of all these abnormalities, the number of secreted collagen molecules is reduced, and many of them are abnormal. In

bone, the abnormal chains and their reduced number lead to defective mineralization of collagen fibrils (see Fig. 13.18).

Molecular Abnormalities of Collagen in Osteogenesis Imperfecta

More than 2000 different pathogenic variants affecting the synthesis or structure of type I collagen have been found in individuals with OI. The clinical heterogeneity of this disease reflects even greater heterogeneity at the molecular level (see Table 13.4). For the type I collagen

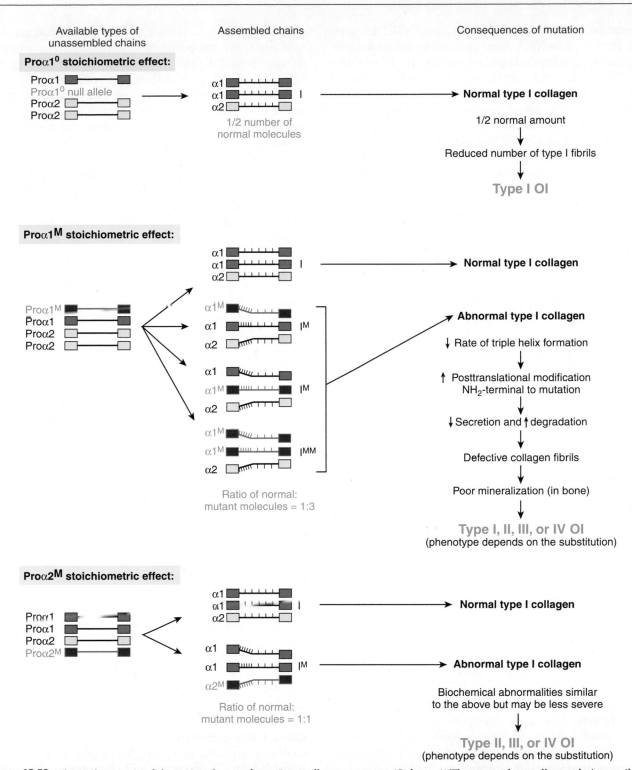

Figure 13.20 **The pathogenesis of the major classes of type I procollagen mutants.** *(Column 1)* The types of procollagen chains available for assembly into a triple helix. Although there are two α1 and two α2 collagen genes/genome, as implied in the left column, twice as many α1 collagen molecules are produced, compared to α2 collagen molecules, as shown in the central column. *(Column 2)* The effect of type I procollagen stoichiometry on the ratio of normal to defective collagen molecules formed in mutants with proα1 chain versus proα2 chain variants. The *small vertical bars* on each procollagen chain indicate posttranslational modifications (see text). *(Column 3)* The effect of variants on the biochemical processing of collagen. *OI,* Osteogenesis imperfecta; *Proα1^M*, a proα1 chain with a missense variant; *Proα2^M*, a proα2 chain with a missense variant; *Proα1^0*, a proα1 chain null allele.

genes, the variants fall into two general classes, those that reduce the amount of type I procollagen made and those that alter the structure of the molecules assembled.

Type I: Diminished Collagen Production. Most individuals with OI type I have variants that result in production by cells of approximately half the normal amount of type I procollagen. Most of these variants result in premature termination codons in one *COL1A1* allele that render the **mRNA** from that allele untranslatable. Because type I procollagen molecules must have two proα1(I) chains to assemble into a triple helix, loss of half the mRNA leads to production of half the normal quantity of type I procollagen molecules, although these molecules are normal (see Fig. 13.20). Missense variants can also give rise to this milder form of OI when the amino acid change is located in the amino terminus. This is because amino terminal substitutions tend to be less disruptive of collagen chain assembly, which can still initiate as usual at the carboxy terminus.

Types II, III, and IV: Structurally Defective Collagens.
The type II, III, and IV phenotypes of OI usually result from variants that produce structurally abnormal proα1(I) or proα2(I) chains (see Fig. 13.20 and Table 13.4). Most of these patients have substitutions in the triple helix that replace a glycine with a bulkier residue that disrupts formation of the triple helix. The specific collagen affected, the location of the substitution, and the nature of the substituting residue are all important phenotypic determinants, but some generalizations about the phenotype likely to result from a specific substitution are nevertheless possible. Thus substitutions in the proα1(I) chain are more prevalent in patients with OI types III and IV and are more often lethal. In either chain, replacement of glycine (a neutral residue) with a charged residue (aspartic acid, glutamic acid, arginine) or large residue (tryptophan) is usually very disruptive and often associated with a severe (type II) phenotype (see Fig. 13.20). Sometimes, a specific substitution is associated with more than one phenotype, an outcome that is likely to reflect the influence of powerful modifier genes.

Novel Forms of Osteogenesis Imperfecta That Do Not Result From Collagen Variants

Seventeen additional forms of clinically defined OI (types V–XXII, or 5–22) do not result from pathogenic variants in type I collagen genes but involve defects in other genes. These 5% of OI subjects with normal collagen genes have either dominant variants in the *IFITM5* gene (encoding interferon-induced transmembrane protein 5) or biallelic variants in any of more than a dozen other genes that encode proteins that regulate osteoblast development and facilitate bone formation or that mediate collagen assembly by interacting with collagens during synthesis and secretion. These genes include, for example, *WNT1*, which encodes a secreted signaling protein, and *BMP1*, which encodes bone morphogenetic protein 1, an inducer of cartilage formation.

The Genetics of Osteogenesis Imperfecta

As just discussed, most of the variants in type I collagen genes that cause OI act in a dominant manner. This group of disorders illustrates the genetic complexities

that result when variants alter structural proteins, particularly those composed of multiple different subunits, or alter proteins that are involved in the folding and transport of collagens to their place of action.

The relatively mild phenotype and dominant inheritance of OI type I are consistent with the fact that although only half the normal number of molecules is made, they are of normal quality (see Fig. 13.20). The more severe consequences of producing structurally defective proα1(I) chains from one allele (compared with producing no chains) partly reflect the stoichiometry of type I collagen, which contains two proα1(I) chains and one proα2(I) chain (see Fig. 13.20). Accordingly, if half the proα1(I) chains are abnormal, three of four type I molecules have at least one abnormal chain; in contrast, if half the proα2(I) chains are defective, only one in two molecules is affected. Variants such as the proα1(I) missense allele (proα1^M) shown in Fig. 13.20 are thus **dominant negative** alleles because they impair the contribution of both the normal proα1(I) chains and the normal proα2(I) chains. In other words, the effect of the mutant allele is amplified because of the trimeric nature of the collagen molecule. Consequently, in dominantly inherited diseases such as OI, it is actually better to have a variant that generates no gene product than one that produces an abnormal gene product. The biochemical mechanism in OI by which the dominant negative effect of dominant negative alleles of the *COL1A1* genes is exerted is one of the best understood in all of human genetics (see Cases 8 and 30 for other examples of dominant negative alleles).

Although variants that produce structurally abnormal proα2(I) chains reduce the number of normal type I collagen molecules by half, this reduction is nevertheless sufficient, in the case of some variants, to cause the severe perinatal lethal phenotype (see Table 13.4). Most infants with OI type II, the perinatal lethal form, have a *de novo* dominant mutation, and consequently there is a very low likelihood of recurrence in the family. In occasional families, however, more than one sibling is affected with OI type II. Such recurrences are usually due to parental **germline** or gonadal mosaicism, as described in Chapter 7.

Clinical Management. If a patient's molecular defect can be determined, increasing knowledge of the correlation between OI genotypes and phenotypes has made it possible to predict, at least to some extent, the natural history of the disease. The treatment of children with the more clinically significant forms of OI is based on physical medicine approaches to increase ambulation and mobility, often in the context of treatment with parenteral bisphosphonates, a class of drugs that act by decreasing bone resorption, to increase bone density and reduce fracture rate. These drugs appear to be less effective in individuals with the recessive forms of OI. The development of better and targeted drugs is a critical issue to improve care.

THE EFFECT OF GENE DUPLICATION AND RETAINED FUNCTION ON PHENOTYPE: SPINAL MUSCULAR ATROPHY

The Phenotypes of Spinal Muscular Atrophy

Spinal muscular atrophy (SMA), an autosomal recessive disease, is the most frequent genetic cause of infant mortality, affecting 1 in 10,000 live births and a carrier rate of 1 in 40 to 50. The disorder leads to progressive loss of the alpha motor neurons of the ventral spinal cord and motor nuclei of the lower brainstem causing hypotonia, muscle weakness, and atrophy of variable severity depending on the underlying genotype. SMA has traditionally been classified into four different phenotypes.

Patients with SMA type 1, which is the most common form (~45% of patients), present with symptoms around 0 to 6 months of age. Clinical presentation includes predominant proximal limb weakness, respiratory insufficiency, and poor feeding. Patients also show signs of intercostal muscle weakness, relative to preserved diaphragm strength, and over time develop a bell-shaped chest deformity with signs of paradoxic breathing. Tongue fasciculations are present, while facial and ocular muscle strength are unaffected. Interestingly, cognitive function is normal to above average. Patients usually do not achieve the ability to sit independently (nonsitters) and have a limited life expectancy.

Type 2 SMA, comprising 30% of cases, presents with muscle weakness by the age of 6 to 18 months. Most patients are able to achieve the ability to sit unsupported (sitters), although they may later lose this ability and are almost never able to stand or walk without support. Patients demonstrate proximal muscle weakness, often more pronounced in the lower extremities, tongue atrophy, and fasciculations. Respiratory insufficiency and dysphagia are common, particularly in more severe phenotypes. Given the significant axial muscle weakness, many patients develop significant scoliosis, which in turn often leads to restrictive lung disease and respiratory insufficiency. Aggressive supportive treatments prior to the onset of disease-modifying therapy led to increased life span, with 68.5% of this historic cohort surviving to age 25.

SMA type 3 (15% of cases) usually shows an onset of symptoms that can present from 18 months to adulthood. Patients are generally able to stand or walk without support (walkers), although some lose this ability with ongoing disease progression. Patients may present with symptoms of proximal weakness such as falls, abnormal gait, and difficulty climbing stairs. In contrast to SMA types 1 and 2, type 3 patients generally have a normal life expectancy and do not develop significant respiratory muscle weakness.

The recent development of disease-modifying therapies has changed the phenotypic landscape significantly, and clinical presentations and disease progression have become more diverse. This has changed previous clinical classifications to focus on the functional status of patients (nonsitters, sitters, walkers) or the response treatment (decline, no change, improvement). Therapeutic approaches are discussed in Chapter 14.

Genetics of Spinal Muscular Atrophy

The *SMN1* gene exhibits a duplication event with subsequent **SNV** in exon 7 of *SMN2* that affects **splicing** (Fig. 13.21). The *SMN2* gene retains about 10% wild-type transcript and is present in zero to four copies in the general population.

With a carrier frequency of 1 in 40 to 50 and an estimated incidence of 1 in 10,000 live births, SMA is the second most common autosomal recessive disorder. On chromosome 5q13, the survival motor neuron protein *SMN1* is reduced in function; however, the modifying *SMN2* gene is maintained. The absence of the *SMN1* gene accounts for most SMA cases. Ninety-five percent of SMA-affected individuals have a homozygous deletion of *SMN1* exon 7 or gene conversion from *SMN1* to *SMN2*, and most of the remaining 5% are compound heterozygotes for an *SMN1* exon 7 deletion and an *SMN1* SNV (see Fig. 13.21: normal in A, variants in B and C). A number of intragenic variants can be detected in the compound heterozygous state with an *SMN1* deletion and can include missense, nonsense, splice site variants, insertions, deletions, and duplications (see Fig. 13.21C). Recurrent variants have been discovered in exons 3 and 6, representing hot spots for small and missense changes, respectively (see Fig. 13.21D). Exon 6 codes for a domain in the protein, which plays a role in protein oligomerization, and individuals with exon 6 missense variants have decreased SMN protein self-oligomerization capacity. The exon 6 p.Tyr272Cys missense variant is the most frequently reported SNV in the *SMN1* gene.

Because both copies of *SMN1* exon 7 are lost in the majority of patients, no phenotype-genotype correlation was initially observed in SMA. The copy number of *SMN2* has now been shown to be a significant modifier of SMA severity. All individuals with SMA have at least one copy of *SMN2*, which generates low amounts of SMN protein but does not fully compensate for the loss of *SMN1*. The *SMN2* gene is unable to create a full transcript because of the presence of the splice variant in exon 7. The copy number varies from zero to three copies in the general population, with around 10% of individuals having no *SMN2*. A fetus that lacks *SMN1* function and has no copies of *SMN2* would presumably be nonviable. The majority of individuals who have type 1 SMA have one to two copies of *SMN2*. The typical number of *SMN2* copies in persons with type 2 SMA is three. Patients with milder type 3 and 4 individuals generally exhibit four or more copies of *SMN2*. These phenotype-genotype correlations have paved the way for developing disease-modifying therapies for SMA (see Chapter 14).

Molecular Testing for Spinal Muscular Atrophy

Screening for a missing or deficient exon 7 is the first step in diagnostic testing in patients, with 95% having a

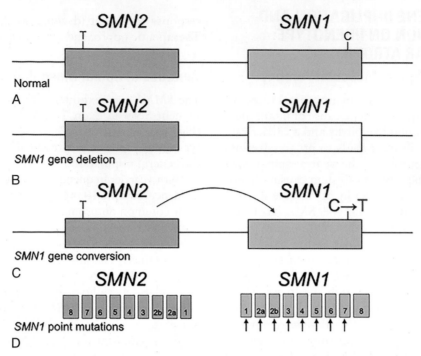

Figure 13.21 (A) A chromosome carrying a normal copy of *SMN1* and *SMN2*. (B) The blank box indicates a deleted gene. A deletion can remove part or all of the *SMN1* gene. (C) The curved arrow represents a conversion. With the C>T transition in *SMN1*, the *SMN1* copy now closely resembles *SMN2* and is considered *SMN2*-like. (D) Point mutations occurring in any of the *SMN1* exons prior to the last exon can affect the SMN protein. (From Keinath MC, Prior DE, Prior TW: Spinal muscular atrophy: Mutations, testing, and clinical relevance, *Appl Clin Genet* 14:11–25, 2021. https://doi.org/10.2147/TACG.S239603)

homozygous lack of *SMN1* exon 7. Several methodologies can detect the absence of *SMN1* exon 7, all based on the c.840C>T variation. One of the most popular techniques as a first deletion test in laboratories is **multiplex ligation-dependent probe amplification (MLPA)**. It is simple to use and highly sensitive and can determine both *SMN1* and *SMN2* copy numbers.

Preimplantation genetic diagnosis and prenatal testing for SMA is available for at-risk couples or due to the presence of abnormal findings on fetal ultrasound, such as decreased fetal movements, contractures *in utero*, or increased **nuchal translucency**. The presence of maternal cell contamination of the fetal specimen may result in a false-negative test result and therefore must be tested and shown to be absent prior to reporting the prenatal test result.

Newborn Screening

The *SMN1* exon 7 deletion test can be used as a reliable confirmatory test for the majority of patients suspected to have SMA and can be reported within 24 hours. The test is highly sensitive (~95%) and nearly 100% specific. Newborn screening for SMA has now been developed and is standard of care in many jurisdictions and is primarily based on real-time **polymerase chain reaction** that detects the common *SMN1* deletion and may also detect *SMN2* copy number on dried blood spots. Follow-up molecular genetic testing confirmation of a positive newborn screening result is always strongly recommended.

NEURODEGENERATIVE DISORDERS

Until recently, the biochemical and molecular mechanisms underlying almost all neurodegenerative diseases were completely obscure. In this section, we discuss three different conditions, each with a different genetic and genomic basis and illustrating different mechanisms of pathogenesis:

- Alzheimer disease
- Disorders of **mitochondrial DNA**
- Diseases due to the expansion of unstable repeat sequences

Alzheimer Disease

One of the most common adult-onset neurodegenerative conditions is Alzheimer disease (AD) (Case 4), introduced in Chapter 9 in the context of complex genetic disorders. AD generally manifests in the sixth to ninth decades, but there are monogenic forms that often present earlier, sometimes as soon as the third decade. The clinical picture of AD is characterized by a progressive deterioration of memory and of higher cognitive functions, such as reasoning, in addition to behavioral changes. These abnormalities reflect degeneration of neurons in specific regions of the cerebral cortex and hippocampus. AD affects ~1.4% of persons in developed countries and is responsible for over 120,000 deaths per year in the United States alone.

The Genetics of Alzheimer Disease

The lifetime risk for AD in the general population is 12.1% in men and 20.3% in women by age 85. Most of the increased risk in relatives of affected individuals is not due to mendelian inheritance; rather, as described in Chapter 9, this familial aggregation results from a complex genetic contribution involving one or more incompletely penetrant genes that act independently, from multiple interacting genes, or from some combination of genetic and environmental factors.

Approximately 7% to 10% of patients, however, have a monogenic highly penetrant form of AD that is inherited in an autosomal dominant manner. In the 1990s, four genes associated with AD were identified (Table 13.5). Pathogenic variants in three of these genes – encoding the β-amyloid precursor protein (βAPP), presenilin 1, and presenilin 2 – lead to autosomal dominant AD. The fourth gene, *APOE*, encodes apolipoprotein E (apoE), the protein component of several plasma lipoproteins. Variants in *APOE* are not associated with monogenic AD. Rather, as we saw in Chapter 9, the ε4 allele of *APOE* modestly increases susceptibility to nonfamilial AD and influences the age at onset of at least some of the monogenic forms (see later).

The identification of the four genes associated with AD has provided great insight not only into the pathogenesis of monogenic AD but also, as is commonly the case in medical genetics, into the mechanisms that underlie the more common form, nonfamilial or sporadic AD. Indeed, overproduction of one proteolytic product of βAPP, called the Aβ peptide, appears to be at the center of AD pathogenesis, and the currently available experimental evidence suggests that the βAPP, presenilin 1, and presenilin 2 proteins all play a direct role in the pathogenesis of AD.

The Pathogenesis of Alzheimer Disease: β-Amyloid Peptide and Tau Protein Deposits

The most important pathologic abnormalities of AD are the deposition in the brain of two fibrillary proteins, β-amyloid peptide (Aβ) and tau protein. The Aβ peptide is generated from the larger βAPP protein (see Table 13.5), as discussed in the next section, and is found in extracellular amyloid or senile plaques in the extracellular space of AD brains. Amyloid plaques contain other proteins besides the Aβ peptide, notably apoE (see Table 13.5). Tau is a microtubule-associated protein expressed abundantly in neurons of the brain. Hyperphosphorylated forms of tau compose the neurofibrillary tangles that, in contrast to the extracellular amyloid plaques, are found within AD neurons. The tau protein normally promotes the assembly and stability of microtubules, functions that are diminished by phosphorylation. Although the formation of tau neurofibrillary tangles appears to be one cause of the neuronal degeneration in AD, variants in the tau gene are associated not with AD but with another autosomal dominant dementia, frontotemporal dementia.

The Amyloid Precursor Protein Gives Rise to the β-Amyloid Peptide

The major features of the βAPP and its corresponding gene are summarized in Table 13.5. βAPP is a single-pass intracellular transmembrane protein found in

TABLE 13.5 Genes and Proteins Associated With Inherited Susceptibility to Alzheimer Disease

Gene	Inheritance	% of FAD	Protein	Normal Function	Role in FAD
PSEN1	AD	50%	Presenilin 1 (PS1): A 5–10 membrane-spanning domain protein found in cell types both inside and outside the brain	Unknown, but required for γ-secretase cleavage of βAPP	May participate in the abnormal cleavage at position 42 of βAPP and its derivative proteins; >100 variants identified in Alzheimer disease
PSEN2	AD	1–2%	Presenilin 2 (PS2): structure similar to PS1, maximal expression outside the brain	Unknown, likely to be similar to PS1	At least 5 missense variants identified
APP	AD	1–2%	Amyloid precursor protein (βAPP): an intracellular transmembrane protein. Normally, βAPP is cleaved endoproteolytically within the transmembrane domain (see Fig. 13.24), so that little of the β-amyloid peptide (Aβ) is formed.	Unknown	β-amyloid peptide (Aβ) is the principal component of senile plaques. Increased Aβ production, especially of the $A\beta_{42}$ form, is a key pathogenic event. Approximately 10 variants have been identified in FAD.
APOE	See Table 13.6	NA	Apolipoprotein E (apoE): a protein component of several plasma lipoproteins. The apoE protein is imported into the cytoplasm of neurons from the extracellular space.	Normal function in neurons is unknown. Outside the brain, apoE participates in lipid transport between tissues and cells. Loss of function causes one form (type III) of hyperlipoproteinemia.	An Alzheimer disease susceptibility gene (see Table 13.6). ApoE is a component of senile plaques.

AD, Autosomal dominant; *FAD*, familial Alzheimer disease; *NA*, not applicable.
Data derived from St. George-Hyslop PH, Farrer LA: Alzheimer's disease and the fronto-temporal dementias: diseases with cerebral deposition of fibrillar proteins. In Scriver CR, Beaudet AL, Sly WS, et al, editors: *The molecular and metabolic bases of inherited disease*, ed 8, New York, 2000, McGraw-Hill; Martin JB: Molecular basis of the neurodegenerative disorders, *N Engl J Med* 340:1970–1980, 1999. Updated in 2022 from ClinVar.

endosomes, lysosomes, the ER, and the Golgi apparatus. It is subject to three distinct proteolytic **fates**, depending on the relative activity of three different proteases: α-secretase and β-secretase, which are cell surface proteases, and γ-secretase, which is an atypical protease that cleaves membrane proteins within their transmembrane domains. The predominant fate of ~90% of βAPP is cleavage by the α-secretase (Fig. 13.22), an event that precludes the formation of the Aβ peptide because α-secretase cleaves within the Aβ peptide domain. The other ~10% of βAPP is cleaved by the β- and γ-secretases to form either the nontoxic $A\beta_{40}$ peptide or the $A\beta_{42}$ peptide. The $A\beta_{42}$ peptide is thought to be neurotoxic because it is more prone to aggregation than its $A\beta_{40}$ counterpart, a feature that makes AD a conformational disease like α1AT deficiency (described previously in this chapter). Normally, little $A\beta_{42}$ peptide is produced, and the factors that determine whether γ-secretase cleavage will produce the $A\beta_{40}$ or $A\beta_{42}$ peptide are not well defined.

In monogenic AD due to missense substitutions in the gene encoding βAPP (*APP*), however, several variants lead to the relative overproduction of the $A\beta_{42}$ peptide. This increase leads to accumulation of the neurotoxic $A\beta_{42}$, an occurrence that appears to be the central pathogenic event of all forms of AD, monogenic or sporadic. Consistent with this model is the fact that patients with Down syndrome, who possess three copies of the *APP* gene (which is on chromosome 21), typically develop the neuropathologic changes of AD by 40 years of age. Moreover, pathogenic variants in the AD genes presenilin 1 and presenilin 2 (see Table 13.5) also lead to increased production of $A\beta_{42}$. Notably, the amount of the neurotoxic $A\beta_{42}$ peptide is increased in the serum of individuals with pathogenic variants in the βAPP, presenilin 1, and presenilin 2 genes; furthermore, in cultured cell systems, the expression of mutant βAPP, presenilin 1, and presenilin 2 increases the relative production of $A\beta_{42}$ peptide by two- to tenfold.

The central role of the $A\beta_{42}$ peptide in AD is highlighted by the discovery of a coding variant (p.Ala673Thr) in the *APP* gene (Fig. 13.23) that protects against both AD and cognitive decline in older adults. The protective effect is likely due to reduced formation of the $A\beta_{42}$ peptide, reflecting the proximity of Thr673 to the β-secretase cleavage site (see Fig. 13.23).

The Presenilin 1 and 2 Genes

The genes encoding presenilin 1 and presenilin 2 (see Table 13.5) were identified in families with autosomal

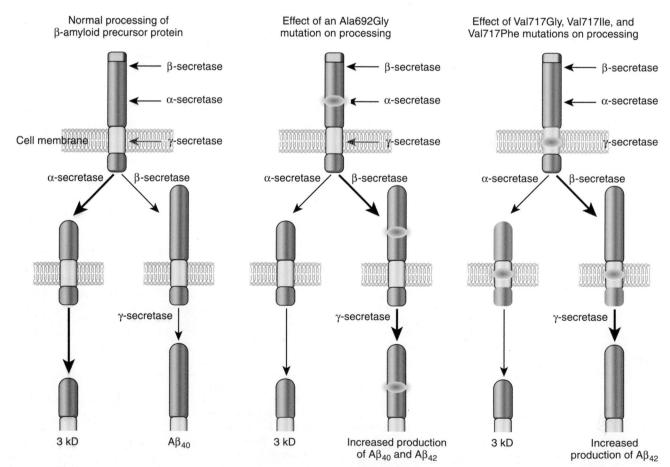

Figure 13.22 The normal processing of β-amyloid precursor protein (βAPP) and the effect on processing of missense variants in the βAPP gene associated with familial Alzheimer disease. The *ovals* show the locations of the missense changes. (Reproduced with permission from Nussbaum RL, Ellis CE: Alzheimer's disease and Parkinson's disease, *N Engl J Med* 348:1356–1364, 2003.)

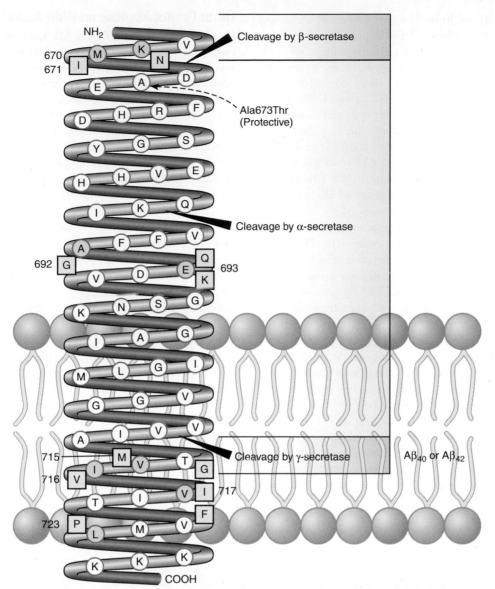

Figure 13.23 The topology of the amyloid precursor protein (βAPP), its nonamyloidogenic cleavage by α-secretase, and its alternative cleavage by putative β-secretase and γ-secretase to generate the amyloidogenic β amyloid peptide (Aβ). Letters are the single-letter code for amino acids in β-amyloid precursor protein, and numbers show the position of the affected amino acid. Normal residues involved in missense variants are shown in *highlighted circles*, whereas the amino acid residues representing various missense pathogenic variants are shown in *boxes*. The mutated amino acid residues are near the sites of β-, α-, and γ-secretase cleavage *(black arrowheads)*. The pathogenic variants lead to the accumulation of toxic peptide $A\beta_{42}$ rather than the wild-type $A\beta_{40}$ peptide. The location of the protective allele Ala673Thr is indicated by the *dashed arrow*. (Reproduced with permission from Nussbaum RL, Ellis CE: Alzheimer's disease and Parkinson's disease, *N Engl J Med* 348:1356–1364, 2003.)

dominant AD. Presenilin 1 is required for γ-secretase cleavage of βAPP derivatives. Indeed, some evidence suggests that presenilin 1 is a critical cofactor protein of γ-secretase. The pathogenic variants in presenilin 1 associated with AD, through an unclear mechanism, increase production of the $A\beta_{42}$ peptide. A major difference between presenilin 1 and presenilin 2 pathogenic variants is that the age at onset with the latter is much more variable (presenilin 1, 35–60 years; presenilin 2, 40–85 years). Indeed, in one family, an asymptomatic octogenarian carrying a presenilin 2 pathogenic variant transmitted the disease to his offspring. The basis of this variation is partly dependent on the number of *APOE* ε4 alleles (see Table 13.5 and later discussion) carried by individuals with a presenilin 2 pathogenic variant; two ε4 alleles are associated with an earlier age at onset than one allele, and one confers an earlier onset than other *APOE* alleles.

The *APOE* Gene Is an Alzheimer Disease Susceptibility Locus

As presented in Chapter 9, the ε4 allele of the *APOE* gene is a major risk factor for the development of AD. The role for *APOE* as a major AD susceptibility locus was suggested by multiple lines of evidence, including linkage to AD in late-onset families, increased association of the ε4 allele with AD patients compared with controls, and the finding that apoE binds to the Aβ peptide. The *APOE* protein has three common forms encoded by corresponding *APOE* alleles (Table 13.6). The ε4 allele is significantly overrepresented in patients with AD (~40% vs ~15% in the general population) and is associated with an early onset of AD (for ε4/ε4 homozygotes, the age at onset of AD is ~10–15 years earlier than in the general population; see Chapter 9). Moreover, the relationship between the ε4 allele and the disease is dose dependent; two copies of ε4 are associated with an earlier age at onset (mean onset before 70 years) than with one copy (mean onset after 70 years). In contrast, the ε2 allele has a protective effect and correspondingly is more common in elderly subjects who are unaffected by AD (see Table 13.6).

The mechanisms underlying these effects are not known, but apoE polymorphisms may influence the processing of βAPP and the density of amyloid plaques in AD brains. It is also important to note that the *APOE* ε4 allele is not only associated with an increased risk for AD; carriers of ε4 alleles can also have poorer neurologic outcomes after head injury, stroke, and other neuronal insults. Although carriers of the *APOE* ε4 allele have a clearly increased risk for development of AD, there is currently no role for screening for the presence of this allele in healthy individuals; such testing has poor positive and negative predictive values and would therefore generate highly uncertain estimates of future risk for AD (see Chapter 19).

TABLE 13.6 Amino Acid Substitutions Underlying the Three Common Apolipoprotein E Polymorphisms

Allele	ε2	ε3	ε4
Residue 112	Cys	Cys	Arg
Residue 158	Cys	Arg	Arg
Frequency in US populations of European ancestry	10%	65%	25%
Frequency in patients with Alzheimer disease	2%	58%	40%
Effect on Alzheimer disease	Protective	None known	30–50% of the genetic risk for Alzheimer disease

These figures are estimates, with differences in allele frequencies that vary with ancestry in control populations, and with age, gender, and ancestry in Alzheimer disease subjects.
Data derived from St. George Hyslop PH, Farrer LA, Goedert M: Alzheimer disease and the frontotemporal dementias: Diseases with cerebral deposition of fibrillar proteins. In Valle D, Beaudet AL, Vogelstein B, et al, editors: The online metabolic & molecular bases of inherited disease (OMMBID). http://www.ommbid.com/

Other Genes Associated With Alzheimer Disease

One significant modifier of AD risk, the *TREM2* gene (which encodes the *t*riggering *r*eceptor *e*xpressed on *m*yeloid cells 2), was identified by whole exome and **whole genome sequencing** in families with multiple individuals affected with AD. Several moderately rare missense coding variants in this gene are associated with a fivefold increase in risk for late-onset AD, making *TREM2* variants the second most common contributor to classic late-onset AD after *APOE* ε4. Statistical analyses suggest that an additional four to eight genes may significantly modify the risk for AD, but their identity remains obscure.

Although case-control association studies (see Chapter 11) of candidate genes with hypothetical functional links to the known biology of AD have suggested more than 100 genes in AD, only one such candidate gene, *SORL1* (sortilin-related receptor 1), has been robustly implicated. Single nucleotide polymorphisms (SNPs) in the *SORL1* gene confer a moderately increased **relative risk** for AD of less than 1.5. The *SORL1*-encoded protein affects the processing of APP and favors the production of the neurotoxic Aβ$_{42}$ peptide from βAPP.

Genome-wide association study analyses (see Chapter 11), on the other hand, have greatly expanded the number of genes believed to be associated with AD, identifying many novel SNPs associated with a predisposition to nonfamilial late-onset forms of AD. The genes implicated by these SNPs and their causal role(s) in AD are presently uncertain.

Overall, it is becoming clear that genetic variants alter the risk for AD in at least two general ways: first, by modulating the production of Aβ, and second, through their impact on other processes, including the regulation of innate immunity, inflammation, and the resecretion of protein aggregates. These latter variants likely modulate AD risk by altering the flux through downstream pathways in response to a given load of Aβ.

DISEASES OF MITOCHONDRIAL DNA (mtDNA)

Neal Sondheimer

The Genetics of mtDNA Disease

The general characteristics of the mtDNA genome and the features of the inheritance of disorders caused by pathogenic variants in this genome were first described in Chapters 2 and 7 but are reviewed briefly here. The small circular mtDNA chromosome is located inside mitochondria and contains only 37 genes (Fig. 13.24). Unlike nuclear chromosomes, different cell types have a wide range in the copy number of mtDNA. The oocyte at fertilization has ~10^6 copies, fibroblasts may have thousands of copies, and red blood cells have none. In addition to encoding two ribosomal RNAs (rRNAs) and 22 **transfer RNAs (tRNAs)**, mtDNA encodes 13 proteins that are subunits of oxidative phosphorylation.

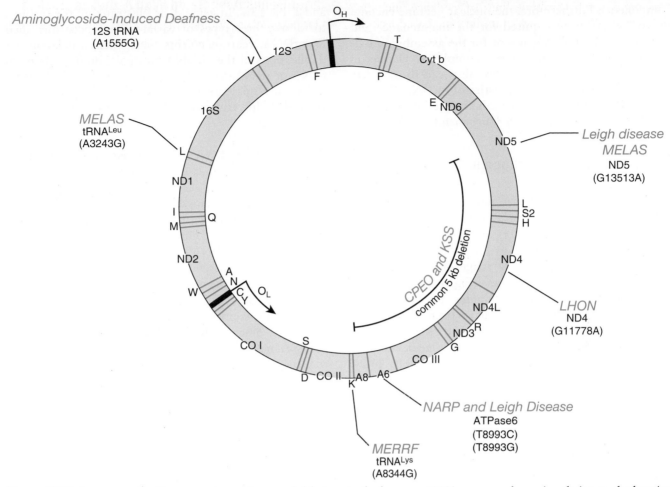

Figure 13.24 Representative disease-causing variants and deletions in the human mtDNA genome, shown in relation to the location of the genes encoding the 22 transfer RNAs (tRNAs), 2 ribosomal RNAs (rRNAs), and 13 proteins of the oxidative phosphorylation complex. O_H and O_L are the origins of replication of the two DNA strands, respectively; 12S, 12S ribosomal RNA; 16S, 16S ribosomal RNA. The locations of each of the tRNAs are indicated by the single-letter code for their corresponding amino acids. The 13 oxidative phosphorylation polypeptides encoded by mitochondrial DNA (mtDNA) include components of complex I: NADH dehydrogenase (ND1, ND2, ND3, ND4, ND4L, ND5, and ND6); complex III: cytochrome b (cyt b); complex IV: cytochrome c oxidase I or cytochrome c (COI, COII, COIII); and complex V: ATPase 6 and 8 (A6, A8). The disease abbreviations used in this figure (e.g., MELAS, MERRF, LHON) are explained in Table 13.7. *CPEO*, Chronic progressive external ophthalmoplegia; *NARP*, neuropathy, ataxia, and retinitis pigmentosa. Variants and annotations from MITOMAP (www.mitomap.org).

Pathogenic variants in mtDNA, and the associated disorders, can be inherited or acquired as somatic mutations. These diseases show distinctive patterns of inheritance due to three features of mtDNA:

- Maternal inheritance
- Homoplasmy and heteroplasmy
- Replicative segregation

The **maternal inheritance** of mtDNA (discussed in greater detail in Chapter 7; see Fig. 7.22) reflects the fact that sperm mtDNA are generally eliminated from the embryo so that mtDNA is inherited entirely from the mother. Paternal inheritance has been well documented in only one instance, and this case may represent a unique failure in the clearance of paternal mtDNA. **Replicative segregation** refers to the fact that the multiple copies of mtDNA in each mitochondrion

replicate and assort randomly among newly synthesized mitochondria, which in turn are distributed randomly between the daughter cells (see Fig. 7.23). This occurs in both mitotic and meiotic divisions and impacts the transmission of **heteroplasmy** between generations (a phenomenon known as a germline bottleneck), which is described in greater detail later.

The 74 polypeptides of the oxidative phosphorylation complex not encoded in the mtDNA are encoded by the nuclear genome, which contains the genes for most of the estimated 1500 mitochondrial proteins. To date, more than 300 nuclear genes are associated with disorders of the respiratory chain. Thus diseases of oxidative phosphorylation arise not only from pathogenic variants in the mitochondrial genome but also from variants in nuclear genes that encode oxidative phosphorylation components. Furthermore, the nuclear genome encodes up to 200 proteins required for the maintenance and expression of mtDNA genes or for the assembly of oxidative phosphorylation protein complexes. Defects in many of these nuclear genes can also lead to disorders with the phenotypic characteristics of mtDNA diseases, but of course the patterns of inheritance in these cases are those typically seen with other mendelian disorders (see Chapter 7).

Diseases Caused by Pathogenic Variants in mtDNA

The sequence of the mtDNA genome and the presence of pathogenic variants in mtDNA have been known for over 4 decades. The disorders are not uncommon, and the prevalence has been shown, in at least one population, to be ~1 per 5000. The range of clinical disease resulting from mtDNA is diverse (Fig. 13.25), although neuromuscular disease predominates. Nearly 100 different disease-related variants have been identified in mtDNA, in addition to more than 100 rearrangements that cause disease. Representative pathogenic variants and the diseases associated are presented in Fig. 13.24

and Table 13.7. In general, as illustrated in the sections to follow, three types of variants have been identified in mtDNA: rearrangements that generate deletions or duplications of the mtDNA molecule, point variants in tRNA or rRNA genes that impair mitochondrial translation, and missense variants in the coding regions of genes that alter the activity of an oxidative phosphorylation protein.

Deletions of mtDNA and Disease. In many cases, mtDNA deletions that cause disease, such as Kearns-Sayre syndrome (see Table 13.7), are inherited from an unaffected mother who carries the deletion in her oocytes but generally not elsewhere, an example of gonadal mosaicism. Under these circumstances, disorders caused by mtDNA deletions appear to be sporadic because oocytes carrying the deletion are relatively rare. In ~5% of cases, the mother may be affected and transmit the deletion. The reason for the low frequency of transmission is uncertain, but it may simply reflect the fact that women with a high proportion of the deleted mtDNA in their germ cells have such a severe phenotype that they rarely reproduce.

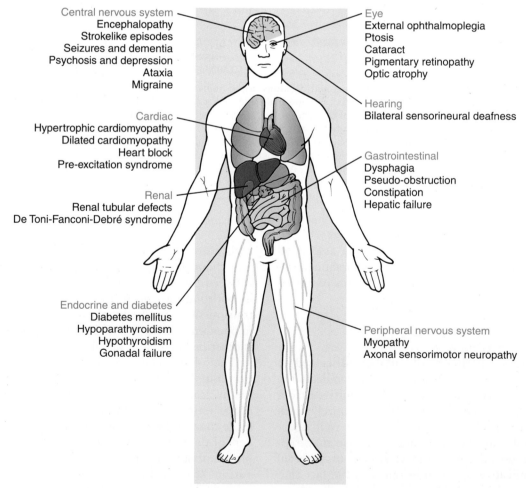

Figure 13.25 The range of affected tissues and clinical phenotypes associated with variants in mitochondrial DNA (mtDNA). (Modified from Chinnery PF, Turnbull DM: Mitochondrial DNA and disease, *Lancet* 354:SI17–SI21, 1999.)

Mitochondrial tRNA and rRNA Are Associated With Disease. Pathogenic variants in the tRNA and rRNA genes of mtDNA are significant because they illustrate that not all disease-causing variants in humans occur in genes that encode proteins (Case 33). Unlike nuclear tRNA and rRNA, which are present at high copy number in the chromosomes, the mitochondrial genes encoding these RNAs exist at unique locations in the genome (see Fig. 13.24) so that single nucleotide variants can disrupt their function. Fifty pathogenic variants have been identified in 15 of the 22 tRNA genes of the mtDNA, and they are the most common cause of oxidative phosphorylation abnormalities in humans (see Fig. 13.24 and Table 13.7).

Pathogenic tRNA variants include 11 different substitutions in the tRNA$^{leu(UUR)}$ gene, some of which, like the m.3243A>G variant, cause a phenotype referred to as MELAS, an acronym for *m*itochondrial *e*ncephalomyopathy with *l*actic *a*cidosis and *s*troke-like episodes (see Fig. 13.24 and Table 13.7); others are associated predominantly with myopathy. The m.3243A>G variant, for reasons that are not entirely clear, is the most commonly observed mitochondrial pathogenic variant in clinical practice. It is only found in a heteroplasmic state, and the homoplasmic state is presumed to be lethal. An example of an rRNA variant causing disease is the m.1555A>G variant in the 12S ribosomal RNA. This variant causes sensorineural prelingual deafness after exposure to aminoglycoside antibiotics and illustrates an important rule for homoplasmic variants, which is that they must either be incompletely penetrant or must allow females to survive to reproduction; otherwise, they would be eliminated from the population.

The Phenotypes of Mitochondrial Disorders

Oxidative Phosphorylation and mtDNA Diseases. Mitochondrial diseases generally affect tissues that depend on intact oxidative phosphorylation to satisfy high demands for metabolic energy. This phenotypic focus reflects the central role of the oxidative phosphorylation complex in the production of ATP. The evidence that mechanisms other than decreased energy production contribute to the pathogenesis of mtDNA diseases is either indirect or weak, but the generation of reactive oxygen species as a byproduct of faulty oxidative phosphorylation may also contribute to the pathology of mtDNA disorders. A substantial body of evidence indicates that there is a **phenotypic threshold effect** associated with mtDNA heteroplasmy (see Fig. 7.23); a critical threshold in the proportion of mtDNA molecules carrying the detrimental variant must be exceeded in cells from the affected tissue before clinical disease becomes apparent. The threshold for the appearance of disease is dependent upon the nature of each variant and its impact on the underlying gene.

The neuromuscular system is most commonly affected by mitochondrial diseases; the consequences can include encephalopathy, myopathy, ataxia, retinal degeneration, and loss of function of the external ocular muscles. Mitochondrial myopathy is characterized by ragged-red (muscle) fibers, a histologic phenotype due to the proliferation of structurally and biochemically abnormal mitochondria in muscle fibers. The spectrum of mitochondrial disease is broad and, as illustrated in Fig. 13.25, may include liver dysfunction, bone marrow failure, pancreatic islet cell deficiency and diabetes, deafness, and other disorders.

TABLE 13.7 **Representative Examples of Disorders due to Variants in Mitochondrial DNA and Their Inheritance**

Disease	Phenotypes	Typical Variant in mtDNA	Homoplasmy vs Heteroplasmy	Inheritance
Leber hereditary optic neuropathy (LHON)	Rapid onset of blindness in young adult life due to optic nerve atrophy; some recovery of vision, depending on the variant. Strong sex bias: ~50% of male carriers have visual loss vs. ~10% of females.	m.1178A>G in the complex I gene *ND4*	Largely homoplasmic	Maternal
Leigh syndrome	Early-onset progressive neurodegeneration with characteristic necrosis of basal ganglia	m.8993T>G in the complex V gene *ATP6*	Heteroplasmic	Maternal
MELAS	Myopathy, mitochondrial encephalomyopathy, lactic acidosis, and stroke-like episodes; may present only as diabetes mellitus and deafness	m.3243A>G in *MT-TL1*, encoding the tRNA$^{leu(UUR)}$	Heteroplasmic	Maternal
MERRF (Case 33)	Myoclonic epilepsy with ragged-red muscle fibers, myopathy, ataxia, sensorineural deafness, dementia	m.8344A>G in *MT-TK*, encoding the tRNA^{lys}	Heteroplasmic	Maternal
Deafness	Aminoglycoside-induced sensorineural deafness	m.1555A>G in *MT-RNR1*, encoding the 12S rRNA	Homoplasmic	Maternal
Kearns-Sayre syndrome (KSS)	Progressive myopathy, progressive external ophthalmoplegia of early onset, cardiomyopathy, heart block, ptosis, retinal pigmentation, ataxia, diabetes	5-kb large deletion (see Fig. 13.24)	Heteroplasmic	Generally sporadic, likely due to maternal gonadal mosaicism

mtDNA, Mitochondrial DNA; rRNA, ribosomal RNA; tRNA, transfer RNA.

BOX 13.2 HETEROPLASMY AND MITOCHONDRIAL DISEASE

Heteroplasmy accounts for three general characteristics of genetic disorders of mtDNA that are of importance to their pathogenesis. These features of the inheritance of heteroplasmic variants greatly complicate the counseling of families affected by mitochondrial disease, and the risk of recurrence of disease cannot be precisely estimated as it is with dominant or recessive disorders.

- *First*, female carriers of disease-causing heteroplasmic mtDNA variants usually transmit some variant mtDNAs to their offspring.
- *Second*, the fraction of variant mtDNA molecules inherited by each child of a carrier mother is not identical in each of her children. This is because the number of mtDNA molecules within each developing oocyte is reduced before being subsequently amplified to the huge total seen in mature oocytes. This restriction and subsequent amplification of mtDNA during oogenesis is termed the **mitochondrial genetic bottleneck**. Consequently, the variability in the percentage of variant-bearing mtDNA molecules seen in the offspring of a mother carrying a mtDNA mutation arises, at least in part, from the sampling of only a subset of the mtDNAs during oogenesis.
- *Third*, despite the variability in the degree of heteroplasmy arising from the bottleneck, mothers with a high proportion of disease-associated mtDNA molecules are more likely to have clinically affected offspring than are mothers with a lower proportion, as one would predict from the distribution of mtDNA ratios through the bottleneck. Nevertheless, even women carrying low proportions of pathogenic mtDNA molecules have some risk for having an affected child because the bottleneck can lead to the sampling and subsequent expansion, by chance, of even a rare mtDNA species.

Unexplained and Unexpected Phenotypic Variation in mtDNA Diseases.

As seen in Table 13.7, heteroplasmy is the rule for many mtDNA diseases. Heteroplasmy leads to an unpredictable and variable fraction of disease-associated mtDNA being present in any particular tissue, undoubtedly accounting for much of the **pleiotropy** and variable **expressivity** of mtDNA mutations (see Box 13.2). An example is provided by the m.3243A>G substitution in the tRNA$^{leu(UUR)}$ gene, previously mentioned in the context of the MELAS phenotype. It also leads to maternally inherited diabetes and deafness in some families, whereas in others it causes a disease called chronic progressive external ophthalmoplegia. Moreover, a very small fraction (<1%) of diabetes mellitus in the general population has been attributed to the m.3243A>G substitution.

Disorders of mtDNA Replication

Because both the nuclear and mitochondrial genomes contribute polypeptides to oxidative phosphorylation, it is not surprising that the phenotypes associated with defects in nuclear genes can be clinically indistinguishable from those due to mitochondrial genes. One additional concept of importance to disease is that the mtDNA itself depends on nuclear genome–encoded proteins for its replication and the maintenance of its integrity.

The medical consequence of this dependency is diseases with mendelian inheritance patterns (dominant or recessive), due to variants in nuclear genes, that have their impact on the mtDNA. An example of this class of disorders is the mtDNA depletion syndromes, which result from pathogenic variants in any of 17 nuclear genes that lead to a reduction in the number of copies of mtDNA (both per mitochondrion and per cell) in various tissues. Some of the affected genes encode proteins required to maintain nucleotide pools or to metabolize nucleotides appropriately in the mitochondrion. One example of a mitochondrial depletion syndrome is Alpers syndrome, which is a recessive disorder caused by pathogenic variants in **DNA polymerase γ (POLG)**. POLG is the DNA-dependent DNA polymerase that replicates mtDNA, and variants in this gene can cause loss of mtDNA but may also lead to excess mutations or rearrangements in mtDNA.

Environmental Influences Modify the Phenotype of mtDNA Diseases.

Although heteroplasmy is a major source of phenotypic variability in mtDNA diseases (see Box), additional factors, including environmental stressors, also play a role. Strong evidence for environmental influence is provided by families carrying variants associated with Leber hereditary optic neuropathy (LHON; see Table 13.7), which is generally homoplasmic (thus ruling out heteroplasmy as the explanation for the observed phenotypic variation). LHON is expressed phenotypically as rapid, painless bilateral loss of central vision due to optic nerve atrophy in young adults (see Table 13.7 and Fig. 13.24).

There is a striking increase in the **penetrance** of the disease in males; ~50% of male carriers but only ~10% of female carriers of an LHON variant develop symptoms. Studies of large numbers of individuals have strongly implicated that cigarette smoking, and possibly alcohol consumption, drives this discrepancy in risk. This suggests that environmental stressors causing oxidative injury may play an important and synergistic role in determining the penetrance of a mitochondrial variant. It has additionally been suggested that interactions with nuclear-encoded variants may also alter the risk of developing LHON symptoms.

Problems in Therapy for mtDNA-Associated Disorders.

Mitochondrial disorders lag other diseases in the development of new therapies based on genetic manipulation. For diseases due to mtDNA there are two critical drivers of this problem. The first is that mitochondrial disease tends to affect many tissues simultaneously, so approaches to correction have to be applied across the whole patient rather than to a single organ or tissue. The second, and more remarkable challenge, is that genetic manipulation of human mtDNA is largely impossible with current technologies. Mitochondria are impermeable to nucleic acids (DNA and RNA), so techniques of mutagenesis that rely on recombination are not effective, even when used on isolated cells in a laboratory. A related challenge is that there are no viruses that infect the mitochondrion, so genetic delivery systems will need to be developed rather than adapted from existing viruses.

DISEASES DUE TO THE EXPANSION OF UNSTABLE REPEAT SEQUENCES

Ryan Yuen

The inheritance pattern of diseases due to unstable repeat expansions was presented in Chapter 7, with emphasis on the unusual genetics of this unique group of almost 60 disorders. These features include the unstable and dynamic nature of the variants, which arise from expansion of repeated sequences within the transcribed region of the affected gene. Examples include the **codon** for glutamine (CAG) in Huntington disease (Case 24) and in most of a group of neurodegenerative disorders called the spinocerebellar ataxias, or the codon for alanine (GCG) in diseases such as oculopharyngeal muscular dystrophy. The expansion can also be of trinucleotides in noncoding regions of RNAs, including CGG in fragile X syndrome (Case 17), GAA in Friedreich ataxia, CUG in myotonic dystrophy 1 (Fig. 13.26), or GCA in glutaminase deficiency.

Although the nucleotide repeat diseases initially described are all due to the expansion of trinucleotide repeats, with the help of advanced genomic technologies, other disorders have been found to result from the

expansion of longer repeats; these include a tetranucleotide (CCTG) in myotonic dystrophy 2 (a close genocopy of myotonic dystrophy 1), a pentanucleotide (ATTCT) in spinocerebellar atrophy 10, an inserted pentanucleotide (TTTCA) in a group of familial adult myoclonic epilepsies, and a hexanucleotide (GGGGCC) in amyotrophic lateral sclerosis. Because the affected gene is passed from generation to generation, the number of repeats may expand to a degree that is pathogenic, ultimately interfering with normal gene expression and function. The intergenerational expansion of the repeats accounts for the phenomenon of **anticipation**: the appearance of the disease at an earlier age or with more severe form as it is transmitted through a family. The biochemical mechanism most proposed to underlie the expansion of unstable repeat sequences is **slipped mispairing** (Fig. 13.27). Remarkably, the repeat expansions appear to occur both in proliferating cells, such as **spermatogonia** (during **meiosis**), and in nonproliferating somatic cells, such as neurons. Consequently, expansion can occur – depending on the disease – during both DNA replication (as shown in Fig. 13.27) and genome maintenance (i.e., DNA repair).

The clinical phenotypes of Huntington disease and fragile X syndrome are presented in Chapter 7 and in Cases 24 and 17, respectively. It has become apparent, particularly with fragile X syndrome, that diseases due to the expansion of unstable repeats are primarily neurologic; the clinical presentations include ataxia, cognitive

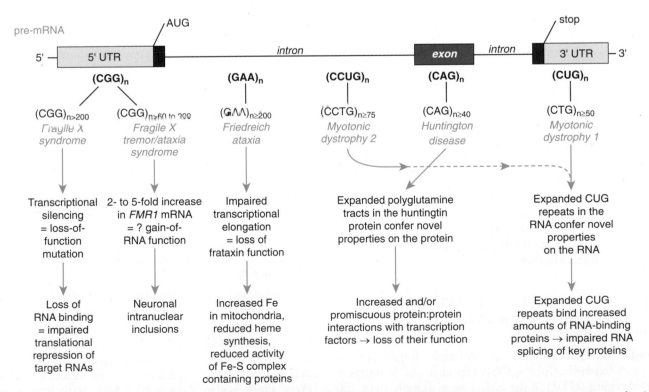

Figure 13.26 The locations of the nucleotide repeat expansions and the sequence of each nucleotide in five representative nucleotide repeat diseases, shown on a schematic of a generic pre–messenger RNA (mRNA). The minimal number of repeats in the DNA sequence of the affected gene associated with the disease is also indicated. The effect of the expansion on the mutant RNA or protein is also indicated. (Based partly on an unpublished figure courtesy John A. Phillips III, Vanderbilt University Nashville.)

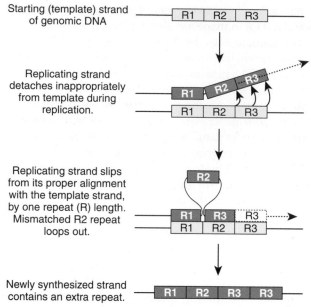

Starting (template) strand of genomic DNA

Replicating strand detaches inappropriately from template during replication.

Replicating strand slips from its proper alignment with the template strand, by one repeat (R) length. Mismatched R2 repeat loops out.

Newly synthesized strand contains an extra repeat.

Figure 13.27 The slipped mispairing mechanism thought to underlie the expansion of unstable repeats, such as the (CAG)$_n$ repeat found in Huntington disease and the spinocerebellar ataxias. An insertion occurs when the newly synthesized strand aberrantly dissociates from the template strand during replication synthesis. When the new strand reassociates with the template strand, the new strand may slip back to align out of register with an incorrect repeat copy. Once DNA synthesis is resumed, the misaligned molecule will contain one or more extra copies of the repeat (depending on the number of repeat copies that slipped out in the misalignment event).

defects, dementia, nystagmus, parkinsonism, and spasticity. Nevertheless, other systems are sometimes involved, as illustrated by some of the diseases discussed here.

The Pathogenesis of Diseases Due to Unstable Repeat Expansions

Diseases of **unstable repeat expansion** are diverse in their pathogenic mechanisms. They can be divided into three main classes, considered in turn in the sections to follow.

- *Class 1*: diseases due to the expansion of noncoding repeats that cause a loss of protein expression
- *Class 2*: disorders resulting from expansions of noncoding repeats that confer novel properties on the RNA
- *Class 3*: diseases due to repeat expansion of a codon such as CAG (for glutamine) that confers novel properties on the affected protein

Class 1: Diseases Due to the Expansion of Noncoding Repeats That Cause a Loss of Protein Expression

Fragile X Syndrome. In the X-linked fragile X syndrome, expansion of the CGG repeat in the 5′ **untranslated region (UTR)** of the *FMR1* gene to more than 200 copies leads to excessive methylation of cytosines in the **promoter**; this **epigenetic** modification of the DNA silences **transcription** of the gene (see Figs. 7.21 and

13.26). Remarkably, the epigenetic silencing appears to be mediated by the variant *FMR1* mRNA itself. The initial step in the silencing of *FMR1* results from the *FMR1* mRNA (containing the transcribed CGG repeat) hybridizing with the complementary CGG-repeat sequence of the *FMR1* gene, to form an RNA:DNA duplex. The mechanisms that subsequently maintain the silencing of the *FMR1* gene are unknown. The loss of the related protein (FMRP) is the cause of the intellectual disability, learning deficits, and nonneurologic features of the clinical phenotype, including postpubertal macroorchidism and connective tissue dysplasia (Case 17). FMRP is an RNA-binding protein that associates with polyribosomes to suppress the translation of proteins from its RNA targets. These targets appear to be involved in cytoskeletal structure, synaptic transmission, and neuronal maturation; **disruption** of these processes is likely to underlie the intellectual disability and learning abnormalities seen in individuals with fragile X. For example, FMRP appears to regulate the translation of proteins required for the formation of synapses because the brains of individuals with the fragile X syndrome have increased density of abnormally long, immature dendritic spines. Moreover, FMRP localizes to dendritic spines, where at least one of its roles is to regulate synaptic plasticity – the capacity to alter the strength of a synaptic connection – a process critical to learning and memory.

Fragile X Tremor/Ataxia Syndrome. Remarkably, in individuals with less pronounced CGG repeat expansion (60–200 repeats) in the *FMR1* gene, causing the clinically distinct fragile X tremor/ataxia syndrome (FXTAS), the pathogenesis is entirely different from that of the fragile X syndrome itself. Although decreased translational efficiency impairs the expression of FMRP in FXTAS, this reduction cannot be responsible for the disease because males with full expansions and virtually complete loss of function of the *FMR1* gene never develop FXTAS. Rather, FXTAS seems to result from the two- to fivefold increase of *FMR1* mRNA in these patients, representing a gain-of-function variant. This pathogenic RNA leads to the formation of intranuclear neuronal inclusions, the cellular signature of the disease.

Class 2: Disorders Resulting From Expansions of Noncoding Repeats That Confer Novel Properties on the RNA

Myotonic Dystrophy. Myotonic dystrophy 1 (DM1) is an autosomal dominant condition with the most **pleiotropic** phenotype of all the unstable repeat expansion disorders. In addition to myotonia, it is characterized by muscle weakness and wasting, cardiac conduction defects, testicular atrophy, insulin resistance, and cataracts; there is also a congenital form with intellectual disability. The disease results from a CTG expansion in the 3′ UTR of the *DMPK* gene, which encodes a protein kinase (see Fig. 13.26). Myotonic dystrophy 2 (DM2) is also an autosomal dominant trait and shares most of the clinical features of DM1, except that there is no associated congenital presentation. DM2 is due to the expansion of a CCTG tetranucleotide in the first intron of the gene encoding zinc finger protein 9 (see Fig. 13.26). The strikingly similar phenotypes of DM1 and DM2 suggest that they have a common pathogenesis. Because the unstable expansions occur within the noncoding regions of two different genes that encode unrelated proteins, the CTG trinucleotide expansion itself (and the resulting expansion of CUG in the mRNA) is thought to underlie an RNA-mediated pathogenesis.

What is the mechanism by which large tracts of the CUG trinucleotide, in the noncoding regions of genes, lead to the DM1 and DM2 phenotypes? The pathogenesis appears to result from the binding of the CUG repeats to RNA-binding proteins. Consequently, the pleiotropy that typifies the disease may reflect the broad array of RNA-binding proteins to which the CUG repeats bind. Many of the RNA-binding proteins sequestered by the excessive number of CUG repeats are regulators of splicing. Indeed, more than a dozen distinct pre-mRNAs have splicing alterations in patients with DM1, including cardiac troponin T (which might account for the cardiac abnormalities) and the insulin receptor (which may explain the insulin resistance). Thus the myotonic dystrophies are referred to as spliceopathies. Knowledge of the abnormal processes underlying DM1 and DM2 is incomplete, but these molecular insights offer hope that a rational small molecule therapy might be developed.

Class 3: Diseases Due to Repeat Expansion of a Codon That Confers Novel Properties on the Affected Protein

Huntington Disease. Huntington disease is an autosomal dominant neurodegenerative disorder associated with chorea, athetosis (uncontrolled writhing movements of the extremities), loss of cognition, and psychiatric abnormalities (Case 24). The pathologic process is caused by the expansion – to more than 40 repeats – of a CAG codon in the *HTT* gene, resulting in long polyglutamine tracts in the protein, huntingtin (see Figs. 7.19 and 7.20). Evidence suggests that the proteins with expanded polyglutamine sequences have novel properties: the expanded tract confers novel features on the protein that damage specific populations of neurons and produce neurodegeneration by unique toxic mechanisms. The most striking cellular hallmark of the disease is the presence of insoluble aggregates of the abnormal protein (as well as other polypeptides) clustered in nuclear inclusions in neurons. The aggregates are thought to result from normal cellular responses to the misfolding of huntingtin that results from the polyglutamine expansion. Dramatic as these inclusions are, however, their formation may be protective rather than pathogenic.

There is no unifying model of the neuronal death mediated by polyglutamine expansion in huntingtin. Many cellular processes are disrupted by expanded huntingtin in its soluble or aggregated form, including transcription, vesicular transport, mitochondrial fission, and synaptic transmission and plasticity. Ultimately, the most critical and primary events in the pathogenesis will be identified, perhaps guided by genetic analyses, leading to correction of the phenotype. For example, expanded huntingtin associates abnormally with a mitochondrial fission protein, GTPase dynamin-related protein 1 (DRP1), leading to multiple mitochondrial abnormalities in individuals with Huntington disease. Remarkably, in mice, these defects are rescued by reducing DRP1 GTPase activity, suggesting both that DRP1 may be a therapeutic target for the disorder and that mitochondrial abnormalities play important roles in Huntington disease.

Despite the substantial progress in identifying novel repeat expansions and our understanding of the molecular events that underlie the pathology of the unstable repeat expansion diseases, we are only beginning to dissect the genetic and pathogenic complexity of these important conditions. It is clear that the use of new genomic technologies and study of animal models are providing critical insights into these disorders. Such insights should soon lead to interventions to prevent or to reverse the pathogenesis of these slowly developing disorders. We begin to explore the concepts relevant to the treatment of disease in the next chapter.

GENERAL REFERENCES

Adam MP, editor: Molecular genetics. In *GeneReviews*, Seattle, 1993–2022, University of Washington. http://www.ncbi.nlm.nih.gov/books/NBK1116/

Hamosh A: *Online mendelian inheritance in man, OMIM.* McKusick-Nathans Department of Genetic Medicine, Baltimore, MD, Johns Hopkins University. http://omim.org/

Strachan T, Read AP: *Human molecular genetics*, ed 5, 2019, Garland Science.

Valle DL, Antonarakis S, Ballabio A, et al, editors: *The online metabolic and molecular bases of inherited disease*, New York, 2019, McGraw Hill. https://ommbid.mhmedical.com

REFERENCES TO SPECIFIC TOPICS

Bettens K, Sleegers K, Van Broeckhoven C: Genetic insights in Alzheimer's disease, *Lancet Neurol* 12:92–104, 2013.

Bird TD: Alzheimer disease overview. In *GeneReviews*, Seattle, 1998, University of Washington. https://www.ncbi.nlm.nih.gov/books/NBK1161/

Blau N, Hennermann JB, Langenbeck U, et al: Diagnosis, classification, and genetics of phenylketonuria and tetrahydrobiopterin (BH4) deficiencies, *Mol Genet Metab* 104:S2–S9, 2011.

Brais B, Bouchard J-P, Xie Y-G, et al: Short GCG expansions in the PABP2 gene cause oculopharyngeal muscular dystrophy, *Nat Genet* 18:164–167, 1998.

Byers PH, Pyott SM: Recessively inherited forms of osteogenesis imperfecta, *Ann Rev Genet* 46:475–497, 2012.

Chamberlin JS: Duchenne muscular dystrophy models show their age, *Cell* 143:1040–1042, 2010.

Chillon M, Casals T, Mercier B, et al: Mutations in the cystic fibrosis gene in patients with congenital absence of the vas deferens, *N Engl J Med* 332:1475–1480, 1995.

Colak D, Zaninovic N, Cohen MS, et al: Promoter-bound trinucleotide repeat mRNA drives epigenetic silencing in fragile X syndrome, *Science* 343:1002–1005, 2014.

Cutting GR: Modifier genes in mendelian disorders: The example of cystic fibrosis, *Ann N Y Acad Sci* 1214:57–69, 2010.

DeJesus-Hernandez M, Mackenzie IR, Boeve BF, et al: Expanded GGGGCC hexanucleotide repeat in noncoding region of C9ORF72 causes chromosome 9p-linked FTD and ALS, *Neuron* 72:245–256, 2011.

Duan D, Goemans N, Takeda S, et al: Duchene muscular dystrophy, *Nat Rev Dis Primers* 7:13, 2021.

Flanigan KM: The muscular dystrophies, *Semin Neurol* 32:255–263, 2012.

Fong LG, Young SG: PCSK9 function and physiology, *J Lipid Res* 49:1152–1156, 2008.

Gall-Duncan T, Sato N, Yuen RKC, et al: Advancing genomic technologies and clinical awareness accelerates discovery of disease-associated tandem repeat sequences, *Genome Res* 32:1–27, 2022.

Gallego D, Leal F, Gámez A, et al: Pathogenic variants of DNAJC12 and evaluation of the encoded cochaperone as a genetic modifier of hyper-phenylalaninemia, *Hum Mutat* 41(7):1329–1338, 2020. https://doi.org/10.1002/humu.24026

Goldstein JL, Brown MS: Molecular medicine: The cholesterol quartet, *Science* 292:1310–1312, 2001.

Gu YY, Harley ITW, Henderson LB, et al: IFRD1 polymorphisms in cystic fibrosis with potential link to altered neutrophil function, *Nature* 458:1039–1042, 2009.

Ishiura H, Doi K, Mitsui J, et al: Expansions of intronic TTTCA and TTTTA repeats in benign adult familial myoclonic epilepsy, *Nat Genet* 50:581–590, 2018.

Janciauskiene SM, Bals R, Koczulla R, et al: The discovery of alpha1-antitrypsin and its role in health and disease, *Respir Med* 105:1129–1139, 2011.

Jonsson T, Atwal JK, Steinberg S, et al: A mutation in APP protects against Alzheimer's disease and age-related cognitive decline, *Nature* 488:96–99, 2012.

Kathiresan S, Melander O, Guiducci C, et al: Six new loci associated with blood low-density lipoprotein cholesterol, high-density lipoprotein cholesterol or triglycerides in humans, *Nat Genet* 40:189–197, 2008.

Keinath MC, Prior DE, Prior TW: Spinal muscular atrophy: mutations, testing, and clinical relevance, *Appl Clin Genet* 14:11–25, 2021. https://doi.org/10.2147/TACG.S239603

Kirkman MA, Yu-Wai-Man P, Korsten A, et al: Gene-environment interactions in Leber hereditary optic neuropathy, *Brain* 132(Pt 9):2317–2326, 2009. https://doi.org/10.1093/brain/awp158

Koopman WJ, Willems PH, Smeitink JA: Monogenic mitochondrial disorders, *N Engl J Med* 366:1132–1141, 2012.

Laine CM, Joeng KS, Campeau PM, et al: WNT1 mutations in early-onset osteoporosis and osteogenesis imperfecta, *N Engl J Med* 368:1809–1816, 2013.

Lopez CA, Cleary JD, Pearson CE: Repeat instability as the basis for human diseases and as a potential target for therapy, *Nat Rev Mol Cell Biol* 11:165–170, 2010.

Moskowitz SM, James F, Chmiel JF, et al: Clinical practice and genetic counseling for cystic fibrosis and CFTR-related disorders, *GeneTests* 10:851–868, 2008.

Ng BG, Freeze HH: Perspectives on glycosylation and its congenital disorders, *Trends Genet* 34(6):466–476, 2018. https://doi.org/10.1016/j.tig.2018.03.002

Nicolau S, Waldrop MA, Connolly AM, et al: Spinal muscular atrophy, *Semin Pediatr Neurol* 37:100878, 2021.

Raal FJ, Santos ED: Homozygous familial hypercholesterolemia: current perspectives on diagnosis and treatment, *Atherosclerosis* 223:262–268, 2012.

Rahaghi FF, Miravitlles M: Long-term clinical outcomes following treatment with alpha 1-proteinase inhibitor for COPD associated with alpha-1 antitrypsin deficiency: A look at the evidence, *Respir Res* 18(1):105, 2017. https://doi.org/10.1186/s12931-017-0574-1

Ramsey BW, Banks-Schlegel S, Accurso FJ, et al: Future directions in early cystic fibrosis lung disease research: An NHLBI workshop report, *Am J Respir Crit Care Med* 185:887–892, 2012.

Renton AE, Majounie E, Waite A, et al: A hexanucleotide repeat expansion in C9ORF72 is the cause of chromosome 9p21-linked ALS-FTD, *Neuron* 72:257–268, 2011.

Schon EA, DiMauro S, Hirano M: Human mitochondrial DNA: Roles of inherited and somatic mutations, *Nat Rev Genet* 13:878–890, 2012.

Selkoe DJ: Alzheimer's disease, *Cold Spring Harb Perspect Biol* 3:a004457, 2011.

Sosnay PR, Siklosi KR, Van Goor F, et al: Defining the disease liability of mutations in the cystic fibrosis transmembrane conductance regulator gene, *Nature Genet* 45:1160–1167, 2013.

Vafai SB, Mootha VK: Mitochondrial disorders as windows into an ancient organelle, *Nature* 491:374–383, 2012.

van Kuilenburg ABP, Tarailo-Graovac M, Richmond PA, et al: Glutaminase deficiency caused by short tandem repeat expansion in GLS, *New Eng J Med* 380:1433–1441, 2019.

Zoghbi HY, Orr HT: Pathogenic mechanisms of a polyglutamine-mediated neurodegenerative disease, spinocerebellar ataxia type 1, *J Biol Chem* 284:7425–7429, 2009.

USEFUL WEBSITES

Variant Databases

ClinVar (an annotated aggregation of variants by gene submitted from clinical labs and researchers): https://www.ncbi.nlm.nih.gov/clinvar

Global Variome Shared LOVD: https://databases.lovd.nl/shared/genes

ClinGen Evidence Repository: https://erepo.clinicalgenome.org/evrepo/

Clinical and functional translation of CFTR (CFTR2 project): http://www.cftr2.org/

Collagen variant database (the osteogenesis imperfecta and Ehlers-Danlos syndrome variant database: http://www.le.ac.uk/genetics/collagen/

Human mitochondrial genome database: https://www.mitomap.org/ MITOMAP

Phenylalanine hydroxylase variant database: http://www.biopku.org/home/pah.asp

The Human Gene Mutation Database: http://www.hgmd.cf.ac.uk/ac/index.php

PROBLEMS

1. One variant allele at the LDL receptor locus (leading to familial hypercholesterolemia) encodes an elongated protein that is ~50,000 Da larger than the normal 120,000-Da receptor. Indicate at least three mechanisms that could account for this abnormality. Approximately how many extra nucleotides would need to be translated to add 50,000 Da to the protein?

2. Comparing autosomal dominant *PSCK9* gain-of-function variants to autosomal dominant variants in the LDL receptor gene, are these phenocopies or genocopies? Explain your answer.

3. In discussing the nucleotide changes in the coding region of the *CFTR* gene, we stated that some of the changes (the missense changes) so far are only "putative" disease-causing variants. What criteria would one need to fulfill before knowing that a nucleotide change is pathogenic and not benign?

continued

PROBLEMS—CONT'D

4. Johnny, 2 years of age, is failing to thrive. Investigations show that although he has clinical findings of CF, his sweat chloride concentration is normal. The sweat chloride concentration is normal in less than 2% of patients with CF. His pediatrician and parents want to know whether DNA analysis can determine whether he indeed has CF.
   a. Would DNA analysis be useful in this case? Briefly outline the steps involved in obtaining a DNA diagnosis for CF.
   b. If he has CF, what is the probability that he is homozygous for the c.1521_1523delCTT (p.Phe508del) variant? (Assume that 95% of CFTR variants could be detected at the time you are consulted and that his parents are from northern Europe, where the Phe508del allele has a frequency of 0.70.)
   c. If he does not have the common variant, does this dis prove the diagnosis? Explain.

5. James is the only person in his kindred affected by DMD. He has one unaffected brother, Joe. DNA analysis shows that James has a deletion in the *DMD* gene and that Joe has received the same maternal X chromosome, but one without a deletion. What genetic counseling would you give the parents regarding the recurrence risk for DMD in a future pregnancy?

6. *DMD* has a high mutation rate but shows no ancestral variation in frequency. Use your knowledge of the gene and the genetics of DMD to suggest why this disorder is equally common in all populations.

7. A 3½-year-old girl, T.N., has increasing difficulty standing up after sitting on the floor. Her serum level of creatine kinase is grossly elevated. Although a female, the presumptive clinical diagnosis is Duchenne muscular dystrophy. Identify three mechanisms that could account for the rare occurrence of DMD in a female.

8. In patients with osteogenesis imperfecta, explain why the missense variants at glycine positions in the triple helix of type I collagen are confined to a limited number of replacement amino acid residues (Ala, Ser, Cys, Arg, Val, Asp).

9. A 2-year-old infant, the child of first-cousin parents, has unexplained developmental delay. A survey of various biochemical parameters indicates that he has a deficiency of four lysosomal enzyme activities. Explain how a single autosomal recessive pathogenic variant might cause the loss of function of four enzyme activities. Why is it most likely that the child has an autosomal recessive condition, if he has a genetic condition at all?

10. The effect of a dominant negative allele illustrates one general mechanism by which changes in a protein cause dominantly inherited disease. What mechanisms are commonly associated with dominance in genes encoding the subunits of multimeric proteins?

11. The clinical effects of pathogenic variants in a housekeeping protein are frequently limited to one or a few tissues, often tissues in which the protein is abundant and serves a specialty function. Identify and discuss examples that illustrate this generalization, and explain why they fit it.

12. The relationship between the site at which a protein is physically present/active and the site of pathological change in a genetic disease may be unpredictable. Give examples of this phenomenon and discuss them.

13. The two pseudodeficiency alleles of hex A are p.Arg247Trp and p.Arg249Trp. What is the probable reason that the missense substitutions of these alleles are so close together in the protein?

14. Why are gain-of-function variants in proteins, as seen with the autosomal dominant *PCSK9* variants that cause hypercholesterolemia, almost always missense variants?

15. What are the possible explanations for the presence of three predominant alleles for Tay-Sachs disease (as well as other lysosomal storage disorders) in Ashkenazi Jews? Does the presence of three alleles, and the relatively high frequency of Tay-Sachs disease in this population, necessarily accord with a heterozygote advantage hypothesis or a founder effect hypothesis?

16. The known loci associated with Alzheimer disease fail to account for the implied genetic contribution to risk. Identify at least three other sources of genetic variation that may account for the genetic contribution to this disorder.

17. The two forms of myotonic dystrophy are characterized by an expansion of a CUG trinucleotide in the RNA, which is thought to lead to an RNA-mediated pathogenesis. Propose a molecular therapy that might counteract the effect of the CUG expansions in the RNAs and that would reduce the binding of RNA-binding proteins to the CUG repeats. Anticipate some possible undesirable effects of your proposed therapy.

CHAPTER 14

The Treatment of Genetic Disease

Ronald Doron Cohn • Ada Hamosh

The understanding of **genetic** disease at a molecular level, as presented in Chapters 11, 12, and 13, is the foundation of rational therapy. In the coming decades, increasing annotation of the human **genome** sequence and the catalogue of human genes, as well as gene, **RNA**, and protein therapy, will have an enormous impact on the treatment of genetic conditions and other disorders. In this chapter we review established therapies as well as new strategies for treating genetic disease. Our emphasis will be on therapies that reflect the genetic approach to medicine, and our focus is on single-gene diseases rather than genetically complex disorders.

The objective of treating genetic disease is to eliminate or ameliorate the effects of the disorder, not only on the patient but also on the patient's family. The importance of educating the patient is paramount – not only to achieve understanding of the disease and its treatment but also to ensure adherence to therapy that may be inconvenient and lifelong. The family must be informed about the **risk** that the disease may occur in other members. Thus **genetic counseling** is a major component of the management of hereditary disorders and will be dealt with separately (see Chapter 17).

For single-gene disorders due to loss-of-function **variants**, treatment is directed to replacing the defective protein, improving its function, or minimizing the consequences of its deficiency. Replacement of the defective **gene** product (RNA or protein) may be achieved by direct administration, cell or organ transplantation, or **gene therapy**. In principle, gene therapy or gene editing will be the preferred mode of treatment of some and perhaps many single-gene diseases once these approaches become routinely safe and effective. However, even when copies of a normal gene can be transferred into the patient to effect permanent cure, the family will need ongoing genetic counseling, **carrier** testing, and prenatal diagnosis, in many cases for several generations.

Recent discoveries promise many more exciting and dramatic therapies for genetic disease. These achievements include the first cures of inherited disorders using gene therapy, the development of novel small molecule therapies that can restore activity to **mutant** proteins, and the ability to prevent the clinical manifestations of previously lethal disorders, including lysosomal storage diseases, by protein replacement therapy.

THE CURRENT STATE OF TREATMENT OF GENETIC DISEASE

Genetic disease can be treated at any level from the mutant gene to the clinical **phenotype** (Fig. 14.1). Treatment at the level of the clinical phenotype includes all the medical or surgical interventions that are not unique to the management of genetic disease. Throughout this chapter we describe the rationale for treatment at each of these levels. The current treatments are not necessarily mutually exclusive and many are used in conjunction to treat certain disorders; however, only gene therapy, gene editing, or cell transplantation can potentially provide cures.

Although powerful advances are being made, the overall treatment of single-gene diseases is presently deficient. Nevertheless, advances in the number of approaches to diagnosis and treatment of inborn errors of metabolism are accelerating (Fig. 14.2). Note, however, that inborn errors are a group of diseases for which treatment is advanced, in general, compared to most other types of **genetic disorders** such as those due, for example, to chromosomal abnormalities, **imprinting** defects, or copy number variation. An encouraging trend over past decades is that treatment is more likely to be successful if the basic biochemical defect is known. In one study, for example, although treatment increased life span in only 15% of all single-gene diseases studied, life span was improved by ~50% in the subset of 57 inborn errors in which the cause was known; significant improvements were also observed for other phenotypes, including growth, intelligence, and social adaptation. Thus research to elucidate the genetic and biochemical bases of hereditary disease has a major impact on the clinical outcome.

The improving but still unsatisfactory state of treatment of monogenic diseases is due to numerous factors, including the following:

- **Gene not identified or pathogenesis not understood.** Although more than 4500 genes have been associated with monogenic diseases, there are still ~16,000 protein coding genes not yet linked to a disease phenotype, and over half of patients undergoing clinical **exome** sequencing do not receive a diagnosis. This fraction will improve over the next decade because of the impact of **whole genome sequencing**

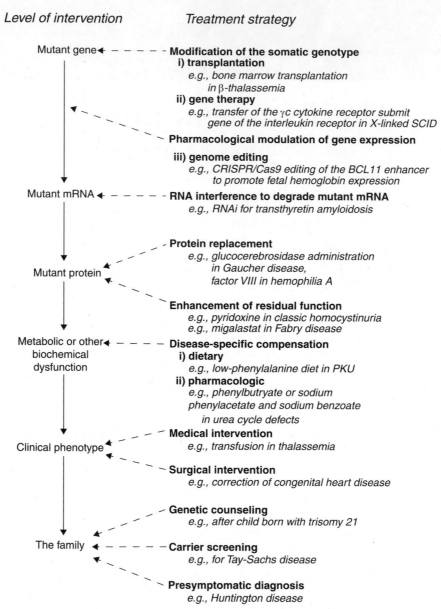

Level of intervention   *Treatment strategy*

Mutant gene ◄ — — — — **Modification of the somatic genotype**
i) transplantation
e.g., bone marrow transplantation
in β-thalassemia
ii) gene therapy
e.g., transfer of the γc cytokine receptor submit
gene of the interleukin receptor in X-linked SCID

Pharmacological modulation of gene expression

iii) genome editing
e.g., CRISPR/Cas9 editing of the BCL11 enhancer
to promote fetal hemoglobin expression

Mutant mRNA ◄ — — — — **RNA interference to degrade mutant mRNA**
e.g., RNAi for transthyretin amyloidosis

Protein replacement
e.g., glucocerebrosidase administration
in Gaucher disease,
factor VIII in hemophilia A

Mutant protein

Enhancement of residual function
e.g., pyridoxine in classic homocystinuria
e.g., migalastat in Fabry disease

Metabolic or other ◄ — — — **Disease-specific compensation**
biochemical   **i) dietary**
dysfunction   *e.g., low-phenylalanine diet in PKU*
ii) pharmacologic
e.g., phenylbutryate or sodium
phenylacetate and sodium benzoate
in urea cycle defects

Medical intervention
e.g., transfusion in thalassemia

Clinical phenotype

Surgical intervention
e.g., correction of congenital heart disease

Genetic counseling
e.g., after child born with trisomy 21

The family ◄ — — — — **Carrier screening**
e.g., for Tay-Sachs disease

Presymptomatic diagnosis
e.g., Huntington disease

Figure 14.1 The various levels of treatment that are relevant to genetic disease, with the corresponding strategies used at each level. For each level, a disease discussed in the book is given as an example. All the therapies listed are used clinically in many centers, unless indicated otherwise. *Hb F*, Fetal hemoglobin; *mRNA*, messenger RNA; *PKU*, phenylketonuria; *RNAi*, RNA interference; *SCID*, severe combined immunodeficiency. (Modified from Valle D: Genetic disease: an overview of current therapy, *Hosp Pract* 22:167–182, 1987.)

and other -omic technologies. However, even when the gene is known, knowledge of the pathophysiologic mechanism is often inadequate and can lag well behind gene discovery. In phenylketonuria (PKU), for example, despite decades of study, the mechanisms by which the elevation in phenylalanine impairs brain development and function are still poorly understood (see Chapter 13).

- **Prediagnostic fetal damage.** Some variants act early in development or cause irreversible pathologic changes before they are diagnosed. These problems can sometimes be anticipated if there is a family history of the genetic disease or if carrier screening identifies couples at risk. In some cases, prenatal treatment is possible (e.g., maternal dexamethasone [a cortisol analog] to prevent virilization in female fetuses known to have **congenital** adrenal hyperplasia).

- **Severe phenotypes are less amenable to intervention.** The initial cases of a disease to be recognized are usually the most severely affected, but they are often less amenable to treatment. In such individuals, the variant frequently leads to the absence of the encoded protein or to a severely compromised mutant protein with no residual activity. In contrast, when the variant is less disruptive, the mutant protein may retain some residual function, and it may be possible to increase the small amount of function sufficiently to have a therapeutic effect, as described later.

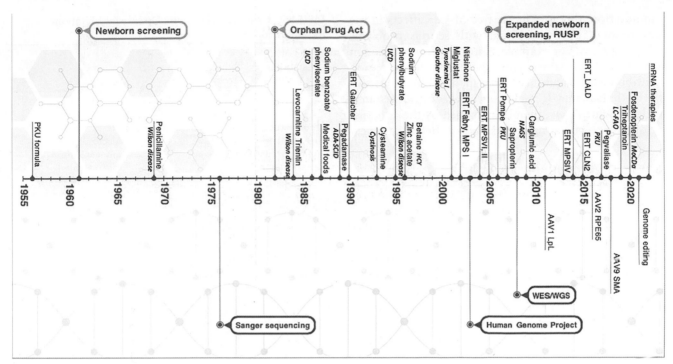

Figure 14.2 Timeline of major developments in the treatment and diagnosis of inborn errors of metabolism (IEM) from 1955 to present. *ADA-SCID*, Adenosine deaminase-severe combined immunodeficiency, *LC-FAO*, long chain fatty acid oxidation defects; *MoCDa*, molybdenum cofactor deficiency type A; *NAGS*, N-acetylglutamate synthetase; *UCD*, urea cycle defects; levocarnitine and medical foods are used to treat many IEMs. (Adapted from Vernon HJ, Manoli I: Milestones in treatments for inborn errors of metabolism: reflections on where chemistry and medicine meet, *Am J Med Genet* 185a:3350–3358, 2021.)

- **The challenge of dominant negative alleles**. For some dominant disorders, the mutant protein interferes with the function of the normal **allele**. The challenge is to decrease the expression or impact of the variant allele or its encoded altered protein specifically, without disrupting expression or function of the normal allele or its normal protein.

SPECIAL CONSIDERATIONS IN TREATING GENETIC DISEASE

Long-Term Assessment of Treatment Is Critical

For treating monogenic diseases, long-term evaluation of cohorts of treated individuals, often over decades, is critical for several reasons. First, treatment initially judged as successful may eventually be revealed to be imperfect; for example, although well-managed children with PKU have escaped severely impaired intellectual development and have normal or nearly normal IQs (see later), they may manifest subtle learning disorders and behavioral disturbances that impair their academic performance in later years.

Second, successful treatment of the pathologic changes in one organ may be followed by unexpected problems in tissues not previously observed to be clinically involved because the patients typically did not survive long enough for the new phenotype to become evident. Galactosemia, a well-known inborn error of carbohydrate metabolism, illustrates this point. This disorder results from an inability to metabolize galactose, a component of lactose (milk sugar), because of the autosomal **recessive** deficiency of galactose-1-phosphate uridyltransferase (GALT).

Affected infants are usually normal at birth but develop gastrointestinal problems, cirrhosis of the liver, and cataracts in the weeks after they are given lactose-containing milk. The pathogenesis is thought to be due to the negative impact of galactose-1-phosphate accumulation on other critical enzymes. If not recognized, galactosemia causes severe intellectual disability and is often fatal. Complete removal of milk from the diet, however, can protect against most of the harmful consequences, although learning disabilities are now recognized to be common, even in well-treated patients. Moreover, despite conscientious treatment, most females with galactosemia have ovarian failure that appears to result from endogenously produced galactose toxicity.

Another example is provided by hereditary retinoblastoma (Case 39) due to **germline** variants in the retinoblastoma *(RB1)* gene (see Chapter 16). Patients successfully treated for the eye tumor in the first years of life are unfortunately at increased risk for development of other independent malignant neoplasms, particularly osteosarcoma, after the first decade of life. Ironically, therefore, treatment that successfully prolongs life provides an opportunity for the manifestation of a previously unrecognized phenotype.

In addition, therapy that is free of side effects in the short term may be associated with serious problems in the long term. For example, clotting factor infusion in hemophilia (Case 21) sometimes results in the formation of antibodies to the infused protein, and blood transfusion in thalassemia (Case 44) invariably produces iron overload, which must then be managed by the administration of iron-chelating agents, such as deferoxamine.

Genetic Heterogeneity and Treatment

The optimal treatment of single-gene defects requires an unusual degree of diagnostic precision; one must often define not only the biochemical abnormality but also the specific gene that is affected. For example, as we saw in Chapter 13, hyperphenylalaninemia can result from variants in either the phenylalanine hydroxylase *(PAH)* gene or in one of the genes that encodes the enzymes required for the synthesis of tetrahydrobiopterin (BH$_4$), the cofactor of the PAH enzyme (see Fig. 13.2). The treatment of these two different causes of hyperphenylalaninemia is entirely different, as shown in Table 13.1.

Allelic heterogeneity (see Chapter 7) may also have critical implications for therapy. Some alleles may produce a protein that is decreased in abundance but has some residual function, so strategies to increase the expression, function, or stability of such a partially functional mutant protein may correct the biochemical defect. This situation is again illustrated by some patients with hyperphenylalaninemia due to variants in the *PAH* gene; the variants in some patients lead to the formation of a mutant PAH enzyme whose activity can be increased by the administration of high doses of the BH$_4$ cofactor (see Chapter 13). Of course, if a patient carries two alleles with no residual function, nothing will be gained by increasing the abundance of the mutant protein. One of the most striking examples of the importance of knowing the specific mutant allele in a patient with a genetic disease is exemplified by cystic fibrosis (CF); the drug ivacaftor (Kalydeco) was approved for treating CF patients carrying any one of only nine of the many hundreds of *CFTR* missense alleles. Further work has resulted in identification of a three-drug regimen that can treat over 90% of CF patients (see later).

TREATMENT BY THE MANIPULATION OF METABOLISM

Presently, the most successful disease-specific approach to the treatment of genetic disease is directed at the metabolic abnormality in inborn errors of metabolism. The principal strategies used to manipulate metabolism in the treatment of this group of diseases are listed in Table 14.1. The necessity for patients with pharmacogenetic diseases, such as glucose-6-phosphate

TABLE 14.1 Treatment of Genetic Disease by Metabolic Manipulation

Type of Metabolic Intervention	Substance or Technique	Disease
Avoidance	Antimalarial drugs	G6PD deficiency
	Isoniazid	Slow acetylators
Dietary restriction	Phenylalanine	PKU
	Galactose	Galactosemia
Replacement	Thyroxine	Monogenic forms of congenital hypothyroidism
	Biotin	Biotinidase deficiency
Diversion	Sodium benzoate/ sodium phenylacetate	Urea cycle disorders
	Drugs that sequester bile acids in the intestine (e.g., colesevelam)	Familial hypercholesterolemia heterozygotes
Enzyme inhibition	Statins PCSK9 inhibitors	Familial hypercholesterolemia heterozygotes
Substrate reduction	Miglustat and eliglustat for Gaucher disease: competitive inhibitors of the first step of glycosylation of ceramide	FDA approved, oral agents, can be instead of enzyme replacement therapy
Receptor antagonism	Losartan	Marfan syndrome
Depletion	LDL apheresis (direct removal of LDL from plasma)	Familial hypercholesterolemia homozygotes

FDA, US Food and Drug Administration; *G6PD,* glucose-6-phosphate dehydrogenase; *LDL,* low-density lipoprotein; *PKU,* phenylketonuria. Updated from Rosenberg LE: Treating genetic diseases: lessons from three children, *Pediatr Res* 27:S10–S16, 1990.

dehydrogenase deficiency (Case 19), to avoid certain drugs and chemicals is described in Chapter 19.

Substrate Reduction

As illustrated by the damaging effects of hyperphenylalaninemia in PKU, enzyme deficiencies may lead to substrate accumulation, with pathophysiologic consequences (see Chapter 13). Strategies to prevent the accumulation of the offending substrate have been one of the most effective methods of treating genetic disease. The most common approach is to reduce the dietary intake of the substrate or of a precursor of it, and presently several dozen disorders – most involving amino acid catabolic pathways – are managed in this way. The drawback is that severe lifelong restriction of dietary protein intake is often necessary, requiring strict adherence to an artificial diet that is onerous for the patient as well as for the family. Nutrients such as 20 essential amino acids cannot be withheld entirely, however; their intake must be sufficient for anabolic needs such as protein synthesis.

A diet restricted in phenylalanine largely circumvents the neurologic damage in classic PKU (see Chapter 13). Children with PKU are normal at birth because the maternal enzyme protects them during prenatal life. Treatment is most effective if begun promptly after diagnosis by newborn screening. Without treatment, irreversible neurologic damage occurs, with the degree of intellectual deficit being directly related to the delay in commencing the low-phenylalanine diet and adherence to it. It is now recommended that patients with PKU remain on a low-phenylalanine diet for life because neurologic and psychiatric (including attention-deficit/hyperactivity disorder, anxiety, and depression) problems develop in many (although perhaps not all) patients if the diet is stopped. However, even PKU patients who have been effectively treated throughout life may have neuropsychologic deficits (e.g., impaired conceptual, visual-spatial, and language skills), despite their having normal intelligence as measured by IQ tests. Nonetheless, treatment produces results vastly superior to the severe intellectual disability that occurs without

treatment. As discussed in Chapter 13, continued and tightly controlled phenylalanine restriction is particularly important in women with PKU during pregnancy to prevent damage to the fetus, even though the fetus is highly unlikely to be affected by PKU.

Substrate Augmentation

Substrate augmentation can either drive an enzyme reaction or stabilize the mutant protein (discussed later). An example of substrate augmentation to drive limited enzyme activity is giving pharmacologic doses of mannose to treat MPI-CDG (CDG1b) (see Chapter 13). High-dose galactose and high-dose manganese are being studied to treat SLC35A2-CDG (CDGIIf) and SLC39A8-CDG (CDGIIn), respectively (Fig. 14.3).

Replacement

The provision of essential metabolites, cofactors, or hormones whose deficiency is due to a genetic disease is simple in concept and often simple in application. Some of the most successfully treated single-gene defects belong to this category. A prime example is provided by congenital hypothyroidism, of which 10%

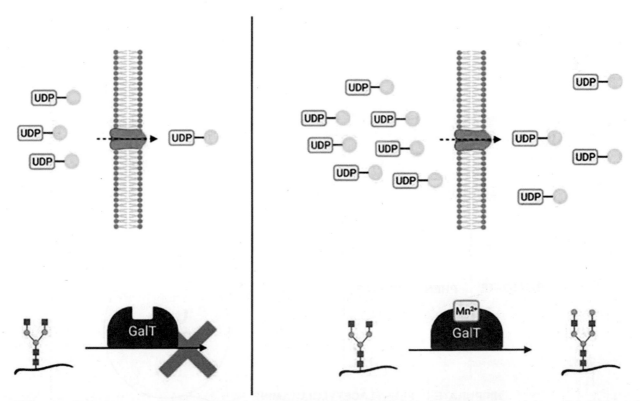

Figure 14.3 **Substrate augmentation.** *(Upper panel)* A treatment for SLC35A2-CDG is high-dose galactose supplementation, where oral supplementation of galactose *(yellow circle)* increases UDP-galactose supplies and thus transport across the defective UDP-galactose transporter SLC35A2. *(Lower panel)* Defects in SLC39A8 lead to a deficiency in manganese *(Mn²⁺)*. Lack of this cofactor impairs the function of galactosyltransferases *(GalT)*. Cofactor supplementation leads to an improved GalT function and thus normalized glycosylation in SLC39A8-CDG (CDG type IIn). (Adapted from Park JH, Marquardt T: Treatment options in congenital disorders of glycosylation, *Front Genet* 12:735348, 2021. https://doi.org/10.3389/fgene.2021.735348.)

to 15% of cases are monogenic in origin. Monogenic congenital hypothyroidism can result from **pathogenic variants** in any one of numerous genes encoding proteins required for the development of the thyroid gland or the biosynthesis or metabolism of thyroxine. Because congenital hypothyroidism from all causes is common (~1 in 4000 neonates), neonatal screening is conducted in many countries so that thyroxine administration may be initiated soon after birth to prevent the severe intellectual deficits that are otherwise inevitable (see Chapter 19).

Diversion

Diversion therapy is the enhanced use of alternative metabolic pathways to reduce the concentration of a harmful metabolite. A major use of this strategy is in the treatment of the urea cycle disorders (Fig. 14.4). The function of the urea cycle is to convert ammonia, which is neurotoxic, to urea, a benign end product of protein catabolism excreted in urine. If the cycle is disrupted by an enzyme defect such as ornithine transcarbamylase deficiency (Case 36), the consequent hyperammonemia cannot be controlled by dietary protein restriction alone. Blood ammonia levels can be reduced to normal, however, by the diversion of excess nitrogen to metabolic pathways that are normally of minor significance, leading to the synthesis of harmless compounds. Thus the administration to hyperammonemic patients of large quantities of sodium benzoate forces the ligation of ammonia with glycine to form hippurate, which is excreted in urine (see Fig. 14.4). Glycine synthesis is thereby increased,

and for each mole of glycine formed, one mole of ammonia is consumed. Additional compounds, sodium phenylbutyrate and glycerol phenylbutyrate, are metabolized to phenylacetate, which then conjugates with glutamine and is excreted as phenylacetylglutamine (PAGN). In this case, each mole of PAGN removes two moles of nitrogen, preventing ammonia accumulation.

A comparable approach is used to reduce cholesterol levels in heterozygotes for **familial** hypercholesterolemia (Case 16) (see Chapter 13). If bile acids are sequestered in the intestine by the oral administration of a compound such as colesevelam and then excreted in feces rather than being reabsorbed, bile acid synthesis from cholesterol increases (Fig. 14.5). The reduction in hepatic cholesterol levels leads to increased production of low-density lipoprotein (LDL) receptors from their single normal LDL receptor gene, increased hepatic uptake of LDL-bound cholesterol, and lower levels of plasma LDL cholesterol. This treatment significantly reduces plasma cholesterol levels because 70% of all LDL receptor uptake of cholesterol occurs in the liver. An important general principle is illustrated by this example: Autosomal **dominant** diseases may sometimes be treated by increasing the expression of the normal allele.

Enzyme Inhibition

The pharmacologic inhibition of enzymes is sometimes used to reduce the impact of metabolic abnormalities in treating inborn errors. This principle is also illustrated by the treatment of heterozygotes of familial

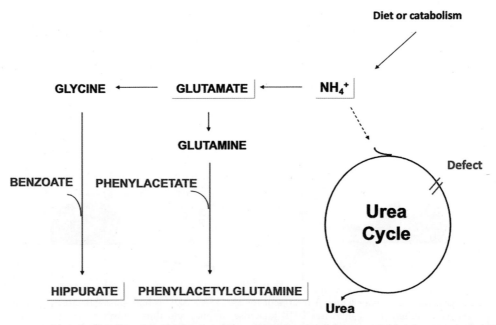

Figure 14.4 The strategy of metabolite diversion. In this example, ammonia cannot be removed by the urea cycle because of a genetic defect of a urea cycle enzyme. The administration of sodium benzoate diverts ammonia to glycine synthesis, and the nitrogen moiety is subsequently excreted as hippurate. The administration of sodium phenylacetate, or it precursors, sodium phenylbutyrate or glycerol phenylbutyrate, diverts ammonia to glutamate synthesis and two nitrogen moieties are then excreted as phenylacetylglutamine.

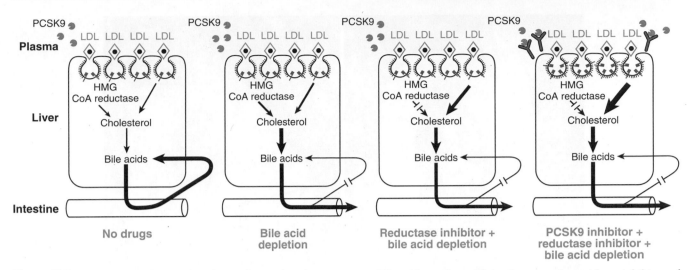

Figure 14.5 Rationale for the combined use of a reagent that sequesters bile acids, such as colesevelam, together with an inhibitor of 3-hydroxy-3-methylglutaryl coenzyme A reductase (HMG CoA reductase) such as a statin, and a PCSK9 inhibitor (green structures) in the treatment of familial hypercholesterolemia heterozygotes. *LDL*, Low-density lipoprotein. (Adapted from Brown MS, Goldstein JL: A receptor-mediated pathway for cholesterol homeostasis, *Science* 232:4, 1986. Copyright by the Nobel Foundation.)

hypercholesterolemia. If a statin, a class of drugs that are powerful inhibitors of 3-hydroxy-3-methylglutaryl coenzyme A reductase, or HMG CoA reductase (the rate-limiting enzyme of cholesterol synthesis), is used to decrease hepatic *de novo* cholesterol synthesis in these patients, the liver compensates by increasing the synthesis of LDL receptors from the remaining intact LDL receptor allele. The increase in LDL receptors typically lowers plasma LDL cholesterol levels by 40% to 60% in familial hypercholesterolemia heterozygotes; used together with colesevelam, the effect is synergistic, and even greater decreases can be achieved (see Fig. 14.5). Inhibition of PCSK9 prevents degradation of LDL receptors, increasing their numbers and thereby further reducing plasma cholesterol by 50% to 60%. PCSK9 inhibitors, approved by the US Food and Drug Administration (FDA) since 2015, are effective as adjunctive therapy in individuals who need additional reduction in cholesterol and are particularly important for those who cannot tolerate statin therapy (5–10%) due to muscle pain.

Receptor Antagonism

In some instances the pathophysiology of an inherited disease results from the increased and inappropriate activation of a biochemical or signaling pathway. In such cases, one therapeutic approach is to antagonize critical steps in the pathway. A powerful example is provided by treatment of an autosomal dominant connective tissue disorder, Marfan **syndrome** (Case 30). The disease results from pathogenic variants in *FBN1*, the gene that encodes fibrillin 1, an important structural component of the extracellular matrix. The syndrome is characterized by many connective tissue abnormalities, such as aortic aneurysm, pulmonary emphysema, and eye lens dislocation (Fig. 14.6).

Unexpectedly, the pathophysiology of Marfan syndrome is only partially explained by the impact of the reduction in fibrillin-1 microfibrils on the structure of the extracellular matrix. Rather, it has been found that a major function of microfibrils is to regulate signaling by the transforming growth factor β (TGFβ), by binding TGFβ to the large latent protein complex of TGFβ. The decreased abundance of microfibrils in Marfan syndrome leads to an increase in the local abundance of unbound TGFβ and in local activation of TGFβ signaling. This increased TGFβ signaling has been suggested to underlie the pathogenesis of many of the phenotypes of Marfan syndrome, particularly the progressive dilation of the aortic root, and aortic aneurysm and dissection, the major cause of death in this disorder. Moreover, a recently recognized group of other vasculopathies, such as nonsyndromic forms of thoracic aortic aneurysm, has also proved to be driven by altered TGFβ signaling.

Angiotensin II signaling is known to increase TGFβ activity, and the angiotensin II type 1 receptor antagonist, losartan, a widely used antihypertensive agent, has been shown to attenuate TGFβ signaling by decreasing the **transcription** of genes encoding TGFβ ligands, receptor subunits, and activators. Treatment with losartan has been found to decrease substantially the rate of aortic root dilation in clinical trials of Marfan syndrome patients, an effect that appears to be largely due to decreased TGFβ signaling.

The novel use of an FDA-approved drug, losartan, to treat a rare inherited disease, Marfan syndrome, represents a paradigm that will be repeated regularly in the future, as small molecule chemical screens to identify compounds with therapeutic potential – including the thousands of FDA-approved drugs – are undertaken to identify safe, effective treatments for other uncommon genetic disorders.

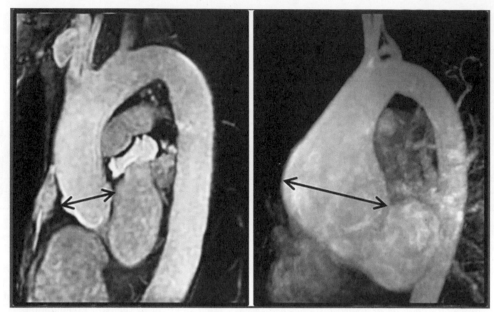

Figure 14.6 Computerized tomography angiograms of the aorta from a control *(left)* and an individual with Marfan syndrome *(right)*. The aortic root diameter is indicated by the arrow. (Courtesy H. Dietz, Johns Hopkins University.)

Depletion

Genetic diseases characterized by the accumulation of a harmful compound are sometimes treated by direct removal of the compound from the body. This principle is illustrated by the treatment of **homozygous** familial hypercholesterolemia. In this instance, for patients whose LDL levels cannot be lowered by other approaches, a procedure called apheresis is used to remove LDL from the circulation. Whole blood is removed from the patient, LDL is removed from plasma by any one of several methods, and the plasma and blood cells are returned to the patient. The use of phlebotomy to alleviate the iron accumulation of hereditary hemochromatosis (Case 20) provides another example of depletion therapy. Chelation of copper using any of several different agents is effective in treating Wilson disease.

TREATMENT TO INCREASE THE FUNCTION OF THE AFFECTED GENE OR PROTEIN

The growth in knowledge of the molecular pathophysiology of monogenic diseases has been accompanied by a small but promising increase in therapies that – at the level of DNA, RNA, or protein – increase the function of the gene affected by the variant. Some of the novel treatments have led to striking improvement in the lives of affected individuals, an outcome that, until recently, would have seemed fanciful. An overview of the molecular treatment of single-gene diseases is presented in Fig. 14.7. These molecular therapies represent one facet of the important paradigm embraced by the concept of individualized or precision medicine,

which is a general one used to describe the diagnosis, prevention, and treatment of a disease – tailored to individual patients – based on a profound understanding of the mechanisms that underlie its etiology and pathogenesis.

Treatment at the Level of the Protein

In many situations, if a mutant protein product is made, it may be possible to increase its function. For example, the stability or function of a mutant protein with some residual function may be further increased. With enzymopathies, the improvement in function obtained by this approach is usually very small, on the order of a few percent, but this increment is often all that is required to restore biochemical homeostasis.

Enhancement of Mutant Protein Function With Small Molecule Therapy

Small molecules are compounds with molecular weights in the few hundreds to thousands. They include vitamins, nonpeptide hormones, and indeed most drugs, whether synthesized by organic chemists or isolated from nature. A strategy for identifying potential drugs is to use high-throughput screening of chemical compound libraries, often containing tens of thousands of known chemicals, against a drug target, such as the protein whose function is disrupted by a variant. As we will discuss, three drugs that are now FDA approved for the treatment of most patients with CF were discovered using such high-throughput screens. Progress in the development of these drugs represents a new frontier with great potential for the treatment of genetic disease.

The Molecular Treatment of Genetic Disease

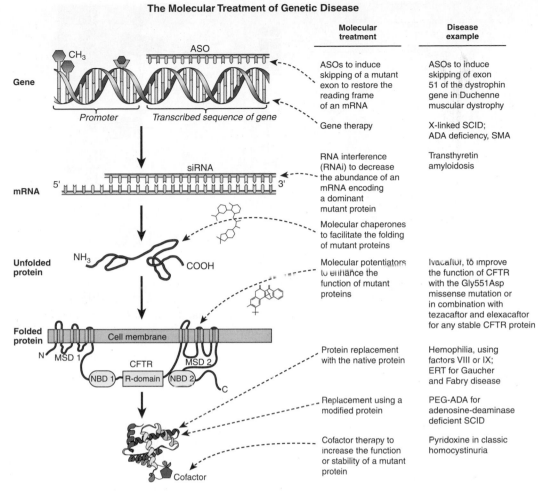

	Molecular treatment	Disease example
	ASOs to induce skipping of a mutant exon to restore the reading frame of an mRNA	ASOs to induce skipping of exon 51 of the dystrophin gene in Duchenne muscular dystrophy
	Gene therapy	X-linked SCID; ADA deficiency, SMA
	RNA interference (RNAi) to decrease the abundance of an mRNA encoding a dominant mutant protein	Transthyretin amyloidosis
	Molecular chaperones to facilitate the folding of mutant proteins	
	Molecular potentiators to enhance the function of mutant proteins	Ivacaftor, to improve the function of CFTR with the Gly551Asp missense mutation or in combination with tezacaftor and elexacaftor for any stable CFTR protein
	Protein replacement with the native protein	Hemophilia, using factors VIII or IX; ERT for Gaucher and Fabry disease
	Replacement using a modified protein	PEG-ADA for adenosine-deaminase deficient SCID
	Cofactor therapy to increase the function or stability of a mutant protein	Pyridoxine in classic homocystinuria

Figure 14.7 **The molecular treatment of inherited disease.** Each molecular therapy is discussed in the text. *ADA*, Adenosine deaminase; *ASO*, antisense oligonucleotide; *ERT*, enzyme replacement therapy; *mRNA*, messenger RNA; *MSD*, membrane-spanning domain; *NBD*, nucleotide-binding domain; *PEG*, polyethylene glycol; *SCID*, severe combined immunodeficiency; *siRNA*, small interfering RNA: *SMA*, spinal muscular atrophy.

Small Molecule Therapy to Allow Skipping Over Nonsense Codons. Nonsense variants account for 11% of deleterious alterations in the human genome. Thousands of small molecules are being examined in laboratories around the world to identify novel non-toxic compounds that facilitate the skipping of nonsense codons, not only for the treatment of CF but also for Duchenne muscular dystrophy (DMD) patients carrying nonsense codons, as well as other diseases. Safe, effective drugs of this type will have a major impact on the treatment of inherited disease.

Small Molecules to Increase the Function of Correctly Trafficked Mutant Membrane Proteins. Amino acid substitutions in membrane proteins may not disrupt the trafficking of the mutant polypeptide to the plasma membrane, but rather interfere with its function at the cell surface. Small molecule screens for new treatments for CF have led this area of drug discovery. Screens for potentiators – molecules that could enhance the

function of mutant CFTR proteins that are correctly positioned at the cell surface – identified ivacaftor, which improves the Cl⁻ transport of some mutant CFTR proteins, such as the p.Gly551Asp *CFTR* missense variant (see Fig. 13.14) that inactivates anion transport; this allele is carried by 4% to 5% of all CF patients. In one clinical trial, patients carrying at least one p.Gly551Asp allele experienced a significant improvement in lung function, weight gain, respiratory symptoms, and a decline in sweat Cl⁻. Ivacaftor is presently FDA approved for the treatment of eight other CFTR missense variants. Although fewer than 200 CF patients in the United States have one of these eight alleles, the allele-specific indications for ivacaftor treatment highlight both the benefits and dilemmas of personalized medicine for genetic disease: Effective drugs can be discovered, but they may be effective only in a relatively small numbers of individuals. Moreover, at present ivacaftor is extremely expensive, costing ~$300,000 per year.

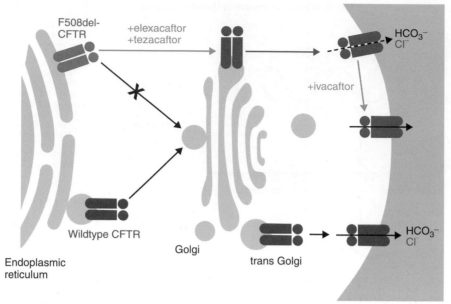

Figure 14.8 Modulators and potentiators to treat cystic fibrosis. Tezacaftor and elexacaftor allow CFTR carrying the F508del variant to traverse the endoplasmic reticulum and Golgi apparatus to reach the cell surface, where ivacaftor prolongs channel open time to allows more chloride ions to leave the cells. Ivacaftor works alone for nine CFTR variants in which channel gating is the main defect. The three-drug combination (marketed in the United States as Trikafta) improves lung function and lowers sweat chloride dramatically.

Small Molecules to Correct the Folding of Mutant Membrane Proteins: Pharmacologic Chaperones. Some variants in membrane proteins may disrupt their ability to fold, pass through the endoplasmic reticulum (ER), and be trafficked to the plasma membrane. These mutant proteins are recognized by the cellular protein quality control machinery, trapped in the ER, and prematurely degraded by the proteasome. The p.Phe508del(F508del) variant of the CFTR protein – which constitutes 68% of all CF causing variants worldwide – is perhaps the best-known example (see Fig. 13.14) of a variant that impairs trafficking of a membrane protein. Over the past decade continuous efforts, including small molecule screens and clinical trials, identified a combination of three modulators, elexacaftor/tezacaftor/ivacaftor, that can correct the folding and trafficking of CFTR carrying the F508del variant or ~200 other CFTR variants. Ivacaftor is a potentiator that improves the function of the CFTR channel once it has made it to the cell membrane. This drug alone was effective in ameliorating lung disease in CF patients with one of nine variants. Elexacaftor and tezacaftor are modulators that improve cellular processing and trafficking of mutant CFTR protein (see Fig. 14.8). Remarkably, this combination is effective in 90% of CF patients (only those who are homozygous or compound **heterozygous** for nonsense variants where no CFTR protein is made cannot be treated with this regimen). Patients with CF treated with elexacaftor/tezacaftor/ivacaftor experience a 70-point decrease in the sweat chloride concentrations and more remarkably a 10% to 14% increase in predicted pulmonary function testing, accompanied by a 63% decline in pulmonary exacerbations. While this treatment is not a cure, it is life changing for individuals

with CF. This example is a milestone in medical genetics because it establishes the principle that molecular chaperones can have dramatic clinical benefits in the treatment of monogenic disease. Nevertheless, the cost of this combination is still ~$300,000 per year.

Small Molecules to Enhance the Function of Mutant Enzymes: Vitamin-Responsive Inborn Errors of Metabolism. The biochemical abnormalities of a number of inherited metabolic diseases may respond, sometimes dramatically, to the administration of large amounts of the vitamin cofactor of the enzyme impaired by the pathogenic variant (Table 14.2). In fact, the vitamin-responsive inborn errors are among the most successfully treated of all genetic diseases. The vitamins used are remarkably nontoxic, generally allowing the safe administration of amounts 100 to 500 times greater than those required for normal nutrition. In homocystinuria due to cystathionine synthase deficiency (see Fig. 13.7), for example, ~50% of patients respond to the administration of high doses of pyridoxine (vitamin B_6, the precursor of pyridoxal phosphate, the cofactor for the enzyme), an example – as we saw earlier in the case of BH_4 administration in PKU – of cofactor responsiveness in a metabolic disease. In most of these responsive patients, free homocysteine completely disappears from the plasma, even though the increase in hepatic cystathionine synthase activity is usually only a few fold, from 1.5% to 4.5% of control activity. The increased pyridoxal phosphate concentrations may stabilize the mutant enzyme or overcome reduced affinity of the mutant enzyme for the cofactor (Fig. 14.9). In any case, vitamin B_6 treatment substantially improves the clinical course of the disease in responsive patients. Nonresponsive patients generally carry null alleles and

TABLE 14.2 Treatment of Genetic Disease at the Level of the Mutant Protein

Strategy	Example	Status
Enhancement of Mutant Protein Function		
Small molecule "correctors" that increase the trafficking of the mutant protein through the ER to the plasma membrane	Tezacaftor and elexacaftor to increase the abundance of the F508del-CFTR protein at the apical membrane of epithelial cells in CF patients	FDA approved and used in combination with ivacaftor; expensive
Small molecule "potentiators" that increase the function at the cell membrane of correctly trafficked membrane proteins	Ivacaftor (VX-770) used alone to enhance the function of specific variant CFTR proteins at the epithelial apical membrane	FDA approved for the treatment of CF patients carrying specific alleles; most effective when used in combination with tezacaftor and elexacaftor; expensive
Vitamin cofactor administration to increase the residual activity of the mutant enzyme	Vitamin B$_6$ for pyridoxine-responsive homocystinuria	Treatment of choice in the 50% of cystathionine synthase patients who are responsive: inexpensive
Protein Augmentation		
Replacement of an extracellular protein	Factor VIII in hemophilia A	Well-established, effective, safe
Extracellular replacement of an intracellular protein	Polyethylene glycol–modified adenosine deaminase (PEG-ADA) in ADA deficiency	Well-established, safe, and effective, but costly; now used principally to stabilize patients before gene therapy or HLA-matched bone marrow transplantation
Replacement of an intracellular protein – cell targeting	β-glucocerebrosidase in nonneuronal Gaucher disease	Well-established; biochemically and clinically effective; expensive

ADA, Adenosine deaminase; *CF*, cystic fibrosis; *ER*, endoplasmic reticulum; *FDA*, US Food and Drug Administration; *HLA*, human leukocyte antigen; *PEG*, polyethylene glycol.

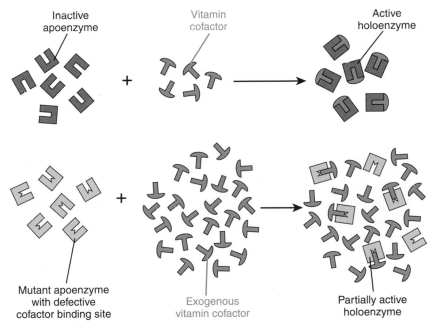

Figure 14.9 **The mechanism of response of a mutant apoenzyme to the administration of its cofactor at high doses.** Vitamin-responsive enzyme defects are often due to variants that reduce the normal affinity (*top*) of the enzyme protein (apoenzyme) for the cofactor needed to activate it. In the presence of the high concentrations of the cofactor that result from the administration of up to 500 times the normal daily requirement, the mutant enzyme acquires a small amount of activity sufficient to restore biochemical normalcy. (Redrawn from Valle D: Genetic disease: an overview of current therapy, *Hosp Pract* 22:167–182, 1987.)

therefore have no residual cystathionine synthase activity to augment.

Small Molecules to Stabilize Mutant Proteins. This class of therapeutics has increased dramatically in recent years and is exemplified not only by known cofactors but also by pharmacologic chaperones. One example is migalastat, which is approved for the treatment of

adults with Fabry disease with specific pathogenic variants in *GLA* that have been shown to be responsive to migalastat in *in vitro* assays of enzyme activity. Other examples include miglustat and eliglustat for Gaucher disease (see Fig. 14.2 and Table 14.1).

Small Molecules to Stabilize Mutant Proteins and Prevent Aggregation. Many conditions are characterized by accumulation of misfolded proteins that aggregate and interfere with cell and tissue function. One example is hereditary amyloidosis due to pathogenic variants in *TTR*, the gene for transthyretin. This condition has highly variable presentation with either polyneuropathy or cardiomyopathy due to amyloid deposition (occasionally both and renal deposition is also possible). Tafamidis is a small molecule that binds to thyroxine binding sites on transthyretin tetramers and inhibits dissociation (>90%) and aggregate formation. This oral agent requires only daily dosing and is most effective when used early in the course of the disease, as it is unable to reverse damage done.

Small Molecules to Drive Enzymatic Reactions. Carglumic acid is a synthetic analogue of *N*-acetylglutamate, which drives expression of carbamoylphosphate synthetase, the first step in the urea cycle. Already approved to treat *N*-acetylglutamate synthetase deficiency, a very rare cause of hyperammonemia, carglumic acid was recently shown to be beneficial in treating acute hyperammonemia in patients with propionic acidemia and methylmalonic acidemia (MMA), where it drives the urea cycle despite the lack of known endogenous defect. The etiology of hyperammonemia in these patients is not clear and is quite unpredictable, but its response to carglumic acid, an oral agent, is welcome when compared with either intravenous sodium benzoate/sodium phenylacetate (Ammonul®) or hemodialysis, which have significant risks.

Protein Augmentation

The principal types of protein augmentation are summarized in Table 14.2. Protein augmentation is a routine therapeutic approach in only a few diseases, all involving proteins whose principal site of action is in the plasma or extracellular fluid. The prime example is the prevention or arrest of bleeding episodes in patients with hemophilia (**Case 21**) by the infusion of plasma fractions enriched for the appropriate factor or with the use of recombinant factor. The decades of experience with this disease illustrate the problems that can be anticipated as new strategies for replacing other, particularly intracellular, polypeptides are attempted. These problems include the difficulty and cost of procuring sufficient amounts of the protein to treat all patients at the optimal frequency, the need to administer the protein at a frequency consistent with its half-life (only 8–10 hours for factor VIII), and the formation of neutralizing antibodies in some patients (5% of classic hemophiliacs).

Enzyme Replacement Therapy: Extracellular Administration of an Intracellular Enzyme

Adenosine Deaminase Deficiency. Adenosine deaminase (ADA) is a critical enzyme of **purine** metabolism that catalyzes the deamination of adenosine to inosine and of deoxyadenosine to deoxyinosine (Fig. 14.10). The pathology of ADA deficiency, an autosomal recessive disease, results entirely from the accumulation of toxic purines, particularly deoxyadenosine, in lymphocytes. A profound failure of both cell-mediated (T-cell) and humoral (B-cell) immunity results, making ADA deficiency one cause of severe combined immunodeficiency (SCID). Untreated patients die of infection within the first 2 years of life. The long-term treatment of ADA deficiency is rapidly evolving, with gene therapy (see later section) now a strong alternative to bone marrow transplantation from a fully **human leukocyte antigen (HLA)** compatible donor. The administration of a modified form of the bovine ADA enzyme, described in the next section, is no longer a first choice for long-term management, but it is an effective stabilizing measure in the short term until these other treatments can be used.

Modified Adenosine Deaminase. The infusion of bovine ADA modified by the covalent attachment of an inert polymer, polyethylene glycol (PEG), is superior in several ways to the use of the unmodified ADA enzyme. First, PEG-ADA largely protects the patient from a neutralizing antibody response (which would remove the ADA from plasma). Second, the modified enzyme remains in the extracellular fluid where it can degrade toxic purines. Third, the plasma half-life of PEG-ADA is

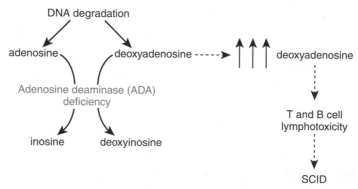

Figure 14.10 Adenosine deaminase *(ADA)* converts adenosine to inosine and deoxyadenosine to deoxyinosine. In ADA deficiency, deoxyadenosine accumulation in lymphocytes is lymphotoxic, killing the cells by impairing DNA replication and cell division to cause severe combined immunodeficiency *(SCID)*.

3 to 6 days, much longer than the half-life of unmodified ADA. Although the near-normalization of purine metabolism obtained with PEG-ADA does not completely correct immune function (most patients remain T lymphopenic), immunoprotection is restored, with dramatic clinical improvement.

The general principles exemplified by the use of PEG-ADA are that (1) proteins can be chemically modified to improve their effectiveness as pharmacologic reagents, and (2) an enzyme that is normally located inside the cell can be effective extracellularly if its substrate is in equilibrium with the extracellular fluid and if its product can be taken up by the cells that require it. A similar approach is used to treat some adults with classic PKU, unresponsive to BH_4 supplementation. Pegvaliase is modified phenylalanine ammonia lyase with PEG added to stabilize. Because it is a bacterial enzyme, it elicits a potent immune response, and the dose must be very slowly titrated up with premedications and an absolute requirement for epinephrine to be available for the daily injection. Pegvaliase has a profound effect on plasma phenylalanine levels lowering them to below treatment range, so careful monitoring is essential. It is contraindicated in pregnancy.

Enzyme Replacement Therapy: Targeted Augmentation of an Intracellular Enzyme. Enzyme replacement therapy (ERT) is now established therapy for nine lysosomal storage diseases, with clinical trials being conducted for several others. Nonneuronal (type 1) Gaucher disease was the first lysosomal storage disease for which ERT was shown to be effective. It is the most prevalent lysosomal storage disorder, affecting up to 1 in 450 Ashkenazi Jews and 1 in 40,000 to 100,000 individuals in other populations (Case 18). This autosomal recessive condition results from deficiency of β-glucocerebrosidase. Loss of this enzyme activity leads to the accumulation of its substrate, the complex lipid glucocerebroside, in the lysosome, where it is normally degraded. The lysosomal accumulation of glucocerebroside, particularly in the macrophages and monocytes of the reticuloendothelial system, leads to gross enlargement of the liver and spleen. Bone marrow is slowly replaced by lipid-laden macrophages (Gaucher cells), leading to anemia and thrombocytopenia. The bone lesions cause episodic pain, osteonecrosis, and substantial morbidity.

Thousands of patients with nonneuronal Gaucher disease have been treated worldwide with β-glucocerebrosidase ERT, with dramatic clinical benefits. ERT results in rapid resolution of anemia and normalization of platelet counts. There is more gradual normalization of liver and spleen size. In severely affected children with failure to thrive, catchup growth occurs after ERT initiation. ERT improves the characteristic skeletal abnormalities and bone density. Early treatment is most effective in preventing irreversible damage to bones.

The success of ERT for nonneuronopathic Gaucher disease provided guidance to the development of enzyme and protein replacement therapy for other lysosomal storage disorders, and other classes of diseases as well, for several reasons. First, this use of ERT highlights the importance of understanding the biology of the relevant cell types. As demonstrated by I-cell disease (see Chapter 13), lysosomal hydrolases such as β-glucocerebrosidase contain posttranslationally added mannose sugars that target the enzyme to the macrophage through a mannose receptor on the plasma membrane. Once bound, the enzyme is internalized and delivered to the lysosome. Thus β-glucocerebrosidase ERT in Gaucher disease targets the protein both to a particular relevant cell and to a specific intracellular address, in this case the macrophage and the lysosome, respectively.

Second, the human enzyme can be produced in abundance from cultured cells expressing the glucocerebrosidase gene, a key factor because this treatment, given as biweekly infusions, must be continuous. Only ~1% to 5% of the normal intracellular enzyme activity is required to correct the biochemical abnormalities in this and other lysosomal storage disorders. Third, the administered β-glucocerebrosidase is not recognized as a foreign antigen because patients with nonneuronal Gaucher disease have small amounts of residual enzyme activity. Unfortunately, however, because β-glucocerebrosidase does not cross the blood-brain barrier, ERT cannot treat the neuronopathic forms of Gaucher disease. Although ERT for any lysosomal disease is very expensive, its success has been a tremendous advance in the treatment of monogenic disorders. It has established the feasibility of directing an intracellular enzyme to its physiologically relevant location to produce clinically significant effects.

Modulation of Gene Expression

Decades ago, the idea that one might treat a genetic disease through the use of drugs that modulate gene expression would have seemed improbable. Increasing knowledge of the normal and pathologic bases of gene expression, however, has made this approach feasible. Indeed, it seems likely that this strategy will become only more widely used as our understanding of gene expression, and how it might be manipulated, increases.

Splicing Modification of the Survival Motor Neuron Gene in Spinal Muscular Atrophy

Spinal muscular atrophy (SMA) is one of the most common autosomal recessive diseases with progressive weakness of skeletal and respiratory muscles, leading to significant disability. The disorder is caused by pathogenic variants in the survival motor neuron 1 *(SMN1)* gene and a consequent decrease in the SMN protein leading to lower motor neuron degeneration (see Chapter 13).

Therapeutic approaches can be subdivided in survival motor neuron (SMN)–dependent gene therapies, which act to modify **splicing** of *SMN2* (nusinersen, small molecules) or replacing the *SMN1* gene (onasemnogene abeparvovec, see later).

Antisense Oligonucleotides to Alter Gene Expression: Nusinersen

Nusinersen was the first drug approved by the FDA in December 2016 and by the European Medical Agency (EMA) in June 2017 for the treatment of SMA. Nusinersen is an **antisense oligonucleotide (ASO)** that promotes the inclusion of exon 7 in **mRNA** transcripts of *SMN2* (see Chapter 13). It binds to an intronic splice-silencing site in **intron** 7 of *SMN2* and inhibits the action of other splice factors, promoting exon 7 incorporation into the mRNA (Fig. 14.11). This mechanism allows the **translation** of a higher level of fully functional SMN protein and was shown to improve survival and pathology in different SMA preclinical studies. Clinical trials for nusinersen demonstrated at times significant efficacy without any major drug-related adverse event. Importantly, ASOs do not cross the blood-brain barrier, so nusinersen must be administered intrathecally. The treatment regimen consists of four injections over 2 months initially, followed by injections every 4 months.

Recently, new data from clinical trials for nusinersen demonstrate long-term safety and efficacy in all patient groups and a significant improvement of survival and motor function. Nearly 100% of SMA type 2 patients were able to sit unsupported after 3 years, with some being able to walk with additional support and 76% of SMA type 3 walking independently.

mRNA Therapy: Risdiplam

Risdiplam (RG7916) is a small molecule splice modulator that was approved by the FDA in 2020 and the EMA in 2021. Risdiplam is an *SMN2* splice modulator and binds to *SMN2* pre-mRNA at two sites (an exon **enhancer** sequence and the 5′ splicing site of exon 7). This leads to stabilization of the ribonucleoprotein complex subsequently promoting exon 7 inclusion and full-length SMN protein production. Risdiplam is a SMN-C class of splice modulators and has been shown to increase full-length SMN protein in preclinical studies of both severe and mild SMA, leading to improved survival and motor phenotypes. Importantly, risdiplam can be administered orally.

Increasing Gene Expression From the Wild-Type or Mutant Locus

Several histone deacetylase inhibitors have been approved by the FDA for treatment of different forms of cancer, including T-cell lymphoma and multiple myeloma. Their use in monogenic disease is still in the early phases of development, but it is an exciting area of research, especially for **epigenetic** disorders (see Chapter 8).

Reducing the Expression of a Dominant Mutant Gene Product: Small Interfering RNAs

The pathology of some inherited diseases results from the presence of a mutant protein that is toxic to the cell, as seen with proteins with expanded polyglutamine tracts (see Chapter 13), as in Huntington disease (Case 24),

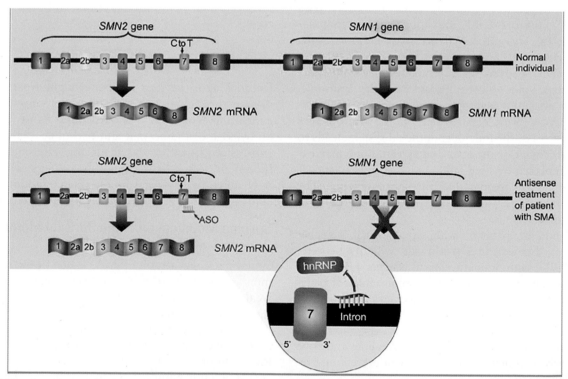

Figure 14.11 The effect of Nusinersen, an antisense oligonucleotide that suppresses exon 7 skipping from the *SMN2* gene, allowing higher levels of full length gene expression. (From Chiriboga CA, Swoboda KJ, Darras BT, et al: Results from a phase 1 study of nusinersen (ISIS-SMN[Rx]) in children with spinal muscular atrophy, *Neurology* 86(10):890–897, 2016. https://doi.org/10.1212/WNL.0000000000002445.)

or with disorders such as the inherited amyloidoses. The autosomal dominant disorder transthyretin amyloidosis is the result of any of more than 100 missense variants in transthyretin, a protein produced mainly in liver, that transports retinol (one form of vitamin A) and thyroxine in body fluids. The major phenotypes are amyloidotic polyneuropathy, due to deposition of the amyloid in peripheral nerves (causing intractable peripheral sensory neuropathy and autonomic neuropathy), and amyloidotic cardiomyopathy, due to its deposition in the heart. Both disorders greatly shorten the life span, and the only prior treatment was hepatic transplantation.

One new approach is provided by a technology called **RNA interference (RNAi)**, which can mediate the degradation of a specific target RNA, such as that encoding transthyretin. Briefly, short RNAs that correspond to specific sequences of the targeted RNA (see Fig. 14.7) – termed **small interfering RNAs (siRNAs)** – are introduced into cells by, for example, lipid nanoparticles or viral **vectors**. Strands of the interfering RNA, ~21 **nucleotides** long, bind to the target RNA and initiate its cleavage. Phase III clinical trials of two compounds, inotersen and patirisen, using an siRNA (encapsulated in injected lipid nanoparticles) directed against transthyretin led to sustained reduction in transthyretin levels and clinical improvements in patients with TTR-polyneuropathy with no significant toxicity. Both agents are now approved for clinical use in many countries and are first-line treatments. The concept of RNAi treatment of an inherited disease is being applied to other diseases where elimination of the mutant gene product is the goal.

Induction of Exon Skipping

Exon skipping refers to the use of molecular interventions to exclude an exon from a pre-mRNA that encodes a **reading frame**–disrupting variant, thereby rescuing expression of the mutant gene. If the number of nucleotides in the excluded exon is a multiple of three, no frame shift will occur and, if the resulting polypeptide with the deleted amino acids retains sufficient function, a therapeutic benefit will result. The most widely studied method of inducing **exon skipping** is through the use of ASOs, which are synthetic 15- to 35-nucleotide single-stranded molecules that can hybridize to specific corresponding sequences in a pre-mRNA (see Fig. 14.7). The clearest example of the potential of this strategy is provided by DMD (see Chapter 13) (Case 14).

The goal of exon skipping in DMD is to convert a DMD pathogenic variant into an in-frame counterpart that generates a functional dystrophin, just as the deletions that allow the production of a partially functioning dystrophin are associated with the milder phenotype of Becker muscular dystrophy (see Fig. 13.15). The distribution of DMD variants is nonrandomly distributed in the gene (see Chapter 13), and thus, remarkably, the skipping of just exon 51 alone would restore the dystrophin reading frame of an estimated 13% of all DMD patients (Fig. 14.12). This exon has therefore been the

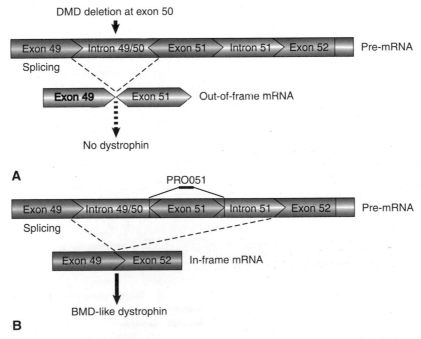

Figure 14.12 Schematic representation of exon skipping. In a patient with Duchenne muscular dystrophy *(DMD)* who has a deletion of exon 50, an out-of-frame transcript is generated in which exon 49 is spliced to exon 51 (A). As a result, a stop codon is generated in exon 51, which prematurely aborts dystrophin synthesis. The sequence-specific binding of the exon-internal antisense oligonucleotide PRO051 interferes with the correct inclusion of exon 51 during splicing so that the exon is actually skipped (B). This restores the open reading frame of the transcript and allows the synthesis of a dystrophin similar to that in patients with Becker muscular dystrophy *(BMD)*. *mRNA*, Messenger RNA. (From van Deutekom JC, Janson AA, Ginjaar IB, et al: Local dystrophin restoration with antisense oligonucleotide PRO051, *N Engl J Med* 357:2677–2686, 2007.)

major focus of exon-skipping drug development. Several clinical trials have established that ASOs that cause skipping of exon 51 can produce significant increases in the number of dystrophin-positive muscle fibers of DMD patients. Moreover, one trial demonstrated stabilization of patient walking ability, but the treatment group was small, so this must be studied in a larger number of subjects. Irrespective of the specific challenges posed by DMD, it will be surprising if exon-skipping strategies do not ultimately play a significant role in the therapy of some inherited disorders.

Creation of a bespoke antisense oligonucleotide, called milasen, was used to treat a single patient with Batten disease to skip an extra exon created by activation of a **cryptic splice site** due to **insertion** of a retrotranspon (see Chapter 4) in *CLN7*. This approach is in clinical trials to treat two types of severe early-onset seizure disorders due to variants in sodium channels.

Genome Editing

Over the last decade molecular biologists have developed methods to introduce site-specific genomic sequence changes into the DNA of intact organisms, including primates. The correction of a mutant gene sequence in its natural DNA context, in a sufficient number of target cells, would be an ideal treatment. This new technology, termed **genome editing**, uses engineered endonucleases containing a DNA-binding domain that will recognize a specific sequence in the genome, such as the sequence in which a missense variant is embedded (Fig. 14.13). Subsequently, a nuclease domain creates a double-stranded break, and cellular mechanisms for homology-directed repair (HDR) then repair the break (see Chapter 4), introducing the **wild-type** nucleotide to replace the mutant one. The template for the HDR must be based on a matching **homologous** wild-type DNA template that is introduced into the target cells

before editing. The most widely used editing approach at present is the *c*lustered *r*egularly *i*nterspaced *s*hort *p*alindromic *r*epeats (CRISPR)/CRISPR-associated (Cas) 9 system, commonly referred to as CRISPR/Cas9 (see Fig. 14.13).

In humans, genome editing offers possibilities for the correction of genetic defects in their natural genomic landscape without the risks associated with the semi-random vector integration of some viral vectors used in gene therapy (see later section).

Genome Editing Approaches for β-thalassemia and Sickle Cell Disease. Genome editing in hematopoietic stem cells (HSCs) can be used as a method to delete an erythroid enhancer of the *BCL11A* gene, thereby blocking its expression in the erythroid cell lineage. As a result, the change from hemoglobin Hb F to Hb A does not occur. Therefore patients retain Hb F instead of the hemoglobin containing a β-thalassemia variant or sickle cell allele (see Chapter 12).

The hemoglobinopathies are the most common genetic defects in the world. These diseases are incurable unless an HSC transplantation is performed from a matched donor. Thus development of effective, safe, and affordable gene therapy for these disorders, the most common being sickle cell disease (SCD) and transfusion-dependent β-thalassemia (TDT), presents an exciting opportunity.

Genome-wide association studies have identified SNVs associated with increased expression of fetal hemoglobin in adults. Some of these SNVs are located in the BCL11A **locus** on **chromosome** 2 and have been shown to cause milder phenotypes in both TDT and SCD. BCL11A is a zinc finger–containing **transcription factor** that represses γ-globin expression and fetal hemoglobin in erythroid cells; the SNVs that are associated with fetal hemoglobin are in an erythroid-specific enhancer

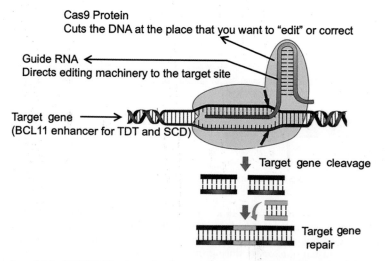

Figure 14.13 The mechanism by which CRISPR/Cas9 works to target, cut, and repair DNA to allow specific genome editing. In this example, the erythroid enhancer of BCL11 is altered to allow continued expression of γ-globin and sustained fetal hemoglobin, which ameliorates sickle cell disease *(SCD)* and transfusion-dependent β-thalassemia *(TDT)*.

and are known to downregulate BCL11A expression and increase the expression of fetal hemoglobin.

Based on these observations, the CRISPR-Cas9 gene editing system was used in hematopoietic stem and progenitor cells (HSPCs) at the erythroid-specific enhancer region of BCL11A to reduce BCL11A expression in erythroid-lineage cells and thereby restore γ-globin synthesis to reactivate production of fetal hemoglobin.

A number of currently ongoing clinical trials use electroporation of CD34+ HSPCs that are obtained from healthy donors and subsequently modified with CRISPR-Cas9 targeting the *BCL11A* erythroid-specific enhancer. The initial reports from these clinical trials demonstrated modification of 80% of the alleles at this locus without evidence of off-target gene editing. Results from two patients, one with TDT and the other with SCD, who were injected with **autologous** CD34+ cells edited with CRISPR-Cas9 targeting the same *BCL11A* enhancer have shown high levels of allelic editing in bone marrow and blood of both patients associated with increased pancellular expression of fetal hemoglobin. These patients were subsequently transfusion independent. The patient with SCD did not show any signs of vasoocclusive episodes suggesting that this approach is safe and effective and presents a novel therapeutic avenue for these patients.

Modification of the Somatic Genome by Transplantation

Transplanted cells retain the **genotype** of the donor, and consequently transplantation can be regarded as a form of **gene transfer therapy** because it leads to a modification of the somatic genome. There are two general indications for the use of transplantation in the treatment of genetic disease. First, cells or organs may be transplanted to introduce wild-type copies of a gene into a patient with pathogenic variants in that gene. This is the case, for example, in homozygous familial hypercholesterolemia (see Chapter 13), for which liver transplantation is an effective but high-risk procedure. The second and more common indication is for cell replacement to compensate for an organ damaged by genetic disease (e.g., a liver that has become cirrhotic in a patient with α$_1$-antitrypsin deficiency). Some examples of the uses of transplantation in genetic disease are provided in Table 14.3.

Stem Cell Transplantation

Stem cells are defined by two properties: (1) their ability to proliferate to form the differentiated cell types of a tissue in vivo, and (2) their ability to self-renew (i.e., to form another stem cell). Embryonic stem cells, which can give rise to the whole organism, are discussed in Chapter 15.

Only three types of stem cells are in clinical use at present: HSCs, which can reconstitute the blood system

TABLE 14.3 Treatment by Modification of the Genome or Its Expression

Type of Modification	Example	Status
RNA interference (RNAi) to reduce the abundance of a toxic or dominant negative protein	RNAi for transthyretin amyloidosis	Safe, effective, expensive
Induction of exon skipping	Use of antisense oligonucleotides to induce skipping of exon 7 in spinal muscular atrophy type I	Safe, effective, very expensive
Gene editing	CRISPR/Cas9 inactivation of the *BCL11* gene in hematopoetic stem cells from individuals with	Investigational; phase II trial successful
Partial modification of the somatic genotype	Bone marrow transplantation in β-thalassemia	Curative with HLA-matched donor; good results overall
By transplantation	Bone marrow transplantation in storage diseases (e.g., Hurler syndrome)	Excellent results in some diseases, even if the brain is affected, such as Hurler syndrome
	Cord blood stem cell transplantation for Hurler syndrome	Excellent results if transplanted before age 2 (the earlier the better)
	Liver transplantation in α$_1$-antitrypsin deficiency	Up to 80% survival over 5 yr for genetic liver disease
By gene transfer into somatic tissues (see Table 14.4)	See Table 14.4	See Table 14.4

Cas, CRISPR-associated; *CRISPR*, clustered regularly interspaced short palindromic repeats; *Hb F*, fetal hemoglobin; *HLA*, human leukocyte antigen.

after bone marrow transplantation; corneal stem cells, which are used to regenerate the corneal epithelium, and skin stem cells. These cells are derived from immunologically compatible donors. The possibility that other types of stem cells will be used clinically in the future is enormous because stem cell research is one of the most active and promising areas of biomedical investigation. Although it is easy to overstate the potential of such treatment, optimism about the long-term future of stem cell therapy is justified.

Hematopoietic Stem Cell Transplantation in Nonstorage Diseases. In addition to its extensive application in the management of cancer, HSC transplantation using bone marrow stem cells is the treatment of choice for a selected group of monogenic immune deficiency disorders, including SCID of any type. Its role in the management of genetic disease in general, however, is less certain and under careful evaluation. For example, excellent outcomes have been obtained with allogeneic HSC transplantation in the treatment of children with β-thalassemia and sickle cell disease. Nevertheless, for each disease that bone marrow transplantation might benefit, its outcomes must be evaluated for many years and weighed against the results obtained with other therapies.

Hematopoietic Stem Cell Transplantation for Lysosomal Storage Diseases

Transplantation of Hematopoietic Stem Cells from Bone Marrow. Bone marrow stem cell transplants are effective in correcting lysosomal storage in many tissues, including (in some diseases) the brain, through the two mechanisms depicted in Fig. 14.14. First, the transplanted cells are a source of lysosomal enzymes that can be transferred to other cells through the extracellular fluid, as discussed in Chapter 13 for I-cell disease. Because bone marrow–derived cells constitute ~10% of the total cell mass of the body, the quantitative impact of enzymes transferred from them may be significant. Second, the mononuclear phagocyte system in tissues is derived from bone marrow stem cells so that, after bone marrow transplantation, this system is of donor origin throughout the body. Of special note are the brain perivascular microglial cells, whose bone marrow origin may partially account for the correction of nervous system abnormalities by bone marrow transplantation in some storage disorders, as we will see next in the case of Hurler syndrome, a lysosomal storage disease due to α-l-iduronidase deficiency.

Bone marrow transplantation corrects or reduces the visceral abnormalities of many storage diseases. For example, a normalization or reduction in the size of the enlarged liver, spleen, and heart seen in Hurler syndrome can be achieved; improvements in upper airway obstruction, joint mobility, and corneal clouding are also obtained. Most rewarding, however, has been the impact of transplantation on the neurologic component of this disease. Patients who have good developmental indices before transplantation and who receive transplants before 24 months of age continue to develop cognitively after transplantation, in contrast to the inexorable loss of intellectual function that otherwise occurs. Interestingly, a **gene dosage** effect is manifested in the donor marrow; children who receive cells from homozygous normal donors appear to be more likely to retain fully normal intelligence than do the recipients of heterozygous donor cells.

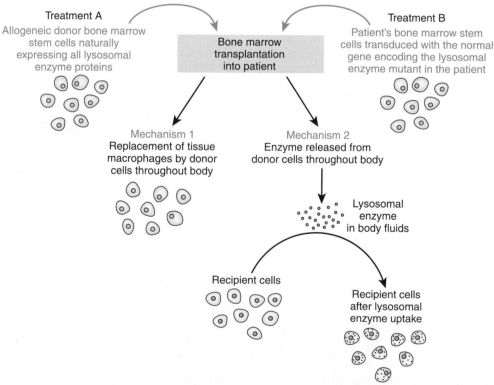

Figure 14.14 The two major mechanisms by which bone marrow transplantation or gene transfer into bone marrow may reduce the substrate accumulation in lysosomal storage diseases. In the case of either treatment, bone marrow transplantation from an allogeneic donor (A) or genetic correction of the patient's own bone marrow stem cells by gene transfer (B), the bone marrow stem cell progeny, now expressing the relevant lysosomal enzyme, expand to repopulate the monocyte-macrophage system of the patient (mechanism 1). In addition, lysosomal enzymes are released from the bone marrow cells derived from the donor or from the genetically modified marrow cells of the patient and taken up by enzyme-deficient cells from the extracellular fluid (mechanism 2).

Transplantation of Hematopoietic Stem Cells from Placental Cord Blood. The discovery that placental cord blood is a rich source of HSCs has made a substantial impact on the treatment of genetic disease. The use of placental cord blood has three great advantages over bone marrow as a source of transplantable HSCs. First, recipients are more tolerant of histoincompatible placental blood than of other allogeneic donor cells. Thus engraftment occurs even if as many as three HLA antigens, cell surface markers encoded by the **major histocompatibility complex** (see Chapter 9), are mismatched between the donor and the recipient. Second, the wide availability of placental cord blood, together with the increased tolerance of histoincompatible donor cells, greatly expands the number of potential donors for any recipient. This feature is of particular significance to patients from minority populations for whom the pool of potential donors is relatively small. Third, the risk for graft-versus-host disease is substantially reduced with use of placental cord blood cells. Cord blood transplantation from unrelated donors appears to be as effective as bone marrow transplantation from a matched donor for the treatment of Hurler syndrome (Fig. 14.15).

Liver Transplantation. For some metabolic liver diseases, liver transplantation is the only treatment of known benefit. For example, the chronic liver disease associated with CF or α1AT deficiency can be treated only by liver transplantation, and together these two disorders account for a large fraction of all the liver transplants performed in the pediatric population. Liver transplantation has now been undertaken for more than two dozen genetic diseases. At present, the 5-year survival rate of all children who receive liver transplants is in the range of 75% to 85%. For almost all of these patients, the quality of life is generally much improved, the specific metabolic abnormality necessitating the transplant is corrected, and in those conditions in which hepatic damage has occurred (such as α1AT deficiency), the provision of healthy hepatic tissue restores growth and normal pubertal development. Liver transplantation is also undertaken as a form of gene replacement in patients with certain inborn errors of metabolism who are at high risk for metabolic decompensation and sudden brain damage or death, but who have no active liver disease. Examples include individuals with urea cycle defects, maple syrup urine disease, propionic acidemia, and MMA. Reports to date indicate a greater than 90% survival and no subsequent metabolic decompensations, although brain and other organ damage sustained prior to transplant does not improve.

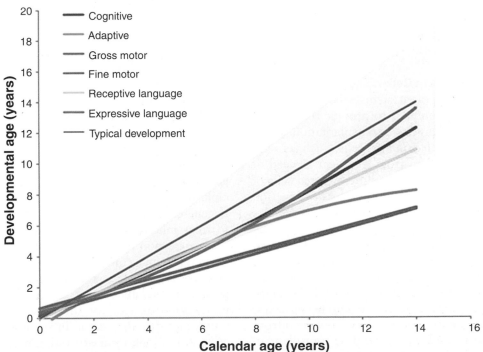

Figure 14.15 Preservation of neurocognitive development in children with Hurler syndrome treated by cord blood transplantation. Neurodevelopmental function of children with Hurler syndrome after umbilical cord blood transplantation compared to that of unaffected children. Age-equivalent scores were used to compare and monitor developmental progress. The colored lines depict the mean developmental curves (i.e., cognitive, adaptive, gross motor, fine motor, receptive language, and expressive language) of the surviving patients. These lines were plotted against the mean typical cognitive growth curve *(gray continuous line)* and approximate variability (95%; *gray area)* observed in typically developing children. Untreated children suffer relentless loss of neurologic and cognitive function with death late in the first or early in the second decade. (From Coletti HY, Aldenhoven M, Yelin K, et al: Long-term functional outcomes of children with Hurler syndrome treated with unrelated umbilical cord blood transplantation, *JIMD Rep* 20:77–86, 2015. https://doi.org/10.1007/8904_2014_395.)

The Problems and the Future of Transplantation.
Two major problems limit the wider use of transplantation for the treatment of genetic disease. First, the mortality after transplantation is still significant, and the morbidity from superimposed infection due to the requirement for immunosuppression and graft-versus-host disease is substantial. Nevertheless, the ultimate goal of transplantation research – transplantation without immunosuppression – comes incrementally closer. The increased tolerance of the recipient to cord blood transplants, compared with bone marrow–derived donor cells, exemplifies the advances in this area.

The second problem with transplantation is the finite supply of organs, cord blood being a singular exception. For example, for all indications, including genetic disease, more than 8000 liver transplants are performed annually in the United States alone, but more than double that number are added to the waiting list each year. In addition, it remains to be demonstrated that transplanted organs are generally capable of functioning normally for a lifetime.

One solution to these difficulties involves the combination of stem cell and either genome editing or gene therapy. Here, a patient's own stem cells would be cultured *in vitro* and either transfected by gene therapy with the gene of interest or corrected by CRISPR/Cas9 editing and returned to the patient to repopulate the affected tissue with genetically restored cells. The identification of stem cells in a variety of adult human tissues and recent advances in gene transfer therapy offer great hope for this strategy.

Induced Pluripotent Stem Cells. The ability to induce the formation of pluripotent stem cells (**iPSCs**) from somatic cells has the potential to provide the optimal solution to both challenges of transplantation posed earlier. In this approach somatic cells, such as skin **fibroblasts**, would be taken from a patient in need of a transplant and induced to form differentiated cells of the organ of interest. For example, the loss-of-function variant in the α1-antitrypsin gene in the fibroblasts cultured from a patient with α1AT deficiency (see Chapter 13) could be corrected either by gene editing (see earlier section) or gene therapy (see later section); the corrected cells could then be induced to form liver-specific iPSCs, which could then be transplanted into the liver of the patient to differentiate into hepatocytes. Alternatively, mature hepatocytes derived *in vitro* from the genetically corrected iPSCs could be transplanted. The great merit of this approach is that the genetically corrected liver cells are derived from the patient's own genome, thus evading immunologic rejection of the transplanted cells as well as graft-versus-host disease. Experimental work in animal models has established that this strategy is capable of correcting inherited disorders. Substantial hurdles with iPSCs must first be overcome, however, including establishing the safety of transplanting cells derived by iPSC methodology and preventing epigenetic modifications in the derived cell type that are not characteristic of wild-type cells of the tissue of interest.

GENE THERAPY

Gene therapy is the introduction of a biologically active gene into a cell to achieve a therapeutic benefit. In 2012, the first gene therapy product was licensed in the United States and Europe for the treatment of lipoprotein lipase deficiency, and gene therapy has now been approved for the treatment of several more disorders; the number in late-stage clinical trials exceed a dozen, some of which are outlined in Table 14.4. These recent successes firmly establish that the treatment of genetic disease at its most fundamental level – the gene – will be increasingly feasible. The goal of gene therapy is to transfer the therapeutic gene early enough in the life of the patient to prevent the pathogenetic events that damage cells. Moreover, correction of the reversible features of genetic diseases should also be possible for many conditions.

In this section, we outline the potential, methods, and probable limitations of gene transfer for the treatment of human genetic disease. The minimal requirements that must be met before the use of gene transfer can be considered for the treatment of a genetic disorder are presented (see Box 14.1).

General Considerations for Gene Therapy

In the treatment of inherited disease, the most common use of gene therapy will be the introduction of functional copies of the relevant gene into the appropriate target cells of a patient with a loss-of-function variant (because most genetic diseases result from such variants).

In these instances, precisely where the transferred gene inserts into the genome of a cell would, in principle, generally not be important (see later discussion). If gene editing (see earlier discussion and Table 14.3) to treat inherited disease becomes routinely possible, then correction of the defect in the mutant gene in its normal genomic context would be ideal and would alleviate concerns such as the activation of a nearby **oncogene** by the regulatory activity of a viral vector or the inactivation of a tumor suppressor due to insertional mutagenesis by the vector. In some long-lived types of cells, stable, long-term expression may not require integration of the introduced gene into the host genome. For example, if the transferred gene is stabilized in the form of an **episome** (a stable nuclear but nonchromosomal DNA molecule, such as that formed by an adeno-associated viral vector, discussed later), and if the target cell is long-lived (e.g., T cells, neurons, myocytes, hepatocytes), then long-term expression can occur without integration.

TABLE 14.4 Examples of Inherited Diseases Treated by Gene Therapy of Somatic Tissues

Disease	Affected Protein (Gene)	Vector, Cell Transduced	Outcome
X-linked SCID	γc-cytokine receptor subunit of several interleukin receptors (IL2RG)	Retroviral vector Allogenic hematopoietic stem cells; new self-inactivating (SIN) vectors that do not promote oncogene expression	Significant clinical improvement in 27 of 32 patients, 5 of whom developed a leukemia-like disorder that was treatable in 4; subsequent efficacy of SIN vectors in short-term follow-up of clinical trials
SCID due to ADA deficiency	Adenosine deaminase (ADA)	Retroviral vector Allogenic hematopoietic stem cells	29 of 40 treated patients are off PEG-ADA enzyme replacement therapy
X-linked adrenoleukodystrophy	A peroxisomal adenosine triphosphate–binding cassette transporter (ABCD1)	Lentiviral vector Autologous hematopoietic stem cells	Apparent arrest of cerebral demyelination in the 17 of 19 boys studied
Spinal muscular atrophy	Survival motor neuron (SMN1)	Adeno-associated virus vector injected IV	Marked improvement in respiratory and skeletal muscle strength in >1800 patients; FDA approved; extremely expensive
Hemophilia B	Factor IX (F9)	Adeno-associated virus vector Patients received a single IV injection	Stable expression of factor IX at 1–7% of normal levels up to 3 yr posttreatment; >20 patients able to stop prophylactic factor IX treatment
Leber congenital amaurosis or early-onset severe retinal dystrophy (one form)	RPE65, a protein required for the cycling of retinoids (vitamin A metabolites) to photoreceptors (RPE65)	Adeno-associated virus vector Retinal pigment epithelial cells	FDA approved for treatment of individuals age 12 mo–65 yr with either congenital or early-onset retinal dystrophy due to pathogenic variants in RPE65

ADA, Adenosine deaminase; *Hb*, hemoglobin; *IV*, intravenous; *PEG*, polyethylene glycol; *SCID*, severe combined immunodeficiency.

BOX 14.1 ESSENTIAL REQUIREMENTS OF GENE THERAPY FOR AN INHERITED DISORDER

- **Identity of the molecular defect**
  The identity of the affected gene must be known.
- **A functional copy of the gene**
  A complementary DNA (cDNA) clone of the gene or the gene itself must be available. If the gene or cDNA is too large for the current generation of vectors, a functional version of the gene from which nonessential components have been removed to reduce its size may suffice.
- **An appropriate vector**
  The most commonly used vectors at present are derived from the adeno-associated viruses (AAVs) or retroviruses, including lentivirus.
- **Knowledge of the pathophysiologic mechanism**
  Knowledge of the pathophysiologic mechanism of the disease must be sufficient to suggest that the gene transfer will ameliorate or correct the pathologic process and prevent, slow, or reverse critical phenotypic abnormalities. Loss-of-function variants require replacement with a functional gene; for diseases due to **dominant negative** alleles, inactivation of the mutant gene or its products will be necessary.
- **Favorable risk-to-benefit ratio**
  A substantial disease burden and a favorable risk-to-benefit ratio, in comparison with alternative therapies, must be present.
- **Appropriate regulatory components for the transferred gene**
  Tight regulation of the level of gene expression is relatively unimportant in some diseases and critical in

others. In thalassemia, for example, overexpression of the transferred gene would cause a new imbalance of globin chains in red blood cells, whereas low levels of expression would be ineffective. In some enzymopathies, a few percent of normal expression may be therapeutic, and abnormally high levels of expression may have no adverse effect.
- **An appropriate target cell**
  Ideally, the target cell must have a long half-life or good replicative potential in vivo. It must also be accessible for direct introduction of the gene or, alternatively, it must be possible to deliver sufficient copies of the gene to it (e.g., through the bloodstream) to attain a therapeutic benefit. The feasibility of gene therapy is often enhanced if the target cell can be cultured *in vitro* to facilitate gene transfer into it; in this case, it must be possible to introduce a sufficient number of the recipient cells into the patient and have them functionally integrate into the relevant organ.
- **Strong evidence of efficacy and safety**
  Cultured cell and animal studies must indicate that the vector and gene construct are both effective and safe. The ideal precedent is to show that the gene therapy is effective, benign, and enduring in a large animal genetic model of the disease in question. At present, however, large animal models exist for only a few monogenic diseases. Genetically engineered or spontaneous mutant mouse models are much more widely available.
- **Regulatory approval**
  Protocol review and approval by an institutional review board are essential. In most countries, human gene therapy trials are also subject to oversight by a governmental agency.

Gene therapy may also be undertaken to inactivate the product of a dominant mutant allele whose abnormal product causes the disease. For example, vectors carrying siRNAs (see earlier section) could, in principle, be used to mediate the selective degradation of a mutant mRNA encoding a dominant negative proα1(I) collagen that causes osteogenesis imperfecta (see Chapter 13).

Gene Transfer Strategies

An appropriately engineered gene may be transferred into target cells by one of two general strategies (Fig. 14.16). The first involves introduction of the gene into cells that have been cultured from the patient ex vivo (i.e., outside the body) and then reintroduction of the cells to the patient after the gene transfer. In the second approach, the gene is injected directly in vivo into the tissue or extracellular fluid of interest (from which it is taken up by the target cells). In some cases, it may be desirable to target the vector to a specific cell type; this is usually achieved by modifying the coat of a viral vector so that only the designated cells bind the viral particles.

The Target Cell

The ideal target cells are stem cells (which are self-replicating) or progenitor cells taken from the patient (thereby eliminating the risk for graft-versus-host disease); both cell types have substantial replication potential. Introduction of the gene into stem cells can result in the expression of the transferred gene in a large population of daughter cells. At present, bone marrow is the only tissue whose stem cells have been successfully targeted as recipients of transferred genes. Genetically modified bone marrow stem cells have been used to cure two forms of SCID, as discussed later. Gene transfer therapy into blood stem cells is also likely to be effective for the treatment of hemoglobinopathies and storage diseases for which bone marrow transplantation has been effective, as discussed earlier.

An important logistical consideration is the number of cells into which the gene must be introduced to have a significant therapeutic effect. To treat PKU, for example, the approximate number of liver cells into which the phenylalanine hydroxylase gene would have to be transferred is ~5% of the hepatocyte mass, or ~10^{10} cells, although this number could be much less if the level of expression of the transferred gene is higher than wild-type. A much greater challenge is gene therapy for muscular dystrophies, for which the gene must be inserted into a significant fraction of the huge number of myocytes in the body to have therapeutic efficacy.

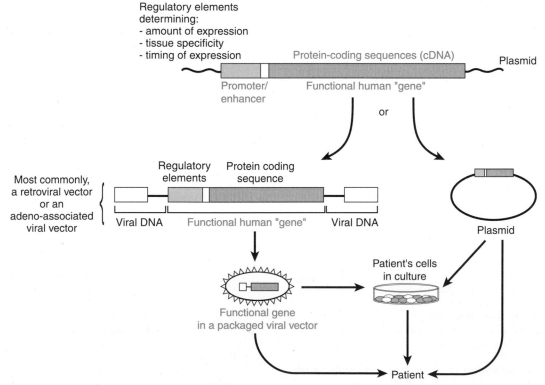

Figure 14.16 **The two major strategies used to transfer a gene to a patient.** For patients with a genetic disease, the most common approach is to construct a viral vector containing the human complementary DNA (cDNA) of interest and to introduce it directly into the patient or into cells cultured from the patient that are then returned to the patient. The viral components at the ends of the molecule are required for the integration of the vector into the host genome. In some instances, the gene of interest is placed in a plasmid, which is then used for the gene transfer.

DNA Transfer Into Cells: Viral Vectors

The ideal vector for gene therapy would be safe, readily made, and easily introduced into the appropriate target tissue, and it would express the gene of interest for life. Indeed, no single vector is satisfactory in all respects for all types of gene therapy, and a repertoire of vectors is required. Here, we briefly review three of the most widely used classes of viral vectors, those derived from retroviruses, adeno-associated viruses (AAVs), and adenoviruses.

One of the most widely used classes of vectors is derived from retroviruses, simple RNA viruses that can integrate into the host genome. They contain only three structural genes, which can be removed and replaced with the gene to be transferred (see Fig. 14.16). The current generation of retroviral vectors has been engineered to render them incapable of replication. In addition, they are nontoxic to the cell, and only a low number of copies of the viral DNA (with the transferred gene) integrate into the host genome. Moreover, the integrated DNA is stable and can accommodate up to 8 kb of added DNA, commodious enough for many genes that might be transferred. A major limitation of many retroviral vectors, however, is that the target cell must undergo division for integration of the virus into the host DNA, limiting the use of such vectors in nondividing cells such as neurons. In contrast, lentiviruses, the class of retroviruses that includes HIV, are capable of DNA integration in nondividing cells, including neurons. Lentiviruses have the additional advantage of not showing preferential integration into any specific gene locus, thus reducing the chances of activating an oncogene in a large number of cells.

AAVs do not elicit strong immunologic responses, a great advantage that enhances the longevity of their expression. Moreover, they infect dividing or nondividing cells to remain in a predominantly episomal form that is stable and confers long-term expression of the transduced gene. A disadvantage is that the current AAV vectors can accommodate inserts of up to only 5 kb, which is smaller than many genes in their natural context.

The third group of viral vectors, adenovirus-derived vectors, can be obtained at high titer, will infect a wide variety of dividing or nondividing cell types, and can accommodate inserts of 30 to 35 kb. However, in addition to other limitations, they have been associated with at least one death in a gene therapy trial through the elicitation of a strong immune response. At present their use is restricted to gene therapy for cancer.

Risks of Gene Therapy

Gene therapy for the treatment of human disease has risks of three general types:

- **Adverse response to the vector or vector-disease combination.** Principal among the concerns is that the patient will have an adverse reaction to the vector or the transferred gene. Such problems should be largely anticipated with appropriate animal and preliminary human studies.

- **Insertional mutagenesis causing malignancy.** The second concern is insertional mutagenesis – that is, the transferred gene will integrate into the patient's DNA and activate a **protooncogene** or disrupt a tumor suppressor gene, leading possibly to cancer (see Chapter 16). The illicit expression of an oncogene is less likely to occur with the current generation of viral vectors, which have been altered to minimize the ability of their promoters to activate the expression of adjacent host genes. Insertional inactivation of a tumor suppressor gene is likely to be infrequent and, as such, is an acceptable risk in diseases for which there is no therapeutic alternative.

- **Insertional inactivation of an essential gene.** A third risk – that insertional inactivation could disrupt a gene essential for viability – will, in general, be without significant effect because such lethal mutations are expected to be rare and will kill only single cells. Although vectors appear to somewhat favor insertion into transcribed genes, the chance that the same gene will be disrupted in more than a few cells is extremely low. The one exception to this statement applies to the germline; an insertion into a gene in the germline could create a dominant disease-causing **mutation** that might manifest in the treated patient's offspring. Such events, however, are likely to be rare and the risk acceptable because it would be difficult to justify withholding, on this basis, carefully planned and reviewed trials of gene therapy from patients who have no other recourse. Moreover, the problem of germline modification by disease treatment is not confined to gene therapy. For example, most chemotherapy used in the treatment of malignant disease is mutagenic, but this risk is accepted because of the therapeutic benefits.

Diseases That Have Been Amenable to Gene Therapy

More than two dozen single-gene diseases have been shown to improve with gene therapy, and a large number of other monogenic disorders are potential candidates for this strategy, including retinal degenerations, hematopoietic conditions such as sickle cell anemia and thalassemia, and disorders affecting liver proteins such as PKU, urea cycle disorders, familial hypercholesterolemia, and α1AT deficiency. Here we discuss several disorders in which gene therapy has been clearly effective, and we highlight some of the challenges associated with this therapeutic approach.

X-linked Severe Combined Immunodeficiency

The SCIDs are due to pathogenic variants in genes required for lymphocyte maturation. Affected individuals fail to thrive and die early in life of infection because they lack functional B and T lymphocytes. The most common form of the disease, X-linked SCID, results from variations in the X-linked gene *IL2RG*, encoding the γc-cytokine receptor subunit of several interleukin receptors. The receptor deficiency causes an early block in T- and natural killer–lymphocyte growth, survival, and **differentiation** and is associated with severe infections, failure to thrive, and death in infancy or early childhood if left untreated. This condition was chosen for a gene therapy trial for two principal reasons. First, bone marrow transplantation cures the disease, indicating that the restoration of lymphocyte expression of *IL2RG* can reverse the pathophysiologic changes. Second, it was believed that transduced cells carrying the transferred gene would have a selective survival advantage over untransduced cells.

The outcome of trials of X-linked SCID has been dramatic and resulted, in 2000, in the first gene therapy cure of a patient with a genetic disease. Subsequent confirmation has been obtained in most patients in subsequent clinical trials (see Table 14.4). Bone marrow stem cells from the patients were infected in culture (ex vivo) with a retroviral vector that expressed the γc cytokine subunit cDNA. A selective advantage was conferred on the transduced cells by the gene transfer. Transduced T cells and natural killer cells populated the blood of treated patients, and the T cells appeared to behave normally. Although the frequency of transduced B cells was low, adequate levels of serum immunoglobulin and antibody levels were obtained. Dramatic clinical improvement occurred, with resolution of protracted diarrhea and skin lesions and restoration of normal growth and development. These initial trials demonstrated the great potential of gene therapy for the correction of inherited disease.

This highly promising outcome, however, came at the cost of **induction** of a leukemia-like disorder in 5 of the 20 treated patients, who developed an extreme lymphocytosis resembling T-cell acute lymphocytic leukemia; 4 of them are now well after treatment of the leukemia. The malignancy was due to insertional mutagenesis: The retroviral vector inserted into the *LMO2* locus, causing aberrant expression of the *LMO2* mRNA, which encodes a component of a transcription factor complex that mediates hematopoietic development. Consequently, trials using integrating vectors in hematopoietic cells must now monitor insertion sites and survey for clonal proliferation. Current-generation vectors are designed to avoid this mutagenic effect by using strategies such as including a self-inactivating or "suicide" gene cassette in the vector to eliminate **clones** of malignant cells. At this point, bone marrow stem cell transplantation remains the treatment of choice for those children with SCID fortunate enough to have a donor with an HLA-identical match. For patients without such a match, autologous transplantation of HSPCs, in which the genetic defect has been corrected by gene

therapy, offers a lifesaving alternative, but one that may not be without risk.

Spinal Muscular Atrophy

SMA is a monogenic defect associated with the loss of SMN protein and became an excellent candidate for gene replacement therapies when it was discovered that systemic delivery of AAV9-based gene transfer via intravenous injection can cross the blood-brain barrier and efficiently transform target cells in the central nervous system, including motor neurons in the spinal cord in mice and nonhuman primates. This changed the assumption that neurologic disorders may not be candidates for gene therapies. Development of the self-complementary AAV9 (scAAV9) vector further improved the efficiency and speed of gene transcription in a number of preclinical experiments. The first gene therapy trial for SMA included 15 infants, 3 with low dose and 12 with high dose. All 15 patients survived to 20 months and did not require respiratory support. Eleven patients reached the motor milestone of sitting unassisted, and two patients were able to walk independently. These data plus additional data released from the successive **phase** II/III trial led to FDA approval in 2019. The main benefits of this method are that a single, one-time injection is required, and the SMN protein becomes systemically expressed. Safety and tolerability, however, have to be strictly monitored as acute hepatotoxicity and sensory neuron toxicity were reported in primates and piglets following high-dose intravenous administration of AAV vectors expressing human SMN. As a result, most individuals require prednisolone therapy to minimize the hepatotoxicity. Another consideration is the reported presence of preexisting anti-AAV9 antibodies in SMA patients, which might influence tolerability and efficacy.

RPE65-associated Retinal Dystrophy

Leber congenital amaurosis (LCA), an autosomal recessive condition, comprises a heterogeneous group of eye diseases that cause nystagmus and significant visual impairment in early infancy and total blindness by the third to fourth decades of life. LCA2 (also known as *RPE65*-LCA) is associated with pathogenic variants of the *RPE65* gene encoding the retinoid isomerohydrolase in the retinal pigment epithelium (RPE), which result in rod-cone–type retinal dystrophy. The gene therapy can be injected directly into the eye's subretinal space, which is an immunoprivileged organ. The majority of studies are conducted on one eye, while the other serves as a control. For *RPE65*-associated retinal dystrophy voretigene neparvovec is a gene therapy that packages the *RPE65* cDNA in an AAV2 vector. This therapy was approved by the FDA in 2017. Follow-up of the original group through 4 years has shown sustained benefit, and additional gene therapy trials are currently underway to treat several other types of LCA.

Hemophilia B

Hemophilia B is an X-linked disorder of coagulation caused by pathogenic variants in the *F9* gene, leading to a deficiency or dysfunction of clotting factor IX (Case 21). The disease is characterized by bleeding into soft tissues, muscles, and weight-bearing joints and occurs within hours to days after trauma. Severely affected subjects, with less than 1% of normal levels of factor IX, have frequent bleeding that causes crippling joint disease and early death. Prophylactic – but not curative – treatment with intravenous factor IX concentrate several times a week is expensive and leads to the generation of inhibitory antibodies.

In 2011, the first successful gene therapy treatment of hemophilia B was reported in six patients using an AAV8 vector that is tropic for hepatocytes, where factor IX is normally produced. After a single infusion of the AAV8-*F9* vector, four patients were able to discontinue prophylactic factor IX infusions, whereas the other two tolerated longer intervals between infusions. The two patients who received the highest dose of the vector had transient asymptomatic increases in liver enzyme levels – which resolved with steroid treatment – indicating that immune-related side effects must remain a concern in future studies. Unfortunately, the AAV vectors cannot accommodate the gene for factor VIII, so other vectors will have to be developed for hemophilia A patients. Apart from this limitation of cargo size, however, AAV-mediated gene therapy targeted to hepatocytes may be applicable to any genetic disease in which production of the protein in the liver is the desired goal.

The Prospects for Gene Therapy

To date, more than 5000 clinical gene therapy trials (the majority are for cancer) have been undertaken worldwide to evaluate both the safety and efficacy of this long-promised and conceptually promising technology. Approximately 775 of these trials were for the treatment of monogenic diseases. The exciting results obtained with gene therapy to date, albeit with small numbers of patients and only a few diseases, validate the optimism behind this immense effort. Although the breadth of applications remains uncertain, it is to be hoped that over the next few decades, gene therapy for both monogenic and genetically complex diseases will contribute to the management of many disorders, both common and rare.

PRECISION MEDICINE: THE PRESENT AND FUTURE OF THE TREATMENT OF MENDELIAN DISEASE

The treatment of single-gene diseases embodies the concept of precision medicine tailored to the individual patient as deeply as any other area of medical treatment. Knowledge of the specific sequence in an individual is central to many of the targeted therapies described in this chapter. The promise of gene therapy for an individual with a **mendelian** disorder must be based on the identification of the responsible gene in each affected individual and on the design of a vector that will deliver the therapeutic gene to the targeted tissue. Similarly, approaches based on gene editing require knowledge of the specific variant to be corrected.

Beyond this, however, precision medicine will frequently require knowledge of the precise allele and of its specific effect on the mRNA and protein. In many cases, the exact nature of the variant will define the drug that will bind to a specific regulatory sequence to enhance or reduce the expression of a gene. In other cases, the variant will dictate the sequence of an **allele-specific oligonucleotide** to mediate the skipping of an exon with a premature **termination codon**, or of an siRNA to suppress a dominant negative allele. A compendium of small molecules will gradually become available to act as chaperones that will rescue mutant proteins from misfolding and proteasomal degradation, or to modulate the activity of mutant proteins.

Genetic treatment is not only becoming more creative but also more precise. The future promises a longer and vastly improved quality life for many patients.

GENERAL REFERENCES

Valle D, Beaudet AL, Vogelstein B, et al, editors: *The online metabolic and molecular bases of inherited disease*, 2019.

Vernon HJ, Manoli I: Milestones in treatments for inborn errors of metabolism: reflections on where chemistry and medicine meet, *Am J Med Genet Part A* 185A:3350–3358, 2021.

REFERENCES FOR SPECIFIC TOPICS

Arora N, Daley GQ: Pluripotent stem cells in research and treatment of hemoglobinopathies, *Cold Spring Harb Perspect Med* 2:a011841, 2012.

Bélanger-Quintana A, Burlina A, Harding CO, et al: Up to date knowledge on different treatment strategies for phenylketonuria, *Mol Genet Metabolism* 104:S19–S25, 2011.

Biffi A, Montini E, Lorioli L, et al: Lentiviral hematopoietic stem cell gene therapy benefits metachromatic leukodystrophy, *Science* 341:1233158, 2013. https://doi.org/10.1126/science.1233158

Birnkrant DJ, Bushby K, Bann CM, et al: Diagnosis and management of Duchenne muscular dystrophy, part 1: Diagnosis, and neuromuscular, rehabilitation, endocrine, and gastrointestinal and nutritional management, *Lancet Neurol* 17:251–267, 2018.

Birnkrant DJ, Bushby K, Bann CM, et al: Diagnosis and management of Duchenne muscular dystrophy, part 2: Respiratory, cardiac, bone health, and orthopaedic management, *Lancet Neurol* 17:347–361, 2018.

Birnkrant DJ, Bushby K, Bann CM, et al: Diagnosis and management of Duchenne muscular dystrophy, part 3: Primary care, emergency management, psychosocial care, and transitions of care across the lifespan, *Lancet Neurol* 17:445–455, 2018.

Cathomen T, Ehl S: Translating the genomic revolution – targeted genome editing in primates, *N Engl J Med* 370:2342–2345, 2014.

Coelho T, Adams D, Silva A, et al: Safety and efficacy of RNAi therapy for transthyretin amyloidosis, *N Engl J Med* 369(9):819–829, 2013.

Daley GQ: The promise and perils of stem cell therapeutics, *Cell Stem Cell* 10:740–749, 2012.

Desnick RJ, Schuchman EH: Enzyme replacement therapy for lysosomal diseases: Lessons from 20 years of experience and remaining challenges, *Ann Rev Genomics Hum Genet* 13:307–335, 2012.

de Souza N: Primer: Genome editing with engineered nucleases, *Nat Methods* 9:27, 2012.

Dong A, Rivella S, Breda L: Gene therapy for hemoglobinopathies: Progress and challenges, *Trans Res* 161:293–306, 2013.

Duan D, Goemans N, Takeda S, et al: Duchenne muscular dystrophy, *Nat Rev Dis Primers* 7:13, 2021.

Gaspar HB, Qasim W, Davies EG, et al: How I treat severe combined immunodeficiency, *Blood* 122:3749–3758, 2013.

Gaziev J, Lucarelli G: Hematopoietic stem cell transplantation for thalassemia, *Curr Stem Cell Res Ther* 6:162–169, 2011.

Goemans NM, Tulinius M, van den Akker JT: Systemic administration of PRO051 in Duchenne's muscular dystrophy, *N Engl J Med* 364:1513–1522, 2011.

Groenink M, den Hartog AW, Franken R, et al: Losartan reduces aortic dilatation rate in adults with Marfan syndrome: A randomized controlled trial, *Eur Heart J* 34:3491–3500, 2013.

Hanna JH, Saha K, Jaenisch R: Pluripotency and cellular reprogramming: facts, hypotheses, unresolved issues, *Cell* 143:508–525, 2010.

Hanrahan JW, Sampson HM, Thomas DY: Novel pharmacological strategies to treat cystic fibrosis, *Trends Pharmacol Sci* 34:119–125, 2013.

High KA: Gene therapy in clinical medicine. In Longo D, Fauci A, Kasper D, editors: *Harrison's principles of internal medicine*, ed 19, New York, 2015, McGraw-Hill.

Huang R, Southall N, Wang Y, et al: The NCGC Pharmaceutical Collection: A comprehensive resource of clinically approved drugs enabling repurposing and chemical genomics, *Sci Transl Med* 3:80ps 16, 2011.

Iftikhar M, Frey J, Shohan MJ, et al: Current and emerging therapies for Duchenne muscular dystrophy and spinal muscular atrophy, *Pharmacol Ther* 220:107719, 2021.

Jarmin S, Kymalainen H, Popplewell L, et al: New developments in the use of gene therapy to treat Duchenne muscular dystrophy, *Expert Opin Biol Ther* 14:209–230, 2014.

Johnson SM, Connelly S, Fearns C, et al: The transthyretin amyloidoses: from delineating the molecular mechanism of aggregation linked to pathology to a regulatory agency approved drug, *J Mol Biol* 421:185–203, 2012.

Kim J, Hu C, El Achkar MC, et al: Patient-customized oligonucleotide therapy for a rare genetic disease, *N Engl J Med* 381(17):1644–1652, 2019. https://doi.org/10.1056/NEJMoa1813279

Li M, Suzuki K, Kim NY, et al: A cut above the rest: Targeted genome editing technologies in human pluripotent stem cells, *J Biol Chem* 289:4594–4599, 2014.

Mallack EJ, Turk B, Yan H, et al: The landscape of hematopoietic stem cell transplant and gene therapy for X-linked adrenoleukodystrophy, *Curr Treat Options Neurol* 21(12):61, 2019. https://doi.org/10.1007/s11940-019-0605-y

Mukherjee S, Thrasher AJ: Gene therapy for primary immunodeficiency disorders: Progress, pitfalls and prospects, *Gene* 525:174–181, 2013.

Nathwani AC, Tuddenham EGD, Rangarajan S: Adenovirus-associated virus vector–mediated gene transfer in hemophilia B, *N Engl J Med* 365:2357–2365, 2011.

Nicolau S, Waldrop MA, Connolly AM, et al: Spinal muscular atrophy, *Semin Pediatr Neurol* 37:100878, 2021.

Okam MM, Ebert BL: Novel approaches to the treatment of sickle cell disease: the potential of histone deacetylase inhibitors, *Expert Rev Hematol* 5:303–311, 2012.

Otsuru S, Gordon PL, Shimono K, et al: Transplanted bone marrow mononuclear cells and MSCs impart clinical benefit to children with osteogenesis imperfecta through different mechanisms, *Blood* 120:1933–1941, 2012.

Peltz SW, Morsy M, Welch EW, et al: Ataluren as an agent for therapeutic nonsense suppression, *Ann Rev Med* 64:407–425, 2013.

Perrine SP, Pace BS, Faller DV: Targeted fetal hemoglobin induction for treatment of beta hemoglobinopathies, *Hematol Oncol Clin North Am* 28:233–248, 2014.

Pillai NR, Stroup BM, Poliner A, et al: Liver transplantation in propionic and methylmalonic acidemia: A single center study with literature review, *Mol Genet Metab* 128(4):431–443, 2019. https://doi.org/10.1016/j.ymgme.2019.11.001

Prasad VK, Kurtzberg J: Cord blood and bone marrow transplantation in inherited metabolic diseases: Scientific basis, current status and future directions, *Br J Haematol* 148:356–372, 2009.

Pritchard AB, Izumi K, Payan-Walters I, et al: Inborn error of metabolism patients after liver transplantation: Outcomes of 35 patients over 27 years in one pediatric quaternary hospital, *Am J Med Genet A* 188(5):1443–1447, 2022. https://doi.org/10.1002/ajmg.a.62659

Ramdas S, Servais L: New treatments in spinal muscular atrophy: An overview of currently available data, *Exp Opin Pharmacother* 21:307–315, 2020.

Ramsey BW, Davies J, McElvaney NG, et al: A CFTR potentiator in patients with cystic fibrosis and the G551D mutation, *N Engl J Med* 365:1663–1672, 2011.

Robinton DA, Daley GQ: The promise of induced pluripotent stem cells in research and therapy, *Nature* 481:295–305, 2012.

Salmaninejad A, Abarghan JY, Qomi BS, et al: Common therapeutic advances for Duchenne muscular dystrophy (DMD), *Int J Neurosci* 131:370–389, 2021.

Sander JD, Joung JK: CRISPR-Cas systems for editing, regulating and targeting genomes, *Nat Biotechnol* 32:347–355, 2014.

Schorling DC, Pechmann A, Kirschner J: Advances in treatment of spinal muscular atrophy – new phenotypes, new challenges, new implications for care, *J Neuromuscul Dis* 7:1–13, 2020.

Sheikh O, Yokota T: Developing DMD therapeutics: A review of the effectiveness of small molecules, stop-codon readthrough, dystrophin gene replacement, and exon-skipping therapies, *Expert Opin Investig Drugs* 30:167–176, 2021.

Sosicka P, Ng BG, Freeze HH: Chemical therapies for congenital disorders of glycosylation, *ACS Chem Biol*, 2021. https://doi.org/10.1021/acschembio.1c00601

Southwell AL, Skotte NH, Bennett CF, et al: Antisense oligonucleotide therapeutics for inherited neurodegenerative diseases, *Trends Mol Med* 18:634–643, 2012.

Tebas P, Stein D, Tang WW, et al: Gene editing of CCR5 in autologous CD4 T cells of persons infected with HIV, *N Engl J Med* 370:901–910, 2014.

van Ommen G-JB, Aartsma-Rus A: Advances in therapeutic RNA-targeting, *Trends Mol Med* 18:634–643, 2012.

Verhaart IEC, Aarsma-Rus A: Therapeutic developments for Duchenne muscular dystrophy, *Nat Rev Neurol* 15:373–386, 2019.

Verma IM: Gene therapy that works, *Science* 341:853–855, 2013.

Xu J, Peng C, Sankaran VG, et al: Correction of sickle cell disease in adult mice by interference with fetal hemoglobin silencing, *Science* 334:993–996, 2011.

USEFUL WEBSITES

Registry and results database of publicly and privately supported clinical studies of human participants conducted around the world: https://clinicaltrials.gov/

Gene Therapy Clinical Trials Worldwide: http://www.wiley.com/legacy/wileychi/genmed/clinical/

PROBLEMS

1. X-linked chronic granulomatous disease (CGD) is characterized by a defect in host defense that leads to severe, recurrent, and often fatal pyogenic infections beginning in early childhood. The X-linked *CGD* locus encodes the heavy chain of cytochrome b, a component of the oxidase that generates superoxide in phagocytes. Because interferon-γ (IFN-γ) enhances the oxidase activity of normal phagocytes, IFN-γ was administered to boys with X-linked CGD to see whether their oxidase activity increased. Before treatment, unlike those of severely affected patients, the phagocytes of some less severely affected patients had small but detectable bursts of oxidase activity, suggesting that their increased activity resulted from greater production of cytochrome b from the affected locus. In these cases, IFN-γ increased the cytochrome b content, superoxide production, and killing

continued

of *Staphylococcus aureus* in the granulocytes. The IFN-γ effect was associated with a definite increase in the abundance of the cytochrome b heavy chain. Presumably, the cytochrome b polypeptide of these patients is partially functional, and its increased expression improved the physiological defect. Describe the genetic differences that might account for the differential response of phagocytes of patients with X-linked CGD to IFN-γ *in vitro*.

2. Identify some of the limitations on the types of proteins that can be considered for extracellular enzyme replacement therapy, as exemplified by polyethylene glycol–adenosine deaminase (PEG-ADA) for ADA deficiency. What makes this approach inappropriate for phenylalanine hydroxylase deficiency? If Tay-Sachs disease caused only liver disease, would this strategy succeed? If not, why? Might Lesch-Nyhan disease be a candidate for this approach?

3. A 3-year-old girl, Rhonda, has familial hypercholesterolemia due to a deletion of the 5′ end of each of her low-density lipoprotein (LDL) receptor genes that removed the promoter and the first two exons. (Rhonda's parents are second cousins.) You explain to the parents that she will require plasmapheresis every 1 to 2 weeks for years. At the clinic, however, they meet another family with a 5-year-old boy with the same disease. The boy has been treated with drugs with some success. Rhonda's parents want to know why she has not been offered similar pharmacologic therapy. Explain.

4. What classes of variants are likely to be found in individuals with homocystinuria who are not responsive to the administration of large doses of pyridoxine (vitamin B_6)? How might you explain the fact that Tom is completely responsive, whereas his first cousin Allan has only a partial reduction in plasma homocysteine levels when he is given the same amount of vitamin B_6?

5. You have isolated the gene for phenylalanine hydroxylase (PAH) and wish ultimately to introduce it into patients with PKU. Your approach will be to culture cells from the patient, introduce a functional version of the gene into the cells, and reintroduce the cells into the patient.
   a. What DNA components do you need to make a functional PAH protein in a gene transfer experiment?
   b. Which tissues would you choose in which to express the enzyme, and why? How does this choice affect your gene construct in (a)?

c. You introduce your version of the gene into fibroblasts cultured from a skin biopsy specimen from the patient. Northern (RNA) blot analysis shows that the messenger RNA (mRNA) is present in normal amounts and is the correct size. However, no PAH protein can be detected in the cells. What kinds of abnormalities in the transferred gene would explain this finding?
   d. You have corrected all the problems identified in (c). On introducing the new version of the gene into the cultured cells, you now find that the PAH protein is present in great abundance, and when you harvest the cells and assay the enzyme (in the presence of all the required components), normal activity is obtained. However, when you add ^{3}H-labeled phenylalanine to the cells in culture, no ^{3}H-labeled tyrosine is formed (in contrast, some cultured liver cells produce a large quantity of ^{3}H-labeled tyrosine in this situation). What are the most likely explanations for the failure to form ^{3}H-tyrosine? How does this result affect your gene therapy approach to patients?
   e. You have developed a method to introduce your functional version of the gene directly into a large proportion of the hepatocytes of patients with PAH deficiency. Unexpectedly, you find that much lower levels of PAH enzymatic activity are obtained in patients in whom significant amounts of the inactive PAH homodimer were detectable in hepatocytes before treatment than in patients who had no detectable PAH polypeptide before treatment. How can you explain this result? How might you overcome the problem?

6. Both variant alleles of an autosomal gene in your patient produce a protein that is decreased in abundance but has residual function. What therapeutic strategies might you consider in such a situation?

7. A Phase III clinical trial is undertaken to evaluate the effectiveness of a small molecule drug that facilitates skipping over nonsense codons. The drug had been shown in earlier trials to have a modest but significant clinical effect in individuals with cystic fibrosis (CF) with at least one *CFTR* nonsense variant. Two individuals with CF each have a nonsense variant in one *CFTR* allele, but at different locations in the reading frame. One patient responds to the drug, whereas the other does not. Discuss how the location of the nonsense variant could account for this differential response.

CHAPTER 15

Developmental Genetics and Birth Defects

Anthony Wynshaw-Boris • Ophir Klein

Knowledge of the principles and concepts of developmental **genetics**, including the mechanisms and pathways responsible for normal human development *in utero*, is essential for the practitioner who seeks to develop a rational approach to the diagnostic evaluation of a patient with a **birth defect**. With an accurate diagnostic assessment in hand, the practitioner can make predictions about prognosis, recommend management options, and provide an accurate **recurrence risk** for the parents and other relatives of the affected child. In this chapter we provide an overview of the branch of medicine concerned with birth defects and review basic mechanisms of embryologic development, with examples of some of these mechanisms and pathways in detail. We present examples of birth defects that result from abnormalities in these processes. Lastly, we show how an appreciation of developmental biology is essential for understanding prenatal diagnosis (see Chapter 18) and **stem cell** therapy as applied to regenerative medicine.

DEVELOPMENTAL BIOLOGY IN MEDICINE
The Public Health Impact of Birth Defects

The medical impact of birth defects is considerable. In 2019, the most recent year for which final statistics are available, the infant mortality rate in the United States was 5.6 infant deaths per 1000 live births; more than 20% of infant deaths were attributed to birth defects (i.e., abnormalities [often referred to as **anomalies**] that are present at birth in the development of organs or other structures). Another 20% of infant deaths may be attributed to complications of prematurity, which can be considered a failure of maintenance of the maternal-fetal developmental environment. Therefore, nearly half of the deaths of infants are caused by derangements of normal development. In addition to mortality, **congenital** anomalies are a major cause of long-term morbidity, intellectual disability, and other dysfunctions that limit the productivity of affected individuals.

Developmental anomalies certainly have a major impact on public health. **Genetic counseling** and prenatal diagnosis, with the option to continue or to terminate a pregnancy, are important for helping individuals faced with a **risk** for serious birth defects in their offspring improve their chances of having healthy children (see Chapter 18). Physicians and other health care professionals must be careful, however, not to limit the public health goal of reducing disease solely to preventing the birth of children with anomalies through voluntary pregnancy termination. Primary prevention of birth defects can be accomplished. For example, recommendations to supplement prenatal folic acid intake, which markedly reduces the incidence of neural tube defects, and public health campaigns that focus on preventing teratogenic effects of alcohol during pregnancy are successful public health approaches to the prevention of birth defects that do not depend on prenatal diagnosis and elective abortion. In the future it is hoped that our continued understanding of the developmental processes and pathways that regulate them will lead to therapies that may improve the morbidity and mortality associated with birth defects.

Dysmorphology and Mechanisms That Cause Birth Defects

Dysmorphology is the study of congenital birth defects that alter the shape or form of one or more parts of the body of a newborn child. Researchers attempt to understand the contribution of both abnormal genes and nongenetic, environmental influences to birth defects, as well as how those genes participate in conserved developmental pathways. The objectives of the medical geneticist who sees a child with birth defects are:
- to diagnose a child with a birth defect,
- to suggest further diagnostic evaluations,
- to give prognostic information about the range of outcomes that could be expected,
- to develop a plan to manage the expected complications,
- to provide the family with an understanding of the causation of the malformation, and
- to give recurrence risks to the parents and other relatives.

To accomplish these diverse and demanding objectives, the clinician must acquire and organize data from the patient, the family history, and published clinical and basic science literature. Medical geneticists work closely with specialists in pediatric surgery, neurology,

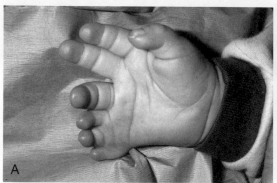
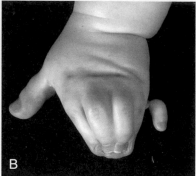

Figure 15.1 **Polydactyly and syndactyly malformations.** (A) Insertional polydactyly. This patient has heptadactyly with insertion of a digit in the central ray of the hand and a supernumerary postaxial digit. This malformation is typically associated with metacarpal fusion of the third and fourth digits. Insertional polydactyly is common in patients with Pallister-Hall syndrome. (B) Postaxial polydactyly with severe cutaneous syndactyly of digits 2 through 5. This type of malformation is seen in patients with Greig cephalopolysyndactyly syndrome. (Images courtesy Dr. Leslie Biesecker, Bethesda, Maryland.)

rehabilitation medicine, and the allied health professions to provide ongoing care for children with serious birth defects.

Malformations, Deformations, and Disruptions

Medical geneticists divide birth defects into three major categories: malformations, deformations, and **disruptions**. We will illustrate the difference between these three categories with examples of three distinct birth defects, all involving the limbs.

Malformations result from intrinsic abnormalities in one or more genetic programs operating in development. An example of a malformation is the extra fingers in the disorder known as Greig cephalopolysyndactyly (Fig. 15.1). This **syndrome**, discussed later in the chapter, results from loss-of-function **variants** in a **gene** for a **transcription factor**, GLI3, which is one component of a complex network of transcription factors and signaling molecules that interact to cause the distal end of the human upper limb bud to develop into a hand with five digits. Because malformations arise from intrinsic defects in genes that specify a series of developmental steps or programs, and because such programs are often used more than once in different parts of the embryo or fetus at different stages of development, a malformation in one part of the body is often but not always associated with malformations elsewhere as well.

In contrast to malformations, deformations are caused by extrinsic factors impinging physically on the fetus during development. They are especially common during the second trimester of development when the fetus is constrained within the amniotic sac and uterus. For example, contractions of the joints of the extremities, known as arthrogryposes, in combination with deformation of the developing skull, occasionally accompany constraint of the fetus due to twin or triplet gestations or prolonged leakage of amniotic fluid (Fig. 15.2). Arthrogryposes have many causes, and some of them are intrinsic malformations due to pathogenic

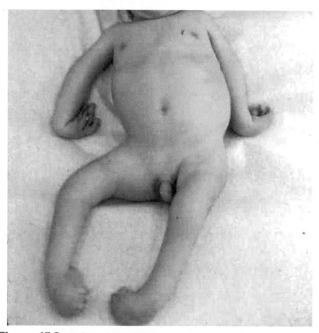

Figure 15.2 Deformation known as congenital arthrogryposis seen with a condition referred to as amyoplasia. There are multiple, symmetric joint contractures due to abnormal muscle development caused by severe fetal constraint in a pregnancy complicated by oligohydramnios. Intelligence is generally normal, and orthopedic rehabilitation is often successful. (Image courtesy Dr. Judith Hall, University of British Columbia, Vancouver, Canada.)

variants. Most deformations apparent at birth either resolve spontaneously or can be treated by external fixation devices to reverse the effects of the instigating cause.

Disruptions, the third category of birth defect, result from destruction of irreplaceable normal fetal tissue. Disruptions are more difficult to treat than deformations because they involve actual loss of normal tissue. Disruptions may be the result of vascular insufficiency, trauma, or teratogens. One example is amnion disruption, the partial amputation of a fetal limb associated with strands of amniotic tissue. Amnion disruption is often recognized clinically by the presence of partial and irregular digit amputations in conjunction with constriction rings (Fig. 15.3).

The pathophysiologic concepts of malformations, deformations, and disruptions are useful clinical guides to the recognition, diagnosis, and treatment of birth defects, but they sometimes overlap. For example, vascular malformations may lead to disruption of distal structures, and urogenital malformations that cause oligohydramnios can cause fetal deformations. Thus a given constellation of birth defects in an individual may represent combinations of malformations, deformations, and disruptions.

Genetic, Genomic, and Environmental Causes of Malformations

Malformations have many causes (Fig. 15.4). **Chromosome** imbalance accounts for ~25%, of which autosomal trisomies for chromosomes 21, 18, and 13 (see Chapter 6) are some of the most common. The clinical application of genome-wide arrays in comparative genomic **hybridization** (**CGH** or **array-CGH**; see Chapter 5) has highlighted small, *de novo* submicroscopic **deletions** and/or duplications, also known as copy number variants (CNVs), in as many as 10% of individuals with birth defects. An additional 20% are caused by variants in single genes, which are being discovered at an increasing pace with the advent of whole **exome** and **genome sequencing**. Some malformations, such as achondroplasia or Waardenburg syndrome, are inherited as autosomal **dominant** traits. Many heterozygotes with birth defects, however, represent new **mutations** that are so severe that they are genetic lethals and are therefore often found to be isolated cases within families (see Chapter 7). Other malformation syndromes are inherited in an autosomal or X-linked **recessive** pattern, such as the Smith-Lemli-Opitz syndrome or the Lowe syndrome, respectively.

Another ~40% of major birth defects have no identifiable cause but recur in families of affected children with a greater frequency than would be expected on the basis of the population frequency and are thus considered to be multifactorial diseases (see Chapter 9). This category includes well-recognized birth defects

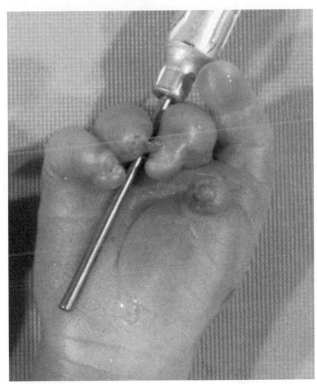

Figure 15.3 Disruption of limb development associated with amniotic bands. This 26-week fetus shows nearly complete disruption of the thumb with only a nubbin remaining. The third and fifth fingers have constriction rings of the middle and distal phalanges, respectively. The fourth digit is amputated distally with a small fragment of amnion attached to the tip. (Image courtesy Dr. Mason Barr, Jr., University of Michigan, Ann Arbor, Michigan.)

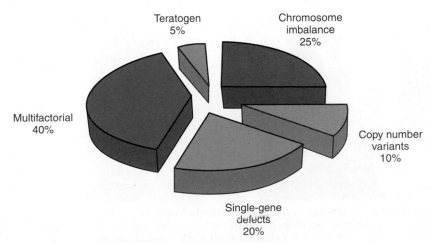

Figure 15.4 The relative contribution of single-gene defects, chromosome abnormalities, copy number variants, multifactorial traits, and teratogens to birth defects.

such as cleft lip with or without cleft palate, and congenital heart defects.

The remaining 5% of birth defects are thought to result from exposure to certain environmental agents—drugs, infections, alcohol, chemicals, or radiation—or from maternal metabolic disorders such as poorly controlled maternal diabetes mellitus or maternal phenylketonuria (see Chapter 13). Such agents are called **teratogens** (derived, inelegantly, from the Greek word for monster plus -*gen*, meaning cause) because of their ability to cause malformations (discussed later in this chapter).

Pleiotropy: Syndromes and Sequences

A birth defect resulting from a single underlying causative agent may result in abnormalities of more than one organ system in different parts of the embryo or in multiple structures that arise at different times during intrauterine life, a phenomenon referred to as **pleiotropy**. The agent responsible for the malformation could be either a **mutant** gene or a **teratogen**. **Pleiotropic** birth defects come about in two different ways, depending on the mechanism by which the causative agent produces its effect. When the causative agent causes multiple abnormalities in parallel, the collection of abnormalities is referred to as a **syndrome**. If, however, a mutant gene or teratogen affects only a single organ system at one point in time, and it is the perturbation of that organ system that causes the rest of the constellation of pleiotropic defects to occur as secondary effects, the malformation is referred to as a **sequence**.

Pleiotropic Syndromes. The autosomal dominant branchio-oto-renal dysplasia syndrome exemplifies a pleiotropic syndrome. It has long been recognized that patients with branchial arch anomalies affecting development of the ear and neck structures are at high risk for having renal anomalies. The branchio-oto-renal dysplasia syndrome, for example, consists of abnormal cochlear and external ear development, cysts and fistulas in the neck, renal dysplasia, and renal collecting duct malformations. The mechanism of this **association** is that a conserved set of genes and proteins are used by mammals to form both the ear and the kidney. The syndrome is caused by **pathogenic variant** in one of three genes—*EYA1*, *SIX1*, or *SIX5*—which encode transcriptional regulators that function in both ear and kidney development. Similarly, the Rubinstein-Taybi syndrome, caused by loss of function in a transcriptional coactivator, results in abnormalities in the **transcription** of many genes that depend on this coactivator being present in a transcription complex for normal expression (Fig. 15.5).

Sequences. In contrast, an example of a sequence is the U-shaped cleft palate and small mandible referred to as the Robin sequence (Fig. 15.6). This sequence comes about because a restriction of mandibular growth before the ninth week of gestation causes the tongue to lie more posteriorly than is normal, interfering with normal closure of the palatal shelves, thereby causing a cleft palate. The Robin sequence can be an isolated birth defect of unknown cause or can be due to extrinsic impingement on the developing mandible by a twin *in utero*. This

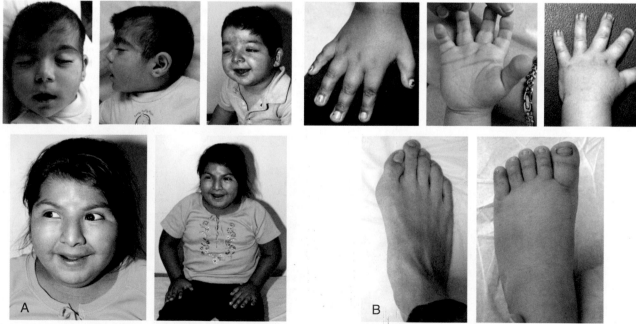

Figure 15.5 Physical characteristics of patients with Rubinstein-Taybi syndrome, a highly variable and pleiotropic syndrome of developmental delay, distinctive facial appearance, broad thumbs and large toes, and congenital heart defects. The syndrome is caused by loss-of-function variants in one of two different but closely related transcriptional coactivators, *CBP* or *EP300*. (A) Distinctive facial features. (B) Appearance of hands and feet. (Reprinted with permission from Jones KL, Jones MC, del Campo M: *Smith's recognizable patterns of human malformation*, ed 7, Philadelphia, 2013, WB Saunders.)

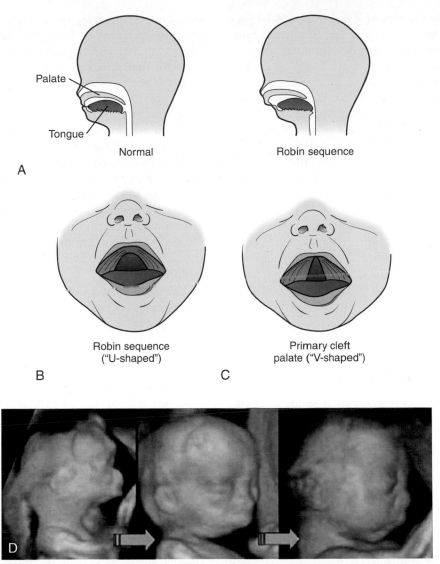

Figure 15.6 (A) Hypoplasia of the mandible and resulting posterior displacement of the tongue lead to the Robin sequence, in which the tongue obstructs palatal closure. (B) Posterior placement of the tongue in the Robin sequence causes a deformation of the palate during development, leading to the constellation of a small chin and a U-shaped cleft palate involving the soft palate and extending into the hard palate. (C) In contrast, primary cleft palate resulting from failure of closure of maxillary ridges is a malformation that begins in the anterior region of the maxilla and extends posteriorly to involve first the hard palate and then the soft palate, and it is often V shaped. (D) The delay in jaw development can be observed by serial three-dimensional fetal scans, from as early as 17 weeks *(left)* to 20 weeks *(middle)* and 29 weeks *(right)*. (A–C, Adapted from Wolpert L: *Principles of development*, New York, 2002, Oxford University Press; D, from Pooh RK, Kurjak A: Recent advances in 3D assessment of various fetal anomalies, *J Ultrasound Obstet Gynecol* 3:1–23, 2009.)

phenotype can also be one of several features of a condition known as Stickler syndrome, in which pathogenic variants in one of six genes encoding subunits of collagen result in an abnormally small mandible as well as other defects in stature, joints, and eyes. The Robin sequence in Stickler syndrome is thought to be a sequence because the mutant collagen gene itself is likely not responsible for the failure of palatal closure; rather, the cleft palate appears to be secondary to the primary defect in jaw growth. Whatever the cause, it is useful to distinguish a cleft palate due to the Robin sequence from other types of cleft palate, which can have differing prognoses and implications for the child and family. Knowledge of

dysmorphology and developmental genetic principles is thus necessary to properly diagnose each condition and to recognize that different prognoses are associated with the different primary causes.

INTRODUCTION TO DEVELOPMENTAL BIOLOGY

The examples introduced briefly in the previous section serve to illustrate the principle that the clinical practice of medical genetics rests on a foundation of the basic science of developmental biology. For this reason, it behooves practitioners to have a working knowledge of some of the basic principles of developmental biology and to be familiar with the ways that abnormal function of genes and pathways affect development and, ultimately, their patients.

Developmental biology is concerned with a single, unifying question: How can a single cell transform itself into a mature organism? In humans, this **transformation** occurs each time a single fertilized egg develops into a human being with more than 10^{13} to 10^{14} cells, several hundred recognizably distinct cell types, and dozens of tissues. This process must occur in a reliable and predictable pattern and time frame.

Developmental biology has its roots in embryology, which was based on observing and surgically manipulating developing organisms. Early animal embryologic studies, carried out in the 19th and early 20th centuries with readily accessible amphibian and avian embryos, determined that embryos developed from single cells and defined many of the fundamental processes of development. Much more recently, the application of molecular biology, genetics, and **genomics** to embryology has transformed the field by allowing scientists to study and manipulate development by a broad range of powerful biochemical and molecular techniques. Of note, the rapid advancement of **next generation sequencing** has allowed the development of single-cell **RNA** sequencing technologies (scRNAseq), which has underscored the transcriptional diversity of cells throughout development and in the adult.

Development and Evolution

A critically important theme in developmental biology is its relationship to the study of evolution. Early in development, the embryos of many species have important similarities. As development progresses, the features shared between species are successively transformed into more specialized features that are, in turn, shared by successively fewer but more closely related species. A comparison of embryologic characteristics among and within evolutionarily related organisms shows that developmental attributes (e.g., fingers) specific to certain groups of animals (e.g., primates) are built on a foundation of less specific attributes common to a larger group of animals (e.g., mammals), which are in turn related to structures seen in an even larger group of animals (e.g., vertebrates). Structures in different organisms are termed **homologous** if they evolved from a structure present in a common ancestor (Fig. 15.7). In the case of the forelimb, the various ancestral lineages of the three species shown in Fig. 15.7, tracing back to their common predecessor, share a common attribute: a functional forelimb. The molecular developmental mechanism that created those limb structures is shared across all three of the contemporary species.

Not all similarity is due to homology, however. Evolutionary studies also recognize the existence of analogous structures, those that appear similar but arose independently of one another, through different lineages that cannot be traced back to a common ancestor with that structure. The molecular pathways that generate analogous structures are often not evolutionarily conserved. In the example shown in Fig. 15.7, the wing structures of the bat and the birds arose independently in evolution to facilitate the task of aerial movement. The evolutionary lineages of these two animals do not share a common ancestor with a primitive wing-like structure from which both bats and birds inherited wings. On the contrary, one can readily see that the birds developed posterior extensions from the limb to form a wing, whereas bats evolved wings by spreading the digits of their forelimbs and connecting them with syndactylous tissue. This situation is termed convergent evolution.

The evolutionary conservation of developmental processes is critically important to studies of human development because the vast majority of such research cannot (for important ethical reasons) be performed in humans (see Chapter 20). Thus, to understand a developmental observation, scientists use animal models to investigate normal and abnormal developmental processes. The ability to extend the results to humans is completely dependent on the evolutionary conservation of mechanisms of development and homologous structures.

GENES AND ENVIRONMENT IN DEVELOPMENT

Developmental Genetics

Development results from the action of genes interacting with environmental cues. The gene products involved include transcriptional regulators, growth factors (diffusible signals that interact with cells and direct them toward specific developmental pathways), the receptors for such factors, structural proteins, intracellular signaling molecules, and many others. It is therefore not surprising that most of the numerous developmental disorders that occur in humans are caused by chromosomal, subchromosomal, or gene variants.

Even though the **genome** is clearly the primary source of information that controls and specifies human development, the role of genes in development is often mistakenly described as a "master blueprint." In reality, however, the genome does not resemble an architect's blueprint that specifies precisely how the materials are to be used, how they are to be assembled, and their final dimensions; it is not a literal description of the final form that all embryologic and fetal structures will take. Rather, the genome specifies a set of interacting proteins and noncoding RNAs (see Chapter 3) that set in motion the processes of growth, migration, **differentiation**, and **apoptosis** that ultimately result, with a high degree of

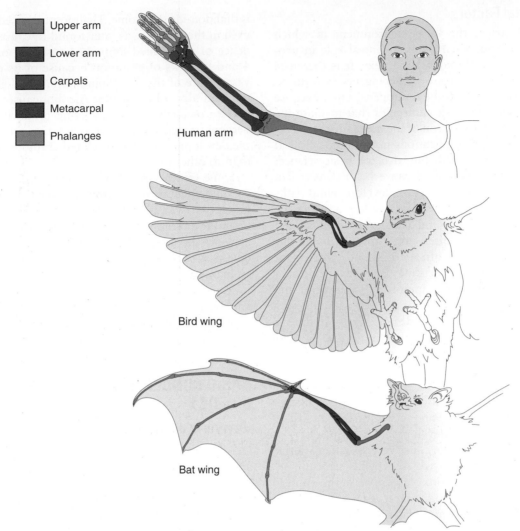

Upper arm
Lower arm
Carpals
Metacarpal
Phalanges

Human arm

Bird wing

Bat wing

Figure 15.7 **Diagram of the upper limb of three species: human, bird, and bat.** Despite the superficially dissimilar appearance of the human arm and hand, the avian wing, and the bat wing, the similarity in their underlying bone structure and functionality reveals the homology of the forelimbs of all three species. In contrast, the two superficially similar wings in the bird and bat are analogous, not homologous structures. Although both the bird and bat wings are used for flying, they are constructed quite differently and did not evolve from a winglike structure in a common ancestor. (Redrawn from Hauk R: *Frequently asked questions about bats*, 2011, Western National Parks Association.)

probability, in the correct mature structures. Thus, for example, there are no genetic instructions directing that the phalanx of a digit adopt an hourglass shape or that the eye be spherical. These shapes arise as an implicit consequence of developmental processes, thereby generating correctly structured cells, tissues, and organs.

Probability

Although genes are the primary regulators of development, other processes must also play a role. That development is regulated but not determined by the genome is underscored by the important role that probability plays in normal development. For example, in the mouse, a pathogenic variant in the *Dishevelled-2* gene produces congenital heart defects in only ~50% of mice who carry the variant, even when such carriers are from inbred strains of mice that are genetically

identical. Thus the 50% **penetrance** of the *Dishevelled-2* variant cannot be explained by different modifying gene variants in the mice affected with heart defects versus the mice who are unaffected. Instead, it appears likely that the *Dishevelled-2* variant shifts the balance of some developmental process by increasing the probability that a threshold for causing congenital heart defects is exceeded, much as we explored in Chapter 9 when discussing complex patterns of inheritance in humans. Thus carrying a *Dishevelled-2* pathogenic variant will not always lead to heart defects, but it sometimes will, and neither the rest of the genome nor nongenetic factors are responsible for development of the defect in only a minority of animals. Probabilistic processes provide a rich source of interindividual variation that can lead to a range of developmental outcomes, some normal and some not.

Environmental Factors

As indicated earlier, the local environment in which a cell or tissue finds itself plays a central role in providing a normal developmental context. It is therefore not unexpected that drugs or other agents introduced from the environment can be teratogens, often because they interfere with intrinsic molecules that mediate the actions of genes. Identification of the mechanism of teratogenesis has obvious implications not only for clinical medicine and public health but also for basic science; understanding how teratogens cause birth defects can provide insight into the underlying developmental pathways that have been disturbed and result in a defect.

Because the molecular and cellular pathways used during development are often not employed in similar developmental processes after adulthood, teratogens that cause serious birth defects may have few or no side effects in adult patients. One important example of this concept is fetal retinoid syndrome, seen in fetuses of pregnant women who took the drug isotretinoin during pregnancy. Isotretinoin is an oral retinoid that is used systemically for the treatment of severe acne. It causes major birth defects when taken by a pregnant woman because it mimics the action of endogenous retinoic acid, a substance that in the developing embryo and fetus diffuses through tissues and interacts with cells, causing them to follow particular developmental pathways.

Different teratogens often cause very specific patterns of birth defects, the risk for which depends critically on the gestational age at the time of exposure, the vulnerability of different tissues to the teratogen, and the level of exposure during pregnancy. One of the best examples is thalidomide syndrome. Thalidomide, a sedative widely used in the 1950s, was later found to cause a high incidence of malformed limbs in fetuses exposed between 4 and 8 weeks of gestation because of its effect on the vasculature of the developing limb. Another example is the fetal alcohol syndrome. Alcohol causes a particular pattern of birth defects involving primarily the central nervous system because it is relatively more toxic to the developing brain and related craniofacial structures than to other tissues.

Some teratogens, such as x-rays, are also **mutagens**. A fundamental distinction between teratogens and mutagens is that mutagens cause damage by creating heritable alterations in genetic material, whereas teratogens act directly and transiently on developing embryonic tissue. Thus fetal exposure to a mutagen can cause an increased risk for birth defects or other diseases (e.g., cancer) throughout the life of the exposed individual and even in his or her offspring, whereas exposure to a teratogen increases the risk for birth defects for current but not for subsequent pregnancies.

BASIC CONCEPTS OF DEVELOPMENTAL BIOLOGY

Overview of Embryologic Development

Developmental biology has its own set of core concepts and terminology that may be confusing or foreign to the student of genetics. We therefore provide a brief summary of a number of key concepts and terms used in this chapter (see Box 15.1).

BOX 15.1 CORE CONCEPTS AND TERMINOLOGY IN HUMAN DEVELOPMENTAL BIOLOGY

Blastocyst: a stage in embryogenesis after the morula, in which cells on the outer surface of the morula secrete fluid and form a fluid-filled internal cavity within which is a separate group of cells, the **inner cell mass**, which will become the fetus itself (see Fig. 15.8 and 15.9).
Chimera: an embryo made up of two or more cell lines that differ in their **genotype**. Contrast with mosaic.
Chorion: membrane that develops from the outer cells of the **blastocyst** and goes on to form the placenta and the outer layer of the sac in which the fetus develops.
Determination: the stage in development in which cells are irreversibly committed to forming a particular tissue.
Dichorionic twins: monozygotic twins arising from splitting of the embryo into two parts, before formation of the blastocyst, so that two independent blastocysts develop.
Differentiation: the acquisition by a cell of novel characteristics specific for a particular cell type or tissue.
Ectoderm: the primary embryonic **germ layer** that gives rise to the nervous system and skin.
Embryo: the stage of a developing human organism between fertilization and 9 weeks of gestation, when separation into placental and embryonic tissues occurs.
Embryogenesis: the development of the embryo.

Embryonic stem cells: cells derived from the inner cell mass that under appropriate conditions can differentiate into all of the cell types and tissues of an embryo and form a complete, normal fetus.
Endoderm: the primary embryonic **germ layer** that gives rise to many of the visceral organs and lining of the gut.
Epiblast: a differentiated portion of the inner cell mass that gives rise to the embryo proper. Human **embryonic stem cells** are considered to be epiblast stem cells.
Fate: the ultimate destination for a cell that has traveled down a developmental pathway.
Fetus: the stage of the developing human between 9 weeks of gestation and birth.
Gastrulation: the stage of development just after implantation in which the cells of the inner cell mass rearrange themselves into the three germ layers.
Germ cell: the cells that are the progenitors of the gametes. These cells are allocated early in development and undergo sex-specific differentiation.
Germ layers: three distinct layers of cells that arise in the inner cell mass, the **ectoderm**, **mesoderm**, and **endoderm**, which develop into distinctly different tissues in the embryo.
Hypoblast: the differentiated portion of the inner cell mass that contributes to fetal membranes (amnion).
Inner cell mass: a group of cells inside the blastocyst destined to become the fetus.

continued

BOX 15.1 CORE CONCEPTS AND TERMINOLOGY IN HUMAN DEVELOPMENTAL BIOLOGY—CONT'D

Mesoderm: the primary embryonic germ layer that gives rise to connective tissue, muscles, bones, vasculature, and the lymphatic and hematopoietic systems.

Monoamniotic twins: monozygotic twins resulting from cleavage of part of the inner cell mass (epiblast) but without cleavage of the part of the inner cell mass that forms the amniotic membrane (hypoblast).

Monochorionic twins: monozygotic twins resulting from cleavage of the inner cell mass without cleavage of the cells on the outside of the blastocyst.

Monozygotic twins: twins arising from a single fertilized egg, resulting from cleavage during embryogenesis in the interval between the first cell division of the zygote and gastrulation.

Morphogen: a substance produced by cells in a particular region of an embryo that diffuses from its point of origin through the tissues of the embryo to form a concentration gradient. Cells undergo **specification** and then **determination** to different **fates**, depending on the concentration of **morphogen** they experience.

Morphogenesis: the creation of various structures during embryogenesis.

Morula: a compact ball of 16 cells produced after four cell divisions of the **zygote**.

Mosaic: an individual who develops from a single fertilized egg but in whom mutation after conception results in cells with two or more genotypes. Contrast with **chimera**.

Mosaic development: a stage in development in which cells have already become committed to the point that removal of a portion of an embryo will not allow normal embryonic development.

Multipotent stem cell: a **stem cell** capable of self-renewal as well as of developing into many different types of cells in a tissue, but not an entire organism. These are often called adult stem cells or tissue progenitor cells.

Organogenesis: the creation of individual organs during **embryogenesis**.

Pluripotent cell: an early stem cell capable of self-renewal as well as of becoming any cell in any embryonic tissue, including the germ cells. **Embryonic stem cells** are **pluripotent**.

Progenitor cell: a cell that is traversing a developmental pathway on its way to becoming a fully differentiated cell.

Regulative development: a stage in development in which cells have not yet become determined so that the cells that remain after removal of a portion of an embryo can still form a complete organism.

Specification: a step along the path of differentiation in which cells acquire certain specialized attributes characteristic of a particular tissue but can still be influenced by external cues to develop into a different type of cell or tissue.

Stem cell: a cell that is capable both of generating another stem cell (self-renewal) and of differentiating into specialized cells within a tissue or an entire organism.

Totipotent cell: a very early stem cell that can form all cell types in a body, plus the extraembryonic, or placental, cells. Embryonic cells within the first couple of divisions after fertilization are the only cells that are totipotent.

Zygote: the fertilized egg, the first step in embryogenesis.

Cellular Processes During Development

During development, cells divide (proliferate), acquire novel functions or structures (differentiate), move within the embryo (migrate), and undergo programmed cell death (often through apoptosis). These four basic cellular processes act in various combinations and in different ways to allow growth and **morphogenesis** (literally, the "creation of form"), thereby creating an embryo of normal size and shape, containing organs of the appropriate size, shape, and location, and consisting of tissues and cells with the correct architecture, structure, and function.

Although growth may seem too obvious to discuss, growth itself is carefully regulated in mammalian development, and unregulated growth is disastrous. The mere doubling (one extra round of cell division) of cell number (hyperplasia) or an increase of cell size (hypertrophy) in an organism can be fatal. Dysregulation of growth of segments of the body can cause severe deformity and dysfunction, such as in hemihyperplasia and other segmental overgrowth disorders. Furthermore, the exquisite differential regulation of growth can change the shape of a tissue or an organ.

Morphogenesis is accomplished in the developing organism by the coordinated interplay of the mechanisms introduced in this section. In some contexts, morphogenesis is used as a general term to describe all of development, but this is formally incorrect because morphogenesis has to be coupled to the process of growth discussed here to generate a normally shaped and functioning tissue or organ.

Human Embryogenesis

This description of human development begins where Chapter 2 ends, with fertilization. After fertilization, the embryo undergoes a series of cell divisions without overall growth, termed cleavage. The single fertilized egg undergoes four divisions to yield the 16-cell morula by day 4 (Fig. 15.8). At day 5, the embryo transitions to become a **blastocyst,** in which cells that give rise to the placenta form a wall, inside of which the cells that will make the embryo itself aggregate to one side into what is referred to as the inner cell mass. This is the point at which the embryo acquires its first obvious manifestation of polarity, an axis of asymmetry that divides the inner cell mass (most of which goes on to form the mature organism) from the embryonic tissues that will go on to form the chorion, an extraembryonic tissue (e.g., placenta) (Fig. 15.9). The inner cell mass then separates again into the epiblast, which will make the embryo proper, and the hypoblast, which will form the amniotic membrane.

The embryo implants in the endometrial wall of the uterus in the interval between days 7 and 12 after fertilization. After implantation, gastrulation occurs, in which

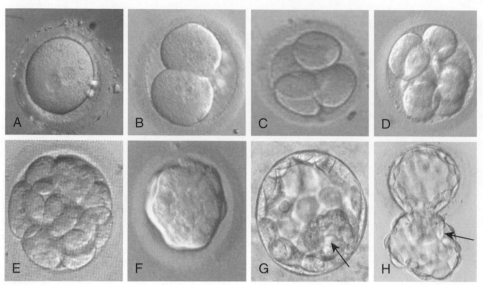

Figure 15.8 **Human development begins with cleavage of the fertilized egg.** (A) The fertilized egg at day 0 with two pronuclei and the polar bodies. (B) A two-cell embryo at day 1 after fertilization. (C) A four-cell embryo at day 2. (D) The eight-cell embryo at day 3. (E) The 16-cell stage later in day 3, followed by the phenomenon of compaction, whereby the embryo is now termed a morula (F, day 4). (G) The formation of the blastocyst at day 5, with the inner cell mass indicated by the arrow. Finally, the embryo *(arrow)* hatches from the zona pellucida (H). (Reprinted with permission from Jones KL: *Smith's recognizable patterns of human malformation,* ed 6, Philadelphia, 2005, WB Saunders.)

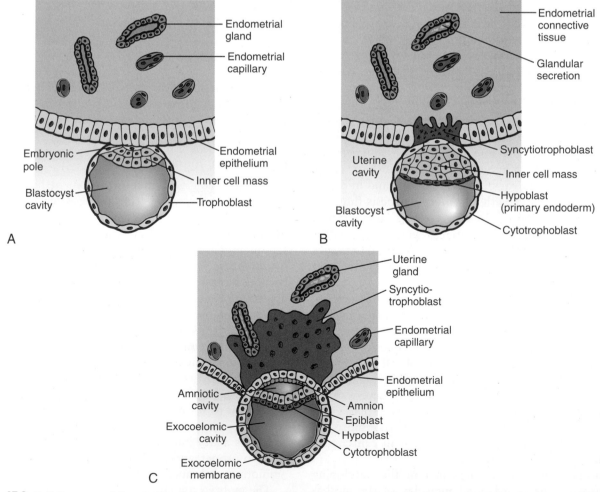

Figure 15.9 **Cell lineage and fate during preimplantation development.** Embryonic age is given in time after fertilization in humans: (A) 6 days, (B) 7 days, (C) 8 days postfertilization. (Reprinted with permission from Moore KL, Persaud TVN: *The developing human: clinically oriented embryology,* ed 6, Philadelphia, 1998, WB Saunders.)

cells rearrange themselves into a structure consisting of three cellular compartments, termed the germ layers, comprising the ectoderm, mesoderm, and endoderm. The three germ layers give rise to different structures. The endodermal lineage forms the central visceral core of the organism. This includes the cells lining the main gut cavity, the airways of the respiratory system, and other similar structures. The mesodermal lineage gives rise to kidneys, heart, vasculature, and structural or supportive functions in the organism. Bone and muscle are nearly exclusively mesodermal and have the two main functions of structure (physical support) and providing physical and nutritive support of the hematopoietic system. The **ectoderm** gives rise to the central and peripheral nervous systems and the skin. During the complicated movements that occur in gastrulation, the embryo also establishes the major axes of the final body plan: anterior-posterior (cranial-caudal), dorsal-ventral (back-front), and left-right axes, which are discussed later.

The next major stages of development involve the initiation of the nervous system, establishment of the basic body plan, and then organogenesis, which occupies weeks 4 to 8. The position and basic structures of all the organs are now established, and the cellular components necessary for their full development are now in place. It is during this **phase** of embryonic development that neural tube defects occur, as we explore next.

Neural Tube Defects

Neural tube defects (NTDs) are among the most common and devastating birth defects. Anencephaly and spina bifida are NTDs that frequently occur together in families and are considered to have a common pathogenesis. In anencephaly, the forebrain, overlying meninges, vault of the skull, and skin are all absent. Many infants with anencephaly are stillborn, and those born alive survive a few hours at most. Approximately two-thirds of affected infants are female. In spina bifida, there is failure of fusion of the arches of the vertebrae, typically in the lumbar region. There are varying degrees of severity, ranging from spina bifida occulta, in which the defect is in the bony arch only, to spina bifida aperta, in which a bone defect is also associated with meningocele (protrusion of meninges) or meningomyelocele (protrusion of neural elements as well as meninges through the defect; see Fig. 18.5).

As a group, NTDs are a leading cause of stillbirth, death in early infancy, and handicap in surviving children. Their incidence at birth is variable, ranging from almost 1% in Ireland to 0.2% or less in the United States. The frequency also appears to vary with social factors and season of birth and oscillates widely over time (with a marked decrease in recent years; see later discussion).

A small proportion of NTDs have known specific causes, for example, amniotic bands (see Fig. 15.3), some single-gene defects with pleiotropic expression, some chromosomal disorders, and some teratogens. Most NTDs, however, are isolated defects of unknown cause.

Maternal Folic Acid Deficiency and Neural Tube Defects. NTDs were long believed to follow a multi-factorial inheritance pattern determined by multiple genetic and environmental factors, as introduced generally in Chapter 9. It was therefore a stunning discovery to find that the single greatest factor in causing NTDs is a vitamin deficiency. The risk for NTDs was found to be inversely correlated with maternal serum folic acid levels during pregnancy, with a threshold of $200\,\mu g/L$, below which the risk for NTD becomes significant. Along with reduced blood folate levels, elevated homocysteine levels were also seen in the mothers of children with NTDs, suggesting that a biochemical abnormality was present at the step of recycling of tetrahydrofolate to methylate homocysteine to methionine (see Fig. 13.7). Folic acid levels are strongly influenced by dietary intake and can become depressed during pregnancy even with a typical intake of $\sim230\,\mu g/day$. The impact of folic acid deficiency is exacerbated by a genetic variant of the enzyme 5,10-methylenetetrahydrofolate reductase (MTHFR), caused by a common missense variant that makes the enzyme less stable than normal. Instability of this enzyme hinders the recycling of tetrahydrofolate and interferes with the methylation of homocysteine to methionine.

The variant **allele** is so common in many populations that between 5% and 15% of the population is **homozygous** for the variant. In studies of infants with NTDs and their mothers, it was found that mothers of infants with NTDs were twice as likely as controls to be homozygous for the allele encoding the unstable enzyme. How this enzyme defect contributes to NTDs and whether the abnormality is a direct result of elevated homocysteine levels, depressed methionine levels, or some other metabolic derangement remains undefined.

Prevention of Neural Tube Defects. There are two approaches to preventing NTDs. The first is to educate women to supplement their diets with folic acid 1 month before conception and continuing for 2 months after conception during the period when the neural tube forms. Dietary supplementation with 400 to $800\,\mu g$ of folic acid per day for women who plan their pregnancies has been shown to reduce the incidence of NTDs by more than 75%. Since 1998, the United States has required cereal products labeled as enriched to be supplemented with $140\,\mu g$ folic acid per $100\,g$ flour as a public health measure to avoid the problem of women failing to supplement their diets individually during pregnancy. The Centers for Disease Control and Prevention estimates that this has reduced the number of infants born with NTDs by 1300 per year.

The second approach is to apply prenatal screening for all pregnancies and offer prenatal diagnosis to high-risk pregnancies. Prenatal diagnosis of anencephaly and most cases of open spina bifida relies on detecting excessive levels of α-fetoprotein (AFP) and other fetal substances in the amniotic fluid and by ultrasonographic scanning, as we shall discuss further in Chapter 18. However, less than 5% of all patients with NTDs are born to women with previous affected children. For this reason, screening of all pregnant women for NTDs by measurements of AFP and other fetal substances in maternal serum is now widespread. Thus we anticipated that a combination of preventive folic acid therapy and maternal AFP screening would provide major public health benefits by drastically reducing the incidence of NTDs, which it has by 35% compared with presupplementation levels.

Human Fetal Development

The embryonic phase of development occupies the first 2 months of pregnancy and is followed by the **fetal phase** of development, which is concerned primarily with the maturation and further differentiation of the components of the organs. For some organ systems, development does not cease at birth. For example, the brain undergoes substantial postnatal development, and limbs undergo epiphyseal growth and ultimately closure after puberty.

The Germ Cell: Transmitting Genetic Information

In addition to growth and differentiation of somatic tissues, the organism must also specify which cells will go on to become the gametes of the mature adult. The germ cell compartment serves this purpose. As described in Chapter 2, cells in the germ cell compartment become committed to undergoing gametogenesis and **meiosis** in order that the species can pass on its genetic complement and facilitate the recombination and random **assortment** of chromosomes. In addition, the sexspecific **epigenetic** imprint that certain genes require must be reset within the germ cell compartment (see Chapters 3, 6, 7, and 8).

The Stem Cell: Maintaining Regenerative Capacity in Tissues

In addition to specifying the program of differentiation that is necessary for development, the organism must also set aside tissue-specific stem cells that can regenerate differentiated cells during adult life. The best-characterized example of these cells is in the hematopoietic system. Among the 10^{11} to 10^{12} nucleated hematopoietic cells in the adult organism are ~10^4 to 10^5 cells that have the potential to generate any of the more specialized blood cells on a continuous basis during a lifetime. Hematopoietic stem cells can be transplanted to other humans and completely reconstitute the hematopoietic system (see Chapter 14). A system of interacting gene products maintains a properly sized pool of hematopoietic stem cells. These regulators permit a balance between the maintenance of stem cells through self-replication and the generation of committed precursor cells that can go on to develop into the various mature cells of the hematopoietic system (Fig. 15.10) (see Box 15.2).

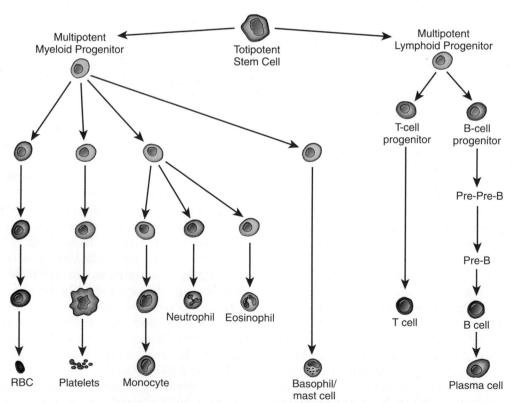

Figure 15.10 **The development of blood cells is a continuous process that generates a full complement of cells from a single, totipotent hematopoietic stem cell.** This hematopoietic stem cell is a committed stem cell that differentiated from a more primitive mesodermal stem cell. *RBC,* Red blood cell. (Reprinted with permission from Stamatoyannopoulos G, Nienhuis AW, Majerus PW, et al: *The molecular basis of blood diseases,* ed 2, Philadelphia, 1994, WB Saunders.)

BOX 15.2 EMBRYONIC STEM CELL TECHNOLOGY

Inner cell mass cells are thought to be capable of forming any tissue in the body. This has been proven in mice but is only suspected of being true in humans, in whom it cannot be tested for obvious ethical reasons. The full developmental potential of inner cell mass cells is the basis of the experimental field of embryonic stem cell technology in mice, a technology that is crucial for generating animal models of human genetic disease (Fig. 15.11). In this

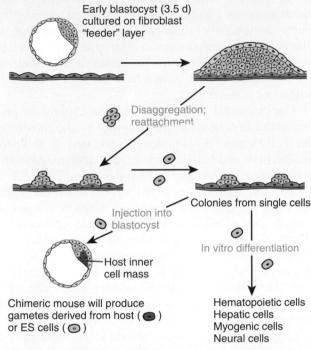

Figure 15.11 Embryonic stem *(ES)* cells are derived directly from the inner cell mass, are euploid, and can contribute to the germline. Cultured ES cells differentiated *in vitro* can give rise to a variety of different cell types.

technique, mouse inner cell mass cells are grown in culture as embryonic stem cells and undergo genetic manipulation to introduce a given mutation into a specific gene. These cells are then injected into the inner cell mass of another early mouse embryo. The mutated cells are incorporated into the inner cell mass of the recipient embryo and contribute to many tissues of that embryo, forming a **chimera** (a single embryo made up of cells from two different sources). If the mutated cells contribute to the **germline** in a chimeric animal, the offspring of that animal can inherit the engineered mutations. The ability of the recipient embryo to tolerate the incorporation of these pluripotent cells, which then undergo specification and can contribute to any tissue in a living mouse, is the converse of **regulative development**, the ability of an embryo to tolerate removal of some cells.

Human embryonic stem cells (hESCs), which probably come from the epiblast, have been made from unused fertilized embryos. hESCs are the subject of intensive research as well as ethical controversy. Although the use of hESCs for cloning an entire human being is considered highly unethical and universally banned, current research is directed toward generating particular cell types from hESCs to provide cellular models of human genetic diseases or to repair damaged tissues and organs, a goal of regenerative medicine.

Induced pluripotent stem cells (iPSCs) are another source of early stem cells that can be cultured and differentiated *in vitro* into particular cell types. Human iPSCs are derived through reprogramming of readily available and ethically uncontroversial somatic cells, such as **fibroblasts**, to very early stem cells through the introduction of certain transcription factors into the cells (e.g., the transcription factors Oct4 [Pou5f1], Sox2, cMyc, and Klf4). This technology makes what were previously inaccessible tissues from patients with genetic disorders, such as cardiac myocytes from patients with cardiomyopathies, or central nervous system neurons from patients with neurodegenerative diseases available for research and, ultimately, perhaps tissue-based therapy using their own gene-corrected iPSCs.

Fate, Specification, and Determination

As an undifferentiated cell undergoes the process of differentiation, it moves through a series of discrete steps in which it manifests various distinct functions or attributes until it reaches its ultimate destination, referred to as its **fate** (e.g., when a precursor cell becomes an erythrocyte, a keratinocyte, or a cardiac myocyte). In the developing organism, these attributes not only vary across the recognizable cell types but also change over time. Early during differentiation, a cell undergoes specification when it acquires specific characteristics but can still be influenced by environmental cues (signaling molecules, positional information) to change its ultimate fate. These environmental clues are primarily derived from neighboring cells by direct cell-cell contact or by signals received at the cell surface from soluble substances, including positional information derived from where a cell sits in a gradient of various morphogens. Eventually a cell either irreversibly acquires attributes or

has irreversibly been committed to acquire those attributes (referred to as **determination**). With the exception of the germ cell and stem cell types just described, all cells undergo specification and determination to their ultimate developmental fate.

Specification and determination involve the stepwise acquisition of a stable cellular phenotype of gene expression specific to the particular fate of each cell—nerve cells make synaptic proteins but do not make hemoglobin, whereas red blood cells do not make synaptic proteins but must make hemoglobin. With the exception of lymphocyte precursor cells undergoing DNA rearrangements in the T-cell receptor or immunoglobulin genes (see Chapter 3), the particular gene **expression profile** responsible for the differentiated cellular phenotype does not result from permanent changes in DNA sequence. Instead, the regulation of gene expression depends on **epigenetic** changes, such as stable transcription complexes, modification of **histones** in **chromatin**, and methylation of DNA (see

Chapters 3 and 8). The epigenetic control of gene expression is responsible for the loss of developmental plasticity, as we discuss next.

Regulative and Mosaic Development

Early in development, cells in many organisms are functionally equivalent and subject to dynamic processes of specification, a phenomenon known as **regulative development**. In regulative development, removal or ablation of part of an embryo can be compensated for by the remaining similar cells. In contrast, later in development, each of the cells in some parts of the embryo has a distinct fate, and in each of those parts, the embryo only appears to be homogeneous. In this situation, known as **mosaic development**, loss of a portion of an embryo would lead to the failure of development of the final structures that those cells were fated to become. Thus the developmental plasticity of the embryo generally declines with time.

Regulative Development and Twinning

That early mammalian development is primarily regulative has been demonstrated by basic embryologic experiments and confirmed by observations in clinical medicine. Identical (monozygotic) twins are the natural experimental evidence that early development is regulative. The most common form of identical twinning occurs in the second half of the first week of development, effectively splitting the inner cell mass into two halves, each of which develops into a normal fetus (Fig. 15.12). Were the embryo even partly regulated by mosaic development at this stage, the twins would develop only partially and consist of complementary parts. This is clearly

not the case because twins are generally completely normally developed and eventually attain normal size through prenatal and postnatal growth.

The various forms of monozygotic twinning demonstrate regulative development at several different stages. Dichorionic twins result from cleavage at the four-cell stage. Monochorionic twins result from a cleaved inner cell mass. Monoamniotic twins result from an even later cleavage, in this case within the bilayered embryo, which then forms two separate embryos but only one extraembryonic compartment that goes on to make the single amnion. All of these twinning events demonstrate that these cell populations can reprogram their development to form complete embryos from cells that, if cleavage had not occurred, would have contributed to only part of an embryo.

The successful application of the technique of **preimplantation diagnosis** (see Chapter 18) also illustrates that early human development is regulative. In this procedure, male and female gametes are harvested from the presumptive parents and fertilized *in vitro* (Fig. 15.13). When these fertilized embryos have reached the eight-cell stage (at day 3), a biopsy microneedle is used to remove one of these cells. The isolated cell with its clearly visible nucleus can then be examined using a variety of appropriate cytogenetic or genomic tests to ascertain if the embryo is suitable for implantation. Embryos composed of the remaining seven cells that are not affected by the disease can then be selected and implanted in the mother. The capacity of the embryo to recover from the biopsy of one of its eight cells is attributable to regulative development. Were those cells removed by biopsy fated to form a particular part or

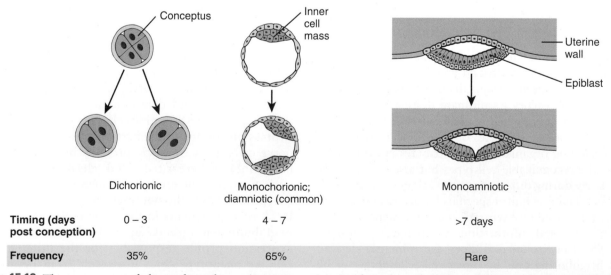

Timing (days post conception)	0 – 3	4 – 7	>7 days
	Dichorionic	Monochorionic; diamniotic (common)	Monoamniotic
Frequency	35%	65%	Rare

Figure 15.12 The arrangement of placental membranes in monozygotic twins depends on the timing of the twinning event. Dichorionic twins result from a complete splitting of the entire embryo, leading to duplication of all extraembryonic tissues. Monochorionic diamniotic twins are caused by division of the inner cell mass at the blastocyst stage. Monoamniotic twins are caused by division of the epiblast but not the hypoblast. (Reprinted with permission from Ogilvie CM, Braude PR, Scriven PN: Preimplantation diagnosis – An overview, *J Histochem Cytochem* 53:255–260, 2005.)

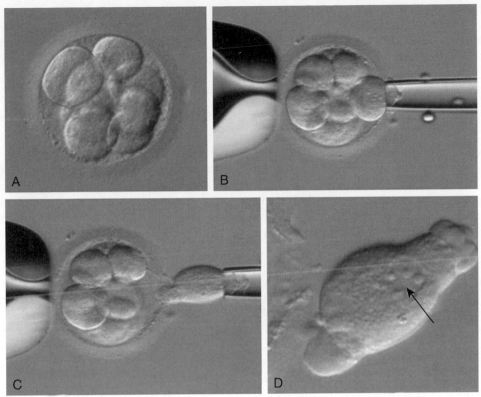

Figure 15.13 Blastomere biopsy of a human cleavage stage embryo. (A) Eight-cell embryo, day 3 after fertilization. (B) Embryo on holding pipette *(left)* with biopsy pipette *(right)* breaching the zona pellucida. (C) Blastomere removal by suction. (D) Blastomere removed by biopsy with a clearly visible single nucleus (indicated by *arrow*).

segment of the body (i.e., governed by mosaic development), one would predict that these parts of the body would be absent or defective in the mature individual. Instead, the embryo has compensatory mechanisms to replace those cells, which then undergo normal development as specified by their neighboring cells.

Mosaic Development

Embryonic development generally proceeds from more regulative to more mosaic development. Typical identical twinning early in development, as mentioned earlier, is an illustration of regulative development. However, later embryo cleavage events result in the formation of conjoined twins, which are two fetuses that share body structures and organs because the cleavage occurred after the transition from regulative to mosaic development, too late to allow complete embryos.

Interestingly, in some adult nonhuman species, ablation of a specific tissue may not limit development. For example, the mature salamander can regenerate an entire tail when it is cut off, apparently retaining a population of cells that can reestablish the **developmental program** for the tail after trauma. One of the goals of research in developmental biology is to understand this process in other species and potentially harness it in practice for human regenerative medicine.

Axis Specification and Pattern Formation

A critical function of the developing organism is to specify the spatial relationships of structures within the embryo. In early development, the organism must determine the relative orientation of a number of body segments and organs, involving the establishment of three axes:

- The head-to-tail axis, termed the cranial-caudal or anterior-posterior axis, is established very early in embryogenesis and is probably determined in certain species by the entry position of the sperm that fertilizes the egg. (It is referred to as the rostral-caudal axis later in development.)

- The dorsal-ventral axis is the second dimension, and here, too, a series of interacting proteins and signaling pathways are responsible for determining dorsal and ventral structures. The morphogen sonic hedgehog (discussed later) participates in setting up the axis of dorsal-ventral polarity along the spinal cord.

- Finally, a left-right axis must be established. The left-right axis is essential for proper heart development and positioning of viscera. It is established by the leftward flow of fluid from motile cilia present in the node where cell migration occurs during gastrulation. Interruption of placement or rotation of these cilia results in randomization of left-right axis determination, termed situs inversus, in which some thoracic and abdominal viscera are on the wrong side of the chest and abdomen, as well as infertility in males. Such ciliary defects can also cause cardiac anomalies.

The three axes that must be specified in the whole embryo must also be specified early in the developing limb. Within the limb, the organism must specify the proximal-distal axis (shoulder to fingertip), the anterior-posterior axis (thumb to fifth finger), and the dorsal-ventral axis (dorsum to palm). On a cellular scale, individual cells also develop an axis of polarity (e.g., the basal-apical axis of the proximal renal tubular cells or the axons and dendrites of a neuron). Thus specifying axes in the whole embryo, in limbs, and in cells is a fundamental process in development.

Once an organismal axis is determined, the embryo then overlays a patterning program onto that axis. Conceptually, if axis formation can be considered as the drawing of a line through an undeveloped mass of cells and specifying which end is to be the head and which end the tail, then patterning is the division of the embryo into segments and the assignment to these segments of an identity, such as head, thorax, or abdomen. The *HOX* genes (discussed in the next section) have major roles in determining the different structures that develop along the anterior-posterior axis. The end result of these pattern specification programs is that cells or groups of cells are assigned an identity related primarily to their position within the organism. This identity is subsequently used by the cells as an instruction to specify how development should proceed.

Pattern Formation and the *HOX* Gene System

The **homeobox (*HOX*) gene** system, first described in the fruit fly *Drosophila melanogaster*, constitutes a paradigm in developmental biology. *HOX* genes are so named because the proteins they encode are transcription factors that contain a conserved DNA-binding motif called the homeodomain. The segment of the gene encoding the homeodomain is called a *homeobox*, thus giving the **gene family** its name, *HOX*.

Many species of animals have *HOX* genes, and the homeodomains encoded by these genes are similar; however, different species contain different numbers of *HOX* genes (e.g., fruit flies contain 8 and humans nearly 40). The 40 human *HOX* genes are organized into four clusters on four different chromosomes. Strikingly, the order of the individual genes within the clusters is conserved across species. The human *HOX* gene clusters (Fig. 15.14) were generated by a series of gene duplication events, conceptually similar to those described in

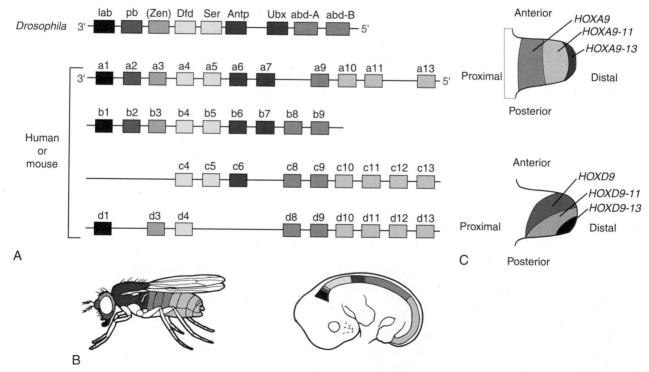

Figure 15.14 Action and arrangement of *HOX* genes. (A) An ancestral *HOX* gene cluster in a common ancestor of vertebrates and invertebrates has been quadruplicated in mammals, and individual members of the ancestral cluster have been lost. (B) The combination of *HOX* genes expressed in adjacent regions along the anteroposterior axis of developing embryos selects a unique developmental fate (as color-coded in the segments of the fly and human embryo). (C) In the developing limbs, different combinations of *HOXA* and *HOXD* genes are expressed in adjacent zones that help specify developmental fate along the proximal-distal and anterior-posterior axes. (From Wolpert L, Beddington R, Brockes J, et al: *Principles of development*, New York, 1998, Oxford University Press. Copyright 1998, Oxford University Press.)

Chapter 12 for the evolution of the globin gene family. Initially, ancient events duplicated the original ancestral *HOX* gene in tandem along a single chromosome. Subsequent duplications of this single set of *HOX* genes and relocation of the new gene set to other locations in the genome resulted in four unlinked *HOX* gene clusters in humans (and other mammals) named *HOXA*, *HOXB*, *HOXC*, and *HOXD*.

Unique combinations of *HOX* gene expression in small groups of cells, located in particular regions of the embryo, help determine the developmental fate of those regions. Just as specific combinations of *HOX* genes from the single *HOX* gene cluster in the fly are expressed along the anterior-posterior axis of the body and regulate different patterns of gene expression and therefore different body structures (see Fig. 15.14), mammals use a number of *HOX* genes from different clusters to accomplish similar tasks. Early, in the whole embryo, HOX transcription factors specify the anterior-posterior axis: the *HOXA* and *HOXB* clusters, for example, act along the rostral-caudal axis to determine the identity of individual vertebrae and somites. Later in development, the *HOXA* and *HOXD* clusters determine regional identity along the axes of the developing limb.

One interesting aspect of *HOX* gene expression is that the order of the genes in a cluster parallels the position in the embryo in which that gene is expressed and the time in development when it is expressed (see Fig. 15.14). In other words, the position of a *HOX* gene in a cluster is collinear with both the timing of expression and the location of expression along the anterior-posterior axis in the embryo. For example, in the *HOXB* cluster, the genes expressed first and in the anterior portion of the embryo are at one end of the cluster; the order of the rest of the genes in the cluster parallels the order in which they are expressed, both by location along the anterior-posterior axis of the embryo and by timing of expression. Although this gene organization is distinctly unusual and is not a general feature of gene organization in the genome (see Chapter 3), a similar phenomenon is seen within another developmentally regulated human gene family, the globin gene cluster (see Chapter 12). In both cases, the association of spatial organization in the genome with temporal expression in development presumably reflects long-range regulatory elements in the genome that govern the epigenetic packaging and accessibility of different genes at different times in the embryo.

The *HOX* gene family thus illustrates several important principles of developmental biology and evolution:
- *First*, a group of genes functions together to accomplish similar general tasks at different times and places in the embryo.
- *Second*, homologous structures are generated by sets of homologous transcription factors derived from common evolutionary predecessors. For example,

flies and mammals have a similar basic body plan (head anterior to the trunk, with limbs emanating from the trunk, cardiorespiratory organs anterior to digestive), and that body plan is specified by a set of genes that were passed down through common evolutionary predecessors.
- *Third*, patterns of expression of these homologues are distinct but overlapping. The intersection of these distinct patterns provides unique combinations of transcription factors that specify cellular diversity. For example, *HOXD9-13* genes are expressed in the most distal part of the developing limb bud (see Fig. 15.14) while *HOXA9-13* are expressed only in the posterior region of the developing limb bud. Cells that express both *HOXD9-13* and *HOXA9-13* are specified into posterior distal limb bud and limb, while cells that express *HOXD9-13* and *HOXA9-11* are specified into more anterior limb bud and limb.
- And *fourth*, although it is not usually the case with genes involved in development, the *HOX* genes show a remarkable genomic organization within a cluster that correlates with their function during development.

CELLULAR AND MOLECULAR MECHANISMS IN DEVELOPMENT

In this section we review the basic cellular and molecular mechanisms that regulate development (see Box 15.3). We illustrate each mechanism with a human birth defect or disease that results from the failure of each of these normal mechanisms.

BOX 15.3 FUNDAMENTAL MECHANISMS OPERATING IN DEVELOPMENT

- Gene regulation by transcription factors
- Cell-cell signaling by direct contact and by morphogens
- **Induction** of cell shape and polarity
- Cell movement
- Programmed cell death

Gene Regulation by Transcription Factors

Transcription factors control development by controlling the expression of other genes, some of which are also transcription factors. Groups of transcription factors that function together are referred to as transcriptional regulatory modules, and the functional dissection of these modules is an important task of the developmental geneticist and, increasingly, of genome biologists. Some transcription factors activate target genes and others repress them. Still other transcription factors have both activator and repressor functions (so-called bifunctional transcription factors); noncoding RNAs such as **microRNAs** also interact with target sequences and can activate or repress gene expression. The recruitment of these various activators and repressors within chromatin can be guided by histone modifications such as acetylation, and the regulation of histone modifications is accomplished by histone acetyltransferases and deacetylases (see Chapter 3). These epigenetic changes to histones are marks that indicate whether a particular gene is likely to be active or inactive. Regulatory modules control development by causing different combinations of transcription factors to be expressed at different places and at different times to direct the spatiotemporal regulation of development. By directing differential gene expression across space and time, the binding of various transcriptional regulatory modules to transcriptional complexes is controlled by histone modifications and is a central element of the development of the embryo.

Transcriptional regulatory complexes are localized into clusters of topologically associating domains (TADs) that allow for loop extrusion of DNA between CTCT sites, bringing otherwise distal gene-regulatory elements (i.e., enhancers and silencers) into 3D proximity of target genes to regulate their expression (see Chapter 3). Such **loops** regulate the communication between gene-regulatory elements and genes by bringing general transcription factors together with the specific transcription factors that are responsible for creating the selectivity of a transcriptional complex (Fig. 15.15). Most general transcription factors are found in thousands of these transcriptional complexes throughout the genome, and although each is essential, their roles in development are nonspecific. Specific transcription factors bind to enhancers and participate in forming active transcription factor complexes, mostly under the control of epigenetic marks of histone modifications, but only in specific cells or at specific times in development, thereby providing the regulation of gene expression that allows developmental processes to be exquisitely controlled.

The importance of transcription factors in normal development is illustrated by an unusual mutation of *HOXD13* that causes synpolydactyly, an **incompletely** dominant condition in which heterozygotes have interphalangeal webbing and extra digits in their hands and feet. Rare homozygotes have similar but more severe abnormalities and have bone malformations of the hands, wrists, feet, and ankles (Fig. 15.16). The *HOXD13* variant responsible for synpolydactyly is caused by expansion of a polyalanine tract in the amino-terminal domain of the protein; the normal protein contains 15 alanines, whereas the mutant protein contains 22 to 24 alanines. The polyalanine expansion that causes synpolydactyly is likely to act by a gain-of-function mechanism (see Chapter 12), as heterozygosity for a *HOXD13* loss-of-function variant has only a mild effect on limb development, characterized by a rudimentary extra digit between the first and second metatarsals and between the fourth and fifth metatarsals of the feet. Regardless of the exact mechanism, this condition demonstrates that a general function for *HOX* genes is to determine regional identity along specific body axes during development.

Morphogens and Cell-to-Cell Signaling

One of the hallmarks of developmental processes is that cells must communicate with each other to develop proper spatial arrangements of tissues and cellular subtypes. This communication occurs through cell signaling mechanisms. These cell-cell communication systems are commonly composed of a cell surface receptor and the molecule, called a ligand, that binds to it. On ligand binding, receptors transmit their signals through intracellular signaling pathways. One of the common ligand-receptor pairs is the fibroblast growth factors and their receptors. There are 23 recognized members of the fibroblast growth factor gene family in the human, and many of them are important in development. The fibroblast growth factors serve as ligands for tyrosine kinase receptors. Abnormalities in fibroblast growth factor receptors cause diseases such as achondroplasia (Case 2) (see Chapter 7) and certain syndromes that involve abnormalities of craniofacial development, referred to as craniosynostoses because they demonstrate premature fusion of cranial sutures in the skull.

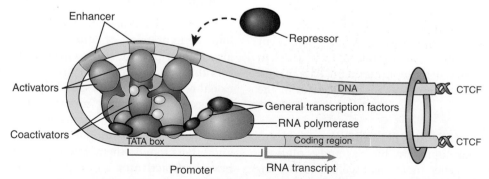

Figure 15.15 Activation of transcription occurs in transcriptional complexes that form loops from topologically associated domains (TADs, see Chapter 3). General transcription factors *(blue)*, and RNA polymerase bind to *cis*-acting sequences closely adjacent to the messenger RNA (mRNA) transcriptional start site; these *cis*-acting sequences are collectively referred to as the promoter. More distal enhancer or silencer elements bind specialized and tissue-specific transcription factors. Coactivator proteins facilitate a biochemical interaction between specialized and general transcription factors. (Redrawn from Tjian R: Molecular machines that control genes, *Sci Am* 272:54–61, 1995.)

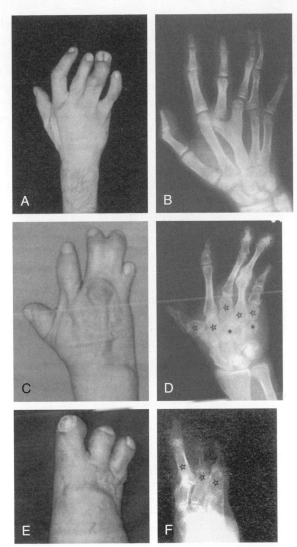

Figure 15.16 An unusual gain-of-function variant in *HOXD13* creates an abnormal protein with a dominant negative effect. Photographs and radiographs show the synpolydactyly phenotype. (A, B) Hand and radiograph of an individual heterozygous for a *HOXD13* variant. Note the branching metacarpal III and the resulting extra digit IIIa. The syndactyly between digits has been partially corrected by surgical separation of III and IIIa-IV. (C, D) Hand and radiograph of an individual homozygous for a *HOXD13* variant. Note syndactyly of digits III, IV, and V and their single knuckle; the transformation of metacarpals I, II, III, and V to short carpal-like bones *(stars)*; two additional carpal bones *(asterisks)*; and short second phalanges. The radius, ulna, and proximal carpal bones appear normal. (E, F) Foot and radiograph of the same homozygous individual. Note the relatively normal size of metatarsal I, the small size of metatarsal II, and the replacement of metatarsals III, IV, and V with a single tarsal-like bone *(stars)*. (Reprinted with permission from Muragaki Y, Mundlos S, Upton J, et al: Altered growth and branching patterns in synpolydactyly caused by mutations in *HOXD13*, *Science* 272:548–551, 1996.)

One of the best examples of a developmental morphogen is hedgehog, originally discovered in *Drosophila* and named for its ability to alter the orientation of epidermal bristles. Diffusion of the hedgehog protein creates a gradient in which different concentrations of the protein cause surrounding cells to assume different fates. In humans, three genes closely related to *Drosophila*

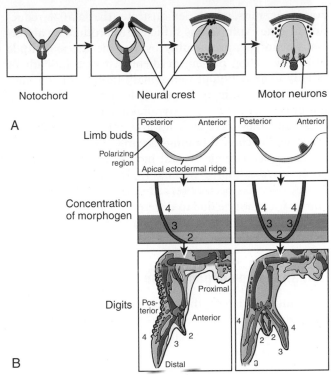

Figure 15.17 (A) Transverse section of the developing neural tube. Sonic hedgehog protein released from the notochord diffuses upward to the ventral portion of the developing neural tube *(brown)*; high concentrations immediately above the notochord induce the floor plate, whereas lower concentrations more laterally induce motor neurons. Ectoderm above (dorsal to) the neural tube releases bone morphogenetic proteins that help induce neural crest development at the dorsal edge of the closing neural tube *(dark purple)*. (B) Morphogenetic action of the sonic hedgehog (SHH) protein during limb bud formation. SHH is released from the zone of polarizing activity (labeled polarizing region in B) in the posterior limb bud to produce a gradient (shown with its highest levels as 4, declining to 2). Mutations or transplantation experiments that create an ectopic polarizing region in the anterior limb bud cause a duplication of posterior limb elements. (A, From Lumsden A, Graham A: Neural patterning: A forward role for hedgehog, *Curr Biol* 5:1347–1350, 1995. Copyright 1995, Elsevier Science; B, from Wolpert L, Beddington R, Brockes J, et al: *Principles of development*, New York, 1998, Oxford University Press.)

hedgehog also encode developmental morphogens; one example is the gene sonic hedgehog *(SHH)*. Although the specific programs controlled by hedgehog in *Drosophila* are very different from those controlled by its mammalian counterparts, the underlying themes and molecular mechanisms are similar. For example, secretion of the SHH protein by the notochord and the floor plate of the developing neural tube generates a gradient that induces and organizes the different types of cells and tissues in the developing brain and spinal cord (Fig. 15.17A). SHH is also produced by a small group of cells in the limb bud known as the **zone of polarizing activity,** which is responsible for establishing the posterior side of the developing limb bud and the asymmetric pattern of digits within individual limbs (see Fig. 15.17B).

Variants that inactivate the *SHH* gene in humans cause birth defects that may be inherited as autosomal dominant traits, which demonstrates that a 50% reduction in gene expression is sufficient to produce an abnormal phenotype, presumably by altering the magnitude of the hedgehog protein gradient. Affected individuals usually exhibit holoprosencephaly (failure of the midface and forebrain to develop), leading to absence of forebrain structures and hypotelorism (closely spaced eyes), and they have cleft lip and palate. On occasion, however, the clinical findings are mild or subtle such as, for example, a single central incisor or partial absence of the corpus callosum (Fig. 15.18). Because variable **expressivity** has been observed in members of the same family, it cannot be due to different variants and instead must reflect the action of modifier genes at other loci, chance, environment, or some combination of all three.

Cell Shape and Organization

Cells must organize themselves with respect to their position and polarity in their microenvironment. For example, kidney epithelial cells must undergo differential development of the apical and basal aspects of their organelles to effect reabsorption of solutes. The acquisition of polarity by a cell can be viewed as the cellular version of axis determination (as discussed in a previous section) with respect to the development of the overall embryo. Under normal circumstances, each renal tubular cell elaborates on its cell surface a filamentous structure, known as a primary cilium. One hypothesis is that the primary cilium is designed to sense fluid flow in the developing kidney tubule and signal the cell to stop proliferating and to polarize. Another hypothesis is that the primary cilium is a sort of cellular antenna that concentrates signal transduction components to facilitate activation or repression of developmental pathways.

There is substantial evidence that the sonic hedgehog signal transduction pathway acts in this fashion. Adult polycystic kidney disease (Case 37) is caused by loss of function of one of two protein components of primary cilia, polycystin 1 or polycystin 2, so that the cells fail to sense

fluid flow or to activate or repress signal transduction pathways properly. As a result, they continue to proliferate and do not undergo the appropriate developmental program of polarization, in which they stop dividing and display polarized expression of certain proteins on either the apical or basal aspect of the tubular epithelial cells (Fig. 15.19). The continued cell division leads to the formation of cysts, fluid-filled spaces lined by renal tubular cells.

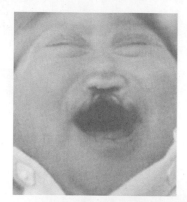

Figure 15.18 Variable expressivity of an *SHH* variant. The mother and her daughter carry the same missense variant in *SHH*, but the daughter is severely affected with microcephaly, abnormal brain development, hypotelorism, and a cleft palate, whereas the only manifestation in the mother is a single central upper incisor. (From Roessler E, Belloni E, Gaudenz K, et al: Mutations in the human Sonic Hedgehog gene cause holoprosencephaly, *Nat Genet* 14:357–360, 1996.)

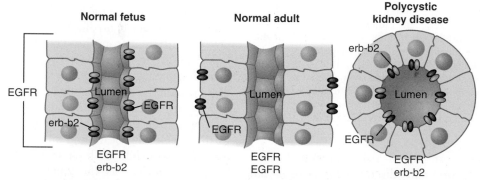

Figure 15.19 Polarization of epidermal growth factor receptor (EGFR) in epithelium from a normal fetus, a normal adult, and a patient with polycystic kidney disease. Fetal cells and epithelial cells from patients with polycystic kidney disease express a heterodimer of EGFR and erb-b2 at apical cell membranes. In normal adults, tubular epithelia express homodimeric complexes of EGFR at the basolateral membrane. (Modified from Wilson PD: Polycystic kidney disease, *N Engl J Med* 350:151–164, 2004. Copyright 2004, Massachusetts Medical Society.)

Cell Migration

Programmed cell movement is essential in development, and one region where it is critical is the central nervous system. The human central nervous system develops from the neural tube, a cylinder of cells created during weeks 4 to 5 of embryogenesis. Much of our knowledge of early development of the central nervous system derives from the mouse and mouse models of neurodevelopmental disorders. Initially, the neural tube is only a single cell layer thick, a pseudostratified columnar epithelium. Once sufficient neuroepithelial cells are produced by vertical and symmetrical division, these cells divide asymmetrically as neural stem cells. These neural stem cells stretch from the apical surface adjacent to the ventricle to the basal surface. The nucleus of these neural stem cells is adjacent to the apical surface in the ventricular cell layer situated adjacent to the ventricle, and the fiber of these cells stretches to the basal or pial

surface as the so-called radial glial cells. When these radial glia (one type of neural stem cells) divide vertically and asymmetrically, they generate new neural stem cells as well as committed neuronal precursors and secondary neural stem cells. These secondary, more basally located neural stem cells can then amplify the number of cells produced from a given radial glial progenitor. Postmitotic neuronal precursors then migrate outward toward the pial surface along the radial glia. The central nervous system is built by waves of migration of these neuronal precursors. The neurons that populate the inner layers of the cortex migrate earlier in development, and each successive wave of neurons passes through the previously deposited, inner layers to form the next outer layer (Fig. 15.20A). The complex interplay of the production of neurons from these neuronal precursors (neurogenesis) and their movement to precise locations (neuronal migration) results in the remarkable and specific wiring of the central nervous system.

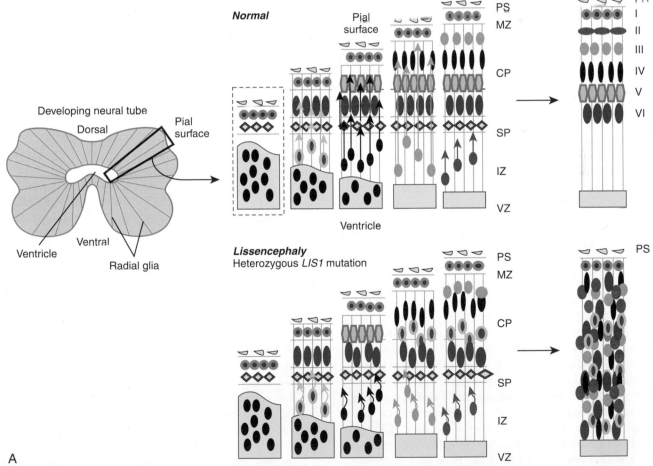

Figure 15.20 (A) The role of neuronal migration in normal cortical development and the defective migration in individuals heterozygous for a *LIS1* mutation causing lissencephaly. *(Top)* A radial slice is taken from a normal developing neural tube of the mouse, showing the progenitor cells at the ventricular zone *(VZ)*. These cells divide, differentiate into postmitotic cells, and migrate radially along a scaffold made up of glia. The different shapes and colors represent the cells that migrate and form the various cortical layers: *IZ*, intermediate zone; *SP*, subplate; *CP*, cortical plate; *MZ*, marginal zone; *PS*, pial surface. The six distinguishable layers of the normal cortex (molecular, external granular, external pyramidal, internal granular, internal pyramidal, multiform) that occupy the region of the cortical plate are labeled I through VI. *(Bottom)* Aberrant migration and failure of normal cortical development seen in lissencephaly.

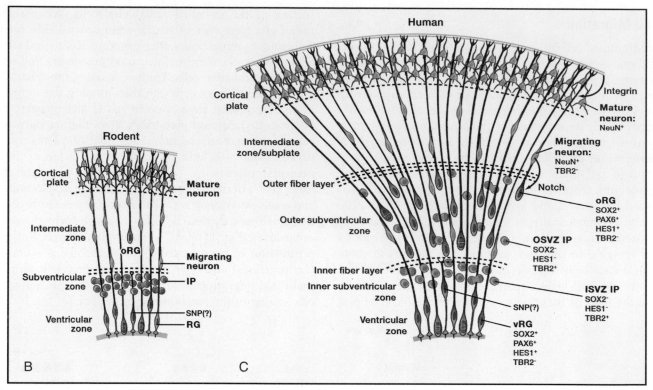

Figure 15.20, cont'd (B, C) The human brain contains expansion of a novel class of early neural precursors termed basal (or outer subventricular zone) radial glia that are attached to the basal (pial) surface but not the apical surface. These cells are found in the mouse, but in very small numbers, while their numbers are greatly expanded in primates, including humans. (A, Diagram modified from Gupta A, Tsai L-H, Wynshaw-Boris A: Life is a journey: A genetic look at neocortical development, *Nat Rev Genet* 3:342–355, 2002. B and C, from Lui JH, Hansen DV and Kriegstein AR. Development and evolution of the human neocortex, *Cell* 146:18–36, 2011.)

More recently, it has been possible to observe the early development of the human brain from fetal tissue obtained from elective pregnancy termination. These studies revealed that the human brain contains expansion of a novel class of early neural precursors termed basal (or outer subventricular zone) radial glia that are attached to the basal (pial) surface, but not the apical surface (see Fig. 15.20B and C). These cells are found in the mouse (Fig. 15.21B), but in very small numbers, while their numbers are greatly expanded in primates including humans (see Fig. 15.21C), leading to the idea that the basal radial glial expansion during primate evolution is a major cause of the increased size of the primate and human brain. The basal radial glia divide horizontally, unlike the ventricular zone radial glia.

Lissencephaly (literally, "smooth brain") is a severe abnormality of brain development causing profound intellectual disability. This developmental defect is one component of the Miller-Dieker syndrome (Case 32), which is caused by a contiguous gene deletion syndrome that involves one copy of the *LIS1* gene on chromosome 17. When there is **heterozygous** loss of *LIS1* function, there is a disruption of both neurogenesis of ventricular and basal radial glia, as well as defective neuronal migration (see Fig. 15.20A). The result is a thickened, hypercellular cerebral cortex with undefined cellular layers and poorly developed gyri, thereby making the surface of the brain appear smooth.

In addition to the neuronal migrations described, another remarkable example of cell migration involves the neural crest, a population of cells that arises from the dorsolateral aspect of the developing neural tube (see Fig. 15.17A). Neural crest cells must migrate from their original location at the dorsal and lateral surface of the neural tube to remarkably distant sites, such as the ventral aspect of the face, the ear, the heart, the gut, and many other tissues, including the skin, where they differentiate into pigmented melanocytes.

Population of the gut by neural crest progenitors gives rise to the autonomic innervation of the gut; failure of that migration leads to the aganglionic colon seen in Hirschsprung disease. The genetics of Hirschsprung disease are complex (see Chapter 9), but a number of key signaling molecules have been implicated. One of the best characterized is the *RET* **protooncogene**. As discussed in Chapter 9, pathogenic variants in *RET* have been identified in ~50% of patients with Hirschsprung disease.

Another example of defects in neural crest development is the group of birth defects known as the Waardenburg syndrome, which includes defects in skin and hair pigmentation, coloration of the iris, and colon innervation (see Fig. 15.21). This syndrome can be caused by pathogenic variants in at least four different transcription factors, each resulting in abnormalities in neural crest development.

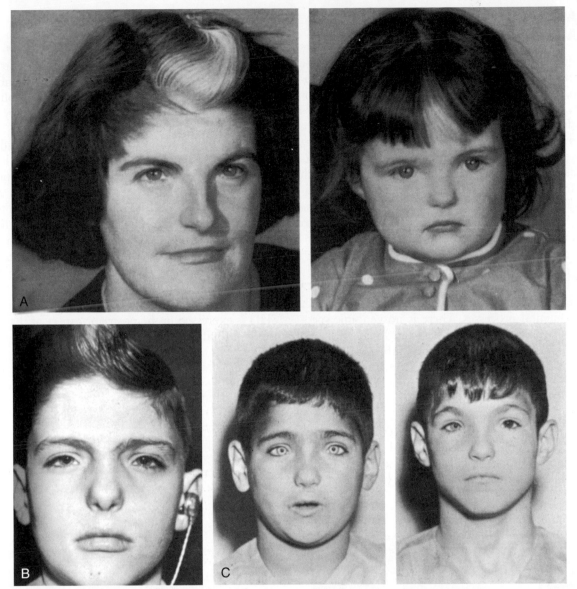

Figure 15.21 **Patients with type I Waardenburg syndrome.** (A) Mother and daughter with white forelocks. (B) A 10-year-old with congenital deafness and white forelock. (C) Brothers, one of whom is deaf. There is no white forelock, but the boy on the right has heterochromatic irides. Pathogenic variants of *PAX3*, which encodes a transcription factor involved in neural crest development, cause type I Waardenburg syndrome. (A, From Partington MW: An English family with Waardenburg's syndrome, *Arch Dis Child* 34:154–157, 1959; B, from DiGeorge AM, Olmsted RW, Harley RD: Waardenburg's syndrome. A syndrome of heterochromia of the irides, lateral displacement of the medial canthi and lacrimal puncta, congenital deafness, and other characteristic associated defects, *J Pediatr* 57:649–669, 1960; C, from Jones KL: *Smith's recognizable patterns of human malformation*, ed 6, Philadelphia, 2005, WB Saunders.)

Programmed Cell Death

Programmed cell death is a critical function in development and is necessary for the morphologic development of many structures. It occurs wherever tissues need to be remodeled during morphogenesis, as during the separation of the individual digits, in perforation of the anal and choanal membranes, or in the establishment of communication between the uterus and vagina.

One major form of programmed cell death is apoptosis. Studies of mice with loss-of-function variants in the *Foxp1* gene indicate that apoptosis is required for the remodeling of the tissues that form portions of the ventricular septum and cardiac outflow tract (endocardial cushions), to ensure the normal positioning of the origins of the aortic and pulmonary vessels. By eliminating certain cells, the relative position of the cushions is shifted into their correct location. It is also suspected that defects of apoptosis underlie some other forms of human congenital heart disease (see Chapter 9), such as the conotruncal heart defects of DiGeorge syndrome caused by deletion of the *TBX1* gene located in chromosome 22q11 (see Chapter 6). Apoptosis also occurs during development of the immune system to eliminate lymphocyte lineages that react to self, thereby preventing autoimmune disease.

INTERACTION OF DEVELOPMENTAL MECHANISMS IN EMBRYOGENESIS

Embryogenesis requires the coordination of multiple developmental processes in which proliferation, differentiation, migration, and apoptosis all play a part. For example, many processes must occur to convert a mass of mesoderm into a heart or a layer of neuroectoderm into a spinal cord. To understand how these processes interact and work together, developmental biologists typically study embryogenesis in a model organism, such as fish, frogs, worms, flies, chicks, mice, or other animal species. The general principles elucidated by these more easily manipulated systems can then be applied to understanding developmental processes in humans.

The Limb as a Model of Organogenesis

The vertebrate limb is a relatively well-studied product of developmental processes. There is no genomic specification for a human arm to be ~1 m long, with one proximal bone, two bones in the forelimb, and 27 bones in the hand. Instead, the limb results from a series of regulated processes that specify development along three axes, the proximal-distal axis, the dorsal-ventral axis, and the anterior-posterior axis (Fig. 15.22).

Limbs begin as protrusions of proliferating cells, the limb buds, along the lateral edge of the mesoderm of the human embryo in the fourth week of development. The location of each limb bud along the anterior-posterior axis of the embryo (head-to-tail axis) is associated with the expression of a specific transcription factor at each location, *TBX4* for the hindlimbs and *TBX5* for the forelimbs, whose expression is induced by various combinations of fibroblast growth factor ligands. Thus the primarily proliferative process of limb bud outgrowth is activated by growth factors and transcription factors.

The limb bud grows primarily in an outward, lateral expansion of the proximal-distal axis of the limb (see Fig. 15.17B). Whereas proximal-distal expansion of the limb is the most obvious process, the two other axes are established soon after the onset of limb bud outgrowth. The anterior-posterior axis is set up soon after limb bud outgrowth, with the thumb considered to be an anterior structure because it is on the edge of the limb facing the upper body. The fifth finger is a posterior structure because it is on the side of the limb bud oriented toward the lower part of the body. During limb formation, the morphogen SHH is expressed in the posterior aspect of the developing limb bud, and its expression level forms a gradient

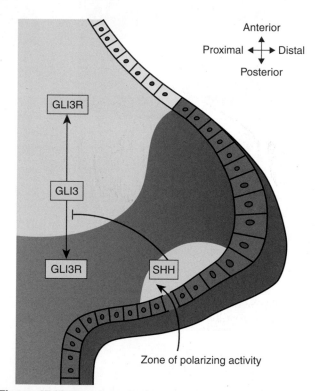

Figure 15.23 Schematic diagram of the anterior-posterior and proximal-distal axes of the limb bud and its molecular components. In this diagram, the anterior aspect is up and the distal aspect is to the right. SHH expression occurs in the zone of polarizing activity of the posterior limb bud. SHH inhibits conversion of the GLI3 transcription factor to GLI3R in the posterior regions of the limb bud. However, SHH activity does not extend to anterior regions of the bud. The absence of SHH allows GLI3 to be converted to GLI3R (a transcriptional repressor) in the anterior limb bud. By this mechanism, the anterior-posterior axis of the limb bud is established with a gradient of GLI3 versus GLI3R. (Modified from Gilbert SF: *Developmental biology*, ed 7, Sunderland, Massachusetts, 2003, Sinauer Associates.)

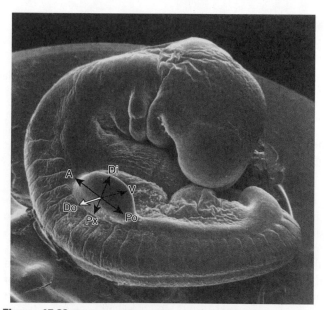

Figure 15.22 This scanning electron micrograph of a 4-week human embryo illustrates the early budding of the forelimb. Overlaid onto the bud are the three axes of limb specification: *Do-V*, dorsal-ventral (dorsal comes out of the plane of the photo, ventral goes into the plane of the photo); *Px-Di*, proximal-distal; and *A-Po*, anterior-posterior. (From Carlson BM: *Human embryology and developmental biology*, ed 3, Philadelphia, 2004, Mosby.)

that is primarily responsible for setting up the anterior-posterior axis in the developing limb (see Fig. 15.17B). Defects in anterior-posterior patterning in the limb cause excessive digit patterning, manifested as polydactyly, or failure of complete separation of developing digits, manifested as syndactyly. The dorsal-ventral axis is also established, resulting in a palm or sole on the ventral side of the hand and foot, respectively.

One can now begin to understand the mechanisms underlying birth defect syndromes by applying knowledge from molecular developmental biology to human disorders. For example, variants in the *GLI3* transcription factor gene cause two pleiotropic developmental anomaly syndromes, the Greig cephalopolysyndactyly syndrome (GCPS) and the Pallister-Hall syndrome (see Fig. 15.1). These two syndromes comprise distinct combinations of limb, central nervous system, craniofacial, airway, and genitourinary anomalies that are caused by perturbed balance in the production of two variant forms of GLI3, referred to as GLI3 and GLI3R, as shown in Fig. 15.23. GLI3 is a component of the SHH signaling pathway. SHH signals, in part, through a cell surface receptor encoded by a gene called *PTCH1*, which is concentrated in the cilium of cells during development. Pathogenic variants in *PTCH1* cause the nevoid basal cell carcinoma syndrome. Also known as Gorlin syndrome, this syndrome comprises craniofacial anomalies and occasional polydactyly that are similar to those seen in GCPS, but in addition, Gorlin syndrome manifests dental cysts and susceptibility to basal cell carcinoma. By considering Gorlin syndrome and GCPS, one can appreciate that the two disorders share phenotypic manifestations precisely because the genes that are mutated in the two disorders have overlapping effects in the same developmental genetic pathway. A third protein in the SHH signaling pathway, the CREB-binding protein, or CBP, is a transcriptional coactivator of the GLI3 transcription factor. Pathogenic variants in *CBP* cause the Rubinstein-Taybi syndrome (see Fig. 15.5),

which also shares phenotypic manifestations with GCPS and Gorlin syndrome.

CONCLUDING COMMENTS

Many other examples of this phenomenon could be cited, but the key points to emphasize are that genes are the primary regulators of developmental processes, their protein products function in developmental genetic pathways, and these pathways are employed in related developmental processes in a number of organ systems. Understanding the molecular basis of gene function, how those functions are organized into modules, and how abnormalities in those modules cause and correlate with malformations and pleiotropic syndromes forms the basis of the modern clinical approach to human birth defects. The understanding of these developmental pathways in great detail may also provide an avenue in the future to devise therapies that target appropriate parts of these pathways.

GENERAL REFERENCES

Barresi MJF, Gilbert SF: *Developmental biology*, ed 12, Sunderland, 2020, Oxford University Press.

Carlson BM: *Human embryology and developmental biology*, ed 6, Philadelphia, 2018, WB Saunders.

Dye FJ: *Dictionary of developmental biology and embryology*, ed 2, New York, 2012, Wiley-Blackwell.

Erickson RP, Wynshaw-Boris AJ, editors: *Epstein's inborn errors of development: the molecular basis of clinical disorders of morphogenesis* ed 3, New York, 2016, Oxford University Press.

Wolpert L, Tickle C: *Principles of development*, ed 4, New York, 2011, Oxford University Press.

REFERENCES SPECIFIC TO PARTICULAR TOPICS

Acimovic I, Vilotic A, Pesl M, et al: Human pluripotent stem cell-derived cardiomyocytes as research and therapeutic tools, *Biomed Res Int* 2014:512831, 2014.

Ross CA, Akimov S: Human induced pluripotent stem cells: Potential for neurodegenerative diseases, *Hum Mol Genet* 23(R1):R17–R26, 2014.

PROBLEMS

1. What is the difference between regulative and mosaic development? What is the significance of these two stages of development for reproductive genetics and prenatal diagnosis?

2. Match the terms in the left-hand column with the terms that best fit in the right-hand column.

   a. Erasure of imprinting during germ cell development
   b. Position-dependent development
   c. Regulative development
   d. Embryonic stem cells

   1. Totipotency
   2. Morphogen
   3. Epigenetic regulation of gene expression
   4. Monozygotic twinning

3. Match the terms in the left-hand column with the terms that best fit in the right-hand column.

   a. Amniotic band
   b. Polydactyly
   c. Inadequate amniotic fluid
   d. Limb reduction
   e. Robin sequence

   1. U-shaped cleft palate
   2. Thalidomide
   3. *GLI3* mutation
   4. Disruption
   5. Deformation

4. What type of diploid cells would not be appropriate nucleus donors in an animal cloning experiment and why?

5. For discussion: Why do some pathogenic variants in transcription factors result in developmental defects even when they are present in the heterozygous state?

CHAPTER 16

Cancer Genetics and Genomics

Michael F. Walsh

Cancer is a common disease. Overall, there are 14 million new cases of cancer diagnosed each year and over 8 million deaths from the disease worldwide. In the United States, there are 250,000 cases each of breast and prostate cancer, 150,000 cases of colon cancer, and over 100,000 cases of lung cancer diagnosed each year. Although cancer is the most common cause of disease-related death in children, pediatric cancer itself is a rare disease in comparison to adult cancer, with 16,000 new cases diagnosed in the United States annually. National costs for cancer care in the United States were estimated to be $190.2 billion in 2015 and $208.9 billion in 2020 (https://progressreport.cancer.gov/after/economic_burden). Identification of persons at increased **risk** for cancer before its development is an important objective of genetics research and clinical care. In the general population as well as in those with a heritable predisposition, early diagnosis and treatment is vital, and both are increasingly reliant on advances in **genome sequencing** and **gene** expression analysis. Historically, in the context of the **genetic** basis of cancer, the focus has been on somatic genetics as most cancer is considered to arise from stochastic acquisition of genetic (and **epigenetic**) events. However, distinguishing **germline** and **somatic** genetics is an important distinction in understanding the pathogenesis of the disease.

GERMLINE VERSUS SOMATIC

Germline refers to the sex cells (gametes) that are used by sexually reproducing organisms to pass on genes from generation to generation. Egg and sperm cells are called germ cells, as opposed to the other cells of the body that are referred to as somatic cells; somatic cells are any cell of the body except sperm and egg cells. **Mutations** in somatic cells can affect the individual, but they are not passed on to offspring.

NEOPLASIA

The word *cancer* originates from the Latin word for crab and refers to the aggressive and malignant forms of **neoplasia**, a disease process characterized by uncontrolled cellular proliferation leading to a mass or tumor. The abnormal accumulation of cells in a neoplasm occurs because of an imbalance between the normal processes of cellular proliferation and cellular attrition. Cells proliferate as they pass through the **cell cycle** and undergo **mitosis**. Attrition, due to programmed cell death (see Chapter 15), removes cells from a tissue. For a neoplasm to be a cancer, however, it must also be malignant, which means that not only is its growth uncontrolled, but it is also capable of invading neighboring tissues that surround the original site (the primary site) and can spread (metastasize) to more distant sites (Fig. 16.1). Tumors that do not invade or metastasize are not cancerous but are referred to as benign tumors, although their abnormal function, size, or location may make them anything but benign to the patient (e.g., disrupting visual pathways, impinging upon nerves or causing vascular stasis and thrombus).

Cancer is not a single disease. Rather, it comes in many forms and degrees of malignancy and varying biologic processes. There are three main classes of cancer:

- Sarcomas, in which the tumor has arisen in mesenchymal tissue, such as bone, muscle, or connective tissue, or in nervous system tissue
- Carcinomas, which originate in epithelial tissue, such as the cells lining the intestine, bronchi, or mammary ducts
- Hematopoietic and lymphoid malignant neoplasms, such as leukemia and lymphoma, which arise in cells of hematopoietic lineage, including bone marrow and the lymphatic system

Within each of the major groups, tumors are classified by site, tissue type, histologic appearance, degree of malignancy, chromosomal **aneuploidy**, and, increasingly, by which gene **variants**, fusions, and abnormalities in gene expression are found in the somatic landscape of the tumor as cataloged in data repositories such as the cBioPortal, COSMIC, PECAN, and Genomic Data Commons (GDC) (Table 16.1).

In this chapter we describe how genetic and genomic studies demonstrate that *cancer is fundamentally a genetic disease* and how cancer evolves because of genetic and environmental factors, as well as distinct patterns of cell turnover at distinct periods over a lifetime. First, we describe genes recognized and implicated

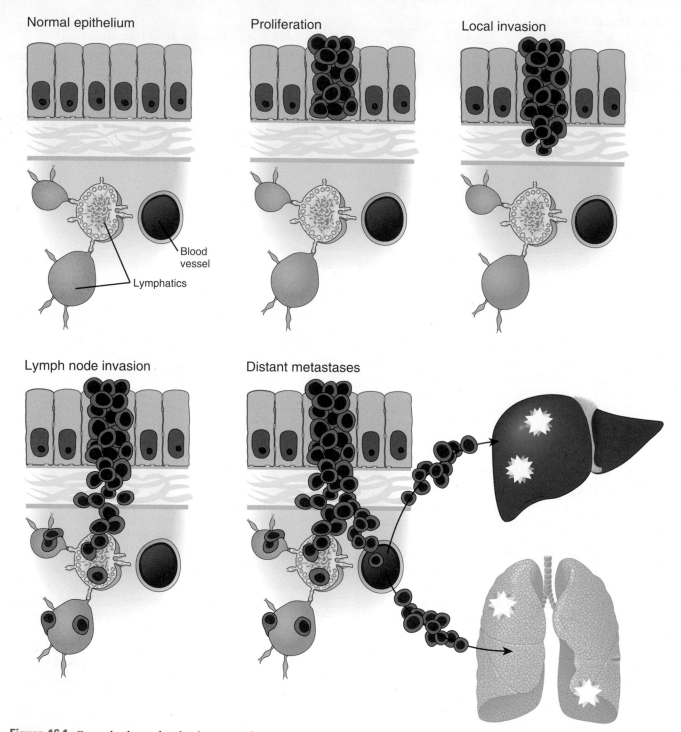

Figure 16.1 **General scheme for development of a carcinoma in an epithelial tissue such as colonic epithelium.** The diagram shows progression from normal epithelium to local proliferation, invasion across the lamina propria, spread to local lymph nodes, and final distant metastases to liver and lung.

in initiating cancer and the mechanisms by which dysfunction of these genes can result in disease. Second, we review heritable cancer **syndromes** and demonstrate how insights gained into their pathogenesis have illuminated the basis of the much more common, **sporadic** forms of cancer. We examine some of the special challenges that such heritable syndromes present for medical geneticists, genetic counselors, and oncologists. Third,

we illustrate ways in which genetics and **genomics** have changed both how we think about the causes of cancer and how we diagnose and treat the disease. The identification of mutations, altered epigenomic modifications, and abnormal gene expression in cancer cells is rapidly expanding our knowledge of why cancer develops and is truly changing approaches to cancer diagnosis and treatment. Furthermore, integrating somatic and germline

TABLE 16.1 Classes of Driver Genes Mutated in Cancer

Genes With Specific Effects on Cellular Proliferation or Apoptosis	Genes With Global Effects on Genome or DNA Integrity or on Gene Expression
Cell-cycle regulation Cell-cycle checkpoint proteins Cellular proliferation signaling • Transcription factors • Receptor and membrane-bound tyrosine kinases • Growth factors • Intracellular serine-threonine kinases • PI3 kinases • G proteins and G protein–coupled receptors • mTOR signaling • Wnt/β-catenin signaling • Transcription factors Differentiation and lineage survival • Transcription factors protecting specific cell lineages • Genes involved in exit from cell cycle into G_0 Apoptosis	Genome integrity • Chromosome segregation • Genome and gene mutation • DNA repair • Telomere stability Gene expression: abnormal metabolites affecting activity of multiple genes/gene products Gene expression: epigenetic modifications of DNA/chromatin • DNA methylation and hydroxymethylation • Chromatin histone methylation, demethylation, and acetylation • Nucleosome remodeling • Chromatin accessibility and compaction (SWI/SNF complexes) Gene expression: posttranscriptional alterations • Aberrant mRNA splicing • MicroRNAs affecting mRNA stability and translation Gene expression: protein stability/turnover

mRNA, Messenger RNA; *mTOR*, mammalian target of rapamycin; *PI3*, phosphatidylinositol-3.

variant data is enabling more rapid interpretations of variants detected in constitutional samples than possible without companion germline sequencing.

GENETIC BASIS OF CANCER

Driver and Passenger Gene Mutations

Applying **next generation sequencing (NGS)** (see Chapter 4) and **RNA** expression studies (see Chapter 3) has provided clarity to understanding the origins of cancer. By aggregating and analyzing thousands of samples obtained from a wide variety of cancer types, researchers continue building **The Cancer Genome Atlas**, a public catalog of variants, epigenomic modifications, and abnormal gene **expression profiles**, which is visualized in the GDC. This endeavor along with Project Genomics Evidence Neoplasia Information Exchange (GENIE) housed in the cBioPortal (https://www.cbioportal.org/) and the Pediatric Cancer Genome Project (PCGP) with illustrated data via the PECAN portal (https://pecan.stjude.cloud/) are tremendous undertakings toward the annotation and classification of genomic variation detected in human cancers. These efforts continue to grow, and findings thus far are extremely informative. The number of mutations present in a tumor can vary from just a few to many tens of thousands. In general, pediatric cancers are more "silent" than adult tumors in terms of the number of mutations detected; however, there are notable exceptions to this trend (e.g., constitutional biallelic **pathogenic variants** in the mismatch repair (MMR) genes result in a very high mutational burden in both pediatric and adult tumors). When identified, this exceptionally high tumor mutational burden indicates a consideration for immunotherapy. Most variants identified through tumor sequencing appear to be random, are not recurrent in particular cancer types,

and likely occurred as the cancer developed rather than directly causing the neoplasia to develop or progress. These are referred to as passenger mutations. However, a subset of a few hundred genes has repeatedly been found to be mutated at a frequency too high to be considered simply passenger in nature. These mutated genes occur in many samples of the same cancer type and often in multiple different types of cancers. They are presumed to be involved in the development or progression of the cancer itself and are therefore referred to as **driver genes**; that is, they harbor mutations (so-called driver mutations) that are likely to be causing a cancer to develop or progress. Although some driver genes are specific to particular tumor types, some, such as those in the *TP53* gene encoding the p53 protein, are found in the vast majority of cancers. Although the most common driver genes are now known, it is likely that additional, less common driver genes will be identified as The Cancer Genome Atlas continues to grow. Another resource in identifying driver genes, (https://cancerhotspots.org/) provides evidence for variants as oncogenic based on gene size, expected **mutation rate**, and cancer types detected. This database is supported by mathematical modeling and statistical rigor to determine the likelihood that a specific variant is oncogenic.

Spectrum of Driver Mutations

Various genomic alterations can act as driver mutations. In some cases, a single **nucleotide** change or small **insertion** or **deletion** can be a driver mutation. Large numbers of cell divisions are required to produce an adult organism of an estimated 10^{14} cells from a single-cell **zygote**. Given a frequency of 10^{-10} replication errors per DNA base per cell division, and an estimated 10^{15} cell divisions during the lifetime of an adult, replication errors alone result in thousands of new single nucleotide or small insertion/deletion variants in the **genome** in every cell of the organism. Some environmental agents, such as carcinogens in cigarette smoke or ultraviolet or X-irradiation, will increase the rate of mutation across the genome. If, by chance, mutations occur in critical driver genes in a particular cell, then the oncogenic process may be initiated and in some instances be evidenced by a tumor signature.

Gross **chromosome** and subchromosomal changes (see Chapters 5 and 6) can also serve as driver mutations. Particular **translocations** or fusions are sometimes highly specific for certain types of cancer and involve specific genes (e.g., the *BCR-ABL* translocation in chronic myelogenous leukemia) (Case 10). In contrast, other cancers can have complex rearrangements in which chromosomes break into numerous pieces and rejoin, forming novel and complex combinations (a process known as **chromothripsis** ["chromosome shattering"]). Finally, large genomic alterations involving many kilobases of DNA can form the basis for loss of function or increased function of one or more driver genes. Large genomic alterations include deletions of a segment of a chromosome or multiplication of a chromosomal segment to produce regions with many copies of the same gene (gene amplification). The nature of these chromosomal events may be driven by somatic or germline events. In the case of fusions, these are nearly always postzygotic events. Complex combinations may be driven by constitutional alterations, for example, in the case of *TP53* germline pathogenic variants associated with chromothripsis in some cancers. Large duplications or deletions may reflect constitutional or somatic origin.

The Cellular Functions of Driver Genes

The nature of some driver mutations comes as no surprise: the mutations directly affect specific genes that regulate processes that are readily understood to be important in oncogenesis. These processes include cell cycle regulation, cellular proliferation, **differentiation** and exit from the cell cycle, growth inhibition by cell-cell contacts, and programmed cell death (**apoptosis**). However, the effects of other driver mutations are not so readily understood and include genes that act more globally and indirectly affect the expression of many other genes. Included in this group are genes encoding products that maintain genome and DNA integrity or genes that affect gene expression, either at the level of **transcription** by epigenetic changes, at the posttranscriptional level through effects on **messenger RNA** (**mRNA**) translation or stability, or at the posttranslational level through their effects on protein turnover (see Table 16.1). Other driver genes affect **translation**, including, for example, genes that encode **noncoding RNAs** from which regulatory **microRNAs** (**miRNAs**) are derived (see Chapter 3). Many miRNAs have been found to be either overexpressed or down-regulated in various tumors, sometimes strikingly so. Because each miRNA may regulate as many as 200 different gene targets, over- or underexpression of miRNAs may have widespread oncogenic effects because many driver genes will be dysregulated. Noncoding miRNAs that impact gene expression and contribute to oncogenesis are referred to as oncomirs. *DICER1* is a gene encoding a protein involved in the production of miRNAs, and germline pathogenic variants in this gene predispose individuals to a number of benign and malignant tumors, including (among others) thyroid cancer, multinodular goiter, Sertoli-Leydig cell tumors, cystic nephroma, and pleuropulmonary blastoma.

Fig. 16.2 outlines how mutations in specific regulators of growth and in global guardians of DNA and genome integrity perturb normal homeostasis (see Fig. 16.2A), leading to a vicious cycle of loss of cell cycle control, uncontrolled proliferation, interrupted differentiation, and defects in apoptosis (see Fig. 16.2B).

Oncogenes and Tumor Suppressor Genes

Both classes of driver genes—those with specific effects on cellular proliferation or survival and those with global effects on genome or DNA integrity (see Table 16.1)—can be further divided into two functional categories depending on how they drive oncogenesis when mutated.

The first category includes **proto-oncogenes**. When mutated in particular ways, these genes become drivers through alterations that lead to excessive levels of activity. Once mutated in this way, driver genes of this type are referred to as activated **oncogenes**. Only a single mutation on one **allele** is typically sufficient for activation. The mutations that activate proto-oncogenes range from highly specific point mutations causing dysregulation or hyperactivity of a protein, to chromosome translocations that drive overexpression of a gene, to gene amplification events that create an overabundance of the encoded mRNA and protein product (Fig. 16.3).

The second, and more common, category of driver genes includes **tumor suppressor genes** (**TSGs**), mutations that cause a loss of expression of proteins necessary to control the development of cancers. To drive oncogenesis, loss of function of a TSG typically requires variants on both alleles. There are many ways that a cell can lose the function of TSG alleles; loss-of-function mechanisms range from missense, nonsense, or frameshift mutations to gene deletions or loss of a part or even an entire chromosome. Loss of function of TSGs can also result from epigenetic transcriptional silencing due to altered **chromatin** conformation or **promoter** methylation (see Chapter 3) or from translational silencing by miRNAs or disturbances in other components of the translational machinery (see Box).

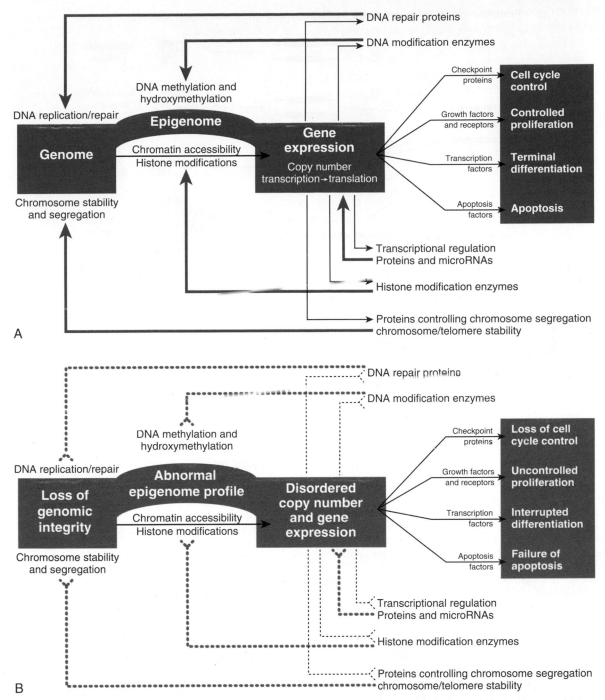

Figure 16.2 (A) Overview of normal genetic pathways controlling normal tissue homeostasis. The information encoded in the genome *(black arrows)* results in normal gene expression, as modulated by the epigenomic state. Many genes provide negative feedback *(purple arrows)* to ensure normal homeostasis. (B) Perturbations in neoplasia. Abnormalities in gene expression *(dotted black arrows)* lead to a vicious cycle of positive feedback *(brown dotted lines)* of progressively more disordered gene expression and genome integrity.

Cellular Heterogeneity Within Individual Tumors

The accumulation of driver mutations does not occur synchronously, in lockstep, in every cell of a tumor. To the contrary, cancer evolves along multiple lineages within a tumor, as chance mutational and epigenetic events in different cells activate proto-oncogenes and cripple the machinery for maintaining genome integrity, leading to more genetic changes in a vicious cycle

of more mutations and worsening growth control. The lineages that experience an enhancement of growth, survival, invasion, and distant spread will come to predominate as the cancer evolves and progresses (see Box 16.1). In this way the original **clone** of neoplastic cells evolves and gives rise to multiple sublineages, each carrying a set of mutations and epigenomic alterations that are different from but overlap with what is carried in other sublineages. The profile of mutations and epigenomic

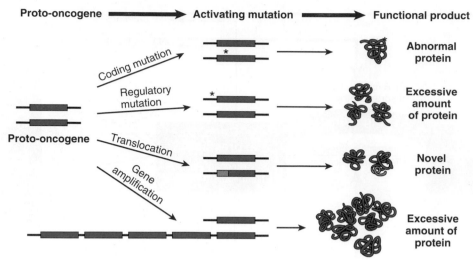

Figure 16.3 Different mutational mechanisms leading to proto-oncogene activation. These include a single point mutation leading to an amino acid change that alters protein function, mutations or translocations that increase expression of an oncogene; a chromosome translocation that produces a novel product with oncogenic properties; and gene amplification leading to excessive amounts of the gene product.

BOX 16.1 GENETIC BASIS OF CANCER

Regardless of whether a cancer occurs sporadically in an individual, purely as a result of **somatic mutation**, or repeatedly in many individuals in a family who share an inherited germline pathogenic variant, cancer is a genetic disease.

- Genes in which mutations cause cancer are referred to as **driver genes**, and the cancer-causing mutations in these genes are driver mutations.
- Driver genes fall into two distinct categories: proto-oncogenes and tumor suppressor genes (TSGs).
- An activated oncogene is a **mutant** allele of a **proto-oncogene**, a class of normal cellular protein-coding genes that promote growth and survival of cells. Activated oncogenes facilitate malignant **transformation** by stimulating proliferation or inhibiting apoptosis. Oncogenes encode proteins such as:
  - Those in signaling pathways that control cell proliferation
  - Transcription factors that control the expression of growth-promoting genes
  - Inhibitors of programmed cell death machinery
- A TSG is a gene in which loss of function through mutation or epigenetic silencing either directly removes normal regulatory controls on cell growth or leads indirectly to such losses through an increased mutation rate or aberrant gene expression. TSGs encode proteins

involved in many aspects of cellular function, including maintenance of correct chromosome number and structure, DNA repair, cell cycle regulation, cellular proliferation, or contact inhibition, just to name a few examples.

- Tumor initiation can be caused by different types of genetic alterations. These include:
  - Activating or gain-of-function mutations, including gene amplification, point mutations, and promoter mutations, that convert one allele of a proto-oncogene into an activated oncogene
  - Ectopic and heterochronic mutations (see Chapter 11) of proto-oncogenes
  - Chromosome translocations leading to gene fusions that cause misexpression of genes or create chimeric genes encoding proteins with novel functional properties
  - Loss of function of both alleles, or a **dominant negative** mutation of one allele, of a TSG
- Tumor progression occurs because of accumulating additional genetic damage, through mutations or epigenetic silencing, of driver genes that encode the machinery that repairs damaged DNA and maintains cytogenetic normality. A further consequence of genetic damage is altered expression of genes that promote vascularization and the spread of the tumor through local invasion and distant metastasis.

---

changes can differ between the primary and its metastases, between different metastases, and even between the cells of the original tumor or within a single **metastasis**. A paradigm for the development of cancer (Fig. 16.4) provides a useful conceptual framework for considering the role of genomic and epigenomic changes in the evolution of cancer, a point we emphasize throughout this chapter. It is a general model that applies to all cancers.

Although the focus of this chapter is on genomic and epigenomic changes within the tumor, the surrounding normal tissue also plays an important role by providing

the blood supply that nourishes the tumor, by permitting cancer cells to escape from the tumor and metastasize, and by shielding the tumor from immune attack. Thus cancer is a complex process, both within the tumor and between the tumor and the normal tissues that surround it.

CANCER IN FAMILIES

Although essentially all individuals are at risk to develop a cancer at some point during their lifetime, many forms of cancer have a higher incidence in relatives of people

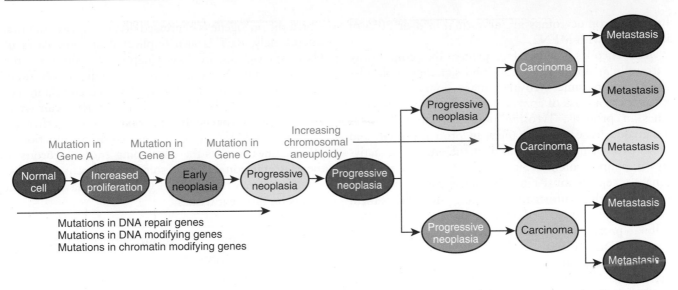

Figure 16.4 **Stages in the evolution of cancer.** Increasing degrees of abnormality are associated with sequential loss of tumor suppressor genes from several chromosomes and activation of proto-oncogenes, with or without a concomitant defect in DNA repair. Multiple lineages, carrying different mutations and epigenomic profiles, occur within the primary tumor itself, between the primary and metastases and between different metastases.

with cancer than in the general population. In some cases, this increased incidence is due primarily to inheritance of a single mutant gene with high **penetrance**. These pathogenic variants result in hereditary cancer syndromes (see, e.g., Cases 7, 29, 39, and 48) following **mendelian** patterns of inheritance that were presented in Chapter 7. Among these syndromes we currently know of ~100 different genes in which pathogenic variants increase the risk for cancer many-fold higher than in the general population. There are also many additional **genetic disorders** that are not usually considered to be hereditary cancer syndromes and yet include some increased predisposition to cancer (Case 6) (e.g., the 10- to 20-fold increased lifetime risk for leukemia in Down syndrome [see Chapter 6]). These clear examples notwithstanding, it is important to emphasize that not all families with an apparently increased incidence of cancer can be explained by known mendelian or clearly recognized genetic disorders. Many of these families likely represent the effects of both shared environment and one or more genetic variants that increase susceptibility and are therefore classified as multifactorial, with **complex inheritance** (see Chapter 9), as will be explored later in this chapter.

Individuals with a hereditary cancer predisposition likely represent at least 15% of all patients with cancer; identification of a genetic basis for their disease has great importance both for clinical management of these families and for understanding cancer in general. Identifying the heritable basis of cancer is important for diagnostics, screening, therapeutics, cascade testing, and family planning. Relatives of individuals with strong hereditary predispositions, in particular when due to pathogenic variants in a single gene, can be offered testing and counseling to provide appropriate reassurance or knowledge about their own risk, guidance on screening and early tumor detection, therapeutic considerations in the context of disease, prenatal and preconception counseling, and testing of other individuals in the family at risk. As is the case with many common diseases, understanding the hereditary forms of cancer provides crucial insights into disease mechanisms that go far beyond the rare hereditary forms themselves. Finally, in multiple studies over the last decade, pathogenic variants in a broad array of cancer predisposition genes have been revealed in agnostic studies, including various cancer populations. These concepts are illustrated in the examples discussed in the sections that follow.

Activated Oncogenes in Hereditary Cancer Syndromes

Multiple Endocrine Adenomatosis, Type 2

The type A variant of multiple endocrine neoplasia, type 2 (MEN2A), is an autosomal **dominant** disorder characterized by a high incidence of medullary carcinoma of the thyroid that is often but not always associated with pheochromocytoma, benign parathyroid adenomas, or both. Patients with the rarer type B variant (MEN2B) have, in addition to younger age of onset of the tumors seen in patients with MEN2A, thickening of nerves and the benign neural tumors, known as neuromas, on the mucosal surface of the mouth and lips and along the gastrointestinal tract.

The pathogenic variants responsible for MEN2 are in the *RET* oncogene. Individuals who inherit an activating variant in *RET* have a greater than 60% chance of developing medullary thyroid carcinoma. Blood tests for thyrocalcitonin or urinary catecholamines synthesized by pheochromocytomas are abnormal in over 90% of individuals with MEN2.

RET encodes a cell-surface protein that contains an extracellular domain that can bind signaling molecules and a cytoplasmic tyrosine kinase domain. Tyrosine kinases are a class of enzymes that phosphorylate tyrosines in proteins. Tyrosine phosphorylation initiates a signaling cascade of changes in protein-protein and DNA-protein interactions and in the enzymatic activity of many proteins (Fig. 16.5). Normally, tyrosine kinase receptors must bind specific signaling molecules to undergo the conformational change that makes them enzymatically active and able to phosphorylate other cellular proteins. The pathogenic variants in *RET* that cause MEN2 increase its kinase activity even in the absence of its ligand (a state referred to as constitutive activation).

The *RET* gene is expressed in many tissues of the body and is required for normal embryonic development of autonomic ganglia and the kidney. It is unclear why germline activating mutations in this proto-oncogene result in particular cancers of distinct histologic types restricted to specific tissues, whereas other tissues in which the oncogene is expressed do not develop tumors. Interestingly, *RET* is also implicated in some cases of Hirschsprung disease (see Chapter 9), although the associated pathogenic variants are usually loss of function, not activating. There are, however, some families in which the same pathogenic variant in *RET* can act as an activated oncogene in some tissues (such as thyroid) and cause MEN2A, and not have sufficient function in other tissues such as the developing enteric neurons of the gastrointestinal tract, resulting in Hirschsprung disease. Thus even the identical variant can have different effects on different tissues.

The Two-Hit Theory of Tumor Suppressor Gene Inactivation in Cancer

As introduced earlier, whereas the proteins encoded by proto-oncogenes promote cancer when activated or overexpressed, mutations in TSGs contribute to malignancy by a different mechanism—namely, the loss of function of both alleles of the gene. The products of many TSGs have now been isolated and characterized, some of which are presented in Table 16.2.

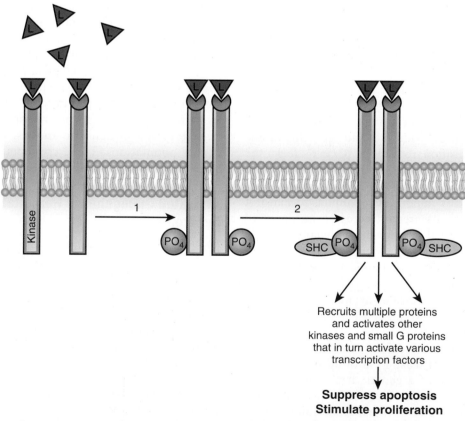

Figure 16.5 Schematic diagram of the function of the Ret receptor, the product of the *RET* proto-oncogene. Upon binding of a ligand (L), such as glial-derived growth factor or neurturin, to the extracellular domain, the protein dimerizes and activates its intracellular kinase domain to autophosphorylate specific tyrosine residues. These then bind the SHC adaptor protein, which sets off multiple cascades of complex protein interactions involving other serine-threonine and phosphatidylinositol kinases and small G proteins, which in turn activate other proteins, ultimately activating certain transcription factors that suppress apoptosis and stimulate cellular proliferation. Pathogenic variants in *RET* that result in the type A variant of multiple endocrine neoplasia, type 2 (MEN2A), cause inappropriate dimerization and activation of its own intrinsic kinase without ligand binding.

The existence of TSG mutations leading to cancer was proposed by Alfred Knudson some five decades ago to explain why certain tumors can occur in either hereditary or sporadic forms (Fig. 16.6) (see discussion in next section). It was suggested that the hereditary form of the childhood cancer retinoblastoma (see next section) might be initiated when a retinal cell in a person **heterozygous** for a germline pathogenic variant in the retinoblastoma TSG (now known to be *RB1*), required to prevent the development of the cancer, undergoes a second somatic event that inactivates the other *RB1* allele.

As a consequence of this second somatic event, the cell loses function of both alleles, giving rise to a tumor. In the sporadic form of retinoblastoma, both alleles are also inactivated, but in this case the inactivation results from two somatic events occurring in the same cell.

This so-called Knudson two-hit model is now widely accepted as the explanation for many hereditary cancers in addition to retinoblastoma, including cancers arising in **familial** adenomatous polyposis (FAP), hereditary breast cancer, neurofibromatosis type 1 (NF1), Lynch syndrome (LS), and Li-Fraumeni syndrome (LFS).

TABLE 16.2 Selected Tumor Suppressor Genes

Gene	Gene Product and Possible Function	Disorders in Which the Gene Is Affected	
		Familial	Sporadic
RB1	p110 Cell cycle regulation	Retinoblastoma	Retinoblastoma, small cell lung carcinomas, breast cancer
TP53	p53 Cell cycle regulation	Li-Fraumeni syndrome	Lung cancer, breast cancer, many others
APC	APC Multiple roles in regulating proliferation and cell adhesion	Familial adenomatous polyposis	Colorectal cancer
VHL	VHL Forms part of a cytoplasmic destruction complex with APC that normally inhibits induction of blood vessel growth when oxygen is present	von Hippel-Lindau syndrome	Clear cell renal carcinoma
BRCA1, BRCA2	BRCA1, BRCA2 Chromosome repair in response to double-stranded DNA breaks	Hereditary breast and ovarian cancer	Breast cancer, ovarian cancer
MLH1, MSH2, MSH6, PMS2, EPCAM	MLH1, MSH2, MSH6, PMS2, EPCAM Repair nucleotide mismatches between strands of DNA	Lynch syndrome	Colorectal cancer

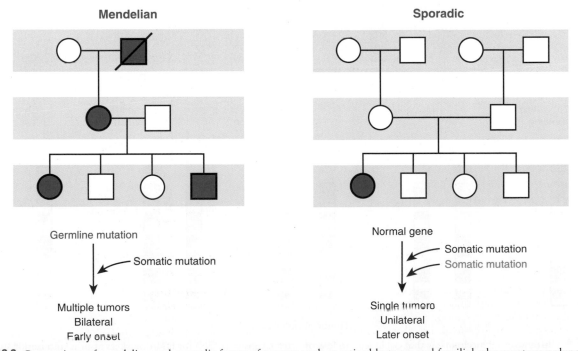

Figure 16.6 Comparison of mendelian and sporadic forms of cancers such as retinoblastoma and familial adenomatous polyposis of the colon. See text for discussion.

Tumor Suppressor Genes in Autosomal Dominant Cancer Syndromes

Retinoblastoma

Retinoblastoma is the prototype of diseases caused by a pathogenic variant in a TSG. It is a rare malignant tumor of the retina in infants, with an incidence of ~1 in 20,000 births (Fig. 16.7) (Case 39). It is the classic example put forth by Knudson, illustrating the role of a germline event leading to earlier age of disease and wider extent (unilateral vs bilateral). Treatment of a retinoblastoma may require removal of the affected eye; however, the advent of intraarterial chemotherapy has allowed many tumors to be effectively treated by local therapy so that vision can be preserved.

Approximately 40% of cases of retinoblastoma are of the heritable form, in which the child (as just discussed and as represented by the family shown in Fig. 16.6) has one germline pathogenic variant in *RB1*, either inherited from a heterozygous parent or which occurred *de novo*, or from a parent with **germline mosaicism** for the *RB1* pathogenic variant (see Chapter 7). In these children, retinal cells, which like all other cells of the body, are already carrying one defective *RB1* allele, suffer a somatic mutation in the other allele, leading to loss of function from both copies of *RB1* and initiating tumor development (Fig. 16.8).

The disorder appears to be inherited as a dominant trait because the large number of primordial retinoblasts and their rapid rate of proliferation make it very likely that a somatic mutation will occur as a second hit

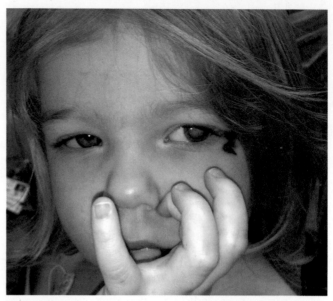

Figure 16.7 Retinoblastoma in a young girl, showing as a white reflex in the affected left eye when light reflects directly off the tumor surface. (Photograph courtesy B. L. Gallie, The Hospital for Sick Children, Toronto.)

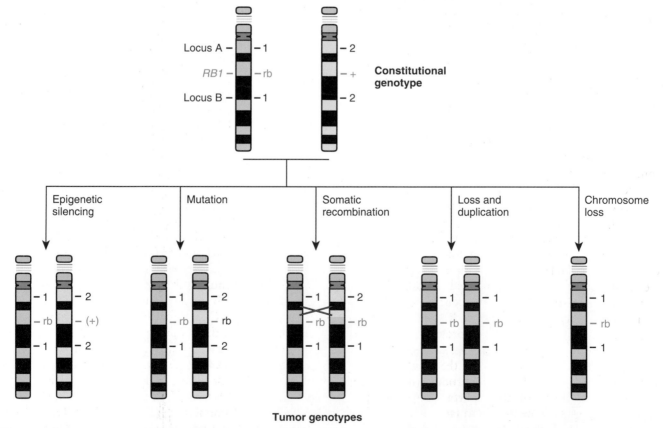

Figure 16.8 Chromosomal mechanisms that could lead to loss of heterozygosity (LOH) for DNA markers at or near a tumor suppressor gene in an individual heterozygous for a germline pathogenic variant. The figure depicts the events that constitute the second hit that leads to retinoblastoma with LOH. Local events such as mutation, gene conversion, or transcriptional silencing by promoter methylation, however, could also cause loss of function of both *RB1* genes without producing LOH. +, Normal allele; *rb*, mutant allele.

in one or more of the retinoblasts already carrying a heterozygous *RB1* pathogenic variant. Because the chance of a second hit is so great, **heterozygotes** for the disorder often have tumors arising at multiple sites, which may be multifocal tumors in one eye or both eyes (bilateral retinoblastoma), as well as less commonly in the pineal gland (referred to as trilateral retinoblastoma). The occurrence of a second hit is, however, a matter of chance and does not occur 100% of the time; thus the **penetrance** of heritable retinoblastoma is high (>90%) but not complete.

The other 60% of cases of retinoblastoma are sporadic; in these cases, both *RB1* alleles in a single retinal cell have been mutated or inactivated independently by chance, and the child does not carry a pathogenic *RB1* variant in the germline. Because two hits in the same cell is a statistically rare event, there is usually only a single clonal tumor: the retinoblastoma is found at one location (unifocal) in one eye only. However, a unilateral tumor does not guarantee that the child does not have the heritable form of retinoblastoma because 15% of patients with unilateral retinoblastoma have a germline pathogenic *RB1* variant. Another difference between hereditary and sporadic tumors is that the average age at onset of the sporadic form is in early childhood—later than in infants with the heritable form (see Fig. 16.6)—reflecting the longer time typically needed for two somatic mutations, rather than one, to occur.

In a few patients with retinoblastoma, the variant responsible is a cytogenetically detectable deletion or translocation of the portion of chromosome 13 containing the *RB1* gene. Such chromosomal changes, if they also disrupt genes adjacent to *RB1*, may cause a contiguous gene deletion syndrome involving varying degrees of developmental delay, **congenital anomalies**, and **dysmorphic features**.

Nature of the Second Hit. Typically, for retinoblastoma as well as for the other hereditary cancer syndromes, the first hit is an inherited pathogenic variant; that is, a change in the DNA **sequence**. The second hit, however, can be caused by a variety of genetic, epigenetic, or genomic mechanisms (see Fig. 16.8). Although it is most often a somatic mutation, loss of function without mutation, such as occurs with epigenetic silencing (see Chapter 3), has been observed. Although a number of mechanisms have been documented, the common theme is loss of function of *RB1*. The *RB1* gene product, p110 Rb1, is a phosphoprotein that normally regulates entry of the cell into the S **phase** of the cell cycle (see Chapter 2). Thus loss of the *RB1* gene and/or absence of the normal *RB1* gene product (by any mechanism) deprives cells of an important checkpoint and allows uncontrolled proliferation (see Table 16.2).

Loss of Heterozygosity. In addition to mutation and epigenetic silencing, a novel and important genomic mechanism was uncovered by geneticists who compared DNA polymorphisms at the *RB1* locus in DNA from normal cells to those in the retinoblastoma tumor from the same patient. Individuals with retinoblastoma who were informative by being heterozygous at polymorphic loci flanking the *RB1* locus in normal tissues (see Fig. 16.8) frequently had tumors with alleles from only one of their two chromosome 13 homologues. This reflected a **loss of heterozygosity (LOH)** in tumor DNA in and around the *RB1* locus. Furthermore, in familial cases, the retained chromosome 13 markers were the ones inherited from the affected parent. Thus, in these cases, LOH represents the second hit. LOH may occur by interstitial deletion, or by mechanisms such as mitotic recombination or **monosomy** 13 due to **nondisjunction** (see Fig. 16.8).

LOH is the most common mutational mechanism by which the function of the remaining normal *RB1* allele is disrupted in heterozygotes, although each of the mechanisms shown in Fig. 16.8 has been documented. LOH is a feature of a number of cancers, both heritable and sporadic, and is often considered evidence for a TSG in the region of LOH.

Hereditary Breast Cancer due to Pathogenic Variants in *BRCA1* or *BRCA2*

Breast cancer is common, with 250,000 women diagnosed annually in the United States alone. It is estimated that ~5% of breast cancer cases are due to a highly penetrant dominantly inherited mendelian predisposition that increases the risk for female breast cancer four- to sevenfold over the 12% lifetime risk observed in the general female population. In these families, one often sees features characteristic of hereditary (as opposed to sporadic) cancer: multiple affected individuals, earlier age at onset, frequent multifocal or bilateral disease or a second independent primary breast tumor, and additional primary cancers in other tissues such as ovary and pancreas.

Although a number of genes in which pathogenic variants cause highly penetrant mendelian forms of breast cancer have been discovered from family studies, the two genes responsible for the majority of all hereditary breast cancers are *BRCA1* and *BRCA2* (Case 7). Together, these two TSGs account for approximately one-half and one-third, respectively, of autosomal dominant familial breast cancer. Thousands of pathogenic variants in both genes have now been catalogued. Pathogenic variants in *BRCA1* and *BRCA2* are also associated with a significant increase in the risk for ovarian and fallopian duct cancer. Moreover, pathogenic variants in *BRCA2* and, to a lesser extent, *BRCA1* also account for 10% to 20% of all male breast cancer and increase the risk for male breast cancer 10- to 60-fold over the 0.1% lifetime risk in the general population (Table 16.3). *BRCA2* is also the most commonly mutated gene observed in men with metastatic prostate cancer.

The gene products of *BRCA1* and *BRCA2* are nuclear proteins contained within the same multiprotein complex. This complex has been implicated in the cellular response to double-stranded DNA breaks, such as those occurring during **homologous** recombination or because of damage to DNA. As might be expected for any TSG, tumor tissue from heterozygotes for *BRCA1* and *BRCA2* pathogenic variants frequently demonstrates LOH with loss of the normal allele. Moreover, germline pathogenic variants in *BRCA1/2* also lead to tumor-specific **phenotypes** in breast and ovarian cancer as reflected by signature 3 or BRCAness characterized by high mutation burden of multiple types.

Penetrance of *BRCA1* and *BRCA2* Pathogenic Variants. Presymptomatic detection of women at risk for breast cancer as a result of any of these susceptibility genes relies on detecting clearly pathogenic variants. For the purposes of patient management and counseling, it would be helpful to know the lifetime risk for development of breast cancer in individuals, whether male or female, carrying particular variants in *BRCA1* and *BRCA2*, compared with the risk in the general population (see Table 16.3). Initial studies showed a greater than 80% risk for breast cancer by the age of 70 years in women heterozygous for *BRCA1* pathogenic variants, with a somewhat lower estimate for *BRCA2* variant carriers. These calculations relied on estimates of cancer risk in female relatives within families ascertained because breast cancer had already occurred many times in the family (i.e., families in which the particular *BRCA1* or *BRCA2* pathogenic variant was highly penetrant).

When similar risk estimates were made from population-based studies, however, in which women carrying *BRCA1* and *BRCA2* pathogenic variants were not selected because they were members of families in which many cases of breast cancer had already developed, the risk estimates were lower and ranged from 40% to 50% by the age of 70 years. The discrepancy between the penetrance of pathogenic variants in families with multiple occurrences of breast cancer and the penetrance in women identified by population screening and not by family history suggests that other genetic or environmental factors must play a role in the ultimate penetrance of *BRCA1* and *BRCA2* pathogenic variants.

In addition to pathogenic variants in *BRCA1* and *BRCA2*, pathogenic variants in other genes can also cause autosomal dominantly inherited breast cancer syndromes, albeit less commonly. These include the LFS, hereditary diffuse gastric and lobular breast cancer, Peutz-Jeghers syndrome, and Cowden syndrome. These conditions have lifetime breast cancer risks that approach those seen in carriers of *BRCA1* or *BRCA2* pathogenic variants, as well as risks for other cancers such as sarcomas, brain tumors, and carcinomas of the stomach, thyroid, and small intestine.

Clinicians faced with a family with multiple affected individuals with breast cancer often look for distinguishing signs in the patient and family history to help guide the choice of which genes to test (see Box 16.2). However, the rapid decline in the cost of gene and **exome** sequencing has allowed the development of gene panels in which multiple genes can be simultaneously analyzed, often at a cost that is equivalent to or even less than what was charged previously to analyze just one or two genes. Many breast and ovarian cancer panels include genes associated with moderately increased risk of breast and ovarian cancer (i.e., *ATM, CHEK2, PALB2, BRIP1, RAD51C,* and *RAD51D*).

Hereditary Colon Cancer

Colorectal cancer, a malignancy of the epithelial cells of the colon and rectum, is one of the most common forms of cancer. It affects ~1.3 million individuals worldwide per year (150,000 of whom are in the United States) and is responsible for ~10% to 15% of all cancer. Most cases are sporadic, but a small proportion of colon cancer cases are familial, among which are two autosomal dominant conditions: FAP and LS, along with their variants.

Familial Adenomatous Polyposis. FAP and its subvariant, Gardner syndrome, together have an incidence of ~1 per 10,000. In FAP, benign adenomatous polyps numbering in the many hundreds develop in the colon

TABLE 16.3 Lifetime Cancer Risks in Carriers of *BRCA1* or *BRCA2* Pathogenic Variants Compared to the General Population

Cancer Type	General Population Risk	Cancer Risk When Pathogenic Variant Present	
		BRCA1	*BRCA2*
Breast in females	12%	50–80%	40–70%
Second primary breast in females	3.5% within 5 yr Up to 11%	27% within 5 yr	12% within 5 yr 40–50% at 20 yr
Ovarian	1–2%	24–40%	11–18%
Male breast	0.1%	1–2%	5–10%
Prostate	15% (N. European origin) 18% (black individuals)	<30%	<39%
Pancreatic (both sexes)	0.50%	1–3%	2–7%

Data from Petrucelli N, Daly MB, Pal T. *BRCA1*- and *BRCA2*-Associated Hereditary Breast and Ovarian Cancer. 1998 Sep 4 [Updated 2022 May 26]. In: Adam MP, Everman DB, Mirzaa GM, et al., editors. GeneReviews® [Internet]. Seattle (WA): University of Washington, Seattle; 1993-2022. Available from: http://www.ncbi. nlm.nih.gov/books/NBK1247/

BOX 16.2 DIAGNOSTIC CRITERIA FOR HEREDITARY CANCER SYNDROMES

Li-Fraumeni Syndrome (LFS): Revised Chompret Criteria

- **Proband** with tumor belonging to LFS tumor spectrum (e.g., soft tissue sarcoma, osteosarcoma, CNS tumor, premenopausal breast cancer, adrenocortical carcinoma) before age 46 years AND at least one first- or second-degree relative with LFS tumor (except breast cancer if proband has breast cancer) before age 56 years or with multiple tumors; OR
- Proband with multiple tumors (except multiple breast tumors), two of which belong to LFS tumor spectrum and first of which occurred before age 46 years; OR
- Patient with adrenocortical carcinoma or choroid plexus tumor (i.e., rhabdomyosarcoma of embryonal anaplastic subtype) or medulloblastoma (SHH subtype) or childhood acute lymphoblastic leukemia (low) hypodiploid, irrespective of family history

Hereditary Diffuse Gastric and Lobular Breast Cancer Syndrome

- Family history of diffuse gastric cancer with two or more cases of gastric cancer, with at least one diffuse gastric cancer diagnosed before age 50 years
- Family with multiple lobular breast cancers

Peutz-Jeghers Syndrome

- Peutz-Jeghers–type hamartomatous polyps in the small intestine as well as in the stomach, large bowel, and extraintestinal sites, including the renal pelvis, bronchus, gallbladder, nasal passages, urinary bladder, and ureters
- Pigmented macules on the face, around oral mucosa and the perianal region, most pronounced in childhood

Cowden Syndrome

- Early-onset breast cancer, particularly before age 40
- Macrocephaly, especially ≥63 cm in males or ≥60 cm in females
- Thyroid cancer, particularly follicular type, before age 50
- Goiter, Hashimoto thyroiditis
- Dysplastic gangliocytoma of the cerebellum (Lhermitte-Duclos disease)
- Intestinal hamartomas
- Esophageal glycogenic acanthosis
- Skin findings of tricholemmomas or penile freckling
- Papillomas of oral cavity

From Bougeard G, Renaux-Petel M, Flaman JM, et al: Revisiting Li-Fraumeni syndrome from TP53 mutation carriers, *J Clin Oncol* 33(21):2345–2352, 2015. https://doi.org/10.1200/JCO.2014.59.5728; Kratz CP, Freycon C, Maxwell KN, et al: Analysis of the Li-Fraumeni spectrum based on an international germline TP53 variant data set: An International Agency for Research on Cancer TP53 database analysis, *JAMA Oncol* 7(12):1800–1805, 2021. https://doi.org/10.1001/jamaoncol.2021.4398

during the first 2 decades of life. In almost all cases, one or more of the polyps become malignant. Surgical removal of the colon (colectomy) prevents the development of colorectal malignancy.

FAP is caused by autosomal dominantly inherited heterozygous loss-of-function variants in a TSG known as *APC* (so-named because the condition used to be called adenomatous polyposis coli). Gardner syndrome is also due to pathogenic variants in *APC* and is therefore allelic to FAP. Patients with Gardner syndrome have, in addition to the adenomatous polyps with malignant transformation seen in FAP, extracolonic anomalies, including osteomas of the jaw and desmoids, which are tumors arising in the muscle of the abdominal wall. Although the relatives of an individual affected with Gardner syndrome who also carry the same *APC* pathogenic variant tend to also show the extracolonic manifestations of Gardner syndrome, the same variant in unrelated individuals has been found to cause only FAP. Thus whether an individual has FAP or Gardner syndrome is not simply due to which pathogenic variant is present in the *APC* gene but is likely affected by variation elsewhere in the genome.

Lynch Syndrome. Approximately 2% to 4% of cases of colon cancer are attributable to LS (Case 29). LS is characterized by autosomal dominant inheritance of colon cancer in **association** with a small number of adenomatous polyps that begin during early adulthood. The number of polyps is generally quite small in comparison to the hundreds to thousands of adenomatous polyps seen with FAP. Nonetheless, polyps in LS have high potential to undergo malignant transformation. Heterozygotes for pathogenic variants in *MLH1*, one of the most penetrant LS genes, have an ~80% lifetime risk for colon cancer; female heterozygotes also have a ~40% risk for endometrial cancer. There are also additional risks of 10% to 20% for cancer of the biliary or urinary tract and the ovary. Sebaceous gland tumors of the skin may be the first presenting sign in LS (in which case it is a variant called Muir-Torre syndrome); thus the presence of such tumors in a patient should raise suspicion of a possible hereditary colon cancer syndrome.

LS results from loss-of-function variants in one of four DNA repair genes (*MLH1, MSH2, MSH6,* and *PMS2*) that encode MMR proteins. Although all four of these genes have been implicated in LS in different families, *MLH1* and *MSH2* are together responsible for the majority of LS, whereas *MSH2* and *PMS2* are often associated with a lesser degree of MMR deficiency and lower penetrance. Like *BRCA1* and *BRCA2*, the LS MMR genes are TSGs involved in maintaining the integrity of the genome. Unlike *BRCA1* and *BRCA2*, however, the LS genes are not involved in double-stranded DNA break repair. Instead, their role is to repair incorrect DNA base pairing (i.e., pairing other than A with T or C with G) that can arise during DNA replication.

At the cellular level, the most striking phenotype of cells lacking MMR proteins is an enormous increase in both point mutations and mutations occurring during replication of simple DNA repeats, such as segments containing a string of the same base, for example $(A)_n$, or a **microsatellite**, such as $(TG)_n$ (see Chapter 4). Microsatellites are believed to be particularly vulnerable to mismatch because slippage of the strand being synthesized on the template strand can occur more readily when a **short tandem repeat** is being synthesized. Such instability, referred to as the **microsatellite instability-positive (MSI+)** phenotype, occurs at two orders of magnitude higher frequency in cells lacking both copies of an MMR gene. The MSI+ phenotype is easily seen in DNA as three, four, or even more alleles of a microsatellite **polymorphism** in a single individual's tumor DNA (Fig. 16.9). It is estimated that cells lacking both copies of an MMR gene may carry 100,000 mutations within simple repeats throughout the genome.

Because of the increased mutation rate in these classes of sequence, loss of function of MMR genes will lead to somatic mutations in other driver genes. Two such driver genes have been isolated and characterized. The first is *APC*, whose normal function and role in FAP were described previously. The second is the gene *TGFBR2*, in which heterozygous germline pathogenic variants primarily cause a connective tissue disorder called Loeys-Dietz syndrome; however, cases of early-onset colon cancer have also been reported. *TGFBR2* encodes transforming growth factor β receptor II, a serine-threonine kinase that inhibits intestinal cell division. Somatically, *TGFBR2* is particularly vulnerable to mutation when MMR proteins are lost because it contains a stretch of 10 adenines encoding three lysines within its coding sequence; deletion of one or more of these As results in a frameshift and loss-of-function mutation. LS is an excellent example of how a gene, like *MLH1*, which has a global effect on mutation rate throughout the genome, can be a **driver gene** through its effect on other genes, such as *TGFBR2*, that are more specifically involved in driving the development of a cancer.

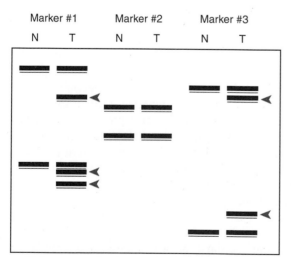

Figure 16.9 Gel electrophoresis of three different microsatellite polymorphic markers in normal *(N)* and tumor *(T)* samples from a patient with a germline pathogenic variant in *MSH2* and microsatellite instability. Although marker 2 shows no difference between normal and tumor tissues, genotyping at markers 1 and 3 reveals extra alleles *(blue arrows)*, some smaller, some larger, than the alleles present in normal tissue.

Pathogenic Variants in Tumor Suppressor Genes Causing Autosomal Recessive Pediatric Cancer Syndromes

As expected from the important role that DNA replication and repair enzymes play in mutation surveillance and prevention, inherited defects that alter the function of DNA repair enzymes can lead to a dramatic increase in the frequency of mutations of all types, including those that lead to cancer.

Pathogenic variants in the LS MMR genes are frequent enough in the population for there to be rare individuals with two (biallelic) germline mutations in one of the LS genes. Although much rarer than autosomal dominant forms of LS just discussed, this condition, known as constitutional MMR deficiency (CMMRD), results in a markedly elevated risk for many cancers during childhood, including colorectal and small bowel cancer, as well as some cancers not associated with LS, such as leukemia and lymphoma and various types of brain tumors. The absence of effective MMR in these tumors leads to high tumor mutational burden and expression of neoantigens, which have been shown to be effective targets for immune checkpoint inhibition (immunotherapy) yielding dramatic tumor responses in some cases. This represents one of the first approaches to targeted therapy for cancers based on underlying germline pathogenic variants.

Several other well-known autosomal **recessive** disorders, including xeroderma pigmentosum (Case 48), ataxia-telangiectasia, Fanconi anemia, and Bloom syndrome, are also due to loss of function of proteins required for normal DNA repair or replication. Patients with these rare conditions have a high frequency of somatic chromosome and **gene mutations** and, as a result, a markedly increased risk for various types of cancer, particularly leukemia or, in the case of xeroderma pigmentosum, skin cancers in sun-exposed areas. Clinically, radiography must be used with extreme caution, if at all, in patients with ataxia-telangiectasia, Fanconi anemia, and Bloom syndrome, and exposure to sunlight must be avoided in patients with xeroderma pigmentosum.

Although these are rare autosomal recessive disorders, heterozygote carriers are common, and some appear to be at increased risk for malignant neoplasia. For example, Fanconi anemia, in which individuals are at risk for congenital anomalies, bone marrow failure, leukemia, and squamous cell carcinoma of the head and neck, is a **chromosome instability syndrome** resulting from biallelic pathogenic variants in one of at least 22 different genes involved in DNA and chromosome repair. In the aggregate, Fanconi anemia has a population frequency of approximately one to five per million, which translates to a **carrier** frequency of approximately one to two per 500. One of these Fanconi anemia genes turns out to be the known hereditary cancer gene *BRCA2*. Others include *BRIP1*, *PALB2*, and *RAD51C* (discussed in the next section), which increase susceptibility to breast cancer in carriers of heterozygote pathogenic variants. Similarly, female heterozygotes for pathogenic variants in *ATM* (the gene responsible for ataxia-telangiectasia) have a twofold increased lifetime risk for breast cancer compared with controls and a fivefold higher risk for breast cancer before the age of 50 years. Thus heterozygotes for germline pathogenic variants in genes related to chromosome instability syndromes constitute a sizable pool of individuals at increased risk for cancer.

Testing for Germline Pathogenic Variants Causing Hereditary Cancer

As introduced earlier, although some sporadic cancers will be truly sporadic and due entirely to somatic mutation(s), other cancers that may appear to be sporadic likely reflect a predisposition to specific cancer(s) due to familial variants in one or more genes. This raises the possibility of using genetic testing to screen for germline pathogenic variants that might inform risk estimates for members of the general population or for families with insufficient family history to implicate a hereditary cancer syndrome. Here we illustrate the issues involved in the case of two common neoplasias: breast cancer and colorectal cancer.

BRCA1 and *BRCA2* Testing

Identification of a germline pathogenic variant in *BRCA1* or *BRCA2* in a patient with breast cancer is of obvious importance for **genetic counseling** and cancer risk management for the patient's children, siblings, and other relatives, who may or may not be at increased risk. Such testing is of course also important for the patient's own management. For instance, in addition to removal of the cancer, a woman found to carry a *BRCA1* pathogenic variant might also choose to have a prophylactic mastectomy of the unaffected breast or a bilateral oophorectomy simultaneously to reduce cancer risk while minimizing the number of separate surgeries and anesthesia exposures. Finding a pathogenic variant in the proband or a first-degree relative would also allow targeted testing in the rest of the family.

Importantly, however, the fraction of all female breast cancer patients whose disease is caused by a germline pathogenic variant in either the *BRCA1* or *BRCA2* gene is small, with estimates that vary between 1% and 3% in populations unselected for family history of breast or ovarian cancer, or for age at onset of the disease. Male breast cancer is 100 times less common than female breast cancer, but when it occurs, the frequency of germline pathogenic variants in hereditary breast cancer genes, particularly *BRCA2*, is ~16%.

Until quite recently, the cost of analysis of *BRCA1* and *BRCA2* was used to justify limiting testing to those patients most likely to be carrying a pathogenic variant, such as all male breast cancer patients and all women younger than 50 years with breast cancer, women with

bilateral breast cancer, or women with first- and second-degree relatives with ovarian cancer or breast cancer. However, as the cost of sequencing falls, and large panels of breast cancer susceptibility genes, including *BRCA1* and *BRCA2*, can now be analyzed for less than it cost previously to sequence just *BRCA1* and *BRCA2*, testing guidelines are inevitably undergoing ongoing reevaluation. Testing at least *BRCA1* and *BRCA2* in all women with high-risk, early-stage, human epidermal growth factor receptor 2 (HER2)–negative breast cancer has gained further support as treatment with PARP inhibitors has been shown to increase survival in individuals with germline *BRCA1/2* pathogenic variants.

Colorectal Cancer Germline Testing

LS is an autosomal dominant cancer predisposition syndrome with up to an 80% lifetime risk of cancer of multiple types. LS patients harbor germline pathogenic variants in the MMR genes (*MLH1*, *MSH2*, *MSH6*, *PMS2*, and *EPCAM* promoter deletion). Only 4% of patients with colon cancer, not selected for a family history of cancer, carry a germline pathogenic variant in one of these genes; an even smaller fraction carry pathogenic variants in *APC*, causing FAP. As with breast cancer, geneticists need to balance the cost and yield of sequencing hereditary colorectal cancer genes in every patient with colon cancer against the obvious importance of finding such a pathogenic variant for the patient and their family. Also of clinical benefit in identifying individuals with LS is the rationale for immunotherapy when tumors exhibit a characteristic high mutational burden.

For LS, clinical factors such as multiple polyps, early age at onset (age <50 years), the location of the tumor in more proximal portions of the colon, multiple synchronous or metachronous colorectal cancers, a family history of colorectal or other cancers (particularly endometrial cancer), and cancer in relatives younger than 50 years of age, all boost the probability that a patient with colon cancer is carrying a pathogenic variant in an MMR gene. Molecular studies of the tumor tissue to look for evidence of the MSI+ phenotype (as discussed earlier in this chapter) or absence of MSH2 and/or MSH6 protein by antibody staining in the tumor also increase the probability that an individual with colorectal cancer carries a germline pathogenic variant in an MMR gene. Unfortunately, loss of MLH1 protein staining in tumors due to promoter methylation is a frequent epigenetic finding in sporadic colon cancers and is therefore much less predictive of LS.

Combining clinical and molecular criteria allows the identification of a subset of colorectal cancer patients in whom the probability of finding a germline pathogenic variant in an MMR gene is much greater than 4%. These patients are clearly the most cost-effective group in which sequencing could be recommended. However, as with all such attempts at cost effectiveness, limiting the number of patients studied to increase the yield of patients with positive results inevitably results in missing a sizable minority

(20%) of patients with LS. Again, the cost of testing must be reevaluated as technology gets less expensive and the therapeutic importance of identifying cancer predisposition is becoming clearer. More detailed discussions of genetic testing will be presented in Chapter 19.

For FAP, the presence of hundreds of adenomatous polyps at an early age, multiple sebaceous adenomas, or the extracolonic manifestations of Gardner syndrome are sufficient to trigger germline testing for an *APC* pathogenic variant. There are, however, certain *APC* pathogenic variants that result in many fewer polyps and no extracolonic features (referred to as attenuated FAP). Attenuated FAP can be confused clinically with LS, but the tumors generally lack MMR defects or microsatellite instability.

FAMILIAL OCCURRENCE OF CANCER

Cancer can also show increased incidence in families without a clear-cut mendelian pattern of inheritance. It is estimated that as many as 20% of all breast cancers occurring in families that lack a clear, highly penetrant mendelian disorder nonetheless have a significant genetic contribution, as revealed by twin and family studies. The observed increase in cancer risk when relatives are affected may be due to pathogenic variants in a single gene but with penetrance that is sufficiently reduced to obscure any mendelian inheritance pattern. For example, pathogenic variants *PALB2* can increase lifetime risk for breast cancer to ~25% by age 55 and ~40% by age 85. A lack of increased breast cancer risk in men with *PALB2* pathogenic variants further obscures the inheritance pattern, although there is a significantly increased risk for pancreatic cancer. Germline pathogenic variants in *BRIP1* and *RAD51C* have similar effects in the setting of ovarian cancer.

The bulk of familial cancer is, however, likely to have a complex etiology caused by both genetic and shared environmental factors (see Chapter 9). The degree of complex familial cancer risk can be assessed by epidemiologic studies that compare how often the disease occurs in relatives versus the general population. The age-specific incidence of many forms of cancer in family members of probands is increased over the incidence of the same cancer in an age-matched cohort in the general population (Fig. 16.10). This increased risk has been observed in individuals whose first-degree relatives (parent, sibling, or child) are affected by a wide variety of different cancers, with an even greater increase in incidence when two first-degree relatives are affected. For example, population-based epidemiologic studies have shown that ~5% of all individuals in North America and Western Europe will develop colorectal cancer in their lifetime, but the lifetime risk is increased two- to threefold if one first-degree relative is affected.

In agreement with the frequently complex inheritance of cancer risk, genome-wide association studies (see Chapter 9) have identified more than 150 mostly common variants associated with a variety of cancers. Prostate cancer, in particular, shows multiple associations with variants in homologous recombination damage genes and with single nucleotide polymorphisms located in the intergenic or intronic regions of over a dozen loci in other genes. However, **odds ratios** for most of these associations are less than 2.0, and many are less than 1.3, therefore accounting for at most 20% of the observed familial risk for prostate cancer. Overall, then, although the role of inherited variants in the genome is clear, we cannot yet explain in detail the increased familial tendencies of most cancers. Whether common variants do not capture all of the risk or there are unrecognized environmental exposures in common between family members remains nonexclusive possibilities.

SPORADIC CANCER

Previously we introduced the concept of activation of oncogenes by a variety of mutational mechanisms (see Fig. 16.3). Here we explore these mechanisms and their effects in greater detail, particularly in the context of sporadic cancers.

Activation of Oncogenes by Point Variation

Many mutated oncogenes were first identified by molecular studies of cell lines derived from sporadic cancers. One of the first activated oncogenes discovered was a mutant *RAS* gene derived from a bladder carcinoma cell line. *RAS* encodes one of a large family of small guanosine triphosphate (GTP)–binding proteins (G proteins) that serve as molecular on-off switches to activate or inhibit downstream molecules. Remarkably, the activated oncogene and its counterpart proto-oncogene differed at only a single nucleotide. The alteration led to synthesis of an abnormal Ras protein that was able to signal continuously, thus stimulating cell division and transforming it into a tumor. *RAS* point mutations, almost exclusively confined to one of three amino acids (12, 13, or 61), are now known in many tumors, and the genes in the *RAS* pathway have been shown experimentally to be the mutational target of known carcinogens, a finding that supports a role for mutated *RAS* pathway genes in the development of many cancers.

To date, nearly 50 human proto-oncogenes have been identified as drivers in sporadic cancer. Only a few of these proto-oncogenes have also been found to be implicated in a hereditary cancer syndrome.

Activation of Oncogenes by Chromosome Translocation or Fusions

As pointed out previously (see Fig. 16.3), oncogene activation is not always the result of a DNA mutation. In some instances, a proto-oncogene is activated by a

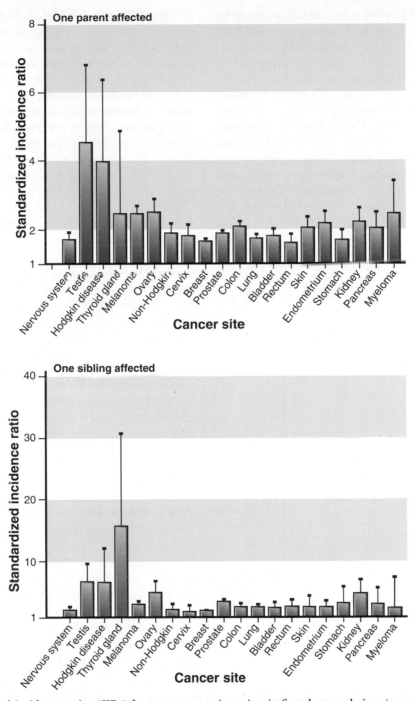

Figure 16.10 Standardized incidence ratios (SIRs) for cancers at various sites in first-degree relatives (parent, sibling, or child) of an affected person. SIR is similar to the relative risk ratio (λ_r) based on prevalence of disease (as described in Chapter 10), except SIR is the ratio of the incidence of cases of cancer in relatives divided by the number expected from the incidence in age-matched controls. Error bars reflect 95% confidence limits on the SIRs. (Adapted from Hemminki K, Sundquist J, Lorenzo Bermejo J: Familial risks for cancer as the basis for evidence-based clinical referral and counseling, *Oncologist* 13:239–247, 2008.)

chromosomal change, typically a translocation. More than 40 oncogenic chromosome translocations have been described to date, primarily in sporadic leukemias and lymphomas but also in a few rare connective tissue sarcomas. Although originally detected only by cytogenetic analysis, such alterations can be detected now by whole genome or RNA sequence analysis, even using **cell-free DNA** in plasma samples from cancer patients.

In some cases, translocation breakpoints lie within the introns of two genes, thereby fusing two genes into one abnormal gene that encodes a chimeric protein with novel oncogenic properties. The best-known example is the translocation between chromosomes 9 and 22, the **Philadelphia chromosome** that is seen in chronic myelogenous leukemia (CML) (Fig. 16.11) (Case 10). The translocation moves the proto-oncogene *ABL1*, a tyrosine kinase, from its normal position on chromosome 9q to a gene of unknown function, *BCR*, on chromosome 22q. The translocation results in the synthesis of a novel, chimeric protein, BCR-ABL1, containing a portion of the normal Abl protein with increased tyrosine kinase activity. The enhanced tyrosine kinase activity of the novel protein encoded by the chimeric gene is the primary event causing the chronic leukemia. Highly effective drug therapies for CML, such as imatinib, have been developed based on inhibition of this tyrosine kinase activity.

In other cases, a translocation activates an oncogene by placing it downstream of a strong, constitutive promoter belonging to a different gene. Burkitt lymphoma

is a B-cell tumor in which the *MYC* proto-oncogene is translocated from its normal position at 8q24 to a position distal to the immunoglobulin heavy chain locus at 14q32 or the immunoglobulin light chain genes on chromosomes 22 and 2. The function of the Myc protein is still not entirely known, but it appears to be a **transcription factor** with powerful effects on the expression of a number of genes involved in cellular proliferation, as well as on telomerase expression (see later discussion). The translocation brings **enhancer** or other transcriptional activating sequences, normally associated with the immunoglobulin genes, near the *MYC* gene (Table 16.4). These translocations allow unregulated *MYC* expression, resulting in uncontrolled cell division.

Telomerase as an Oncogene

Another type of oncogene is the gene encoding **telomerase**, a **reverse transcriptase** that is required to synthesize the hexamer repeat TTAGGG, a component of **telomeres** at the ends of chromosomes. Telomerase is needed because, during normal semiconservative replication of DNA (see Chapter 2), **DNA polymerase** can only add nucleotides to the 3' end of DNA and cannot complete the synthesis of a growing strand all the way to the very end of that strand on the chromosome arm; thus, in the absence of a specific mechanism to allow replication of telomeres, the end of each **chromosome arm** would shorten significantly with each and every cell division.

In human germline cells and embryonic cells, telomeres contain ~15 kb of the telomeric repeat. As cells differentiate, telomerase activity declines in somatic tissues; as telomerase function is lost, telomeres shorten, with a loss of ~35 bp of telomeric repeat DNA with each cell division. After hundreds of cell divisions, the chromosome ends become damaged, leading cells to stop dividing and enter G_0 of the cell cycle; the cells will ultimately undergo apoptosis and die.

In contrast, in highly proliferative cells of tissues such as bone marrow, telomerase expression persists, allowing self-renewal. Similarly, telomerase persistence is

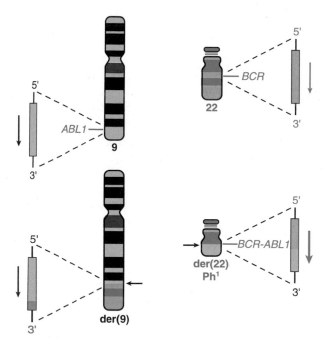

Figure 16.11 The Philadelphia chromosome translocation, t(9;22) (q34;q11). The Philadelphia chromosome (Ph¹) is the derivative chromosome 22, which has exchanged part of its long arm for a segment of material from chromosome 9q that contains the *ABL1* oncogene. Formation of the chimeric *BCR-ABL1* gene on the Ph¹ chromosome is the critical genetic event in the development of chronic myelogenous leukemia.

TABLE 16.4 Characteristic Chromosome Translocations in Selected Human Malignant Neoplasms

Neoplasm	Chromosome Translocation	Percentage of Cases	Proto-oncogene Affected
Burkitt lymphoma	t(8;14)(q24;q32)	80	*MYC*
	t(8;22)(q24;q11)	15	
	t(2;8)(q11;q24)	5	
Chronic myelogenous leukemia	t(9;22)(q34;q11)	90–95	*BCR-ABL1*
Acute lymphocytic leukemia	t(9;22)(q34;q11)	10–15	*BCR-ABL1*
Acute lymphoblastic leukemia	t(1;19)(q23;p13)	3–6	*TCF3-PBX1*
Acute promyelocytic leukemia	t(15;17)(q22;q11)	≈95	*RARA-PML*
Chronic lymphocytic leukemia	t(11;14)(q13;q32)	10–30	*BCL1*
Follicular lymphoma	t(14;18)(q32;q21)	≈100	*BCL2*

Based on Croce CM: Role of chromosome translocations in human neoplasia, *Cell* 49:155–156, 1987; Park M, van de Woude GF: Oncogenes: Genes associated with neoplastic disease. In Scriver CR, Beaudet AL, Sly WS, et al, editors: *The molecular and metabolic bases of inherited disease*, ed 6, New York, 1989, McGraw-Hill, pp 251–276; Nourse J, Mellentin JD, Galili N, et al: Chromosomal translocation t(1;19) results in synthesis of a homeobox fusion mRNA that codes for a potential chimeric transcription factor, *Cell* 60:535–545, 1990; Borrow J, Goddard AD, Sheer D, et al: Molecular analysis of acute promyelocytic leukemia breakpoint cluster region on chromosome 17, *Science* 249:1577–1580, 1990.

observed in many tumors, which permits tumor cells to proliferate indefinitely. In some cases, increased telomerase activity results from chromosome or gene mutations that directly up-regulate the telomerase gene; in others, telomerase may be only one of many genes whose expression is altered by a transforming oncogene, such as *MYC*. The extent of oncogenesis resulting from disorders of telomere biology is still being recognized, as evidenced by classic telomere syndromes in which telomere attrition is a characteristic associated with cancer, and in disorders in which there is alternative lengthening of telomeres.

Loss of Tumor Suppressor Genes in Sporadic Cancer

TP53 and *RB1* in Sporadic Cancers

Although LFS, caused by dominantly inherited germline pathogenic variants in *TP53*, is a rare familial syndrome, somatic mutation of *TP53* is one of the most common genetic alterations seen in sporadic cancer (see Table 16.2). Mutations in *TP53*, deletion of the segment of chromosome 17p that includes *TP53*, or loss of the entire chromosome 17 are frequently seen in a wide range of sporadic cancers. These include breast, ovarian, bladder, cervical, esophageal, colorectal, skin, and lung carcinomas; glioblastoma; osteogenic sarcoma; and hepatocellular carcinoma. *TP53* is the most commonly mutated gene in cancer.

The retinoblastoma gene *RB1* is also frequently mutated in many sporadic cancers. For example, 13q14 LOH in human breast cancers is associated with loss of *RB1* mRNA in the tumor tissue. In other cancers, the *RB1* gene is intact and its mRNA appears to be at or near normal levels, yet the Rb1 protein is deficient. This anomaly has now been explained by the recognition that *RB1* can be down-regulated in association with overexpression of the oncomir *miR-106a*, which targets *RB1* mRNA and blocks its translation.

CYTOGENETIC CHANGES IN CANCER

Aneuploidy and Aneusomy

As introduced in Chapter 5, cytogenetic changes are hallmarks of cancer, whether sporadic or familial, particularly in later and more malignant or invasive stages of tumor development. Constitutional chromosomal abnormalities also predispose to cancer, as in Down syndrome (acute lymphoblastic leukemia and acute myeloid leukemia), Turner syndrome (germ cell tumors), and Klinefelter (germ cell tumors, breast cancer). Somatic cytogenetic alterations suggest that a critical element of cancer progression includes defects in genes involved in maintaining chromosome stability and integrity and ensuring accurate mitotic **segregation**.

Initially, most of the cytogenetic studies of tumor progression were carried out in leukemias because the tumor cells were amenable to being cultured and karyotyped by standard methods. For example, when CML, with the t(9;22) Philadelphia chromosome, evolves from the typically indolent chronic phase to a severe, life-threatening blast crisis, there may be several additional cytogenetic abnormalities, including numeric or structural changes, such as a second copy of the 9;22 translocation chromosome or an **isochromosome** 17q. In advanced stages of other forms of leukemia, other translocations are common. In contrast, a vast array of chromosomal abnormalities is seen in most solid tumors. Cytogenetic abnormalities found repeatedly in a specific type of cancer are likely to be driver events involved in the initiation or progression of the malignant neoplasm. A current focus of cancer research is to develop a comprehensive cytogenetic and genomic definition of these abnormalities, many of which result in enhanced proto-oncogene expression or the loss of TSG alleles. Medulloblastoma is a salient example of this comprehensive molecular and cytogenetic characterization for which four distinct types are described: SHH, Wnt, Group 3, and Group 4. Each has characteristic clinical features and distinct treatment-related outcomes. Genome sequencing is replacing cytogenetic analysis in many instances because it provides a level of **sensitivity** and precision well beyond detection of cytologically visible genome changes. Furthermore, RNA (cDNA) fusion detection utilizing NGS is also commonly deployed to detect somatic oncogenic fusions, and technologies now exist that enable detection of fusions without prior knowledge of the fusion partner or translocation breakpoints.

Gene Amplification

In addition to translocations and other rearrangements, another cytogenetic aberration seen in many cancers is gene amplification, a phenomenon in which many additional copies of a segment of the genome are present in the cell (see Fig. 16.3). Gene amplification is common in cancers, including neuroblastoma, squamous cell carcinoma of the head and neck, colorectal cancer, and malignant glioblastomas of the brain. Amplified segments of DNA are readily detected by **comparative genome hybridization** or genome sequencing and appear as two types of cytogenetic change in routine chromosome analysis: **double minutes** (very small accessory chromosomes) and **homogeneously staining regions** that do not band normally and contain multiple, amplified copies of a particular DNA segment. How and why double minutes and homogeneously staining regions develop are poorly understood, but amplified regions are known to include extra copies of proto-oncogenes such as the genes encoding Myc, Ras, and epithelial growth factor receptor, which stimulate cell growth, block apoptosis, or both. For example, amplification of the *MYCN* proto-oncogene encoding N-Myc is an important clinical indicator of prognosis in the childhood cancer neuroblastoma. *MYCN* is amplified more than 200-fold in 40% of advanced stages of neuroblastoma; despite aggressive treatment, only 30% of patients with advanced disease survive 3 years. In contrast, *MYCN* amplification is found in only 4% of early-stage neuroblastoma, and the 3-year survival is 90%. Amplification of genes encoding the targets of chemotherapeutic agents has also been implicated as a mechanism for the development of drug resistance in patients previously treated with chemotherapy.

THE ROLE OF EPIGENETICS IN CANCER

Some cancers (e.g., breast or prostate) are readily diagnosed based on the organ in which they arise. Other cancer types (such as central nervous system [CNS] or sarcomas) are more difficult to diagnose. Tumors in these tissue types may have similar histologies but very different biologic and prognostic characteristics. Distinguishing these can be addressed using **DNA methylation (DNAm)** analysis. Another difficult scenario addressed by DNAm is cancer originating from an unknown primary: disease that is metastatic at diagnosis, but the primary cancer it arose from is unclear.

DNAm analysis is increasingly incorporated into the diagnostic investigation of various cancers due to its precision in defining specific tumor types, especially those that evade definition by other types of molecular and pathologic analyses (i.e., some brain tumors). For these situations, DNAm analysis is likely superior to gene expression signatures and is closer to application in clinical practice. DNAm signatures can also aid in risk assessment, diagnosis, and prognostication.

Cancer, although conventionally considered a genetic disorder, typically involves genome-wide epigenetic dysregulation, including alterations to DNAm, histone modifications, **chromatin remodeling**, and microRNA. These changes can support the development of cancer by a variety of mechanisms. There is generalized DNAm dysregulation in cancer, which contributes to tumor development in a variety of ways. Generally, CpG islands near gene promoters will gain methylation, which can be associated with changes in that gene's expression. Conversely, hypomethylation events are more common but not associated with specific genomic features. It is unclear whether hypomethylation in cancer plays a functional role, but it appears to be related to genome instability, manifested through cytogenetic events such as aneuploidy. Furthermore, silencing of certain critical homeostatic genes (e.g., DNA repair genes) can lead to MMR deficiency and hypermutability.

Further genome-wide alterations in DNAm can also be downstream consequences of variants in chromatin modifier genes (e.g., genome-wide hypermethylation due to *DNMT3A* gain of function or *TET2* loss of function). Finally, loss-of-function sequence variants in epigenetic regulators have been identified as a hallmark of etiology in several cancers: in certain hematologic malignancies and variants in epigenetic regulators, including *MLL1* and *CBP/p300*, which normally mediate lineage **specification**/differentiation and cause blocks in transitions to correct **commitment** pathways, resulting in proliferation of undifferentiated cells that manifest as leukemia. In brain tumors, *H3-K27M* plays a role in midline glioma development. Epigenetic changes involving chromosome 11p15.5 predispose to Wilms tumor and hepatoblastoma, as in Beckwith-Wiedemann syndrome (Case 6).

Improved Diagnostic Yield with Methylation Testing

The introduction of genome-wide DNAm profiling of tumors has been transformative in diagnostics. Importantly, DNAm-based tumor classification is as reliable as gene expression; it has emerged as a promising approach to differentiate tumor types and to improve diagnostics and prognostics. This is exemplified by CNS tumors and sarcomas, which can be more precisely defined by DNAm profiling than with traditional pathologic subgroups. This results from DNAm not only providing data about the current state of cellular modification but defining the tumor's cell type of origin. It appears that the state of cell differentiation at the time of tumor initiation remains relatively stable during tumor development/progression. Furthermore, DNAm, as a method of tumor subgrouping, provides a means to classify medulloblastoma subgroups for clinical trials and therapy modification. The World Health Organization (WHO) now recognizes medulloblastoma as four different diseases based on these subgroups initially defined by DNAm.

Therapies Targeting Epigenetic Modifications

Epigenetic changes are reversible and therefore represent a viable target for therapeutic intervention. In the cancer realm, DNAm signatures are not only used for treatment **selection**, based on optimized diagnostics, but also to identify new treatment targets. Significant progress has been made in the development of pharmaceutical agents that target **histones** and DNAm. Some, including DNA methyltransferase inhibitors, which reverse aberrant hypermethylation, have been approved for clinical use for treatment of a variety of cancers, including hematologic malignancies and solid tumors. There are several other epigenetic agents currently available as standard-of-care cancer treatments. Romidepsin, a histone deacetylase, has been approved by the US Food and Drug Administration for cutaneous T-cell lymphoma—a painful and disfiguring condition. Positive response rates are ~30%, and the median duration of response is longer than 1 year.

As these epigenetic drugs are not curative, they are frequently combined with other treatments, including classic chemotherapies and immune checkpoint inhibitors, to broaden response rates among patients. In summary, although epigenetic therapies are still a work in progress, chromatin remains an important therapeutic target for investigation.

One of the biggest limitations of epitargeted drug therapies is that they target epigenetic marks nonspecifically; there need to be more tailored therapies to reduce harm and improve outcomes.

APPLYING GENOMICS TO INDIVIDUALIZE CANCER THERAPY

Genomics is already having a major impact on diagnostic precision and optimization of therapy in cancer. In this section we describe how one such approach, gene expression profiling, is used to guide diagnosis and treatment.

Gene Expression Profiling and Clustering to Identify Signatures

Comparative **hybridization** techniques can be used to simultaneously measure the level of mRNA expression of some or all of the genes in any human tissue sample.

A measurement of mRNA expression in a sample of tissue constitutes a gene **expression profile** specific to that tissue. Fig. 16.12 depicts a hypothetical, idealized situation of eight samples, four from each of two types of tumor, A and B, profiled for 100 different genes. The expression profile derived from expression arrays for this simple example is already substantial, consisting of 800 expression values. In a real expression profiling experiment, however, hundreds of samples may be analyzed for the expression of all human genes, producing a massive data set of millions of expression values. Organizing the data and analyzing them to extract key information are challenging problems that have inspired the development of sophisticated statistical and bioinformatic tools. Using such tools, one can organize the data to find groups of genes whose expression seems to correlate (i.e., increase or decrease together) between and among the samples. Grouping genes by their patterns of expression across samples is termed clustering.

Clusters of gene expression can then be tested to determine if any correlate with particular characteristics of the samples of interest. For example, profiling might indicate that a cluster of genes with a correlated expression profile is found more frequently in samples from tumor A than from tumor B, whereas another cluster of genes with a

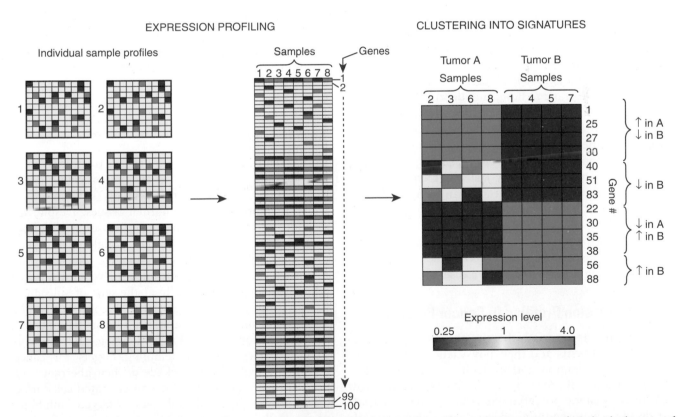

Figure 16.12 Schematic of an idealized gene expression profiling experiment of eight samples and 100 genes. *(Left)* Individual arrays of gene sequences spotted on glass or silicon chips are used for comparative hybridization of eight different samples relative to a common standard. *Red* indicates decreased expression compared with control, *green* indicates increased expression, and *yellow* is unchanged expression. (In this schematic, *red, yellow,* and *green* represent decreased, equal, or increased expression, whereas a real experiment would provide a continuous quantitative reading with shades of red and green.) *(Center)* All 800 expression measurements are organized so that the relative expression for each gene (1–100) is put in order vertically in a column under the number of each sample. *(Right)* Clustering into signatures involves only those 13 genes that showed correlation across subsets of samples. Some genes have reciprocal (high vs low) expression in the two tumors; others show a correlated increase or decrease in one tumor and not the other.

correlated expression profile is more frequent in samples derived from tumor B than from tumor A. Clusters of genes whose expression correlates with each other and with a particular set of samples constitute an expression signature characteristic of those samples. In the hypothetical profiles in Fig. 16.12, certain genes have a correlated expression that serves as a signature for tumor A; tumor B has a signature derived from the correlated expression of a different subset of these 100 genes.

Application of Gene Signatures

The application of gene expression profiles to characterize tumors is useful in several ways.

- First, it increases our ability to discriminate between different tumors in ways that complement the standard criteria applied by pathologists to characterize tumors, such as histologic appearance, cytogenetic markers, and expression of specific marker proteins. Once distinguishing signatures for different tumor types (e.g., tumor A vs tumor B) are defined using known samples, the expression pattern of unknown tumor samples can then be compared with the expression signatures for tumor A and tumor B and classified as A-like, B-like, or neither, depending on how well their expression profiles match the signatures of A and B. Pathologists have used expression profiling to make difficult distinctions between tumors that require very different management approaches. These include distinguishing large B-cell lymphoma from Burkitt lymphoma, differentiating primary lung cancers from squamous cell carcinomas of the head and neck metastatic to lung, and identifying the tissue of origin of a cryptic primary tumor whose metastasis gives too little information to allow its classification.
- Second, different signatures may be found to correlate with known clinical outcomes, such as prognosis, response to therapy, or any other outcome of interest. If validated, such signatures can be applied prospectively to help guide therapy in newly diagnosed patients.
- Finally, for basic research, clustering may reveal previously unsuspected connections of functional importance among genes involved in a disease process.

Gene Expression Profiling in Cancer Prognosis

Choosing the appropriate therapy for most cancers is difficult for patients and their physicians alike because recurrence is common and difficult to predict. Better characterization of each patient's cancer as to **recurrence risk** and metastatic potential would clearly be beneficial for deciding between more or less aggressive courses of surgery and/or chemotherapy. For example, in breast cancer—although presence of the estrogen and progesterone receptors, amplification of the *HER2* oncogene, and absence of metastatic tumor in lymph nodes found on dissection of axillary lymphatics are strong predictors of better response to therapy and prognosis—they

are still imprecise. Expression profiling (Fig. 16.13) is opening up a promising new avenue for clinical decision making in the management of breast cancer, as well as in other cancers, including lymphoma, prostate cancer, and metastatic adenocarcinomas of diverse tissue origins (lung, breast, colorectal, uterine, and ovarian).

Gene expression profiling of various sets of genes is clinically available for use in the management of breast, colon, and ovarian cancer; which genes and how many are included in the profile depends on the tumor type and vendor. Although the **clinical utility** and cost effectiveness continue to be debated (see Chapter 19), there is a general consensus that combinations of clinical and gene expression data in patients newly diagnosed with cancer will provide better prospective estimates of prognosis and improved guidance of therapy. It is hoped that by improving the accuracy of prognosis with tumor expression profiling, oncologists can better tailor therapy and minimize exposure to toxic drugs when possible.

The fact that prognosis for practically every patient could be associated with a particular combination of clinical features, genome sequence, and expression signatures underscores a crucial point about cancer: each person's cancer is a unique disorder. The genomic and gene expression **heterogeneity** among patients who all carry the same cancer diagnosis should not be surprising. *Every patient is unique in the genetic variants carried, including those variants that will affect how the cancer develops and the body responds to it.* Moreover, the **clonal evolution** of a cancer implies that chance mutational and epigenetic events will likely occur in different and unique combinations in every patient's particular cancer.

Targeted Cancer Therapy

Until recently, most nonsurgical cancer treatments relied on cytotoxic agents, such as chemotherapeutic agents or radiation, designed to preferentially kill tumor cells while attempting to spare normal tissues. Despite tremendous successes in curing such diseases as childhood acute lymphocytic leukemia and Hodgkin lymphoma, most cancer patients in whom complete removal of the tumor with surgery is not possible achieve remission, not cure, of their disease, usually at the cost of substantial toxicity from cytotoxic agents. The discovery of specific driver genes and their mutations in cancers has opened a new avenue for precisely targeted, less toxic treatments. Activated oncogenes are tempting targets for cancer therapy through direct blockade of their aberrant function. This can include blocking an activated cell surface receptor by monoclonal antibodies, or targeted inhibition of intracellular constitutive kinase activity with drugs designed to specifically inhibit their enzymatic activities.

The proof of principle for this approach was established with the development of imatinib, a highly effective inhibitor of a number of tyrosine kinases, including the ABL1 kinase in CML. Prolonged remissions of this disease have been seen, in some cases with apparently

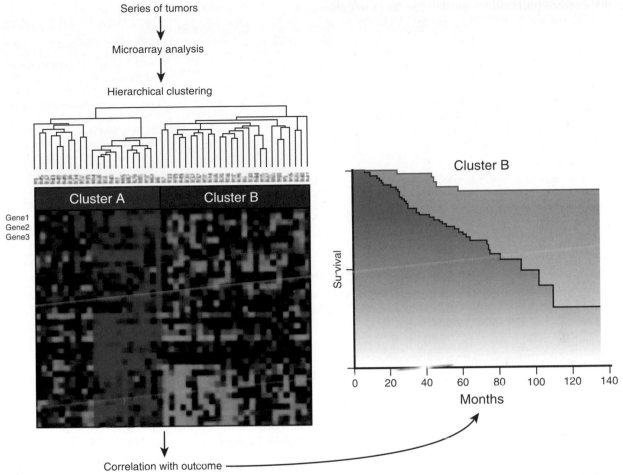

Figure 16.13 Expression patterns for a series of genes (along the vertical axis at *left*) for series of patient tumors, with the tumors arranged along the horizontal axis at *top* so that tumors with more similar expression patterns are grouped more closely together. The tumors appear to generally cluster into two groups, which are then correlated with long-term survival. (Adapted from Reis-Filho J, Pusztai L: Gene expression profiling in breast cancer: Classification, prognostication, and prediction, *Lancet* 378:1812–1823, 2011.)

indefinite postponement of the transformation into a virulent acute leukemia (blast crisis) that so often meant the end of a CML patient's life. Additional kinase inhibitors have been developed to target other activated oncogene driver genes in a variety of tumor types. Furthermore, constitutional pathogenic variants have been the impetus for targeted therapies (e.g., *BRCA1/BRCA2, MLH1, MSH2, MSH6, PMS2, VHL1, NF1*) (Table 16.5).

The initial results with targeted therapies, although very promising in some cases, have not led to permanent cures in most patients largely because tumors develop resistance to the targeted therapy. The outgrowth of resistant tumors is not surprising. First, as previously discussed, cancer cells are highly mutable, and their genomes undergo recurrent mutation. Even if only a small minority of cells acquire resistance through either mutation of the targeted oncogene itself or a compensatory mutation elsewhere, the tumor can progress even in the face of oncogene inhibition. Newer compounds that can overcome drug resistance are being developed and used in clinical trials. Ultimately, combination therapy that targets different driver genes may be required, based on the idea that a tumor cell is less likely to develop resistance in multiple unrelated pathways targeted by a combination of agents.

CANCER AND THE ENVIRONMENT

Although the theme of this chapter emphasizes the genetic basis of cancer, there is no contradiction in considering the role of environment in carcinogenesis. By environment, we mean exposure to a wide variety of different types of agents—food, natural and artificial radiation, chemicals, and even viruses and bacteria that are colonizing the gut. The risk for cancer shows significant variation among different populations and even within the same population in different environments. For example, gastric cancer is almost three times as common among Japanese people in Japan as among Japanese people living in Hawaii or Los Angeles.

In some cases, environmental agents act as mutagens that cause somatic mutations; the somatic mutations, in turn, are responsible for carcinogenesis. According to some estimates based chiefly on data from the aftermath of the atomic bombings of Hiroshima and Nagasaki, as much as 75% of the risk for cancer may be environmental

TABLE 16.5 Cancer Treatments Targeted to Specific Driver Oncogenes

Tumor Type	Driver Gene and Mutation	Representative FDA-Approved Targeted Therapeutic	Mechanism of Action
Breast cancer	Amplified *HER2*	Trastuzumab	Anti-HER2 monoclonal antibody
Breast cancer, ovarian, prostate, pancreatic	*BRCA1/BRCA2*	Olaparib	PARP inhibitor
Colon cancer	Mismatch repair *MLH1, MSH2, MSH6, PMS2*	Nivolumab, pembrolizumab	Targeting neoantigens induced by hypermutable state
Renal tumors	*VHL*	Belzutifan	HIF2α inhibitor
Malignant peripheral nerve sheath tumors	*NF1*	Selumetinib	Kinase inhibitor blocks RAS pathway signaling by inhibiting MEK, downstream of RAS
Non–small cell lung cancer	Activated *EGFR*	Gefitinib	Tyrosine kinase inhibitor
Chronic myelogenous leukemia and gastrointestinal stromal tumor	Activated receptor tyrosine kinases *AB1, KIT*, and *PDGF*	Imatinib, nilotinib, and dasatinib	Tyrosine kinase inhibitor
Non–small cell lung cancer	Translocated *ALK*	Crizotinib	Tyrosine kinase inhibitor
Neuroblastoma	Activated *ALK*		
Melanoma	Activated *MEK*	Trametinib	Serine-threonine kinase inhibitor
Melanoma	Activated *BRAF* kinase	Vemurafenib	Serine-threonine kinase inhibitor

ALK, Anaplastic lymphoma kinase; *EGFR*, epidermal growth factor receptor; *FDA*, US Food and Drug Administration; *HER2*, human epidermal growth factor receptor 2; *MEK*, mitogen-activated extracellular signal-regulated kinase; *PDGF*, platelet-derived growth factor.

in origin. In other cases there appears to be a **correlation** between certain exposures and risk for cancer, such as the benefits of dietary fiber or low-dose aspirin therapy in lowering colon cancer risks. The nature of environmental agents that increase or reduce the risk for cancer, the assessment of the additional risk associated with exposure, and ways of protecting the population from such hazards are matters of strong public concern.

Radiation

Ionizing radiation is known to increase the risk for cancer. Everyone is exposed to some degree of ionizing radiation through background radiation (which varies greatly from place to place) and medical exposure. The risk is dependent on the age at exposure, being greatest for children younger than 10 years and for older adults.

Although there are still large areas of uncertainty about the magnitude of the effects of radiation (especially low-level radiation) on cancer risk, some information can be gleaned from events involving large-scale release of radiation into the environment. The data for survivors of the Hiroshima and Nagasaki atomic bombings, for example, show a long latency period, in the 5-year range for leukemia but up to 40 years for some tumors. In contrast, there has been little increase in cancer detectable among populations exposed to ionizing radiation by the more recent nuclear accident at Chernobyl, with the exception of a significant five- to sixfold increase in thyroid cancer among the most heavily exposed children living in Belarus. The increase in thyroid cancer is almost certainly caused by the radioactive iodine (^{131}I) that was present in the nuclear material released from the damaged reactor and was taken up and concentrated within the thyroid gland.

Chemical Carcinogens

Interest in the carcinogenic effect of chemicals dates back at least to the 18th century, when the high incidence of scrotal cancer in young chimney sweeps was noticed. Today there is concern about many possible chemical carcinogens, especially tobacco, components of the diet, industrial carcinogens, and toxic wastes. Documentation of the risk of exposure is often difficult, but the level of concern is such that all clinicians should have a working knowledge of the subject and be able to distinguish between well-established facts and areas of uncertainty and debate.

The precise molecular mechanisms by which most chemical carcinogens cause cancer are still the subject of extensive research. One illustrative example of how a chemical carcinogen may contribute to the development of cancer is that of hepatocellular carcinoma, the fifth most common cancer worldwide. In many parts of the world, hepatocellular carcinoma occurs at increased frequency because of ingestion of aflatoxin B1, a potent carcinogen produced by a mold found on peanuts. Aflatoxin has been shown to mutate a particular base in the *TP53* gene, causing a G to T mutation in **codon 249**, thus converting an arginine codon to serine in the critically important p53 protein. This mutation is found in nearly half of all hepatocellular carcinomas in patients from parts of the world in which there is a high frequency of contamination of food by aflatoxin, but it is not found in similar cancers in patients whose exposure to aflatoxin in food is low. The p.Arg249Ser variant in *p53* enhances hepatocyte growth and interferes with the growth control and apoptosis associated with **wild-type** *p53*; LOH of *TP53* in hepatocellular carcinoma is associated with a more malignant appearance of the cancer. Although aflatoxin B1 alone is capable of causing hepatocellular carcinoma, it can also act synergistically with chronic hepatitis B and C infections.

A more complicated situation occurs with an exposure to complex mixtures of chemicals, such as the many known or suspected carcinogens and mutagens found in cigarette smoke. The epidemiologic evidence is overwhelming that cigarette smoke increases the risk for lung cancer and throat cancer, as well as other cancers. Cigarette smoke contains polycyclic hydrocarbons that are converted to highly reactive epoxides that cause mutations by directly damaging DNA. The relative importance of these substances and how they might interact in carcinogenesis are still being elucidated.

The case of cigarette smoking also raises another interesting issue. Why do only some cigarette smokers get lung cancer? Increasingly heritable underpinnings are becoming understood. The association between cancer and cigarette smoking provides an important example of the interaction between environmental and genetic factors to either enhance or prevent the carcinogenic effects of chemicals. The enzyme aryl hydrocarbon hydroxylase (AHH) is an inducible protein involved in the metabolism of polycyclic hydrocarbons, such as those found in cigarette smoke. AHH converts hydrocarbons into an epoxide form that is more easily excreted by the body but is also carcinogenic. AHH activity is encoded by members of the *CYP1* family of cytochrome P450 genes (see Chapter 19). The *CYP1A1* gene is inducible by cigarette smoke, but the inducibility is variable in the population because of different common variants at the *CYP1A1* locus. People who carry a high-inducibility variant, particularly those who are smokers, appear to be at an increased risk for lung cancer, with odds ratios of 4 to 5 compared to individuals without the cancer-susceptibility *CYP1A1* variant. On the other hand, homozygotes for the recessive low-inducibility variant appear to be less likely to develop lung cancer, possibly because their AHH is less effective at converting the hydrocarbons to highly reactive carcinogens.

Similarly, individuals **homozygous** for common variants in the *CYP2D6* gene that reduce the activity of another cytochrome P450 enzyme appear to be more resistant to the potential carcinogenic effects of cigarette smoke or occupational lung carcinogens (e.g., asbestos or polycyclic aromatic hydrocarbons). Normal or ultrafast metabolizers, on the other hand, who carry variants that increase the activity of the Cyp2D6 enzyme, have a fourfold greater risk for lung cancer than do slow metabolizers. This risk increases to 18-fold among persons exposed routinely to lung carcinogens. A similar association has been reported for bladder cancer.

Although the precise genetic and biochemical basis for the apparent differences in cancer susceptibility within the normal population remains to be determined, these associations could have significant public health consequences and may point eventually to a way of identifying persons who are genetically at a higher risk for the development of cancer.

ACKNOWLEDGMENT

We thank David Malkin, Rosanna Weksberg and Elise Fiala for contributing to this chapter.

GENERAL REFERENCES

https://www.annualreviews.org/doi/full/10.1146/annurevge nom-110320-121752 --- scaling genetic counseling in genomic era
https://www.nature.com/articles/nm.4333 somatic landscape
https://www.nature.com/articles/s41586-020-1943-3 tumor signature
https://www.nejm.org/doi/full/10.1056/nejmoa1508054 peds germline frequency
https://pubmed.ncbi.nlm.nih.gov/28873162/ adult germline frequency
https://www.nature.com/articles/s43018-021-00172-1 pediatric pediatric translation
https://pubmed.ncbi.nlm.nih.gov/34133209/ adult translation
https://ascopubs.org/doi/full/10.1200/JCO.19.02010 cascade testing
https://ascopubs.org/doi/full/10.1200/JCO.22.00995 regulation

SPECIFIC REFERENCES

Bouffet E, Larouche V, Campbell BB, et al: Immune checkpoint inhibition for hypermutant glioblastoma multiforme resulting from germline biallelic mismatch repair deficiency, *J Clin Oncol* 34(19):2206–2211, 2016. https://doi.org/10.1200/JCO.2016.66.6552

Bougeard G, Renaux-Petel M, Flaman JM, et al: Revisiting Li-Fraumeni syndrome from TP53 mutation carriers, *J Clin Oncol* 33(21):2345–2352, 2015. https://doi.org/10.1200/JCO.2014.59.5728

Chen P-S, Su J-L, Hung M-C: Dysregulation of microRNAs in cancer, *J Biomed Sci* 19:90, 2012.

Chin L, Anderson JN, Futreal PA: Cancer genomics, from discovery science to personalized medicine, *Nat Med* 17:297–303, 2011.

Di Leva G, Garofalo M, Croce CM: MicroRNAs in cancer, *Annu Rev Pathol Mech Dis* 9:287–314, 2014.

Fiala, EM, Jayakumaran, G, Mauguen, A, et al: Prospective pan-cancer germline testing using MSK-IMPACT informs clinical translation in 751 patients with pediatric solid tumors. *Nat Cancer* 2, 357–365 (2021). https://doi.org/10.1038/s43018-021-00172-1

Kiplivaara O, Aaltonen LA: Diagnostic cancer genome sequencing and the contribution of germline variants, *Science* 339:1559–1562, 2013.

Kratz CP, Freycon C, Maxwell KN, et al: Analysis of the Li-Fraumeni spectrum based on an international germline TP53 variant data set: an International Agency for Research on Cancer TP53 database analysis, *JAMA Oncol* 7(12):1800–1805, 2021. https://doi.org/10.1001/jamaoncol.2021.4398

Lal A, Panos R, Marjanovic M, et al: A gene expression profile test to resolve head & neck squamous versus lung squamous cancers, *Diagn Pathol* 8:44, 2013.

Reis-Filho J, Pusztai L: Gene expression profiling in breast cancer: Classification, prognostication, and prediction, *Lancet* 378:1812–1823, 2011.

Stadler ZK, Maio A, Chakravarty D, et al: Therapeutic Implications of Germline Testing in Patients With Advanced Cancers. *Journal of Clinical Oncology* 2021 39:24, 2698–2709.

Watson IR, Takahashi K, Futreal PA, et al: Emerging patterns of somatic mutations in cancer, *Nat Rev Genet* 14:703–718, 2013.

Wogan GN, Hecht SS, Felton JS, et al: Environmental and chemical carcinogenesis, *Semin Cancer Biol* 14:473–486, 2004.

Wong MW, Nordfors C, Mossman D, et al: BRIP1, PALB2, and RAD51C mutation analysis reveals their relative importance as genetic susceptibility factors for breast cancer, *Breast Cancer Res Treat* 127:853–859, 2011.

Zhang J, Walsh MF, Wu G, et al: Germline mutations in predisposition genes in pediatric cancer. *N Engl J Med.* (2015) 373:2336–46. https://doi.org/10.1056/NEJMoa1508054.

USEFUL WEBSITES

The Cancer Genome Atlas http://cancergenome.nih.gov/abouttcga/overview
cBioPortal   https://www.cbioportal.org/
PECAN   https://pecan.stjude.cloud/
COSMIC   https://cancer.sanger.ac.uk/cosmic
CIVIC   https://civicdb.org/welcome
ClinVar   https://www.ncbi.nlm.nih.gov/clinvar/
Genomic Data Commons https://gdc.cancer.gov/
GENIE   https://www.aacr.org/professionals/research/aacr-project-genie/aacr-project-genie-data/

PROBLEMS

1. An individual with retinoblastoma has a single tumor in one eye; the other eye is free of tumors. What steps would you take to try to determine whether this is sporadic or heritable retinoblastoma? What is the empiric likelihood the child has an *RB1* germline variant that is likely pathogenic or pathogenic? What genetic counseling would you provide? What information should the parents have before a subsequent pregnancy? Are there subsequent cancer risks?

2. Discuss possible reasons why colorectal cancer is predominantly an adult cancer, whereas retinoblastoma affects children. In which pediatric syndromes have colorectal cancers been reported?

3. Many tumor types are characterized by the presence of an isochromosome for the long arm of chromosome 17. Provide a possible explanation for this finding. In which constitutional cancer syndrome might there be an increase of this finding?

4. Many children with Fanconi anemia have limb defects. If an affected child requires surgery for the abnormal limb, what special considerations arise?

5. Margaret, whose sister has premenopausal bilateral breast cancer, has a greater risk for developing breast cancer herself than Wilma, whose sister has premenopausal breast cancer in only one breast. Both Margaret and Wilma, however, have a greater risk than does Elizabeth, who has a completely negative family history. Discuss the role of molecular testing in these women. What would their breast cancer risks be if a pathogenic *BRCA1* or *BRCA2* variant were found in the affected relative? What if no pathogenic variants were found? What are the differences between recommendations for screening individuals with pathogenic variants in moderate versus highly penetrant breast cancer predisposition breast cancer genes?

6. Propose a theory for why hereditary cancer syndromes, inherited as autosomal dominant diseases, are rarely caused by activated oncogenes; rather, by germline pathogenic variants in tumor suppressor genes.

CHAPTER 17

Genetic Counseling and Risk Assessment

Carolyn Dinsmore Applegate • Jodie Marie Vento

GENETIC COUNSELING

In this chapter, we present the fundamentals of the practice of **risk** estimation, which is a key component of the larger landscape of **genetic counseling**. Genetic counseling is defined as the process of helping people understand and adapt to the medical, psychological, and **familial** implications of **genetic** contributions to disease. Genetic counseling integrates the interpretation of family and medical histories, risk assessment, education, and counseling to promote informed choice and adaptation to the risk or condition. As technology and **genomics** have evolved, so has the definition of genetic counseling and the roles of professionals working in clinical genetics.

CLINICAL GENETICS

Clinical genetics is concerned with the diagnosis and management of the medical, social, and psychological aspects of hereditary conditions. As in all other areas of medicine, it is essential in clinical genetics to do the following:

- Make a correct diagnosis, which often involves laboratory testing, including genetic testing to find the pathogenic variants(s) responsible.
- Recommend appropriate treatment and management, including referrals to other specialist providers as needed.
- Help the affected person and family members understand and come to terms with the nature and consequences of the risk or condition.

Just as the unique feature of genetic conditions is its tendency to recur within families, the unique aspect of clinical genetics is its focus on both the patient and on members of the patient's family, both present and future. All providers performing genetic counseling have a responsibility to do the following:

- Empower patients to inform other family members of their potential risk.
- Offer testing to provide the most precise risk assessments possible for other family members.
- Explain what approaches are available to the patient and family members to modify these risks.

Finally, genetic counseling is not limited to the provision of information and identification of individuals at risk for manifestation of a genetic condition, rather, it is a process of exploration and communication. Genetic counselors define and address the complex psychosocial issues associated with a genetic condition in a family and provide psychologically oriented counseling to help individuals adapt and adjust to the impact and implications of the condition in the family. For this reason, genetic counseling may be most effectively accomplished through ongoing contact with the family as the medical or social issues become relevant to the lives of those involved.

The Profession of Genetic Counseling

Genetic counseling can be provided by genetic counselors, physicians, and genetic nurses. However, in the United States, Canada, the United Kingdom, and a few other countries, genetic counseling services are often provided by genetic counselors or genetic nurses, professionals specially trained in genetics and counseling, who serve as members of a health care team. Genetic counseling in the United States and Canada is a self-regulating health profession with its own board (the American and Canadian Boards of Genetic Counseling, respectively) for certification of practitioners and the Accreditation Council for Genetic Counseling for accreditation of training programs. Nurses with genetics expertise are certified through a separate process and organization. In the United States, many states license genetic counselors to provide clinical services. State-based licensing of medical providers serves as a measure to protect the public from unqualified providers by setting a standard for minimum education and training requirements and sets the state-specific scope of practice.

Genetic counselors and genetic nurses play an essential role in clinical genetics, participating in many aspects of the investigation and management of genetic conditions. A genetic counselor provides genetic counseling directly to individuals, helps patients and families deal with the many psychological and social issues that arise during genetic counseling, and continues in a supportive role and as a source of information after the clinical investigation and formal counseling have been completed. Genetic counselors are also active in the field of genetic testing; they serve as liaison between the referring physicians, the diagnostic laboratories, and the families themselves. Their special expertise is valuable to clinical laboratories because explaining and interpreting genetic testing to patients and referring physicians often requires a sophisticated knowledge of genetics and genomics as well as excellent communication skills.

Historically, genetic counseling was primarily performed in pediatric and prenatal clinical settings. However, increased understanding of the genetic contribution to medical conditions and the increased availability of genetic testing has increased the need for genetic counseling in many other medical specialties. For example, many genetic counselors now work in the specialties of oncology and cardiology, among others. Similarly, the unique training in genetics and genomics, biomedical technology, and psychosocial counseling received by genetic counselors allows genetic counselors to fulfill roles outside of patient care, such as research, marketing, and product development.

Common Indications for Genetic Counseling

Table 17.1 lists some of the most common situations that lead people to pursue genetic counseling. Individuals seeking genetic counseling (referred to as the **consultands**) may themselves have a genetic condition, or they may be the parents of an affected child or have relatives with a potential or known genetic condition. Additionally, consultands may seek genetic counseling in the pretesting setting to determine if they want to pursue genetic testing and in the posttesting setting for explanation and implications of results. Another important aspect of genetic counseling is to help individuals and their families adapt and strengthen their own abilities to manage the risk and impact of a genetic condition through supportive counseling. Genetic counseling is an integral part of prenatal testing (see Chapter 18) and of genetic testing and some screening programs (discussed in Chapter 19).

Established standards of medical care require that providers of genetic services obtain a history that includes family and ancestry information, inquire as to possible consanguinity, advise patients of the genetic risks to them and other family members, offer genetic testing or prenatal diagnosis when indicated, and outline the various treatment or management options for reducing the risk for disease. Although genetic counseling case management must be individualized for each consultand's needs and situation, a standard approach can be summarized (Table 17.2). The process of genetic counseling incorporates education, facilitating decision making and providing emotional support. This approach is necessary to support autonomy and to encourage shared decision making.

Psychosocial Considerations

Genetic counselors have expertise in psychosocial assessment, communication, and counseling techniques. The psychosocial domain includes the emotional, cognitive, familial, social, economic, and cultural beliefs of those involved. A challenging diagnostic journey or a new medical diagnosis often impacts all of these areas of the psychosocial domain. As discussed later in the chapter, uncertainty can be a particularly challenging experience for patients and their families. Patients and families receiving a genetic diagnosis experience many normal reactions that can include grief, guilt, shame, isolation, frustration, and psychological challenges such as anxiety and depression relating to chronic management of a condition that may be medically and psychosocially complex. Genetic counselors often help patients and their families understand and adapt to the medical, psychological, and familial implications of genetic

---

TABLE 17.1 Common Indications for Genetic Counseling

- Personal history or family history of a hereditary condition, such as cystic fibrosis, fragile X syndrome, congenital heart defect, hereditary cancer, or diabetes
- Previous child with multiple congenital anomalies, intellectual disability, or an isolated birth defect such as neural tube defect or cleft lip and palate
- Pregnancy at risk for a chromosomal or hereditary condition
- Consanguinity
- Teratogen exposure, such as to occupational chemicals, medications, alcohol
- Repeated pregnancy loss or infertility
- Newly diagnosed medical condition with genetic etiology
- Before pursuing genetic testing and after receiving results
- As follow-up for a positive result of a newborn test, as with phenylketonuria
- Carrier screening
- A positive first- or second-trimester maternal serum screen, a noninvasive prenatal screen by cell-free fetal DNA analysis, or abnormal fetal ultrasound examination results

---

TABLE 17.2 Genetic Counseling Case Management

Case Management
- Contracting (goal-setting and alignment)
- Clinical History
  - Family history
  - Medical and developmental history
  - Personal and familial genetic testing results
  - Laboratory, radiologic tests or additional assessments
- Risk Assessment and Counseling
  - Natural history
  - Inheritance patterns and associated recurrence risk
- Shared Decision Making
  - Genetic testing options and considerations
  - Review of management and treatment options
  - Referral to appropriate medical providers for diagnosis and management
- Psychosocial Considerations
  - Psychosocial assessment and support
  - Focused counseling
  - Connection to community, advocacy, and support resources

contributions to medical conditions and provide ongoing psychosocial assessment and counseling throughout the lifespan of the patient. Genetic counselors can be particularly helpful during periods of new challenges and transitions. Identifying individualized resources and sources of support is an important tenet of genetic counseling encounters. Many individuals have the strength to deal personally with such challenges; they may even prefer receiving bad news to remaining uninformed, and they make their own decisions based on the most complete and accurate information they can obtain. Other individuals require much more support and may need referral for psychotherapy. The extensive psychological aspects of genetic counseling are beyond the scope of this book, but several texts cited in the General References at the end of this chapter examine this important topic.

RISK ASSESSMENT

As noted, risk assessment is a key component of the larger genetic counseling process. Genetic counseling is much more than simply determining and providing a numerical risk to a consultand—in fact, it is the combination of counseling and communication skills with expertise in genetics principles and risk estimation that provides the unique niche of genetic counselors in the health care system. In this section we provide the fundamental principles and practice of risk assessment used by geneticists and genetic counselors.

FAMILY HISTORY RISK ASSESSMENT

The assessment of risk in genetic counseling begins with the personal and family medical histories. Family history collection can aid in identifying patterns of inheritance, establishing rapport with the patient and family, distinguishing genetic risk factors from other environmental risk factors, and determining medical surveillance for at-risk relatives. Applying the known rules of **mendelian** inheritance introduced in Chapter 7 allows the clinician to provide an assessment of risk for the condition in relatives of affected individuals (Fig. 17.1). Family history is also important when a clinician assesses the risk for complex conditions, as discussed in Chapter 9 and elsewhere in this book. Family history is also critical for determining when genetic and genomic testing is indicated.

Even in the absence of a recognizable pattern of mendelian inheritance or genetic testing, the family history can be a useful clinical tool. As discussed in Chapter 9, the more first-degree relatives one has with a complex trait and the earlier in life the medical condition occurs in a family member, the greater the load of susceptibility genes and environmental exposures likely to be present in the patient's family. Thus consideration of family history can lead to the designation of a patient as being at high risk for a particular medical condition based

on family history. For example, a male with three male first-degree relatives with prostate cancer has an 11-fold greater **relative risk** for development of the medical condition than a man with no such family history.

Determining that an individual is at increased risk based on family history can have an impact on individual medical care. For example, if there is family history information about a first-degree relative with colon cancer, that is sufficient to trigger the initiation of colon cancer screening by colonoscopy at the age of 40 years, or 10 years before the earliest diagnosis of colorectal cancer. This contrasts with the recommendation that people at average risk of colorectal cancer start regular screening at age 45. The increase in risk is even more pronounced if two or more relatives have had the same medical condition, an empirical observation that has driven standards of clinical care for screening in this condition. This family history information could also lead to genetic testing for a condition such as Lynch **syndrome**, which if present could have more significant medical care implications.

Although it is an indirect method of assessing the contribution of an individual's own genetic variants to health and disease susceptibility, the family history is a useful tool to provide individuals with a diagnosis, risk assessment, education, and psychosocial support. Direct detection of genetic risk factors and demonstrating that they are valid for guiding health care is a major challenge in applying genomics to medicine, as we will take up in Chapter 19.

Genetic counselors often refer a patient and family with a genetic condition or morphologic anomaly to family and patient support groups. These organizations, which can be focused either on a single medical condition or on a group of conditions, can help those concerned to share their experience, to learn how to deal with the day-to-day problems caused by the condition, to hear of new developments in therapy or prevention, and to promote research into the condition. Many support groups have internet and social media sites, through

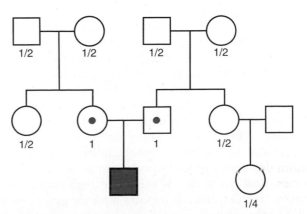

Figure 17.1 Pedigree of a family with an **autosomal recessive** condition. The probability of being a carrier is shown beneath each individual symbol in the pedigree.

BOX 17.1 GENETIC COUNSELING AND RISK ASSESSMENT

One component of genetic counseling is to provide information and support to families at risk for having, or who already have, members with genetic conditions. Genetic counseling helps the family or individual to do the following:

- Comprehend the medical facts, including the diagnosis, the probable course of the condition, and the available management.
- Understand the way heredity contributes to the condition and the inheritance risks for themselves and other family members.
- Understand the available reproductive options for mitigating genetic risks.
- Identify those values, beliefs, goals, and relationships affected by the risk for, or presence of, hereditary condition.
- Choose the course of action that seems most appropriate to them in view of their risk, their family goals, and their ethical and religious standards.
- Make the best possible adjustment to the condition or to the inheritance risks for that condition, or both, by providing supportive counseling to families and making referrals to appropriate specialists, social services, and family and patient support groups.

TABLE 17.3 Factors That Impact Risk Perception

- Seriousness of the condition
- Personal attributes: age, education, gender, coping style, risk tolerance, optimism, having a living affected child, desire for children
- Beliefs about etiology, prognosis, and risk management options
- Stress and perceptions of vulnerability
- Familial experience with the condition
- Sense of "likeness" with the affected family member
- Level and accuracy of knowledge
- Heightened media attention

From Uhlmann WR, Schuette JL, Yashar B: A guide to genetic counseling, ed 2, New York, 2009, Wiley-Liss.

which patients and families give and receive information and advice, ask and answer questions, and obtain much needed emotional support. Similar condition-specific, self-help organizations are active in many nations around the world.

RISK COMMUNICATION AND PERCEPTION

One of the primary responsibilities of a genetic counselor is to communicate risk effectively. Most individuals can appreciate the concept of risk; however, acceptable risk thresholds and communication preferences are highly individual and may vary depending upon the circumstances. The multifaceted process of risk communication involves calculating the risks, tailored communication, and engaging patients in guided and informative conversations (see Box 17.1). There are many factors that impact the risk communication process. Some of these factors include the ability to internalize and retain risk information, one's own perception of risk, the impact of fear, distress or anxiety, and patient preference for the format of risk information (e.g., percentage vs proportions). Many adults have limited numeracy, with only 10% of adults scoring in upper levels of numeric understanding. Therefore, assuming individuals can both understand and utilize complex numeric risk to make health decisions can lead to suboptimal counseling outcomes. Risk perception is subject to both internal and external factors, and it is important for the genetic counselor to thoughtfully consider and explore these factors throughout the communication process (Table 17.3). Goal alignment in patient encounters can help to ground

these challenging conversations. A critical part of the genetic counseling process is to accurately ascertain the consultand's questions and needs. The consultand's goal(s) for the session may be very different from that of the provider and may involve complex family dynamics, profound existential questions, or more pragmatic questions such as deciding about genetic testing or choosing among various management options.

In some circumstances qualitative risk descriptions may be helpful; however, they should be used cautiously. Adding qualitative descriptors such as "high" or "low" when describing risk can inadvertently add subjective bias. Presenting both sides of a risk figure can be a useful and balanced strategy. For example, in a couple who is **heterozygous** for a recessively inherited condition, one could explain there is a 25% chance of an affected offspring and a 75% chance that the offspring would not be affected with each pregnancy. Lastly, checking patient understanding is a key strategy to assess confusion, misinformation, and/or perceptions about risk information that has been presented. There are several studies about patient empowerment that demonstrate that the genetic counseling process of supporting autonomy and decision making is often more impactful than the risk number itself.

DETERMINING RECURRENCE RISKS

The estimation of recurrence risks is an important component of genetic counseling. Ideally, it is based on knowledge of the genetic nature of the condition in question and on the **pedigree** of the family being counseled. The consultand whose risk for a genetic condition is to be determined is usually a relative of a **proband**, such as a sibling of an affected child or a living or future child of an affected adult. In some families, especially for some traits inherited in an autosomal **dominant** or X-linked pattern, it may also be necessary to estimate the risk for more remote relatives.

When a condition is known to have single-**gene** inheritance, the **recurrence risk** for specific family members can usually be determined from basic mendelian principles (see Fig. 17.1; also see Chapter 7). On the other hand, risk calculations may be less than straightforward if there is reduced **penetrance** or variability of expression, or if the condition is frequently the result of a *de novo* **variant**, as in many conditions with X-linked and autosomal dominant inheritance. Laboratory tests that give uncertain results can add further complications. Under these circumstances, mendelian risk estimates can sometimes be modified by means of applying the method of bayesian probability to the pedigree (see later), which considers information about the family that may increase or decrease the underlying mendelian risk. In fact, bayesian probability is widely used across all domains of the medical diagnostic process. Here we show the application of this fundamental principle to genetic risk assessment and diagnosis for conditions with mendelian inheritance.

In contrast to single-gene conditions, the underlying mechanisms of inheritance for most chromosomal or medical conditions cannot be calculated through use of basic genetic principles because of many unknown factors that are involved. For most complex genetic conditions, risk also cannot be assessed in this way, although rapid advances in **polygenic risk scores** will lead to advances in the near future. For these conditions, estimates of recurrence risk are based on previous experience, known as **empirical risk** (Fig. 17.2). This approach to risk assessment is useful if there are reliable data on the frequency of recurrence of the condition in families and if the **phenotype** is not heterogeneous. However, if a phenotype has etiologic **heterogeneity** and phenocopies with widely different risks, estimation of the recurrence risk is hazardous at best. In a later section, the estimation of recurrence risk in some typical clinical situations, both straightforward and more complicated, is considered.

GENERAL PRINCIPLES OF RISK ESTIMATION

Risk estimations are calculations based on the family and medical history information from the consultand and other family members, diagnostic and testing data, and the state of current knowledge. While the soundness of the fundamental principles of genetics and probability upon which such estimates are based is assured, it is essential for the clinician to recognize the limitations of such risk estimates. Family history recall is rarely complete or completely correct. Diagnostic and test data may be historical with little documentation. Knowledge of genetic conditions is changing constantly. Therefore it is essential when calculating risk estimates to make reasonable assumptions about these source data. The clinician should specify these assumptions and limitations so that changes in such understanding can lead to revised estimates in the future.

Risk Estimation by Use of Mendel's Laws When Genotypes Are Fully Known

The simplest risk estimates pertain to conditions with simple mendelian inheritance patterns and apply to families in which the relevant genotypes of all family members are known or can be inferred. For example, if both members of a couple are known to be heterozygous carriers of a condition with autosomal **recessive** inheritance because of **carrier** testing, the risk (probability) is one in four with each pregnancy that the child will inherit two pathogenic alleles and manifest the condition (Fig. 17.3A). Even if the couple were to have six unaffected children (see Fig. 17.3B), the risk in the seventh, eighth, or ninth, pregnancy would still be one in four for each pregnancy.

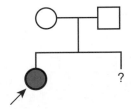

Figure 17.2 Empirical risk estimates in genetic counseling. A family with no other positive family history has one child affected with a condition known to be multifactorial or chromosomal. What is the recurrence risk? If the child is affected with spina bifida, the empirical risk to a subsequent child is ~4%. If the child has Down syndrome, the empirical risk for recurrence would be ~1% if the karyotype is trisomy 21, but it may be substantially higher if one of the parents is a carrier of a robertsonian translocation involving chromosome 21 (see Chapter 6).

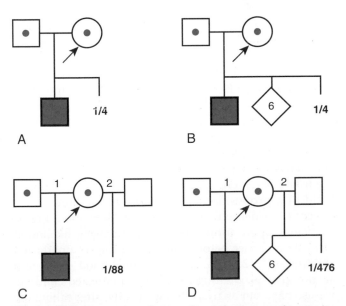

Figure 17.3 Series of pedigrees showing autosomal recessive inheritance with contrasting recurrence risks. (A, B) The genotypes of the parents are known. (C) The genotype of the consultand's second partner is inferred from the carrier frequency in the population. (D) The inferred genotype is modified by additional pedigree information. *Arrows* indicate the consultand. Numbers indicate recurrence risk in the consultand's next pregnancy.

Risk Estimation by Use of Conditional Probability When Alternative Genotypes Are Possible

In contrast to the simple case just described, situations arise in which the genotypes of the relevant individuals in the family are not definitively known; the risk for recurrence will be very different, depending on whether the consultand is a carrier of a pathogenic **allele** of a gene. For example, the chance that a woman, who has an offspring with cystic fibrosis (CF), with her first partner might have a subsequent affected child depends on the chance that her next partner is a carrier of a pathogenic allele in the gene that causes CF, *CFTR* (see Fig. 17.3C). The likelihood that the partner is a carrier depends on his ancestry (see Chapter 10). For the general US non-Hispanic white (a US census category) population, this likelihood is ~1 in 22. Therefore the chance that a known carrier and her unrelated partner would have an affected first child is the product of these probabilities, or $\frac{1}{22} \times \frac{1}{4} = \frac{1}{88}$ (~1.1%).

Of course, if the second partner actually were a carrier, the chance that the child of two carriers would be a **homozygote** or a **compound heterozygote** for the pathogenic CF alleles is one in four. If the second partner were not a carrier, then the chance of having an affected child is very low < (<<1%). Suppose, however, that one cannot test the second partner's carrier status directly. A carrier risk of 1 in 22 is the best estimate one can make for individuals of his ancestry who have no family history of CF, when carrier testing is not possible. This person either is a carrier or is not, but the problem is that we do not know. In this situation, the more opportunities the male in Fig. 17.3C (who may or may not be a carrier of a pathogenic allele) has to pass on the pathogenic allele and fails to do so, the less likely it would be that he is indeed a carrier. Thus if the couple were to come for counseling already with six children, none of whom is affected (see Fig. 17.3D), it would seem reasonable, intuitively, that the man's chance of being a carrier should be less than the 1 in 22 risk that the childless male partner in Fig. 17.3C was assigned based on the population carrier frequency. In this situation, we apply **bayesian analysis** (based on Bayes's theorem on probability published in 1763), a method that measures the likelihood of a proposition before and after accounting for a piece of evidence that bears on that likelihood. In this particular application, the second partner's likelihood of being a carrier before considering the six unaffected children is 1/22. To calculate his likelihood of being a carrier after accounting for the six unaffected children, we use bayesian analysis. In Fig. 17.3D, after taking the six unaffected children into account, the chance that the second partner is a carrier is 1 in 119, and the chance that this couple would have a child with CF is therefore 1 in 476, not 1 in 88, as calculated in Fig. 17.3C. Some examples of the use of bayesian analysis for risk assessment in pedigrees are examined in the following section.

Bayesian Analysis Using Conditional Probability

To illustrate the application of bayesian analysis, consider the pedigrees shown in Fig. 17.4. In Family A, the mother II-1 is an obligate carrier for the bleeding disorder hemophilia A, which is inherited in an X-linked recessive pattern because her father was affected. Her risk for transmitting the pathogenic factor VIII *(F8)* allele responsible for hemophilia A is 1 in 2, and the fact that she has already had four unaffected sons does not reduce this risk. Bayesian analysis cannot be used to adjust the mother's risk since her **genotype** is known. Thus the risk that the consultand (III-5) is a carrier of a pathogenic *F8* allele is 1 in 2 because she is the daughter of a known carrier

In Family B, however, the consultand's mother (individual II-2) may or may not be a carrier, depending on whether she has inherited a pathogenic *F8* allele from her mother, I-1. Bayesian analysis can be used to adjust the consultand's risk since the mother's genotype is not known and alternative genotypes are possible. If III-5 were the only child of her mother, III-5's risk for being a carrier would be 1 in 4, calculated as $\frac{1}{2}$ (her mother's risk for being a carrier) $\times \frac{1}{2}$ (her risk for inheriting the pathogenic allele from her mother). Short of testing III-5 directly for the pathogenic allele, we cannot tell whether she is a carrier. In this case, however, the fact that III-5 has four unaffected brothers is relevant because every

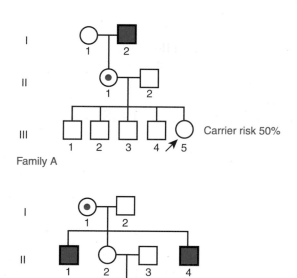

Figure 17.4 Modified risk estimates in genetic counseling. The consultands in the two families are at risk for having a son with hemophilia A. In Family A, the consultand's mother is an obligate heterozygote; in Family B, the consultand's mother may or may not be a carrier. Application of bayesian analysis reduces the risk for being a carrier to only ~3% for the consultand in Family B but not the consultand in Family A. See text for derivation of the modified risk.

time II-2 had a son, the chance that the son would be unaffected is only 1 in 2 if II-2 were a carrier, whereas it is a near certainty (probability = 1) that the son would be unaffected if II-2 were, in fact, not a carrier at all. With each son, II-2 has, in effect, tested her carrier status by placing herself at a 50% risk for that son to be affected. To have four unaffected sons is a **conditional probability** that reduces the likelihood that her mother is a carrier. Bayesian analysis allows one to take this kind of indirect information into account in calculating whether II-2 is a carrier, thus modifying the consultand's risk for being a carrier. In fact, as we show in the next section, her carrier risk is far lower than 50%.

Identify the Possible Scenarios

To translate this intuition into actual risk calculation, we use a bayesian probability calculation. First, we list all possible alternative genotypes that may be present in the relevant individuals in the pedigree (Fig. 17.5). In this case there are three scenarios, each reflecting a different combination of alternative genotypes:

A. II-2 is a carrier, but the consultand is not.
B. II-2 and the consultand are both carriers.
C. II-2 is not a carrier, which implies that the consultand could not be one either because there is no variant allele to inherit.

Why do we not consider the possibility that the consultand is a carrier even though II-2 is not? We do not list this scenario because it would require the occurrence of two *de novo* pathogenic variants in the same gene independently in the same family, one inherited by the affected males (II-1 and II-4) and one in the consultand, a scenario that is so unlikely that it does not significantly change the resulting risk estimate.

First, we draw the three possible scenarios as pedigrees (as in Fig. 17.5) and write down the probability of individual II-2's being a carrier or not. This is referred to as her prior probability because it depends simply on her risk for carrying a variant allele inherited from her known carrier mother, I-1, and it has not been modified (conditioned) at all by her own reproductive history.

Next, we write down the probabilities that individuals III-1 through III-4 would be unaffected under each scenario. These probabilities are different, depending on whether II-2 is a carrier or not. If she is a carrier (situations A and B), then the chance that individuals III-1 through III-4 would all be unaffected is the chance that each did not inherit II-2's variant *F8* allele, which is 1 in 2 for each of her sons or $(\frac{1}{2})^4$ for all four. In situation C, however, II-2 is not a carrier, so the chance that her four sons would all be unaffected is 1 because II-2 does not have a variant *F8* to pass on to any of them. These are called **conditional probabilities** because they are probabilities based on the conditions of each scenario, II-2 is a carrier or II-2 is not a carrier.

Similarly, we can write down the probability that the consultand (III-5) is a carrier. In A, she did not inherit the variant allele from her carrier mother, with a probability of 1 in 2. In B, she did inherit the variant allele (probability = ½). In C, her mother is not a carrier, and so III-5 has essentially a 100% chance of not being a carrier. Multiply the prior and conditional probabilities together to form the joint probabilities for each situation, A, B, and C.

Finally, we determine what fraction of the total joint probability is represented by any scenario of interest; this is called the posterior probability of each of the three situations. Because III-5 is the consultand and

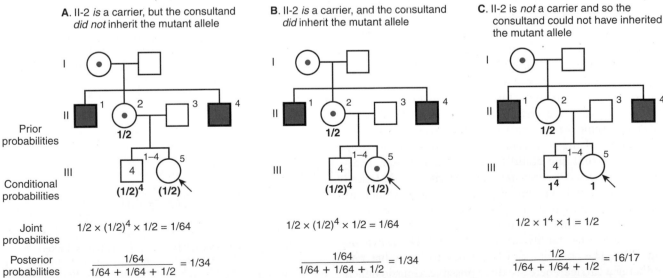

Figure 17.5 Conditional probability used to estimate carrier risk for a consultand in a family with hemophilia in which the prior probability of the carrier state is determined by mendelian inheritance from a known carrier at the top of the pedigree. These risk estimates, based on genetic principles, can be further modified by considering information obtained from family history, carrier detection testing, or molecular genetic methods for direct detection of the pathogenic variant in the affected boy, with use of bayesian calculations. (A–C) The three mutually exclusive situations that could explain the pedigree.

wants to know her risk for being a carrier, we need the posterior probability of situation B, which is:

$$\frac{\dfrac{1}{64}}{\dfrac{1}{64} + \dfrac{1}{64} + \dfrac{1}{2}} = \frac{1}{34} = \approx 3\%$$

If we wish to know the chance that II-2 is a carrier, we add the posterior probabilities of the two situations in which she is a carrier, A and B, to get a carrier risk of 1 in 17, or ~6%.

If III-5 were also to have unaffected sons, her carrier risk could also be modified downward by a bayesian calculation. However, if II-2 were to have an affected child, then she would have proved herself a carrier, and III-5's risk would thus become 1 in 2. Similarly, if III-5 were to have an affected child, then she must be a carrier, and bayesian analysis would no longer be necessary.

Bayesian analysis may seem to some like mere statistical maneuvering. However, the analysis allows the clinician to quantify what seemed to be intuitively likely from inspection of the pedigree: the fact that the consultand had four unaffected brothers provides support for the hypothesis that her mother is not a carrier. The analysis having been performed, the final risk that III-5 is a carrier can be used in genetic counseling. The risk that her first child will have hemophilia A is $\frac{1}{34} \times \frac{1}{4}$, or less than 1%. This risk is appreciably below the prior probability estimated without considering the genetic evidence provided by her brothers and demonstrates the importance of using all available information to assess the risk.

Bayesian Probability in Zero Reproductive Fitness and X-Linked Inheritance

Because conditions with X-linked recessive inheritance are manifested in the **hemizygous** male, an isolated occurrence (no family history) of such a condition may represent either a *de novo* **pathogenic variant** (in which case the mother is not a carrier) or inheritance of a pathogenic allele from his unaffected carrier mother; we do not consider the chance of gonadal **mosaicism** for the pathogenic variant in the mother (see Chapter 7). Estimation of the recurrence risk depends on knowing the chance that she could be a carrier. Bayesian analysis can be used to estimate carrier risks in X-linked conditions that have zero reproductive **fitness** such as Duchenne muscular dystrophy (DMD) and severe ornithine transcarbamylase deficiency.

Consider the family at risk for DMD shown in Fig. 17.6. The consultand, III-2, wants to know her risk for being a carrier. There are three possible scenarios, each with dramatically different risk estimates for the family:

A. III-1's condition may be the result of a *de novo* pathogenic variant. In this case, his sister and maternal aunt are not at significant risk for being a carrier.

B. His mother, II-1, is a carrier, but her condition is the result of a *de novo* pathogenic variant. In this case, his sister (III-2) has a ~1 in 2 risk for being a carrier, but his maternal aunt is at population risk for being a carrier because his grandmother, I-1, is not a carrier.

C. His mother is a carrier who inherited a pathogenic allele from her carrier mother (I-1). In this case, all the female relatives have either a 1 in 2 or a 1 in 4 risk for being carriers.

How can we use conditional probability to determine the carrier risks for the female relatives of III-1 in this pedigree? If we proceed as we did previously with the hemophilia family in Fig. 17.4, what do we use as the prior probability that individual I-1 is a carrier? We do not have pedigree information, as we did in the hemophilia pedigree, from which to calculate these prior probabilities. We can, however, use some simple assumptions that the frequency of the condition is unchanging (see Chapter 10), and the *de novo* **mutation rate** per **chromosome** is equal in males and females to estimate the prior probability (see Box 17.2).

$$H = (\frac{1}{2} \times H) + \mu + \mu = H/2 + 2\mu$$

BOX 17.2 PRIOR PROBABILITY THAT A FEMALE IN THE POPULATION IS A CARRIER OF A GENETICALLY LETHAL CONDITION WITH X-LINKED RECESSIVE INHERITANCE

Suppose H is the population frequency of female carriers of an X-linked lethal condition. Assume H is constant from generation to generation.

Suppose the mutation rate at this X-linked locus in any one gamete = μ. Assume μ is the same in males and females. Mutation rate μ is a small number, in the range of 10^{-4} to 10^{-6} (see Chapter 4).

Then, there are three mutually exclusive ways that any female could be a carrier:

1. She inherits a variant allele from a carrier mother = $\frac{1}{2} \times H$. or
2. She receives a newly pathogenic allele on the X she receives from her mother = μ. *or*
3. She receives a newly pathogenic allele on the X she receives from her father = μ.

The chance a randomly ascertained female is a carrier is the sum of the chance that she inherited a preexisting variant and the chance that she received a new pathogenic variant from her mother or from her father.

$$H = (\frac{1}{2} \times H) + \mu + \mu = H/2 + 2\mu$$

Solving for H, you get the chance that a random female in the population is a carrier of a particular X-linked condition = 4μ. Note that half of this 4μ, 2μ, is the probability she is a carrier by inheritance, and the other 2μ is the probability that she is a carrier by a *de novo* pathogenic variant.

The chance a random female in the population is *not* a carrier is $1 - 4\mu \cong 1$ (because μ is a very small number).

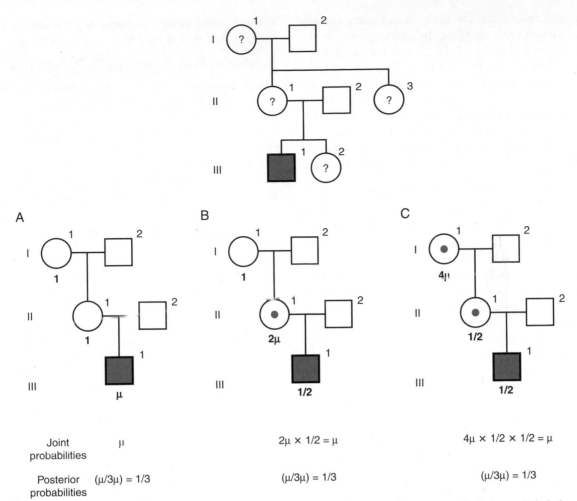

Figure 17.6 Conditional probability used to determine carrier risks for females in a family with an X-linked genetic lethal condition in which the prior probability of being a carrier has to be calculated by assuming that the carrier frequency is not changing from generation to generation, and that the mutation rates are the same in males and females. *(Top)* Pedigree of a family with an X-linked genetic lethal condition. *(Bottom)* The three mutually exclusive situations that could explain the pedigree. (A) The proband is a new pathogenic variant. (B) The mother of the proband is a new pathogenic variant. (C) The mother of the proband inherited the pathogenic variant from her carrier mother, the grandmother of the proband.

Now we can use this value 4μ from the Box as the prior probability that a woman is a carrier of an X-linked lethal condition (see Fig. 17.6). For the purpose of calculating the chance that II-1 is a carrier, we ignore the female relatives II-3 and III-2 because there is nothing known about them, such as phenotype, laboratory testing, or reproductive history, that could serve as a conditional probability that would affect the likelihood that II-1 is a carrier.

- A. III-1 is a *de novo* pathogenic variant with probability μ. His mother and grandmother are both noncarriers, each of which has a probability of $1 - 4\mu \cong 1$. The joint probability is $\mu \times 1 \times 1 = \mu$.
- B. I-1 is a noncarrier, and so II-1 must be the product of a maternal or paternal *de novo* pathogenic variant and not a carrier by inheritance because we are specifying in scenario B that I-1 is not a carrier. The chance that a female will be a carrier by *de novo* pathogenic variant only is $\mu + \mu = 2\mu$ (and not 4μ). The joint probability is therefore $2\mu \times \frac{1}{2} = \mu$.

- C. Individuals I-1 and II-1 are both carriers. As explained in the Box, the chance that I-1 is a carrier has a prior probability of 4μ. For II-1 to be a carrier, she must have inherited the variant allele from her mother, which has probability 1 in 2. In addition, the chance that II-1 has passed the variant allele on to her affected son is also 1 in 2. The joint probability is therefore $4\mu \times \frac{1}{2} \times \frac{1}{2} = \mu$.

The posterior probabilities are now easy to calculate as $\mu/(\mu + \mu + \mu) = \frac{1}{3}$ each for scenarios A, B, and C. A key feature of this calculation is that since μ is in both the numerator and the denominator, they cancel and thus the fact that μ varies among various genes does not matter—the 1/3 risk of being a carrier is the same. The affected boy has a 1 in 3 chance of being affected because of a *de novo* pathogenic variant (situation A), whereas his mother II-1 is a carrier in both B and C and therefore has a $\frac{1}{3} + \frac{1}{3} = \frac{2}{3}$ chance of being a carrier. The grandmother, I-1, is a carrier only in C, and so her chance of being a carrier is 1 in 3.

With these risk figures for the core individuals in the pedigree, we can then calculate the carrier risks for the female relatives II-3 and III-2. III-2's risk for being a carrier is $\frac{1}{2} \times$ [the chance II-1 is a carrier] $= \frac{1}{2} \times \frac{2}{3} = \frac{1}{3}$. The risk that II-3 is a carrier is $\frac{1}{2} \times$ [the chance I-1 is a carrier] $= \frac{1}{2} \times \frac{1}{3} = \frac{1}{6}$. In all of these calculations, for the sake of simplicity, we do not include the small but very real possibility of **germline** or somatic mosaicism. In a real genetic counseling situation, however, the possibility of mosaicism must be communicated to the family.

Conditions With Incomplete Penetrance

To estimate the recurrence risk for conditions with incomplete penetrance, the probability that an apparently unaffected person is heterozygous for the gene variant in question must be considered. Fig. 17.7 shows a pedigree of split hand malformation, which has autosomal dominant inheritance with incomplete penetrance (discussed in Chapter 7). An estimate of penetrance can be made from a single pedigree if it is large enough, or from a review of published pedigrees; we use 70% in our example. Thus a heterozygote for a pathogenic variant that causes split hand malformation has a 30% chance of not showing the phenotype. The pedigree shows several people who must be heterozygous for the variant gene but do not manifest it (i.e., in whom the condition is not penetrant), I-1 or I-2 (assuming no somatic or **germline mosaicism**) and II-3. The other unaffected family members may or may not be heterozygous for the variant gene.

If III-4, the daughter of a known affected heterozygote, is the consultand, there are two possibilities (Fig. 17.8). First, she may have not inherited the variant allele from her affected mother or, second, she may have inherited it but is not manifesting the phenotype because of incomplete penetrance. In A, III-4 has a prior probability of 1 in 2 of not being heterozygous for the variant. If she is not heterozygous for the variant, she has an essentially 100% chance of not manifesting the phenotype, so the joint probability for A is $\frac{1}{2} \times 1 = \frac{1}{2}$ or 0.5. In B, III-4 is heterozygous for the variant, also with prior probability 1 in 2. Here, we must apply the conditional probability that she is heterozygous for the variant but does not manifest the phenotype, which has probability of 1 − penetrance = 1 − 0.7 = 0.3, so the joint probability for B is $\frac{1}{2} \times 0.3 = 0.15$. The posterior probability that III-4 is heterozygous for the variant

without manifesting the phenotype is therefore (0.15)/(0.15 + 0.5) = $\frac{3}{13}$ = ≈23%.

Conditions With Age-Specific Penetrance

Many conditions with autosomal dominant inheritance show a late age at onset, beyond the age of reproduction. Thus, it is not uncommon in risk assessment to ask whether a person of reproductive age, who is at risk though asymptomatic for such a condition, harbors the pathogenic variant. One example of such a condition is a rare, familial form of Parkinson disease (PD) inherited in an autosomal dominant pattern with age-specific penetrance.

Consider the pedigree in Fig. 17.9 in which the consultand, an asymptomatic 35-year-old man, wishes to know his risk for PD. His prior risk for having inherited the PD pathogenic variant from his affected grandmother is 1 in 4. Considering that perhaps only 5% of persons with this rare form of PD have symptoms at his age, he would not be expected to have signs of the condition even if he had inherited the variant allele. The more significant aspect of the pedigree, however, is that the consultand's

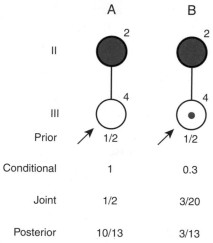

	A	B
Prior	1/2	1/2
Conditional	1	0.3
Joint	1/2	3/20
Posterior	10/13	3/13

Figure 17.8 Conditional probability calculation for the risk for the carrier state in the consultant in Fig. 17.7. There are two possibilities: either she is not a carrier (A) or she is a carrier (B). Her failure to demonstrate the phenotype lowers her carrier risk from the prior probability of 1 in 2 (50%) to 3 in 13 (23%).

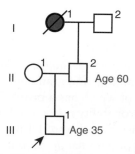

Figure 17.9 Age-modified risks for genetic counseling in dominant Parkinson disease. That the consultand's father is asymptomatic at the age of 60 years reduces the consultand's final risk for carrying the gene to ~12.5%. That the consultand himself is asymptomatic reduces the risk only slightly because most patients carrying the pathogenic allele for this disease will be asymptomatic at the age of 35 years.

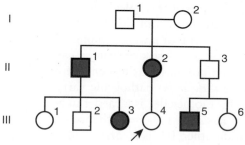

Figure 17.7 Pedigree of family with split hand deformity and lack of penetrance in some individuals.

father (II-2) is also asymptomatic at the age of 60 years, an age by which perhaps two-thirds of persons with this form of PD have symptoms and one-third do not.

As shown in Fig. 17.10, there are three possibilities:

A. His father did not inherit the variant allele, so the consultand is not at risk.
B. His father inherited the pathogenic variant and is asymptomatic at the age of 60 years, but the consultand did not.
C. His father inherited the variant allele and is asymptomatic. The consultand inherited it from his father and is asymptomatic at the age of 35 years.

The father's chance of having the variant allele (situations B and C) is 25%; the consultand's chance of having the variant allele (situation C only) is 12%. Providing these recurrence risks in genetic counseling requires careful follow-up. If, for example, the consultand's father were to develop symptoms of PD, the risks would change dramatically.

EMPIRICAL RECURRENCE RISKS

Counseling for Complex Conditions

Genetic counselors deal with many conditions that are not single-gene diseases. Instead, counselors may be called on to provide risk estimates for complex medical condition with a strong genetic component and familial clustering, such as cleft lip and palate, **congenital** heart disease, meningomyelocele, psychiatric illness, and coronary artery disease (see Chapter 9). In these situations the risk for recurrence in first-degree relatives of affected individuals may be increased over the background incidence of the condition in the population. For most of these conditions, however, knowledge is still emerging about the relevant underlying genetic variants or how they interact with each other or with the environment to cause these conditions.

As the information gained through the **Human Genome Project** is applied to the problem of medical conditions with **complex inheritance**, physicians, genetic counselors, and other health professionals will have more of the information they need to provide accurate molecular diagnosis and risk assessment and to develop rational preventive and therapeutic measures. In the meantime, however, clinicians must rely on empirically derived risk figures to give patients and their relatives some answers to their questions about their risk and how to manage that risk. Recurrence risks are estimated empirically by studying as many families with the condition as possible and observing how frequently the condition recurs. The observed frequency of a recurrence is taken as an empirical recurrence risk. With time, research should make empirical recurrence risks obsolete, replacing them with individualized assessments of risk based on knowledge of a person's polygenic risk score and environmental exposures.

Another area in which empirical recurrence risks must be applied is for chromosomal abnormalities (see Chapter 6). When one member of a couple is carrying a chromosomal or **genome** abnormality, such as a balanced **translocation** or a chromosomal **inversion**, the risk for a liveborn, chromosomally unbalanced child depends on a number of factors. These include the following:

- Whether the couple was ascertained through a previous liveborn child with a chromosome abnormality, in which case a viable offspring with the chromosome abnormality is clearly possible, or the **ascertainment** was through chromosome or genome studies for infertility or recurrent miscarriage
- The chromosomes involved, which region of the chromosome was affected, and the size of the regions that could be potentially trisomic or monosomic in the fetus
- Whether the mother or father is the carrier of the balanced translocation or inversion

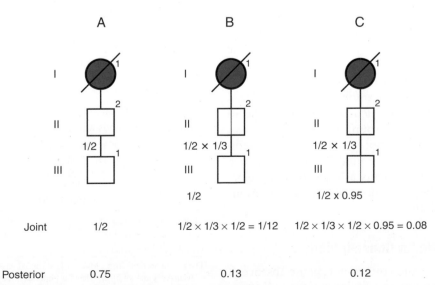

Figure 17.10 Three scenarios pertaining to the Parkinson disease pedigree in Fig. 17.9. Individual II-2 is a nonpenetrant carrier (*vertical line* inside the symbol) in scenarios B and C. Individual III-1 is a nonpenetrant carrier in scenario C.

These factors must all be considered when empirical recurrence risks are determined for a couple in which one member is carrying a balanced translocation or a seemingly normal genomic **copy number variant**.

Empirical recurrence risks are also applied when both parents are chromosomally normal but have a child with, for example, **trisomy** 21. In this case, the age of the mother plays a major role in that, in a woman younger than 30 years, recurrence risk for trisomy 21 is ~5 per 1000 and the risk for any chromosome abnormality is ~10 per 1000 as opposed to the population risk of ~1.6 per 1000 live births. Over age 30, however, the age-specific risk becomes the dominant factor, and the fact of a previously affected child with trisomy 21 plays much less of a role in determining recurrence risk.

Clinicians must use caution in applying empirical risk figures to a particular family. First, empirical estimates are an average over what is undoubtedly a group of heterogeneous conditions with different mechanisms of inheritance. In any one family, the real recurrence risk may be higher or lower than the average. Second, empirical risk estimates use history to make predictions about future occurrences; if the underlying biologic causes are changing through time, data from the past may not be accurate for the future.

For example, neural tube defects (myelomeningocele and anencephaly) occur in ~3.3 per 1000 live births in the US of European ancestry. If, however, a couple has a child with a neural tube defect, the risk in the next pregnancy has been shown to be 40 per 1000 (13 times higher). The risks remained elevated compared with the general population risk for more distantly related individuals; a second-degree relative (e.g., a nephew or niece) of an individual with a neural tube defect was found to have a 1.7% chance of a similar **birth defect**. Thus, as we saw in Chapter 9, neural tube defects manifest many of the features typical of multifactorial inheritance. However, these empirical recurrence risks were calculated before widespread folic acid supplementation. With folate supplementation before conception and during early pregnancy, these recurrence risk figures have fallen dramatically (see Chapter 9). This is not because the allelic variants in the families have changed but rather because a critical environmental factor has changed.

Finally, it is important to emphasize that empirical figures are derived from a particular population, and so the data from one ancestry group, socioeconomic class, or geographic location may not be accurate for an individual from a different background. Nonetheless, such figures are useful when patients ask genetic counselors to give a best estimate for recurrence risk for conditions with complex inheritance.

Genetic Counseling for Consanguinity

In counseling a consanguineous couple, in the absence of a family history for a known condition with autosomal recessive inheritance, we use empirical risk figures for the offspring, based on population surveys of congenital **anomalies** in children born to first-cousin couples compared with nonconsanguineous couples (Table 17.4).

These results provide empirical risk figures in the counseling of first cousins. The relative risk for a genetic condition in the offspring is higher for related than for unrelated parents: approximately double in the offspring of first cousins, compared with baseline risk figures for any abnormality of 15 to 20 per 1000 for any child, regardless of consanguinity. This increased risk is not exclusively for single-gene conditions with autosomal recessive inheritance but includes the entire spectrum of single-gene and complex conditions. However, any couple, consanguineous or not, who has a child with a congenital anomaly is at greater risk for having another affected child in a subsequent pregnancy.

These risk estimates for consanguinity may be slightly inflated given they are derived from communities in which first-cousin marriages are widespread and encouraged. These are societies in which the **degree of relationship** (coefficient of **inbreeding**) between two first cousins may be greater than the theoretical $\frac{1}{16}$ due to multiple other lines of relatedness (see Chapter 10). Furthermore, these same societies may also limit marriages to individuals from the same clan, leading to substantial population **stratification**, which also increases the rate of conditions with autosomal recessive inheritance beyond what might be expected based on variant allele frequency alone (see Chapter 10).

REPRODUCTIVE OPTIONS

Many families seek genetic counseling to ascertain the risk for heritable conditions in their children and to learn about possible options. All reproductive options available to the family should be stated, though the discussion may be focused on one or two of the options depending on the family's desires and values. Prenatal diagnosis is an option when the pathogenic variant(s) of the genetic condition are known or for conditions that can be diagnosed by biochemical or cytogenetic tests (see Chapter 18). Similarly, preimplantation genetic

TABLE 17.4 Incidence of Birth Defects in Children Born to Nonconsanguineous and First-Cousin Couples

	Incidence of First Birth Defect in Sibship (per 1000)	Incidence of Recurrence of Any Birth Defect in Subsequent Children in Sibship (per 1000)
First-cousin marriage	36	68
Nonconsanguineous marriage	15	30

Data from Stoltenberg C, Magnus P, Skrondal A, et al: Consanguinity and recurrence risk of birth defects: a population-based study, Am J Med Genet 82:424–428, 1999.

testing is an option when the pathogenic variant(s) causing a genetic condition in a family are known (see Chapter 18). When a parent has an autosomal dominant or X-linked condition, use of a **gamete** donor can significantly reduce the chance to have a child with a genetic condition. Use of a sperm donor for couples at risk to have a child with an autosomal recessive is a viable reproductive option, assuming that the sperm donor, whether anonymous or designated, has been screened for the genetic condition in question, with negative test results. Use of an egg donor can also be offered to reduce the risk for chromosome abnormality in families who are concerned about maternal age-related **aneuploidy** or in families with mitochondrial conditions caused by pathogenic variants in the **mitochondrial DNA**. Adoption is also an option for families that want a child or more children. Similarly, for couple's wanting to experience pregnancy, receipt of an embryo donated by another couple is an available family planning option. Lastly, if the parents do not plan to have additional children, contraception may be the best option, and they may need information about possible procedures or an appropriate referral. Discussions around family planning can elicit strong emotions, so discussions are best approached in a sensitive manner that elicits the family's personal and cultural desires and values.

GENETIC COUNSELING IN THE ERA OF GENOMIC MEDICINE

Molecular and Genome-Based Diagnostics

Recent advances in molecular technology have led to increased diagnostic rates across all areas of clinical genetics allowing providers to make more accurate/precise diagnoses and perform more specific risk assessment. With our expanding knowledge of the genes involved in hereditary conditions and the rapidly falling cost of DNA sequencing, direct detection of pathogenic variants in a patient's or family member's **genomic DNA** to make a molecular diagnosis has become standard of care for many conditions. DNA samples for analysis are available from such readily accessible tissues as a blood sample, buccal swab or saliva sample, but also from tissues obtained by more invasive testing, such as **chorionic villus sampling** or **amniocentesis** (see Chapter 18).

Genetic test results for mendelian disorders generally report the identified variants as being pathogenic, likely pathogenic, **variant of uncertain significance** (**VUS**), likely benign, or benign. This five-category scale is in fact a probabilistic assertion by the testing laboratory of the likelihood that the variant is causally associated with the condition. Specifically:
Pathogenic means ≥99% likely
Likely pathogenic means ≥90% to <99% likely
VUS means ≥10% to <90% likely

Likely benign means ≥1% to <10%
Benign means <1%

These likelihoods of pathogenicity are in fact also derived from bayesian probability. Clinical genetic and genomic laboratory analysts start their analysis with a prior probability of pathogenicity and then evaluate a host of distinct variant attributes (e.g., the frequency in affected cases vs controls, computer modeling of the effect of variant, inheritance patterns in affected families), which serve as conditional probabilities to yield a posterior probability of pathogenicity, expressed in terms of the five-category scale just described.

Pretest Counseling and Informed Consent

For the purpose of informed consent, molecular genetic testing can generally be divided into two categories based on the reporting criteria of a particular test: **genome-wide testing** and targeted/focused testing. Although this is an artificial distinction and does not account for differences in genomic technology, this categorization is useful to highlight the unique and overlapping elements of pre- and posttest genetic counseling. Examples of genome-wide testing include chromosomal microarrays, clinical **exome** sequencing, and clinical **genome sequencing**. Pretest informed consent and counseling for this type of genomic test result should include a review of the five possible testing results and likelihood of each outcome: positive, negative, VUS, expected secondary findings, and unexpected secondary, or incidental, findings.

Positive Results

A positive result means that a pathogenic variant was identified in a gene that corresponds to the patient's phenotype or genetic condition. In some cases, a positive result may only be a partial positive, meaning that only part of the patients' phenotype or clinical presentation can be attributed to the identified gene and variant(s). The likelihood of a positive result depends on the detection rate of the test, though this may be adjusted to account for differences in detection among certain categories of conditions and patient populations. Chromosome microarrays identify a pathogenic copy number variant in about 15% to 20% of individuals with developmental delay, intellectual disability, and/or multiple congenital anomalies. Studies of clinical exome sequencing have found detection rates ranging between 25% and 40% with childhood-onset neurologic disease having closer to 40% detection rate and adults with nonneurologic indications having lower detection rates of 11% to 14%. Depending on the setting and circumstances of the patient and family, a positive result can be perceived as good news or bad news, though many individuals and families will show a combination of evolving positive and negative psychological reactions. A positive result typically allows the genetics provider to counsel on specific recurrence risk and offer targeted familial testing, as appropriate, to family members. A positive result also allows the genetics provider to share medical management and preventive or screening recommendations as well as provide anticipatory guidance about the natural history of the condition.

Negative Results

A negative result means that no pathogenic or likely pathogenic variant(s) were detected in a gene that corresponds to the patient's phenotype or genetic condition. The most important point for patients and families to understand about a negative test result is that this does not exclude a genetic etiology for the condition presenting in the individual or family. Explanations for negative genome-wide test results can include (1) technical limitations in the ability to detect certain variants (e.g., noncoding or intronic variants or intermediate size deletions/duplications), (2) knowledge-based limitations, specifically the phenotypic result of pathogenic variants is only known for ~5000 of our ~20,000 genes, or (3) complex genetic etiologies, such as multifactorial and **epigenetic** conditions. Like a positive result, a negative result can be perceived as good news or bad news depending on the setting and circumstances. Recurrence risk counseling after a negative result relies on assessment of the family history and applying mendelian inheritance patterns and empiric recurrence risks as appropriate. Clinical exome and genome sequencing generate large amounts of **sequence** data with the final report highlighting variants in genes associated with the clinical phenotype. Negative genome-wide tests offer the opportunity for ongoing analysis or timed reanalysis of the sequence data generated. As sequencing technologies improve, it often becomes necessary to repeat sequencing to maximize detection rates. However, some studies suggest that negative results are more likely due to our incomplete knowledge of gene-phenotype relationships, such that over time, reanalysis of existing data is more likely to result in a positive test result than utilizing new sequencing technologies.

Variants of Uncertain Significance (VUS)

As the number of genes being tested increases, the number of differences between an individual's sequence and that of a reference sequence also increases; consequently, many variants will be found whose pathogenetic significance is unknown (i.e., VUS). This is particularly the case for missense variants that result in the substitution of one amino acid for another in the encoded protein. Exome sequencing and genome sequencing find more than 100,000 variants, many of which will not have enough evidence to be classified as benign or pathogenic. The identification of a VUS alone should not be used to inform clinical management or decision making (e.g., a prophylactic mastectomy should not be considered based on the finding of a VUS in the *BRCA2* gene alone). In some circumstances, testing of family members can aid in **segregation** and analysis of the suspected pathogenicity of the variant. Absent that, it is not recommended to test family members for

a VUS to determine whether they inherited the genetic predisposition to the condition in the family or for prenatal diagnosis to determine whether a fetus has or does not have a genetic condition. Although these are guiding principles, there are some instances when additional clinical information is available that may change the clinicians' classification of variant even when the laboratory classification may not change. These cases require careful consideration with multidisciplinary input from the care team, laboratory, and family. It is important to inform individuals about the likelihood and clinical significance of finding a VUS as individuals naturally assume that if a variant was reported that it must be clinically significant. It is also important to encourage families to follow up with their provider(s) and the laboratory since, over time, additional population, familial segregation studies, and functional data become available that allow for reclassification of VUSs. Reclassification of a variant may change management and familial testing recommendations.

Secondary Findings

Secondary findings refer to the generation of information from sequencing that is not related to the indication for testing. This can occur due to the agnostic nature of the sequence generation and is inherent to the process of genome-wide testing. Clinical exome and genome sequencing can identify variants in all genes, not just those that are relevant to the reported phenotype. Therefore, the American College of Medical Genetics and Genomics (ACMG) has provided a policy statement for reporting of secondary findings. These guidelines state that during informed consent, individuals undergoing testing should be given the choice whether to receive secondary findings. The ACMG provides a list of genes that meet criteria for actionability and updates the list periodically. Additionally, ACMG recommends limiting reporting to variants that are classified as likely pathogenic and pathogenic. In pretest discussions with families, it is important to review the benefits and implications of such findings on the individual's and family's medical care, potential for negative psychological impacts (e.g., stress, anxiety), altered family dynamics, and insurance implications. It is important to highlight that the variants that are recommended for reporting are known to have effective medical interventions that can significantly reduce morbidity and mortality.

Incidental Findings

Secondary findings that result inherently from the process, sometimes referred to as incidental findings, include the potential to identify consanguinity and misattributed maternity or paternity. Consanguinity can be identified on chromosome microarrays that use single **nucleotide polymorphism**–based methods through the identification of multiple regions with **loss of heterozygosity** (also known as regions or runs of homozygosity) as well as exome and genome sequencing, which will show an increased rate of **homozygous** variants. When parental samples are submitted for duo or trio exome/genome sequencing, which is preferred to augment interpretation and reduce the number of VUSs, misattributed paternity or maternity will be identified. Discussion of these possible outcomes of testing prior to testing allows individuals and families to be fully informed about the advantages and risks associated with this testing to make a truly informed choice to proceed with or decline testing. Verbalizing these possible findings also allows the individual or family to share with the provider any concerns, and in some cases testing strategy or results disclosure planning may be adjusted.

Phenotype-driven tests interrogate a subset of genes and variants that are limited to those genes and variants associated with the phenotype of interest. Examples include multigene panels, single-gene sequencing, and targeted variant and familial variant testing. Pretest consent for this category of testing still requires a review of the detection rate, possible outcomes, and limitations. A major difference between genome-wide testing and targeted phenotype-driven testing is that secondary findings are unlikely to be reported in targeted testing; however, as technology advances and laboratory reporting criteria evolve, secondary findings may be reported more frequently. With phenotype-driven tests, it is important to review that an individual may have a pathogenic variant in a gene not included on the panel and that each testing technology will have technical limitations that could cause a variant within a gene included on the panel to be missed. Additionally, since new gene-phenotype relationships are constantly being described, testing may need to be repeated in the future.

Cascade Testing

When a pathogenic variant has been identified in a family, it is recommended to offer at-risk relatives targeted testing for the variant identified, a process called cascade testing. Targeted testing of family members who have the phenotype or genetic condition is often done to confirm the presumed presence of the pathogenic variant in that individual. Family members who are not known to have the phenotype or genetic condition (i.e., asymptomatic individuals) are identified through risk assessment and are offered presymptomatic testing. As is true for any medical test, individuals should be offered as a choice whether to undergo genetic testing and should be engaged in a discussion of the positive implications of such findings on the individual's medical care, the small but real potential for negative psychological impacts (e.g., stress, anxiety), altered family dynamics, and insurance implications. Alternatives to testing, including the risks and benefits of each alternative, should be explored. Alternative options to presymptomatic testing may include delaying or deferring testing to a later time and/or following medical management or surveillance guidelines based on family history without

a confirmation of the pathogenic variant. Special consideration should be taken when the at-risk individual is a minor. It is generally recommended to defer presymptomatic testing of a minor until the age that medical intervention is recommended to begin and to engage the minor in the decision-making process at a level that is developmentally appropriate.

Another important aspect of how to use molecular and genome-based diagnostic testing in families is the **selection** of the best person(s) to test. If the consultand is also the affected proband, then molecular testing is appropriate. If, however, the consultand is an unaffected, at-risk individual, with an affected relative serving as the indication for having genetic counseling, it is best to test the affected person rather than the consultand, if logistically possible. This is because a negative test in the unaffected consultand is an uninformative negative; that is, we do not know if the test was negative because (1) the gene or variant responsible for the condition in the proband was not covered by the test, or (2) the consultand in fact did not inherit a variant that could have been detected had the pathogenic variant been identified in the affected proband in the family. Once the variant or variants responsible for a particular condition are found in the proband, then the other members of the family no longer need comprehensive gene sequencing to assess that particular risk. The DNA of family members can be assessed with less expensive testing only for the presence or absence of the specific pathogenic variants already found in the family. If a family member tests negative under these circumstances, the test is a true negative that eliminates any elevated risk due to this person having an affected relative.

Proper Interpretation of Genetic and Genomic Testing

The key to proper interpretation and use of genetic and genomic testing is to recognize its probabilistic nature (see earlier). Unfortunately, genetic and genomic testing have been mischaracterized by some as being deterministic: that one's **fate** is wholly determined by one's gene variants. In fact, genetic and genomic testing performance characteristics are exactly analogous to any other medical test. All medical tests have higher **positive predictive values** in diagnostic settings as opposed to screening settings. This is another implication of bayesian probability because in a diagnostic setting, the prior probability of disease is much higher than it is in a screening setting. Just as for any other medical test, genetic and genomic testing are context dependent, and the clinician must take that context into account when determining the next steps for their patient. Genetic and genomic testing is a powerful tool, and when coupled with proper risk assessment and genetic counseling, patients can be provided with medical information that can be life saving and life altering.

GENERAL REFERENCES

Buckingham L: *Molecular diagnostics: fundamentals, methods and clinical applications*, ed 2, Philadelphia, 2011, F.A. Davis and Co.

Clarke A, Murray A, Sampson J: *Harper's practical genetic counseling*, ed 8, Boca Raton, 2019, CRC Press. http://doi.org/10.1201/9780367371944

Gardner RJM, Sutherland GR, Shaffer LG: *Chromosome abnormalities and genetic counseling*, ed 4, Oxford, 2011, Oxford University Press.

LeRoy BS, McCarthy P, Veach NP: *Genetic counseling practice, advanced concepts and skills*, ed 2, New York, 2021, Wiley Blackwell.

Uhlmann WR, Schuette JL, Yashar B: *A guide to genetic counseling*, ed 2, New York, 2009, Wiley-Liss.

Young ID: *Introduction to risk calculation in genetic counseling*, ed 3, New York, 2007, Oxford University Press.

REFERENCES FOR SPECIFIC TOPICS

Alfares A, Aloraini T, Subaie LA, et al: Whole-genome sequencing offers additional but limited clinical utility compared with reanalysis of whole-exome sequencing, *Genet Med* 20(11):1328–1333, 2019. https://doi.org/10.1038/gim.2018.41

Biesecker LG, Green RC: Diagnostic clinical genome and exome sequencing, *N Engl J Med* 370:2418–2425, 2014.

Borle K, Morris E, Inglis A, et al: Risk communication in genetic counseling: exploring uptake an perceptions of recurrence numbers, and their impact on patient outcomes, *Clin Genet* 94(2):239–245, 2018.

Brock JA, Allen VM, Keiser K, et al: Family history screening: use of the three generation pedigree in clinical practice, *J Obstet Gynaecol Can* 32:663–672, 2010.

Guttmacher AE, Collins FS, Carmona RH: The family history—more important than ever, *N Engl J Med* 351:2333–2336, 2004.

Miller DT, Adam MP, Aradhya S, et al: Consensus statement: chromosomal microarray is a first-tier clinical diagnostic test for individuals with developmental disabilities or congenital anomalies, *Am J Hum Genet* 86:749–764, 2010.

Miller DT, Lee K, Chung WK, et al: ACMG SF v3.0 list for reporting of secondary findings in clinical exome and genome sequencing: a policy statement of the American College of Medical Genetics and Genomics (ACMG), *Genet Med* 23(8):1381–1390, 2021. https://doi.org/10.1038/s41436-021-01172-3

National Society of Genetic Counselors: Genetic testing of minors for adult-onset conditions, position statement. https://www.nsgc.org/Policy-Research-and-Publications/Position-Statements/Position-Statements/Post/genetic-testing-of-minors-for-adult-onset-conditions

Online Mendelian Inheritance in Man, OMIM®. McKusick-Nathans Institute of Genetic Medicine, Johns Hopkins University (Baltimore, MD), {date}. World Wide Web. https://omim.org/statistics/geneMap

Posey JE, Rosenfeld JA, James RA, et al: Molecular diagnostic experience of whole-exome sequencing in adult patients, *Genet Med* 18(7):678–685, 2016. https://doi.org/10.1038/gim.2015.142

Resta R, Biesecker BB, Bennett RL, et al: A new definition of genetic counseling: National Society of Genetic Counselors' Task Force Report, *J Genet Couns* 15(2):77–83, 2006.

Retterer K, Juusola J, Cho MT, et al: Clinical application of whole-exome sequencing across clinical indications, *Genet Med* 18(7):696–704, 2016. https://doi.org/10.1038/gim.2015.148

Richards S, Aziz N, Bale S, et al: Standards and guidelines for the interpretation of sequence variants: a joint consensus recommendation of the American College of Medical Genetics and Genomics and the Association for Molecular Pathology, *Genet Med Off J Am Coll Med Genet* 17(5):405–424, 2015. https://doi.org/10.1038/gim.2015.30

Sheridan E, Wright J, Small N, et al: Risk factors for congenital anomaly in a multiethnic birth cohort: an analysis of the Born in Bradford study, *Lancet* 382:1350–1359, 2013.

Yang Y, Muzny DM, Reid JG, et al: Clinical whole-exome sequencing for the diagnosis of mendelian disorders, *N Engl J Med* 369:1502–1511, 2013.

Zhang VW, Wang J: Determination of the clinical significance of an unclassified variant, *Methods Mol Biol* 837:337–348, 2012.

PROBLEMS

1. Meera's maternal grandfather, Dhruv, had congenital stationary night blindness (CSNB), which also affected Dhruv's maternal uncle, Jay; the family history appears to fit an X-linked inheritance pattern. (There are also autosomal dominant and recessive forms.) Whether Dhruv's mother was affected is unknown. Meera and Steven have a daughter, Elsie, and sons, Zack and Peter, all unaffected by CSNB. Elsie is planning to have children and wonders whether she might be a carrier of a serious eye condition. Sketch the pedigree, and answer the following.

   a. What is the chance that Elsie is a carrier of X-linked CSNB?

   b. An ophthalmologist reviews the clinical notes from the affected individuals and considers that they were more likely to have had an autosomal form of the disorder, rather than X-linked. There is no evidence that Meera's mother, Rosemary, was affected. On this basis, what is the chance that Elsie is a carrier for an autosomal form of CSNB?

2. A deceased boy, Nathan, was the only member of his family with Duchenne muscular dystrophy (DMD). He is survived by two sisters, Norma (who has a daughter, Olive) and Nancy (who has a daughter, Odette). His mother, Molly, has two sisters, Maud and Martha. Martha has two unaffected sons and two daughters, Nora and Nellie. Maud has one daughter, Naomi. No carrier tests are available because the variant in the affected boy remains unknown.

   a. Sketch the pedigree, and calculate the posterior risks for all these females, using information provided in this chapter.

   b. Suppose prenatal diagnosis by DNA analysis is available only to women with more than a 2% risk that a pregnancy will result in a son with DMD. Which of these women would not qualify?

3. What is the probability of 13 successive male births? What is the probability of 13 successive births of a single sex? What is the probability that after 13 male births, the 14th child will be a boy?

4. Let H be the population frequency of carriers of hemophilia A. The incidence of hemophilia A in males (I) equals the chance that a maternal *F8* gene has a new pathogenic variant (μ) *plus* the chance it was inherited as a preexisting variant from a carrier mother ($\frac{1}{2} \times H$). Adding these two terms gives $I = \mu + (\frac{1}{2} \times H)$. H is the sum of the chance a reproducing affected father ($I \times f$) (where f is the fitness of hemophilia) transmits his variant *plus* the chance of a new paternal pathogenic variant (μ) *plus* the chance of a new maternal pathogenic variant (μ) *plus*

the chance of inheriting a variant from a carrier mother ($\frac{1}{2} \times H$). Adding these four terms gives $H = (I \times f) + \mu + \mu + (\frac{1}{2})H$.

a. If hemophilia A has a fitness (f) of ~0.70—that is, hemophiliacs have ~70% as many offspring as do controls—then what is the incidence of affected males? Of carrier females? (Answer in terms of multiples of the mutation rate.) If a woman has a son with an isolated case of hemophilia A, what is the risk that she is a carrier? What is the chance that her next son will be affected?

b. For DMD, $f = 0$. What is the population frequency of affected males? Of carrier females?

c. Color blindness is thought to have normal fitness ($f = 1$). What is the incidence of carrier females if the frequency of color blind males is 8%?

5. Ira and Margie each have a sibling affected with cystic fibrosis.

a. What are their prior risks for being carriers?

b. What is the risk for their having an affected child in their first pregnancy together?

c. They have had three unaffected children and now wish to know their risk for having an affected child before considering genetic testing. Using bayesian analysis to take into consideration that they have already had three unaffected children, calculate the chance that their next child will be affected.

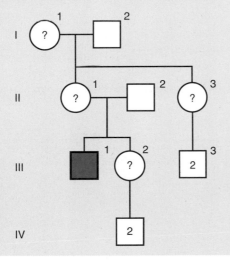

6. A 30-year-old woman with myotonic dystrophy comes in for genetic counseling. Her son, age 14 years, shows no symptoms, but she wishes to know whether he will be affected with this autosomal dominant condition later in life. Approximately half of individuals carrying the gene with a pathogenic variant are asymptomatic before the age of 14 years. What is the risk that the son will eventually develop myotonic dystrophy? Should you test the child for the expanded repeat in the gene for myotonic dystrophy?

7. A couple arrives in your clinic with their 7-month-old son, who has been moderately developmentally delayed from birth. The couple is contemplating having additional children, and you are asked whether this could be a genetic condition.

a. Is this possible, and if so, what pattern or patterns of inheritance would fit this story?

b. On taking a detailed family history, you learn that both parents' families were originally from the same small village in northern Italy. How might this fact alter your assessment of the case?

c. You next learn that the mother has two sisters and five brothers. Both sisters have developmentally delayed children. How might this alter your assessment of the case?

8. A couple returns for genetic counseling to discuss their genetic test results for Tay Sachs disease. Their daughter (Ananya) has symptoms consistent with Tach-Sachs disease. Additionally, Ananya had near-absent HEX A enzymatic activity and *HEXA* sequencing that identified one pathogenic variant and one variant of unknown significance (VUS). Parental testing revealed that both the pathogenic variant and VUS were maternally inherited. What is the interpretation of this result?

CHAPTER 18

Preconception and Prenatal Screening and Diagnosis

Angie Child Jelin • Ignatia B. Van den Veyver

The goal of preconception and prenatal screening and diagnosis is to inform women and couples about the risks for **genetic** disorders and birth defects in their fetus during a future or ongoing pregnancy. In recent years, advances in technology have led to new cost-effective strategies for preconception **genetic screening**, preimplantation genetic testing, and sensitive prenatal **aneuploidy** screening. Women and couples should be counseled about these options (see Chapter 17) starting before a pregnancy so they can make informed decisions about the testing and screening they wish to pursue and about management options depending on test results.

Couples who learn before a pregnancy that they are at increased **risk** for having a child with a significant **birth defect** or **genetic disorder** can choose to undergo preimplantation genetic testing, pursue a pregnancy with donor gametes, or elect to forego having children. When an increased risk is discovered during pregnancy, prenatal genetic diagnosis can confirm the presence or absence of the genetic disorder in the fetus. If the fetus is found to be affected, parents and providers can use this information to plan for appropriate prenatal and perinatal management, psychological preparation of the family, early postnatal treatment, in some cases prenatal treatment, and some parents may choose to terminate the pregnancy. Absence of the genetic condition in the fetus will provide reassurance.

Preconception screening addresses the risk for genetic disorders in a future pregnancy through family history, such as a previous affected child, and by offering the option of parental **carrier** screening for a growing number of autosomal **recessive** and X-linked conditions. If not already performed preconceptionally, carrier screening can also be offered during pregnancy.

Prenatal screening uses maternal blood samples and ultrasonography to noninvasively assesses the risk for certain common genetic disorders (e.g., chromosomal aneuploidies), common birth defects (e.g., neural tube defects [NTDs]), and structural anomalies in pregnancies not otherwise known to be at an increased risk for these conditions. Screening tests are designed to be inexpensive with sufficiently low risk to make them suitable for cost-effective screening of all pregnant individuals in a population. They do not provide a diagnostic answer about whether an abnormality is present but are intended to find those with pregnancies at higher risk relative to the background and offer them follow-up diagnostic testing.

Prenatal diagnosis is the term applied to performing genetic testing on a fetal sample to determine if the fetus is affected with a genetic disorder. It is traditionally offered when the risk for a genetic disorder is increased because of the previous birth of an affected child, a family history of the disorder, a positive parental carrier test, or when a prenatal screening indicates an increased risk. Prenatal diagnosis, which is meant to provide a definitive answer as to whether the fetus is affected, requires a procedure such as **chorionic villus sampling** (**CVS**) or **amniocentesis** (see later in this chapter) to directly acquire fetal or placental cells for analysis.

The purpose of this chapter is to discuss the various approaches to preconception and prenatal screening and diagnosis and to review the methodologies and indications as currently being used in this rapidly changing field. The reader is cautioned, however, that because of technologic advances in the methods available for assessing the fetus and the fetal **genome**, standards of care in prenatal screening and diagnosis evolve rapidly.

PRENATAL SCREENING METHODS

Prenatal screening has traditionally relied on ultrasonography combined with measurements of proteins and hormones (referred to as analytes) whose levels in maternal serum are altered when a fetus is affected by a **trisomy** or NTD. Prenatal genetic screening took a great leap forward with the discovery that in addition to these analytes, maternal serum and plasma also contain **cell-free DNA**, of which a fraction is fetal in origin. Sequencing of cell-free DNA from maternal plasma with advanced technologies (see later in this chapter) has made noninvasive screening for trisomies more sensitive and accurate compared to serum analyte screening.

Screening for Neural Tube Defects

An estimated 95% of infants with NTDs are born into families with no prior history of this malformation. The first developed noninvasive serum analyte-based screening test measures the amount of maternal serum α-fetoprotein (MSAFP) to identify pregnancies at increased risk for a fetal open NTD, including open spina bifida, anencephaly, and encephalocele not covered by skin. These are associated with high amounts of **AFP** in the amniotic fluid. AFP is a fetal glycoprotein produced mainly in the liver, secreted into the fetal circulation, and excreted through the fetal kidneys (see also Amniocentesis, later). AFP also leaks into the amniotic fluid when the fetal skin is breached. Because AFP enters the maternal bloodstream via the placenta, membranes, and maternal-fetal circulation, MSAFP is also elevated, which is the basis for using MSAFP measurements at ~16 weeks (15–21 weeks) to screen for open NTDs. There is considerable overlap between the range of MSAFP concentrations in unaffected pregnancies and those where the fetus has an open NTD (Fig. 18.1), and the **sensitivity** of MSAFP screening to detect an increased risk for fetal open NTDs depends on statistically defined cutoff values. As shown in Fig. 18.1, if the cutoff for an elevated concentration is defined as 2.5 multiples of the median (MoM) value in unaffected pregnancies (which is 1 MoM), one can estimate that 80% of fetuses with open NTDs are detected and 20% remain undetected. However, lowering the cutoff to improve sensitivity would be at the expense of reduced **specificity**, thereby increasing the number of unaffected pregnancies that would be interpreted as high risk (false-positive rate). An elevated MSAFP concentration is not specific to a pregnancy with an open NTD. As listed in Table 18.1, there are many other causes of high MSAFP, most of which can be distinguished from open NTDs by fetal ultrasonography, which should be offered when MSAFP is increased. Combining MSAFP screening with detailed diagnostic ultrasonography approaches the accuracy for the detection of open NTDs of ultrasonography combined with amniocentesis to measure AFP in amniotic fluid. Thus it is acceptable to offer ultrasound examination (at 18 weeks) paired with an MSAFP assay to first-degree, second-degree, or more distant relatives of individuals with NTDs instead of amniocentesis. MSAFP measurement has now become integrated in a second trimester multiple serum analyte screen for fetal trisomies (see later), but far more women now have first trimester trisomy screening with serum analytes and ultrasound, or more recently with cell-free DNA analysis. Thus providers should remember to offer these women screening for open NTDs by ultrasound with or without MSAFP. Currently, in expert centers, NTDs are increasingly diagnosed by a screening anatomy ultrasound alone, without MSAFP.

Screening for Down Syndrome and Other Aneuploidies

Although the **association** between advancing maternal age and increased risk for major trisomies is well known, more than 70% of children with autosomal trisomies are born to women without risk factors. The

TABLE 18.1 Findings Associated With Elevated α-Fetoprotein Concentration

Gestational age older than calculated	Urinary obstruction*
Spina bifida*	Polycystic kidney*
Anencephaly*	Absent kidney*
Congenital skin defects*	Congenital nephrosis*
Abdominal wall defects*	Other renal anomalies*
Gastrointestinal defects*	Osteogenesis imperfecta*
Liver necrosis	Fetal growth restriction*
Cloacal exstrophy*	Oligohydramnios*
Cystic hygroma*	Multiple gestation*
Fetal demise*	Decreased maternal weight
Sacrococcygeal teratomas*	Fetal bleeding*

All listed findings can result in elevated maternal serum α-fetoprotein (MSAFP).
*Indicates causes of elevated AFP level that can be seen by ultrasonographic examination.

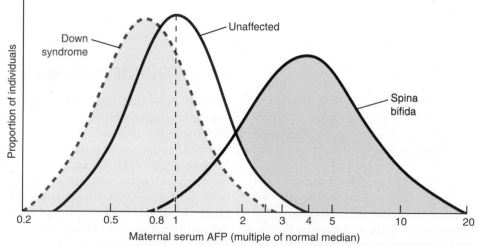

Figure 18.1 Maternal serum α-fetoprotein *(AFP)* concentration, expressed as multiples of the median, in normal fetuses, fetuses with open neural tube defects, and fetuses with Down syndrome. (Redrawn from Wald NJ, Cuckle HS: Recent advances in screening for neural tube defects and Down syndrome. In Rodeck C, editor: *Prenatal diagnosis*, London, 1987, Bailliére Tindall, pp 649–676.)

unexpected finding that the concentration of MSAFP, measured during the second trimester to screen for NTDs, was lower in women who carried pregnancies with autosomal trisomies, particularly trisomies 18 and 21, led to its investigation as a screening analyte for Down syndrome (**trisomy 21**); however, MSAFP concentrations of unaffected pregnancies and Down syndrome pregnancies overlap too much (see Fig. 18.1) for MSAFP to be a useful screening analyte on its own. Since then more sensitive and specific trisomy screening strategies have been developed that combine different serum analytes in the first or second trimester with specific ultrasound measurements. About 10 years ago analysis of cell-free DNA in maternal plasma was introduced. Cell-free DNA screening can be done at any gestational age after 10 weeks and is more sensitive and specific for aneuploidy screening than serum analyte screening. The most recent guidance states that all pregnant women should be informed about the option of cell-free DNA analysis along with other screening and testing, but the less costly serum analyte screening is still used for women at low or average risk for fetal aneuploidy. Thus all these different screening options will be explained in more detail later.

First Trimester Screening

First trimester screening is ideally performed between 11 and 13 completed weeks of gestation and relies on measuring the levels of pregnancy-associated plasma protein A (PAPP-A) and the hormone human chorionic gonadotropin (hCG), either as total hCG or as its free β subunit in maternal serum. PAPP-A levels are below the normal range in all trisomies; hCG (or free β-hCG) is higher in trisomy 21 but lower in the other trisomies (Table 18.2). These analyte measurements are combined with the ultrasonographic measurement of the **nuchal translucency (NT)**, defined as the thickness of the echo-free space between the skin and the soft tissue overlying the dorsal aspect of the cervical spine caused by subcutaneous edema of the fetal neck (Fig. 18.2A). An increase in NT is commonly seen in fetuses with trisomies 21, 13, and 18 and in 45,X (see Fig. 18.2B). Sonographers performing NT measurements used for first trimester screening must obtain and maintain special certification, and the size must be determined with reference to gestational age. An enlarged NT in fetuses with a normal **karyotype** is associated with an increased risk for other genetic conditions and birth defects. The most common ones are listed in Table 18.3.

TABLE 18.2 Performance of First and Second Trimester Screening Tests

| | First Trimester Screen | | | | | Second Trimester Screen | | | | | |
	NT	PAPP-A	Free β-hCG	SPR	DR	uE₃	AFP	hCG	Inhibin A	SPR	DR
Trisomy 21	↑	↓	↑	5%	85–90%	↓	↓	↑	↑	5%	80%
Trisomy 18	↑	↓	↓	5%	90–95%*	↓	↓	↓	—	5%	60–70%
Trisomy 13	↑	↓	↓	5%	90–95%*	↓	↓	↓	—	n/a	n/a
NTD	—	—	—	n/a	n/a	—	↑↑	—	—	5%	80–85%

Up and down arrows indicate direction of change in measurement compared to average.

AFP, α-fetoprotein; *β-hCG*, human chorionic gonadotropin β subunit; *DR*, detection rate; *NT*, nuchal translucency; *PAPP-A*, pregnancy-associated plasma protein A; *SPR*, screen positive rate; *uE₃*, unconjugated estriol.

*Indicates combined trisomy 13/18 detection rate.

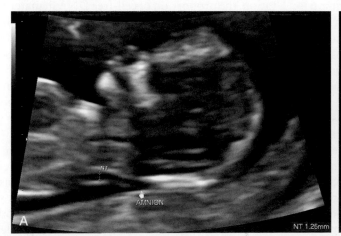
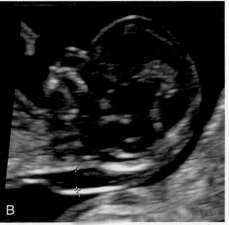

Figure 18.2 First trimester nuchal translucency (NT) measurement. The NT is a dark, echo-free zone beneath the skin in an ultrasonographic sagittal section through the fetus and is marked by two yellow "+" signs. The average NT size is 1.2 mm at 11 weeks of gestation (95th percentile up to 2 mm) and 1.5 mm at 14 weeks of gestation (95th percentile up to 2.6 mm). (A) Normal NT measurement of 1.25 mm. (B) Increased NT measurement associated with a greatly increased risk for Down syndrome. (Images courtesy of Wesley Lee, MD, Baylor College of Medicine, Houston, Texas.)

TABLE 18.3 Common Causes of Increased Nuchal Translucency Thickness

- Chromosomal aneuploidy:
  - Trisomies 21, 13, or 18
  - Monosomy X
  - Other rare aneuploidies
- Triploidy
- Pathogenic copy number variants
- Congenital heart defects
- Rasopathies
- Skeletal dysplasias
- Other single-gene disorders

Second Trimester Screening

Second trimester screening for trisomies 21 and 18 is usually accomplished by measuring hCG levels in combination with three other analytes: MSAFP, unconjugated estriol (uE3), and inhibin A. This battery of tests is referred to as a quadruple screen. MSAFP and uE3 are lower than average when the fetus has a trisomy 21 or 18, whereas hCG is higher with fetal trisomy 21 but lower with trisomy 18, and inhibin A is higher with fetal trisomy 21 but not significantly affected in trisomy 18 (see Table 18.2). These analyte levels are affected by other factors, including ancestry, smoking, maternal diabetes, multiple pregnancy, and pregnancy conceived by *in vitro* fertilization (IVF), and laboratories generally adjust for these variables. Extremely low levels of uE3 may be indicative of rare genetic conditions such as steroid sulfatase deficiency or Smith-Lemli-Opitz syndrome. Second trimester screening is generally reserved for low-risk patients who missed the window for first trimester screening. For standard first and second trimester screening a cutoff of screen positive rate of 5% results in the detection rates of first and second trimester screening shown in Table 18.2.

Integrated Screening Strategies

Different strategies for combining the results of first trimester and second trimester screening to increase the ability to detect pregnancies with autosomal trisomies, particularly trisomy 21, have also been developed. In one approach, integrated screening, women undergo first trimester screening with serum analytes with or without NT, followed by second trimester serum screening, and the results are combined to provide a more precise risk estimate, but only after the second trimester result is available. The integrated screening strategy has the highest overall sensitivity of analyte-based screening and can detect up to 95% of all Down syndrome cases with an ~5% false-positive rate. Sensitivity for other trisomies is in the 90% to 95% range, with a low false-positive rate of less than 1%. This strategy is less attractive to women because they have to wait until the second trimester for their screening result. More stepwise variations also exist, wherein women found to be at highest risk after the first trimester screen are offered diagnostic

TABLE 18.4 Sensitivity, Specificity, Positive and Negative Predictive Values of Cell-Free DNA Screening for Chromosomal Abnormalities

	DR (%)	FPR (%)	PPV (%)[a]			NPV (%)[†]		
Age (y)			25	35	40	25	35	40
Trisomy 21	99.7*	0.04*	51	79	93	>99	>99	>99
Trisomy 18	97.9*	0.04*	15	39	69	>99	>99	>99
Trisomy 13	99.0*	0.04*	7	21	50	>99	>99	>99
Monosomy X	95.8*	0.14*	41	41	41	>99	>99	>99
Other SCA*	100*	0.04*	-	-	-	-	-	-
XXY	-	-	29	30	52	>99	>99	>99
XXX	-	-	27	28	45	>99	>99	>99
XYY	-	-	25	25	25	>99	>99	>99

DR, Detection rate; *FPR*, false-positive rate (1-specificity); *NPV*, negative predictive value; *PPV*, positive predictive value; *SCA*, sex chromosome aneuploidy. DRs and FPRs are from Gil MM, Accurti V, Santacruz B, et al: Analysis of cell-free DNA in maternal blood in screening for aneuploidies: Updated meta-analysis, *Ultrasound Obstet Gynecol* 50:302–314, 2017.
*Other SCA include 47,XXY, 47,XXX, 47,XYY.
[†]PPV and NPV were calculated using the Perinatal Quality Foundation's NIPT/ Cell Free DNA Screening Predictive Value Calculator (www.perinatalquality. org/Vendors/NSGC/NIPT/).

testing and those not at increased risk or more moderate risk are offered a second trimester screen, followed by combined interpretation of the first and second trimester screening results.

Noninvasive Prenatal Screening by Analysis of Cell-Free Fetal DNA

All individuals have fragmented DNA in their blood that is not contained in the nucleus of cells but free floating and can be assayed from plasma or serum. The discovery that during pregnancy maternal plasma contains fetal cell-free DNA derived from trophoblast cells of the placenta, which have the same genome as the fetus, has drastically changed the approach to prenatal screening for fetal chromosomal anomalies. After 10 weeks of gestation, the proportion of cell-free DNA in maternal blood that is derived from trophoblast, referred to as fetal fraction, is ~5% to 20%. The circulating cell-free DNA can be analyzed using high-throughput DNA sequencing technologies to noninvasively evaluate whether the fetus has aneuploidy. This led to the introduction and rapid expansion of cell-free DNA-based **noninvasive prenatal screening (NIPS)** (also known as noninvasive prenatal testing [NIPT]) for trisomies 21, 13, and 18, with sensitivities and specificities approaching 99% for trisomy 21 (Table 18.4). A growing number of commercial NIPS tests on the market assess variable combinations of testing for these common aneuploidies, combined with sex **chromosome** abnormalities (see Table 18.4), other rare autosomal aneuploidies, and selected microdeletions. A few providers also offer genome-wide analysis of copy number gains and losses. Cell-free DNA can also be used to detect **Y chromosome** sequences for the purposes of determining fetal sex.

Analyzing cell-free DNA for aneuploidy detection is done in different ways, but the common principle is to detect the small increased amount of total cell-free DNA from a particular chromosome if the fetus has trisomy. In one approach, referred to as the counting approach, total cell-free DNA is subjected to **next generation sequencing**, and millions of molecules of DNA are each mapped to its particular chromosome of origin (Fig. 18.3). The number of molecules that map to each chromosome is counted, without knowing which of the fragments are fetal and which are maternal. Because chromosome 21 constitutes ~1.5% of total DNA in the genome, ~1.5% of total fragments should be assigned to chromosome 21 if the fetus and mother have two normal copies of chromosome 21. If, however, the fetus has trisomy 21, more sequences than expected will map to chromosome 21, and this can be measured relative to the number of sequences that map to an appropriate reference chromosome or to the full set of chromosomes not including chromosome 21. Similar calculations can be used for the other autosomal trisomies and for sex chromosome aneuploidies. Other commonly used approaches evaluate not only the amount of cell-free DNA coming from each chromosome but also take into account differences in the **nucleotide sequence** between the maternal and fetal DNA (polymorphisms) to assign whether the sequenced DNA comes from the maternal or the fetal DNA.

Although cell-free DNA provides a substantial improvement in sensitivity and specificity of screening for fetal trisomies (particularly trisomy 21), it remains a screening test, not a diagnostic test. A result that indicates the fetus is at increased risk for a chromosomal abnormality should be confirmed by diagnostic testing, either via CVS or amniocentesis (presented later in this chapter). If prenatal diagnostic testing is declined, it should be confirmed on a blood sample obtained from the infant after birth. Furthermore, the accuracy by which NIPS can predict that the fetus is affected by a chromosomal abnormality, calculated as the **positive**

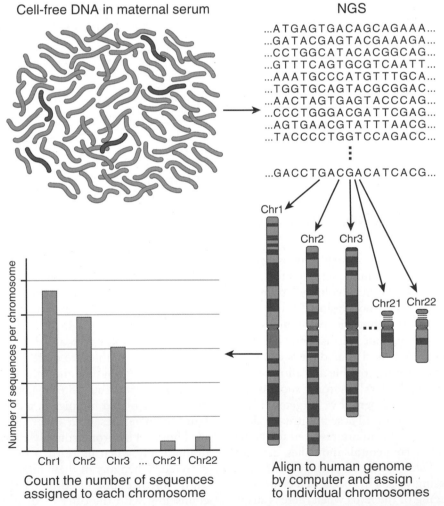

Figure 18.3 Schematic diagram of noninvasive prenatal screening for trisomies by analysis of cell-free DNA in maternal blood. Fetal component of maternal plasma cell-free DNA is shown in *red*; maternal contribution is in *blue*. Millions of molecules of DNA are sequenced and assigned to each chromosome by computerized alignment against the human genome. Highly accurate measurements of small but significant increases in the fraction of molecules assigned to chromosome 13, 18, 21, or X compared to a reference indicate increased risk for trisomy of each of these chromosomes.

predictive value (PPV) varies. The PPV depends on the prevalence of the condition tested for, and PPV for common trisomies is lower for younger women but is not affected by age for **monosomy** X (see Table 18.4). The accuracy by which NIPS correctly predicts that a fetus is unaffected, the **negative predictive value (NPV)**, is greater than 99% for all aneuploidies, as there are far more unaffected fetuses in the population in all age groups. PPVs are typically lower for rarer conditions, such as rare autosomal trisomies and microdeletions and duplications. Therefore the current recommendation in the United States and many other countries is that NIPS is not recommended for screening for conditions other than the common aneuploidies (trisomies 21, 13, 18). As the technology continues to improve and more data are accumulated, this guidance may change in the future. For example, newer data on screening performance for 22q11.2 deletions are promising.

Other Current and Future Applications of Cell-Free Fetal DNA Analysis

Cell-free fetal DNA in maternal plasma is also used to **genotype** the fetus at the *RH* locus and to determine fetal sex. In some countries, noninvasive tests for a growing number of single-gene disorders in high-risk pregnancies are already available (Table 18.5), and noninvasive cell-free DNA sequencing tests for small panels of genes have been introduced already but with still limited validation, and cell-free DNA-based sequencing of the entire fetal genome has been explored on a research basis. Refinements in the analysis of cell-free DNA will likely make noninvasive testing for many other genetic disorders available in the future.

Prenatal Detection of Fetal Congenital Anomalies by Ultrasonography

High-resolution, real-time ultrasonography is widely used for assessment of fetal viability, fetal number, fetal size, gestational age, amniotic fluid volume, and evaluation of fetal and placental morphology. Most basic ultrasonography exams are done via two-dimensional (2D) ultrasound imaging, but ultrasound in three dimensions (3D) (Fig. 18.4) and four dimensions (4D) (which is 3D over time) is also possible and allows more detailed examination of the fetal anatomy such as, for example, for fetal echocardiography (targeted ultrasound exam on the fetal heart). These are usually done in advanced imaging centers and are reserved for better definition of suspected **congenital** anomalies detected by 2D sonography. Fetal magnetic resonance imaging (MRI) is also increasingly used in specialized centers for high-resolution imaging of the fetus when there is suspicion for conditions that are difficult to detect by ultrasound or need more detailed evaluation (see Fig. 18.4). Studies investigating the safety indicate that prenatal ultrasonography and fetal MRI are not harmful to the

TABLE 18.5 Cell-Free DNA Assays Developed for Single-Gene Disorders

Clinically Available*
- Achondroplasia
- Apert syndrome
- Congenital adrenal hyperplasia
- Crouzon syndrome
- Cystic fibrosis
- Duchenne and Becker muscular dystrophy
- Blood group genotyping (RHD/RHCE; Kell)
- Thanatophoric dysplasia
- Torsion dystonia
- Spinal muscular atrophy
- Selected familial known mutation analysis
- cfDNA screening tests for small panels of genes**

Examples of Reported Assay Development†
- Fraser syndrome
- Hemoglobinopathies (sickle cell, thalassemias)
- Hemophilia A and B
- Huntington disease
- Leber congenital amaurosis
- Polycystic kidney disease
- Propionic acidemia
- Methylmalonic acidemia
- Retinitis pigmentosa

*Only in certain countries, primarily United Kingdom.
†Incomplete list.
**Commercially available in some countries, limited clinical validity data.
Modified from Van den Veyver IB, Chitty LS: Noninvasive prenatal diagnosis and screening for monogenic disorders using cell-free DNA. In Milunsky A, Milunsky JM, editors, *Genetic disorders and the fetus: Diagnosis, prevention and treatment*, ed 8, New York, 2021, John Wiley & Sons, Ltd.

fetus or mother. As equipment and techniques used by ultrasonographers continue to improve, the detection of many malformations by routine ultrasonography in the second trimester (optimally around 18–20 weeks of gestation), and increasingly also in the late first trimester continues to improve (Fig. 18.5; see also Fig. 18.4).

Prenatal Ultrasonographic Findings with Fetal Chromosomal Abnormalities

A number of findings on prenatal ultrasonography are associated with chromosomal aneuploidy, including trisomies 21, 18, and 13; 45,X; and many other abnormal karyotypes (Tables 18.6 and 18.7). Some are soft sonographic markers that are more common in fetuses with common aneuploidies, and others are major congenital anomalies (see Table 18.6). Many of these can also be present as isolated findings in a chromosomally normal fetus or in fetuses with other genetic conditions. The likelihood of a chromosomally abnormal fetus increases dramatically when more than one fetal abnormality is detected. When any of these findings are detected, referral for further specialized prenatal imaging and genetic counseling with the offer of diagnostic genetic testing, usually by amniocentesis, are indicated (see later). If no chromosomal abnormalities are identified, single-gene disorders or multifactorial etiologies for the congenital anomalies should be considered.

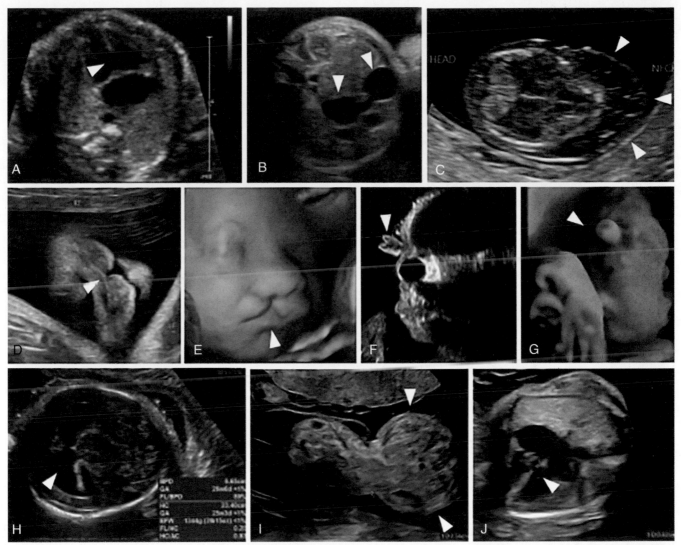

Figure 18.4 Examples of advanced imaging of fetal anomalies that can be present with chromosomal disorders. (A–C) Some features of trisomy 21: (A) atrioventricular septum defect of the heart; (B) double bubble sign with duodenal atresia; (C) cystic hygroma (also high risk of 45,X). (D–H) Some features of trisomy 13: (D, E) 2D and 3D views of cleft lip; (F, G) 2D and 3D views of proboscis in a fetus with holoprosencephaly; (H) monoventricle in holoprosencephaly. (I–K) Some features of trisomy 18: (I) ventricular septum defect; (J) large omphalocele containing liver. (*Arrowheads* point to defects in each panel.) (Images courtesy Wesley Lee, Baylor College of Medicine, Houston, Texas.)

Prenatal Ultrasonography for Single-Gene and Multifactorial Disorders

Prenatal ultrasonography can detect certain features that are highly suggestive of specific single-gene disorders. This can be useful when prenatal DNA testing is not possible because the patient declines the amniocentesis procedure or when a sample or specific prenatal genetic test is otherwise unavailable. For example, skeletal dysplasias such as osteogenesis imperfecta or thanatophoric dysplasia can present with distinct features on prenatal ultrasound. Recognizing the prenatal presentation of common genetic syndromes can also be helpful in deciding which genetic test—a specific **gene** test, gene panel, or whole **exome** analysis—to offer, based on the combined anomalies that are detected. However, ultrasonography cannot identify disorders with phenotypes that

either develop only after birth or that are not detectable by imaging, such as metabolic disorders or syndromes that present primarily with intellectual disability.

Ultrasound examination can be used to determine fetal sex as early as 13 weeks of gestation. This may help with the prenatal diagnosis of certain X-linked recessive disorders (e.g., hemophilia) for women who are carriers and at increased risk of having an affected son (see Chapter 7). Fetal chromosomal sex can now also be screened by cell-free DNA analysis as early as 10 weeks of gestation.

Ultrasonography can also identify isolated abnormalities that may recur in families and are believed to have multifactorial inheritance, including NTDs (see Fig. 18.5), cleft lip and palate (see Fig. 18.4), congenital heart defects (Fig. 18.5), and others. Fetal

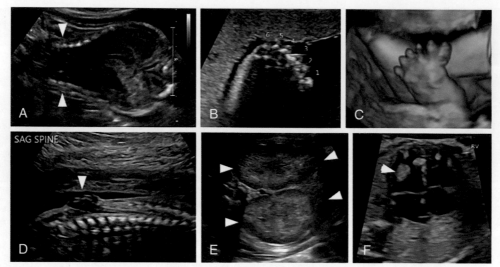

Figure 18.5 Additional examples of advanced imaging of fetal anatomy in other disorders. (A) Narrow chest in fetus with lethal osteogenesis imperfecta. (B, C) 2D and 3D views of polydactyly of feet. (D) Sagittal view of lumbar spine with meningomyelocele sac. (E) Large echogenic kidneys can be seen in fetuses with infantile polycystic kidney disease. (F) Cardiac rhabdomyomas can be seen in fetuses with tuberous sclerosis. (Images courtesy Wesley Lee, Baylor College of Medicine, Houston, Texas.)

TABLE 18.6 Typical Major Congenital Anomalies Visible on Prenatal Ultrasonography of Fetuses With Common Aneuploidies

Trisomy 21	Trisomy 13	Trisomy 18	Monosomy X
50% have findings	80–90% have findings	80–90% have findings	Up to 90% have findings
Cystic hygroma	Cystic hygroma	Cystic hygroma	Cystic hygroma
CHD (VSD, AVSD)	CHD	CHD (polyvalvular disease)	CHD (HLHS, aortic coarctation)
Duodenal atresia	Polydactyly	Clenched fist	Renal anomalies (horseshoe kidney)
Wide gap between first and second toe	Holoprosencephaly	Omphalocele	Hydrops
	Omphalocele	Rocker bottom feet	Foot edema
	Cleft lip / palate	Fetal growth restriction	

Other defects are also commonly found, but those listed are more typical or can be seen at higher frequency.
AVSD, Atrioventricular septum defect; *CHD,* congenital heart defect (multiple types of CHD possible; more typical ones are listed in parentheses); *HLHS,* hypoplastic left heart syndrome; *VSD,* ventricular septum defect.

TABLE 18.7 Some Examples of Indications for Fetal Echocardiography*

Maternal Indications (% Risk for Congenital Heart Defect)
• Insulin-dependent diabetes mellitus (3–5%)
• Phenylketonuria (15%)
• Teratogen exposure
• Thalidomide (10% if 20–36 days postconception)
• Phenytoin (2–3%)
• Alcohol (25% with fetal alcohol syndrome)
• Maternal congenital heart disease (5–10% for most lesions)
• Pregnancy conceived by *in vitro* fertilization
Fetal Indications
• Abnormal general fetal ultrasound examination results
• Arrhythmia
• Chromosome abnormalities
• Nuchal thickening
• Nonimmune hydrops fetalis
Familial Indications
• Mendelian syndromes
• Paternal congenital heart disease (2–5%)
• Previously affected child with congenital heart lesion (2–4%, higher for certain lesions)

*This list is not comprehensive, and indications vary between centers.

echocardiography is also available at many centers for a detailed assessment of pregnancies at risk for a congenital heart defect. Table 18.7 shows some common indications for prenatal echocardiography.

PRENATAL DIAGNOSTIC PROCEDURES

To perform definitive prenatal diagnosis, diagnostic procedures that retrieve **fetal cells** are required. The two most common ones are amniocentesis to retrieve amniotic fluid, performed from 15 weeks of gestation onwards, and CVS to retrieve a small sample of placental villi, usually done between 11 and 13 completed weeks of gestation. When amniocentesis is not technically possible, or for specific indications, fetal cord blood sampling or late CVS or placental biopsies can be done instead.

Amniocentesis

Technique

During amniocentesis a needle is inserted transabdominally under continuous ultrasound visualization into the amniotic sac to remove a sample of amniotic fluid (Fig. 18.6A). The amniotic fluid contains fetal cells that can be cultured or from which DNA can be prepared without prior culture and used for diagnostic tests. Before amniocentesis, ultrasonography is used to assess fetal viability, gestational age (by measuring biometric parameters such as head circumference, abdominal circumference, and femur length), the number of fetuses,

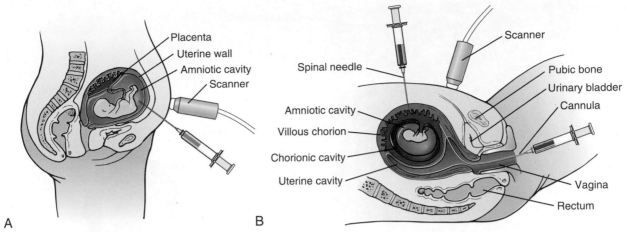

Figure 18.6 **Prenatal diagnostic procedures.** (A) Amniocentesis. A needle is inserted transabdominally into the amniotic cavity, and a sample of amniotic fluid (usually ~20 mL) is withdrawn by syringe for diagnostic studies (e.g., chromosome studies, enzyme measurements, or DNA analysis). Ultrasonography is routinely performed before or during the procedure. (B) Chorionic villus sampling. Two alternative approaches are drawn: transcervical (by means of a flexible cannula) and transabdominal (with a spinal needle). In both approaches, success and safety depend on use of ultrasound imaging.

volume of amniotic fluid, fetal anatomic structures, and position of the fetus and placenta to allow the optimal approach for needle **insertion**. Amniocentesis is typically performed between 16 and 20 weeks of gestation but can be done any time after 15 weeks.

Different types of tests can be done on amniotic fluid. Fetal chromosome analysis by karyotype and chromosomal **microarray** analysis (CMA) are the standard genetic tests when there is an increased risk for chromosomal conditions based on screening or presence of fetal congenital anomalies. When there is an increased risk for single-gene disorders based on family history or because of distinct findings on prenatal ultrasound, sequencing of genes, gene panels, or the fetal exome can also be done (see Laboratory Studies, later).

When an amniocentesis is done between 16 and 20 weeks, the concentration of AFP in amniotic fluid (AFAFP) can be measured by a relatively simple and inexpensive immunoassay to detect fetal open NTDs that can be an added test on second trimester amniotic fluid samples retrieved for other indications. If the AFAFP level is above the normal range for a particular gestational age, targeted ultrasound is recommended to look for an open NTD and other causes of high AFAFP (see Table 18.1). When the AFAFP assay is used together with ultrasonography at 18 to 19 weeks of gestation, ~99% of fetuses with open spina bifida and virtually all fetuses with anencephaly are identified. Other tests sometimes done on amniotic fluid samples include studies to detect viral infections or, less frequently, metabolic studies.

Complications

The major complication associated with midtrimester amniocentesis at 16 to 20 weeks of gestation is a 1 in 909 risk for inducing miscarriage over the baseline risk of pregnancy loss of ~1% to 2% for any pregnancy at this stage of gestation. Other complications are rare, including leakage of amniotic fluid, infection, and injury to the fetus by needle puncture. Early amniocentesis performed between 10 and 14 weeks is no longer recommended because of an increased risk for amniotic fluid leakage, a threefold increased risk for spontaneous abortion, and an approximately six- to sevenfold increased risk for talipes equinovarus (clubfeet), over the 0.1% to 0.3% population risk. Early amniocentesis has now been replaced by CVS.

Chorionic Villus Sampling

Technique

For CVS a small amount of placental villi (5–40 μg) is removed between weeks 10 and 14 of pregnancy (see Fig. 18.6B). Chorionic villi consist of a mesenchymal core that contains capillaries and are covered by a layer of trophoblast cells, which are derived from the extraembryonic part of the early developing embryo (Fig. 18.7) and are a ready source of fetal tissue. As with amniocentesis, ultrasonographic scanning is used before CVS to determine the best approach, and the procedure is performed under continuous ultrasound visualization. CVS can be performed transabdominally with a needle or transcervically with a flexible catheter that is advanced into the placenta. The major advantage of CVS over amniocentesis is that results are available at an early stage of pregnancy, thus reducing the period of uncertainty and allowing termination, if it is elected, to be performed earlier. However, AFAFP cannot be assayed at this stage, and evaluation for a possible open NTD thus must be done by other methods, including MSAFP screening and ultrasonography.

The success of chromosome analysis by karyotype or CMA is the same as with amniocentesis (>99%).

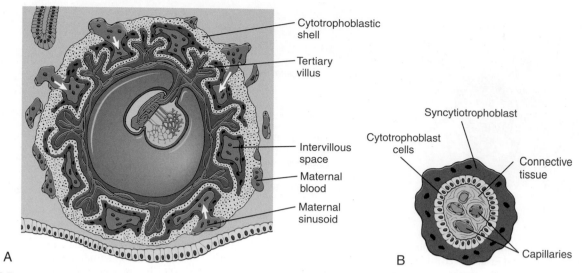

Figure 18.7 **Development of the tertiary chorionic villi and placenta.** (A) Cross-section of an implanted embryo and placenta at ~21 days. (B) Cross section of a tertiary villus showing establishment of circulation in mesenchymal core, cytotrophoblast, and syncytiotrophoblast. (From Moore KL: *The developing human: Clinically oriented embryology*, ed 4, Philadelphia, 1988, WB Saunders.)

However, ~1% of CVS yield ambiguous results because of chromosomal **mosaicism** (including true mosaicism and **pseudomosaicism**; described later in this chapter). In these situations, follow-up with amniocentesis may be recommended to establish whether the fetus has a chromosomal abnormality.

Complications

In prenatal diagnostic centers experienced with CVS, the rate of procedure-related fetal loss is about 1 in 450, only slightly increased over the baseline risk of 2% to 5%, and approximating the risk of amniocentesis. Although there were initial reports of an increase in the frequency of birth defects, particularly limb reduction defects, after CVS, this has not been confirmed in large series of CVS procedures performed after 10 weeks of gestation by experienced physicians.

Indications for Prenatal Diagnosis by Amniocentesis or Chorionic Villus Sampling

There are several well-accepted indications for prenatal testing by amniocentesis or CVS (see Box 18.1). The most common indication for invasive prenatal diagnosis is to test for Down syndrome (trisomy 21) and the more severe autosomal trisomies, 13 and 18. For this reason, advanced maternal age is a common reason for referral for prenatal diagnosis by amniocentesis or CVS. Other reasons include increased risk for an affected fetus because of a family history of a specific genetic condition, a positive maternal screening test result, or other well-defined risk factors. Current clinical guidelines no longer support using only maternal age as an indication for invasive testing for aneuploidies. The American College of Obstetricians and Gynecologists (ACOG) has now recommended that amniocentesis or CVS be made available to all women regardless of age along with

screening options by the noninvasive methods described earlier. It is also considered appropriate that if a woman elects to undergo testing for fetal chromosomal abnormalities by amniocentesis or CVS, to perform not only karyotype but also CMA (see Chapter 5 and later in this chapter) on the extracted fetal DNA.

There are also numerous single-gene disorders for which testing is available. Couples known to be at risk for any of these disorders in their fetus can be offered genetic counseling and prenatal testing by amniocentesis or CVS. Whether or not a couple considers the risk for a genetic condition in their fetus sufficiently burdensome to justify an invasive procedure is a personal decision each woman makes for herself. It is important to stress in counseling that invasive prenatal diagnosis cannot be used to rule out all possible fetal abnormalities.

LABORATORY STUDIES

Methods to Detect Fetal Chromosomal Abnormalities

Karyotype Analysis

Either amniocentesis or CVS can provide fetal cells for karyotyping (see Chapter 5). Preparation and analysis of chromosomes from cultured amniotic fluid cells or cultured chorionic villi require 10 to 14 days, although chorionic villi can also be used for karyotyping after short-term incubation. This short-term incubation using rapid **metaphase** analysis of villous **cytotrophoblast** tissue provides a result more quickly, but it has lower resolution and a higher rate of mosaicism (see later) that can render interpretation difficult. With long-term culture, the cultured cells from which the karyotype is obtained come from the mesenchymal core of the villus (see Fig. 18.7), which is embryologically more closely related to the developmental lineages that give rise to the fetus. Some

BOX 18.1 PRINCIPAL INDICATIONS FOR PRENATAL DIAGNOSIS BY AMNIOCENTESIS OR CHORIONIC VILLUS SAMPLING

- *The pregnant woman or couple wishes diagnostic testing*
  Although limited at one time to a pregnant woman with no increased risk other than advanced maternal age, some current professional guidelines call for diagnostic testing (amniocentesis or CVS) to be offered to all couples.
- *Increased risk as determined by* **maternal serum screening***, ultrasound examination, and noninvasive prenatal screening test of cell-free DNA*
  Genetic assessment and further testing are recommended when fetal abnormalities are suspected based on routine screening by maternal serum screening and fetal ultrasound examination.
- *Previous child with de novo chromosomal aneuploidy or other genomic imbalance*
  Although the parents of a child with chromosomal aneuploidy may have normal chromosomes themselves, in some situations there is still an increased risk for a chromosomal abnormality in a subsequent child. For example, if a woman at 30 years of age has a child with Down syndrome, her **recurrence risk** for any chromosomal abnormality is ~1 per 100, compared with the age-related population risk of ~1 per 390. Parental mosaicism is one possible explanation for the increased risk, but in most cases the mechanism of the increased risk is unknown.
- *Presence of structural chromosomal or genome abnormality in one of the parents*
  The risk for a chromosome abnormality in a child varies according to the type of abnormality and sometimes the parent of origin. The greatest risk, 100% for Down

syndrome, occurs only if either parent has a 21q21q **robertsonian translocation** (see Chapter 6).
- *Family history of a genetic disorder that may be diagnosed or ruled out by biochemical or DNA analysis*
  Most of the disorders in this group are caused by single-gene defects with 25% or 50% recurrence risks. Cases in which the parents have been diagnosed as carriers after a carrier screening test, rather than after the birth of an affected child, are also in this category. Mitochondrial disorders pose special challenges for prenatal diagnosis.
- *Family history of an X-linked disorder for which there is no specific prenatal diagnostic test*
  When there is no alternative method, the parents of a boy affected with an X-linked disorder may use fetal sex determination to help them make decisions about their pregnancy because the recurrence risk may be as high as 50% for male children. For X-linked disorders for which prenatal diagnosis by DNA analysis is available, DNA analysis is the preferred method of testing. Note that if **familial** increased risk is known before pregnancy, preimplantation genetic testing (see later) with the transfer to the uterus of only those embryos determined to be unaffected for the disorder in question is an option.
- *Risk for a neural tube defect (NTD)*
  First-degree relatives (and second-degree relatives at some centers) of patients with NTDs are eligible for amniocentesis because of an increased risk for having a child with NTD. However, as described in this chapter, most open NTDs can be detected by ultrasound and amniocentesis is no longer commonly done to confirm or exclude NTDs by assaying AFP levels but instead is done to determine whether a fetus with NTD has an associated chromosomal abnormality.

laboratories use both techniques, but if only one is used, long-term culture is therefore the technique of choice. The resolution of chromosome spreads prepared from prenatal samples is lower than from other tissues, but segmental abnormalities of 7 to 10 **Mb** and larger should be readily visible, depending on the region involved.

Chromosomal abnormalities are detected in 10% to 30% of pregnancies with fetal congenital anomalies, and this number is higher when multiple malformations are present. The karyotypes most often seen in fetuses ascertained by abnormal ultrasonographic findings are the common autosomal trisomies (21, 18, and 13) and 45,X (Turner syndrome). The presence of a cystic hygroma is associated with aneuploidy in more than 50% of cases, most commonly 45,X, but it can also occur in Down syndrome and trisomy 18, or in fetuses with normal karyotypes.

Fluorescence *In Situ* Hybridization

Fluorescence *in situ* hybridization (FISH) (see Chapter 5) makes it possible to rapidly screen **interphase** nuclei in fetal cells for the common aneuploidies of chromosomes 13, 18, 21, X, and Y immediately after amniocentesis or CVS, with a result available usually in 1 to 2 days. This can be useful when rapid information is needed if time-sensitive decisions regarding pregnancy management

and delivery planning could be affected by a trisomy diagnosis (e.g., when a growth-restricted fetus is suspected to have trisomy 18). Because FISH only provides limited information, it should always be followed by a more definitive test, karyotype, or CMA. Although still offered, FISH is now less commonly used because CMA can provide more definitive results with only a slightly longer turnaround time of 5 to 7 days. In some countries outside the United States, rapid aneuploidy testing on CVS or amniotic fluid samples is done by quantitative **polymerase chain reaction** (**PCR**) amplification of unique regions on chromosomes 13, 18, and 21.

Chromosomal Microarray Analysis

CMA (see Chapter 5) is increasingly replacing karyotyping for prenatal diagnosis. Copy number variants (CNVs), including chromosomal aneuploidy and segmental imbalances, such as duplications, triplications, deletions, or marker chromosomes (see Chapter 4), can be detected at much higher resolution by CMA than can be accomplished even with high-resolution karyotyping. Although ACOG has advised that CMA, rather than karyotyping, should be the first-line test when a fetal abnormality is detected by ultrasonography and recommends that all women having invasive testing be given the option to have CMA, the Society of Obstetricians and Gynaecologists of Canada still recommends CMA as a second-tier test following a normal karyotype.

For some findings a karyotype is still needed (e.g., to determine whether a copy number gain for chromosome 21 is the result of a trisomy or an unbalanced robertsonian **translocation**). CMA also does not detect balanced translocations and balanced inversions, but these are more rarely the cause of fetal congenital anomalies or syndromes. The current data support that a prenatal CMA can identify a clinically significant **CNV** about 1% to 1.7% of the time, and when a CMA is done for fetal congenital anomalies this number goes up to 6% to 7% overall and to over 10% when there are multiple congenital anomalies. About 1% to 2% of the time CMA can identify **variants of uncertain significance (VUS)**, or findings that indicate presence of a condition in the fetus that was not suspected. These can make counseling complex and are discussed in more detail later.

Sequencing to Detect Chromosomal Abnormalities

Some laboratories outside the United States are beginning to use low-coverage **whole genome sequencing** with counting of fragments aligned to each chromosome to determine the copy number of entire chromosomes (aneuploidy) or chromosomal segments as a low-cost, high-throughput alternative method to CMA. This is not used in the United States for prenatal diagnosis but is the method of choice for preimplantation genetic testing for aneuploidy (see later).

Fetal DNA Sequencing and Fetal Genome Analysis

As the molecular basis for an increasing number of genetic disorders is determined (see Chapter 12), many conditions that were not previously detectable prenatally by other means can now be diagnosed by analyzing fetal DNA. Any technique used for direct **variant** analysis can be used for prenatal diagnosis on a fetal DNA sample extracted from amniotic fluid or CVS samples or from cell cultures derived from these samples. Three main modalities that can be used are single-gene testing, either by sequencing or targeted analysis for a known variant, gene panel sequencing, or sequencing of the exome or genome. Because not 100% of the exome (all exons) or genome (all **genomic DNA**) can be sequenced, we refer to these as **exome sequencing (ES)** and **genome sequencing** rather than whole exome or whole genome sequencing.

Single-Gene Testing and Gene Panel Sequencing for Prenatal Diagnosis

When there is a known familial **pathogenic variant** for which the fetus is at risk, or a recognizable fetal condition, such as thanatophoric dysplasia, a lethal skeletal dysplasia caused by only a few different pathogenic variants, a specific targeted molecular test can be done

to determine if that variant is detected in the fetal DNA. These tests are highly accurate, but such clinical presentations are relatively rare. More commonly, fetal anomalies detected by ultrasonography are suggestive for a class of genetic disorders. In those situations, a gene panel sequencing test, which analyzes a variable number of genes that have been associated with that class of disorders (e.g., a broad skeletal dysplasia panel), can be done. These panels have limitations. They are usually designed based on gene-disease relationships that are recognized postnatally, but the prenatal phenotypes for the same conditions may not be well known or may differ from those observed postnatally. In addition, the gene content of these panels needs to be kept up to date with the rapidly growing knowledge of gene-disease relationships. Participation of medical geneticists or genetic counselors, whose role it is to stay informed about these rapid changes, is essential for counseling and **selection** of such tests for prenatal diagnosis. This type of genetic testing is reserved for pregnancies found to be at increased risk and not for routine screening or testing.

Exome Sequencing and Genome Sequencing for Prenatal Diagnosis

In addition to the above mentioned limitations of gene panels for sequencing of DNA from fetuses diagnosed with congenital anomalies, it is increasingly recognized that the genetic basis for many fetal anomalies, in particular those that lead to fetal or neonatal demise, are not yet known. Furthermore, some prenatally diagnosed fetal anomalies may be caused by variants in genes known to cause a different **phenotype** postnatally, which is referred to as prenatal phenotype expansion. For these reasons and because of its success in diagnosing genetic conditions postnatally, multiple studies have investigated the benefit of prenatal ES of fetal DNA for pregnancies complicated with fetal anomalies for which standard testing by CMA has not yielded a diagnosis. A few large studies have demonstrated that in these circumstances the diagnostic rate is between 8.5% and 13%, but in some more selected series that include pregnancies with stronger suspicion for a single gene disorder, it is higher, ranging from ~20% to 40%, or up to 80% in very selected series with fetal skeletal dysplasias. Much more research is needed on the impact of prenatal exome sequencing on the care of pregnancies and newborns, but professional societies are now supporting its clinical use for selected pregnancies when a diagnosis cannot otherwise be made. This test should be offered by genetics providers who are familiar with prenatal genetics and the complexities of such testing and who are skilled at counseling pregnant individuals and their partners about its benefits and limitations. With exome sequencing there is a substantially higher chance of detecting unwanted findings such as VUS, incidental and secondary findings, including possible diagnosis of adult-onset disorders, and unexpected paternity (see upcoming discussion). The analysis of exome sequences is more complex and time consuming, and it may take longer to obtain results than for prenatal CMA and karyotypes. To speed up variant interpretation, prenatal exome sequencing is primarily done in trios, where the parental DNAs are also sequenced and analyzed to help interpret the variants found in the fetal DNA.

More recently, trio genome sequencing is also being studied for prenatal diagnosis. While it is more comprehensive, evaluating both noncoding and coding regions of DNA as well as including the possibility of copy number analysis, the information obtained from genome sequencing is even more complex. Prenatal genome sequencing is a rapidly evolving area that bears watching closely in the years ahead, with increasingly important ethical and policy implications for the practice of fetal medicine and prenatal genetics.

Biochemical Assays for Metabolic Diseases

Although any disorder for which the genetic basis and responsible genetic variant(s) are known can be diagnosed prenatally by DNA analysis, more than 100 metabolic disorders can also be diagnosed by biochemical analysis of chorionic villus tissue or cultured amniotic fluid cells. A few rare conditions can even be identified directly by assaying a substance in amniotic fluid. Most metabolic disorders are rare in the general population but have a high recurrence risk since most are autosomal recessive conditions. Because each condition is rare, the experience of the laboratory performing the prenatal diagnostic testing is important and it should be done at specialized centers. Whenever possible, a biochemical assay on directly sampled chorionic villus tissue (as opposed to cultures) is preferred to avoid misinterpretation of results due to the expansion in culture of contaminating maternal cells. Access to a cultured cell line from an affected individual in the family is highly advisable so that the laboratory can confirm its ability to detect the biochemical abnormality in the **proband** before the assay is attempted in CVS or amniotic fluid cells from the pregnancy at risk. Many metabolic disorders cannot be diagnosed prenatally by enzyme assays because the enzyme is not expressed in amniocytes or chorionic villi or a reliable biochemical assay is not available. For these, DNA sequencing should be performed.

Biochemical tests have one advantage over DNA: they can detect abnormalities caused by any **mutant allele** that has a significant effect on the protein function. This is particularly significant for disorders with a high degree of **allelic heterogeneity**, genes in which pathogenic variants occur in regions that are not routinely sequenced, or by a high proportion of new mutations (see Chapter 12). In addition, biochemical testing may be the only option for prenatal diagnosis if the causative mutations in the family are unknown.

Problems in Prenatal Chromosome Analysis and Gene Sequencing

Mosaicism

Mosaicism refers to the presence of two or more cell lines in an individual or tissue sample (see Chapter 7). Because invasive prenatal techniques, particularly CVS, sample extraembryonic tissues of the placenta, and not the fetus itself, mosaicism found in cultured fetal cells may be difficult to interpret. The prenatal geneticist must determine if the fetus is truly mosaic and understand the clinical significance of any apparent mosaicism.

Cytogeneticists distinguish three levels of mosaicism in amniotic fluid or CVS cell cultures based on the number of cells with mosaicism and the number of colonies from which they arise. Mosaicism detected in multiple colonies from several different primary cultures is considered true mosaicism. Postnatal studies have confirmed that true mosaicism in culture is associated with a high risk that mosaicism is present in the fetus. The probability varies with different situations. However, mosaicism for structural aberrations of chromosomes, for example, is hardly ever confirmed. Mosaicism involving several cells or colonies of cells from a single primary culture is difficult to interpret, but it is generally thought to reflect **pseudomosaicism** that has arisen in culture. When mosaicism is restricted to only a single cell, it is also considered to reflect pseudomosaicism and is typically disregarded.

Maternal cell contamination (MCC; see later) can explain some cases of apparent mosaicism in which both XX and XY cell lines are present. This is more common in products of conception from miscarriages and in long-term CVS cultures than in amniotic fluid cell cultures because chorionic villi and maternal tissue are anatomically closely associated (see Fig. 18.6).

In CVS studies, mosaic discrepancies between the karyotypes found in the cytotrophoblast, villous stroma, and fetus have been reported in 1% to 2% of pregnancies studied at 10 to 11 weeks of gestation. **Confined placental mosaicism (CPM)** is mosaicism that is present in the placenta but not in the fetus (Fig. 18.8). CPM can be the result of a trisomic cell line arising postzygotically in the placenta, in which case the fetus will always be **diploid**. Another mechanism for CPM is trisomy rescue (see Chapter 6), where the **zygote** has trisomy, but postzygotically during one of the cell divisions one of the copies of the trisomic chromosome is lost, establishing diploid normal cell lineages, alongside the trisomic cells. Occasionally, a liveborn infant or fetus with nonmosaic trisomy 13 or trisomy 18 has been reported in a pregnancy with placental mosaicism for the trisomic cell line and a normal diploid cell line. It has been proposed that the placental diploid cell line improves the probability of intrauterine survival of a trisomic fetus. When trisomy rescue results in a diploid fetus, it raises the concern that the fetus could have retained two copies of a chromosome from the same parent, resulting

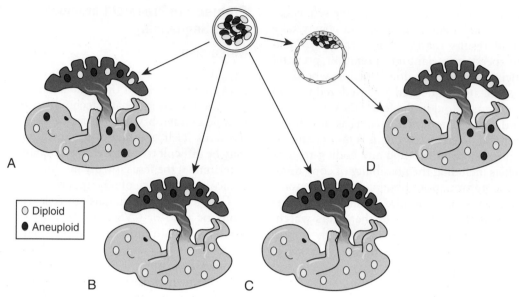

Figure 18.8 The different types of mosaicism that may be detected by prenatal diagnosis. (A) Generalized mosaicism with diploid *(yellow)* and abnormal aneuploid *(blue)* cell lineages affecting both the fetus and placenta. (B) Confined placental mosaicism with diploid and aneuploid cells in the placenta and a diploid fetus. (C) Mosaicism with only aneuploid cells in the placenta and a diploid fetus. (D) Mosaicism confined to the fetus with a diploid placenta. (Modified from Kalousek DK: Current topic: Confined placental mosaicism and intrauterine fetal development, *Placenta* 15:219–230, 1994.)

in **uniparental disomy (UPD)** (see Chapter 6). This can affect all chromosomes but is particularly concerning for chromosomes 7, 11, 14, or 15, which contain imprinted genes. For example, two maternal copies of chromosome 15 cause Prader-Willi syndrome, and two paternal copies are associated with Angelman syndrome (see Chapter 6). Thus when there is CPM for these chromosomes, tests should be done to exclude UPD.

Because CMA uses pooled DNA from tissues or cultured cells and does not examine individual cells the way karyotyping does, it is less sensitive for detection of mosaicism. Mosaicism in which 10% of the cells are aneuploid is difficult to detect as a copy number change by CMA, whereas 10% mosaicism will be detected with greater than 99% probability when 50 cells are examined by karyotype. CMA is even less sensitive for detecting mosaicism for a CNV of only a segment of a chromosome unless it is present in more than 20% to 25% of the cells.

Confirmation and interpretation of apparent mosaicism are difficult challenges in genetic counseling for prenatal diagnosis when mosaicism is identified during an amniocentesis because clinical outcome information on the different types and extents of mosaicism can be limited. Further studies such as cordocentesis (fetal blood sampling) may provide some guidance, but the interpretation can remain uncertain. If mosaicism is identified at the time of CVS, parents can be reassured if follow-up amniocentesis results is normal and UPD is excluded (see earlier), particularly if the prenatal ultrasound demonstrates normal growth and no congenital anomalies are visualized. Parents should be counseled in advance of the possibility for mosaicism and that its interpretation could be uncertain. After birth, an effort should be made

to verify any abnormal chromosome findings suspected on the basis of prenatal diagnosis. Confirmation of mosaicism, or lack thereof, may prove helpful with respect to medical management as well as for genetic counseling of the specific couple and other family members.

Culture Failure and Maternal Cell Contamination

Prenatal diagnosis is time sensitive, and culture failure, which is fortunately very rare, can be a concern. When a CVS culture fails to grow, there is time to repeat the chromosome study with amniocentesis. If an amniotic fluid cell culture fails, either repeated amniocentesis or cordocentesis could be offered, depending on fetal age. MCC is another potential risk of prenatal sampling. During cell culture, contaminating maternal cells could outgrow the fetal cells. MCC can be suspected when there are XX cell lines with a male pregnancy and is common in CVS cultures as a consequence of the intimate association between chorionic villi and the maternal tissue (see Fig. 18.6). To minimize the risk for MCC, maternal decidua present in a CVS must be carefully dissected and removed, but this does not always eliminate every cell of maternal origin. A maternal blood sample can also be utilized to confirm or refute MCC through parallel genotyping of the DNA from the maternal and fetal sample with use of polymorphisms.

Unexpected Findings: Variants of Uncertain Significance, Incidental and Secondary Findings

On occasion, prenatal chromosome analysis performed primarily to rule out aneuploidy reveals some other unusual chromosome finding (e.g., a rare chromosomal **rearrangement**, a **marker chromosome** [see Chapter 5], and now more commonly a VUS on CMA or exome sequencing and genome sequencing).

Unbalanced or *de novo* structural rearrangements may cause serious fetal abnormalities (see Chapter 6). If a parent carries a balanced structural rearrangement (e.g., a balanced translocation) that is present in unbalanced form in the fetus (unbalanced translocation), the consequences for the fetus can be serious. If a fetus has a structural chromosomal rearrangement that is also present in one of the parents, it is more likely to be a benign change without untoward consequences, but there are exceptions to this. They include variable **expressivity** and involvement of a region of the genome that contains imprinted genes.

CMA has a higher chance of detecting VUS than a karyotype analysis, which is one reason why it has been more selectively used for pregnancies with fetal anomalies rather than as a first-line test. As experience and knowledge of CNV in the human genome improves (see Chapter 4), the medical relevance of an increasingly greater fraction of CNVs will become clearer. The incidence of VUS with CMA has dropped to levels close to what is seen with a karyotype, justifying replacing fetal karyotyping by CMA for nearly all indications.

Exome sequencing and genome sequencing remain tests for second-line evaluation of pregnancies with fetal anomalies for which a genetic etiology is not identified by CMA. They both have a higher chance for detecting VUS, which can be mitigated by limiting prenatal analysis to genes relevant for the sonographic phenotype or family history. When a VUS is identified, analysis of parental data from trio sequencing may help with interpretation.

Incidental findings of pathogenic or likely pathogenic variants that are unrelated to the fetal phenotype but may cause a different serious condition can occasionally be discovered in the sequence of the fetal or parental samples. It is recommended that significant incidental findings related to serious childhood disorders in the fetal sample are reported. However, the reporting of parental findings (e.g., a variant that increases the risk for late-onset conditions such as cancer) often involves the option for parents to opt out of obtaining parental results. Secondary findings are pathogenic and likely pathogenic variants in a list of genes curated by the ACMG to be associated with diseases for which the discovery of these variants could result in health care measures that benefit the individual. In general, patients should be given the option to opt out of receiving secondary findings.

PRECONCEPTION GENETIC SCREENING AND TESTING

Parental Carrier Screening for Autosomal Recessive and X-Linked Disorders

Preconception screening refers to the evaluation of parents for the risk for genetic disorders in their future children before the pregnancy. This is the optimal time to offer and perform carrier screening, but it is infrequently done preconceptionally. Therefore risks for autosomal recessive and X-linked single-gene disorders and carrier screening should also be addressed in prenatal counseling. The approach to carrier screening has evolved over time. It initially relied on targeted screening for a few diseases, based on individual risk factors assessed through family history, such as a prior affected child, the presence of **consanguinity**, and information on the ancestry of the prospective parents. With the currently available high-throughput laboratory methods, cost-effective rapid sequencing of many genes is now available and allows for a more equitable approach to carrier screening with larger panels of genes. The ACMG now recommends that carrier screening is offered to all preconception or pregnant patients and their reproductive partners in an ancestry and population neutral fashion. They recommend using a panel with genes for 97 autosomal recessive and 16 X-linked conditions with a carrier frequency at or greater than 1/200 to be offered to all pregnant patients while reserving larger panels with additional disease genes for patients with possible consanguinity or when warranted based on family or medical history.

Couples who are carriers for pathogenic or likely pathogenic variants that increase the risk for inherited recessive or X-linked disease in their current or future pregnancy should be offered appropriate counseling about reproductive options and residual risk. Preconceptionally, they can consider preimplantation genetic testing for monogenic disorders (PGT-M) (see later), use of donor eggs or sperm, adoption, or the option to forgo having children. They can also choose to conceive and have CVS or amniocentesis during the pregnancy or testing of the infant at the time of birth.

Preimplantation Genetic Testing

PGT, formerly referred to as preimplantation genetic diagnosis (PGD), is performed on *in vitro* fertilized embryos prior to embryo transfer (Fig. 18.9). PGT offers couples at significant risk for a specific genetic disorder or aneuploidy in their offspring an option to manage reproductive risks that avoid pregnancy termination. In the most commonly used approach, **blastocyst** biopsy (see Fig. 18.9), women have to undergo IVF. They first undergo ovarian stimulation and retrieval of ~10 or fewer oocytes in the stimulated cycle. The oocytes are then fertilized *in vitro* and cultured for 5 to 6 days until the blastocyst stage. At that time, 5 to 10 cells are retrieved from the trophectoderm, which develops into the future placenta, without disrupting the **inner cell mass**, which will develop into the fetus (see Chapter 15). PGT was initially done by blastomere biopsy on eight-cell–stage embryos, but trophectoderm biopsy on blastocysts, which provides more cellular material and apparently greater accuracy, is now preferred. Usually,

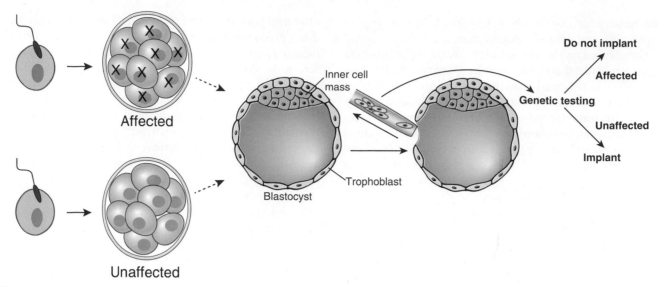

Figure 18.9 Preimplantation genetic diagnosis. After ovarian stimulation, oocytes are retrieved and fertilized *in vitro*. The fertilized embryos are incubated for 5 to 6 days, to the blastocyst stage, and about 5 to 10 cells are removed from the trophectoderm, which will develop into the placenta. These cells will be used for genetic testing for chromosomal abnormalities or single-gene disorders. In this example, the embryo (labeled *X*) will not be transferred. Only embryos that are unaffected will be transferred into the patient's uterus to establish a pregnancy.

biopsied embryos are frozen while the molecular diagnosis proceeds. One of the embryos that are found not to carry the genetic abnormality in question can then be transferred and allowed to implant in a future cycle, as is routinely done after IVF. Affected embryos are discarded. Data currently available suggest that there are no detrimental effects to embryos that have undergone biopsy.

There are three types of PGT: PGT monogenic (M) evaluates for single-gene disorders, PGT aneuploidy (A) evaluates for whole chromosome abnormalities, and PGT structural rearrangements (SR) is used to detect structural chromosomal abnormalities such as translocations. PGT-M is utilized to detect known pathogenic variants in specific genes that were previously found in a family member with a genetic disorder or through parental carrier screening. It involves PCR amplification followed by a method to detect the variant. Because of the small amount of starting material, analysis of linked polymorphic markers is often included to improve accuracy.

Initially, FISH and later microarray analysis were used to detect chromosome abnormalities, but more recently laboratories have switched primarily to next generation sequencing methods to detect CNVs for PGT-A and unbalanced translocations (see Chapters 4 and 5). PGT-A is now offered to women undergoing IVF to increase the live birth rate by only selecting **euploid** embryos for transfer. The American Society of Reproductive Medicine recommends offering PGT-A to all infertile women, but research is ongoing to fully establish the **clinical utility** of PGT-A.

Despite technologic improvements in recent years, there are limitations to PGT. These include mosaicism

and challenges with detecting *de novo* mutations, microdeletions, and duplications. Because with PGT diagnoses are made on small numbers of cells, women who have PGT-M and PGT-SR should be offered confirmatory CVS or amniocentesis during ensuing pregnancies. Because of the small risk (~2–3%) for false-positive and false-negative results with PGT-A, it is considered good practice to offer prenatal aneuploidy screening for pregnancies conceived by IVF with PGT-A. Although PGT was developed to avoid the ethical, religious, and psychological difficulties with pregnancy terminations, ethical dilemmas remain related to the disposition of affected embryos and remaining frozen healthy embryos after parents have completed their family.

FETAL SURGICAL AND MEDICAL INTERVENTIONS

The number of conditions for which fetal surgical or medical interventions are available has expanded significantly in the last 4 decades and is frequently impacted by ethical considerations related to the underlying genetic etiology of the fetal condition in need of treatment. Fetal therapy began in the 1960s with intrauterine transfusion for anemia, particularly in the setting of fetal Rh alloimmunization. This was followed by insertion of shunts to drain excess fluid from the fetus into the amniotic cavity. Shunts are still used for some cases of fetal uropathy (e.g., to drain urine when there is bladder outlet obstruction or to drain large pleural effusions). Laser ablation of communicating placental vessels for twin-twin transfusion syndrome started in the 1990s, and laser procedures for this condition have now become standard of care. For some cases of evolving hypoplastic left heart syndrome, aortic valvuloplasty and now balloon septostomy and atrial septostomy are done in expert centers. After a multicenter randomized controlled trial, the Management of Myelomeningocele Study (MOMS) showed improved outcomes after intrauterine surgical repair of fetal myelomeningocele (spina bifida); this option is now available at selected centers. In recent years the approach has transitioned from open to laparoscopic repair. A subset of fetuses with congenital diaphragmatic hernia have improved outcomes after a balloon is placed inside the trachea with the goal to improve growth and expansion of the fetal lungs. The balloon is removed prior to controlled delivery. Finally, investigation is underway to examine the value of serial amnioinfusions to treat early-onset anhydramnios for fetuses with nonfunctioning kidneys.

In addition to these mechanical fetal procedures, a number of *in utero* medical therapies are being adopted. Fetal arrhythmias are treated with maternally administered antiarrhythmia medications such as digoxin and sotalol. Sirolimus has established efficacy in the treatment of severe cases of fetal rhabdomyomas. *In utero* **stem cell** transplantation and **gene therapy** trials are underway for conditions such as osteogenesis imperfecta and hemoglobinopathies.

The disorders and congenital anomalies for which these fetal interventions can provide benefit can be caused by genetic defects. Therefore multidisciplinary approaches to evaluation and decision making that include prenatal genetic counseling and assessment are recommended prior to any such procedures. Debate remains as to the depths of investigation that should be undertaken, and a fetal karyotype is recommended as the minimum requirement for some procedures, which contrasts with general recommendations for CMA as a primary genetic test for major congenital anomalies. Post-test counseling after genetic test results are available should include multidisciplinary discussion about the risks, benefits, and alternatives of pursuing a fetal procedure.

GENETIC COUNSELING FOR PRECONCEPTION AND PRENATAL DIAGNOSIS AND SCREENING

Most prenatal and reproductive genetic counselors practice in the setting of a prenatal diagnosis program. The professional staff of a prenatal diagnosis program (physician, nurse, and genetic counselor) must obtain an accurate family history and determine whether other previously unsuspected genetic problems should be considered on the basis of family history or ancestry. Pretest and posttest counseling is recommended when genetic screening or testing is considered, including carrier screening, PGT, and prenatal screening and diagnosis.

For carrier screening and testing, until recently, ancestry was utilized to assess the need for carrier testing for a small number of X-linked or autosomal

recessive conditions that are more prevalent in certain populations. Such disorders include thalassemias in individuals of Mediterranean or Asian background, sickle cell anemia in people of African descent, and various disorders that are more prevalent in people of Ashkenazi Jewish ancestry. Because it is becoming increasingly difficult to assign a single background to each individual, use of broader carrier screening panels, in which individuals are tested for a large array of genetic disorders irrespective of apparent or stated ancestry, is now recommended.

The complexities posed by the availability of so many different prenatal screening and testing options include the distinction between screening and diagnostic testing, the many different and distinctive indications for testing, the subtleties of interpretation of test results, and the personal, ethical, religious, and social considerations that enter into reproductive decision making. They make providing prenatal genetic services challenging, and prospective parents considering prenatal genetic screening or diagnosis should be provided with understandable information that will allow them to make informed decisions about which conditions to test or screen and whether they give or withhold consent for diagnostic procedures. Prenatal genetic counseling for women considering CVS or amniocentesis usually addresses several different points (see Box 18.2).

Screening tests avoid the risk of a diagnostic procedure but do not give a yes/no diagnostic answer. They provide a risk estimate for a disorder relative to the background risk. The cutoff for a positive screen is set to balance sensitivity and specificity, and screening tests generally allow higher false-negative rates than would be acceptable for a diagnostic test to keep false-positive rates to a reasonable level, generally below 5%. Advances in laboratory technology, both for screening and diagnostic tests, have led to testing options that are both more accurate and more expansive, providing information for a growing number

---

BOX 18.2 COUNSELING FOR CHORIONIC VILLUS SAMPLING OR AMNIOCENTESIS

- The reason/indication for testing and alternative options (screening)
- The risk that the fetus will be affected with the condition tested
- The nature and prognosis of the genetic condition (or categories of conditions) tested
- The risks and limitations of the procedures to be used
- The possible need for a repeated procedure in the event of a failed attempt
- The type of genetic testing performed
- The chance that the test will find the genetic cause
- The time required before a report can be issued
- The possibility of an uninterpretable result or a variant of unknown significance
- The possibility of incidental and/or secondary findings and the option to opt out of being informed of these findings

of genetic conditions. This has made prenatal genetic counseling and parental decision making on which option to choose more complex. Although it is clear that cell-free DNA-based screening for Down syndrome is far more sensitive than maternal serum screening, we now know that CVS or amniocentesis coupled with CMA, a test that surveys the entire genome for aneuploidy and smaller imbalances (deletions and duplications), can detect a significant chromosomal abnormality in 1% to 1.7% of all pregnancies and in 6% of pregnancies with structural fetal abnormalities found on prenatal ultrasound. The latest data also support that amniocentesis and CVS are safer than previously thought. This has led to recommendations that this prenatal diagnostic test be offered to all women. Thus prenatal genetic counseling must inform women of all options and support them in decisions that balance their desire to know genetic information about their pregnancy with their willingness to undergo a procedure and the decisions they would make with this information.

As with counseling for any genetic test, in addition, the couple must be advised that if a result is difficult to interpret, further tests and consultation may be required. After they are available, genetic counselors review the laboratory results and may seek clarification as indicated by clinical cytogeneticists or molecular geneticists. Result disclosure requires informing the patient of the implications of the results, recommending any additional testing that is needed to clarify the results, and discussing implications for other family members. Variants of uncertain clinical significance are often reported, along with the possibility of future reclassification. Incidental and secondary findings are reported if the patient did not opt out of receiving these results. Genetic counselors also discuss in generalized terms the implications of the results on future management of the pregnancy and infant after birth. For certain conditions, the availability of fetal therapy can be discussed, along with suggestions for appropriate subspecialist referrals depending on the specific findings. Providers can address options regarding continuation or termination of the pregnancy within the legal limitations of their location of practice while always respecting the personal thoughts of patients on whether this is an acceptable path for them.

For parents at increased risk for a genetic condition in their children, the principal goal and benefit of PGT and prenatal genetic diagnosis is to be able to consider pregnancies that they might otherwise not have considered. PGT offers them a means to avoid pregnancies with an affected fetus, while through prenatal diagnosis they can learn early in a pregnancy if the fetus has the condition, allowing them to make an informed decision about whether to continue the pregnancy. For parents at low or average risk of having a child with a genetic disorder, the great majority of prenatal genetic screens and follow-up diagnostic tests ultimately end in reassurance. The primary objective of prenatal diagnosis is to determine whether the fetus is affected or unaffected with the disorder in question. Irrespective of the reason why testing is pursued, parents should be informed about all available options in the event of an abnormal result. Diagnosis of an affected fetus will allow parents to prepare emotionally and medically for the management of a newborn with a disorder. Termination of pregnancy is one choice they can make, but it is important parents understand that by undertaking prenatal diagnosis there is no implied obligation to terminate a pregnancy in the event of an abnormal result.

In closing, prenatal genetic screening and diagnosis is a rapidly evolving discipline. Standards of care in this field will continue to be modified and refined because of the fast-paced technologic advances in methods available for assessing the fetus and the fetal genome, the ongoing discussions on social and ethical norms, and the varying governmental policies concerning prenatal diagnosis in different cultures and countries around the globe.

GENERAL REFERENCES

Gardner RJM, Amor DJ: *Gardner and Sutherland's chromosome abnormalities and genetic counseling*, ed 5, New York, 2018, Oxford University Press.

Milunsky A, Milunsky J: *Genetic disorders and the fetus: Diagnosis, prevention, and treatment*, ed 8, Chichester, West Sussex, England, 2021, Wiley-Blackwell.

Norton M, Kuller J, Dugoff L: *Perinatal genetics*, ed 1, St. Louis, 2019, Elsevier.

SPECIFIC REFERENCES

Adzick NS, Thom EA, Spong CY, et al: A randomized trial of prenatal versus postnatal repair of myelomeningocele, *N Engl J Med* 364:993–1004, 2011.

American College of Obstetricians and Gynecologists Committee on Practice Bulletins–Obstetrics: Practice Bulletin No. 187: Neural tube defects, *Obstet Gynecol* 130:e279–e290, 2017.

American College of Obstetricians and Gynecologists Committee on Genetics: Committee Opinion No. 799: preimplantation genetic testing, *Obstet Gynecol* 135:e133–e137, 2020.

American College of Obstetricians and Gynecologists: Practice Bulletin No. 162: Prenatal diagnostic testing for genetic disorders, *Obstet Gynecol* 127:e108–e122, 2016.

American College of Obstetricians and Gynecologists Committee on Practice Bulletins–Obstetrics: Committee on Genetics; Society for Maternal-Fetal Medicine: Practice Bulletin No. 226: Screening for fetal chromosomal abnormalities, *Obstet Gynecol* 136:e48–e69, 2020.

Armour CM, Dougan SD, Brock JA, et al: Canadian College of Medical Geneticists: Practice Guideline: Joint CCMG-SOGC recommendations for the use of chromosomal microarray analysis for prenatal diagnosis and assessment of fetal loss in Canada, *J Med Genet* 55:215–221, 2018.

Bianchi DW, Chiu RWK: Sequencing of circulating cell-free DNA during pregnancy, *N Engl J Med* 379:464–473, 2018.

Bianchi DW, Parker RL, Wentworth J, et al: DNA sequencing versus standard prenatal aneuploidy screening, *N Engl J Med* 370:799–808, 2014.

Deprest J, Benachi A, Gratacos E, et al: Randomized trial of fetal surgery for moderate left diaphragmatic hernia, *N Engl J Med* 385:119–129, 2021.

Deprest J, Nicolaides K, Benachi A, et al: Randomized trial of fetal surgery for severe left diaphragmatic hernia, *N Engl J Med* 385:107–118, 2021.

Fan HC, Gu W, Wang J, et al: Non-invasive prenatal measurement of the fetal genome, *Nature* 487:320–324, 2012.

Grati FR, Ferreira J, Benn P, et al: Outcomes in pregnancies with a confined placental mosaicism and implications for prenatal screening using cell-free DNA, *Genet Med* 22:309–316, 2020.

Gregg AR, Aarabi M, Klugman S, et al: ACMG Professional Practice and Guidelines Committee: Screening for autosomal recessive and X-linked conditions during pregnancy and preconception: A practice resource of the American College of Medical Genetics and Genomics (ACMG), *Genet Med* 23:1793–1806, 2021.

Gregg AR, Edwards JG: Prenatal genetic carrier screening in the genomic age, *Sem Perinatol* 42:303–306, 2018.

Harris S, Gilmore K, Hardisty E, et al: Ethical and counseling challenges in prenatal exome sequencing, *Prenat Diagn* 38:897–903, 2018.

Kardon G, Ackerman KG, McCulley DJ, et al: Congenital diaphragmatic hernias: From genes to mechanisms to therapies, *Dis Model Mech* 10:955–970, 2017.

Kitzman J, Snyder M, Ventura M, et al: Noninvasive whole-genome sequencing of a human fetus, *Sci Transl Med* 4(137):137ra76, 2012.

Lord J, McMullan D, Eberhardt R, et al: Prenatal exome sequencing analysis in fetal structural anomalies detected by ultrasonography (PAGE): A cohort study, *Lancet* 393(10173):747–757, 2019.

Malone FD, Canick JA, Ball RH, et al: First-trimester and second-trimester screening, or both, for Down's syndrome, *N Engl J Med* 353:2001–2011, 2005.

McArthur SJ, Leigh D, Marshall JT, et al: Blastocyst trophectoderm biopsy and preimplantation genetic diagnosis for familial monogenic disorders and chromosomal translocations, *Prenat Diagn* 28:434–442, 2008.

Monaghan KG, Leach NT, Pekarek D, et al: The use of fetal exome sequencing in prenatal diagnosis: A points to consider document of the American College of Medical Genetics and Genomics (ACMG), *Genet Med* 22:675–680, 2020.

Nassr AA, Erfani H, Fisher JE, et al: Fetal interventional procedures and surgeries: A practical approach, *J Perinat Med* 46:701–715, 2018.

Petrovski S, Aggarwal V, Giordano J, et al: Whole-exome sequencing in the evaluation of fetal structural anomalies: A prospective cohort study, *Lancet* 393(10173):758–767, 2019.

Pratt M, Garritty C, Thuku M, et al: Application of exome sequencing for prenatal diagnosis: A rapid scoping review, *Genet Med* 22:1925–1934, 2020.

Vossaert L, Chakchouk I, Zemet R, et al: Overview and recent developments in cell-based noninvasive prenatal testing, *Prenat Diagn* 41:1202–1214, 2021.

Wapner RJ, Martin CL, Levy B, et al: Chromosomal microarray versus karyotyping for prenatal diagnosis, *N Engl J Med* 367:2175–2184, 2012.

Zhang J, Li J, Saucier J, et al: Non-invasive prenatal sequencing for multiple mendelian monogenic disorders using circulating cell-free fetal DNA, *Nat Med* 25:439–447, 2019.

PROBLEMS

1. Match the term in the top section with the appropriate comment in the bottom section.
   a. Cell-free DNA
   b. 10th week of pregnancy
   c. Cordocentesis
   d. Mosaicism
   e. 16th week of pregnancy
   f. α-fetoprotein in maternal serum
   g. Aneuploidy
   h. Cystic hygroma
   i. Amniotic fluid

   _____ method of obtaining fetal blood for karyotyping

   _____ usual time at which amniocentesis is performed

   _____ increased level when fetus has NTD

   _____ contains fetal cells viable in culture

   _____ major cytogenetic problem in prenatal diagnosis

   _____ ultrasonographic diagnosis indicates possible Turner syndrome

   _____ risk increases with maternal age

   _____ earliest time at which CVS can be performed

   _____ used to screen for aneuploidy starting at 10 weeks of gestation

2. A couple has a child with Down syndrome, who has a 21q21q translocation inherited from the mother. Could prenatal diagnosis be helpful in the couple's next pregnancy? Explain.

3. Cultured cells from a chorionic villus sample show two cell lines: 46,XX and 46,XY. Does this necessarily mean the fetus is abnormal? Explain.

4. What two main types of information about a fetus can be indicated (although not proven) by assay of AFP, hCG, and uE3 in maternal serum during the second trimester?

5. A young woman consults a geneticist during her first pregnancy. Her brother was previously diagnosed with Duchenne muscular dystrophy and had since died. He was the only affected person in her family. The woman had been tested biochemically and found to have elevated creatine kinase levels, indicating she is a carrier of the disease. Unfortunately, no DNA analysis had been conducted on the woman's brother to determine what type of altered *DMD* gene he had.
   a. What other testing can be done on her to evaluate her risk for a child with DMD?
   b. Can information from that test be used to diagnose her pregnancy?

6. Discuss the relative advantages and disadvantages of the following diagnostic procedures, and cite types of disorders for which they are indicated or not indicated: amniocentesis, CVS, first trimester maternal serum screening, second trimester screening, noninvasive screening of cell-free fetal DNA (NIPS).

7. A second trimester anatomy ultrasound exam is performed on a 30-year-old primigravida and reveals the following findings: Congenital diaphragmatic hernia, short femur at the 5th percentile, small ventricular septal defect. No other anomalies are found. You counsel her about the risk for chromosomal abnormalities and she agrees to have an amniocentesis. CMA and karyotype results are unremarkable.
   a. What follow-up test can you offer at this time? Discuss the next level of testing and consider what you should tell her about the benefits, detection rates, potential risks associated with this level of testing? Does the patient have options about disclosing certain types of information?
   b. What treatment options can you counsel her about for this defect, and how would you consider genetic testing results in the decision for treatments?

CHAPTER 19

Application of Genomics to Medicine and Individualized Health Care

Ronald Doron Cohn • Iris Cohn

The last several chapters have been dedicated to introducing various aspects of the applications of modern **genomics** to the practice of medicine. In Chapter 16 we described powerful new genomic technologies, such as identifying the **variants** in a tumor and profiling its pattern of **RNA** expression, which are used for determining prognosis and choosing appropriate targeted therapies for individuals with cancer. In Chapter 17 we discussed how modern genomic approaches are expanding our capabilities in **risk** assessment and **genetic counseling** for those dealing with heritable disease. Chapter 18 focused on prenatal genetics and the advances in prenatal diagnosis made possible by genomics.

In this chapter we explore other applications of genomics to individualized health care: screening asymptomatic individuals for susceptibility to disease in them or their family members and applying that knowledge to improve health care. We first describe population screening and present one of the best-established and highly successful forms of **genetic screening**: the detection of abnormalities in newborns at high risk for preventable illness. We then present some basic concepts and applications of **pharmacogenomics** and how knowledge of individual variation affecting drug therapy can improve therapeutic efficacy and reduce adverse events. Finally, we discuss screening of persons for **genetic** susceptibility based on their **genome sequence**, reviewing some of the concepts and methods of **genetic epidemiology** commonly used to evaluate screening for susceptibility genotypes.

GENETIC SCREENING IN POPULATIONS

Genetic screening is a population-based method to identify persons with increased susceptibility to a particular genetic disease. Screening at the population level is not to be confused with testing for affected persons or for carriers already identified because of family history, as we explored in Chapter 17. Although family history is a very useful tool (Fig. 19.1), no one except an identical twin shares all variants with another family member. Family history is only an indirect means of assessing the contribution that an individual's own combination of genetic variants might make to disease. Family history

is also an insensitive indicator of susceptibility, as it depends on disease being overt in the relatives of the individual concerned.

The challenge going forward is to screen populations, independent of family history and independent of clinical status, for variants relevant to health and disease and to apply this information to make risk assessments that can be used to improve the health care of an individual and the family.

The objective of population screening is to examine all members of a designated population, regardless of family history. Applying the information derived requires demonstration that genetic risk factors are valid indicators of actual risk in an individual and, if valid, that such information is useful in guiding health care. Genetic screening for disease susceptibility is an important public health activity that will become more significant as more and better screening tests become available.

Newborn Screening

The best-known population screening efforts in genetics are government-supported or -mandated programs that identify presymptomatic infants with diseases for which early treatment can prevent, or at least ameliorate the consequences. For newborn screening, the anticipated disease is generally not assessed by directly determining the genotype. Instead, in most instances, asymptomatic newborns are screened for abnormal levels of various substances in the blood. Abnormalities thus identified trigger further evaluation to confirm or rule out the presence of a disorder. One exception to this paradigm of using a biochemical measurement to detect a disease-causing **genotype** is screening for abnormalities in hearing, in which the **phenotype** itself is the target of screening and intervention (see later). While typically using blood taken from a heelstick, more recent newborn screening expansion has included bedside testing to detect conditions such as hearing loss and cardiac disease. The latter 2 conditions are now included in the U.S. federally recommended uniform screening panel (RUSP)2 and are included in some programs in other parts of the worl

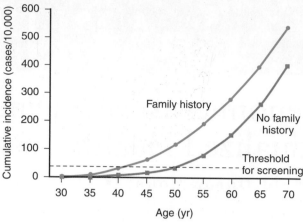

Figure 19.1 Cumulative incidence (per 10,000) of colon cancer versus age in individuals with and without a family history of the disease. Data from Fuchs CS, Giovannucci EL, Colditz GA, et al: A prospective study of family history and the risk of colorectal cancer, *N Engl J Med* 331:1669–1674, 1994.

Many of the general issues concerning genetic screening are highlighted by newborn screening programs. A **determination** of the appropriateness of newborn screening for any particular condition is based on a standard set of criteria involving **clinical validity** and **clinical utility** (see Box 19.1). The design of newborn screening tests includes keeping false-negative rates low so that true-positive cases are not missed, without making the test so nonspecific as to drive the false-positive rate unacceptably high. False-positive results cause

BOX 19.1 GENERAL CRITERIA FOR AN EFFECTIVE NEWBORN SCREENING PROGRAM

Analytic Validity

- A rapid and economic laboratory test is available that detects the appropriate metabolite.

Clinical Validity

- The laboratory test is highly sensitive (no false negatives) and reasonably specific (few false positives). **Positive predictive value** is high.

Clinical Utility

- Treatment is available.
- Early institution of treatment, before symptoms become manifest, reduces or prevents severe illness.
- Routine observation and physical examination will not reveal the disorder in the newborn – a test is required.
- The condition is frequent and serious enough to justify the expense of screening; that is, screening is cost effective.
- The public health system infrastructure is in place to inform the newborn's parents and physicians of the results of the screening test, to confirm the test results, and to institute effective treatment and counseling.

unnecessary anxiety to the parents and increase costs, because more unaffected infants have to be recalled for retesting. At the other extreme, false-negative results vitiate the purpose of a screening program. In deciding whether to institute screening for any given condition, consideration must be given to the ability of the public health system infrastructure to handle the care of affected newborns so identified through such screening.

The prototype condition that satisfies all of these criteria is phenylketonuria (see Chapter 13). For decades, finding elevated levels of phenylalanine in a spot of blood on filter paper obtained soon after birth has been the mainstay of neonatal screening for phenylketonuria and other forms of hyperphenylalaninemia. Currently, this applies throughout North America and Europe, most of Latin America and much of Asia Pacific (see Chapter 13). A positive screen result, followed by definitive confirmation of the diagnosis, leads to the institution of dietary phenylalanine restriction early in infancy, thereby preventing irreversible intellectual disability.

Two other conditions that are widely targeted for newborn screening are **congenital** hearing loss and congenital hypothyroidism. Newborn screening for hearing loss is mandated throughout the United States and Canada. Approximately half of all congenital deafness is due to single-gene defects (Case 13). Infants found to have hearing impairments by newborn screening are offered intervention with sign language, cochlear implants, and other communication aids early in life, meant to improve their long-term language skills and intellectual abilities beyond those seen if the impairment is discovered later in childhood. Screening for congenital hypothyroidism, a disorder whose genetic basis is known in only 10 to 15% of cases, but is easily treatable, is universal in the United States and Canada and routine in many other countries. Thyroid hormone replacement therapy started early in infancy completely prevents the severe and irreversible intellectual disability caused by congenital hypothyroidism. Thus, both hypothyroidism and congenital hearing loss easily fulfill the criteria for newborn screening.

A number of other disorders, such as galactosemia, sickle cell disease (Case 42), biotinidase deficiency (see Chapter 13), severe combined immunodeficiency, and congenital adrenal hyperplasia (see Chapter 6), are part of many or most neonatal screening programs. Which disorders should be the target of newborn screening varies among jurisdictions. In the United States, Recommended Universal Screening Panel (RUSP) is a national guideline listing conditions for which the U.S. Secretary of Health and Human Services recommends all newborns be tested.

Standards for newborn screening differ widely around the globe. Which disorders should be the target of newborn screening varies from province to province in Canada without a national consensus. As of 2022, the United Kingdom's national program to screen newborns across all jurisdictions included just nine disorders.

Tandem Mass Spectroscopy

For many years, most newborn screening was performed by a test specific for each individual condition. For example, phenylketonuria screening was based on a microbial or a chemical assay that tested for elevated phenylalanine level. This situation has changed dramatically with the application of the technology of tandem mass spectrometry (TMS). Not only can a neonatal blood spot be examined accurately and rapidly for an elevation of phenylalanine, with fewer false positives than with the older testing methods, but TMS analysis can simultaneously detect a few dozen other biochemical disorders. Some of these, such as homocystinuria (see Chapter 13) or maple syrup urine disease, were already being screened for by individual tests (Table 19.1). TMS, however, does not replace the disease-specific testing methods for other disorders currently included in some newborn screening, such as galactosemia, biotinidase deficiency, congenital adrenal hyperplasia, and sickle cell disease.

TMS also provides a reliable method for newborn screening for some disorders that fit the criteria for screening but had no reliable newborn screening program in place. For example, medium-chain acyl-CoA dehydrogenase (MCAD) deficiency is a disorder of fatty acid oxidation that is usually asymptomatic but manifests clinically when the patient becomes catabolic. Detection of MCAD deficiency at birth can be lifesaving. Affected infants and children are at very high risk for life-threatening hypoglycemia in early childhood during the catabolic stress caused by an intercurrent illness, such as a viral infection; nearly 25% of children with undiagnosed MCAD deficiency will die with their first episode of hypoglycemia. The metabolic derangement can be successfully managed if it is treated promptly. In MCAD deficiency, alerting parents and physicians to the risk for metabolic decompensation is the primary goal of screening. The children are healthy between attacks and do not require daily management other than avoidance of prolonged fasting.

TMS provides a rapid test for many disorders for which newborn screening is already being done or

TABLE 19.1 Disorders Detectable by Tandem Mass Spectrometry

A. Amino Acid Disorders
- Classical phenylketonuria (PKU)
- Variant PKU
- Guanosine triphosphate cyclohydrolase 1 (GTPCH) deficiency (biopterin deficiency)
- 6-pyruvoyl-tetrahydropterin synthase (PTPS) deficiency (biopterin deficiency)
- Dihydropteridine reductase (DHPR) deficiency (biopterin deficiency)
- Pterin-4α-carbinolamine dehydratase (PCD) deficiency (biopterin deficiency)
- Argininemia/arginase deficiency
- Argininosuccinic acid lyase deficiency (ASAL deficiency)
- Citrullinemia, type I/argininosuccinic acid synthetase deficiency (ASAS deficiency)
- Citrullinemia, type II (citrin deficiency)
- Gyrate atrophy of the choroid and retina
- Homocitrullinuria, hyperornithinemia, hyperammonemia (HHH)
- Homocystinuria/cystathionine beta-synthase deficiency (CBS deficiency)
- Methionine adenosyltransferase deficiency (MAT deficiency)
- Maple syrup urine disease (MSUD)
- Prolinemia
- Tyrosinemia, types I, II, III, and transient
- Ornithine transcarbamylase deficiency (OTC deficiency)
- Remethylation defects (MTHFR, MTR, MTRR, Cbl D v1, Cbl G deficiencies)

B. Organic Acid Disorders
- 2-methyl-3-hydroxybutyryl-CoA dehydrogenase deficiency
- 2-methylbutyryl-CoA dehydrogenase deficiency
- 3-hydroxy-3-methylglutaryl-CoA lyase deficiency (HMG CoA lyase deficiency)
- 3-methylcrotonyl-CoA carboxylase deficiency (3MCC deficiency)

- 3-methylglutaconic aciduria (MGA), type I (3-methylglutaconyl-CoA hydratase deficiency)
- Beta-ketothiolase (BKT) deficiency
- Ethylmalonic encephalopathy (EE)
- Glutaric acidemia type-1 (GA-1)
- Isobutyryl-CoA dehydrogenase deficiency
- Isovaleric acidemia (IVA)
- Malonic aciduria
- Methylmalonic acidemia, mut −
- Methylmalonic acidemia, mut 0
- Methylmalonic acidemia (Cbl A, B)
- Methylmalonic acidemia (Cbl C, D)
- Multiple carboxylase deficiency (MCD)
- Propionic acidemia (PA)

C. Fatty Acid Oxidation Disorders
- Carnitine transporter deficiency
- Carnitine-acylcarnitine translocase deficiency (CAT deficiency)
- Carnitine palmitoyltransferase deficiency-type 1 (CPT-1 deficiency)
- Carnitine palmitoyltransferase deficiency-type 2 (CPT-2 deficiency)
- Long chain hydroxyacyl-CoA dehydrogenase deficiency (LCHAD deficiency)
- Medium chain acyl-CoA dehydrogenase deficiency (MCAD deficiency)
- Medium/short chain L-3-hydroxy acyl-CoA dehydrogenase deficiency (M/SCHAD deficiency)
- Multiple acyl-CoA dehydrogenase deficiency (MAD deficiency)/glutaric acidemia type-2 (GA-2)
- Short chain acyl-CoA dehydrogenase deficiency (SCAD deficiency)
- Trifunctional protein deficiency (TFP deficiency)
- Very long chain acyl-CoA dehydrogenase deficiency (VLCAD deficiency)
- Formiminoglutamic acid (FIGLU) disorder

Cbl, Cobalamin; *MTHFR*, methylene tetrahydrofolate reductase; *MTR*, 5-methyltetrahydrofolate-homocysteine methyltransferase; *MTRR*, methionine synthase reductase.
Modified from California Newborn Screening Program, http://www.cdph.ca.gov/programs/nbs/Documents/NBS-DisordersDetectable011312.pdf.

can easily be justified. TMS also identifies infants with inborn errors—such as ethylmalonic acidemia—that have not generally been the targets of newborn screening because of their rarity and difficulty of providing definitive therapy to prevent the progressive neurologic impairment. TMS can also identify abnormal metabolites whose significance for health are uncertain. For example, short-chain acyl-CoA dehydrogenase (SCAD) deficiency, another disorder of fatty acid oxidation, is most often asymptomatic, although a few individuals may have difficulties with episodic hypoglycemia. Thus, a positive TMS screen result is not particularly predictive of developing symptomatic SCAD later in life. Although TMS can identify many metabolic disorders, does the benefit of detecting disorders such as SCAD deficiency outweigh the negative impact of raising parental concern for most newborns whose test result is positive but who will never be symptomatic? Thus not every disorder detected by TMS fits the criteria for newborn screening. Some public health experts argue that only those metabolites of proven clinical relevance should be reported to parents and physicians.

PHARMACOGENOMICS

One area of medicine that is receiving a lot of attention for potential application of genomics to individualized medical care is pharmacogenomics: the study of how genetic variation among individuals affects the response to medication therapy. The development of a genetic profile that predicts efficacy, toxicity, or an adverse drug reaction is likely to have clinical significance. It allows health care professionals to choose a drug from which the patient will benefit—by reducing the risk for an adverse event—or to decide on a dosage that ensures adequate therapy and minimizes complications.

The US Food and Drug Administration (FDA) has recognized the importance of pharmacogenetic variation in individual response to drug treatment by including pharmacogenetic information on the labels that come with a broad range of pharmaceuticals (Table 19.2). As with all other aspects of personalized medicine, however, the cost effectiveness of such testing must be proved if it is to become part of accepted medical care.

There are two ways that genetic variation affects drug therapy. The first is the effect of variation on **pharmacokinetics**; that is, the rate at which the body absorbs, transports, metabolizes, or excretes drugs and/or their metabolites. The second is the variation affecting pharmacodynamics; that is, differences in the way the body responds to a drug. This can involve biochemical, physiologic, and molecular effects of drugs on the body and can include receptor binding (including **sensitivity**) and chemical interactions.

The terms **pharmacogenetics** and pharmacogenomics can be used interchangeably, although historically

TABLE 19.2 Gene-Drug Combinations for Which There Is Pharmacogenetic Information in Their US Food and Drug Administration Package Inserts*

Gene	Drug(s)
CYP2C19	Clopidogrel, voriconazole, omeprazole, pantoprazole, esomeprazole, diazepam, nelfinavir, rabeprazole
CYP2C9	Celecoxib, warfarin
CYP2D6	Atomoxetine, venlafaxine, risperidone, tiotropium bromide inhalation, tamoxifen, timolol maleate, fluoxetine, cevimeline, tolterodine, terbinafine, tramadol and acetaminophen, clozapine, aripiprazole, metoprolol, propranolol, carvedilol, propafenone, thioridazine, protriptyline, tetrabenazine, codeine
DPYD	Capecitabine, fluorouracil
G6PD	Rasburicase, dapsone, primaquine, chloroquine
HLA-B*1502	Carbamazepine
HLA-B*5701	Abacavir (Case 1)
NAT	Rifampin, isoniazid, and pyrazinamide; isosorbide dinitrate and hydralazine hydrochloride
TPMT	Azathioprine, thioguanine, mercaptopurine
UGT1A1	Irinotecan, nilotinib
VKORC1	Warfarin

*Constitutional variants only; chemotherapy whose usage is affected by somatic variants are not included.

pharmacogenetics referred to variations in a single gene influencing drug response and pharmacogenomics referred to the sum total of all relevant genetic variation that determine drug behavior.

Variation in Pharmacokinetic Response

Variation in Drug Metabolism: The Example of Cytochrome P-450

The human cytochrome P-450 proteins are a large family of at least 57 different functional enzymes, each encoded by a different CYP gene. The cytochromes P-450 are grouped into 18 families according to amino acid sequence homology. They code for enzymes. Three of these families, CYP1, CYP2, and CYP3, are particularly active in the detoxification of exogenous chemicals (xenobiotics), such as drugs. Four cytochrome P-450 genes (CYP2C9, CYP2C19, CYP2D6, and CYP3A4/5) are especially important because the enzymes they encode are responsible for the metabolism of about 75 to 80% of all commonly used drugs (Fig. 19.2).

For many drugs, the action of a cytochrome P-450 is to begin the process of detoxification through a series of reactions (oxidation) that render the drug less active and easier to excrete. Some drugs, however, are themselves inactive prodrugs whose conversion into an active metabolite by a cytochrome P-450 is required for the drug to have any therapeutic effect.

Many of the CYP genes important for drug metabolism (including CYP2C9, CYP2C19, CYP2D6, CYP3A4, and CYP3A5) are highly polymorphic, with alleles that result in absent, decreased, or increased enzyme activity. Variants affect the rate at which many drugs are metabolized, with real functional consequences for how individuals respond to drug therapy. As one example, *CYP2D6*, the primary cytochrome in the metabolism of more than 70 different drugs, has dozens of reduced, absent, or increased activity alleles, leading to normal, poor, intermediate, or ultrafast metabolism (see table on metabolizer phenotypes). Missense variants decrease the activity of this cytochrome; alleles with no activity are caused by **splicing** or frameshift variants. In contrast, the *CYP2D6*1XN* **allele** is actually a series of **copy number variant** alleles in which the *CYP2D6* gene is present in three, four, or more copies on one **chromosome**. Predictably, these larger copy number variants produce high levels of the enzyme. There are dozens more alleles that do not affect the function of the protein and are considered to be **wild type**. Various combinations of these four classes of alleles produce quantitative differences in metabolizing activity, resulting in four main phenotypes: normal (also called extensive) metabolizers, intermediate

metabolizers, poor metabolizers, and ultrafast metabolizers (Fig. 19.3).

Depending on whether a drug is itself an active compound or is a prodrug that requires activation by a cytochrome P-450 enzyme to have its pharmacologic effect, poor metabolizers may either accumulate toxic levels of the drug or fail to have therapeutic efficacy because of poor activation of a prodrug. In contrast, ultrafast metabolizers are at risk for being undertreated by a drug with doses inadequate to maintain blood levels in the therapeutic range, or they may suffer overdose due to too rapid conversion of a prodrug to its active metabolite. For example, codeine is a weak narcotic drug that exerts most of its analgesic effect on conversion to morphine, a bioactive metabolite with a 10-fold higher potency. This conversion is carried out by the *CYP2D6* enzyme. Poor metabolizers—quite common in some populations, carrying loss-of-function alleles at the *CYP2D6* locus fail to convert codeine to morphine, thereby receiving little therapeutic benefit; in contrast, ultrafast metabolizers can become rapidly intoxicated with low doses of codeine. A number of children have died from codeine overdoses due to having an ultrafast metabolizer phenotype.

As with many forms of genetic variation (see Chapter 10), the frequency of many of the alleles in the cytochromes P-450 differs among different populations (Table 19.3). For example, a slow metabolizing phenotype for *CYP2D6* that is present in 1 in 14 individuals of European ancestry is rare in Asia and nearly absent in Native Americans and Pacific Islanders. Similarly, slow metabolizing alleles at *CYP2C19* show striking population variability, with 1 in 33 individuals of European descent but nearly 1 in 6 Asians having slow metabolism. These differences in the frequency of poor and ultrarapid metabolizers are important for the delivery of individualized genetic medicine in heterogeneous populations.

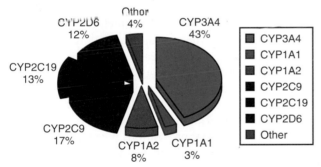

Figure 19.2 Contribution of individual cytochrome P-450 enzymes to drug metabolism. Modified with permission from Guengerich F: Cytochrome P450s and other enzymes in drug metabolism and toxicity, *AAPS J* 8:E101–E111, 2006.

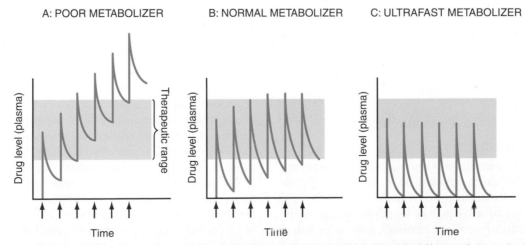

Figure 19.3 Serum drug levels after repeated doses of a drug (*arrows*) in three individuals with different phenotypic profiles for drug metabolism. (A) Poor metabolizer accumulates drug to toxic levels. (B) Normal (extensive) metabolizer reaches steady-state levels within the therapeutic range. (C) Ultrafast metabolizer fails to maintain serum levels within the therapeutic range.

Metabolizer Phenotypes Arising from Various Combinations of *CYP2D6* Alleles

Metabolizer Status	Alleles and Activity	Anticipated Response (compared to average world population)
Normal (extensive)	Two normal activity alleles One normal activity allele and one decreased activity allele One increased activity allele and one decreased functional allele	Typical metabolism
Intermediate	One normal activity allele and one nonfunctional activity allele Two decreased activity alleles One decreased activity allele and one non-functional activity allele	Decreased metabolism
Poor	Two nonfunctional activity alleles	Little or no metabolism
Ultrarapid	Two increased activity alleles	Increased metabolism

TABLE 19.3 Frequency of Poor *CYP2D6* and *CYP2C19* Metabolizers in Various Population Groups

Origin of Population	Population Frequency of Poor Metabolizers (%)	
	CYP2D6	*CYP2C19*
Sub-Saharan Africa	3.4	4.0
Native American	0	2
Asian	0.5	15.7
European	7.2	2.9
Middle Eastern/North Africa	1.5	2.0
Pacific Islander	0	13.6

Data from Burroughs VJ, Maxey RW, Levy RA: Racial and ethnic differences in response to medicines: towards individualized pharmaceutical treatment, *J Natl Med Assoc* 94(Suppl):1–26, 2002.

Clinical pharmacogenetics—the use of genetic data to guide drug therapy decisions, is supported by professional societies such as the Clinical Pharmacogenetics Implementation Consortium (CPIC), the Royal Dutch **Association** for the Advancement of Pharmacy–Pharmacogenetic Working Group (DPWG), the Canadian Pharmacogenomic Network for Drug Safety, and others. They established guidance on pharmacogenes to provide actionable recommendations for the use of genomic information in a consistent manner. Additionally, the FDA has recognized the importance of pharmacogenetic variation in individual response to drug treatment by including pharmacogenetic information on the labels that come with a broad range of pharmaceuticals (see Table 19.2). As with all other aspects of individualized medicine, further cost-effectiveness studies of such testing must be provided if it is to become part of accepted medical care.

Variation in Pharmacodynamic Response

Malignant Hyperthermia

Malignant hyperthermia is a rare autosomal **dominant** condition in which there may be a dramatic adverse response to the administration of many commonly used inhalational anesthetics (e.g., halothane) and depolarizing muscle relaxants (e.g., succinylcholine). Soon after **induction** of anesthesia, a patient develops life-threatening fever, sustained muscle contraction, and attendant hypercatabolism. The fundamental physiologic abnormality in the disease is an elevation of the level of ionized calcium in the sarcoplasm of muscle. This increase leads to muscle rigidity, elevation of body temperature, rapid breakdown of muscle (rhabdomyolysis), and other abnormalities. The condition is an important, if not a common cause of death during anesthesia. The incidence is 1 in 50,000 adults undergoing anesthesia but for unknown reasons is 10-fold higher in children.

Malignant hyperthermia is most frequently associated with pathogenic variants in a gene called *RYR1*, encoding an intracellular calcium ion channel. However, variants in *RYR1* account for only approximately half of cases of malignant hyperthermia. At least five other loci have now been identified, one of which is the *CACNA1S* gene, which encodes the α_1 subunit of a dihydropyridine-sensitive calcium channel. Precisely why the abnormalities in calcium handling in muscle found with *RYR1* or *CACNA1S* variants make the muscle sensitive to inhalation anesthetics and muscle relaxants and precipitate malignant hyperthermia is unknown.

The need for special precautions when at-risk persons require anesthesia is obvious. Cooling blankets, muscle relaxants, and cardiac antiarrhythmics may all be used to prevent or reduce the severity of the response if an unsuspected attack occurs, and alternative anesthetics can be given to patients at risk. Pharmacogenomics guidelines are available to help guide clinical decision making.

Adverse Drug Reactions

The majority (75–80%) of adverse drug events result from predictable, nonimmunologic drug toxicities such as overdoses caused by medication errors, renal or hepatic disease, or drug-drug interactions. Most nonpredictable adverse drug events are thought to have a genetic component related to drug-gene interactions that contribute to about one-third of potential major or substantial drug interactions that occur in patients.

Of these, ~25 to 50% are true IgE-mediated drug hypersensitivity reactions (HSRs), including life-threatening anaphylaxis characterized by sudden onset of laryngeal edema, leading to occlusion of the airway, marked hypotension, and cardiac arrhythmias.

The remaining 50 to 75% of adverse drug reactions are genetically determined nonallergic immune reactions (i.e., HSR). These manifest as widespread damage to skin and mucous membranes, referred to as Stevens-Johnson syndrome (SJS) and (in its more serious extreme form), toxic epidermal necrolysis (TEN) (Case 1). Although rare, TEN is a very serious adverse drug reaction that causes denuding of large areas of skin and carries a mortality rate of 30 to 40%. There is a strong **correlation** between particular drugs and certain **human leukocyte antigen (HLA)** alleles in the **major histocompatibility complex** (see Chapter 9) that result in SJS and TEN. For example, individuals who take the retroviral drug abacavir and carry the *HLA-B*5701* allele have a 50% risk for SJS or TEN, leading to the introduction of *HLA-B*5701* typing as a standard of care screening tool prior to prescribing abacavir. Because ~5 to 8% of Europeans carry the *HLA-B*5701* allele, the risk for a severe drug reaction in abacavir-treated patients from this population is especially significant. *HLA-B*5701* screening has a **negative predictive value** of 100% and a positive predictive value of 47.9% for immunologically confirmed HSR (i.e., positive result on epicutaneous patch testing 6 to 10 weeks after clinical diagnosis), as demonstrated by one study. A similar situation exists with the use of the antiseizure medication carbamazepine and *HLA-B*1502*, which is present in (see Table 19.3).

PHARMACOGENOMICS AS A COMPLEX TRAIT

The examples of pharmacogenomics provided in this chapter primarily involve variation at single genes and its effect on drug treatment. In truth, most drug response is a complex trait. A drug may have its effect directly or through more active metabolites, each of which may then be metabolized by different pathways and exert its effects on various targets. Thus, variants at more than one locus may interact, synergistically or antagonistically, either to potentiate or to reduce the effectiveness of a drug or to increase its toxic side effects. Further research is required to create a comprehensive **pharmacogenomic** profile that takes into account multiple genetic variants as well as other factors, to offer precise and predictive information to guide drug therapy. Other factors include environmental effects, interactions within the biologic system, disease state, and drug interactions, The ultimate goal is for a patient to receive the best drug at the right dose and avoid potentially dangerous side effects. We expect pharmacogenomics to become increasingly important in the delivery of individualized, precision medicine in the years ahead.

SCREENING FOR GENETIC SUSCEPTIBILITY TO DISEASE

Genetic Epidemiology

Epidemiologic studies of risk factors for disease rely on population studies that measure disease prevalence or incidence and determine whether certain risk factors (e.g., genetic, environmental, social) are more prevalent in individuals with disease than those without. **Genetic epidemiology** is concerned with how genotypes and environmental factors interact to increase or decrease susceptibility to disease. Epidemiologic studies generally follow one of three different strategies: case-control, cross-sectional, and cohort design (see Box 19.2).

BOX 19.2 STRATEGIES USED IN GENETIC EPIDEMIOLOGY

- **Case-control:** Individuals with and without the disease are selected, and the genotypes and environmental exposures of individuals in the two groups are determined and compared.
- **Cross-sectional:** A random sample of the population is selected and divided into those with and without the disease, and their genotypes and environmental exposures are determined and compared.
- **Cohort:** A sample of the population is selected and observed for some time to ascertain who does or does not develop disease, and their genotypes and environmental exposures are determined and compared. The cohort may be selected at random or may be targeted to individuals who share a genotype or an environmental exposure.

Cohort and cross-sectional studies not only capture information on the **relative risk** conferred by different genotypes but, if they are random population samples, also provide information on the prevalence of the disease and the frequency of the various genotypes under study. A randomly selected **cohort study**, in particular, is the most accurate and complete approach, in that phenotypes that take time to appear have a better chance of being detected and scored; they are, however, more expensive and time consuming. Cross-sectional studies, on the other hand, suffer from underestimation of the frequency of the disease. First, if the disease is rapidly fatal, many of those with disease and carrying a risk factor will be missed. Second, if the disease shows age-dependent **penetrance**, some individuals carrying a risk factor will not be scored as having the disease. Case-control studies, on the other hand, allow researchers to efficiently target individuals, particularly with relatively rare phenotypes for which very large sample sizes would be needed in a cross-sectional or cohort study. However, unless a study is based on complete **ascertainment** of individuals with a disease (e.g., in a population register or surveillance program) or uses a random sampling scheme, a **case-control study** cannot capture information on the population prevalence of the disease.

Disease Association

A genetic disease association is the relationship in a population between a susceptibility or protective genotype and a disease phenotype (see Chapter 10). The susceptibility or protective genotype can be an allele (in either a **heterozygote** or a **homozygote**), a genotype at one locus, a **haplotype** containing alleles at neighboring loci, or even combinations of genotypes at multiple unlinked loci. Whether a disease association between genotype and phenotype is statistically significant can be determined from standard statistical tests, such as the chi-square test; whereas, how strongly associated the genotype and phenotype are is given by the **odds ratio** or **relative risk**, as discussed in Chapter 10. The relationship between some of these concepts is best demonstrated by means of a 2 × 2 table.

Determination of the Predictive Value of a Test

Genotype	Disease		
	Affected	Unaffected	Total
Susceptibility genotype present	a*	b	a + b
Susceptibility genotype absent	c	d	c + d
Total	a + c	b + d	a + b + c + d = N

Frequency of the susceptibility genotype = (a + b)/N

Disease prevalence = (a + c)/N (with random sampling or a complete population survey)

Relative Risk:

$$= \frac{a/(a + b)}{c/(c + d)}$$

$$RR = \frac{\text{Disease prevalence in carriers of susceptibility genotype}}{\text{Disease prevalence in noncarriers of susceptibility genotype}}$$

Sensitivity: Fraction of individuals with disease who have the susceptibility genotype = a/(a + c)

Specificity: Fraction without disease who do not have the susceptibility genotype = d/(b + d)

Positive predictive value: Proportion of individuals with the susceptibility genotype who have or will develop a particular disease = a/(a + b)

Negative predictive value: Proportion of individuals without the susceptibility genotype who do not have or will not develop a particular disease = d/(c + d)

*The values of a, b, c, and d are derived from a random sample of the population, divided into those with and without the susceptibility genotype, and then examined for the disease (with or without longitudinal follow-up, depending on whether it is a cross-sectional or cohort study) (see later).

Clinical Validity and Utility

Finding the genetic contributions to health and disease is of obvious importance for research into underlying disease etiology and pathogenesis, as well as for identifying potential targets for intervention and therapy. In medical practice, however, whether to screen individuals for increased susceptibilities to illness depends on the clinical validity and clinical utility of the test. That is, how predictive of disease is a positive test, and how useful is it to have this information?

Clinical Validity

Clinical validity is the extent to which a test result is predictive for disease. Clinical validity is captured by the two concepts of positive predictive value and negative predictive value. The **positive predictive value** is the frequency with which a group of individuals who test

positive have or will develop the disease. For **mendelian** disorders, the positive predictive value of a genotype is the penetrance. Conversely, the **negative predictive value** is the frequency with which a group of individuals who test negative are free of disease and remain so. When faced with a unique patient, the practitioner of individualized genetic medicine needs to know more than just whether there is an association and its magnitude (i.e., relative risk or odds ratio). It is important to know clinical validity (i.e., how well the test predicts the presence or absence of disease).

Susceptibility Testing Based on Genotype

The positive predictive value of a genotype that confers susceptibility to a particular disease depends on the relative risk for disease conferred by one genotype over another and on the prevalence of the disease. Fig. 19.4 provides the positive predictive value for genotype frequencies ranging from 0.5% (rare) to 50% (common), which confer a relative risk that varies from low (2-fold) to high (100-fold), when the prevalence of the disease ranges from relatively rare (0.1%) to more common (5%). As the figure shows, the value of the test as a predictor of disease increases substantially when one is dealing with a common disorder due to a relatively rare susceptibility genotype that confers a high relative risk, compared with the risk for individuals who do not carry the genotype. The converse is also clear; testing for a common genotype that confers a modest relative risk is of limited value as a predictor of disease.

We will illustrate the use of the 2 × 2 table in assessing the role of susceptibility alleles in a common disorder, colorectal cancer. Shown in the following Box are data from a population-based study of colorectal cancer risk conferred by common variant in the *APC* gene (see Chapter 16) that changes isoleucine to lysine at position 1307 of the protein (p.Ile1307Lys). This variant has an allele frequency of ~3.1% among those of Ashkenazi Jewish ancestry, which means that ~1 in 17 such individuals is a heterozygote (and 1 in 1000 are **homozygous**) for the allele. The prevalence of colon cancer among this population is 1%. The common p.Ile1307Lys variant confers a 2.4-fold increased risk for colon cancer relative to individuals without the allele. However, the small positive predictive value (≈2%) means that an individual who tests positive for this allele has only a 2% chance of developing colorectal cancer. If this had been a cohort study that allowed complete ascertainment of everyone in whom colorectal cancer was going to develop, the penetrance would, in effect, be only 2%.

Clinical Utility

The clinical utility of a test is more difficult to assess than clinical validity because it has different meanings for different people. In its narrowest sense, the clinical

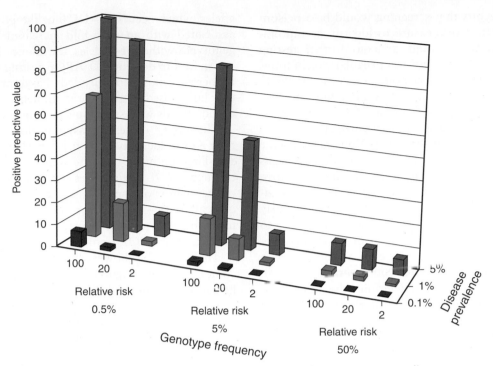

Figure 19.4 Theoretical positive predictive value calculations for a susceptibility genotype for a disease, over a range of genotype frequencies, disease prevalences, and relative risks for disease conferred by the genotype.

BOX 19.3 THE P.ILE1307LYS ALLELE OF THE *APC* GENE AND COLON CANCER

	Colon Cancer		
Allele	Affected	Unaffected	Total
Lys1307	7	310	317
Ile1307	38	4142	4180
Total	45	4452	4497

- Relative Risk $= \dfrac{\text{Disease prevalence in allele carriers}}{\text{Disease prevalence in non-carriers}}$

$$= \frac{7/317}{38/4180} = 2.4$$

- **Sensitivity:** Fraction of individuals with colon cancer who have the Lys1307 allele = 7/45 = 16%
- **Specificity:** Fraction without colon cancer who do not have the Lys1307 allele = 4142/4452 = 93%
- **Positive predictive value:** Fraction of individuals with the Lys1307 allele who develop colon cancer = 7/317 = 2%
- **Negative predictive value:** Fraction of individuals without the Lys1307 allele who do not develop colon cancer = 99%

Data from Woodage T, King SM, Wacholder S, et al: The APC I1307K allele and cancer risk in a community-based study of Ashkenazi Jews, *Nat Genet* 20:62–65, 1998.

utility of a test is that the result is medically actionable; that is, the result will change medical care for an individual and, as a consequence, will improve the outcome of care, both medically and economically. At the other end of the spectrum is the broader definition as any piece of information an individual might wish to have, for any reason, including simply for the sake of knowing.

In a person who tests positive for the *APC* Ile1307Lys allele, how does a positive predictive value of 2% translate into clinical utility for medical practice? (see Box 19.3) One critical factor is a public health economic one: can the screening be shown to be cost effective? Is the expense of the testing outweighed by improving health outcomes while reducing health care costs, disability, and loss of earning power? In the example of screening for the APC p.Ile1307Lys allele in those of Ashkenazi ancestry, more frequent screening or the use of different approaches to screening for colon cancer may be effective. Screening methods (occult stool blood testing vs fecal DNA testing, or sigmoidoscopy vs full colonoscopy) differ in expense, sensitivity, **specificity**, and potential for hazard; deciding which regimen to follow has important implications for the person's health and health care costs.

Even with demonstrable clinical validity and actionable clinical utility, to demonstrate that testing improves health care is not always straightforward. For example, 1 in 200 to 1 in 250 individuals of European ancestry are homozygous for a p.Cys282Tyr variant in the *HFE* gene associated with hereditary hemochromatosis: a disorder characterized by iron overload that can silently lead to extensive liver damage and cirrhosis (Case 20, Chapter 7, Chapter 11). A simple intervention – regular phlebotomy to reduce total body iron stores – can prevent hepatic cirrhosis. The susceptibility genotype is common, and 60 to 80% of p.Cys282Tyr homozygotes show biochemical evidence of increased body iron stores. This suggests that screening would be a reasonable and cost-effective measure to identify asymptomatic individuals who should undergo further testing and, if indicated, the institution of regular phlebotomy. However, most p.Cys282Tyr homozygotes (>90–95%) remain clinically asymptomatic, leading to the argument that the positive predictive value of *HFE* gene testing for liver disease in hereditary hemochromatosis is too low to justify population screening. Nonetheless, some of these largely asymptomatic individuals do have signs of clinically occult fibrosis and cirrhosis on liver biopsy, indicating that the Cys282Tyr homozygote may actually be at a higher risk for liver disease than previously thought. Thus, some argue for population screening to identify individuals in whom regular prophylactic phlebotomy should be instituted. The clinical utility of such population screening remains controversial and will require additional research to determine the natural history of the disease and whether the silent fibrosis and cirrhosis seen on liver biopsy represent the early stages of a progressive illness. As of 2019, guidelines recommend screening of transferrin levels to look for any cause of iron overload, rather than HFE testing, due to the very low penetrance.

APOE testing in Alzheimer disease (AD) (Chapter 13) (Case 4) is another example of the role of a careful assessment of clinical validity and clinical utility in applying genetic testing to individualized medicine. Heterozygotes for the ε4 allele of the *APOE* gene are at two- to three-fold increased risk for development of AD, compared with individuals without an *APOE* ε4 allele. *APOE* ε4/ε4 homozygotes are at eight-fold increased risk. An analysis of both the clinical validity and clinical utility of *APOE* testing, including calculation of the positive predictive value for asymptomatic and symptomatic individuals, is shown in Table 19.4.

As can be seen from these positive predictive values for asymptomatic people aged 65 to 74 years, a single ε4 allele is not a strong predictor of whether AD will develop, despite the three-fold increased risk conferred for the disease. Thus, most individuals **heterozygous** for an ε4 allele identified through *APOE* testing as being at increased risk will not develop AD. Even with two ε4 alleles, which occurs in ~1.5% of the population and is associated with an eight-fold increased risk relative to genotypes without ε4 alleles, the chance is still less than one in four to develop AD. *APOE* testing for the ε4 allele is, therefore, not recommended in asymptomatic individuals but is used by some practitioners in the evaluation of individuals with symptoms and signs of dementia.

The utility of testing asymptomatic individuals at their *APOE* locus to assess risk for AD is also controversial. First, knowing that one is at increased risk for AD through *APOE* testing does not lead to any preventive or therapeutic options. Thus, under a strict definition of clinical utility – that is, the result is actionable and leads to changes in medical management – there would be little value in *APOE* testing for AD risk.

There may be, however, positive and negative outcomes of testing that are psychological or economic in nature and more difficult to assess than the purely clinical factors. For example, testing positive for a susceptibility genotype could empower individuals with knowledge of their risks as they make important life decisions. On the other hand, it has been suggested that knowing of an increased risk through *APOE* testing might cause significant emotional and psychological distress. However, careful studies of the impact of receiving *APOE* genotype information have shown little harm in appropriately counseled individuals with a family history of AD who wished to know this information. Finally, individuals who test negative for the ε4 alleles could be falsely reassured that they are at no increased risk for the disorder, despite having a positive family history or other risk factors for dementia. Balancing all of these considerations, *APOE* testing is still not recommended in asymptomatic individuals, even in light of such a strong genotype-disease association, because of the low positive predictive value and lack of clinical utility, rather than because such information is harmful.

As in all of medicine, the benefits and costs for each component of individualized genetic medicine need to be clearly demonstrated and continually reassessed. The requirement for constant reevaluation is obvious: imagine how the recommendations for *APOE* testing, despite its low positive predictive value, might change

TABLE 19.4 Clinical Validity and Utility of *APOE* Population Screening and Diagnostic Testing for Alzheimer Disease

	Population Screening	Diagnostic Testing
Clinical validity	Asymptomatic individuals aged 65–74 yr	Individuals aged 65–74 yr with symptoms of dementia
	Population prevalence of AD = 3%	Proportion of dementia patients with AD = ≈60%
	PPV given ε2/ε4 or ε3/ε4 = 6%	PPV given ε2/ε4 or ε3/ε4 = ≈75%
	PPV given ε4/ε4 = 23%	PPV given ε4/ε4 = ≈98%
Clinical utility	No intervention possible to prevent disease	Increases suspicion that another, potentially treatable cause of dementia may be present
	Psychological distress for most people with ε4 alleles who are not likely to develop AD	Reduces unnecessary testing
	False reassurance for those without ε4 alleles	

Positive predictive value (PPV) calculations are based on a population prevalence of Alzheimer disease (AD) of ~3% in individuals aged 65–74 years, an allele frequency for the ε4 allele in those of European ancestry of 10–15%, a relative risk of ~3 for one ε4 allele, and a relative risk of ~20 for two ε4 alleles.

if a low-risk and inexpensive medical intervention were discovered that could prevent or significantly delay the onset of dementia.

Heterozygote Screening

In contrast to screening for genetic disease in newborns or for genetic susceptibility in individuals, screening for carriers of mendelian disorders has, as its main purpose, the identification of individuals who are themselves healthy but are at substantial risk (25% or higher) to have children with a severe autosomal **recessive** or X-linked illness. The principles of heterozygote screening are shown in the accompanying (see Box 19.4).

Until recently, heterozygote screening programs focused on particular population groups in which the frequency of variant alleles is high. In contrast to newborn screening, as discussed previously in this chapter, heterozygote screening is voluntary and focuses on individuals who identify themselves as members of particular high-risk groups. Heterozygote screening has been used extensively for a battery of disorders for which **carrier** frequency is relatively high: Tay-Sachs disease (Case 43) (the prototype of carrier screening) (see Chapter 13), Gaucher disease, and Canavan disease in the Ashkenazi Jewish population; sickle cell disease (Case 42) in the black population of North America; and β-thalassemia (Case 44) in high-incidence areas, especially in Cyprus and Sardinia, or in extended consanguineous families from Pakistan (see Chapter 12).

Carrier screening for cystic fibrosis (Case 12) has become standard of care for couples contemplating a pregnancy. As discussed in Chapter 13, more than 2000 different disease-causing variants have been described in the *CFTR* gene. Although the vast majority of disease-causing variants in *CFTR* can be readily detected with greater than 99% sensitivity when the entire gene is sequenced, such an approach for every couple seeking preconception carrier testing would be expensive if carried out on a population-wide basis, particularly in individuals with low prior probability of carrying a variant. Current recommendations are to report pathogenic and likely-pathogenic variants identified by sequencing or targeted testing. Targeted testing panels range from the most frequent 23 variants found in persons of European

ancestry—as proposed by the American College of Medical Genetics and Genomics (ACMG), to considerably more extensive panels with more than 60 distinct variants that include those identified in populations with lower frequencies of disease, such as of African or Asian ancestry. Because this approach is intended to find only the most frequent variants, their sensitivity is around (88 to 90%) in individuals of European descent and 64 to 72% among those of African descent.

The classification-based reporting technique involves giving individuals comprehensive cystic fibrosis testing that includes an evaluation of all the exonic coding regions and +/−2 bp proximal splice junctions of the *CFTR* gene, as well as reporting on all pathogenic and likely-pathogenic variants for classic cystic fibrosis. **Sanger sequencing** has long been employed in medical laboratories for the study of *CFTR* because of its accuracy, precision, and simplicity of use. The analysis of *CFTR* using next-generation sequencing approaches is now successful, although there is still a danger of false negatives and positives. Furthermore, certain regions may need Sanger sequencing to detect variants. **Multiplex ligation-dependent probe amplification** (MLPA see Chapter 5) continues to be an efficient method to detect large deletions and duplications in the *CFTR* gene, and commercial reagents exist.

Regardless of the test indication, all *CFTR* variants should be classified using ACMG sequence variant classification criteria. Information from *CFTR* variant databases can be used to inform those variant classifications.

As the cost of variant detection using next-generation sequencing has fallen, it has become much less compelling to restrict carrier screening to a small number of alleles common in certain ancestral groups in genes that are known to be associated with disease. It is possible now to expand carrier screening beyond disorders common to particular groups, such as cystic fibrosis, sickle cell trait, or thalassemia, to include carrier status for more than 400 autosomal recessive and X-linked disorders. With sequencing instead of allele-specific detection methods, there is no longer any limit to which genes and which alleles in these genes can (theoretically) be detected. Rare variant alleles in genes associated with known disease will be found, thereby raising the sensitivity of carrier detection methods. Sequencing, however, can uncover variants—particularly missense changes, of uncertain significance in genes whose role in the disease may be known or unknown. Unless great care is taken in assessing the clinical validity of rare variants detected by sequencing, the frequency of false-positive carrier test results will increase.

The impact of carrier screening in lowering the incidence of a genetic disease can be dramatic. Carrier screening for Tay-Sachs disease in the Ashkenazi Jewish population began in some communities in 1969. Screening followed by prenatal diagnosis, when indicated, has already lowered the incidence of Tay-Sachs

---

BOX 19.4 CRITERIA FOR HETEROZYGOTE SCREENING PROGRAMS

- High frequency of carriers, at least in a specific population
- Availability of an inexpensive and dependable test with very low false-negative and false-positive rates
- Access to genetic counseling for couples identified as heterozygotes
- Availability of prenatal or preimplantation genetic diagnosis
- Acceptance and voluntary participation by the population targeted for screening

disease by 65 to 85% in this group. In contrast, attempts to screen for carriers of sickle cell disease in the US Black community have been less effective, with little impact on the incidence of the disease. The success of carrier screening programs for Tay-Sachs disease, as well as the relative failure for sickle cell anemia, underscores the importance of community consultation, community engagement, and the availability of genetic counseling and prenatal or preimplantation genetic diagnosis as critical requirements for an effective program.

INDIVIDUALIZED GENOMIC MEDICINE

More than a century ago, British physician-scientist Archibald Garrod proposed the concept of **chemical individuality**, in which each of us differs in our health status and susceptibility to various illnesses because of our individual genetic makeup. Indeed, in 1902, he wrote:

> … the factors which confer upon us our predisposition and immunities from disease are inherent in our very chemical structure, and even in the molecular groupings which went to the making of the chromosomes from which we sprang.

The goal of individualized **genomic medicine** is to use knowledge of an individual's genetic variants relevant to maintaining health or treating illness as a routine part of medical care.

Now, more than a hundred years after Garrod's visionary pronouncement, in the era of human genomics, we have the means to assess an individual's genotype at every locus by genome sequencing (**whole genome sequencing [WGS]**). WGS is a comprehensive test capable of detecting nearly all DNA variation in a genome. WGS can identify the 7000 diseases described in the Online Mendelian Inheritance in Man database (www.omim.org) that have a known molecular basis. These include those we have discussed extensively in this textbook, such as cystic fibrosis, Duchenne muscular dystrophy, **familial** hypercholesterolemia, and hemophilia. Patients may present with unusual constellations of features, or with common conditions such as autism spectrum disorder, cardiomyopathy, congenital heart disease, epilepsy, cancer, schizophrenia, or dementia, although this list is not comprehensive. WGS is broader in scope than other commonly used genetic tests (see Box 19.5), and data can be analyzed in both hypothesis-driven and hypothesis-generating ways. For these reasons, WGS will most certainly eclipse **exome** sequencing, large next-generation sequencing gene panel tests, and chromosomal **microarray** analysis in the future.

Genome sequencing is a 3-stage process. First, a medical geneticist or other health care professional obtains the required information on the patient's phenotype and family history. Second, a clinical laboratory geneticist analyzes the genome data. Third, a physician compares the genetic findings to the clinical manifestation to assess the diagnostic fit or associated risk. The overall goal of interpreting a genetic variant is to explain it in the

---

BOX 19.5 OVERVIEW OF SELECTED CLINICAL GENETIC TEST MODALITIES

For phenotypes with known genetic **heterogeneity**, the following tests are commonly employed in clinical practice:
- Chromosomal microarray analysis: a genome-wide test that typically detects only copy number variations (i.e., chromosome imbalances).
- Next-generation sequencing gene panel test: a targeted test focusing on a predefined list of genes, which typically detects only exonic sequence-level variants, deletions or duplications in those genes.
- Exome sequencing: a genome-wide test that typically detects only exonic sequence-level variants, or a subset of exon-level deletions or duplications (CNVs).
- Genome sequencing (also whole genome sequencing or WGS): this approach offers myriad advantages as a single comprehensive test. Current short-read genome sequencing can reliably detect sequence, structural and copy number variations, both within and outside of exons, as well as clinically relevant short **tandem repeats**, pseudogenes and **mitochondrial DNA** variation.

---

context of all or part of the clinical manifestation. The main aim of genome sequencing as a clinical diagnostic test is to identify these variations. Some laboratories in North America will also search for secondary findings, which are disease-causing variants in genes associated with medically actionable conditions that are unrelated to the initial intent for testing.

The procedure of sequencing is safe; however, possible negative consequences are tied to how results are interpreted and disclosed. First, genome sequencing may be misinterpreted as a diagnostic that can answer all clinical questions. The clarity in clinical data and family history is still essential for interpreting findings. A positive result does not necessarily explain all of the patient's characteristics, and a negative test does not indicate that there was no genetic component nor invalidate an obvious clinical diagnosis. Second, because of ongoing understanding and the characterization of new information, the classification of a genetic variant may change over time. The majority of ancient peoples other than Europeans are under-represented in the big-scale reference databases of genomic variation that guide interpretation; thus, misdiagnosis is a risk for these people who needs to be taken into consideration. Third, genetic test results might provide information about the person, their family members, or their connections to one another that was not previously considered. These facts underscore the need for thorough pre- and post-test counseling and qualified genetics professionals.

The majority of the data come from prospective clinical trials testing in clinically diverse populations with anticipated rare genetic diseases. Primary outcome measures are frequently diagnostic yield or time to diagnosis. Clinical usefulness and cost-effectiveness are desirable secondary outcomes. Genome sequencing has a greater diagnostic yield than exome sequencing and chromosomal microarray analysis, while being increasingly price competitive. Different phenotype categories are associated with different diagnostic yields. For individuals with severe-to-profound intellectual disability, such yields can be less than 10%, but they can be as much as 50% or greater for other indications.

Genome sequencing with a rapid turnaround time is most commonly utilized in neonatal and pediatric intensive care settings.

In children and adults with suspect genetic conditions that have high genetic heterogeneity, genome sequencing is expected to become a first-tier test (i.e., a broad genetic differential diagnosis with many candidate genes or loci) instead of the second-tier technique it has typically been used for so far. This will cut down on the time it takes to conduct several genetic tests. Genomic testing may reveal pharmacogenetic profiles, reproductive carrier status information, and genetic risk profiles for later-onset diseases. The use of genome sequencing as a preventative health tool in seemingly healthy people is uncertain at this time, but it has tremendous potential for the future.

Ongoing research is needed to examine the clinical usefulness, cost-effectiveness, and possible unintended future consequences of genome sequencing in our healthcare system. In certain circumstances, the added yield of genome sequencing over exome sequencing is modest; nevertheless, this gap will increase with improvements in data analysis and bigger data sets to compare against. The **anticipation** of additional clinically relevant information arising from as-yet-unexplored areas of the genome is also driving investments in genome sequencing technology. Ensuring equitable access to care informed by the DNA code, irrespective of postal code, is a challenge in many countries and needs to be a priority for policy-makers.

PRECISION CHILD HEALTH

Precision Child Health (PCH) refers to a concept and movement to transform pediatric health care through the integration of data from all domains of a child's determinants of health (genes, biology, environment). This must go along with patient-reported perceptions of their health and objectively measured physiology in order to predict, prevent, diagnose, and treat disease in a targeted, individualized way. Application of **bioinformatics**, computing tools, and advanced statistical approaches applied to these integrated data resources will support the evaluation and discovery of rapid, accurate, and cost-effective diagnostics, individualized therapies, and enhanced drug safety and efficacy. Insights unlocked by PCH will fuel the next generation of data-guided quality improvement initiatives and preventative care. This strategy has the potential to radically transform our approach to healthcare delivery by unlocking efficiencies, decreasing preventable harm, and enhancing our approaches to patient-centered care that will eventually be extrapolated to all of medicine.

GENERAL REFERENCES

Feero WG, Guttmacher AE, Collins FS: Genomic medicine—an updated primer, *N Engl J Med* 362:2001–2011, 2010.

Ginsburg G, Willard HF, editors: Genomic and personalized medicine, ed 2, vols 1 & 2, New York, 2012, Elsevier.

Kitzmiller JP, Groen DK, Phelps MA, et al: Pharmacogenomic testing: relevance in medical practice, *Cleve Clin J Med* 78:243–257, 2011.

Schrodi SJ, Mukherjee S, Shan Y, et al: Genetic-based prediction of disease traits: prediction is very difficult, especially about the future, *Frontiers Genet* 5:1–18, 2014.

REFERENCES FOR SPECIFIC TOPICS

Amstutz U, Carleton BC: Pharmacogenetic testing: time for clinical guidelines, *Pharmacol Ther* 89:924–927, 2011.

Bardolia C, Matos A, Michaus V, et al: Utilizing pharmacogenomics to reduce adverse drug events, *Am J Biomed Sci Res*, 2020. https://biomedgrid.com/pdf/AJBSR.MS.ID.001638.pdf

Bennett MJ: Newborn screening for metabolic diseases: saving children's lives and improving outcomes, *Clin Biochem* 47(9):693–694, 2014.

Deignan JL, Astbury C, Cutting GR, et al: CFTR variant testing: a technical standard of the American College of Medical Genetics and Genomics (ACMG), *Gen Med Off J Am Coll Med Genet* 22(8):1288–1295, 2020. https://doi.org/10.1038/s41436-020-0822-5

Dorschner MO, Amendola LM, Turner EH, et al: Actionable, pathogenic incidental findings in 1,000 participants' exomes, *Am J Hum Genet* 93:631–640, 2013.

Ferrell PB, McLeod HL: Carbamazepine, HLA B*1502 and risk of Stevens-Johnson syndrome and toxic epidermal necrolysis: US FDA recommendations, *Pharmacogenomics* 9:1543–1546, 2008.

Green RC, Roberts JS, Cupples LA, et al: Disclosure of APOE genotype for risk of Alzheimer's disease, *N Engl J Med* 361:245–254, 2009.

Ingelman-Sundberg M, Rodriguez-Antona C: Pharmacogenetics of drug-metabolizing enzymes: implications for a safer and more effective drug therapy, *Philos Trans R Soc Lond B Biol Sci* 360:1563–1570, 2005. https://doi.org/10.1098/rstb.2005.1685

Johnston JJ, Dirksen RT, Girard T, et al: Variant curation expert panel recommendations for RYR1 pathogenicity classifications in malignant hyperthermia susceptibility, *Gen Med Off J Am Coll Med Genet* 23(7):1288–1295, 2021. https://doi.org/10.1038/s41436-021-01125-w

Karczewski KJ, Daneshjou R, Altman RB: Pharmacogenomics, *PLoS Comput Biol* 8(12):e1002817, 2012.

Kohane IS, Hsing M, Kong SW: Taxonomizing, sizing, and overcoming the incidentalome, *Genet Med* 14:399–404, 2012.

Mallal S, Phillips E, Carosi G, et al: HLA-B*5701 screening for hypersensitivity to abacavir, *N Engl J Med* 358:568–579, 2008.

Mayo Clinic Laboratories: Test ID: CARBR. https://www.mayoclinicclabs.com/test-catalog/Overview/610048#Clinical-and-Interpretive.

McCarthy JJ, McLeod HL, Ginsburg GS: Genomic medicine: a decade of successes, challenges and opportunities, *Sci Transl Med* 5: 189sr4, 2013.

Mounzer K, Hsu R, Fusco JS, et al: HLA-B*57:01 screening and hypersensitivity reaction to abacavir between 1999 and 2016 in the OPERA® observational database: a cohort study, *AIDS Res Ther* 16:1, 2019. https://doi.org/10.1186/s12981-019-0217-3

PharmGKB: Annotation of CPIC guideline for desflurane and CACNA1S, RYR1. https://www.pharmgkb.org/chemical/PA164749136/guidelineAnnotation/PA166180457

PharmGKB: Dosing guidelines. https://www.pharmgkb.org/guidelinesRelling MV, Klein TE: CPIC: clinical pharmacogenetics implementation consortium of the pharmacogenomics research network, *Clin Pharmacol Ther* 89(3):464–467, 2011.

Topol EJ: Individualized medicine from prewomb to tomb, *Cell* 157:241–253, 2014.

Urban TJ, Goldstein DB: Pharmacogenetics at 50: genomic personalization comes of age, *Sci Transl Med* 6:220ps1, 2014.

Zanger UM, Schwab M: Cytochrome P450 enzymes in drug metabolism: regulation of gene expression, enzyme activities, and impact of genetic variation, *Pharm Ther* 138:103–141, 2013. https://doi.org/10.1016/j.pharmthera.2012.12.007

Zhu Y, Swanson KM, Rojas RL, et al: Systematic review of the evidence on the cost-effectiveness of pharmacogenomics-guided treatment for cardiovascular diseases, *Genet Med* 22:475–486, 2020. https://doi.org/10.1038/s41436-019-0667-y

PROBLEMS

1. In a population sample of 1 million Europeans, idiopathic cerebral vein thrombosis (iCVT) occurred in 18, consistent with an expected rate of 1 to 2 per 100,000. All the individuals were tested for factor V Leiden (FVL). Assuming an allele frequency of 2.5% for FVL, how many homozygotes and how many heterozygotes for FVL would you expect in this sample of 1 million people, assuming Hardy-Weinberg equilibrium? Among the individuals affected with iCVT, two were heterozygotes for FVL and one was homozygous for FVL.

    a. Set up a 3 × 2 table for the association of the homozygous FVL genotype, the heterozygous FVL genotype, and the wild-type genotype for iCVT.

    b. What is the relative risk for iCVT in a FVL heterozygote versus in the wild-type genotype?

    c. What is the risk in a FVL homozygote versus in wild type?

    d. What is the sensitivity of testing positive for either one or two FVL alleles for iCVT?

    e. What is the positive predictive value of being homozygous for FVL? Heterozygous?

2. In a population sample of 100,000 European women taking oral contraceptives, deep venous thrombosis (DVT) of the lower extremities occurred in 100, consistent with an expected rate of 1 per 1000. Assuming an allele frequency of 2.5% for factor V Leiden (FVL), how many homozygotes and how many heterozygotes for FVL would you expect in this sample of 100,000 women, assuming Hardy-Weinberg equilibrium? Among the affected individuals, 58 were heterozygotes for FVL and three were homozygous for FVL. Set up a 3 × 2 table for the association of the homozygous FVL genotype, the heterozygous FVL genotype, and the wild-type genotype for DVT of the lower extremity. What is the relative risk for DVT in a FVL heterozygote using oral contraceptives versus in women with the wild-type genotype taking oral contraceptives? What is the risk in a FVL homozygote versus in wild type? What is the sensitivity of testing positive for either one or two FVL alleles for DVT while taking oral contraceptives? Finally, what is the positive predictive value for DVT of being homozygous for FVL while taking oral contraceptives? Heterozygous?

3. What steps should be taken when a newborn phenylketonuria (PKU) screening test comes back positive?

4. Newborn screening for sickle cell disease can be performed by hemoglobin electrophoresis or high-performance liquid chromatography (HPLC), which separates hemoglobin A and S, thereby identifying individuals who are heterozygotes as well as those who are homozygotes for the sickle cell variant. What potential benefits might accrue from such testing? What harms?

5. Toxic epidermal necrolysis (TEN) and the Stevens-Johnson syndrome (SJS) are two related, life-threatening skin reactions that occur in ~1 per 100,000 individuals in China, most commonly as a result of exposure to the antiepileptic drug carbamazepine. These conditions carry a significant mortality rate of 30 to 35% (TEN) and 5 to 15% (SJS). It was observed that individuals who suffered this severe immunologic reaction carried a particular major histocompatibility complex class 1 allele, *HLA-B*1502*, as do 8.6% of the Chinese population. In a retrospective cohort study of 145 patients who received carbamazepine therapy, 44 developed either TEN or SJS. Of these, all 44 carried the *HLA-B*1502* allele, whereas only three of those who received the drug without incident were *HLA-B*1502* positive. What is the sensitivity, specificity, and positive predictive value of this allele for TEN or SJS in individuals receiving carbamazepine?

6. A 21-month-old boy with ventricle atrioventricular septal defect and complete pulmonary atresia and history of thrombotic event was put on standard warfarin dosing, with a goal INR (international normalized ratio) of 2.5 to 3. After a second warfarin dose, the INR level rose to 8. Parents took the child to the emergency room where he was observed overnight. Upon review of his pharmacogenomics data, it was found that the patient was warfarin sensitive, as he was a poor metabolizer for the metabolizing enzyme CYP2C9. Warfarin is broken down in the liver by CYP2C9 enzyme to its inactive metabolites. Absent or low CYP2C9 enzyme activity reduces the clearance rates of warfarin. Warfarin exhibits its anticoagulant effect by inhibiting the Vitamin K epoxide reductase (VKORC1) enzyme. VKORC1 converts vitamin K into its active form, which is needed to produce clotting factors. Certain genetic variants in the *VKORC1* gene may decrease the level of active vitamin K, thus causing fewer clotting factors to be available.

    Conclusion: Much lower starting dose would have been sufficient.

    Question: Review the most common variants in the *CYP2C9* gene among different populations.

7. A 10-year-old male with eosinophilic esophagitis (EoE) was prescribed lansoprazole: 15 mg orally twice daily. EoE is a chronic immune system disease in which eosinophils build up in the lining of the esophageal tract. Damaged esophageal tissue can lead to difficulty swallowing or cause food impaction and poor appetite. Currently, proton pump inhibitors with/without budesonide slurry are the standard of care for this condition. After 3 months, this child did not show any improvement of symptoms. Pharmacogenomics testing was requested. The metabolizing enzyme CYP2C19 is mainly responsible for the breakdown of proton pump inhibitors such as lansoprazole, omeprazole and pantoprazole. This patient was found to an ultra-rapid CYP2C19 metabolizer. He breaks down lansoprazole much faster than the world population average, leading to a much-decreased plasma concentration, with therapeutic failure. He was switched to rabeprazole which is less influenced by the CYP2C19 metabolizer status.

    Conclusion: After another 4 months, patient underwent an endoscopy which revealed evidence of healing of the esophageal tract.

    Question: Which other health condition can be influenced by genetic changes in the *CYP2C19* gene?

CHAPTER 20

Ethical and Social Issues in Genetics and Genomics

Bartha Maria Knoppers • Ma'n H. Zawati

Human genetics and **genomics** are having a major impact in all areas of medicine and across all age groups and in emerging fields such as epigenetics, cellular genomics, and pathogen genomics. The importance will only grow as knowledge increases and the power and reach of sequencing technologies improves. At the same time, no single area of medical practice raises as many challenging ethical, social, and policy issues in so many areas of medicine across a broad a spectrum of age groups, including the fetus, neonates, children, prospective parents, and adults.

Numerous categories of information are affected by genetics and genomics, ranging from ancestry and personal heritage to the diagnosis of treatable or untreatable disease to explanations for **familial** traits to concerns about what has been or might be passed on to the next generation and to the meaning of **polygenic risk scores** (PRSs). Some of these were introduced in previous chapters; others are presented in this chapter. But, as we shall see, they all pose ethical, legal, social, personal, and policy challenges. And if that is true today, it will become only more commonplace in the years and decades ahead, as **genome** sequences (and the data-rich landscape of genomic and medical information) become available for hundreds of millions of individuals worldwide.

The ethical and social issues raised by these new capabilities are especially relevant to decisions in the area of reproduction (see Chapter 18) because of the absence of a societal consensus. The damaging legacy of **eugenics** (discussed later in this chapter) still hangs over discussions of reproductive genetics, now especially timely in light of the ability to evaluate the **sequence** of fetal genomes and to perform **gene therapy** and editing. Finally, privacy and security concerns also loom large because **genetic** and genomic information, even in the absence of any other demographic information, may still render individuals and their personal sensitive health information uniquely identifiable. Yet, we share DNA variation with our family members and indeed with all of humanity. Thus privacy concerns need to be balanced against the benefits that could be derived from making personal genetic information available to other family members and to society at large.

In this chapter we review some of the most challenging ethical and societal issues arising from the application of genetics and genomics to medicine. These relate to prenatal diagnosis, presymptomatic testing, familial genetic information, and the policy challenges arising from the discovery of genetic variants that confer increased risk for conditions that are found incidental to diagnostic testing for another Indication.

PRINCIPLES OF BIOMEDICAL ETHICS

Four cardinal principles are frequently considered in any discussion of ethical issues in medicine:
- **Respect for individual autonomy**, safeguarding an individual's rights to control own medical care and medical information, free of coercion
- **Beneficence**, doing good
- **Nonmaleficence**, not harming, preventing harm
- **Justice**, ensuring that all individuals are treated equally and fairly

Complex ethical issues arise when these principles are perceived to be in conflict with one another. The role of ethicists working at the interface between society and medical genetics is to weigh and balance conflicting demands, each of which has a claim to legitimacy based on one or more of these cardinal principles.

ETHICAL DILEMMAS ARISING IN MEDICAL GENETICS

In this section we focus our discussion on some of the ethical dilemmas arising in medical genetics, dilemmas that will only become more difficult and complex as genetics and genomics research expands our knowledge (Table 20.1). The list of issues discussed in this chapter is by no means exhaustive, nor are the issues necessarily independent of one other.

Prenatal Genetic Testing

Geneticists are frequently asked to help couples use prenatal diagnosis or assisted reproductive technology to avoid having offspring with a serious hereditary

TABLE 20.1 Major Ethical and Policy Issues in Medical Genetics

Genetic Testing
- Prenatal diagnosis, especially for nondisease traits or sex
- Testing asymptomatic adults for genotypes that predispose to late-onset disease
- Testing asymptomatic children for genotypes that predispose to adult-onset diseases
- Secondary and incidental findings and the right "not to know" about clearly deleterious variants that will cause diseases that could be ameliorated or prevented if the risk were known

Privacy of Genetic Information
- Duty to warn and permission to warn family members

Misuse of Genetic Information
- Insurance/employment discrimination based on an employee's genotype
- Discrimination in life and health insurance underwriting based on a person's genotype

Genetic Screening
- Expansion of screening programs
- Privacy

disorder. For some hereditary disorders, prenatal diagnosis remains controversial, particularly when the diagnosis leads to a decision to terminate the pregnancy for a disease that causes various kinds of physical or intellectual disabilities but is not fatal in infancy. Prenatal diagnosis is equally controversial for adult-onset disorders, particularly ones that may be managed or treated. The debate is still ongoing in the community of persons who have a physical or intellectual disability and deaf patients and their families (to name only a few examples) about whether prenatal diagnosis and abortion for these disorders are ethically justified. Other areas of ethical debate include seeking prenatal diagnosis to avoid recurrence of a disorder associated with a mild or cosmetic defect or for putative genetic enhancement, such as genetic variants affecting muscle physiology and therefore athletic prowess. The dilemma lies in attempting to balance, on the one hand, respect for the autonomy of reproductive decision making about the kind of family they wish to have versus, on the other hand, an assessment of how aborting a fetus affected with a disability might be viewed by the broader community of persons with a disability.

The dilemma also arises when a couple makes a request for prenatal diagnosis in a pregnancy that is at risk for what most people would not consider a disease or disability at all. Particularly difficult is prenatal diagnosis for **selection** of sex for reasons other than reducing the risk for **sex-limited** or X-linked disease. Some genetics professionals are concerned that couples are using assisted reproductive technologies, such as *in vitro* **fertilization** and blastomere biopsy, or prenatal sex **determination** by ultrasonography and abortion, to balance the sexes of the children in their family or to avoid having children of one or the other sex for sociocultural and economic reasons prevalent in their societies. There are already clear signs of a falling ratio of female to male infants from 0.95 to less than 0.85 in certain areas of the world where male children are more highly prized. Some countries explicitly prohibit sex selection by law (absent a link to the presence of a genetic condition).

Many of these dilemmas have so far been more theoretical than real. For example, surveys of couples with deafness or achondroplasia show that the couples are concerned about having children who are not deaf or do not have achondroplasia. The vast majority would not actually use prenatal diagnosis and abortion to avoid having children who do not share their conditions. Moreover, as we will see, somatic **gene** editing will increase the range of interventions and treatments for children and the range of parental and pediatric choices.

Yet, in the future, particular alleles and genes that contribute to complex traits, such as intelligence, personality, stature, and other physical characteristics, will likely be identified. Will such nonmedical criteria be viewed as a justifiable basis for prenatal diagnosis? Some might argue that parents are already expending tremendous effort and resources on improving the environmental factors that contribute to healthy, successful children. They might therefore ask why they should not try to improve the genetic factors as well. Others consider prenatal selection for particular desirable genes a dehumanizing step that treats children simply as commodities fashioned for their parents' benefit. Does a health professional have, on the one hand, a responsibility or, on the other hand, any right to intervene in the decision of a couple concerning the "seriousness" of a disorder?

There is little consensus among geneticists as to where or even whether one can draw the line in deciding what constitutes a trait serious enough to warrant prenatal testing. Preimplantation testing of embryos not only moves these dilemmas earlier in time but to date has faced less public scrutiny.

Genetic Testing for Predisposition to Disease

Another area of medical genetics and genomics in which ethical dilemmas frequently arise is genetic testing of asymptomatic individuals for diseases that may have an onset in life later than the age at which the molecular testing is to be performed. The ethical principles of respect for individual autonomy and beneficence are central to testing in this context. At one end of the spectrum is testing for late-onset, highly penetrant neurologic disorders, such as Huntington disease (see Chapter 13) (Case 24). For such diseases, individuals carrying a **variant allele** may be asymptomatic but will almost certainly develop a devastating illness later in life for which there is currently little or no treatment. For these asymptomatic individuals, is knowledge of the test result more beneficial than harmful, or vice versa? There is no simple answer. Studies demonstrate that some individuals at risk for Huntington disease choose not to undergo testing and would rather not know their risk, whereas others choose to undergo testing. Those who choose testing and test positive have been shown to sometimes have a transient period of depression, but with few suffering severe depression, and many report positive benefits in terms of the knowledge provided to make life decisions about marriage and choice of career. Those who choose testing and are found not to carry the trinucleotide expansion allele report positive benefits of relief, but they can also experience negative emotional responses due to guilt for no longer being at risk for a disease that either affects or threatens to affect many of their close relatives. In any case, the decision to undergo testing is a highly personal one that must be made only after thorough review of the issues with a genetics professional.

The balance for or against testing of unaffected, at-risk individuals shifts when testing indicates a predisposition to a disease for which intervention and early treatment are available. For example, in autosomal **dominant** hereditary breast cancer, individuals carrying various pathogenic variants in *BRCA1* or *BRCA2* have a 50% to 90% chance of developing breast or ovarian cancer (see Chapter 16) (Case 7). Identification of **heterozygous** carriers would be of benefit because individuals at risk could choose to undergo more frequent surveillance or have preventive surgery, such as mastectomy, oophorectomy, or both, recognizing that these measures can reduce but not completely eliminate the increased risk for cancer. What if surveillance and preventive measures were more definitive, as they are in familial adenomatous polyposis, for which prophylactic colectomy is a proven preventive measure (see Chapter 16)? Moreover, upon testing for any predisposing gene variant(s), individuals incur the risk for serious psychological distress, stigmatization in their social lives, and possible discrimination in insurance and employment (see later). How are respect for a patient's autonomy, the physician's duty not to cause harm, and the physician's desire to prevent illness to be balanced in these different situations?

Geneticists would all agree that the decision to be tested or not to be tested is not one made in a vacuum. The patient must make an informed decision using all available information concerning the risk for and severity of the disease, the effectiveness of preventive and therapeutic measures, and the potential harm that could arise from testing.

Genetic Testing of Asymptomatic Children

Ethical issues in the testing of asymptomatic individuals take on a further degree of complexity when such testing involves minor children (generally, <18 years), particularly children too young to even give assent. There are several reasons why parents may wish to have their children tested for a disease predisposition. Testing asymptomatic children for alleles that predispose to disease can be beneficial, even life saving, if interventions that decrease morbidity or increase longevity are available. One example is testing the asymptomatic sibling of a child with medium-chain acyl-CoA dehydrogenase deficiency (see Chapter 19) (Case 31).

However, a minority have argued that even in situations where there are currently no clear medical interventions that might benefit the child, it is the parents' duty to inform and prepare their children for the future possibility of development of a serious illness. The parents may also seek this information for their own family planning or to avoid what some parents consider the corrosive effects of keeping important information about their children from them. Testing children, however, carries the same risks for serious psychological damage, stigmatization, and certain kinds of insurance discrimination as does testing adults (see later). Children's autonomy—their ability to make decisions for themselves about their own genetic constitution—must also now be balanced with the desire of parents to obtain and use such information.

A different but related issue arises in testing children for the **carrier** state of a disease that poses no threat to their health but places them at risk for having affected children. Once again, the debate centers on the balance between respect for children's autonomy in regard to their own procreation when they could choose as adults and the desire on the part of well-meaning parents to educate and prepare children for the difficult decisions and risks that lie ahead once they reach childbearing age.

Most bioethicists believe (and the American College of Medical Genetics and Genomics [ACMG] agrees) that predictive pediatric genetic testing should generally be deferred until a child is sufficiently mature, unless an intervention in childhood would reduce mortality or morbidity. Testing for adult-onset conditions should likewise typically be deferred until the child reaches a sufficient level of maturity. The European Society of Human Genetics echoes this view, suggesting that genetic testing decisions that affect children should be approached with a certain degree of caution. Minors, as soon as their maturity and degree of understanding permit, should have their perspectives taken into account and should be permitted to decide personally whether to undergo asymptomatic genetic testing when they are sufficiently well informed and capable of understanding the test and its consequences. The Canadian College of Medical Geneticists (CCMG) takes a slightly different approach, noting that while asymptomatic pediatric testing might sometimes be in the best interests of the child, but testing for adult-onset conditions should generally be deferred until such children are competent to consent to such testing on their own behalf. In exceptional circumstances, parents may insist that the asymptomatic testing of a child be carried out. The CCMG notes that physicians are not obliged to carry out such testing if it is not in the best interests of the child concerned.

Gene Therapy

Genetic testing inevitably raises the possibility of gene therapy. Such therapy is subject to much public scrutiny as a potential option for patients living with serious, and even incurable, diseases. This technology promises to replace genes that cause medical problems with genes that do not, or even "turn off" genes in the body that cause illness. Beyond the safety and consent issues, gene therapy raises other ethical, legal, and social concerns. As a new and expensive therapy, we need to think about how and who determines whether a condition is serious enough for its use, what uses are for therapy versus enhancement, and how do we make sure that everyone has access to it?

However, the main debate is the difference between somatic and **germline** gene therapy. Somatic therapies target genes in specific cells, such as lungs or skin cells, and cannot be passed on to a person's children. On the other hand, germline therapies make changes in reproductive cells (e.g., egg or sperm cells), correcting genes that are subsequently inherited by future generations. While germline therapy could prevent future generations in a family from having a particular genetic condition and could eliminate certain serious diseases altogether from society (e.g., Huntington disease), this therapy could have unexpected effects on the future child to be born. Finally, gene therapy could be used to select or enhance different human characteristics (e.g., height, intelligence, athletic skills), which may result in society being less accepting of people who are different or have a certain disability. While somatic therapies are beginning to be used on patients (e.g., spinal muscular atrophy, sickle cell), no country has decided to allow germline therapy. But the debate continues and will require considering the views of communities, patients, and families, as well as the ethical and legal issues and the possible long-term effects for society.

Incidental and Secondary Findings From Exome and Whole Genome Sequencing

Another area of controversy has arisen in patients who have given consent for **exome** or **whole genome sequencing** (ES/WGS) to find a genetic basis for their undiagnosed diseases (see Chapter 19). Laboratories searching the exomes or genomes of such patients usually develop a primary candidate gene list based on the **phenotype** of the patient. The laboratory considers deleterious variants in these genes as their primary findings (i.e., the results that are actively being sought as the primary target of the testing). In the process of analyzing an exome or genome, however, pathogenic variants may be discovered incidentally in genes known to be associated with diseases unrelated to the phenotype for which the sequencing test was originally conducted. If the pathogenic variants uncovered as incidental findings cause serious diseases that can be ameliorated or prevented, then is there benefit of drawing up a list of genes that every laboratory doing ES/WGS would deliberately analyze in every patient, even though they are not relevant to the primary goal of finding the genetic cause for a patient's unexplained disease? Pathogenic and likely pathogenic variants in this list of genes would be secondary findings that would be sought regardless of whether the patient wishes to know these results, because the patient's providers deem the benefit of knowing is so compelling for the patient's health that it outweighs the requirement of patient autonomy, to be able to choose what kind of information the patient wants to know.

The ACMG has drawn up a list of secondary findings that a laboratory should seek. The current list (SF v3.0) includes 73 genes, most of which are involved in serious hereditary cancer and cardiovascular syndromes that are (1) life threatening, (2) not readily diagnosable before the onset of symptoms, and (3) preventable or treatable. The secondary finding gene list is subject to ongoing refinement and will presumably grow over time. Furthermore, whether a given gene variant should always be a secondary finding that must be sought is also undergoing reevaluation. The current ACMG recommendation is that patients should be provided with appropriate counseling and then given the opportunity prior to testing to agree or to refuse to have such secondary findings looked for and reported. Other jurisdictions take a wide variety of approaches to the return of individual findings. The European Union's General Data Protection Regulation (GDPR), for example, maintains a right of access to genetic data that works to facilitate the return of individual results and secondary findings. In France, the *Code de la Santé Publique* requires subjects to consent that findings associated with severe genetic abnormalities be returned. German policy documents are somewhat more sweeping, requiring the return of any medically relevant findings. Other countries, Israel and Italy, for example, require that any returned information be accompanied by access to **genetic counseling**. In June 2021, the Global Alliance for Genomics and Health released an international policy document on the return of clinically actionable findings in genomics research. Among other things, the policy emphasizes the importance of adhering to clear research protocols, upfront resourcing of any commitments to return findings, and linking return to current clinical practices and standards of care.

Newborn Screening

Although newborn screening programs with implicit parental consent following notification (see Chapter 19) are one of the great triumphs of modern genetics in improving public health and considered to be in the best interests of the child, questions about newborn screening programs still arise in some countries. First, should parents be asked to provide active consent or can they simply be offered the opportunity to opt out of the program? Second, who has access to samples and data, and how can we make sure that samples are not used for purposes other than the screening tests for which they were collected and for which consent was given (or at least, not withheld)? In the United States, these questions came to a head in the area of newborn screening in the state of Texas in 2019 when a group of parents of children sued the state because blood spots obtained through an opt-out process for newborn screening had been diverted to the Department of Defense and private companies and used for purposes other than newborn screening, without parental consent. Texas agreed to destroy their collection of more than 5 million blood spots. In doing so, the state lost samples that could have been used for legitimate purposes, such as developing new newborn screening tests and for quality control of current testing efforts. Increasingly, distinctions are being made between the right of the at-risk, asymptomatic newborn to be found via screening, followed by testing and treatment and the need for parental permissions.

It should be noted that children have their own right to the "highest attainable standard of health" and their interests are "primary" according to the 1989 Convention on the Rights of the Child. Thus, many countries continue to notify parents about newborn screening but do not require an explicit, written consent. The same does not hold, however, as concerns further storage or use for research progress where parental permission is usually required.

Polygenic Risk Scores

PRSs provide individuals with a risk level for developing a range of disorders and diseases to which there is a genetic contribution. Through algorithms, PRSs give the **relative risk** level for a particular disease but are unable to assign an absolute lifetime risk measurement. PRS testing is capable of identifying risk scores for a wide range of conditions, from breast cancer to type 2 diabetes, schizophrenia to atrial fibrillation. Fundamentally, PRS testing depends on the comparison of individual genotyping results with **genome-wide association study** data. Insofar as many large-scale genomic research projects are not demographically representative of populations apart from those with European ancestry, it is likely that the risk categories are not generalizable and that benefits of PRS testing will not be equitably distributed. PRS also raises issues of communication and understanding of their meaning by health professionals and patients alike.

PRIVACY OF GENETIC INFORMATION

Legal protections for genetic information are not uniform across the globe or even within different jurisdictions in the same country. In the United States, the primary set of regulations governing the privacy of health information, including genetic information, is the Privacy Rule of the Health Insurance Portability and Accountability Act (HIPAA). The HIPAA rule sets criminal and civil penalties for disclosing such information without authorization to others, including other providers, except under a defined set of special circumstances.

When it was enacted in 2018, Europe's GDPR upended the privacy rules to which genetic information are subject, both within and outside of Europe. In particular, the GDPR created a context-specific and risk-based approach to data protection, permitting a limited degree of flexibility for the processing of personal data in the scientific research context. Different data processing standards apply in the GDPR depending on whether individual data are identifiable, pseudonymized (i.e., coded), or anonymized. Anonymized data are not considered to be personal data, since data of this kind cannot be directly associated with an identifiable person. The GDPR explicitly recognizes that genetic data fall within the special category of sensitive personal data, though it is unclear at present how genetic data might be distinguished within the text of the GDPR from the biologic materials from which it is obtained. There is additional disagreement about how sensitive genetic data can best be protected and yet still shared for research and care. It is not clear, for example, whether genetic data can be fully anonymized within the meaning of the GDPR. Neither are international transfers of such data clearly addressed or facilitated.

Privacy Issues for Family Members in a Family History

Patients are free to provide their physicians with a complete family medical history or communicate with their physicians about conditions that run in the family. Privacy legislation does not prevent individuals from gathering medical information about their family members or from deciding to share this information with their health care providers, but it is best to openly address this need for shared familial data with one's patient.

This information becomes part of the individual's medical record and is treated as "protected health information" about the individual but often is not protected health information for the family members included in the medical history. In other words, often only patients, and not their family members, may exercise their privacy rights to their own family history information in the same fashion as any other information in their personal medical records, including the ability to elect to control disclosure to others.

Duty to Warn and Permission to Warn Family Members

A patient's desire to have medical information kept confidential is one facet of the concept of patient autonomy, in which patients have the right to make their own decisions about how their individual medical information is used and communicated to others. Medical confidentiality is also an ethical and legal norm. Genetics, however, more than any other branch of medical practice, is concerned with both the patient and the family. A serious ethical and legal dilemma can arise in the practice of genetic medicine when patients' insistence that their medical information be kept strictly private restrains the geneticist from letting other family members know about their risk for a condition, even when such information could be beneficial to their own health and the health of their children (see Box 20.1). In this situation, is the genetics practitioner obligated to respect patient autonomy by keeping information confidential, or is the practitioner permitted or, more forcefully, does the practitioner have a duty to inform other family members and/or their providers? Is there a duty to warn? If so, is informing patients that they should share the information with relatives sufficient to discharge the practitioner's duty?

Judges have ruled in a number of court cases in the United States on whether or not a health care practitioner is permitted or is even required to override a patient's wishes for confidentiality. The precedent-setting case was not one involving genetics. In the 1976 State Supreme Court case in California, *Tarasoff v. the Regents of the University of California*, judges ruled that a psychiatrist who failed to warn law enforcement that his client had declared an intention to kill a young woman was liable in her death. The judges declared that this situation is no different from one in which physicians have a duty to protect the contacts of a patient with a contagious disease by warning them that the patient has the disease, even against the express wishes of the patient. In the realm of genetics, a duty to warn was mandated in a case in New Jersey, *Safer v. Estate of Pack* (1996), in which a panel of three judges concluded that a physician had a duty to warn the daughter of a man with familial adenomatous polyposis of her risk for colon cancer. The Court found that "there is no essential difference between the type of genetic threat at issue here and the menace of infection, contagion, or a threat of physical harm." They added that the duty to warn relatives is not automatically fulfilled by telling the patient that the disease is hereditary and that relatives need to be informed. Along similar lines, the 2001 *Molloy v. Meier* case in the Minnesota Supreme Court found that physicians may owe a duty to warn to third parties who are not patients of the physician, in particular to expecting mothers with respect to genetic risks to their future children. The *Molloy* case

---

BOX 20.1 CASE STUDIES DUTY TO WARN: PATIENT AUTONOMY AND PRIVACY VERSUS PREVENTING HARM TO FAMILY MEMBERS

A woman first presents with an autosomal dominant disorder at the age of 40 years, undergoes testing, and is found to carry a particular variant in a gene known to be causative of this disorder. She is planning to discuss the results with her teenage daughter but insists that her younger adult half-siblings (from her father's second marriage after her mother's and father's divorce) not be told that they might be at risk for this disorder and that testing is available. How does a practitioner reconcile the obligation to respect the patient's right to privacy with a desire not to cause her relatives harm by failing to inform them of their risk?

There are many questions to answer in determining whether "a serious threat to another person's health or safety" exists to justify unauthorized disclosure of risk to a relative.

Clinical Questions

- What is the **penetrance** of the disorder, and is it age dependent? How serious is the disorder? Can it be debilitating or life threatening? How variable is the **expressivity**? Are there interventions that can reduce the risk for disease or prevent it altogether? Is this a condition that will be identified by routine medical care, once it is symptomatic, in time for institution of preventive or therapeutic measures?
- The risk to half-siblings of the patient is either 50% or negligible, depending on which parent passed the variant allele to the patient. What does the family history reveal, if anything, about the parent in common between the patient and her half-siblings? Is the patient's mother still alive and available for testing?

Counseling Questions

- Was the patient informed at the time of testing that the results might have implications for other family members? Did she understand in advance that she might be asked to warn her relatives?
- What are the reasons for withholding the information? Are there unresolved issues, such as resentment, feelings of abandonment, or emotional estrangement, that are sources of psychological pain that could be addressed for her own benefit as well as to help the patient clarify her decision making?
- Are the other family members already aware of the possibility of this hereditary disease, and have they made an informed choice not to seek testing themselves? Would the practitioner's warning be seen as an unwarranted intrusion of psychologically damaging information, or would their risk come as a complete surprise?

Legal and Practical Questions

- Does the practitioner have the information and resources required to contact all the half-siblings without the cooperation of the patient?
- Could the practitioner have reached an understanding, or even a formal agreement, with the patient in advance of testing that she would help in informing her siblings? Would asking for such an agreement be seen as coercive and lead to the patient's depriving herself of the testing she needs for herself and her children?
- What constitutes adequate discharge of the practitioner's duty to warn? Is it sufficient to provide a form letter for the patient to show to relatives that discloses the absolute minimal amount of information needed to inform them of a potential risk?

bears a degree of resemblance to the *Watters v. White* case decided by the Quebec Court of Appeal in 2012. The central dispute in that case surrounded the failure of two physicians to provide a warning to relatives of their patients about the possibility their children would inherit a serious **genetic disorder**. After a decision at trial finding the physicians had not met their obligation to warn, the Court of Appeal overturned, finding, among other things, that the duty to warn operates only in the presence of a clear risk to third parties. Yet, in the genetics context, probabilistic risks are often not clear. In the United Kingdom, the 2020 *ABC v. St George's Healthcare NHS Trust* case addressed a similar set of facts. In that case, the UK High Court found that a claimant alleging breach of a duty to warn of genetic risk could recover against a health care provider if, on balance, the need to warn relatives of the risk of disease appears to outweigh the wishes of the affected individual. This decision suggests that health care providers might in some circumstances be obliged to warn relatives of risk of a serious genetic disorder even against a patient's wishes.

Several modern commenters diverge slightly from this perspective, arguing that while physicians may have an ethical duty to provide warnings to third parties, this ethical duty is usually most appropriately discharged by assisting and encouraging their patients to provide warnings to their family members.

ARTIFICIAL INTELLIGENCE AND INCREASED DIGITIZATION

Hardly any field is as affected by the increasingly significant influence of artificial intelligence (AI) and digitization as genomics. AI systems in genomics research, for example, are capable of sifting through massive volumes of data, assessing linkages, determining patterns, and making novel findings that promise to translate into treatments and prevention that improve human health. The digitization of health information makes it easier than ever to share health genomic data. Cloud computing, for example, provides a secure and efficient mechanism for making genomic data widely available for research, similarly working to accelerate discoveries in the field. Applications of AI and digitization in genomics are many. But the use of AI techniques and increased reliance on digitization also presents a range of challenges, notably that many of these technologies draw on datasets that may work to entrench biases that preexist in the health care system. AI systems that have been trained on data derived from personal health might be especially susceptible to this issue. It is well documented that care access and health outcomes are not equitably distributed across populations. To the extent that AI models learn to make important decisions on the basis of data drawn from contexts in which bias is preexisting, these systems may learn to replicate factors that caused unequal outcomes. AI and digitization also raise substantial concerns about data privacy. As both trends depend on the processing of data drawn from large collections, it may be that certain permutations might lead to the identification of individuals or to data breaches where appropriate safeguards are not maintained.

Guidelines from international health organizations, individual national health policy groups, and professional medical organizations are not unanimous on this issue, but some countries have legally mandated communication to at-risk family members. Furthermore, in the United States, the inconsistent case law from state courts must also be considered with respect to legislative and regulatory mandates.

Contrary to widespread belief in the United States, the HIPAA Privacy Rule permits a physician to disclose protected health information about a patient to another health care provider who is treating a family member of the physician's patient without the individual's authorization, unless the patient has explicitly chosen to impose additional restrictions on the use or disclosure of such protected health information. For example, an individual who has obtained a genetic test may request that the health care provider not disclose the test results. If the health care provider agrees to the restriction, HIPAA prevents disclosing such information without authorization to providers treating other family members who are seeking to identify their own genetic health risks. However, the health care provider should discuss such restrictions with the patient in advance of doing the test and is not obligated to agree to the requested restriction.

In France, Article 15 of a newly adopted statute on bioethics has express provisions on familial recontact, including that physicians must inform patients subject to genetic testing that there may be certain risks associated with failing to share genetic information with their relatives. Physicians prescribing tests for a serious genetic abnormality are obliged to enter an agreement with their patient for the possible communication of results identifying the tested abnormality. The tested patient is encouraged to contact potentially affected relatives for whom they are able to obtain contact information. Such communication may be delegated to the physician. Where a diagnosed individual refuses to communicate the diagnosis of a severe genetic abnormality, for which preventative measures are justified, the bioethics statute further requires that a physician communicate the diagnosis in question to the *Conseil national pour l'accès aux origines personnelles*. The *Conseil* then informs potentially affected relatives of the diagnosed person.

Although the genetics practitioner is most knowledgeable about the clinical aspects of the disease, the relevance of the family history, and the family risk assessment, the many legal and ethical controversies surrounding a possible duty to warn suggest that consultation with legal and bioethics experts is advisable should a conflict arise over the release of a patient's medical information.

USE OF GENETIC INFORMATION BY EMPLOYERS AND INSURERS

The fourth major ethical principle is justice—the requirement that everyone be able to benefit equally from progress in medical genetics. Justice is a major concern in the area of the use of genetic information in employment and health insurance. Whether healthy individuals could be denied employment or health insurance because they carry a genetic predisposition to disease was not a settled issue in the United States until passage of the landmark Genetic Information Nondiscrimination Act (GINA) of 2008. Under this act, private employers with 15 or more employees are prohibited from deliberately seeking or using genetic information, including family history, to make an employment decision because genetic information was not considered to be relevant to an individual's current ability to work. Similarly, GINA prohibits most group health insurers from denying insurance or adjusting group premiums based on the genetic information of members of the group.

Significantly, GINA does not apply to life, disability, and long-term care insurance. Insurers that sell such products insist that they must have access to all pertinent genetic information about individuals that they themselves have when making a decision to purchase one of these policies. Life insurance companies calculate their premiums on the basis of actuarial tables of age-specific survival averaged over the population; premiums will not cover losses if individuals with private knowledge that they are at higher risk for disease conceal this information and buy extra life or long-term disability insurance, a practice referred to as **adverse selection**. If adverse selection were widespread, the premiums for the entire population would have to increase so that in essence, the entire population would be subsidizing the increased coverage for a minority. Adverse selection is likely to be a real phenomenon in some circumstances; in one study of asymptomatic individuals tested for the *APOE* ε4 allele, those who chose to know that they tested positive were found to be nearly six times more likely to purchase extra long-term care insurance than those who did not choose to know their *APOE* **genotype**. Knowledge that one carried an *APOE* ε4 allele did not, however, affect life, health, or disability insurance purchases. There must be, however, a clear distinction between what are already phenotypic manifestations of a disease, such as hypertension, hypercholesterolemia, and diabetes mellitus, and what are predisposing alleles, such as *BRCA1* mutations (see Chapter 16) and *APOE* ε4 alleles (see Chapters 9 and 13), that may never result in overt disease in the individual who carries such an allele.

At present, there is little evidence that life insurance companies have actually engaged in discriminatory underwriting practices on the basis of genetic testing. Nevertheless, the fear of such discrimination, and the negative impact that discrimination would have on people obtaining clinical testing for their own health benefit as well as on their willingness to participate in genetic research, has led to proposals to ban the use of genetic information in life insurance. In the United Kingdom, for example, life insurance companies have voluntarily agreed to an extended moratorium on the use of genetic information in most life underwriting, except when large policies are involved, or, in the specific case of Huntington disease, for which disclosure of a positive test result by the patient is required.

Countries outside of the United States take a variety of statutory approaches on discrimination as concerns life and disability insurance. In 2017, Canada, a country with universal health care, adopted the Genetic Non-Discrimination Act. The Act prohibits employers and insurance providers from requiring genetic testing. Insurers in particular are prohibited from requiring the provision of genetic test results as a provision of coverage. Certain jurisdictions, including France, adopt a broad-based human rights approach to prohibiting genetic discrimination. Others have adopted moratoria in certain applications of genetic testing in an effort to curb potential discrimination. The United Kingdom and Australia have taken this approach. Still other jurisdictions, such as Japan, rely on existing legal frameworks to prevent genetic discrimination. Importantly, countries with national health care systems may not face substantial problems with genetic discrimination in health insurance though it may affect life and disability insurance as well as employment, hence attracting regulation. For most countries, there is widespread agreement that genetic discrimination should not be permitted in insurance and employment.

EUGENIC AND DYSGENIC EFFECTS OF MEDICAL GENETICS

The Issue of Eugenics

The term **eugenics**, introduced by Darwin's cousin Francis Galton in 1883, refers to the improvement of a population by selection of only its "best" specimens for breeding. Plant and animal breeders have followed this practice since ancient times. In the late 19th century, Galton and others began to promote the idea of using selective breeding to improve the human species, thereby initiating the eugenics movement, which was widely advocated for the next half-century. The ideal qualities that the eugenics movement sought to promote through the encouragement of certain kinds of human breeding were more often than not defined by social, ethnic, and economic prejudices and fed by antiimmigrant and racist sentiments in society. What we now would consider a lack of education was described then as familial "feeble-mindedness"; what we now would call rural poverty was considered by eugenicists to be hereditary "shiftlessness." The scientific difficulties in determining whether traits or characteristics are heritable and to what extent heredity contributes to a trait were badly overestimated because most human traits, even those with some genetic component, are complex in their inheritance pattern and are influenced strongly by environmental factors. Thus, by the middle of the last century, many scientists began to appreciate the theoretical and ethical difficulties associated with eugenics programs.

Eugenics is commonly thought to have been largely discredited when it was resurrected and used in Nazi Germany as a justification for mass murder. However, it should be pointed out that in North America and Europe, involuntary sterilization of institutionalized individuals deemed to be mentally incompetent or disabled was carried out under laws passed in the early part of the 20th century in support of eugenics and was continued for many years after the Nazi regime was destroyed.

Genetic Counseling and Eugenics

Genetic counseling, with the aim of helping patients and their families manage the pain and suffering caused by genetic disease, should not be confounded with the eugenic goal of reducing the incidence of genetic disease or the frequency of alleles considered deleterious in the population. Helping patients and families come to free and informed decisions, particularly concerning reproduction, without coercion, forms the basis for the concept of nondirective counseling (see Chapter 17). Nondirectiveness asserts that individual autonomy is paramount and must not to be subordinated to reducing the burden of genetic disease on society or to a theoretical goal of "improving the **gene pool**." Some, however, have argued that true nondirective counseling is a myth, often acclaimed but not easy to accomplish because of the personal attitudes and values the counselor brings to the counseling session. Moreover, patients often explicitly request more directed guidance.

Nonetheless, despite the difficulties in attaining the ideal of nondirective counseling, the ethical principles of respect for autonomy, beneficence, nonmaleficence, and justice remain at the heart of all genetic counseling practice, particularly in the realm of individual reproductive decision making.

The Issue of Dysgenics

The opposite of eugenics is dysgenics, a deterioration in the health and well-being of a population by practices that allow the accumulation of deleterious alleles. In this regard, the long-term impact of activities in medical genetics that can affect gene frequencies and the incidence of genetic disease may be difficult to predict.

In the case of some single-gene defects, medical treatment can have a dysgenic effect by reducing selection against a particular genotype, thereby allowing the frequency of harmful genes and consequently of disease to increase. The effect of relaxed selection is likely to be more striking for autosomal dominant and X-linked disorders than for autosomal **recessive** disorders, in which the majority of variant alleles is found in silent heterozygous carriers.

For example, if successful treatment of Duchenne muscular dystrophy were to be achieved, the incidence of the disease would rise sharply because the *DMD* genes of the affected males would then be transmitted to all their daughters. The effect of this transmission would be to greatly increase the frequency of carriers in the population. In contrast, if all persons affected with cystic fibrosis could survive and reproduce at a normal rate, the incidence of the disease would rise from 1 in 2000 to only ~1 in 1550 over 200 years. Common genetic disorders with **complex inheritance**, discussed in Chapter 9, could theoretically also become more common if selection were removed, although it is likely that as with autosomal recessive diseases, most of the many susceptibility alleles are distributed among unaffected individuals. Consequently, reproduction by affected persons would have little effect on susceptibility allele frequencies.

As prenatal diagnosis (see Chapter 18) becomes widespread, increasing numbers of pregnancies in which the fetus has inherited a genetic defect may be terminated. The effect on the overall incidence of disease is quite variable. In a disorder such as Huntington disease, prenatal diagnosis and pregnancy termination would have a large effect on the incidence of the responsible gene. For most other severe X-linked or autosomal dominant disorders, some reduction might occur, but the disease will continue to recur owing to new mutations. In the case of autosomal recessive conditions, the effect on the frequency of the mutant allele, and consequently of the disease, of aborting all affected pregnancies would be small because most of these alleles are carried silently by heterozygotes.

One theoretical concern is the extent to which pregnancy termination for genetic reasons is followed by reproductive compensation—that is, by the birth of additional, unaffected children, many of whom are carriers of the deleterious gene. Some families with X-linked disorders have chosen to terminate pregnancies in which the fetus was male, but of course daughters in such families, although unaffected, may be carriers. Thus reproductive compensation has the potential long-term consequence of increasing the frequency of the genetic disorder that led to the loss of an affected child.

GENETICS AND GENOMICS IN MEDICINE

The 20th century will be remembered as the era that began with the rediscovery of Mendel's laws of inheritance and their application to human biology and medicine, continued with the discovery of the role of DNA in heredity, and culminated in the completion of the **Human Genome Project**. At the beginning of the 21st century, the human species has, for the first time:
- An increasingly complete representative sequence of its own DNA
- A comprehensive, albeit likely incomplete, inventory of its genes
- A vigorous ongoing effort to identify and characterize variants in DNA sequence and copy number

- A rapidly expanding knowledge base that includes diverse populations and in which various diseases and disease predispositions will be attributable to such variation
- Powerful new sequencing technologies that allow sequencing of an exome or genome at a tiny fraction of the cost of the first human genome sequence

With such knowledge comes powerful capabilities as well as great responsibilities. Ultimately, genetics and genomics in medicine is not about knowledge for its own sake, but for the sake of sustaining wellness, improving health, relieving suffering, and enhancing human dignity. The challenge confronting us all, both future health professionals and members of society at large, is to make sure that the advances in human genetics and genomics knowledge and technology are used responsibly, fairly, and humanely.

ACKNOWLEDGMENTS

The authors (Bartha Maria Knoppers and Ma'n H. Zawati) would like to acknowledge the contributions of the original authors of this chapter. They would also like to acknowledge the assistance of Michael Lang and Minh Thu Nguyen, both Academic Associates at the Centre of Genomics and Policy in McGill University's Faculty of Medicine and Health Sciences. Ma'n H. Zawati acknowledges the generous support of the Fonds de recherche du Québec-Santé Junior 1 Research Scholar program.

GENERAL REFERENCES

Beauchamp TL, Childress JF: *Principles of biomedical ethics*, ed 5, New York, 2001, Oxford University Press.

Gostin LO, Wiley LF: *Public health law and ethics*, ed 3, Oakland, 2018, University of California Press.

Kevles D: *In the name of eugenics: genetics and the uses of human heredity*, Cambridge, 1995, Harvard University Press.

Milunsky A, Milunsky JM, editors: *Genetic disorders and the fetus— Diagnosis, prevention, and treatment* ed 8, Oxford, 2021, Wiley Blackwell.

REFERENCES FOR SPECIFIC TOPICS

American Academy of Pediatrics: Policy statement: ethical and policy issues in genetic testing and screening of children, *Pediatrics* 131:620–622, 2013.

Biesecker LG: Incidental variants are critical for genomics, *Am J Hum Genet* 92:648–651, 2013.

Borry P: Genetic testing in asymptomatic minors, *Eur J Hum Gen* 17:711–719, 2009.

Canadian Pediatric Society: Guidelines for genetic testing of healthy children, *Paediatr Child Health* 8(1):42–45, 2003.

Elger B, Michaud K, Mangin P: When information can save lives: the duty to warn relatives about sudden cardiac death and environmental risks, *Hastings Center Report* 40:39–45, 2010.

Global Alliance for Genomics and Health: 2021 policy on clinically actionable genomic research results POL 007, v1.0, 2021.

HIPAA regulations on family history. http://www.hhs.gov/ocr/privacy/hipaa/faq/family_medical_history_information/index.html.

Human Cell Atlas: Ethics Toolkit, Pediatric Template Consent Form, v. 1.0 (2022). https://docs.google.com/document/d/11-B68-wO5rlOuzOKxA9vMaD7Tonhb7W8/edit.

Joly Y: Looking beyond GINA: policy approaches to address genetic discrimination, *Ann Rev Genomics Hum Genet* 21:491–507, 2020.

Kleiderman E, Ravitsky V, Knoppers BM: The 'serious' factor in germline modification. *J Med Ethics* 45:508–513, 2019.

Knoppers BM, Doerr M, Wallace S, et al: Pediatric Consent to Genetic Research: Clauses, Global Alliance for Genomics and Health, 2021. <https://www.ga4gh.org/wp-content/uploads/Pediatric-Consent-to-Genetic-Research_-Clauses-1.pdf>.

Knoppers BM, Isasi R, Caulfield T, et al: Human gene editing: revisiting Canadian policy, *NPJ Regen Med* 2:3, 2017.

Knoppers BM, Kekesi-Lafrance K: The genetic family as patient? *Am J Bioethics* 20(6):77–80, 2020.

Knoppers BM, Thorogood A, Zawati MH: Letter: relearning the 3 R's? Reinterpretation, recontact, and return of genetic variants, *Genet Med*, 2019.

MacEwen JE, Boyer JT, Sun KY: Evolving approaches to the ethical management of genomic data, *Trends Genet* 29:375–382, 2013.

Martin AR: Clinical use of current polygenic risk scores may exacerbate health disparities, *Nat Genet* 51:584–591, 2019.

McGuire AL, Joffe S, Koenig BA, et al: Point-counterpoint, *Ethics and genomic incidental findings*, *Science* 340:1047–1048, 2013.

Middleton A: Professional duties are now considered legal duties of care within genomic medicine, *Eur J Human Genet* 28:1301–1304, 2020.

Offit K, Thom P: Ethicolegal aspects of cancer genetics, *Cancer Treat Res* 155:1–14, 2010.

Rothstein M: Reconsidering the duty to warn genetically at-risk relatives, *Genet in Med* 20:285–290, 2018.

Shabani M, Borry P: Rules for processing genetic data for research purposes in view of the new EU General Data Protection Regulation, *Eur J Hum Gen* 26(2):149–156, 2018.

Thorogood A, Zawati MH, Knoppers BM: Oversight, governance, and policy for making decisions about return of individual genomic findings, *Sec Find Genom Res Trans Appl Genomics* 29–41, 2020.

Visscher PM, Gibson G: What if we had whole-genome sequence data for millions of individuals? *Genome Med* 5:80, 2013.

Yurkiewicz IR, Korf BR, Lehmann LS: Prenatal whole-genome sequencing—Is the quest to know a fetus's future ethical? *N Engl J Med* 370:195–197, 2014.

Zawati MH, Thorogood A: The physician who knew too much: a comment on Watters v White, *Health L J* 21:1–27, 2014.

PROBLEMS

1. A couple with two children is referred for genetic counseling because their younger son, age 12 years, has a movement disorder for which testing for juvenile Huntington disease (**Case 24**) is being considered. What are the ethical considerations for the family in testing?

2. A research project screened more than 40,000 consecutive, unselected births for the number of X chromosomes and the presence of a Y chromosome and correlated the sex chromosome karyotype with the sex assigned by visual inspection in the newborn nursery. The purpose of the project was to observe infants with sex chromosome abnormalities (see Chapter 6) prospectively for developmental difficulties. What are the ethical considerations in carrying out this project?

3. In the case described in the Box in the section on duty to warn, consider what might be your course of action if you were the genetic counselor and the disease in question were the following: hereditary breast and ovarian cancer due to *BRCA1* mutations (see Chapter 16) (**Case 7**); malignant hyperthermia due to *RYR1* (ryanodine receptor) variants (see Chapter 19); early-onset, familial Alzheimer disease due to a *PSEN1* (presenilin 1) variant (see Chapter 13) (**Case 4**); neurofibromatosis due to *NF1* variants (see Chapter 7) (**Case 34**); or type II diabetes mellitus.

4. Draw up a list of a dozen genes and disorders that you believe should be analyzed and reported if they emerge as secondary findings during ES/WGS for undiagnosed diseases. Explain how and why you chose each of these dozen genes and conditions.

Clinical Case Studies Illustrating Genetic Principles

These 49 clinical vignettes illustrate genetic and genomic principles in the practice of medicine. Each vignette is followed by a brief explanation or description of the disease and its etiology, pathophysiology, phenotype, management, and inheritance. These explanations and descriptions are based on current knowledge and understanding; therefore, like most things in medicine and science, they are subject to refinement and change as our knowledge and understanding evolve. The description of each case uses standard medical terminology; student readers therefore may need to consult a medical dictionary for explanations. Each vignette is also followed by a few questions that are intended to initiate discussion of some basic genetic or clinical principles illustrated by the case.

The cases are not intended to be definitive or comprehensive or to set a standard of care; rather, they are simply illustrations of the application of genetic and genomic principles to the practice of medicine. Although the cases are loosely based on clinical experience, all individuals and medical details presented are fictitious.

Ronald Cohn, Stephen Scherer, Ada Hamosh

CASE PRESENTATIONS

Acknowledgement: We thank Stacy Hewson and Students in the MSc Genetic Counselling Program, University of Toronto (Class of 2023) for assistance with creating some of the pedigree drawings for these reports.

1 ABACAVIR-INDUCED STEVENS-JOHNSON SYNDROME/ TOXIC EPIDERMAL NECROLYSIS (MIM 608579) (Genetically Determined Immunological Adverse Drug Reaction)

Autosomal Dominant

Iris Cohn

PRINCIPLES

- Pharmacogenetic test that has been widely adopted as standard of care
- Significant positive and negative predictive values
- Population differences in the frequency of the predisposing allele

MAJOR PHENOTYPIC FEATURES

- Widespread red/purple patches on the skin and mucosal membranes (eye, mouth, genitalia) 10 to 14 days after beginning antiretroviral treatment with abacavir.
- Skin sloughing of greater than 30% of body surface area is referred to as toxic epidermal necrolysis; a similar rash but with sloughing of less than 10% of body surface area is referred to as Stevens-Johnson syndrome.

HISTORY AND PHYSICAL FINDINGS

P.R., a 37-year-old German man, was admitted to the hospital with shortness of breath and confusion and found to have both *Pneumocystis carinii* pneumonia and *Toxoplasma gondii* encephalitis. These opportunistic infections occur commonly in the setting of newly diagnosed human immunodeficiency virus (HIV)-1 acquired immunodeficiency syndrome (AIDS). His CD4 cell count was 2/mm³ and HIV-1 viral load was 120,000 copies/mL. Treatment with trimethoprim-sulfamethoxazole was started, and he was started on antiretroviral therapy (ART) that included the nucleoside analogue reverse transcriptase inhibitor, abacavir. His encephalitis and pneumonia cleared, and he was discharged from the hospital on oral antiparasitic treatment.

Two weeks after beginning ART, P.R. presented with a nonfebrile, generalized macular rash involving his palms and mouth. His blood pressure was 130/60 mm Hg, temperature was 37.1°C, pulse was 88 beats/min, he was breathing 15 breaths/min, and oxygen saturation was 96% on room air. He had a disseminated cutaneous eruption of discrete dark red macules on 90% of the body surface area, a detachment of 5% of the epidermis, genital ulcerations, erosive stomatitis, and conjunctival lesions with hyperemia but without keratitis or corneal erosions. The application of minor pressure to the skin resulted in sloughing of the skin (Nikolsky sign).

Skin biopsy was compatible with Stevens-Johnson syndrome (SJS). Because of previous reports of cutaneous hypersensitivity reactions with abacavir treatment, the drug was stopped, and he was transferred to a burn unit, monitored for further skin sloughing, and treated with supportive care. The epidermis began to heal over the next week, and the skin lesions resolved completely within 3 weeks. His ART was changed to a combination of protease inhibitors and different nucleoside analogue reverse transcriptase inhibitors without recurrence of the skin reaction. His viral load decreased to undetectable, and the CD4 count returned to normal.

One year later, when the increased susceptibility to SJS with abacavir therapy was shown to depend on human leukocyte antigen (HLA) genotype, he had HLA typing and was found to carry the SJS-abacavir susceptibility allele HLA-B*5701.

BACKGROUND

Adverse drug reactions are defined as harmful reactions caused by normal use of a drug at correct doses. The majority (75–80%) of all adverse drug reactions are caused by predictable, nonimmunological effects, some of which are due to genetically determined pharmacokinetic or pharmacodynamic differences between individuals. The remaining 20 to 25% of adverse drug events are caused by largely unpredictable effects that may or may not be immune mediated. Immune-mediated reactions account for 5 to 10% of all drug reactions and represent true drug hypersensitivity, with immunoglobulin E–mediated drug allergies with hives or laryngeal swelling, falling into this category. A different kind of skin reaction – a generalized maculopapular rash – is also common in response to certain medications, including sulfa drug antibiotics.

One particularly dangerous drug-induced hypersensitivity reaction is T-cell mediated damage to skin and mucous membranes, referred to as Stevens-Johnson syndrome (SJS), and its more serious extreme manifestation, toxic epidermal necrolysis (TEN) (Fig. C.1.1). Both SJS and TEN are characterized by malaise and fever, followed by rapid appearance of red/purple patches on the skin, which progress to sloughing of the skin, similar to what is seen with a thermal burn. Mucosal membranes (eye, mouth, genitalia) are frequently affected. In SJS, skin sloughing involves less than 10% of body surface area, whereas TEN involves sloughing of greater than 30% of the body surface area.

Histological features in the skin in drug-induced SJS/TEN patients include epidermal necrosis, in some cases extending through the full thickness of the epidermis as seen with thermal burn, individual keratinocyte apoptosis, subepidermal bullae, and dense dermal infiltrates with lymphocytes, as well as a substantial number of eosinophils or neutrophils.

The mortality rate in SJS/TEN ranges from 10 to 30%. Although SJS and TEN represent only a small fraction of all immune-mediated drug reactions, they are particularly severe and can be life threatening.

Pathogenesis

SJS/TEN is mediated by cytotoxic T cells. Drugs or their reactive metabolites, which are considered foreign antigens, bind to T cell receptors and further activate immune response. Molecular immunological studies have elucidated

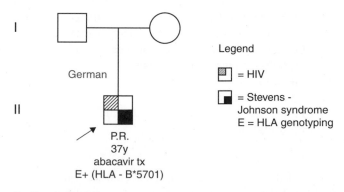

Pedigree Case 1

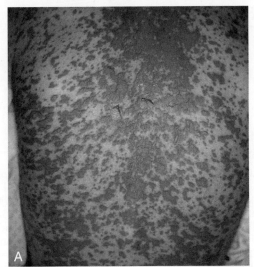

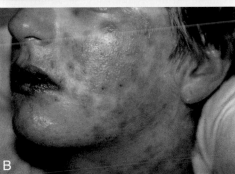

Figure C.1.1 (A) Numerous coalescing dusky lesions with flaccid bullae and multiple sites of epidermal detachment involving 10 to 30% of skin surface. This extent of epidermal detachment is in the "zone of overlap" between Stevens-Johnson syndrome and toxic epidermal necrolysis. (B) Stevens-Johnson syndrome, showing involvement of lips and mucous membranes of the mouth. ((A) from French LE, Prins C: Erythema multiforme, Stevens-Johnson syndrome and toxic epidermal necrolysis. In Bolognia JL, Jorizzo JL, Schaffer JV, editors: *Dermatology*, ed 3, Philadelphia, 2012, Elsevier, pp 319–333. © 2012, Elsevier Limited. All rights reserved. (B) from Armstrong AW: Erythema multiforme, Stevens-Johnson syndrome, and toxic epidermal necrolysis. In Schwarzenberger K, Werchniak AE, Ko CJ, editors: *General dermatology*, Philadelphia, 2009, Elsevier, pp 23–28. © 2009, Elsevier Limited. All rights reserved.)

why T-cell–mediated hypersensitivity occurs in individuals with the HLA-B*5701 allele treated with abacavir. In HLA-B*5701–expressing cells cultured in the presence of abacavir, up to 25% of the peptides present in the antigen-presenting groove of their class I cell-surface antigen-presenting molecules are novel self-peptides that are not seen in the absence of abacavir. Abacavir appears to interact specifically with segments of the HLA-B*5701 peptide-binding groove, altering its binding properties. This alteration allows HLA-B*5701 to present novel peptides that happen to have a much higher cross-reactivity to self, including skin antigens. Drugs precipitate over 50% of SJS cases and up to 95% of TEN cases.

Management

Discontinuation of the offending drug and transfer to a burn unit for supportive care are the mainstays of treatment. Other therapies such as systemic corticosteroids and intravenous immunoglobulin have been suggested but have not to date been proven to be either beneficial or harmful.

TABLE C.1.1

Population	Frequency of the HLA-B*5701 Allele (%)
European	5–8
African American	2.5
Chinese	0–2
South Indian	5–20
Thai	4–10

Prevention

The specificity of the HLA-B*5701 test is high. Studies of large cohorts of individuals treated with abacavir have demonstrated that approximately 50% of those carrying an HLA-B*5701 allele will develop drug-induced hypersensitivity reactions such as SJS or TEN, whereas none of those without this antigen will develop these conditions. In immunologically confirmed subjects with abacavir-induced hypersensitivity reactions, the prevalence of the HLA-B*5701 allele is nearly 100%. This data led some health care authorities such as the U.S. Food and Drug Administration, Health Canada, and European Medicines Agency to require screening for carriage of the HLA-B*5701 allele prior to initiating abacavir treatment independent of ancestry with the guidance that abacavir should not be used in patients known to carry the HLA-B*5701 allele. Other countries such as Japan recommend but do not mandate HLA-B*5701 testing for their population.

The number of new abacavir users needed to genotype to prevent one case of abacavir-induced hypersensitivity reactions is 14 to 90 in people of European ancestry, but the same is around 10 times higher in African Americans.

INHERITANCE

As with all HLA alleles (see Chapter 9), inheritance is autosomal codominant.

The frequency of the HLA-B*5701 allele (and therefore the risk for abacavir-induced SJS and TEN) differs greatly among various populations (see Table C.1.1).

Similar associations between SJS or TEN and other HLA alleles have been seen with the antiepileptic drug carbamazepine (HLA-B*1502), the uric acid–lowering drug allopurinol (HLA-B*5801) used for gout, and other commonly used medications.

QUESTIONS FOR SMALL GROUP DISCUSSION

1. Suggest a mechanism by which SJS/TEN might arise in individuals with different HLA-B alleles when exposed to different drugs.
2. Why might there be different frequencies of various HLA-B alleles in different ancestral groups?

REFERENCES

Downey A, Jackson C, Harun N, et al: Toxic epidermal necrolysis: Review of pathogenesis and management, *J Am Acad Dermatol* 66:995–1003, 2012.

Mallal S, Phillips E, Carosi G, et al: HLA-B*5701 screening for hypersensitivity to abacavir, *N Engl J Med* 358:568–579, 2008.

Manson LE, Swen JJ, Guchelaar HJ. Diagnostic test criteria for HLA genotyping to prevent drug hypersensitivity reactions: a systematic review of actionable HLA recommendations in CPIC and DPWG guidelines, *Frontiers in pharmacology*, 2020 Sep 23;11:567048.

Martin MA, Kroetz DL: Abacavir pharmacogenetics—from initial reports to standard of care, *Pharmacotherapy* 33:765–775, 2013.

Mockenhaupt M, Viboud C, Dunant A, et al: Stevens-Johnson syndrome and toxic epidermal necrolysis: Assessment of medication risks with emphasis on recently marketed drugs: The EuroSCAR-study, *J Invest Dermatol* 128(1):35–44, 2008.

ACHONDROPLASIA (MIM 100800) (*FGFR3* Pathogenic Variant)
Autosomal Dominant

Julie Hoover-Fong

PRINCIPLES

- Gain-of-function variants
- Advanced paternal age
- De novo mutation

MAJOR PHENOTYPIC FEATURES

- Age at onset: Prenatal
- Rhizomelic short stature
- Macrocephaly
- Spinal cord compression

HISTORY AND PHYSICAL FINDINGS

P.S., a 30-year-old healthy woman, was 27 weeks pregnant with her first child. A fetal ultrasound examination at 26 weeks gestation identified a female fetus with macrocephaly (>97.5%ile for gestation) and rhizomelia (shortening of proximal segments of extremities; <2.5 %ile for gestation). P.S.'s spouse was 45 years of age and healthy; he had three healthy children from a previous relationship. Neither parent had a family history of skeletal dysplasia, birth defects, or genetic disorders. The obstetrician explained to the parents that their fetus had features of achondroplasia. The infant girl was delivered at 38 weeks gestation by cesarean section due to cephalopelvic disproportion. She had the physical features of achondroplasia including frontal bossing, macrocephaly, midface hypoplasia, lumbar kyphosis, limited elbow extension, rhizomelia, trident hands, brachydactyly, and axial and appendicular hypotonia. Radiographs showed characteristic features of achondroplasia, including shortened long bones of the upper and lower extremities, generalized metaphyseal flaring, square iliac bones, lucency of the proximal femora, and interpedicular narrowing of the lumbar vertebrae. Based on these features, sequencing was undertaken of the fibroblast growth factor receptor 3 gene (*FGFR3*). This identified the common c.1138 G>A variant found in achondroplasia, which leads to a glycine to arginine substitution at codon 380 (p.Gly380Arg).

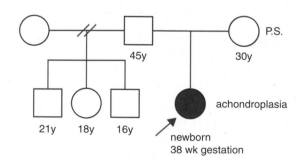

Pedigree Case 2

BACKGROUND
Disease Etiology and Incidence

Achondroplasia (MIM 100800), the most common type of short stature skeletal dysplasia or dwarfism, is an autosomal dominant disorder caused by specific pathogenic variants in *FGFR3*. Two pathogenic variants, c.1138 G>A (≈98%) and c.1138 G>C (1–2%), account for more than 99% of cases of achondroplasia, and both result in the p.Gly380Arg substitution. Guanine at position c.1138 in the *FGFR3* gene is one of the most mutable nucleotides identified in *any* human gene. Approximately 20% of all people with achondroplasia inherited the condition from an affected parent. The remaining 80% have a *de novo* pathogenic variant that occurs exclusively in the father's germline, increasing in frequency with advanced paternal age (>35 years) (see Chapters 4 and 10). Achondroplasia has an incidence of 1 in 15,000 to 1 in 40,000 live births and affects those of all ancestries.

Pathogenesis

FGFR3 is a transmembrane tyrosine kinase receptor that binds fibroblast growth factors. Binding of fibroblast growth factors to the extracellular domain of FGFR3 activates the intracellular tyrosine kinase domain of the receptor and initiates a signaling cascade. In endochondral bone, FGFR3 activation inhibits proliferation of chondrocytes within the growth plate and thus helps coordinate the growth and differentiation of chondrocytes with the growth and differentiation of bone progenitor cells.

The *FGFR3* pathogenic variants associated with achondroplasia are gain-of-function changes that cause ligand-independent activation of FGFR3. Such constitutive activation of FGFR3 inappropriately inhibits chondrocyte proliferation within the growth plate and consequently leads to shortening of the long bones as well as to abnormal differentiation of other bones.

Phenotype and Natural History

Patients with achondroplasia present at birth with rhizomelic shortening of the arms and legs, relatively long trunk as compared to the limbs, trident configuration of the hands, and macrocephaly with midface hypoplasia and prominent forehead (Fig. C.2.1). Birth growth parameters (i.e., length, weight, head circumference) typically overlap those of average stature infants. However, in the first few months of life, length rapidly falls below the average stature curve while head circumference accelerates to the 95%ile and above.

In general, individuals with achondroplasia have normal intelligence, although most have delayed motor development, which arises from a combination of hypotonia, hyperextensible joints (although the elbows have limited extension and rotation), and mechanical difficulty balancing their large heads. Motor delays that exceed expected achondroplasia-specific milestones may be related to foramen magnum stenosis and brainstem compression.

Abnormal growth of the skull and facial bones results in midface hypoplasia, a small cranial base, and small cranial foramina. The midface hypoplasia causes dental crowding, obstructive apnea, and otitis media. Narrowing of the foramen magnum causes compression of the brainstem at the

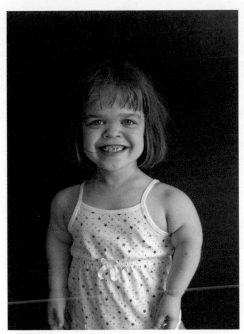

Figure C.2.1 Irina, who has achondroplasia, representing Little People of America (www.lpaonline.org). Beyond the grin, note her short arms with rhizomelia – meaning specific shortening of the upper portion of the extremities – as well as her macrocephaly. Photograph by Rick Guidotti, Positive Exposure (www.positiveexposure.org).

craniocervical junction in approximately 10 to 20% of individuals. If unrecognized and untreated, critical craniocervical compression may cause central apnea, weakness, hypotonia, quadriparesis, failure to thrive, and even sudden death in up to 5% in the first year of life. Other medical complications include obesity, hypertension, lumbar spinal stenosis that worsens with age, and genu varum.

Management

Suspected on the basis of clinical features, the diagnosis of achondroplasia is usually confirmed by clinical and radiographic findings. DNA testing for *FGFR3* pathogenic variants can be helpful in ambiguous cases but is usually not necessary for the diagnosis to be made.

Throughout life, management should focus on the anticipation and treatment of the complications of achondroplasia. During infancy, early assessment for central and obstructive sleep apnea with polysomnography and critical cervicomedullary compression by MRI in conjunction with careful, serial neurologic examinations and developmental assessments are essential. Treatment of patients with brainstem compression by decompression of the craniocervical junction usually results in marked improvement of neurological function. In early childhood, patients also must be monitored for chronic otitis media, hearing deficits, obstructive apnea, and thoracolumbar kyphosis. During later childhood and through early adulthood, patients must be monitored for symptomatic spinal stenosis, symptomatic genu varum, obesity, hypertension, dental crowding, and chronic otitis media and treated as necessary. Treatment of the spinal stenosis usually requires surgical decompression and sometimes stabilization of the spine. Obesity is difficult to prevent and control and often complicates the management of obstructive apnea and joint and spine problems.

It is essential to be physically active and exercise dietary discretion to avoid obesity. These individuals should avoid activities in which there is risk for injury to the craniocervical junction, such as collision sports, use of a trampoline, diving from diving boards, and vaulting in gymnastics.

Both growth hormone therapy and surgical lengthening of the legs and arms have been promoted for treatment of short stature in patients with achondroplasia. Both therapies remain controversial. Recently, there have been clinical trials of injectable and oral medications to increase growth in individuals with achondroplasia. ClinicalTrials.gov is a publicly available database that outlines such clinical trials and provides relevant links to those medications that are kj approved by the U.S. Food and Drug Administration.

In addition to the management of their medical issues, people with achondroplasia may need help with social adjustment because of the psychological impact of their appearance and physical differences. It is also important to share information about adaptive equipment (i.e., to drive, toilet independently) and how to advocate in school and work settings to make their environment accessible. Support groups often assist by providing interaction with similarly affected peers and social awareness programs.

Inheritance

For average stature parents with a child with achondroplasia, the risk for recurrence is low but probably higher than that for the general population because of possible germline mosaicism. Gonadal mosaicism for achondroplasia has been documented, but rarely. For relationships in which one partner has achondroplasia and the other is of average stature, each pregnancy has a 50% chance of inheriting achondroplasia because it is an autosomal dominant disorder with full penetrance. For relationships in which both partners have achondroplasia, each pregnancy has a 50% chance of inheriting achondroplasia, a 25% chance of inheriting achondroplasia from both parents (i.e., double dominant or homozygous achondroplasia, which is lethal), and a 25% chance of being of average stature. Cesarean section is required for all pregnant individuals with achondroplasia, regardless of the stature of the fetus.

Prenatal testing for achondroplasia is possible through testing of fetal DNA obtained via chorionic villus sampling or amniocentesis or by cell-free DNA in maternal blood. Preimplantation testing may be carried out after in vitro fertilization if both partners have achondroplasia and are seeking to implant an embryo without both parental *FGFR3* variants (see Chapter 18). Recognition of achondroplasia by ultrasound is unlikely at the time of the usual anatomy scan (i.e., around 18–20 weeks gestation) but features may be detectable in a third trimester ultrasound. Conversely, if long bone shortening or other skeletal anomalies are apparent by the time of the anatomy scan, the fetus likely has a more severe and potentially lethal skeletal dysplasia, such as thanatophoric dysplasia.

QUESTIONS FOR SMALL GROUP DISCUSSION

1. Name other disorders that increase in frequency with increasing paternal age. What types of variants are associated with these disorders?
2. Discuss possible reasons that the *FGFR3* mutations c.1138 G>A and c.1138 G>C occur exclusively during spermatogenesis.
3. Marfan syndrome, Huntington disease, and achondroplasia arise as a result of dominant gain-of-function variants. Compare and contrast the pathological mechanisms of these gain-of-function variants.
4. In addition to achondroplasia, gain-of-function variants in *FGFR3* are associated with hypochondroplasia and thanatophoric dysplasia. Explain how the phenotypic severity of these three disorders correlates with the level of constitutive FGFR3 tyrosine kinase activity.

REFERENCES

Hoover-Fong JE, Alade AY, Hashmi SS, Hecht JT, Legare JM, Little ME, Liu C, McGready J, Modaff P, Pauli RM, Rodriguez-Buritica DF, Schulze KJ, Serna ME, Smid CJ, Bober MB: Achondroplasia Natural History Study (CLARITY): A multicenter retrospective cohort study of achondroplasia in the United States, *Genet Med* 23(8):1498–1505, 2021. https://doi.org/10.1038/s41436-021-01165-2. Epub 2021 May 18. PMID: 34006999; PMCID: PMC8354851. ***This article provides an overview of the natural history of a US cohort of 1374 patients with achondroplasia.***

Hoover-Fong J, Scott CI, Jones MC: Committee on Genetics: Health supervision for people with achondroplasia, *Pediatrics* 145(6):e20201010, 2020. https://doi.org/10.1542/peds.2020-1010. PMID: 32457214. ***This article includes age-specific anticipatory guidance for patients with achondroplasia, growth charts and other resources.***

Pauli RM: Achondroplasia: A comprehensive clinical review, *Orphanet J Rare Dis* 14(1):1, 2019. https://doi.org/10.1186/s13023-018-0972-6. PMID: 30606190; PMCID: PMC6318916. ***This article includes Dr. Ireland's developmental chart for achondroplasia, growth charts and other resources.***

AGE-RELATED MACULAR DEGENERATION (MIM 603075)
(Complement Factor H Variants)

Mandeep Singh • Christopher B. Toomey

PRINCIPLES

- Complex inheritance
- Predisposing and resistance alleles, at several loci
- Gene-environment (smoking) interaction

MAJOR PHENOTYPIC FEATURES

- Age at onset: >50 years
- Drusen in the macula is the hallmark of early and intermediate stages
- Late stage is characterized by atrophy of the retinal pigment epithelium (in the nonexudative or "dry" form) and choroidal neovascularization (in the exudative or "wet" form)
- Loss of central vision occurs in the late stage

HISTORY AND PHYSICAL EXAMINATION

C.D., a 57-year-old woman, presents to her ophthalmologist for routine eye examination. She has not been evaluated in five years. She reports no change in visual acuity but has noticed that it takes her longer to adapt to changes in ambient illumination. Her mother was blind from age-related macular degeneration by her 70s. C.D. smokes a pack of cigarettes per day. On retinal examination, she has many drusen, which are yellow deposits found beneath the retinal pigment epithelium. A few of these drusen are large. She is told that she has features of intermediate age-related macular degeneration, which may cause progressive loss of central vision over time and, eventually, legal blindness. Although there is no specific treatment for this disorder, smoking cessation and oral administration of a nutritional supplement that includes vitamin C, vitamin E, lutein, zeaxanthin, copper, and zinc are recommended as steps she can take to slow the progression of disease.

BACKGROUND

Disease Etiology, Incidence, and Role of Complement Factor H Variants

Age-related macular degeneration (AMD, MIM 603075) is a progressive degenerative disease of the macula: the region of the retina responsible for central vision, which is critical for fine visual acuity (e.g., reading). AMD is one of the most common forms of blindness in older adults. Early signs occur in 30% of all individuals older than 75 years and approximately 20% of these individuals have severe disease with visual loss. AMD is rarely found in individuals younger than 55 years. Up to 50% of the population-attributable genetic risk is associated with a common haplotype in the complement factor H gene (*CFH*), which is, in turn, highly associated with a coding variant, p.Tyr402His. In addition to the common *CFH* haplotype, a rare variant in the *CFH* gene – p.Arg1210Cys – shows high penetrance for AMD. Common variants in three other genes in the alternative complement pathway – factor I (*CFI*), C2/factor B (*CFB*), and complement component 3 (*C3*) – have been linked to AMD risk (see Chapter 11).

Pathogenesis

AMD is broadly classified into three categories: early, intermediate, and late. The late stage is further divided into "dry" (atrophic) and "wet" (neovascular or exudative) types. Early and intermediate AMD are characterized by drusen: the clinical and pathological hallmark lesion of AMD. Drusen are acellular lipid and protein-rich deposits that occur in the extracellular matrix separating the retinal pigmented epithelial (RPE) cells from the choriocapillaris in the macula.

As AMD progresses to the late stage, cases with thinning and loss of RPE tissue in focal or patchy areas are classified as dry AMD. In approximately 10% of affected individuals, RPE remodeling occurs at the site of large, soft drusen. Generally, damage occurs to the choriocapillaris and RPE cells due to oxidative stress and complement activation. The loss of the choriocapillaris and RPE cells results in photoreceptor degeneration in the macula, causing central vision loss. Late AMD cases with invasion of the subretinal space by new and leaky blood vessels that grow in from the choroid (i.e., choroidal neovascularization) are classified as wet AMD. These vessels are fragile; they break and bleed in the retina, causing hemorrhage and/or exudation, thus also causing vision loss.

Drusen contain complement factors, including complement factor H (CFH). Both the common p.Tyr402His and rare p.Arg1210Cys occur in glycosaminoglycan binding domains of the CFH protein. It is proposed that the CFH p.Tyr402His change is a functional variant that affects CFH binding to glycosaminoglycans, causing increased lipid and protein deposition in Bruch's membrane. Genetic risk factors in other complement and lipid metabolism pathways, and environmental factors, including smoking and diet, appear to alter the pathobiology of AMD by altering lipid metabolism, oxidative stress, and/or inflammation.

Phenotype and Natural History

AMD leads to changes in the central retina that are readily apparent by ophthalmoscopy (Fig. C.3.1). In early and intermediate AMD, people can experience a decrease in contrast sensitivity and dark adaptation. In late AMD, loss of central vision occurs, making reading and driving difficult or impossible. Visual loss is generally slowly progressive in the dry form of AMD. In contrast, in the wet form, CNV can lead to bleeding and exudation under the retina and cause rapid vision loss. Peripheral vision is usually preserved in both dry and wet AMD.

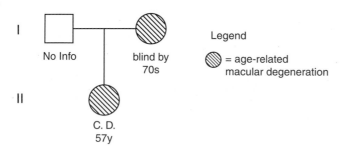

I No Info   blind by 70s

II C. D. 57y

Legend

= age-related macular degeneration

Pedigree Case 3

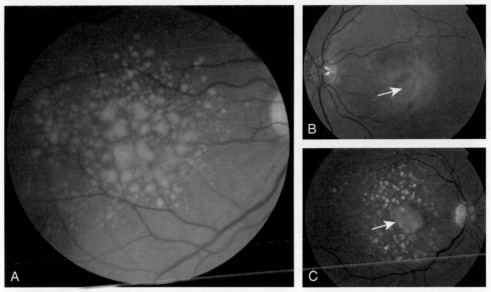

Figure C.3.1 Phenotypic features of AMD. (A) Funduscopic image of numerous large, soft drusen in and around the region of the fovea (intermediate dry AMD). (B) Neovascularization (wet AMD) and scarring in the region of the fovea (*arrow*). (C) Area of thinning and loss of retinal tissue at the fovea ("geographic atrophy" in late dry AMD; *arrow*). (Courtesy Alan Bird, Moorfields Eye Hospital, London.)

Management

Retinal imaging, using retinal angiography and optical coherence tomography, is often used to establish the diagnosis of wet versus dry AMD. There is no specific treatment for dry AMD. Smoking cessation is strongly indicated. Large clinical trials have suggested that, for individuals with extensive medium-sized or one large drusen, the use of a supplement that includes vitamins C and E, lutein, zeaxanthin, copper, and zinc can slow progression of disease. Cases with established retinal and RPE atrophy may be candidates for stem cell therapy in the future, should such a treatment be successfully developed and approved. For wet AMD, serial injections of antivascular endothelial growth factor agents into the vitreous can improve vision and dramatically slow the rate of visual loss.

Inheritance

The role of both genetic and environmental influences is demonstrated by twin studies. Concordance in monozygotic twins of 37% is far below the 100% expected for a purely genetic trait, but it is still significantly greater than the 19% concordance in dizygotic twins. This indicates a prominent genetic contribution to the disorder. First-degree relatives of AMD patients are at a 4.2-fold greater risk for disease compared with that of the general population. Thus, AMD falls into the category of a genetically complex common disease. Despite ample evidence for familial aggregation in AMD, most affected individuals are in families without a clear Mendelian pattern of inheritance.

QUESTIONS FOR SMALL GROUP DISCUSSION

1. How could variants in a complement factor account for a disease limited to the eye?
2. Genome-wide association studies often show many common variants associated with risk of developing disease in each gene, including the common haplotype of CFH in AMD. How do we determine which of such variants are functional?
3. Suggest other types of proteins that could be implicated in AMD.

REFERENCES

Arroyo JG: Age-related macular degeneration. http://uptodate.com.

Fritsche LG, Fariss RN, Stambolian D, *et al*: Age-related macular degeneration: Genetics and biology coming together, *Ann Rev Genomics Hum Genet* 15:5.1–5.21, 2014.

Holz FG, Schmitz-Valkenberg S, Fleckenstein M: Recent developments in the treatment of age-related macular degeneration, *J Clin Invest* 124:1430–1438, 2014.

Ratnapriya R, Chew EY: Age-related degeneration—clinical review and genetics update, *Clin Genet* 84:160–166, 2013.

Singh MS, MacLaren RE: Stem cell treatment for age-related macular degeneration: The challenges, *Investig Ophthalmol Vis Sci* 59(4):AMD78–AMD82, 2018.

Toomey CB, Johnson LV, Bowes Rickman CB: Complement factor H in AMD: Bridging genetic associations and pathobiology, *Prog Retin Eye Res* 62:38–57, 2018.

ALZHEIMER DISEASE (MIM 104300)

Multifactorial or Autosomal Dominant

Peter St George-Hyslop

PRINCIPLES

- Variable expressivity
- Genetic heterogeneity
- Gene dosage
- Toxic gain of function
- Risk modifier

MAJOR PHENOTYPIC FEATURES

- Age at onset: middle to late adulthood
- Dementia
- β-Amyloid plaques
- Neurofibrillary tangles
- Amyloid angiopathy

HISTORY AND PHYSICAL FINDINGS

L.W. was an older woman with dementia. Eight years before her death, she and her family noticed a deficit in her short-term memory. Initially they ascribed this to the forgetfulness of "old age". Her cognitive decline continued, however, and progressively interfered with her ability to drive, shop, and look after herself. L.W. did not have findings suggestive of thyroid disease, vitamin deficiency, brain tumor, drug intoxication, chronic infection, depression, or strokes; magnetic resonance imaging of her brain showed diffuse cortical atrophy. L.W.'s brother, father, and two other paternal relatives had died with dementia in their 70s. A neurologist explained to L.W. and her family that normal aging is not associated with dramatic declines in memory or judgment and that declining cognition with behavioral disturbance and impaired daily functioning suggested a clinical diagnosis of familial dementia, possibly Alzheimer disease. The suspicion of Alzheimer disease was supported by her apolipoprotein E genotype: *APOE* ε4/ε4. L.W.'s condition deteriorated rapidly during the next year, and she died in hospice at 82 years of age. Her autopsy confirmed the diagnosis of Alzheimer disease.

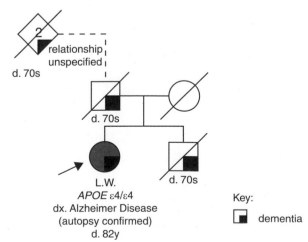

L.W.
APOE ε4/ε4
dx. Alzheimer Disease
(autopsy confirmed)
d. 82y

Key:

▣ dementia

Pedigree Case 4

BACKGROUND

Disease Etiology and Incidence

Approximately 10% of persons older than 70 years have dementia, and approximately half of them have Alzheimer disease (AD, MIM 104300). AD is a genetically heterogeneous disease; less than 5% of affected persons have early-onset familial disease, 15 to 25% have late-onset familial disease, and 75% have sporadic disease. Approximately 10% of familial AD exhibits autosomal dominant inheritance; the remainder exhibits multifactorial inheritance.

Current evidence suggests that defects of β-amyloid precursor protein metabolism play a central role in causing the neuronal dysfunction and death observed with AD. Consistent with this hypothesis, pathogenic variants associated with early-onset autosomal dominant AD have been identified in the β-amyloid precursor protein gene (*APP*), the presenilin 1 gene (*PSEN1*), and the presenilin 2 gene (*PSEN2*) (see Chapter 13). The prevalence of variants in these genes varies widely, depending on the inclusion criteria of the study. Of those with early-onset autosomal dominant AD, 20 to 70% have pathogenic variants in *PSEN1*, 1 to 2% in *APP*, and less than 5% in *PSEN2*.

No fully penetrant mendelian causes of late-onset AD have been identified; however, both familial AD and sporadic late-onset AD are strongly associated with allele ε4 at the apolipoprotein E gene (*APOE*; see Chapters 9 and 13). The frequency of ε4 is 12% to 15% in normal controls compared with 35% in all cases with AD and 45% in those with a family history of dementia.

There is evidence for at least 20 additional AD loci in the genome. A significant proportion of these genes (e.g., *TREM2*, *ABI3*, *PLCG2*) are expressed in microglia. This latter observation has caused revision of concepts surrounding the role of microglia in AD pathogenesis. It was previously thought that their activation was simply a reaction to neuronal death and release of membrane debris. However, the discovery of risk alleles in *TREM2*, *ABI3* and resistance alleles in *PLCG2* forces a reconsideration and suggests that microglia may in fact play a central role. Finally, there have been associations between AD and various marker variants in many other genes.

Pathogenesis

As discussed in Chapter 13, β-amyloid precursor protein (βAPP) undergoes endoproteolytic cleavage to produce peptides with neurotrophic and neuroprotective activities. Cleavage of βAPP within the endosomal-lysosomal compartment produces a carboxyl-terminal peptide of 40 amino acids ($A\beta_{40}$); the function of $A\beta_{40}$ is unknown. In contrast, cleavage of APP within the endoplasmic reticulum or *cis*-Golgi produces a carboxyl-terminal peptide of 42 or 43 amino acids ($A\beta_{42/43}$). $A\beta_{42/43}$ readily aggregates and is neurotoxic in vitro and possibly in vivo. Patients with AD have a significant increase in $A\beta_{42/43}$ aggregates within their brains. Variants in *APP*, *PSEN1*, and *PSEN2* increase the relative or absolute production of $A\beta_{42/43}$. Approximately 1% of all cases of AD occur in individuals with Down syndrome, who overexpress βAPP (because the gene for βAPP is on chromosome 21) and, thus, $A\beta_{42/43}$. The increased risk of AD imparted by the *APOE* ε4 allele is clear, but the mechanism is uncertain.

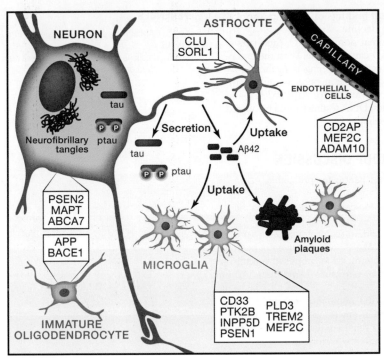

Figure C.4.1 A neurofibrillary tangle (*left*) and a neuritic plaque (*right*) observed on histopathological examination of the brain of an individual with Alzheimer disease. (Courtesy D. Armstrong, Baylor College of Medicine and Texas Children's Hospital, Houston.)

AD is a central neurodegenerative disorder, especially of cholinergic neurons of the hippocampus, neocortical association area, and other limbic structures. Neuropathological changes include cortical atrophy, extracellular neuritic plaques, intraneuronal neurofibrillary tangles (Fig. C.4.1), and amyloid deposits in the walls of cerebral arteries. The neuritic plaques contain many different proteins, including $A\beta_{42/43}$ and apolipoprotein E. The neurofibrillary tangles are composed predominantly of hyperphosphorylated tau protein. Tau helps maintain neuronal integrity, axonal transport, and axonal polarity by promoting the assembly and stability of microtubules.

Phenotype and Natural History

AD is characterized by a progressive loss of cognitive function, including recent memory, abstract reasoning, concentration, language, visual perception, and visual-spatial function. Beginning with a subtle failure of memory, AD is often attributed initially to benign "forgetfulness." Some people perceive their cognitive decline and become frustrated and anxious, whereas others are unaware. Eventually they are unable to work, and they require supervision. Social etiquette and superficial conversation are often retained surprisingly well. Ultimately, most individuals develop rigidity, mutism, and incontinence and are bedridden. Other symptoms associated with AD include agitation, social withdrawal, hallucinations, seizures, myoclonus, and parkinsonian features. Death usually results from malnutrition, infection, or heart disease.

Aside from the age at onset, early-onset AD and late-onset AD are clinically indistinguishable. Pathogenic variants in *PSEN1* cause a fully penetrant phenotype and usually cause rapidly progressive disease, with a mean onset at 45 years. Variants in *APP* cause a less penetrant disorder with rate of AD progression similar to that of late-onset AD; the age at onset ranges from the 40s to early 60s. Variants in *PSEN2* with reduced penetrance, usually cause slowly progressive disease with onset ranging from 40 to 75 years. In contrast to early-onset AD, late-onset AD develops after 60 to 65 years of age; the duration of disease is usually 8 to

10 years, although the range is 2 to 25 years. For both late-onset AD and AD secondary to *APP* alleles, the *APOE* allele ε4 is a dose-dependent modifier of onset; that is, the age at onset varies inversely with the number of copies of the ε4 allele (see Chapter 9).

Management

Except for members of families segregating an AD-associated variant, those with dementia can be definitively diagnosed with AD only by autopsy; however, with rigorous adherence to diagnostic criteria and implementation of an increasing array of biomarkers from cerebrospinal fluid (e.g., phosphorylated forms of tau) and neuroimaging (e.g., amyloid and tau positron emission tomography and magnetic resonance imaging), a clinical suspicion of AD is confirmed by neuropathological examination 80 to 90% of the time. The accuracy of the clinical suspicion increases to 97% if the individual is homozygous for the *APOE* ε4 allele.

Because no curative therapies are available for AD, treatment is focused on the amelioration of associated behavioral and neurological problems. Approximately 10 to 20% of individuals have a modest decrease in the rate of cognitive decline if they are treated early in the disease course with agents that increase cholinergic activity.

Inheritance

Old age, family history, female sex, and Down syndrome are the most important risk factors for AD. In Western populations, the empirical lifetime risk for AD is 5%. An individual with a first-degree relative in whom AD developed after 65 years has a three- to six-fold increase in risk for AD. Someone with a sibling in whom AD developed before 70 years and an affected parent has a risk increased by seven- to nine-fold. *APOE* testing may be used as a diagnostic adjunct in individuals seeking evaluation for signs and symptoms suggestive of dementia but is generally not used for predictive testing for AD in asymptomatic patients (see Chapter 19).

Individuals with Down syndrome have an increased risk for AD. After the age of 40 years, nearly all those with Down syndrome have neuropathological findings of AD, and approximately 50% manifest cognitive decline.

For families segregating autosomal dominant AD, each person has a 50% risk for inheriting an AD-causing allele. With the exception of some *PSEN2* variants, genetic counseling is facilitated by full penetrance and relatively consistent age at onset within a family. Currently, clinical DNA testing is available for *APP*, *PSEN1*, and *PSEN2*, as well as several other genes; DNA testing should be offered only in the context of genetic counseling.

QUESTIONS FOR SMALL GROUP DISCUSSION

1. Why is the *APOE* genotype not useful for predicting AD in asymptomatic individuals?
2. Why is AD usually a neuropathological diagnosis? What is the differential diagnosis for AD?
3. Variants of *MAPT*, the gene encoding tau protein, cause frontotemporal dementia; however, *MAPT* variants have not been detected in AD. Compare and contrast the proposed mechanisms by which abnormalities of tau cause dementia in AD and frontotemporal dementia.
4. Approximately 30% to 50% of the population risk for AD is attributed to genetic factors. What environmental factors are proposed for the remaining risk? What are the difficulties with conclusively identifying environmental factors as risks?

REFERENCES

Bird TD: Alzheimer disease overview. http://www.ncbi.nlm.nih.gov/books/NBK1161/.

Karch CM, Cruchaga C, Goate AM: Alzheimer's disease genetics: From the bench to the clinic, *Neuron* 83:11–26, 2014.

16p11.2 DELETION SYNDROME (MIM 611913)

Autosomal Dominant or De Novo

Jacob A.S. Vorstman

PRINCIPLES

- Genomic recombination locus
- Copy number variant (benign and pathogenic), recombination
- Variant of uncertain significance
- Mirror phenotype effect
- Variable penetrance and pleiotropy

MAJOR PHENOTYPIC FEATURES

- Decreased intellectual functioning relative to unaffected family members; in ~20% meeting criteria for intellectual disability.
- Impaired social and communication skills in 20 to 25%, meeting criteria for autism spectrum disorder (ASD)
- Minor dysmorphic features, macrocephaly
- Hypotonia (50%) and seizures (24%)

HISTORY AND PHYSICAL FINDINGS

M.L., a 3-year-old boy, was referred to a medical genetics clinic to identify the cause of his speech delay. Pregnancy and birth were uneventful. He walked at about 14 months of age and spoke his first words at 30 months. At 3 years, he had five words. His parents felt that he understood more than he could communicate, although his receptive language was also delayed. M.L. had no other issues of medical concern, and his family history was noncontributory. A physical examination revealed minor dysmorphic features, including mild macrocephaly (98th percentile), simple, low-set ears, a single transverse palmar crease on the left hand, and bilateral 2/3/4 toe syndactyly. His parents described him as a "loner"; he preferred to play alone rather than with his siblings or peers. Behaviors of concern included becoming very agitated with loud noises or irritating textures, such as his shirt tag, and throwing tantrums when his routine was changed. He was interested only in cars and preferred to play with their wheels or place them in groups rather than race them. The geneticist ordered a chromosome microarray and fragile X DNA studies, due to his developmental delay with autistic features and mild dysmorphic features. The fragile X DNA test result was normal.

The chromosomal (SNP) microarray revealed two copy number variants: a 550-kb deletion at 16p11.2 (pathogenic) and a 526-kb duplication at 21q22.12 (a variant of uncertain significance). Given the presence of a pathogenic variant associated with neurodevelopmental outcomes, a full developmental assessment was performed, confirming diagnoses of developmental delay and ASD – both annotated as 'related to the 16p11.2 deletion'. Parental studies showed that M.L.'s mother had the 21q duplication, but the 16p11.2 deletion was *de novo*. The family was counseled that the 16p11.2 deletion was likely the cause of M.L.'s autistic features and delays, and that the 21q22.12 duplication was likely a benign variant.

BACKGROUND

Pathogenesis

The 16p11.2 region is marked by several low copy repeats (LCRs; see Chapter 6), which render this region vulnerable to recurrent *de novo* deletions or duplications. This is similar to other genomic regions where *de novo* CNVs recur, such as 22q11.2 and 15q11-13. During replication, the DNA misaligns on these LCRs, causing nonallelic homologous recombination (NAHR) and consequent deletion or duplication of the DNA between the LCRs.

Disease Etiology and Incidence

At 16p11.2, a distinction is made between CNVs mediated by the distal LCRs (e.g., LCR1–LCR3, also called breakpoints [BPs], leading to deletions or duplications of ~550kb) and CNVs of ~600kb, mediated by the proximal LCR4 and LCR5 (Fig. C.5.1). While CNVs in both the proximal and distal 16p11.2 regions are associated with clinically neurodevelopmental phenotypes – including developmental delay and ASD – those affecting the proximal (LCR4–LCR5) region are more frequent (~6–16/10,000 population) than those of the distal (LCR1–LCR3) region (~4–6/10,000 population). Both deletions and duplications of the proximal 16p11.2 region are among the most frequently identified genetic causes of ASD, collectively amounting to ~0.4 to 0.8% of individuals with ASD. In addition, both the proximal 16p11.2 duplication and the distal 16p11.2 deletion are associated with an increased risk for schizophrenia.

Phenotype and Natural History

CNVs at 16p11.2 – both proximal and distal – show variable penetrance. Phenotypes associated with the duplications are generally less severe than those with deletions; consequently, the duplications are more often recognized as inherited than are the deletions. In addition, a remarkable phenotypic "mirror effect" is observed in carriers of CNVs in this region: those with deletions have obesity and increased head circumference, whereas those with duplications have decreased head circumference and body weight.

The proximal 16p11.2 microdeletion syndrome is characterized by susceptibility to neurodevelopmental disorders, including speech/language impairment (>70%), motor

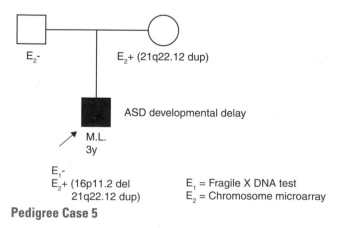

E₂- ☐————○ E₂+ (21q22.12 dup)

■ M.L. ASD developmental delay
3y

E₁-
E₂+ (16p11.2 del
21q22.12 dup)

E₁ = Fragile X DNA test
E₂ = Chromosome microarray

Pedigree Case 5

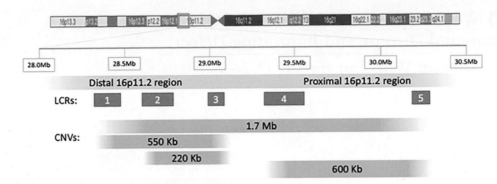

Figure C.5.1 Schematic overview of the 16p11.2 region. Low copy repeats (*LCRs*, *orange boxes*) in this region mediate the recurrent deletions or duplications of different sizes (light orange bars). A distinction is made between 16p11.2 distal CNVs (LCR1–LCR3, including the smaller LCR2–LCR3 variant), and the 16p11.2 proximal CNVs mediated by LCRs 4 and 5.

coordination difficulties (~60%), developmental delay eventually diagnosed as learning disorder and/or intellectual disabilities (~20%), and ASD (20–25%). The penetrance of the proximal 16p11.2 deletion can also be evaluated dimensionally (rather than categorically) while comparing the observed phenotype to that expected given their first-degree family members. For example, from a categorical perspective, ~20% of individuals with this deletion meet the criteria for intellectual disability. Taking the alternative approach, the deletion is associated with a cognitive level (IQ) of (average) 1.7 standard deviations below those of parents and/or siblings without the deletion. In other words, while the categorical penetrance for "intellectual disability" is said to be "incomplete" (~20%), the dimensional penetrance – conceptualized as "negative impact on expected cognitive function" – may be considered (almost) complete.

The proximal 16p11.2 deletion also exemplifies the phenomenon of pleiotropy; that is, the association with both neurodevelopmental and somatic phenotypes, as observed with many other high-impact pathogenic variants. For example, seizures are somewhat more common in these individuals than in the general population. Some with this deletion have aortic valve abnormalities; a majority of individuals do not have heart malformations.

Management

Because of the higher prevalence of developmental delay/intellectual disability and ASD in individuals with 16p11.2 microdeletions, referral to a developmental pediatrician, child psychiatrist, or clinical psychologist is recommended. This would facilitate developmental assessment and placement into appropriate early intervention services, such as physical, occupational, and speech therapies. Social, behavioral, and educational interventions are also available for children with ASDs. An echocardiogram and/or electrocardiogram should be considered, to look for aortic valve or other structural heart anomalies, and referral to a pediatric neurologist should be made if there is suspicion of seizure activity. Weight management and nutritional support should be provided because of the increased risk for obesity.

Inheritance

The proximal 16p11.2 deletion is usually *de novo* but can be inherited from a parent. When *de novo*, the recurrence risk is less than 5%, taking into account the likelihood of gonadal mosaicism in a parent. If one parent also carries the deletion, recurrence risk for the deletion is 50% for each subsequent pregnancy.

Therefore, appropriate genetic counseling depends upon parental studies when a 16p11.2 abnormality is diagnosed in a child. However, due to pleiotropy and variable expression, a child who inherits the deletion may not be affected with the same features as in the proband. A carrier sibling may exhibit intelligence and behavior in the normal range. However, these evaluations may change when considering the penetrance dimensionally, and in the context of what was expected given familial functioning in these domains (see discussion above).

QUESTIONS FOR SMALL GROUP DISCUSSION

1. Name other recurring microdeletion/microduplication disorders caused by LCRs. Are the principles of variable penetrance and pleiotropy relevant to these as well? Can you give examples?

2. In performing microarray testing and whole-exome sequencing, what are some results that may give rise to ethical dilemmas? How would you counsel patients with these types of results, before and after the testing is ordered?

3. Deletions of a particular genomic region are typically more severe than duplications of the same region. In what situations would a duplication create a greater health risk than a deletion?

4. Why was a karyotype not ordered for this patient? Is there ever an indication for a karyotype? If so, what is it/are they?

REFERENCES

Chung WK, Roberts TPL, Sherr EH, Green Snyder LA, Spiro JE: 16p11.2 deletion syndrome, *Curr Opin Genet Dev* 68:49–56, 2021.

Marshall CR, Howrigan DP, Merico B: Contribution of copy number variants to schizophrenia from a genome-wide study of 41,321 subjects, *Nat Gene* 49(1):27–35, 2017. https://doi.org/10.1038/ng.3725

Miller DT, Nasir R, Sobeih MM, *et al*: 16p11.2 Microdeletion. http://www.ncbi.nlm.nih.gov/books/NBK11167/

Moreno-De-Luca A, Evans DW, Boomer KB, *et al*: The role of parental cognitive, behavioral, and motor profiles in clinical variability in individuals with chromosome 16p11.2 deletions, *JAMA Psychiatry* 72(2):119–126, 2015.

Simons VIP Consortium: Simons Variation in Individuals Project (Simons VIP): A genetics-first approach to studying autism spectrum and related neurodevelopmental disorders, *Neuron* 73:1063–1067, 2012.

Unique, the Rare Chromosomal Disorder Support Group. http://www.rarechromo.org

Weiss LA, Shen Y, Korn JM, *et al*: Association between microdeletion and microduplication at 16p11.2 and autism, *N Engl J Med* 358:667–675, 2008.

BECKWITH-WIEDEMANN SYNDROME (MIM 130650)
(Uniparental Disomy and Imprinting Defect)

Chromosomal With Imprinting Defect

Rosanna Weksberg

PRINCIPLES

- Multiple pathogenic mechanisms
- Imprinting
- Uniparental disomy
- Somatic mosaicism
- Assisted reproductive technology

MAJOR PHENOTYPIC FEATURES

- Age at onset: prenatal
- Prenatal and postnatal overgrowth
- Macroglossia
- Omphalocele
- Visceromegaly
- Ear Creases and Pits
- Hemihyperplasia
- Embryonal tumors in childhood
- Renal abnormalities
- Adrenocortical cytomegaly
- Neonatal hypoglycemia

HISTORY AND PHYSICAL FINDINGS

A.B., a 27-year-old gravida 1/para 0 woman, presented to a prenatal diagnostic center for detailed ultrasonography and genetic counseling at 19 weeks gestation, after a prior routine ultrasound examination revealed a male fetus, large for gestational age with possible omphalocele. The pregnancy, the first for each of his parents, was achieved without assisted reproductive technology. After confirmation by detailed ultrasonography, the family was counseled that the fetus had a number of findings suggestive of Beckwith-Wiedemann syndrome. The family history was negative for features of this syndrome. The couple declined invasive prenatal diagnostic testing by amniocentesis. The baby, B.B., was delivered by cesarean section at 37 weeks with a birth weight of 9 pounds, 2 ounces, and a notably large placenta. Omphalocele was noted, as were macroglossia, hemihyperplasia involving the right leg, and ear lobe creases.

A genetics consultant made a clinical diagnosis of Beckwith-Wiedemann syndrome. Hypoglycemia was detected on day 2 and B.B. was treated with intravenous glucose for 1 week, following which the hypoglycemia resolved and no further treatment was required. The findings on cardiac evaluation were normal, and the omphalocele was surgically repaired without difficulty.

MS-MLPA (methylation-specific multiplex ligation-dependent probe amplification) testing of the chromosome 11p15 region detected no genomic alterations. DNA methylation was normal at both the telomeric and centromeric imprinting control centers, IC1 and IC2, respectively. The parents were counseled that a normal molecular result for MS-MLPA for chromosome 11p15 is found in the peripheral blood of ~20% of individuals with a clinical diagnosis of Beckwith-Wiedemann syndrome and that is most likely due to somatic mosaicism for a chromosome 11p15 molecular change (e.g., chromosome 11p15 uniparental disomy). They agreed to MS-MLPA testing of an independent tissue (buccal cells from a cheek swab) to assess for somatic mosaicism for a chromosome 11p15 molecular alteration.

Given the clinical diagnosis of Beckwith-Wiedemann syndrome, which is associated with an increased risk for embryonal tumors (most commonly Wilms tumor and hepatoblastoma), tumor surveillance was discussed. Specifically, measurement of serum alpha-fetoprotein level was recommended every 3 months for the first 4 years as a screen for hepatoblastoma. Abdominal ultrasound examination was recommended every 3 months to 8 years of age.

At a follow-up visit, the family was informed that the second MS-MLPA test on the buccal cells demonstrated methylation changes at both chromosome 11p15 imprinting control centers; that is, gain of methylation at IC1 and loss of methylation at IC2. This result is consistent with somatic mosaicism for chromosome 11p15 paternal uniparental disomy and confirmed the clinical diagnosis of Beckwith-Wiedemann syndrome. The family was counseled that somatic mosaicism for 11p15 results from a postzygotic error and therefore the recurrence risk for future pregnancies would be low.

BACKGROUND

Disease Etiology and Incidence

Beckwith-Wiedemann syndrome (BWS, MIM 130650) is a syndrome that is usually sporadic but is inherited in an autosomal dominant manner in approximately 15% of cases. BWS affects approximately 1 in 13,700 live births.

BWS results from an imbalance in the expression of imprinted genes that map to two imprinted domains in the chromosome 11p15 region. These genes include *KCNQ1OT1* and *H19*, which encode noncoding RNAs (see Chapters 3 and 8), and *CDKN1C* and *IGF2*, encoding proteins that regulate growth. The transcriptional regulation of *H19* and *IGF2* in the telomeric imprinted domain is controlled by a differentially methylated imprinting center, IC1, which supports monoallelic maternal expression of *H19* and monoallelic paternal expression of *IGF2*. In the centromeric imprinted domain, the expression of *KCNQ1OT1* and *CDKN1C* is regulated by imprinting center 2 (IC2), which maintains monoallelic paternal expression of *KCNQ1OT1* and monoallelic maternal expression of *CDKN1C*. Proteins

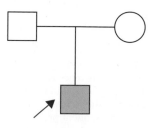

Pedigree Case 6.

known to be relevant to the pathogenesis of BWS include IGF2—an insulin-like growth factor that *promotes* growth—and CDKN1C—a cell cycle suppressor that *constrains* cell division and growth.

Unbalanced expression of the 11p15 imprinted genes can occur through a number of mechanisms. Approximately 5% of individuals with BWS have gain of methylation at IC1; imprinting defects that disrupt IC1 may have concomitant microdeletions. The majority (~50%) of BWS cases have loss of methylation at IC2, which leads to loss of expression of the maternal *CDKN1C* allele. Genomic alterations can be associated with imprinting defects at IC2 but are less common than in individuals with imprinting defects at IC1. In approximately 20% of individuals with BWS, paternal uniparental isodisomy of 11p15 results in loss of maternal *CDKN1C* expression and increased *IGF2* expression. Individuals with segmental uniparental disomy of 11p15 have mosaicism for this alteration as the somatic recombination event leading to segmental uniparental disomy in BWS occurs after conception. Therefore, testing of tissues other than blood may be required to demonstrate the presence of chromosome 11p15 isodisomy. Pathogenic variants in the maternal *CDKN1C* allele are found in 5% to 10% of sporadic cases and in 40% of families with autosomal dominant BWS. A relatively small number of individuals with BWS have a detectable chromosomal abnormality, such as maternal translocation, inversion of chromosome 11, or duplication of paternal chromosome 11p15. As noted above, approximately 20% of individuals with BWS have no alteration detectable on currently available testing. Undetected somatic mosaicism for chromosome 11p15 alterations likely accounts for a significant proportion of these cases.

Pathogenesis

During normal gamete formation and early embryonic development, different patterns of DNA methylation are established in males and females at the two primary imprinting centers on chromosome 11p15, that is, IC2 and IC1, associated with the *KCNQOT1* gene in imprinted domain 2 and the *H19* gene in imprinted domain 1, respectively (Chapter 8). Abnormal imprinting in BWS is usually tested by analysis of DNA methylation at the CpG islands in IC1 and IC2. In those with BWS, a chromosome 11p15 MS-MLPA test detects a variety of molecular changes including microdeletions and microduplications as well as *loss of* methylation of the maternal IC2. This results in reduced *CDKN1C* expression and *gain of* methylation of the maternal IC1, which decreases *H19* expression, resulting in excess *IGF2* expression. Inappropriate *IGF2* expression from both parental alleles can explain some of the overgrowth seen in BWS. Similarly, loss of expression of the maternal copy of *CDKN1C* removes a constraint on fetal growth. Sequence analysis is required to detect pathogenic variants of *CDKN1C*. Such variants are not detected by the MS-MLPA assay and they are not associated with methylation changes at IC1 or IC2. SNP-based microarray analysis can be used to detect some 11p15 copy number variants; for example, larger genomic alterations such as duplications of 11p15. Rare families have balanced translocations of 11p15 that can be associated with BWS, likely due to changes in chromatin that impact accessibility to regulatory elements/transcription factors in the centromeric imprinted domain. These cases usually do not demonstrate methylation alterations detectable by MS-MLPA.

Phenotype and Natural History

BWS is associated with prenatal and postnatal overgrowth. Up to 50% of affected individuals are premature and large

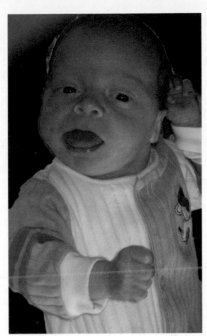

Figure C.6.1 Characteristic macroglossia in a 4-month-old male infant with Beckwith-Wiedemann syndrome. The diagnosis was made soon after birth on the basis of the clinical findings of macrosomia, macroglossia, omphalocele, a subtle ear crease on the right, and neonatal hypoglycemia. Organomegaly was absent. Karyotype was normal, and molecular studies showed hypomethylation of the *KCNQ1OT1* gene. (Courtesy Rosanna Weksberg and Cheryl Shuman, Hospital for Sick Children, Toronto, Canada.)

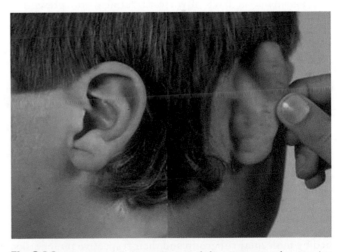

Fig C.6.2 Characteristic anterior ear lobe creases and posterior helical ear pits in a child with Beckwith-Wiedemann syndrome.

for gestational age at birth. The placentas are large and pregnancies are frequently complicated by polyhydramnios. Additional features in infants with BWS may variably include omphalocele, macroglossia (Fig. C.6.1), ear creases and/or ear pits (Fig. C.6.2), neonatal hypoglycemia, and, rarely, cardiomyopathy, all of which contribute to increased neonatal mortality. Neonatal hypoglycemia is typically mild and transient, but sometimes more severe hypoglycemia. Congenital renal malformations are also common and some individuals with BWS develop elevated urinary calcium levels with nephrocalcinosis and nephrolithiasis in childhood/adolescence. Hyperplasia of various body segments (hemihyperplasia) or of selected organs may be present at birth and may become more or less evident over time. Development is typically normal in individuals with BWS unless they have an unbalanced chromosome abnormality, a brain malformation (which is very rare), or a history of a serious neonatal hypoglycemic event and/or other perinatal complications.

Children with BWS have an increased risk for the development of embryonal tumors, particularly Wilms tumor and hepatoblastoma but also neuroblastoma, rhabdomyosarcoma, adrenocortical carcinoma, and others. The overall risk for neoplasia in children with BWS is approximately 7.5%. Most hepatoblastomas present by 4 years and Wilms tumor by 8 years of age. Although there is evidence of epi-genotype-phenotype correlations for some features of BWS, the clinical phenotype is highly variable, even within specific molecular subgroups. This variability is driven, in part, by somatic mosaicism, most commonly for 11p15 paternal uniparental disomy, but also for other molecular subgroups. Individuals with positive molecular alterations involving 11p15 may present with multiple features or with a single feature of BWS. Some with molecularly confirmed BWS may present with an omphalocele prenatally, or with hemihyperplasia in a child with macrosomia, or an embryonal tumor in childhood or medullary cystic kidney disease and hemihyperplasia in adulthood. There are some important phenotype-epigenotype-genotype correlations with respect to tumor types and risks for these tumors. The risk for Wilms tumor is highest for individuals with IC1 gain of methylation and 11p15 UPD and lower for those with IC2 loss of methylation.

Management

Management of BWS involves treatment of presenting symptoms, such as management of hypoglycemia. Special feeding techniques or speech therapy may be required due to the macroglossia. Surgical intervention may be indicated for abdominal wall defects, macroglossia, and leg length discrepancies.

Surveillance for embryonal tumors is essential because these can be fast-growing and potentially fatal neoplasias. The current recommendations for tumor surveillance include serial ultrasound examination every 3 months (specifically, abdominal ultrasound for the first four years followed by renal ultrasound to 8 years) and measurement of serum alpha-fetoprotein level for hepatoblastoma every 3 months for the first 4 years. However, there are some variations in these recommendations across different centers. In particular, there are significant differences with respect to which children are offered such surveillance. In some centers in the United Kingdom and Europe, children are stratified by molecular subgroup and their respective tumor risks, so that only those at highest risk (e.g., IC1 gain of methylation and chromosome 11p15 UPD) are offered tumor surveillance. However, in most centers in North America and internationally, tumor surveillance (as outlined above) is offered to all children with BWS regardless of their molecular test results, including those with no identified molecular alteration. After the age of 8 years, tumor development is uncommon; however, renal ultrasound examination is suggested annually or biennially through to midadolescence, in light of the increased risk for nephrocalcinosis, medullary sponge kidney disease, and renal calculi.

In the prenatal clinic when fetal ultrasound detects a BWS-associated finding such as omphalocele, prenatal diagnostic testing, including epigenetic testing for methylation status, may be offered. Somatic mosaicism should be considered in the interpretation of test results. At present, epigenetic testing is more reliable when undertaken on amniocytes than on chorionic villus samples, since the methylation status of the 11p15 imprinting centers can vary in early pregnancy.

Inheritance

The recurrence risk for siblings and offspring of children with BWS depends on the molecular etiology defined in the BWS proband. Imprinting defects that are postzygotic or limited to epigenetic alterations without an associated genetic alteration are usually *de novo* occurrences with low risks of recurrence. For BWS cases that have an associated genetic alteration (e.g., pathogenic variants in *CDKN1C*, microduplications or microdeletions, chromosome abnormalities), predicted risks are based on standard genetic risks for transmission of the genomic alteration. Results of parental testing may be relevant for defining risk estimates for siblings. The predicted phenotype in the offspring is dependent on the sex of the individual transmitting the genomic alteration, due to parent of origin-specific imprinting (see Chapter 8, Fig. 8.4). Specific prenatal testing is possible for families with a defined BWS-associated heritable genomic alteration.

Beckwith-Wiedemann Syndrome and Assisted Reproductive Technologies

Assisted reproductive technologies (ART), such as in vitro fertilization (IVF) and intracytoplasmic sperm injection, have become commonplace, accounting now for >1% of all births in many countries. Retrospective studies demonstrate an increased incidence of BWS in children conceived using ART, compared to those conceived naturally. The risk for BWS after IVF is increased several-fold over that in the general population (1 in 10,000), although the absolute risk is low (~1/2500). The rates of other imprinting disorders, specifically, Angelman syndrome, Prader-Willi syndrome, and Russell-Silver syndrome, are also increased with ART. The reason for the increased incidence of imprinting defects with ART is likely an error in early developmental epigenetic reprogramming.

QUESTIONS FOR SMALL GROUP DISCUSSION

1. Discuss possible reasons for embryonal tumors in BWS. Why would these decline in frequency with age?
2. Discuss reasons why imprinted genes frequently affect fetal size. Name another condition associated with uniparental disomy for another chromosome.
3. Besides imprinting defects, discuss other genetic disorders that may cause infertility and yet can be passed on by means of ART.
4. Discuss how, in addition to pathogenic sequence variants in the genes implicated in BWS, an epigenetic alteration in the imprinting locus control region could cause BWS.

REFERENCES

Brioude F, Kalish JM, Mussa A, *et al*: Expert consensus document: Clinical and molecular diagnosis, screening and management of Beckwith-Wiedemann syndrome: an international consensus statement, *Nat Rev Endocrinol* 14:229, 2018.

Cortessis VK, Azadian M, Buxbaum J, *et al*: Comprehensive meta-analysis reveals association between multiple imprinting disorders and conception by assisted reproductive technology, *J Assist Reprod Genet* 35(6):943–952, 2018. https://doi.org/10.1007/s10815-018-1173-x

Kalish JM, Doros L, Helman LJ, Hennekam R, Kuiper RP, Maas SM, Maher ER, Nichols KE, Plon SE, Porter CC, Rednam S, Schultz K, States LJ, Tomlinson GE, Zelley K, Druley T: Surveillance recommendations for children with overgrowth syndromes and predisposition to Wilms tumors and hepatoblastoma, *Clin Cancer Res* 23(13):e115–e122, 2017. https://doi.org/10.1158/1078-0432.CCR-17-0710

Shuman C, Beckwith JB, Weksberg R: Beckwith-Wiedemann syndrome, *GeneReviews*. http://www.ncbi.nlm.nih.gov/books/NBK1394/

HEREDITARY BREAST AND OVARIAN CANCER
(MIM 604370, 612555) (*BRCA1* and *BRCA2* Pathogenic Variants)

Autosomal Dominant

Amy Finch • Steve Narod

PRINCIPLES

- Tumor-suppressor gene
- Incomplete penetrance and variable expressivity
- Founder effect

MAJOR PHENOTYPIC FEATURES

- Age at onset: adulthood
- Breast cancer
- Ovarian and fallopian tube cancer
- Prostate cancer
- Multiple primary cancers

HISTORY AND PHYSICAL FINDINGS

S.M., a 35-year-old previously healthy woman, was referred to the cancer genetics clinic by her breast surgeon after being diagnosed with breast cancer. She was of Ukrainian ancestry. She was concerned about her risk for the development of a second cancer and her daughter's risk for developing cancer. Her mother had ovarian cancer and her aunt also had breast cancer (Fig. C.7.1). The genetic counselor explained that the family history of cancer was suggestive of an inherited predisposition and calculated that the proband's risk for carrying a pathogenic variant in a cancer susceptibility gene (*BRCA1, BRCA2, PALB2, CHEK2, ATM, BARD1, RAD51D, RAD51C or BRIP1*) was 80% using the CanRiskTool. S.M. chose to pursue panel genetic testing, which showed that she had a premature termination (protein truncating) pathogenic variant in one *BRCA2* allele that had been previously detected in other individuals with breast cancer. During the discussion of the results, S.M. inquired whether her 6- and 7-year-old girls should be tested. The genetic counselor explained that because the variant posed little risk in childhood, the decision to have genetic testing was better left until the children were 18 and were old enough to decide on the utility of testing. S.M. agreed.

S.M. communicated her results to her family members, showing them the letter that the genetic counselor had written summarizing the findings. Five adult relatives elected to have predictive testing, and four (three females and one male) were found to be carriers of the same variant; one cousin pursued prophylactic bilateral mastectomy at age 40. The risk for cancers at other sites was also discussed with all carriers.

BACKGROUND

Disease Etiology and Incidence

The prevalence of *BRCA1* pathogenic variants is approximately 1 in 500 and for *BRCA2* is approximately 1 in 350, with higher frequencies in some populations due to founder effects. Variants in major cancer predisposition genes account for 3 to 10% of cases of breast cancer. Those in *BRCA1* or *BRCA2* account for the majority of hereditary breast cancer cases but only a small fraction of breast cancer overall (see Chapter 16). Germline variants in *BRCA1 or BRCA2* account for approximately 18% of unselected serous ovarian cancer, the most prevalent histologic type.

Pathogenesis

BRCA1 and *BRCA2* encode ubiquitously expressed nuclear proteins that are believed to maintain genomic integrity by regulating DNA repair, transcriptional transactivation, and the cell cycle.

Despite the ubiquitous expression of *BRCA1* and *BRCA2*, mutation of these genes predisposes predominantly to breast and ovarian cancers. Loss of *BRCA1* or *BRCA2* function probably permits the accumulation of other variants that contribute to neoplastic progression.

Tumor formation in carriers of *BRCA1* or *BRCA2* germline variants follows the two-hit hypothesis; that is, both alleles of either *BRCA1* or *BRCA2* lose function in tumor cells (see Chapter 16). Somatic loss of function by the second allele can occur by a variety of mechanisms, including loss of heterozygosity, intragenic mutation, or promoter hypermethylation. Because of the high frequency with which the second allele of *BRCA1* or *BRCA2* loses function, families segregating a germline *BRCA1* or *BRCA2* variant exhibit autosomal dominant inheritance of neoplasia.

The population prevalence of individual *BRCA1* or *BRCA2* germline variants varies from country to country and there are several founder effects. Among those of Ashkenazi Jewish ancestry, the *BRCA1* c.185delAG (c.68_69delAG) and c.5382insC (c.5266dupC) variants and the *BRCA2* c.6174delT (c.5946delT) variant are founder alleles, with prevalences of 1%, 0.4%, and 1.2%, respectively. In most circumstances, it is warranted to test only for these three variants in Jewish women. In Iceland, the *BRCA2* c.999del5 (c.771_775del) variant has a prevalence of 0.6% and accounts for the majority of *BRCA2* variants. Among those with breast cancer, the highest reported prevalence of pathogenic variants is in the Bahamas, accounting for 23% of all breast cancer in the country.

Phenotype and Natural History

Patients with *BRCA1* or *BRCA2* germline variants have an increased risk for several cancers (see Table C.7.1). In addition to the increased risk for ovarian, fallopian tube, and female breast cancers, *BRCA1* variant alleles confer an increased risk for pancreatic cancer. Germline *BRCA2* variants increase the risk for prostate, pancreatic, melanoma, and male breast cancers. Prostate cancer in men who carry a *BRCA2* variant is associated with more aggressive disease.

Among female carriers of a *BRCA1* germline variant, the penetrance of breast cancer is about 75% and the penetrance of ovarian and fallopian tube cancer is about 40%. Among female carriers of a *BRCA2* germline variant, the penetrance of breast cancer is about 70% and the penetrance of ovarian and fallopian tube cancer is about 20%. The cumulative risk for contralateral breast cancer for both *BRCA1* and *BRCA2* female carriers at 20 years after initial diagnosis is significant, at approximately 40% and 25%, respectively.

Management

Current recommendations for women with a germline *BRCA1* or *BRCA2* pathogenic variant include frequent breast examinations as well as breast imaging studies (mammography and MRI). Total bilateral mastectomy may reduce the risk for breast cancer by more than 90%, although the risk is not abolished, because some breast tissue often remains. Similarly, bilateral salpingo-oophorectomy may reduce the risk for

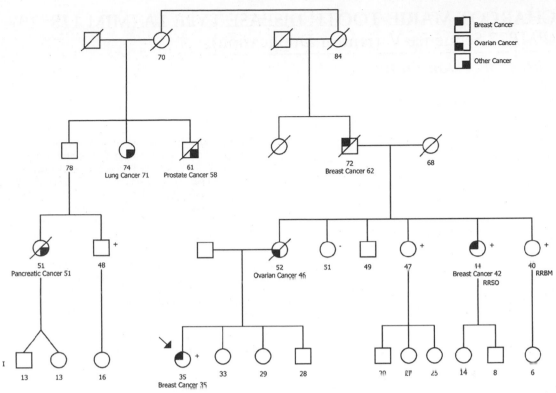

Figure C.7.1 The proband S.M. is indicated by an arrow. Shaded symbols indicate a diagnosis of cancer. Ages are shown directly below the symbol. A *plus sign* identifies carriers of the *BRCA2* pathogenic variant, and a *minus sign* identifies noncarriers as determined by DNA sequencing. Cancer diagnoses are followed by the age of diagnosis. RRBM, risk-reducing bilateral mastectomy; RRSO, risk-reducing salpingo-oophorectomy.

TABLE C.7.1 Cumulative Risk (%) by Age 70 Years

	Female		Male		Female and Male
	Breast Cancer	Ovarian and Fallopian Tube Cancer	Breast Cancer	Prostate Cancer	Pancreatic Cancer
General population	8–10	1.5	<0.1	10	1.5
BRCA1 carriers	60–69	39–58	~1	21*	≤5
BRCA2 carriers	48–73	13–29	7	27**	5–10

*Cumulative risk (%) to age 75.
**Cumulative risk to age 85 is estimated to be up to 60%.

ovarian cancer and fallopian tube cancer by more than 80%; a small risk for primary peritoneal cancer remains. Management of at-risk males includes frequent prostate and breast examinations and laboratory tests for evidence of prostate cancer. In families with known germline variants, molecular analysis can focus surveillance or prophylaxis on members carrying the variant allele.

Inheritance

In Western populations, the cumulative female breast cancer incidence is 1 in 200 at 40 years, 1 in 50 at 50 years, and 1 in 10 by 70 years. Family history is one of the most important risk factors for breast cancer. Those with a first-degree relative in whom breast cancer developed after 55 years have a 1.6-fold relative risk for breast cancer; the relative risk increases to 2.3 if the breast cancer developed in the family member before 55 years and to 3.8 if it developed before 45 years. If the first-degree relative had bilateral breast cancer, the relative risk is 6.4.

Children of an individual with a *BRCA1* or *BRCA2* germline variant have a 50% risk for inheriting that variant. Because of incomplete penetrance and variable expressivity, the development and onset of cancer cannot be precisely predicted.

QUESTIONS FOR SMALL GROUP DISCUSSION

1. At what age and under what conditions might testing of an at-risk child be appropriate?
2. What is the risk for development of prostate cancer in a son if a parent carries a pathogenic *BRCA1* germline variant? A *BRCA2* germline variant?
3. How should a report of "no pathogenic variant detected by sequencing" be interpreted and counseled? What are the various possibilities? How do we counsel unaffected female relatives of women who have no variant detected?

REFERENCES

Chen J, Bae E, Zhang L, *et al*: Penetrance of breast and ovarian cancer in women who carry a, BRCA1/2 Mutation and Do Not Use Risk-Reducing Salpingo-Oophorectomy: An Updated Meta-Analysis. *JNCI Cancer Spectr* 4(4):pkaa029, 2020.

Domchek SM, Robson ME: Update on genetic testing in gynecologic cancer *J Clin Oncol* 37(27):2501–2509, 2019.

Donenberg I, Lunn J, Curling D, *et al*: A high prevalence of BRCA1 mutations among breast cancer patients from the Bahamas, *Breast Cancer Res Treat* 125(2):591–596, 2011. https://doi.org/10.1007/s10549-010-1156-9

Daly MB, Pal T, Berry MP *et al*.: Genetic/Familial High-Risk Assessment: Breast, Ovarian, and Pancreatic V2. 2021.

NCCN: Clinical Practice Guidelines in Oncology, *J Natl Compr Canc Netw.* 2021 Jan 6;19(1):77–102. https://doi.org/10.6004/jnccn.2021.0001

Nyberg T, Frost D, Barrowdale D, *et al*: Prostate cancer risks for male BRCA1 and BRCA2 mutation carriers: A prospecti...

CHARCOT-MARIE-TOOTH DISEASE TYPE 1A (MIM 118220)
(*PMP22* Sequence Variant or Duplication)

Autosomal Dominant

James R. Lupski

PRINCIPLES

- Genetic heterogeneity
- Gene dosage
- Recombination between repeated DNA sequences
- Reciprocal recombination

MAJOR PHENOTYPIC FEATURES

- Age at onset: childhood to adulthood
- Progressive distal weakness
- Distal muscle wasting
- Hyporeflexia
- Intrinsic muscle wasting of hands and feet
- gait disturbance
- pes cavus/pes planus
- Distal symmetric polyneuropathy (DSP)

HISTORY AND PHYSICAL FINDINGS

During the past few years, J.T., an 18-year-old woman, had noticed a progressive decline in her strength, endurance, and ability to run and walk. She also complained of frequent leg cramps exacerbated by cold, and recent difficulty stepping over objects and climbing stairs. She did not recollect a precedent illness, or give a history suggestive of an inflammatory process, such as myalgia, fever, or night sweats. No other family members had similar problems or a neuromuscular disorder. On examination, J.T. was thin and had atrophy of her lower legs, mild weakness of ankle extension and flexion, absent ankle reflexes, reduced patellar reflexes, footdrop as she walked, and enlarged peroneal nerves. She had difficulty walking on her toes and could not walk on her heels. The findings from her examination were otherwise normal. She had graduated high school and had no neurocognitive issues during childhood. As part of her evaluation, the neurologist requested several studies, including nerve conduction velocities (NCVs). J.T.'s NCVs were abnormal on both sides of her body; her median NCV was 25 m/sec (normal, >43 m/sec). Results of a subsequent nerve biopsy showed segmental demyelination, myelin sheath hypertrophy (redundant wrappings of Schwann cells around nerve fibers), and no evidence of inflammation.

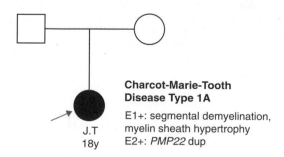

Charcot-Marie-Tooth Disease Type 1A

E1+: segmental demyelination, myelin sheath hypertrophy
E2+: *PMP22* dup

J.T
18y

Key
E1: nerve biopsy
E2: *PMP22* duplication test

Pedigree Case 8

The neurologist explained that these results were strongly suggestive of a demyelinating neuropathy such as type 1 Charcot-Marie-Tooth (CMT) disease, also known as hereditary motor and sensory neuropathy type 1. Explaining that the most common cause of type 1 CMT disease (CMT1) is a duplication of the peripheral myelin protein 22 gene (*PMP22*) – the CMT1A duplication – the neurologist requested targeted DNA testing for this duplication. This test confirmed that J.T. had a duplicated *PMP22* allele and type 1A Charcot-Marie-Tooth disease. She was informed of the diagnosis and counseled that any pregnancy of hers would have a 50% recurrence risk and that, given different reproductive options (see Chapter 17), she would benefit from a session with prenatal genetic counselor prior to planning a pregnancy.

BACKGROUND

Disease Etiology and Incidence

The CMT disorders are a genetically heterogeneous group of hereditary neuropathies involving chronic motor and sensory polyneuropathy, characterized as a distal symmetric polyneuropathy (DSP). CMT has been subdivided according to patterns of inheritance, neuropathological changes, and clinical features. By definition, type 1 CMT (CMT1) is an autosomal dominant demyelinating neuropathy; it has a prevalence of approximately 15 in 100,000 and is genetically heterogeneous. CMT1A, which represents 70 to 80% of CMT1, is caused by increased dosage of *PMP22* secondary to duplication of the *PMP22* locus in chromosome 17p12. *De novo* duplications account for 20 to 33% of CMT1A cases; of these, more than 90% arise during male meiosis.

Pathogenesis

PMP22 is an integral membrane tetraspan glycoprotein. Within the peripheral nervous system, PMP22 is found in compact but not in noncompact myelin. The function of PMP22 has not been fully elucidated, but evidence suggests that it plays a key role in myelin compaction.

Either dominant negative sequence variants within *PMP22* or increased dosage of PMP22 can cause this peripheral polyneuropathy. Increased dosage of PMP22 arises by tandem duplication of a 1.5-Mb region in 17p11.2 flanked by repeated DNA sequences that are approximately 98% identical. Misalignment of these flanking repeat elements during meiosis can lead to unequal crossing over and formation of one chromatid with a duplication of the 1.5-Mb region and another with the reciprocal deletion. (The reciprocal deletion causes the disease hereditary neuropathy with pressure palsies [HNPP].) An individual inheriting a chromosome with the duplication will have three copies of a normal *PMP22* gene and thus overexpress PMP22 (see Chapter 6).

Overexpression of PMP22 or expression of dominant negative forms of PMP22 results in an inability to form and to maintain compact myelin. Nerve biopsy specimens from severely affected infants show a diffuse paucity of myelin, and nerve biopsy specimens from more mildly affected patients show segmental demyelination and myelin sheath hypertrophy. The mechanism by which PMP22 overexpression causes this pathological process remains unclear, but evidence suggests

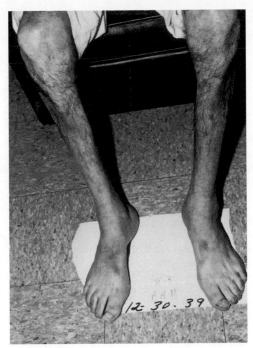

Figure C.8.1 Distal leg muscle wasting in an older man with the *PMP22* duplication. (Courtesy J. R. Lupski, Department of Molecular and Human Genetics, Baylor College of Medicine, Houston.)

that potential protein aggregation and the stimulation of the unfolded protein response may play some role.

The muscle weakness and atrophy observed in CMT1 result from muscle denervation secondary to axonal degeneration. Longitudinal studies of patients have shown an age-dependent reduction in the nerve fiber density that correlates with the development of disease symptoms. In addition, evidence in murine models suggests that myelin is necessary for maintenance of the axonal cytoskeleton. The mechanism by which demyelination alters the axonal cytoskeleton and affects axonal degeneration has not been completely elucidated.

Phenotype and Natural History

CMT1A has nearly full penetrance, although the severity, onset, and progression of CMT1 vary markedly within and among families; variation can even be observed in identical twins. Many affected individuals do not seek medical attention, either because their symptoms are not noticeable or because their symptoms are accommodated easily. On the other hand, others have severe disease that is manifested in infancy or in childhood.

Symptoms of CMT1A usually develop in the first two decades of life; onset after 30 years of age is rare. Typically, symptoms begin with an insidious onset of slowly progressive weakness and atrophy of the distal leg muscles and mild sensory impairment (Fig. C.8.1). The weakness of the feet and legs leads to abnormalities of gait, a dropped foot, and eventually foot deformities (*pes cavus* and hammer toes, but *pes planus* can occur in 10–15% of patients) and loss of balance; it rarely causes individuals to lose their ability to walk. Weakness of the intrinsic hand muscles usually occurs late in the disease course and, in severe cases, causes claw hand deformities because of imbalance between flexor and extensor muscle strength. Hand weakness can manifest as difficulties with buttons or zippers and reduced grip strength. Other associated findings include

decreased or absent reflexes, upper extremity ataxia and tremor, scoliosis, and palpably enlarged superficial nerves. On occasion, the phrenic and autonomic nerves are also involved.

In electrophysiological studies, the hallmark of CMT1A is the uniform slowing of NCVs in all nerves and nerve segments, on both sides of the body, and as a result of demyelination. The full reduction in NCVs is usually present by 2 to 5 years of age, although clinically apparent symptoms may not be manifested for many years.

Management

Although the diagnosis of CMT1 is suspected because of clinical, electrophysiological, and pathological features, a definitive diagnosis often depends on the detection of a pathogenic genomic variant. Inflammatory peripheral neuropathies are frequently difficult to distinguish from CMT1 and HNPP. Before the advent of molecular testing, many patients with inherited neuropathies were treated with immunosuppressants and experienced the associated morbidity without improvement of their neuropathy. All forms of CMT appear to cause an increased susceptibility to neurotoxicity of vincristine; treatment of childhood acute lymphocytic leukemia that yields subsequent acute paralysis may elicit a family history of CMT or a parent with CMT signs or symptoms.

Molecular therapies for several forms of CMT are now becoming available. Paralleling disease progression, therapy generally follows three stages: strengthening and stretching exercises to maintain gait and function, use of orthotics and special adaptive splints, and orthopedic surgery. Further deterioration may require use of ambulatory supports such as canes and walkers or, in rare, severely affected cases, a wheelchair. All should be counseled to avoid exposure to neurotoxic medications and chemicals.

Inheritance

Because the *PMP22* duplication and most *PMP22* single nucleotide variants are autosomal dominant with fully penetrant phenotype, each child of an affected parent has a 50% chance for development of CMT1A. The variable expressivity of the *PMP22* duplication and *PMP22* variants, however, makes prediction of disease severity challenging.

QUESTIONS FOR SMALL GROUP DISCUSSION

1. Genomic deletions and duplications frequently arise by recombination between repetitive sequences within the human genome (see Chapter 6). Name three disorders caused by deletion after presumed recombination between repetitive sequences. Which of these deletions are associated with a reciprocal duplication? What does the identification of a reciprocal duplication suggest about the mechanism of recombination? Does the absence of a reciprocal duplication suggest that it does not exist or that it has just not yet been defined?

2. In general, genomic duplications are associated with less severe disease than genomic deletions. Duplication of a *PMP22* allele, however, usually causes more severe disease than deletion of a *PMP22* allele does. Discuss possible reasons for this.

3. Name two other diseases that are caused by a gene dosage effect.

REFERENCES

Bird TD: Charcot-Marie-Tooth neuropathy type 1. http://www.ncbi.nlm.nih.gov/books/NBK1205/

Harel T, Lupski JR: Charcot-Marie-Tooth disease and pathways to molecular based therapies, *Clin Genet* 86:422–431, 2014.

CHARGE SYNDROME (MIM 214800) (*CHD7* Disorder)

Autosomal Dominant

Donna Martin

PRINCIPLES

- Pleiotropy
- Haploinsufficiency
- Association versus syndrome

MAJOR PHENOTYPIC FEATURES

- Coloboma of the iris, retina, optic disc, or optic nerve
- Heart defects
- Atresia of the choanae
- Retardation of growth and development
- Genital abnormalities
- Ear anomalies
- Facial palsy
- Cleft lip
- Tracheoesophageal fistula

HISTORY AND PHYSICAL FINDINGS

Baby girl E.L. was the product of a full-term pregnancy to a 34-year-old gravida 1, para 1 mother after an uncomplicated pregnancy. At birth, it was noted that E.L.'s right ear was cupped and posteriorly rotated. Because of feeding difficulties, she was placed in the neonatal intensive care unit. Placement of a nasogastric tube was attempted but was unsuccessful in the right naris, demonstrating unilateral choanal atresia. A geneticist determined that she might have CHARGE syndrome. Further evaluation included echocardiography, which revealed a small atrial septal defect; ophthalmological examination demonstrated a retinal coloboma in the left eye. The atrial septal defect was repaired surgically without complications. E.L. failed the newborn hearing screen and was subsequently diagnosed with mild to moderate sensorineural hearing loss. Gene sequencing and deletion/duplication analysis for variants in the gene associated with CHARGE syndrome, *CHD7*, demonstrated a c.5418 C>G heterozygous pathogenic variant in exon 26, predicted to result in a premature termination codon (p.Tyr1806X). Variant analyses in E.L.'s parents were negative, indicating that the variant had occurred *de novo*. Consequently, the family was advised that the recurrence risk in future pregnancies was low but still possible due to parental germline mosaicism. At 1 year of age, E.L. was moderately delayed in gross motor skills and had speech delay. Her height and weight were at the 5th percentile, and head circumference was at the 10th percentile. Yearly follow-up was planned.

BACKGROUND

Disease Etiology and Incidence

CHARGE syndrome (MIM 214800) is an autosomal dominant condition with multiple congenital malformations caused, in most individuals tested, by pathogenic variants in the *CHD7* gene. CHARGE syndrome affects roughly 1 in 10,000 individuals worldwide. However, expanded genetic testing has revealed *CHD7* pathogenic variants in atypical cases, leading to recognition of broader phenotypes in *CHD7*-related disorders.

Pathogenesis

The *CHD7* gene, located at 8q12, is a member of the superfamily of chromodomain helicase DNA-binding (CHD) genes. The proteins in this family are predicted to affect chromatin structure and gene expression in early embryonic development. The *CHD7* gene is expressed broadly in many fetal and adult tissues, including the eye, cochlea, brain, central nervous system, intestine, skeleton, heart, and kidney. Over 500 heterozygous nonsense and missense pathogenic variants in the *CHD7* gene, as well as deletions in the 8q12 region encompassing *CHD7*, have been demonstrated in individuals with CHARGE syndrome, indicating that haploinsufficiency for the gene causes the disease. Most pathogenic variants are novel, although a few hot spots for variants in the gene exist. Some individuals with CHARGE syndrome have no identifiable pathogenic variant in *CHD7*, suggesting that pathogenic variants in other loci or in noncoding regions may underlie the condition.

Phenotype and Natural History

The acronym CHARGE (*c*oloboma, *h*eart defects, *a*tresia of the choanae, *r*etardation of growth and development, *g*enital abnormalities, *e*ar anomalies)—encompassing the most common features of the condition—was coined by dysmorphologists to describe an association of abnormalities of unknown etiology and pathogenesis seen together more often than would be expected by chance. With the discovery of *CHD7* pathogenic variants in CHARGE, the condition is now considered to be a dysmorphic syndrome with a characteristic pattern of causally related anomalies (see Chapter 15). A clinical diagnosis of CHARGE is made when two of the following major diagnostic criteria are met: (1) ocular coloboma (affecting the iris, retina, choroid, or disc with or without microphthalmia), (2) choanal atresia (unilateral or bilateral; stenosis or atresia) or cleft palate, (3) abnormal external, middle or inner ears, including hypoplastic semicircular canals, and (4) pathogenic *CHD7* variant. Multiple other features are commonly observed in CHARGE and *CHD7*-related disorders, including cranial nerve anomalies (with unilateral or bilateral

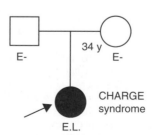

E+ : *CHD7* c.5418C>G (p.Tyr1806X)

Key:
E = *CHD7* targeted sequence, del/dup analysis

Pedigree Case 9

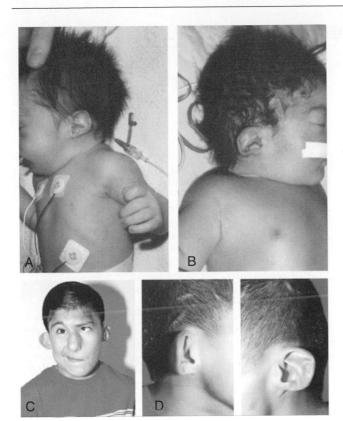

Figure C.9.1 Ear and eye anomalies in individuals with CHARGE syndrome. (*From Jones K: Smith's recognizable patterns of human malformation, ed 6, Philadelphia, 2005, Elsevier.*)

facial palsy or swallowing problems), congenital heart defect, growth deficiency, and tracheoesophageal fistula or esophageal atresia. (see Figure C.9.1.)

Perinatal or early infant mortality (before 6 months of age) is seen in approximately half of affected individuals and appears to be correlated with the most severe congenital anomalies, including bilateral posterior choanal atresia and congenital heart defects. Gastroesophageal reflux is a significant cause of morbidity and mortality. Feeding problems are also common; as many as 50% of adolescent and adult individuals require gastrostomy tube placement. Delayed puberty is found in the majority of individuals with CHARGE syndrome. Developmental delay or intellectual disability can occur, ranging from mild to severe, and behavioral abnormalities (including hyperactivity, sleep disturbances, and obsessive-compulsive behavior) are frequent. As CHD7 variant testing delineates more individuals with CHARGE, the features of the condition may become better defined and the phenotypic spectrum widened.

Management

If CHARGE syndrome is suspected, thorough evaluation is warranted for possible choanal atresia or stenosis (unilateral), congenital heart defect, central nervous system abnormalities, renal anomalies, hearing loss, and feeding difficulties. Management consists of surgical correction of malformations and supportive care. Developmental evaluation is an important component of follow-up. With the availability of testing for CHD7 pathogenic variants, a molecular diagnosis can be made in at least 70-80% of individuals. With broader application of next generation sequencing, CHD7 variants are increasingly likely to be uncovered through gene panel, exome, or genome wide sequencing approaches. SEMA3E pathogenic variants are found and may be another rare cause of the syndrome.

Inheritance

Almost all cases of CHARGE syndrome are due to new dominant pathogenic variants, with the majority arising in the paternal germline. Recurrence risk is therefore low for future offspring. There have been reported cases of monozygotic twins having CHARGE, as well as families with multiple affected siblings (male and female). The latter situation is consistent with parental germline mosaicism; unaffected or mildly affected individuals may also have somatic mosaicism for pathogenic CHD7 variants. If a pathogenic variant in CHD7 is found in an affected individual and both parents test negative for the variant, the recurrence risk for future offspring is thought to be less than 5%. For an affected individual, the risk of recurrence in his or her offspring is 50%.

QUESTIONS FOR SMALL GROUP DISCUSSION

1. Explain the difference between an association and a syndrome. Give an example of a common association.
2. By what mechanism could haploinsufficiency for a chromodomain protein cause the pleiotropic effects of CHARGE syndrome?
3. Why would you counsel the parents of a child with a proven *de novo* pathogenic variant in CHD7 of a 5% recurrence risk? Would the risk change if their next child were affected?

REFERENCES

Hale CL, Niederriter AN, Green GE, Martin DM: Atypical phenotypes associated with pathogenic CHD7 variants and a proposal for broadening CHARGE syndrome clinical diagnostic criteria, *Am J Med Genet A* 170A:344–354, 2016.

Hus P, Ma A, Wilson M, *et al*: CHARGE syndrome: a review, *J Paediatr Child Health* 50:504–511, 2014.

Janssen N, Bergman JE, Swertz MA, *et al*: Mutation update on the CHD7 gene involved in CHARGE syndrome, *Hum Mutat* 33:1149–1160, 2012.

Pauli S, von Velsen N, Burfeind P, *et al*: CHD7 mutations causing CHARGE syndrome are predominantly of paternal origin, *Clin Genet* 8:234–239, 2012.

van Ravenswaaij-Arts, C.M., Hefner, M., MS, Kim Blake, K., and Martin, D.M.: CHD7 Disorder. Available from: https://www.ncbi.nlm.nih.gov/books/NBK1117/

CHRONIC MYELOGENOUS LEUKEMIA (MIM 608232)
(*BCR-ABL1* Oncogene)
Somatic Mutation

Johann Hitzler

PRINCIPLES

- Chromosomal abnormality
- Oncogene activation
- Fusion protein
- Molecularly targeted cancer therapy based on inhibition of a constitutively active fusion tyrosine kinase

MAJOR PHENOTYPIC FEATURES

- Age at onset: middle to late adulthood
- Leukocytosis
- Splenomegaly
- Fatigue and malaise

HISTORY AND PHYSICAL FINDINGS

E.S., a 45-year-old woman, presented to her family physician for her annual checkup. She had been in good health and had no specific complaints. On examination, she had a palpable spleen tip but no other abnormal findings. Results of her complete blood count unexpectedly showed an elevated white blood cell count of 31×10^9/L and a platelet count of 650×10^9/L. The peripheral blood smear revealed basophilia and immature granulocytes. Her physician referred her to the oncology department for further evaluation. Her bone marrow was found to be hypercellular, with an increased number of myeloid and megakaryocytic cells and an increased ratio of myeloid to erythroid cells. Cytogenetic analysis of her marrow identified several myeloid cells with a Philadelphia chromosome, der(22) t(9;22)(q34;q11.2). Her oncologist explained that she had chronic myelogenous leukemia in the chronic phase (CP-CML), which, although indolent now, had a substantial risk of progressing to life-threatening leukemia in the next few years. She was also advised that, while previously, this disease was only curable by allogeneic stem cell transplantation, newly developed oral drug therapy with tyrosine kinase inhibitors (TKI) is now used as first line treatment. TKI targets the function of the oncogene in chronic myelogenous leukemia and can achieve long-lasting remissions and a near-normal life expectancy in most patients.

BACKGROUND
Disease Etiology and Incidence

Chronic myelogenous leukemia (CML, MIM 608232) is a clonal myeloproliferative disorder that is characterized by the accumulation of transformed, initially mature-appearing cells of myeloid lineage cells in blood and bone marrow. Transformation of a pluripotent hematopoietic stem cell occurs by expression of the *BCR-ABL1* oncogene generated by the t(9;22)(q34;q11). CML accounts for 15% of adult leukemia and has an incidence of 1 to 2/100,000 individuals; the age-adjusted incidence is higher in men than in women (1.3 to 1.7 vs 1.0).

Pathogenesis

Approximately 95% of patients with CML have a Philadelphia chromosome (see Chapter 16); the remainder have complex or variant translocations. The Abelson protooncogene 1 (*ABL1*)

encodes a nonreceptor tyrosine kinase and maps to 9q34; the breakpoint cluster region gene (*BCR*), which encodes a phosphoprotein, maps to 22q11. During the formation of the Philadelphia chromosome, the *ABL1* gene is disrupted in intron 1 and the *BCR* gene in one of three breakpoint cluster regions; the *BCR* and *ABL1* gene fragments are joined head to tail on the derivative chromosome 22 (Fig. C.10.1). The *BCR-ABL1* fusion gene on the derivative chromosome 22 generates a fusion protein that varies in size according to the length of the BCR peptide attached to the amino terminus. (Three principal size forms in CML are the predominant p210, as well as p190 and p230.)

To date, the normal functions of ABL1 and BCR have not been clearly defined. ABL1 has been conserved well throughout metazoan evolution. It is found in both the nucleus and cytoplasm and as a myristoylated product associated with the inner cytoplasmic membrane. The relative abundance of ABL1 in these compartments varies among cell types and in response to stimuli. ABL1 participates in the cell cycle, stress responses, integrin signaling, and neural development. The functional domains of BCR include a coiled-coil motif for polymerization with other proteins, a serine-threonine kinase domain, a GDP-GTP exchange domain involved in the regulation of Ras

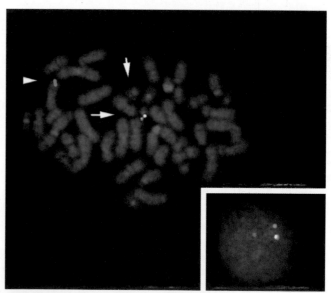

Figure C.10.1 FISH analysis in metaphase and interphase (*inset*) cells for the detection of the t(9;22)(q34;q11.2) in CML. The DNA is counterstained with DAPI. The probe is a mixture of DNA probes specific for the *BCR* gene (*red*) at 22q11.2 and for the *ABL1* gene (*green*) at 9q34. In cells with the t(9;22), a green signal is observed on the normal chromosome 9 (*arrowhead*) and a red signal on the normal chromosome 22 (*short arrow*). As a result of the translocation of *ABL1* to the der(22) chromosome, a yellow fusion signal (*long arrow*) is observed from the presence of both green and red signals together on the Philadelphia chromosome. (Courtesy M. M. LeBeau and H. T. Abelson, University of Chicago.)

family members, and a guanosine triphosphatase–activating domain for regulating Rac and Rho GTPases.

Expression of ABL1 does not result in cellular transformation, whereas expression of the BCR-ABL1 fusion protein does. Transgenic mice expressing BCR-ABL1 develop acute leukemia at birth, and infection of normal mice with a retrovirus expressing BCR-ABL1 causes a variety of acute and chronic leukemias, depending on the genetic background. In contrast to ABL1, BCR-ABL1 has constitutive tyrosine kinase activity and is confined to the cytoplasm, where it avidly binds actin microfilaments. BCR-ABL1 phosphorylates several cytoplasmic substrates and thereby activates signaling cascades – such as RAS/RAF/MEK/ERK, PI3K/AKT/mTOR, and JAK2/STAT5 – that control growth and differentiation and possibly adhesion of hematopoietic cells. Unregulated activation of these signaling pathways results in unregulated proliferation of the hematopoietic stem cell, release of immature cells from the marrow, and ultimately CML.

As CML progresses, it becomes increasingly aggressive. During this evolution, tumor cells of 50 to 80% of patients acquire additional chromosomal changes (trisomy 8, i(17q), or trisomy 19), another Philadelphia chromosome, or both. In addition to the cytogenetic changes, tumor-suppressor genes (e.g., *TP53*, *CDKN2A*, *RB1*), oncogenes (e.g., *RUNX1*, *NRAS*, *KRAS*, Wnt/beta-catenin pathway), and genes important in epigenetic regulation (e.g., *ASXL1*, *TET2*) (see Chapter 8) are also frequently mutated during the progression of CML.

Phenotype and Natural History

CML is a biphasic or triphasic disease. The initial or chronic stage is characterized by an insidious onset, with subsequent development of fatigue, malaise, weight loss, and minimal to moderate splenic enlargement. Over time, CML typically evolves to an accelerated phase and then to a blast crisis, although some patients progress directly from the chronic phase to the blast crisis. CML progression includes development of additional chromosomal abnormalities within tumor cells, progressive leukocytosis, anemia, thrombocytosis or thrombocytopenia, increasing splenomegaly, fever, and bone lesions. Blast crisis is an acute leukemia in which the blasts can be myeloid, lymphoid, erythroid, or undifferentiated. The accelerated phase is intermediate between the chronic phase and blast crisis.

Approximately 85% of patients are diagnosed in the chronic phase. Depending on the study, the median age at diagnosis ranges from 45 to 65 years, although all ages, including children and adolescents, can be affected. Untreated, the rate of progression from the chronic phase to blast crisis is approximately 5 to 10% during the first 2 years and then 20% per year subsequently. Because blast crisis is rapidly fatal, demise parallels progression to blast crisis. A major goal of CML treatment is the prevention of progression from the chronic to advanced stage.

Management

Recognition of the constitutive activation of the BCR-ABL1 fusion kinase as the molecular basis of CML led to the development of several generations of BCR-ABL1 TKIs, including imatinib (FDA approved in 2001), dasatinib, nilotinib, bosutinib, and ponatinib. TKIs are now the first line of treatment for CML. More than 85% of patients have a clear cytogenetic response after imatinib therapy, with disappearance of the t(9;22) in cells obtained by bone marrow aspirates. Response to daily and continued treatment with TKI is monitored by measurement of *BCR-ABL1* transcripts in the blood by quantitative RT-PCR. Results are compared to a standardized

baseline and expressed as a ratio (% on the International Scale, IS). Patients who do not meet milestones of *BCR-ABL1* transcript reduction at defined time points (e.g., 3, 6, 12 months) are investigated, by sequencing, for TKI resistance due to single nucleotide variants of the BCR-ABL1 kinase domain; they can be treated with a second-line TKI, depending on the mutational profile. Complete cytogenetic response corresponds to at least a 2-log reduction of *BCR-ABL1* transcripts ($\leq$1% IS). A major molecular response consists of at least a 3-log reduction ($\leq$0.1% IS) and is associated with a very low probability of CML progression. TKIs, however, have to be administered daily and may be associated with side effects that decrease quality of life (e.g., fatigue, muscle cramps). In addition to progression-free survival, an important goal of treatment of CML is to define subsets of patients who may be able to stop TKI treatment after several years. Depth and duration of molecular response (as assayed every 3–6 months by qRT-PCR) help to define this subset. Treatment of patients in blast crisis, in which blasts may have a myeloid or lymphoid phenotype, remains a challenge. It includes evaluation of patients for allogeneic stem cell transplantation (SCT), considering the fitness of the patient and donor availability. Success of SCT depends on the stage of CML, the age and health of the patient, the bone marrow donor (related vs unrelated), the preparative regimen, the development of graft-versus-host disease, and the posttransplantation treatment, which may include a TKI. Much of the long-term success of SCT depends on a graft versus-leukemia effect, that is, a graft-versus-host response directed against the leukemic cells. After SCT, patients are monitored frequently for relapse, by RT-PCR to detect *BCR-ABL1* transcripts, and treated as necessary.

Patients in blast crisis are treated with TKI, chemotherapy and, if possible, SCT. The outcome of these therapies for blast crisis remains poor.

Inheritance

Because CML arises from a somatic mutation that is not found in the germline, the risk for a patient to pass the disease to his or her children is zero. Due to the risk of teratogenicity, treatment with TKI is contraindicated during pregnancy.

QUESTIONS FOR SMALL GROUP DISCUSSION

1. Discuss three mechanisms of protooncogene activation in human cancer.
2. Neoplasias graphically illustrate the effects of the accumulation of somatic variants; however, other less dramatic diseases arise, at least in part, through the accumulation of somatic variants. Discuss the effect of somatic mutation on aging.
3. Many variants arising from somatic mutation and cytogenetic rearrangements are never detected because the cells containing them do not have a selective advantage. What advantage does the Philadelphia chromosome confer?
4. Name other cancers caused by fusion genes resulting in oncogene activation. Which others have been successfully targeted?

REFERENCES

Braun TP, Eide CA, Druker BJ: Response and resistance to BCR-ABL1-targeted therapies, *Cancer Cell* 37(4):530–542, 2020.

Hehlmann R: Chronic myeloid leukemia in 2020, *HemaSphere* 4(5):e468, 2020.

Zhou T, Medeiros LJ, Hu S: Chronic myeloid leukemia: Beyond BCR-ABL1, *Curr Hematol Malig Rep* 13(6):435–445, 2018.

INFLAMMATORY BOWEL DISEASE (MIM 266600)

Xiao P. Peng

PRINCIPLES

- Multifactorial – genetic susceptibility, host exposures and commensals, epithelial integrity
- Age-related variability in penetrance and effect size

MAJOR PHENOTYPIC FEATURES

- Location dependent, but any segment of the intestinal tract may be involved
  - Abdominal pain, hematochezia, diarrhea, obstruction, fistulas, abscesses
- Extraintestinal manifestations including inflammation of the joints, eyes, and skin
- Crohn disease
  - Transmural ulceration and granulomas, leading to strictures and fistulas
  - Patchy involvement, typically of terminal ileum; small and large bowel may be affected
- Ulcerative colitis
  - Diffuse friability and superficial erosions starting in rectum and extending proximally in a continuous manner
  - Inflammation restricted to the mucosa and submucosa of the colon

HISTORY AND PHYSICAL FINDINGS

P.L., a 26-year-old male, was referred to outpatient Genetics clinic by his gastroenterologist for evaluation of his personal and family history of IBD and other autoimmune concerns. He reported a 2-year history of progressively worsening weight loss, severe nonbloody diarrhea, and acute-on-chronic abdominal pain and nausea with ongoing steroid dependence and refractory to multiple biologics. In infancy, he was diagnosed with milk protein allergy, then celiac disease, but gluten was reintroduced into his diet at age 6 without issue. He had lifetime eczema and was diagnosed with type 1 diabetes (T1DM) at age 14. His infection history was notable for a few "chest infections" in childhood and two episodes of mild shingles after natural chickenpox infection. Family history is shown in Figure C.11.1. Physical examination revealed severe popliteal eczema and diffuse lower abdominal tenderness to palpation without palpable masses or organomegaly.

Treatment-naive studies included a peripheral blood count showing leukocytosis and microcytic hypochromic anemia and blood chemistries showing low albumin and globulin levels. Immunophenotyping found low IgG and mildly elevated IgE levels, suboptimal vaccine responses, and mildly low CD4+T cell and natural killer cell numbers. Computerized tomography scan showed mucosal inflammation extending from distal ileum to ascending colon. Upper endoscopy and colonoscopy with biopsy revealed transmural ulceration of the distal ileum with ulceration of the ileocecal junction, consistent with Crohn disease.

Exome sequencing (for P.L., his brother, M.L., and both parents) identified a hemizygous maternally inherited FOXP3 missense variant in P.L. and M.L., as well as a paternally

inherited NOD2 variant (p.Arg702Trp) in M.L. The former was consistent with P.L.'s history of multisystem immune dysregulation; he was referred to Immunology, who started him on sirolimus with good effect, while stem cell transplant was explored for both brothers. Counseling provided to M.L. and his father regarding their shared NOD2 risk allele is detailed below; this was considered to contribute to M.L.'s early age of IBD onset and his father's history of gastrointestinal (GI) and extra-GI problems. More extensive family history-taking identified additional affected relatives who would benefit from genetic counseling and cascade testing.

BACKGROUND

Disease Etiology and Incidence

Inflammatory bowel disease (IBD, MIM 266600) is a chronic systemic inflammatory disease predominantly affecting the GI tract, which has been traditionally classified into three subgroups: Crohn disease (CD), ulcerative colitis (UC), and unclassified. Northern Europe and North America harbor the highest worldwide incidence and prevalence of IBD. There is a particularly high incidence in Northern Europeans and individuals of Ashkenazi Jewish descent (incidence 3.2/1000), though historically low rates in Asia, Africa, and South America are changing with increased industrialization. Both UC and CD show bimodal incidence, with ~12 to 20% of individuals developing symptoms before age 20.

Evolving Genetic Paradigms of Inheritance

IBD is a multifactorial disorder associated with an increasingly diverse range of genetic and environmental contributions. Both CD and UC show familial clustering and increased concordance for closer degrees of kinship, but reported rates differ significantly across studies. Genome-wide association studies (GWASs) thus far have identified ~300 loci linked to adult-onset IBD, many of which overlap with pediatric-onset IBD and other autoimmune and autoinflammatory conditions. The majority of these common genetic risk alleles have small effects (odds ratio <1.5) and explain only approximately 13% and 8% of the variance in disease heritability for CD and UC, respectively. Exome sequencing studies have also contributed an expanding list of rare monogenic variants with Mendelian inheritance patterns for IBD and associated conditions. Thus IBD-associated loci fall along a spectrum of allele frequencies and effect sizes – from more penetrant, rare monogenic etiologies to more common alleles associated with reduced penetrance (Fig. C.11.2), as seen in the case above.

Pathogenesis

Nearly 100 causative genes and loci have been associated with robust IBD risk to date, including long-held associations with developmental syndromes such as Down syndrome, Turner syndrome (Case 47), and chr22q11 deletion syndrome (Case 22). Some monogenic IBD lesions specifically impair GI homeostasis and function, while others cause inborn

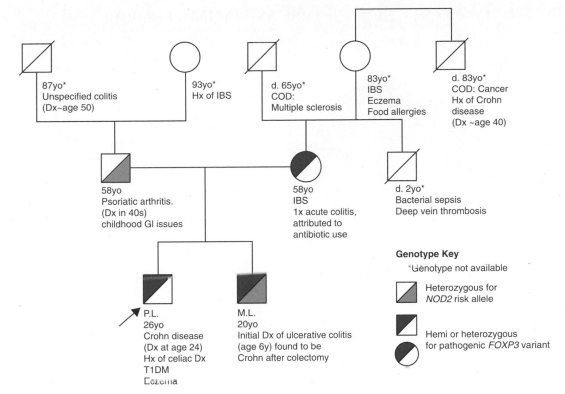

Figure C.11.1 Three-generation family history. *COD*, cause of death; *Dx*, diagnosis; *GI*, gastrointestinal; *Hx*, history; *IBS*, irritable bowel syndrome; *T1DM*, type 1 diabetes mellitus; *yo*, years old.

errors of immunity with pleiotropic multi-organ involvement. Identification of these monogenic etiologies has helped shed light on pathogenesis of the more "typical" polygenic etiologies, suggesting not only overlapping mechanisms but also shared potential therapies.

NOD2, the first gene associated with susceptibility to Crohn disease (CD) [MIM:266600], highlights the importance of host immune tolerance and interactions with the intestinal microbiota to IBD pathogenesis. Three common *NOD2* variants – R702W, G908R, and 1007fs – are individually associated with two- to four-fold increased risk for CD, but the risk increases to 17-fold for biallelic combinations. All three variants are located within the leucine-rich repeat domain of the NOD2 protein, which triggers inflammatory responses upon binding to bacterial components. Between 30 and 50% of those with CD in the Western hemisphere carry disease-associated *NOD2* variants, but the low penetrance (<10%) associated with even the highest-risk *NOD2* genotypes and their lack of association with CD in Asian or African populations points to as-yet-unidentified genetic or environmental factors.

Phenotype and Natural History

CD can occur anywhere along the GI mucosa, with patches of granulomatous inflammation penetrating the wall of the intestine to involve all layers of the bowel (transmural). Strictures, fistulous tracks, and abscesses are frequent, and the mucosa evolves a "cobblestone" appearance over time. In contrast, mucosal inflammation in UC begins at the rectum and progresses continuously to the proximal colon, leading to edema, ulcers, bleeding, and electrolyte losses. Pancolitis is seen in ~15% of patients. In chronic UC, the rigid colon loses its haustral markings, leading to a "lead-pipe" appearance.

Even without treatment, individuals with IBD show immune deficits such as suboptimal vaccine memory, but they are also predisposed to extraintestinal inflammation of the skin, eyes, and bones and other comorbidities. Age of onset, severity, progression, family history, and endoscopic and systemic findings help distinguish monogenic from polygenic forms of IBD. Importantly, age does not rule out the possibility of monogenic etiologies, as genes historically associated with early-onset disease, such as *FOXP3* in this case, are increasingly identified in older patients.

Management

Currently, there is no cure for IBD, so the goals of treatment include induction and maintenance of remission, minimization of mucosal injury, bowel loss and adverse effects, and quality of life improvement. Four main therapeutic categories have traditionally been used: Corticosteroids, antiinflammatory drugs, immunosuppressive agents, and immune modulators. Some therapies currently under investigation target specific steps in the pathogenesis of IBD, while others are also being studied for use in other disorders with which IBD shares overlapping pathophysiologies. Identification of a monogenic etiology may inform additional management approaches. Hematopoietic stem-cell transplantation (HSCT) can be curative for some monogenic forms of IBD, but other strategies such as gene therapy or metabolic modulation may also be considered. Finally, regardless of etiology, vigilance must always be maintained regarding the potential for GI malignancy.

Inheritance

The empirical risk for development of IBD is not compatible with classic autosomal recessive or dominant inheritance, but is high compared with the risk in the general population (the relative risk ratio, λs, for siblings is between 10 and 30 (see Chapters 9 and 17)). Genetic epidemiological data,

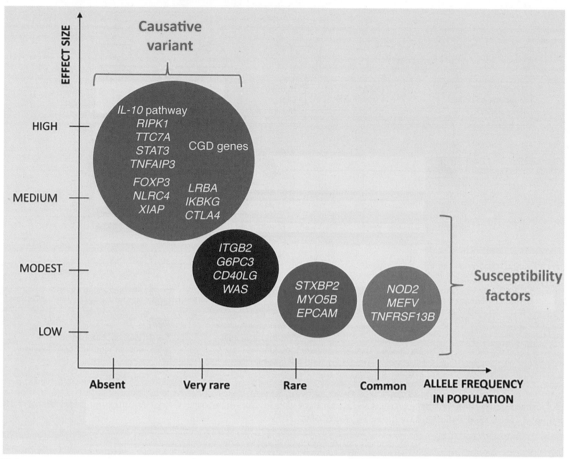

Figure C.11.2 McCarthy/Manolio model of the current IBD genetic landscape. Some examples of IBD-associated genes are plotted showing the range of allelic effect sizes and frequencies with which they are typically associated; *CGD*, chronic granulomatous disease.

including from twin studies, support classification of IBD as a disorder with a strong genetic contribution but with complex inheritance.

QUESTIONS FOR SMALL GROUP DISCUSSION

1. Discuss the host factors that play a role in IBD.
2. What are some features in an individual's personal and family history that would make you more suspicious of a monogenic IBD etiology?
3. What clinical and functional tests would you obtain to assess for a potentially monogenic IBD etiology? How would these inform your molecular testing strategy?
4. How should a family member of a patient with CD who is found to have one of the *NOD2* variants be counseled? Should the testing be performed and reported? Why or why not?

KEY REFERENCES

Bianco AM, Girardelli M, Tommasini A: Genetics of inflammatory bowel disease from multifactorial to monogenic forms, *World J Gastroenterol* 21(43):12296–12310, 2015. https://doi.org/10.3748/wjg.v21.i43.12296 PMID: 26604638; PMCID: PMC4649114.

Bolton C, Smillie CS, Pandey S, Elmentaite R, Wei G, Argmann C, Aschenbrenner D, James KR, McGovern DPB, Macchi M, Cho J, Shouval DS, Kammermeier J, Koletzko S, Bagalopal K, Capitani M, Cavounidis A, Pires E, Weidinger C, McCullagh J, Arkwright PD, Haller W, Siegmund B, Peters L, Jostins L, Travis SPL, Anderson CA, Snapper S, Klein C, Schadt E, Zilbauer M, Xavier R, Teichmann S, Muise AM, Regev A, Uhlig HH: An integrated taxonomy for monogenic inflammatory bowel disease, *Gastroenterology* S0016-5085(21):03737-9, 2021. https://doi.org/10.1053/j.gastro.2021.11.014. Epub ahead of print. PMID: 34780721.

Economou M, Trikalinos TA, Loizou KT, Tsianos EV, Ioannidis JP: Differential effects of NOD2 variants on Crohn's disease risk and phenotype in diverse populations: A metaanalysis, *Am J Gastroenterol* 99(12):2393–2404, 2004. https://doi.org/10.1111/j.1572-0241.2004.40304.x. PMID: 15571588.

Nambu R, Warner N, Mulder DJ, Kotlarz D, McGovern DPB, Cho J, Klein C, Snapper SB, Griffiths AM, Iwama I, Muise AM: A systematic review of monogenic inflammatory bowel disease, *Clin Gastroenterol Hepatol* S1542-3565(21):00331-1, 2021. https://doi.org/10.1016/j.cgh.2021.03.021. Epub ahead of print. PMID: 33746097; PMCID: PMC8448782.

Somineni HK, Nagpal S, Venkateswaran S, Cutler DJ, Okou DT, Haritunians T, Simpson CL, Begum F, Datta LW, Quiros AJ, Seminerio J, Mengesha E, Alexander JS, Baldassano RN, Dudley-Brown S, Cross RK, Dassopoulos T, Denson LA, Dhere TA, Iskandar H, Dryden GW, Hou JK, Hussain SZ, Hyams JS, Isaacs KL, Kader H, Kappelman MD, Katz J, Kellermayer R, Kuemmerle JF, Lazarev M, Li E, Mannon P, Moulton DE, Newberry RD, Patel AS, Pekow J, Saeed SA, Valentine JF, Wang MH, McCauley JL, Abreu MT, Jester T, Molle-Rios Z, Palle S, Scherl EJ, Kwon J, Rioux JD, Duerr RH, Silverberg MS, Zwick ME, Stevens C, Daly MJ, Cho JH, Gibson G, McGovern DPB, Brant SR, Kugathasan S: Whole-genome sequencing of African Americans implicates differential genetic architecture in inflammatory bowel disease, *Am J Hum Genet* 108(3):431–445, 2021. https://doi.org/10.1016/j.ajhg.2021.02.001. Epub 2021 Feb 17. PMID: 33600772; PMCID: PMC8008495.

CYSTIC FIBROSIS (MIM 219700) (*CFTR* Pathogenic Variants)

Autosomal Recessive

Karen Raraigh

PRINCIPLES

- Variation in variant frequency by ancestry
- Variable expressivity
- Tissue-specific expression of variants
- Genetic and environmental modifiers

MAJOR PHENOTYPIC FEATURES

- Age at onset: neonatal to adulthood
- Progressive pulmonary disease
- Exocrine pancreatic insufficiency
- Obstructive azoospermia
- Elevated sweat chloride concentration
- Growth failure
- Meconium ileus

HISTORY AND PHYSICAL FINDINGS

L.G., a 13-day-old male infant, was referred to the CF pediatric specialty clinic for evaluation and consultation following a positive newborn screen for cystic fibrosis (CF). L.G. was born after an uncomplicated pregnancy and underwent routine newborn screening in his home state. His immunoreactive trypsinogen (IRT) level was elevated at 102 ng/mL and his newborn screening sample was therefore reflexed to a *CFTR* genotyping panel, which identified one *CFTR* variant: c.613C>T (aka P205S). The combination of an elevated IRT and one identified *CFTR* variant is considered a positive newborn screen for CF, and L.G. was referred for diagnostic sweat testing at 10 days of age. His results were 71 mmol/L and 75 mmol/L (normal, <30 mmol/L; indeterminate, 30–59 mmol/L), a level consistent with CF.

L.G.'s parents reported no concerns about his health prior to learning the newborn screening result. He regained his birth weight, was feeding well, and had normal stooling. During the clinic visit, L.G.'s weight, height, and head circumference all plotted within the normal range and his physical examination

was unremarkable. Discussion focused on the typical disease progression of CF, treatment and management, and details regarding L.G.'s *CFTR* variant. The P205S variant is associated with pancreatic sufficiency and confers a degree of residual CFTR function, making it amenable to treatment with CFTR modulator therapy.

Following the visit, additional genetic testing was ordered to identify L.G.'s second causal *CFTR* variant. Full *CFTR* sequencing and deletion/duplication analysis confirmed the finding of P205S and identified a common exon deletion: CFTRdele2,3. Parental testing later confirmed that the variants were in *trans*.

During L.G.'s evaluation, his parents reported no known family history of CF, nor had they undergone CF carrier screening. They reported that they are of Spanish/Irish (maternal) and Russian (paternal) ancestry and denied consanguinity. They have a 3-year-old daughter (S.G.) who is generally healthy but has a history of lingering cough after respiratory infections and has previously been hospitalized with bronchitis. Given L.G.'s recent diagnosis, sweat testing and genetic analysis were performed on his sister. Her sweat chloride levels were 78 and 80 mmol/L and genetic testing identified the same two *CFTR* variants found in L.G., confirming a CF diagnosis. Notably, S.G. was born when the family's home state was using an IRT-IRT algorithm for CF newborn screening, in which the threshold for IRT elevation is higher and no genetic testing is performed.

BACKGROUND

Disease Etiology and Incidence

Cystic fibrosis (CF, MIM 219700) is an autosomal recessive disorder of epithelial ion transport caused by variation in the CF transmembrane conductance regulator gene (*CFTR*) (see Chapter 13). Although CF has been observed in all ancestral backgrounds, it is most common in individuals of northern European ancestry. The live birth incidence of CF ranges from

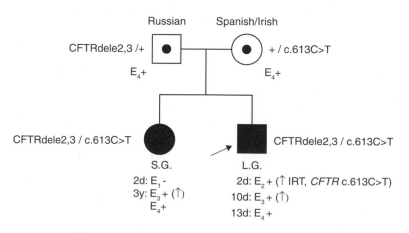

Russian — CFTRdele2,3 /+ ☐● E$_4$+

Spanish/Irish — +/ c.613C>T ○● E$_4$+

CFTRdele2,3 / c.613C>T
S.G.
2d: E$_1$ -
3y: E$_3$ + (↑)
E$_4$+

CFTRdele2,3 / c.613C>T
L.G.
2d: E$_2$ + (↑ IRT, *CFTR* c.613C>T)
10d: E$_3$ + (↑)
13d: E$_4$ +

Key:

◆ cyctic fibrosis (pancreatic sufficient)

E$_1$ = newborn screen IRT-IRT
E$_2$ = newborn screen IRT-DNA
E$_3$ = sweat chloride test
E$_4$ = *CFTR* sequence, deletion/duplication test

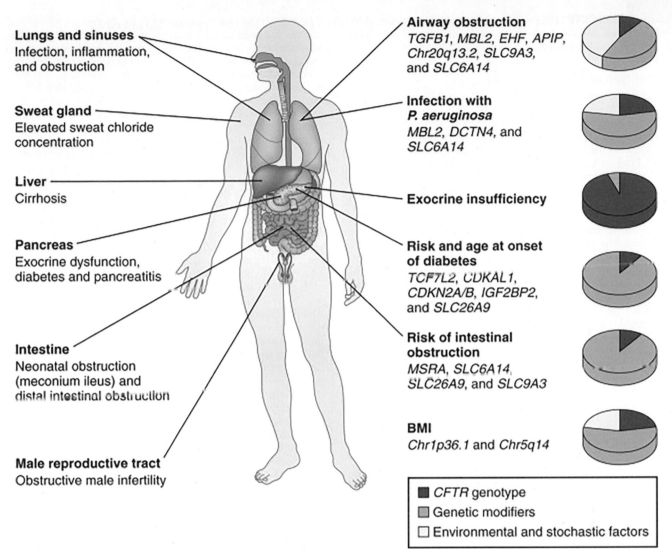

Lungs and sinuses
Infection, inflammation, and obstruction

Sweat gland
Elevated sweat chloride concentration

Liver
Cirrhosis

Pancreas
Exocrine dysfunction, diabetes and pancreatitis

Intestine
Neonatal obstruction (meconium ileus) and distal intestinal obstruction

Male reproductive tract
Obstructive male infertility

Airway obstruction
TGFB1, MBL2, EHF, APIP, Chr20q13.2, SLC9A3, and *SLC6A14*

Infection with *P. aeruginosa*
MBL2, DCTN4, and *SLC6A14*

Exocrine insufficiency

Risk and age at onset of diabetes
TCF7L2, CDKAL1, CDKN2A/B, IGF2BP2, and *SLC26A9*

Risk of intestinal obstruction
MSRA, SLC6A14, SLC26A9, and *SLC9A3*

BMI
Chr1p36.1 and *Chr5q14*

- ■ *CFTR* genotype
- ▨ Genetic modifiers
- ☐ Environmental and stochastic factors

Figure C.12.1 Cardinal features of cystic fibrosis (*CF*) and relative contribution of genetic modifiers to variation in select cystic fibrosis traits. A diagnosis of CF is based on the presence of clinical findings shown on the left, along with an elevated sweat chloride concentration (>60 mM). The degree of organ system dysfunction varies considerably among affected individuals. Genetic modifiers and nongenetic factors both contribute to airway obstruction and infection with Pseudomonas aeruginosa – two traits that define lung disease in CF. CF transmembrane conductance regulator (*CFTR*) genotype is the primary determinant of the degree of pancreatic exocrine dysfunction. The presence of *CFTR* variants associated with severe pancreatic exocrine dysfunction is essentially a prerequisite for the development of diabetes and intestinal obstruction. In the setting of severe endocrine dysfunction, genetic modifiers determine when, and if, diabetes occurs and whether neonatal intestinal obstruction occurs. Genetic variation plays the predominant part in nutritional status as assessed by body mass index. (From Hiatt, PW, Mann, MC, Moffett, KS. *Feigin and Cherry's textbook of pediatric infectious diseases*, 2019. © 2019.)

1 in 313 among the Hutterites of southern Alberta, Canada, to 1 in 90,000 among the Asian population of Hawaii. Among US individuals identified as white, the incidence is 1 in 3200.

Pathogenesis

CFTR is an anion channel that conducts chloride and bicarbonate. It is regulated by ATP and by phosphorylation by cAMP-dependent protein kinase. CFTR facilitates the maintenance of hydration of airway secretions through the transport of chloride and inhibition of sodium uptake (see Chapter 13). Dysfunction of CFTR can affect many different organs, particularly those that secrete mucus, including the upper and lower respiratory tracts, pancreas, biliary system, male genitalia, intestine, and sweat glands (Fig. C.12.1).

The dehydrated and viscous secretions in the lungs of individuals with CF interfere with mucociliary clearance,

inhibit the function of naturally occurring antimicrobial peptides, provide a medium for growth of pathogenic organisms, and obstruct airflow. Within the first months of life, these secretions and the bacteria colonizing them initiate an inflammatory reaction. The release of inflammatory cytokines, host antibacterial enzymes, and bacterial enzymes damages the bronchioles. Recurrent cycles of infection, inflammation, and tissue destruction decrease the amount of functional lung tissue and eventually lead to respiratory failure.

Loss of CFTR chloride transport into the pancreatic duct impairs the hydration of secretions and leads to the retention of exocrine enzymes in the pancreas. Damage from these retained enzymes eventually causes fibrosis of the pancreas.

CFTR also regulates the uptake of sodium and chloride from sweat as it moves through the sweat duct. In the absence of functional CFTR, the sweat has an increased sodium chloride content, and this is the basis of the historical "salty baby syndrome" and the diagnostic sweat chloride test.

Phenotype and Natural History

CF classically manifests in early childhood, although approximately 4% of patients are diagnosed in adulthood; 15 to 20% of patients present at birth with meconium ileus, and the remainder present with chronic respiratory complaints (rhinitis, sinusitis, obstructive lung disease), poor growth, or both later in life. The poor growth results from a combination of increased caloric expenditure because of chronic lung infections and malnutrition from pancreatic exocrine insufficiency. About 5 to 15% of individuals with CF do not develop pancreatic insufficiency. More than 95% of males with CF are azoospermic due to congenital bilateral absence of the vas deferens. The progression of lung disease is the chief determinant of morbidity and mortality. Most patients die of respiratory failure and right ventricular failure secondary to the destruction of lung parenchyma and high pulmonary vascular resistance (cor pulmonale); the current median age of survival is over 50 years in North America and other regions of the world.

In addition to CF, variation within *CFTR* has been associated with a spectrum of diseases, including isolated obstructive azoospermia, idiopathic pancreatitis, disseminated bronchiectasis, allergic bronchopulmonary aspergillosis, atypical sinopulmonary disease, and asthma. In certain individuals, such conditions may be diagnosed as CFTR-related disorders, indicating modest loss of CFTR function that does not result in enough symptoms to meet the clinical diagnostic criteria for CF. These conditions may be associated with heterozygous variants within a single *CFTR* allele or – like CF – may be observed only when variants are present in both *CFTR* alleles. A direct causative role for pathogenic *CFTR* alleles has been established for some, but not all of these disorders.

Correlation between specific *CFTR* variant alleles, their resulting level of CFTR dysfunction, and CF disease severity exists for pancreatic insufficiency and sweat chloride. Secondary variation or other variants within a *CFTR* allele may alter the efficiency of splicing or protein maturation, thereby expanding the spectrum of disease associated with some variants. In addition, some variants in *CFTR* cause disease manifestations only in certain tissues; for example, some affecting the efficiency of splicing have a greater effect on Wolffian duct derivatives than in other tissues because of a tissue-specific need for full-length transcript and protein. Environmental factors, such as exposure to cigarette smoke or inequities in access to healthcare, markedly worsen the severity of lung disease among individuals with CF.

Management

Because over 2000 different variants have been described across the *CFTR* gene, the diagnosis of CF is usually based on clinical criteria and sweat chloride concentration, though a genetic diagnosis following identification of two CF-causing variants in *trans* is permitted as long as sweat chloride concentration is used as a confirmatory measure. Sweat chloride concentrations are normal in 1 to 2% of patients with CF; in these individuals, an abnormal nasal transepithelial potential difference measurement is usually diagnostic of CF.

Currently there are no curative treatments for CF, although improved symptomatic management has increased the average longevity from early childhood to over 50 years of age in some countries. The estimated life expectancy is predicted to increase even more with widespread use of newly developed small molecule therapies (termed CFTR modulators) that target the basic defect causing CF, by correcting or enhancing the function of CFTR protein-bearing specific variants. Modulators primarily increase lung function and decrease sweat chloride, with additional benefits observed in other aspects of health and quality of life. For those ineligible for such modulator intervention, or when used in addition, medical therapy has the following objectives: clearance of pulmonary secretions; control of pulmonary infection; pancreatic enzyme replacement; adequate nutrition; and prevention of intestinal obstruction. Although medical therapy slows the progression of pulmonary disease, the only effective treatment of respiratory failure in CF is lung transplantation. Pancreatic enzyme replacement and supplementation of fat-soluble vitamins treat the malabsorption effectively; because of increased caloric needs and anorexia, however, many patients also require caloric supplements. Therapies that act on the DNA or RNA level, including gene editing or replacement, are also under development. Most patients also require extensive counseling to deal with the psychological effects of having a chronic life-limiting disease.

Newborn screening for CF has been implemented in all 50 US states, in all Canadian provinces and territories, in Australia, and throughout parts of Europe. Such detection in the newborn period prevents the malnutrition seen in clinically undiagnosed pancreatic insufficient patients and allows early initiation of other treatments. Long-term effects of newborn screening for CF on survival and on progression of pulmonary disease are emerging, so far indicating a modest but significant decrease in CF-related mortality in children. Most CF newborn screening protocols utilize IRT – a pancreatic enzyme precursor measured from dried blood spot – as the first-tier test and progress to another IRT measurement and/or screening for specific *CFTR* variants as a second tier. Sweat chloride testing is performed on infants with a positive CF newborn screening result and typically either confirms or refutes a CF diagnosis. When a diagnosis remains equivocal after *CFTR* genotyping and sweat chloride testing, an infant may be labeled as having CFTR-related metabolic syndrome or CF screen positive, inconclusive diagnosis (CRMS/CFSPID) and followed at regular intervals to monitor for the development of CF symptoms.

Inheritance

Carrier frequency for CF varies greatly among ancestral groups. For North Americans who do not have a family history of CF and are of northern European ancestry, the empirical probability for each to be a carrier is approximately 1 in 29; for each child of such a couple, the likelihood of CF is therefore 1 in 3200. For couples who already have an affected child, the probability for future children to have CF is 1 in 4 (25%). In 1997, a U.S. National Institutes of Health consensus conference recommended offering CF carrier testing to all pregnant women and couples considering a pregnancy in the United States. The American College of Obstetrics and Gynecology adopted and have periodically reaffirmed those recommendations. Carrier screening has traditionally been performed using a panel of verified disease-causing variants but tests based on next-generation sequencing – many of which screen for CF among several hundred other genetic conditions – are increasing in popularity. These more comprehensive tests offer a greater carrier detection rate within some populations, particularly among individuals not of European ancestry. They may also detect variants of uncertain significance, making risk assessment challenging.

Prenatal diagnosis of CF is based on identification of disease-causing *CFTR* variants in DNA from fetal tissue, such as chorionic villi or amniocytes; use of cell-free fetal DNA to detect monogenic diseases such as CF is also an emerging screening tool. Effective identification of affected fetuses usually requires that the variants responsible for CF in a family have already been identified.

QUESTIONS FOR SMALL GROUP DISCUSSION

1. Newborn screening for CF can be performed by testing IRT alone or by IRT followed by variant screening. Discuss the risks and benefits of adding *CFTR* variant screening to a newborn screening panel.

2. The most common CF-causing variant is c.1521_1523delCTT (p.Phe508del, aka F508del); it accounts for approximately 70% of all pathogenic *CFTR* alleles worldwide. For a couple of northern European origin, of whom each tests negative for F508del, what is the likelihood that a child of theirs will have CF? What if one tests positive and the other tests negative for F508del?

3. What constitutes disease: a pathogenic variant(s) in a gene or the phenotype caused by that variant? Does the detection of a variant in the *CFTR* gene of an individual with congenital bilateral absence of the vas deferens mean they have CF?

REFERENCES

Boyle MP, de Boeck K: A new era in the treatment of cystic fibrosis: Correction of the underlying CFTR defect, *Lancet Respir Med* 1:158–163, 2013.

Burgener EB, Moss RB: Cystic fibrosis transmembrane conductance regulators: Precision medicine in cystic fibrosis, *Curr Opin Pediatr* 30(3):372–377, 2018.

Clinical and Functional Translation of CFTR (CFTR2). https://cftr2.org

Cutting GR: Cystic fibrosis genetics: From molecular understanding to clinical application, *Nat Rev Genet* 16(1):45–56, 2015.

Farrell PM, White TB, Ren CL, et al: Diagnosis of cystic fibrosis: Consensus guidelines from the Cystic Fibrosis Foundation, *J Pediatr* 181S:S4–S15, 2017.

Shteinberg M, Haq IJ, Polineni D, et al: Cystic fibrosis, *Lancet* 397(10290):2195–2211, 2021.

Sosnay PR, Siklosi KR, Van Goor F, et al: Defining the disease liability of variants in the cystic fibrosis transmembrane conductance regulator gene, *Nat Genet* 45(10):1160–1167, 2013.

Tewkesbury DH, Robey RC, Barry PJ: Progress in precision medicine for cystic fibrosis: A focus on CFTR modulator therapy, *Breathe (Sheff)* 17(4):210112, 2021.

HEARING LOSS (NonSyndromic) (MIM 220290) (*GJB2* Pathogenic Variants)

Autosomal Recessive

Heidi L. Rehm

PRINCIPLES

- Allelic heterogeneity with both dominant and recessive inheritance patterns
- Newborn screening
- Cultural sensitivity in counseling

MAJOR PHENOTYPIC FEATURES

- Congenital hearing loss in the recessive form
- Progressive childhood hearing loss in the dominant form

HISTORY AND PHYSICAL FINDINGS

R.K. and J.K. are a couple referred to the genetics clinic by their ear, nose, and throat specialist because their 6-week-old daughter, B.K., was diagnosed with congenital hearing loss. The child was initially identified by routine neonatal hearing screening (evoked otoacoustic emissions testing) and then underwent formal auditory brainstem response (ABR) testing, which demonstrated moderate hearing impairment.

Both of B.K.'s parents are of European ancestry. Neither parent has a personal or family history of hearing difficulties in childhood, although the father thought that his aunt might have had some hearing difficulties in her old age. B.K. was the product of a full-term, uncomplicated pregnancy.

On examination, B.K. was nondysmorphic. There was no evidence of craniofacial malformation affecting the pinnae or external auditory canals. Tympanic membranes were visible and normal. Ophthalmoscope examination was limited because of the patient's age, but no abnormalities were seen. There was no goiter. Skin was normal.

Laboratory testing revealed a hearing loss of 60 dB bilaterally in the middle- and high-frequency ranges (500–2000 Hz and >2000 Hz). Electrocardiography results were normal.

DNA from B.K. was examined by targeted testing for variants in the *GJB2* gene. She was found to be homozygous for the common frameshift variant, c.35delG, in the *GJB2* gene. The counselor could thus reassure the parents that B.K.'s hearing loss

was nonsyndromic, and no further investigations to look for other syndromic features would be needed. Knowledge of the genetic cause would be helpful in planning the next steps for B.K. The couple were advised that the likelihood of recurrence of this form of hearing loss was 25% for any of their future offspring together. Genetic testing could be offered to members of their extended families who might wish to be informed.

BACKGROUND

Disease Etiology and Incidence

Approximately 1 in 500 to 1000 neonates has clinically significant congenital hearing impairment, which arises either from defects of the conductive apparatus in the middle ear or from neurological defects. Approximately one-third to one-half of congenital hearing loss has a genetic etiology. Of the hereditary forms, approximately three-quarters are nonsyndromic, characterized by hearing loss alone; one-quarter is syndromic, that is, associated with other manifestations.

Among inherited forms of nonsyndromic hearing loss, pathogenic variants of *GJB2* are the most common cause, although variants in over 100 other genes can also lead to nonsyndromic hearing loss. Pathogenic *GJB2* variants cause DFNB1 hearing loss (MIM 220290), which accounts for half of congenital nonsyndromic autosomal recessive hearing loss, as well as DFNA3 hearing loss (MIM 601544), a rare form of childhood-onset, progressive, autosomal dominant hearing loss. The c.35delG variant accounts for approximately two-thirds of identified autosomal recessive pathogenic *GJB2* variants in populations of European ancestry, but not in other ancestry groups. Among those of Chinese ancestry, for example, a different *GJB2* variant – c.235delC – is more common, causing DFNB1 hearing loss.

Pathogenesis

The *GJB2* gene encodes connexin 26, one of a family of proteins that form gap junctions. Gap junctions create pores between cells, allowing exchange of ions and passage of electrical currents between cells. Connexin 26 is highly expressed in the cochlea – the inner ear organ that transduces sound waves to electrical impulses. The failure to form functional gap junctions results in loss of cochlear function but does not affect the vestibular system or auditory nerve.

Phenotype and Natural History

Autosomal recessive hearing loss due to pathogenic *GJB2* variants is usually congenital and may be mild to profound (Fig. C.13.1). About 5% of such infants have hearing that is normal at birth but declines rapidly thereafter. Cognitive deficits are *not* a component of the disorder if the hearing impairment is detected early and the child is referred for proper management to allow the development of spoken or sign language.

Autosomal dominant hearing loss due to *GJB2* variants also occurs. It has an early childhood onset and is associated with progressive, moderate to severe, high-frequency sensorineural hearing loss. Like the autosomal recessive disease, it is not associated with cognitive deficits.

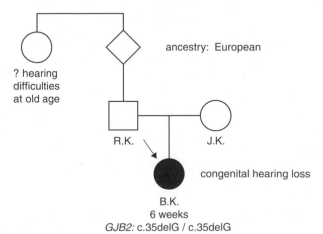

ancestry: European

? hearing difficulties at old age

R.K.   J.K.

congenital hearing loss

B.K.
6 weeks
GJB2: c.35delG / c.35delG

Pedigree Case 13

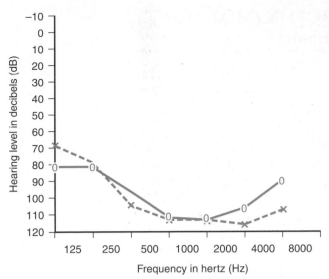

Figure C.13.1 Profound hearing loss in a child homozygous for pathogenic variants in the *GJB2* gene. X and O represent left and right ear, respectively. Normal hearing level is 0 to 20 dB throughout the frequency range. (Audiogram courtesy Virginia W. Norris, Gallaudet University.)

Management

The diagnosis of congenital hearing loss is usually made through newborn screening. Newborn screening is carried out either by measuring otoacoustic emissions, which are sounds caused by internal vibrations from within a normal cochlea, or by automated ABR, which detects electrical signals in the brain generated in response to sound. With the introduction of universal newborn screening, the average age at diagnosis has fallen to 3 to 6 months, allowing early intervention with hearing aids and other forms of therapy. Infants in whom therapy is initiated before 6 months of age show better language development compared with infants identified at an older age.

As soon as hearing loss is identified, the child needs to be referred for early intervention, regardless of the cause of the hearing loss. By consulting with professionals such as audiologists, otolaryngologists, and speech pathologists about the benefits and the drawbacks of different options, parents can be helped to choose intervention approaches that seem best for their families. Age-appropriate, intensive language therapy with sign language and spoken language with hearing assistance with hearing aids can be instituted as early as possible. For those children whose hearing loss is profound and not able to be augmented with hearing aids, parents can be offered the option of an early cochlear implant: a device that directly stimulates the cochlear nerve. Use of cochlear implants before 3 years of age is associated with better oral speech and language outcomes than when implanted later in childhood.

During the newborn period, clinically distinguishing between some forms of syndromic and nonsyndromic hearing loss is difficult because some syndromic features – such as the goiter in Pendred syndrome or the retinitis pigmentosa in any of the Usher syndromes – may have onset late in childhood or adolescence. However, a definitive diagnosis is often important for prognosis, management, and counseling; therefore, genetic testing for variants in the *GJB2* gene, as well as in other genes, is key to such a diagnosis. Importantly, distinguishing among nonsyndromic forms of hearing loss is often critical for selecting proper therapy.

Inheritance

The form of severe congenital hearing loss caused by loss-of-function variants in *GJB2* (DFNB1) is inherited in a typical autosomal recessive manner. Unaffected parents are typically both carriers of one normal and one altered gene. Offspring of two carrier parents each has one chance in four to have hearing loss due to biallelic variants in *GJB2*. Prenatal diagnosis by direct detection of familial variant(s) is available.

A small number of pathogenic variants in *GJB2* lead to dominant nonsyndromic hearing loss. In these cases, the likelihood that an offspring of an affected parent will be hearing impaired is 50%.

QUESTIONS FOR SMALL GROUP DISCUSSION

1. Why might certain missense variants in *GJB2* cause *dominant* hearing loss, whereas another variant (frameshift) results in *recessive* hearing loss?
2. What special considerations and concerns might arise in providing genetic counseling to a hearing-impaired couple about the likelihood that a child of theirs would be similarly affected by hearing loss? What is meant by the term *Deaf culture*?
3. Genetic testing detects only a single heterozygous pathogenic variant in many families presumed to have autosomal recessive hearing loss secondary to *GJB2* defects. Also, many sequence variants have been detected in the *GJB2* gene that have uncertain significance. If a couple with a congenitally hearing-impaired child presented to you and genetic testing detected a single heterozygous pathogenic *GJB2* sequence variant inherited from only one normal hearing parent, how would you counsel them regarding recurrence risk and genetic etiology? Would your counseling be different if the sequence variant were of uncertain significance?
4. Why might a child with a cochlear implant learn sign language in addition to spoken language?
5. Because variants in many different genes can underlie recessive forms of nonsyndromic hearing loss, discuss various approaches to molecular diagnosis of the gene responsible in any given case: *GJB2* testing, testing a panel of known hearing loss-associated genes, exome sequencing, or genome sequencing.

REFERENCES

Duman D, Tekin M: Autosomal recessive nonsyndromic deafness genes: A review, *Front Biosci* 17:2213–2236, 2012.

Li MM, Tayoun AA, DiStefano M, Arti P, Rehm HL, Robin NH, Schaefer AM, Yoshinaga-Itano C, ACMG Professional Practice and Guidelines Committee: Clinical evaluation and etiologic diagnosis of hearing loss: A clinical practice resource of the American College of Medical Genetics and Genomics (ACMG), *Genet Med.* https://www.sciencedirect.com/science/article/abs/pii/S1098360022007134

Shearer AE, Hidebrand MS, Smith RJH: Hereditary hearing loss and deafness overview. http://www.ncbi.nlm.nih.gov/books/NBK1434/

Shearer AE, Smith RJ: Genetics: Advances in genetic testing for deafness, *Curr Opin Pediatr* 24:679–686, 2012.

Smith RJH, Jones MKN: Nonsyndromic hearing loss and deafness, DFNB1. http://www.ncbi.nlm.nih.gov/books/NBK1272/

Vona B, Muller T, Nanda I, et al: Targeted next-generation sequencing of deafness genes in hearing-impaired individuals uncovers informative mutations, *Genet Med* 10.945–953, 2014.

DUCHENNE MUSCULAR DYSTROPHY (MIM 310200)
(Dystrophin [*DMD*] Pathogenic Variants)

X-Linked

Ronald Doron Cohn

PRINCIPLES

- High frequency of new mutation
- Allelic heterogeneity
- Manifesting carriers
- Phenotypic variability

MAJOR PHENOTYPIC FEATURES

- Age at onset: childhood
- Muscle weakness
- Calf pseudohypertrophy
- Mild intellectual compromise
- Elevated serum creatine kinase level

HISTORY AND PHYSICAL FINDINGS

A.Y., a 6-year-old boy, was referred to a pediatric neurologist by his primary care provider for mild developmental delay. He had difficulty climbing stairs, running, and participating in vigorous physical activities; he had decreased strength and endurance. His parents, two brothers, and one sister (S.Y.) were all healthy; no other family members were similarly affected. On examination, A.Y. had difficulty jumping onto the examination table, a Gowers sign (sequence of maneuvers for rising from the floor; Fig. C.14.1), proximal weakness, a waddling gait, tight heel cords, and apparently enlarged calf muscles. His serum creatine kinase level was 50-fold higher than normal. Because the history, physical examination findings, and elevated creatine kinase level strongly suggested a myopathy, A.Y. was referred to the neurogenetics clinic for further evaluation. Results of his muscle biopsy showed marked variation of muscle fiber size, fiber necrosis, fat and connective tissue proliferation, and no staining for dystrophin. Based on these results, A.Y. was given a provisional diagnosis of Duchenne muscular dystrophy, and he was tested for deletions of the dystrophin gene (*DMD*); he was found to have a deletion of exons 45 through 48. Subsequent testing showed his mother (M.Y.) to be a carrier. The family was therefore counseled that the risk for future sons to be affected was 50%. For any daughter, the likelihood to be affected was low but dependent on skewing of X inactivation; the likelihood to be a carrier would be 50%. Using the same DNA test, prenatal diagnosis could be undertaken for any future pregnancy.

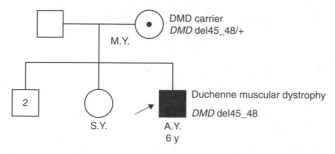

Counseling and carrier testing for S.Y. was offered, but to be deferred until age appropriate. Because M.Y.'s carrier status placed her at a high risk for cardiac complications, she was referred for a cardiac evaluation.

BACKGROUND
Disease Etiology and Incidence

Duchenne muscular dystrophy (DMD, MIM 310200) is an X-linked progressive myopathy caused by pathogenic variants within the *DMD* gene. It has an incidence of approximately 1 in 3500 male births.

Pathogenesis

DMD encodes dystrophin, an intracellular protein that is expressed predominantly in smooth, skeletal, and cardiac muscle as well as in some brain neurons (see Chapter 13). In skeletal muscle, dystrophin is part of a large complex of sarcolemma-associated proteins that confers stability to the sarcolemma (see Fig. 13.16).

DMD variants that cause DMD include large deletions (60–65%), large duplications (5–10%), and small deletions, insertions, or nucleotide changes (25–30%). Most large deletions occur in one of two hot spots. Nucleotide changes occur throughout the gene, predominantly at CpG dinucleotides. *De novo* mutations occur with comparable frequency during oogenesis and spermatogenesis; most of the *de novo* large deletions arise during oogenesis, whereas most of the *de novo* nucleotide changes arise during spermatogenesis.

Variants causing a dystrophin null phenotype are associated with more severe muscle disease than are *DMD* alleles expressing partially functional dystrophin. No consistent genotype-phenotype correlation has been defined for the intellectual impairment.

Phenotype and Natural History
Males

DMD is a progressive myopathy resulting in muscle degeneration and weakness. Beginning with the hip girdle muscles and neck flexors, the muscle weakness progressively involves the shoulder girdle and distal limb and trunk muscles. Although occasionally manifesting in the newborn period with hypotonia or failure to thrive, male patients usually present between the ages of 3 and 5 years with gait abnormalities. By 5 years of age, most affected boys use a Gowers maneuver (see Fig. C.14.1) and have calf pseudohypertrophy, that is, enlargement of the calf through replacement of muscle by fat and connective tissue. By 12 years of age, most are confined to a wheelchair and have – or are developing – contractures and scoliosis. Due to improvement in disease management of respiratory and cardiac complications, the disease trajectory of individuals with DMD has changed from a life-limiting to a life-threatening disease; most now reach adulthood, beyond the age of their 20s.

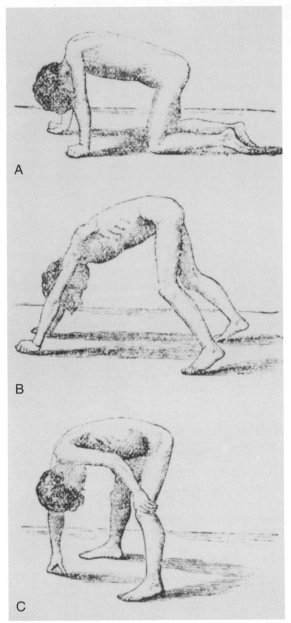

Figure C.14.1 Drawing of a boy with Duchenne muscular dystrophy rising from the ground, illustrating the Gowers maneuver. (From Gowers WR: *Pseudohypertrophic muscular paralysis. A clinical lecture*. London, 1879, J. and A. Churchill.)

Nearly 95% of individuals with DMD have some cardiac compromise (dilated cardiomyopathy, electrocardiographic abnormalities, or both), and 84% have demonstrable cardiac involvement at autopsy. Chronic heart failure develops in nearly 50% of these individuals. Rarely, cardiac failure is the presenting complaint for patients with DMD.

Individuals with DMD have an average IQ approximately one standard deviation below the mean, and nearly one-third have some degree of intellectual disability. The basis of this impairment has not been established. Furthermore, it has now been established that those with DMD have a higher incidence of mental health problems.

Females

The age at onset and the severity of DMD in females depend on the degree of skewing of X inactivation (see Chapter 6). If the X chromosome carrying the variant *DMD* allele is active in most cells, females may develop signs of DMD. Regardless of whether they have clinical symptoms of skeletal muscle weakness, most carrier females have cardiac abnormalities, such as dilated cardiomyopathy, left ventricle dilatation, and electrocardiographic changes.

Management

The diagnosis of DMD is based on family history and either DNA analysis or, in rare circumstances, muscle biopsy to test for immunoreactivity for dystrophin. Given the frequency of deletions involving *DMD*, the first approach is often with multiplex ligation-dependent amplification (MLPA), a technology that readily identifies deletions and duplications and can evaluate all 79 exons in the dystrophin gene associated with DMD. Being semiquantitative, MLPA is also effective in detecting duplications and for carrier testing of females, neither of which can be done using multiplex PCR. If no pathogenic deletion is found, exome or genome sequence analysis of *DMD* may be considered.

Carrier testing should be offered to at-risk females, at an age that is deemed appropriate according to current local professional guidelines.

Currently, there are no curative treatments for DMD, although improved symptomatic management has increased the average longevity from late childhood to early adulthood. The objectives of therapy are slowing of disease progression, maintenance of mobility, prevention and correction of contractures and scoliosis, weight control, and optimization of pulmonary and cardiac function. Glucocorticoid therapy is now considered standard of care, slowing the progression of DMD for several years. Several experimental therapies, including gene transfer, are under investigation. There are now a number of clinical trials that target conventional gene therapy with delivery of a microdystrophin construct. Furthermore, some newly developed drugs that enable exon skipping and restore a shorter but functional dystrophin have now been approved for treatment. Most patients and families also require extensive counseling to deal with the psychological effects of having a chronic disease with a life-threatening disease trajectory.

Inheritance

One-third of mothers who have a single affected son will themselves not be carriers of a pathogenic variant in the *DMD* gene (see Chapter 17). For the approximately 30 to 35% of DMD families with a single nucleotide or small indel variant, carrier determination has proved difficult in the past because of the large number of exons in the dystrophin gene. Advances in DNA sequencing, however, have made targeted exome sequencing much more effective. Counseling of recurrence risk must take into account the high rate of germline mosaicism (currently estimated to be 14%).

If a mother is a carrier, each son has a 50% risk for DMD and each daughter has a 50% risk of inheriting the *DMD* allele. Reflecting the random nature of X chromosome inactivation, daughters inheriting the *DMD* allele have a low risk for DMD; however, for reasons not fully understood, their risk for cardiac abnormalities may be as high as 50 to 60%. If the mother of an affected son is apparently not a carrier by DNA testing, there is still a chance (~7%) that another son will have DMD due to germline mosaicism (see Chapter 7). Counseling and possibly the offer of prenatal diagnosis are indicated for these mothers.

QUESTIONS FOR SMALL GROUP DISCUSSION

1. What features define a condition as being genetically lethal? Is DMD considered a genetic lethal condition today?

2. Discuss what mechanisms may cause a gender bias in different types of mutation. Name several diseases other than DMD in which this occurs. In particular, discuss the mechanism and high frequency of mutation at CpG dinucleotides during spermatogenesis.

3. How is the rate of germline mosaicism determined for a disease? Name several other diseases with a high rate of germline mosaicism.

4. Contrast the phenotype of Becker muscular dystrophy with DMD. What is the postulated basis for the milder phenotype of Becker muscular dystrophy?

REFERENCES

Darras BT, Miller DT, Urion DK: Dystrophinopathies. http://www.ncbi.nlm.nih.gov/books/NBK1119/

Fairclough RJ, Wood MJ, Davies KE: Therapy for Duchenne muscular dystrophy: Renewed optimism from genetic approaches, *Nat Rev Genet* 14:373–378, 2013.

Shieh PB: Muscular dystrophies and other genetic myopathies, *Neurol Clin* 31:1009–1029, 2013.

MONOGENIC DIABETES (MIM 600496) (Single Gene Pathogenic Variants Impacting Pancreatic Islet β Cell Development and/or Function)

Multifactorial

Farid Mahmud

PRINCIPLES

- Heterogenous group of monogenic conditions
- Key distinguishing clinical phenotypes
- Frequently misdiagnosed as more common forms of diabetes, type 1 or type 2
- Appropriate genetic diagnosis impacts monitoring and therapies

MAJOR PHENOTYPIC FEATURES

- Age at onset: neonatal/infantile (neonatal diabetes) through adulthood
- Variable: asymptomatic (incidental lab finding) to hyperglycemia, with symptoms including polyuria, polydipsia, polyphagia
- Some forms have associations with neurodevelopmental dysfunction, renal/hepatic disease

HISTORY AND PHYSICAL FINDINGS

M.M., a 14-year-old boy, was referred to the genetics clinic for counseling. He was diagnosed with diabetes 1 year ago at his local hospital after presenting to the emergency room with a 2-week history of polyuria and polydipsia and a 2 kg weight loss. At the time of diagnosis, his weight was 55 kg, height 167 cm, body mass index (weight in kilograms/[height in meters]²) was 20, and he presented with a random blood sugar of 12.3 mmol/L with large amounts of glucose but negative ketones detected in his urine. There were no other medical or surgical problems. The family was told he had type 1 diabetes and he was started on long acting (basal) insulin as well as insulin with meals (prandial/bolus insulin). Since that time and despite being on low doses of insulin, he has been having significant challenges managing his blood sugars and experiencing regular hypoglycemic episodes with activity. There is a strong family history of diabetes. His mother, S.M., was diagnosed 6 months ago with diabetes, which is being treated with dietary and lifestyle modification, and she had gestational diabetes treated with insulin with both of her pregnancies. S.M. is lean with a normal BMI of 20. M.M.'s maternal aunt, maternal uncle, and maternal grandfather all have diabetes treated with a variety of medications and insulin. Given the strong family history of diabetes, S.M. requested testing to confirm M.M.'s diagnosis, as she strongly felt that diabetes "ran in his family" and may have a genetic cause. He did have testing for insulin autoantibodies which were negative; his local medical team deemed this inconsistent with the type 1 diabetes diagnosis, thus prompting the referral to Genetics for further assessment. Given the strong, multigenerational family history of diabetes, as well as early onset in non-obese family members and negative autoantibody testing, testing for monogenic diabetes with a multiplexed sequencing panel was undertaken. The results showed that he had a missense variant in an exon of the *HNF1A* gene, consistent with HNF1A-MODY (maturity-onset diabetes of the young). Results were shared with M.M. and his family, with a discussion that this form of monogenic diabetes

can be treated with other medications. In collaboration with his diabetes care team, his insulin was discontinued and he was started on low-dose oral sulfonylurea. M.M. was seen in follow-up; his blood glucose levels have normalized and he is playing soccer regularly without any issues. S.M. was also tested and she had the same *HNF1A* variant as M.M. and testing is underway with other family members.

BACKGROUND

Disease Etiology and Incidence

Monogenic forms of diabetes are caused by single gene variants and comprise 1 to 5% of all cases of diabetes in children and adults. While this represents a minority of diabetes cases overall, the known etiology of the many forms of monogenic diabetes (more than 15 have been described) allows for an individualized, or precision approach to diagnosis and treatment.

HNF1A-MODY is the most commonly reported subtype, comprising 30 to 65% of monogenic diabetes cases. Given the wide range of monogenic diabetes subtypes, a description of the most common form of monogenic diabetes (HNF1A-MODY) with key clinical characteristics is reviewed here, and the reader may refer to the selected references for a more detailed description of other types.

Pathogenesis

Monogenic diabetes is a heterogeneous group of conditions, each with a specific impact on the pancreatic islet β cell, ranging from impairing pancreatic development to dysfunction and impairments in insulin secretion. The *HNF1A* gene, originally described as coding for a hepatic nuclear factor, encodes transcription factors present in many tissues. HNF1A-MODY is caused by pathogenic variants in *HNF1A*, which is located at 12q24.2, with autosomal dominant inheritance due to HNF1α haploinsufficiency. Hepatocyte nuclear factor 1α is a tissue-specific transcription factor; loss-of-function (LOF) variants result in the monogenic diabetes phenotype. DNA variants, including missense, frame shift, nonsense, splicing mutations, in-frame amino acid deletions, insertions, duplications, and partial and whole-gene deletions, have been described. Loss of HNF1α function results in impairments of pancreatic beta cell development and insulin secretion. In addition, HNF1α regulates a sodium-glucose cotransporter in the kidney (SGLT2), which is responsible for renal reabsorption of glucose. All of these contribute to the diabetes phenotype.

Phenotype and Natural History

Diabetes risk increases with age and *HNF1A* variant carriers may have normal blood sugars during childhood, although glycosuria has been reported. Diabetes symptoms often manifest during adolescence or young adulthood with classic symptoms of polyuria, polydipsia, and weight loss, with characteristic glycosuria in the absence of ketosis. Treatment at this stage is warranted and described below. Patients with HNF1A-MODY can experience diabetes-related microvascular complications and it is important that they receive regular follow-ups and meet recommended diabetes glycemic targets.

Heightened clinical suspicion for monogenic types of diabetes, such as HNF1A-MODY, are clearly described in the case of M.M. These include several key clinical pearls that discriminate monogenic diabetes from the more common types of diabetes. These include onset of diabetes prior to age 25 years and a family history of diabetes consistent with autosomal dominant inheritance, with diabetes in at least 2 generations of multiple family members also diagnosed at a young age, and the absence of obesity or clinical features of type 2 diabetes. Absence of pancreatic antibodies and low insulin requirements are additional diagnostic features.

Management

Treatment of genetically confirmed HNF1A-MODY may depend upon the severity of glycemia at diagnosis. In instances where isolated glycosuria is identified and blood glucose and hemoglobin A1c levels are within the normal range (less than 6%), dietary counseling and ongoing monitoring may be required. In those with elevated glucose, oral sulfonylurea medications are recommended. These agents act on the pancreatic beta cell to increase insulin secretion and allow for more stable glycemia. As described in this case, many patients are misdiagnosed and are successfully switched from insulin to sulfonylureas. Use of glucagon-peptide 1 receptor agonists and insulin has been described in adulthood. Sodium-glucose cotransporter 2 inhibitors (SGLT2i) should not be used.

Inheritance

As a mostly autosomal dominant condition, there is a 50% chance of the affected gene being passed on from a parent at conception. This means each child has a 1 in 2 chance of

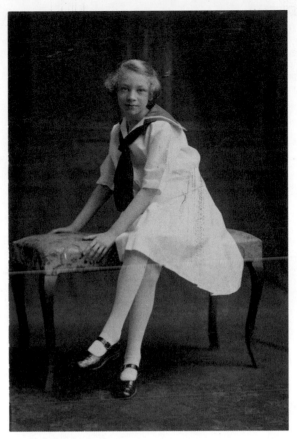

Figure C.15.1 Elsie Needham, October 1922. The first child to recover from coma via the use of insulin. Elsie was admitted to the Hospital for Sick Children in a diabetic coma. She was treated with insulin by Drs. F. G. Banting and Gladys Boyd, head of the Hospital's new diabetic clinic. Elsie was revived from her coma, regained her strength, and recovered sufficiently to be back at school in January. (Courtesy, Thomas Fisher Rare Book Library, University of Toronto.)

inheriting the variant allele, and if they have inherited the affected gene, they will go on to develop diabetes. Children and brothers and sisters of people with HNF1A-MODY who have inherited the same change in *HNF1A* have a 63% chance of developing diabetes by the age of 25 years and a 96% chance by the age of 55 years. Family members of an individual known to have HNF1A-MODY should be aware of the symptoms of diabetes and have their HbA1c measured. Because other types of diabetes such as type 1 and type 2 diabetes are common in the population, it is important that family members with diabetes also have genetic testing.

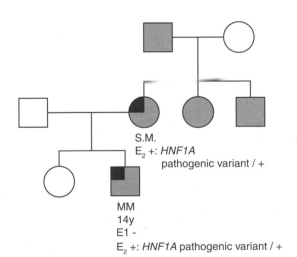

Key

■ = Diabetes

■ = Maturity-onset diabetes of the young (MODY)

E1 = insulin auto-antibody test

E2 = Multiplex sequencing panel for monogenic diabetes

Pedigree Case 15

QUESTIONS FOR SMALL GROUP DISCUSSION

1. Discuss the difficulties of identifying monogenic diabetes.
2. What are some important clinical features of monogenic forms of diabetes?
3. Discuss the underlying mechanisms of HNF1A-MODY in causing diabetes?
4. Discuss the implications of the identification of monogenic diabetes on treatment for the individual and family.

REFERENCES

Broome DT, Pantalone KM, Kashyap SR, Philipson LH: Approach to the patient with MODY-monogenic diabetes, *J Clin Endocrinol Metab* 106(1):237–250, 2021.

Hattersley AT, Greeley SAW, Polak M, Rubio-Cabezas O, Njølstad PR, Mlynarski W, Castano L, Carlsson A, Raile K, Chi DV, Ellard S, Craig ME: ISPAD Clinical Practice Consensus Guidelines 2018: The diagnosis and management of monogenic diabetes in children and adolescents, *Pediatr Diabetes* 19(Suppl 27):47–63, 2018.

Riddle MC, Philipson LH, Rich SS, Carlsson A, Franks PW, Greeley SAW, Nolan JJ, Pearson ER, Zeitler PS, Hattersley AT: Monogenic diabetes: From genetic insights to population-based precision in care. Reflections from a *Diabetes Care* Editors' Expert Forum, *Diabetes Care* 43(12):3117–3128, 2020.

16 FAMILIAL HYPERCHOLESTEROLEMIA (MIM 143890)
(Low-Density Lipoprotein Receptor [*LDLR*] Variants)

Autosomal Semidominant

Robert A. Hegele

PRINCIPLES

- Genetic complexity
- Founder effects
- Cascade screening
- Polygenic influences

MAJOR PHENOTYPIC FEATURES

- Age at onset: heterozygote – early to middle adulthood; homozygote – childhood
- Hypercholesterolemia
- Atherosclerotic cardiovascular disease (ASCVD)
- Xanthomas
- Xanthelasmas
- Arcus corneae

HISTORY AND PHYSICAL FINDINGS

A 34-year-old male truck driver of Irish ancestry was referred from the cardiology unit to the lipid clinic for dyslipidemia management. At age 29, routine bloodwork had shown a markedly elevated plasma low-density lipoprotein (LDL) cholesterol (C) level of 8.22 mmol/L or 318 mg/dL (normal <3 mmol/L or 130 mg/dL). He received no medical advice at that time, despite a family history of premature coronary heart disease (CHD): his father and two paternal uncles had elevated cholesterol and each died of a myocardial infarction (MI) before age 50. At age 34, the patient had suffered an acute MI. Physical examination showed bilateral Achilles tendon xanthomas and bilateral arcus corneae. Angiography showed widespread coronary arterial disease requiring placement of three stents.

The lipid clinic advised a reduced fat diet and daily medication for secondary prevention of CHD, including a high-intensity statin and a cholesterol absorption inhibitor. Six months post MI, his LDL-C was improved but was still above target for a patient with CHD. An injectable monoclonal antibody inhibitor self-administered subcutaneously every 2 weeks was added, and 8 weeks later, his LDL-C was 1.24 mmol/L or 48 mg/dL, which was now at the desired target level. DNA analysis initiated by the lipid clinic, using a targeted gene panel for dyslipidemias, showed a pathogenic heterozygous splice acceptor site variant in intron 14 of the *LDLR* gene. Cascade screening of his immediate family, including targeted *LDLR* gene analysis, found that his 12-year-old daughter had elevated LDL-C and the same *LDLR* variant, but that other first-degree relatives were unaffected.

BACKGROUND

Etiology and Incidence

Familial hypercholesterolemia (FH, MIM 143890) is an autosomal semidominant disorder of lipoprotein metabolism. FH results from pathogenic variants in one of three genes governing the function of the LDL receptor pathway – most commonly the *LDLR* gene itself – resulting in accumulation of high plasma levels of LDL-C (Table C.16.1). The prevalence of heterozygous FH (HeFH) is 1 in 250 to 300 in most populations, with well-known founder populations including among Quebecois, Christian Lebanese, and Afrikaners.

Pathogenesis and Genetic Basis

LDL is a species of spheroidal, macromolecular lipoproteins that carry lipids within plasma; others include high-density

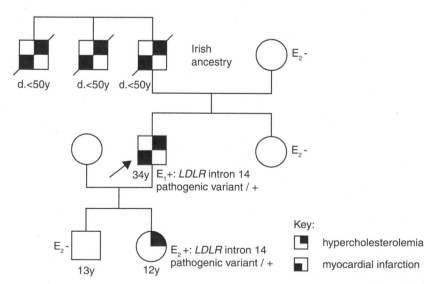

Irish ancestry

d.<50y d.<50y d.<50y

E₂-

34y E₁+: *LDLR* intron 14 pathogenic variant / +

E₂-

E₂-

13y

12y E₂+: *LDLR* intron 14 pathogenic variant / +

Key:
- hypercholesterolemia
- myocardial infarction

E₁ = dyslipidemia gene panel test
E₂ = cascade test: targeted *LDLR* variant

TABLE C.16.1 Causal Genes for Familial Hypercholesterolemia

Inheritance	Causative Gene/Location	MIM Numbers	Comments
Semidominant	*LDLR*/19p13.3	143890, 606945	80–90% of cases
	APOB/2p24-p23	144010, 107730	5–10% of cases
	PSCK9/1p32.3	603776, 607786	<2% of cases
Recessive	*LDLRAP1*/1p36-p35	603813, 605747	<1% of cases

TABLE C.16.2 Clinical Scoring Systems for Heterozygous Familial Hypercholesterolemia

		Simon Broome Register	Dutch Lipid Clinic Network	Canadian Criteria
Biochemical criteria	TC (mmol/L)	>7.5 (A) (a) >6.7 (C) (a)	—	—
	LDL-C (mmol/L)	>4.9 (A) (a) >4.0 (C) (a)	>8.5 (8) 6.5–8.4 (5) 5.0–6.4 (3) 4.0–4.9 (1)	>4 (C) (a) >4.5 (18–39 years) (a) >5 (>40 years) (a) >8.5 (b)
Physical findings	Personal	TX (b)	TX (6) AC* (4)	TX (c)
	Family	TX (b)	TX/AC (2)	
Family history	CAD	MI <50 yr in 2 relatives; or <60 yr in 1 relative (d)	Premature CAD** (2) Premature CVD/PVD**	Premature CAD in ≥1 relative** (d)
	LDL-C (mmol/L)	>7.5 in 1 or 2 relative (e)	Child with LDL-C >95th percentile (2)	≥1 relative with high LDL-C (d)
	Genetics	—	—	FH pathogenic variant in ≥1 family member
Genetics		*LDLR*, *PCSK9*, or *APOB* pathogenic variant (c)	*LDLR*, *PCSK9*, or *APOB* pathogenic variant (8)	*LDLR*, *PCSK9*, or *APOB* pathogenic variant (c)
Diagnosis		Definite: a + b or c Probable: a + d OR a + e	Definite: >8 Probable: 6–8 Possible: 3–5	Definite: (a + c) OR b Probable: a + d

*Arcus cornealis (AC) when age <45 years; **age <55 years in men, age <60 years in women; A, adult ≥ 18 years; C, child < 18 years. *CAD*, coronary artery disease; *CVD*, cerebrovascular disease; *LDL-C*, plasma low-density lipoprotein cholesterol concentration; *MI*, myocardial infarction; *PVD*, peripheral vascular disease; *TC*, plasma total cholesterol concentration; *TX*, tendon xanthoma (Adapted from Berberich AJ, Hegele RA: The complex molecular genetics of familial hypercholesterolaemia, *Nat Rev Cardiol* 16:9–20, 2019).

lipoprotein (HDL), very-low-density lipoprotein (VLDL), and chylomicrons. Chronically high LDL-C levels accelerate the growth of arterial wall plaques that can rupture and cause occlusions, leading to premature atherosclerotic cardiovascular disease (ASCVD) end points, including MI, stroke, and peripheral arterial disease.

About 75% of plasma cholesterol is transported within LDL particles, which are cleared by LDL receptors (LDLRs). The LDLR is a 160 kD transmembrane glycoprotein of 839 amino acids, expressed on all cell surfaces but especially on hepatocytes. The LDLR binds apolipoprotein (apo) B-100, the sole protein of LDL. The receptor-ligand complex is internalized via receptor-mediated endocytosis that also requires the LDLR adaptor protein type 1 (LDLRAP1). The cholesterol is retained, but the LDLR recycles to the cell surface to mediate uptake of additional LDL particles – a process that occurs repeatedly until the receptor is degraded by proprotein convertase subtilisin kexin type 9 (PCSK9).

Increased LDL-C levels in FH patients result from either (1) reduced LDLR activity, usually caused by different classes of pathogenic *LDLR* variants (MIM 606945); (2) defective apo B-100 resulting from pathogenic *APOB* variants located within the LDLR binding domain (MIM #144010 and 107730); or (3) hyperactivity of PCSK9 from gain-of-function *PCSK9* variants, resulting in rapid degradation that reduces LDLR numbers (MIM #603776 and 607786).

Pathogenic variants in *LDLR*, *APOB*, and *PCSK9* follow semidominant inheritance; that is, the heterozygote's phenotype is intermediate in severity between those of an individual with biallelic pathogenic variants and one with two normal alleles. Pathogenic variants associated with FH occur across all *LDLR* functional domains; 5 to 10% are copy number variants (CNVs), mostly large deletions. More than 3000 pathogenic *LDLR* variants are archived in the ClinVar database, accounting for 80 to 90% of all HeFH cases. A few dozen pathogenic *APOB* variants – particularly p.Arg3527Cys – account for 5 to 10% of cases, while several missense gain-of-function variants in *PCSK9* account for most of the remainder. Very occasionally, individuals with pathogenic variants in other dyslipidemia genes, such as *ABCG5/8* (sitosterolemia; MIM 618666), *APOE* (dysbetalipoproteinemia; MIM 617347), or *LIPA* (lysosomal acid lipase deficiency; MIM 278000) can present atypically with a phenotype that resembles HeFH. Diverse types of pathogenic variants in all these genes can be detected using next-generation DNA sequencing.

Among *LDLR* variants, individuals with a CNV, splicing variant, or nonsense variant tend to have more severe LDL-C elevation compared to those with a missense variant. LDL-C levels are also strongly influenced by polygenic effects, meaning that common nonpathogenic single-nucleotide variant genotypes with individually small effects on LDL-C act additively to raise LDL-C levels above a threshold suggestive of HeFH. For instance, among lipid clinic patients referred with LDL-C >5 mmol/L or 200 mg/dL, 20 to 40% have polygenic predisposition instead of monogenic HeFH. With polygenic predisposition, elevated LDL-C levels aggregate in families but do not follow clear inheritance patterns. ASCVD in individuals with polygenic elevated LDL-C is more severe than in those with normal lipids but less severe than in those with monogenic HeFH. Background polygenic effects also exacerbate LDL-C elevation in individuals with a pathogenic HeFH variant.

ASCVD risk in untreated HeFH patients is >80% by age 70. Environment, sex, and genetic background modify the effect of *LDLR* mutations on LDL-C levels and ASCVD risk. For instance, individuals of Chinese ancestry with HeFH living in China rarely have xanthomas and cardiovascular disease, whereas those who immigrated to Western societies express clinical manifestations similar to those of HeFH heterozygotes of European origin.

Homozygous FH is a clinical shorthand term for an individual who has inherited two pathogenic variants (i.e., biallelic FH) due either to identical or different variants on both alleles of the same gene, or to two different variants in two different genes (i.e., digenic inheritance). This is seen in ~1 in 300,000 people. In addition to the three genes with causal FH variants, there is a true autosomal recessive subtype of homozygous FH – with normal parental lipid profiles – caused by biallelic variants in *LDLRAP1*. Such individuals have xanthomas expressed in the first decade, extremely elevated LDL-C, and high risk of premature ASCVD and aortic disease, which can be fatal.

Phenotype and Diagnosis

Biochemical hypercholesterolemia is often the only clinical finding when HeFH is diagnosed. At all ages, plasma LDL-C concentration is >95th percentile in most HeFH patients. A generation ago, characteristic clinical features such as arcus corneae, xanthelasmas, and extensor tendon xanthomas were detected by clinicians in >50% of HeFH patients. Recently, however, such findings have been reported in <20% of patients. This could reflect increased detection of patients on the milder end of the spectrum or, perhaps, the impact of earlier treatment.

Diagnostic algorithms for HeFH include the Dutch Lipid Clinic Network Criteria, the Simon Broome Register Criteria (UK), and the Canadian FH Diagnostic Criteria (see Table C.16.2). Each set of criteria tallies and give weights to clinical, biochemical, and genetic features, yielding a score that translates to a "possible," "probable," or "definite" diagnosis of HeFH. The most consistent features of HeFH are elevated LDL-C and a family history of dyslipidemia or early ASCVD. DNA analysis is not necessary to diagnose HeFH, but a pathogenic variant yields the highest score in all algorithms. While HeFH accounts for 2 to 5% of those with hypercholesterolemia in the general population, a pathogenic DNA variant is seen in 30 to 60% of patients referred to a lipid clinic with suspected HeFH and LDL-C >5 mmol/L. Among those with LDL-C >8 mmol/L, >95% have a pathogenic variant.

Management

Treatment guidelines for HeFH focus on reduction of LDL-C. For primary prevention of ASCVD in HeFH patients, many clinical guidelines recommend reducing LDL-C by >50% from baseline levels. In contrast, for secondary prevention of ASCVD, LDL-C target levels are much stricter, usually requiring ≥2 medications.

All HeFH patients benefit from counseling on diet and physical activity to maintain appropriate body weight. Advice on modification of risk factors – such as smoking, diabetes, and hypertension – should be implemented where appropriate. Nonpharmacologic lifestyle measures reduce LDL-C by 10 to 20% and improve efficacy of medical therapy. Drug treatment centers on oral inhibition of 3-hydroxy-3-methylglutaryl coenzyme A reductase using high-intensity statin drugs. Most guidelines recommend initiating treatment as early as possible.

To achieve LDL-C goals, HeFH patients frequently require a second agent, usually ezetimibe, an oral inhibitor of cholesterol absorption. Older lipid-lowering drugs, that is, bile acid sequestrants and niacin, have side effects and limited efficacy and are infrequently prescribed. However, recently approved agents that inhibit PCSK9 via either biweekly injections of monoclonal antibodies or semiannual injections of a small interfering RNA are efficacious and well tolerated. As access improves, these agents should become part of the standard of care for HeFH patients.

For homozygous FH individuals, the above therapies have limited efficacy since they all require functional LDLRs, which these patients lack. The standard of care for those with homozygous FH is weekly or biweekly extracorporeal LDL removal by apheresis. Orphan drug treatments for homozygous FH include lomitapide and evinacumab, which are both extremely costly.

Inheritance and Screening

In practical terms, HeFH behaves as a typical fully penetrant autosomal dominant condition: each child of an affected parent has a 50% chance of inheriting the pathogenic variant. Approaches to finding new HeFH cases are population-wide screening and cascade screening. With the former, for every 1000 infants screened for hypercholesterolemia at birth, 4 HeFH cases are detected; follow-up parental screening detects an additional 4 HeFH cases; that is, 8 new cases/1000 screened individuals. In contrast, biochemical or DNA cascade screening of relatives of a clinically identified case has a higher case-finding rate: 50%, 25%, and 12.5% of first-, second-, and third-degree relatives, respectively.

QUESTIONS FOR SMALL GROUP DISCUSSION

1. Discuss mechanisms by which pathogenic variants in *LDLR, APOB, PCSK9,* and *LDLRAP1* each cause hypercholesterolemia.
2. How essential is finding a pathogenic variant to the diagnosis and treatment of HeFH?
3. While biologic treatments for HeFH have clear benefits, what potential issues of access or health equity do you see?
4. Is universal screening or cascade screening the best approach for finding new cases of HeFH?

REFERENCES

Berberich AJ, Hegele RA: The complex molecular genetics of familial hypercholesterolaemia, *Nat Rev Cardiol* 16:9–20, 2019.

Cuchel M, Bruckert E, Ginsberg HN, *et al*: Homozygous familial hypercholesterolaemia: new insights and guidance for clinicians to improve detection and clinical management. A position paper from the Consensus Panel on Familial Hypercholesterolaemia of the European Atherosclerosis Society, *Eur Heart J* 35:2146–2157, 2014.

Defesche JC, Gidding SS, Harada-Shiba M, *et al*: Familial hypercholesterolaemia, *Nat Rev Dis Primers* 3:17093, 2017. https://doi.org/10.1038/nrdp.2017.93

Nordestgaard M, Chapman MJ, Humphries SE, *et al*: Familial hypercholesterolaemia is underdiagnosed and undertreated in the general population: Guidance for clinicians to prevent coronary heart disease: Consensus statement of the European Atherosclerosis Society, *Eur Heart J* 34:3478–3490, 2013.

17 FRAGILE X SYNDROME (MIM 300624), FRAGILE X–ASSOCIATED TREMOR/ATAXIA SYNDROME (FXTAS) (MIM 300623), and FRAGILE X–ASSOCIATED PRIMARY OVARIAN INSUFFICIENCY (FXPOI) (MIM 311360) (Pathogenic *FMR1* Repeat Expansion)

X-Linked

Weiyi Mu

PRINCIPLES

- Trinucleotide repeat expansion
- Somatic mosaicism
- Sex-specific anticipation
- DNA methylation

MAJOR PHENOTYPIC FEATURES

- Age at onset: fragile X syndrome – childhood; FXPOI – early to middle adulthood; FXTAS – late adulthood
- Fragile X syndrome: intellectual disability, neuropsychiatric features, craniofacial features
- FXPOI: primary ovarian insufficiency
- FXTAS: cerebellar ataxia, intention tremor, cognitive decline; premorbid features may include higher risk for neuropsychiatric disorders such as anxiety and depression, termed fragile X–associated neuropsychiatric disorders (FXAND)

HISTORY AND PHYSICAL FINDINGS

R.L., a 6-year-old boy, was referred to the developmental pediatrics clinic for evaluation of intellectual disability and hyperactivity. He needs to repeat kindergarten due to disruptive and inattentive behaviors, as well as poor speech and motor skills. His development was delayed, but he had not lost developmental milestones: he sat by 10 to 11 months, walked by 20 months, and spoke two or three clear words by 24 months.

He had otherwise been in good health. His mother had mild childhood learning disabilities, and a maternal aunt has had 10 years of unexplained infertility. The maternal grandfather has a longstanding history of depression and anxiety and had recent onset gait impairment and now uses a cane. The findings from R.L.'s physical examination were normal except for hyperactivity. The physician recommended several tests, including a chromosomal microarray, thyroid function studies, and targeted analysis for Fragile X Syndrome using trinucleotide repeat-primed PCR. Diagnostic analysis was notable for more than 200 CGG repeats in *FMR1*, consistent with a diagnosis of fragile X syndrome. After the diagnosis was established in R.L., additional family members were offered testing to determine repeat length. R.L.'s mother was found to have a full mutation (>200 CGG repeats), and his maternal aunt and maternal grandfather were each found to have 102 CGG repeats (premutation range), establishing the diagnosis of Fragile X–Associated Primary Ovarian Insufficiency (FXPOI) and Fragile X Tremor/Ataxia Syndrome (FXTAS), respectively.

BACKGROUND

Disease Etiology and Prevalence

Fragile X syndrome (MIM 300624) is an X-linked neurodevelopmental disorder caused by pathogenic variants in the *FMR1* gene on Xq27.3 (see Chapter 13). The estimated

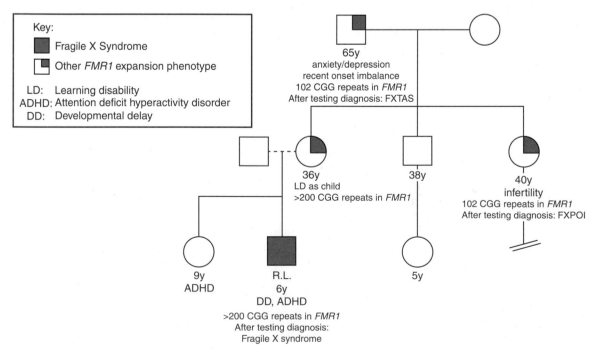

Key:

■ Fragile X Syndrome

◨ Other *FMR1* expansion phenotype

LD: Learning disability
ADHD: Attention deficit hyperactivity disorder
DD: Developmental delay

65y
anxiety/depression
recent onset imbalance
102 CGG repeats in *FMR1*
After testing diagnosis: FXTAS

36y
LD as child
>200 CGG repeats in *FMR1*

38y

40y
infertility
102 CGG repeats in *FMR1*
After testing diagnosis: FXPOI

9y
ADHD

R.L.
6y
DD, ADHD
>200 CGG repeats in *FMR1*
After testing diagnosis:
Fragile X syndrome

5y

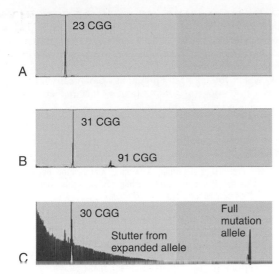

Figure C.17.1 Polymerase chain reaction (*PCR*) analysis of *FMR1* CGG repeat number in a normal male (A), a premutation female (B), and a full mutation female (C). The number of CGG repeats is on the x-axis, and fluorescence intensity is on the y-axis. Normal and premutation ranges are boxed in *gray*; full mutation range is boxed in *pink* with characteristic stutter from the repeat-targeted primer in the *gray box*. (Courtesy Lori Bean and Katie Rudd, Emory Genetics Laboratory, Emory University, Atlanta, Georgia.)

prevalence of a full mutation (expansion) is 1.4/10,000 males and 0.9/10,000 females. The disorder is a leading genetic cause for intellectual disability as well as autism spectrum disorder among males. The estimated prevalence of a premutation (i.e., in the size range vulnerable to further expansion) is 1 in 850 males and 1 in 300 females.

Pathogenesis

The *FMR1* gene product, FMRP, is expressed in many cell types but most abundantly in neurons. The FMRP protein is involved in cortical development and neuronal synapse plasticity and functions to inhibit dendritic protein translation. Brains of individuals with fragile X syndrome exhibit abnormally long and thin dendritic spines.

More than 99% of *FMR1* pathogenic variants are expansions of a (CGG)n repeat sequence in the 5'-untranslated region of the gene (see Chapter 13). In normal alleles of *FMR1*, the number of CGG repeats ranges from 6 to ~44. In disease-causing expanded alleles (full mutations), the number of repeats is more than 200. Alleles with more than 200 CGG repeats usually have hypermethylation of the CGG repeat sequence and the adjacent *FMR1* promoter (Fig. C.17.1). In Fragile X Syndrome, hypermethylation epigenetically inactivates the *FMR1* promoter, causing a loss of FMRP expression.

FMR1 full mutations arise from premutation alleles (of approximately 55–200 CGG repeats) almost exclusively with maternal transmission of an expanded *FMR1* allele; premutations often shorten with paternal transmission. Full mutations do not arise directly from normal alleles. Because the length of an unstable CGG repeat increases each generation when it is transmitted by a female, increasing proportions of affected offspring are usually observed in later generations of an affected family. This phenomenon is referred to as genetic anticipation (see Chapter 7). The risk for premutation expansion to

a full mutation increases as the repeat length of the premutation increases (see Fig. 7.21). Intermediate alleles (also known as "gray zone" alleles) of 45-54 CGG repeats may expand to the premutation range in the next generation but have a very low risk to expand to the full mutation range. Individuals with intermediate alleles have not been shown conclusively to have associated disease.

In disorders associated with *FMR1* premutation (FXPOI, FXTAS, FXAND), there is a different mechanism of molecular pathogenisis. Rather than epigenetic gene silencing, repeat-associated non-AUG (RAN) translation occurs: overabundant mRNA transcription resulting in noncanonical protein synthesis, aggregation, and cell death.

Phenotype and Natural History

Fragile X syndrome causes moderate intellectual disability in affected males and mild intellectual deficits in affected females. Most affected individuals also have behavioral and psychiatric features, including hyperactivity, hand flapping or biting, temper tantrums, poor eye contact, and autistic features. The physical features of males vary in relation to puberty; before puberty, they have somewhat large heads but few other distinctive features, whereas after puberty, they frequently have more distinctive features (long face with prominent jaw and forehead, large ears, and macroorchidism). Additional systemic symptoms may include hypotonia, gastrointestinal disorders, seizures, musculoskeletal features including joint laxity, and cardiovascular features including aortic root dilation. Individuals with Fragile X Syndrome have a normal life span.

Nearly all males and up to 50% of females who inherit a full mutation will have Fragile X Syndrome. The severity of the phenotype depends on repeat length mosaicism and repeat methylation (Fig. C.17.1). Because full mutations are mitotically unstable, some individuals have a mixture of cells with repeat lengths ranging from premutation to full mutation (repeat length mosaicism). Some also have a mixture of cells, with and without methylation of the CGG repeat (repeat methylation mosaicism). In addition, in females, the phenotype is dependent on the degree of skewing of X chromosome inactivation (see Chapter 6).

Premutations predispose to FXAND, FXTAS, and FXPOI (the last for female carriers only). Female carriers of premutations are at a 20% risk for premature ovarian insufficiency and amenorrhea. In addition, individuals with premutations are at risk for FXTAS. FXTAS manifests as late-onset, progressive cerebellar ataxia and intention tremor. Affected individuals may also have loss of short-term memory, executive function, and cognition as well as parkinsonism, peripheral neuropathy, lower limb proximal muscle weakness, and autonomic dysfunction. Penetrance of FXTAS is age and sex dependent, with increasing incidence over time, becoming manifest in 45% of males and 17% of females with premutations over age 50 years. Additionally, 50% of individuals with premutations have neuropsychiatric disorders, including anxiety, depression, ADHD, substance use disorder, chronic pain, and fibromyalgia – collectively termed Fragile X–Associated Neuropsychiatric Disorders (FXAND).

Management

No curative treatments are currently available for *FMR1* disorders. Therapy focuses on early diagnosis and symptomatic management, including but not limited to: early intervention and behavioral therapy for individuals with neurodevelopmental features, psychiatric evaluation and treatment for those with neuropsychiatric disorders, fertility evaluation and intervention for women with FXPOI, and neurological evaluation and intervention for individuals with FXTAS.

Inheritance

The risk that the offspring of an individual with a premutation will be affected is determined by the biological sex of the individual, the size of the allele, and the sex of the fetus. Empirically, the risk to the child of a female intermediate allele carrier can be as high as 50% for each male child and 25% for each female child but depends on the size of the mother's allele. Empiric risk tables are available for each maternal individual repeat size range. The risk for the offspring of a woman with an intermediate allele to have a premutation range allele is 14%. Prenatal testing is available by use of fetal DNA derived from chorionic villi or amniocytes.

QUESTIONS FOR SMALL GROUP DISCUSSION

1. Fragile X syndrome, Myotonic dystrophy, Friedreich ataxia, Huntington disease, and several other disorders are caused by expansion of repeat sequences. Contrast the mechanisms or proposed mechanisms by which expansion of the repeat causes disease for each of these disorders. Why do some of these disorders show anticipation, whereas others do not?

2. The sex bias in transmission of *FMR1* alleles is believed to arise because FMRP expression is necessary for production of viable sperm. Compare the sex bias in transmitting Fragile X syndrome and Huntington disease. Discuss mechanisms that could explain biases in the transmitting sex for various diseases.

3. How would you counsel a biological female (46,XX) seeking preconception counseling, with routine carrier testing showing that she has 33 and 55 CGG repeats in *FMR1*? What is the risk for expansion to full mutation in her next pregnancy? What disorders is she at risk for?

4. How would you counsel a pregnant woman carrying a 46,XY fetus with 60 repeats? A 46,XX fetus with 60 repeats? A 46,XX fetus with more than 200 repeats?

REFERENCES

Hagerman RJ, Protic D, Rajaratnam A: Fragile X-associated neuropsychiatric disorders (FXAND), *Front Psychiatry* 9:564, 2018. https://doi.org/10.3389/fpsyt.2018.00564 eCollection 2018. https://fragilex.org/

Kraan CM, Godler DE, Amor DJ: Epigenetics of fragile X syndrome and fragile X-related disorders, *Dev Med Child Neurol* 61(2):121–127, 2019. https://doi.org/10.1111/dmcn.13985

Musci TJ, Moyer K: Prenatal carrier testing for fragile X: Counseling issues and challenges, *Obstet Gynecol Clin North Am* 37(1):61–70, 2010. Table of Contents. https://doi.org/10.1016/j.ogc.2010.03.004. PMID: 20494258.

Saul RA, Tarleton JC: *FMR1*-related disorders. http://www.ncbi.nlm.nih.gov/books/NBK1384/

Spector E, Behlmann A, Kronquist K, *et al*: Laboratory testing for fragile X, 2021 revision: A technical standard of the American College of Medical Genetics and Genomics (ACMG), *Genet Med* 23(5):799–812, 2021. https://doi.org/10.1038/s41436-021-01115-y. Epub 2021 Apr 1.

GAUCHER DISEASE TYPE I (Non-Neuronopathic) (MIM 230800) (*GBA* Pathogenic Variants)

Autosomal Recessive Lysosomal Storage Disease

Shira G. Ziegler

PRINCIPLES

- Variable expressivity
- Asymptomatic homozygotes
- Symptomatic carriers

MAJOR PHENOTYPIC FEATURES

- Age at onset: childhood or early adulthood
- Hepatosplenomegaly
- Anemia
- Thrombocytopenia
- Bone pain
- Short stature

CASE PRESENTATION

An 8-year-old girl of Ashkenazi Jewish ancestry presented to the Genetics clinic with easy bleeding and bruising, excessive fatigue, short stature, and enlarged abdomen. Complete blood count showed pancytopenia, skeletal survey demonstrated Erlenmeyer flask deformity, and abdominal ultrasound revealed hepatosplenomegaly. Her parents were healthy and had a 6-year-old son without known medical concerns. Neither parent had a family history of blood disease, bone anomalies, or liver and spleen disease. The patient's maternal grandfather developed Parkinson disease at age 65. Given the proband's clinical history and physical exam findings, a blood test specific for glucocerebrosidase enzyme activity was sent and results showed reduced activity. Reflex targeted genetic testing identified a homozygous p.Asn409Ser (formerly known as p.N370S) variant in *GBA*. Her parents, brother, and maternal grandfather were subsequently found to be heterozygous carriers for the p.Asn409Ser variant. The proband was started on bimonthly enzyme replacement therapy, which normalized her blood counts and led to reduction of her hepatosplenomegaly.

BACKGROUND

Disease Etiology and Incidence

Gaucher disease encompasses a continuum of clinical features ranging from a perinatal lethal disorder to an asymptomatic type. Type 1 (nonneuronopathic) Gaucher disease (MIM 230800) is the most prevalent lysosomal storage disorder as well as the most common Gaucher disease phenotype, accounting for more than 90% of all Gaucher disease patients. It is an autosomal recessive disorder caused by biallelic pathogenic variants in the *GBA* gene, resulting in glucocerebrosidase deficiency. Type 1 Gaucher disease has a prevalence worldwide of 1 in 50,000 to 1 in 100,000, but it is as high as approximately 1 in 855 in the Ashkenazi Jewish population.

Clinical Characteristics

Gaucher disease is traditionally classified into three broad phenotypic categories: type 1, nonneuronopathic disease; type 2 (MIM 230900), a fulminant neuronopathic disease with onset before 1 year and a rapidly progressive course with death by 2 to 4 years; and type 3 (MIM 231000), chronic neuronopathic disease, which often has a more slowly progressive course with survival into the third or fourth decade. Other categories identified include a perinatal-lethal form (MIM 608013) associated with collodion skin abnormalities and/or nonimmune hydrops fetalis and a cardiovascular form (MIM 231005) associated with calcification of the aortic and mitral valves, mild splenomegaly, corneal opacities, and supranuclear ophthalmoplegia.

Type 1 Gaucher disease typically presents with bone disease, cytopenias, hepatosplenomegaly, and occasional coagulation abnormalities and lung involvement (Fig. C.18.1). Bone disease ranges from asymptomatic osteopenia to focal lytic or sclerotic lesions and osteonecrosis. Bone involvement, which can lead to acute or chronic bone pain, is usually the most

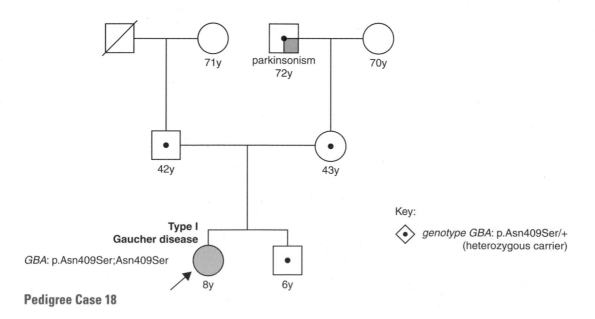

Type I
Gaucher disease

GBA: p.Asn409Ser;Asn409Ser

Key:

◇ *genotype GBA*: p.Asn409Ser/+
(heterozygous carrier)

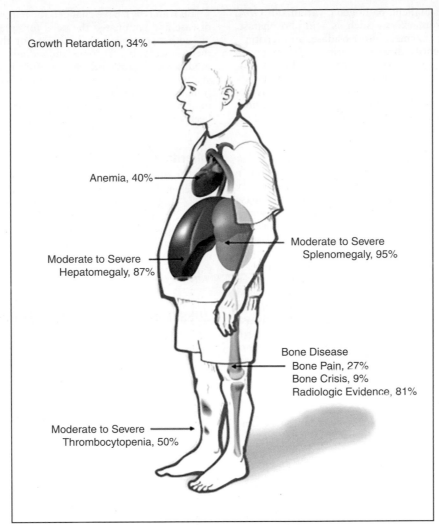

Figure C.18.1 Prevalence of affected organ involvement in Gaucher disease among children at diagnosis. Growth retardation refers to patients below the 5th percentile for height. Radiologic evidence of bone disease may indicate Erlenmeyer flask deformity, marrow infiltration, osteopenia, avascular necrosis, infarction, and/or new fractures. Anemia is defined according to age and sex references for hemoglobin concentrations as follows: less than 11 g/dL for boys 12 years and older; less than 10 g/dL for girls 12 years and older; less than 9.5 g/dL for children aged 2 to younger than 12 years; less than 8.5 for children aged 6 months to younger than 2 years; and less than 9.1 g/dL for infants younger than 6 months. Hepatomegaly (liver volume in multiples of normal size predicted for body weight [MN]) is defined as moderate (>1.25–2.5 MN) to severe (>2.5 MN). Splenomegaly (spleen volume in multiples of normal) is defined as moderate (>5–15 MN) to severe (>15 MN). Thrombocytopenia is defined as moderate (platelet count, 60 × 10³/μL to >120 × 10³/μL) to severe (platelet count, <60 × 10³/μL). (From The Clinical and Demographic Characteristics of Nonneuronopathic Gaucher Disease in 887 Children at Diagnosis *Arch Pediatr Adolesc Med*. 2006;160(6):603-608. https://doi.org/10.1001/archpedi.160.6.603)

debilitating aspect of type I Gaucher disease. Conventional radiographs may reveal undertubulation (Erlenmeyer flask deformity) in the distal femur and endosteal scalloping as a sign of bone marrow infiltration. The spleen is usually enlarged and leads to hypersplenism, which can cause secondary pancytopenia. Anemia, thrombocytopenia, and leukopenia may be present simultaneously or independently. While usually secondary to the status of the spleen, the cytopenias can also be due to infiltration of the marrow. The liver is also typically enlarged but does not usually progress to cirrhosis or hepatic failure. There is a wide range of coagulation factor abnormalities that can lead to a bleeding diathesis, most commonly epistaxis. Interstitial lung disease and pulmonary arterial hypertension can also be observed.

While there is no definitive genotype-phenotype correlation among patients with type 1 Gaucher disease, in general, individuals who are homozygous for the p.Asn409Ser (formerly known as p.N370S) or p.Arg535His (formerly known as p.R486H) variants tend to have milder disease and might be asymptomatic. Individuals with at least one p.Asn409Ser allele do not develop primary neuronopathic forms for Gaucher disease.

There is a striking association between *GBA* variants and Parkinson disease. Pathogenic *GBA* variants have been identified in 5 to 10% of individuals with Parkinson disease, suggesting that obligate heterozygotes – who are considered asymptomatic carriers – have an increased risk of developing Parkinson disease (approximately 20- to 30-fold the risk of an individual in the general population).

Diagnosis

The diagnosis of Gaucher disease is established by measuring glucocerebrosidase enzyme activity in peripheral blood leukocytes (affected individuals have 0–15% of normal levels) and/or identification of biallelic pathogenic variants in *GBA*. Increased activity of biomarkers – such as acid phosphatase, angiotensin-converting enzyme, chitotriosidase, and ferritin – can also be used to identify disease severity and response to treatment. Subsequent genetic testing may be relatively targeted to common variants in *GBA*, particularly if the family is of Ashkenaki Jewish descent. Otherwise, it may involve sequencing *GBA*, or possibly a multigene panel that includes *GBA*. If only one sequence variant is found, deletion/duplication analysis may follow.

Pathogenesis

Gaucher disease is caused by dysfunction of the constitutive enzyme, glucocerebrosidase, which cleaves a glucose moiety from the lipid glucocerebroside. Defects in glucocerebrosidase lead to the accumulation of glucocerebroside within lysosomes of macrophages, inducing their transformation into Gaucher cells. Under light microscopy, these cells are typically enlarged, with eccentric nuclei and condensed chromatin and cytoplasm with a heterogenous "crumpled tissue paper" appearance. Gaucher cells mainly infiltrate the bone marrow, liver, and spleen, in addition to other organs, and are considered the primary instigators of disease pathogenesis. To explain the increased incidence of Parkinson disease in Gaucher disease carriers, it has been demonstrated that defective glucocerebrosidase activity compromises lysosomal protein degradation, causing accumulation of α-synuclein and resulting in neurotoxicity, specifically in the substantia nigra.

Management

Since 1993, when recombinant glucocerebrosidase became available, enzyme replacement treatment (ERT) has remarkably improved the clinical outcome of individuals with Gaucher disease. Particularly, hepatosplenomegaly and hematological abnormalities show notable improvement under ERT in those with both the nonneuronopathic and chronic neuronopathic types. ERT is currently the standard treatment for nonneuronopathic Gaucher disease, notably decreasing levels of biomarkers (including chitotriosidase, acid phosphatase, and angiotensin-converting enzyme). However, because the recombinant enzyme cannot cross the blood-brain barrier, it cannot prevent neurological deterioration in those with neuronopathic Gaucher disease.

Substrate reduction therapy (SRT), another therapeutic option, aims to restore metabolic homeostasis by limiting the amount of substrate precursor synthesized to a level that can still be effectively cleared by an altered glucocerebrosidase enzyme with residual hydrolytic activity. SRT is approved for individuals with mild to moderate type 1 Gaucher disease and decreases or mildly improves bone involvement and pancytopenia. There are preclinical studies currently testing SRT analogs that might be efficacious for primary CNS involvement.

ERT and SRT have changed the natural history of Gaucher disease and eliminated the need for splenectomy in individuals with hypersplenism, but costs of these treatments make them inaccessible to some. Individuals not receiving disease-modifying therapy and certain other individuals may require symptomatic treatment, including partial or total splenectomy, transfusion of blood products, analgesics for bone pain, and joint replacement surgery. Bone marrow transplant has largely been superseded by ERT and SRT.

Inheritance

For unaffected parents with a child affected with type 1 Gaucher, the risk for recurrence in their future children is 25%. Targeted analysis for pathogenic *GBA* variants can also be used to detect carriers. Since there are some asymptomatic homozygotes, carrier testing might incidentally identify such individuals. Prenatal or preimplantation genetic diagnosis is also available for families with known pathogenic *GBA* variants.

QUESTIONS FOR SMALL GROUP DISCUSSION

1. Name and discuss other disorders for which enzyme replacement therapy has been used.
2. How do the pathogenic variants in *GBA* affect mRNA and protein production?
3. The reason for the high rate of asymptomatic homozygotes for the p.Asn409Ser (formerly known as p.N370S) variant in *GBA* is unknown. What possible explanations might there be for this finding?

REFERENCES

Desnick RJ, Schuchman EH: Enzyme replacement therapy for lysosomal diseases: Lessons from 20 years of experience and remaining challenges, *Annu Rev Genomics Hum Genet* 13:307–335, 2012.

Mazzulli JR, Xu YH, Sun Y, Knight AL, McLean PJ, Caldwell GA, Sidransky E, Grabowski GA, Krainc D: Gaucher disease glucocerebrosidase and α-synuclein form a bidirectional pathogenic loop in synucleinopathies, *Cell* 146(1):37–52, 2011. https://doi.org/10.1016/j.cell.2011.06.001. Epub 2011 Jun 23. PMID: 21700325; PMCID: PMC3132082.

Mignot C, Gelot A, De Villemeur TB: Gaucher disease, *Handb Clin Neurol* 113:1709–1715, 2013.

Pastores GM, Hughes DA: Gaucher disease. http://www.ncbi.nlm.nih.gov/books/NBK1269/

Sidransky E, Nalls MA, Aasly JO, *et al*: Multicenter analysis of glucocerebrosidase mutations in Parkinson's disease, *N Engl J Med* 361(17):1651–1661, 2009. https://doi.org/10.1056/NEJMoa0901281

GLUCOSE-6-PHOSPHATE DEHYDROGENASE DEFICIENCY
(MIM 300908) (*G6PD* Pathogenic Variants)

X-Linked

PRINCIPLES

- Balancing selection
- Pharmacogenetics

MAJOR PHENOTYPIC FEATURES

- Age at onset: neonatal
- Hemolytic anemia
- Neonatal jaundice

HISTORY AND PHYSICAL FINDINGS

L.M., a previously healthy 5-year-old boy, presented to the emergency department febrile, pale, tachycardic, tachypneic, and minimally responsive; his physical examination was otherwise normal. The morning before presentation, he had been in good health, but during the afternoon, he had abdominal pain, headache, and fever and his urine was cola colored; by late evening, he was tachypneic and incoherent. He had not ingested any medications or known toxins (ultimately results of a urine toxicology screen were negative). Results of other laboratory tests showed massive nonimmune intravascular hemolysis and hemoglobinuria. After fluid resuscitation and red cell transfusions, L.M. was admitted to the hospital; the hemolysis resolved without further intervention. L.M. was of Greek ancestry. His parents were unaware of a family history of hemolysis, although his mother (M.M.) had some cousins in Europe with a "blood problem." Further inquiry revealed that the morning before admission, L.M. had been eating fava beans from the garden. The physician explained to the parents that L.M. was probably deficient in glucose-6-phosphate dehydrogenase (G6PD) and that because of this, he had become ill after eating fava beans (favism). Subsequent measurement of L.M.'s erythrocyte G6PD activity confirmed that he had G6PD deficiency. The parents were counseled concerning L.M.'s risk for acute hemolysis after exposure to certain drugs and toxins and given a list of compounds that L.M. should avoid (including fava beans). The genetic counselor discussed with the couple that M.M. was almost certainly a carrier for a variant in *G6PD* and might wish to be tested, in case she might have low activity due to strongly skewed X inactivation. The counselor described the possible outcomes for any future children of M.M. (as detailed below). They were encouraged to share this information with their extended families, who might wish to pursue their own testing.

BACKGROUND

Disease Etiology, Incidence, and Prevalence

G6PD deficiency (MIM 300098), a hereditary predisposition to hemolysis, is an X-linked disorder of antioxidant homeostasis that is caused by any of nearly 200 defined pathogenic variants, mostly single-nucleotide, in the *G6PD* gene (MIM 305900). It is the most common human enzyme defect known and increasing in incidence, to >7.5 million cases per year (2017), affecting almost 5% of the world population. As of 2019, it had the largest worldwide incidence and prevalence of all inherited erythrocyte disorders. The highest incidence is in

Africa. In areas in which malaria is endemic, G6PD deficiency has a prevalence of 5% to 35%; in nonendemic areas, it has a prevalence of less than 0.5% (Fig. C.19.1). Like sickle cell disease (see Case 42), G6PD deficiency appears to have reached a substantial frequency in some areas because it confers some resistance to malaria and thus a survival advantage to individuals heterozygous or hemizygous for G6PD deficiency (see Chapter 10). Studies of the potential protective effect of G6PD deficiency alleles have yielded complex results, due to differences between *Plasmodium falciparum* and *P. vivax* malaria, their respective world distributions, and the diverse effects and world distributions of different variant alleles of *G6PD*.

Pathogenesis

G6PD is the first enzyme in the hexose monophosphate shunt, a pathway critical for generating nicotinamide adenine dinucleotide phosphate (NADPH). NADPH is required for the regeneration of reduced glutathione. Within erythrocytes, reduced glutathione is used for the detoxification of oxidants produced by the interaction of hemoglobin and oxygen and by exogenous factors such as drugs, infection, and metabolic acidosis.

Most G6PD deficiency arises because variants in the X-linked *G6PD* gene decrease the catalytic activity or the stability of G6PD, or both. When G6PD activity is sufficiently depleted or deficient, insufficient NADPH is available to regenerate reduced glutathione during times of oxidative stress. This results in the oxidation and aggregation of intracellular proteins (Heinz bodies) (see Fig. 12.8) and the formation of rigid erythrocytes that readily hemolyze.

With the more common aberrant *G6PD* alleles, which cause the protein to be unstable, deficiency of G6PD within erythrocytes worsens as erythrocytes age. Because erythrocytes do not have nuclei, new G6PD mRNA cannot be synthesized; thus, erythrocytes are unable to replace G6PD as it is degraded. During exposure to an oxidative stress episode, therefore, hemolysis begins with the oldest erythrocytes and progressively involves younger erythrocytes, depending on the severity of the oxidative stress.

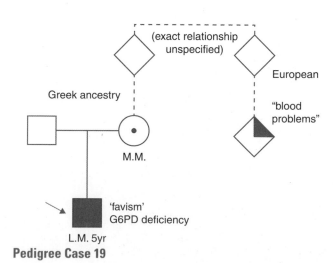

Pedigree Case 19

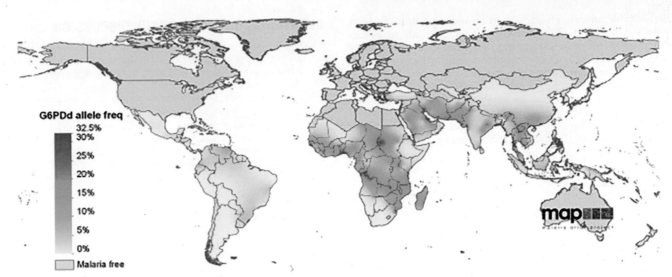

Figure C.19.1 (Seidlein, L, Auburn, S, Espino, F, Shanks, D, Cheng, Q, McCarthy, J, Baird, K, Moyes, Howes, R, Menard, D, Bancone, G, Winasti-Satyagraha, A, Vestergaard, I , Green, J, Domingo, G, Yeung, Sh, Price, R: Review of key knowledge gaps in glucose-6-phosphate dehydrogenase deficiency detection with regard to the safe clinical deployment of 8-aminoquinoline treatment regimens: A workshop report, *Malar J* 12:112, 2013. https://doi.org/10.1186/1475-2875-12-112)

Phenotype and Natural History

As an X-linked disorder, G6PD deficiency affects males predominantly and most severely. Rare symptomatic females have a skewing of X chromosome inactivation such that the X chromosome carrying the variant *G6PD* allele is the active X in erythrocyte precursors (see Chapter 6).

The severity of G6PD deficiency depends not only on sex but also on the specific G6PD variants. The World Health Organization has designated five classes, according to enzyme activity. The most severe of the commonly found G6PD variants is the Mediterranean (*G6PD* Med) genotype (*G6PD* c.563 C>T). Recent evidence indicates a strong protective effect of this variant against *P. vivax* malaria. The common ("A-") genotype (*G6PD* c.292 G>A) is prevalent in sub-Saharan African populations (see Fig. C.19.1) where *P. falciparum* predominates; its protective effect against *P. vivax* is much less than with *G6PD* Med. In individuals with *G6PD* Med, enzyme activity decreases to insufficient levels 5 to 10 days after erythrocytes appear in the circulation, whereas in those with the *G6PD* A⁻ genotype, G6PD activity becomes insufficient 50 to 60 days after erythrocytes appear. Most erythrocytes are thus susceptible to hemolysis in patients with severe forms of G6PD deficiency, such as *G6PD* Med, but only 20 to 30% are susceptible in patients with *G6PD* A⁻ variants.

G6PD deficiency most commonly manifests as either neonatal jaundice or acute hemolytic anemia. The peak incidence of neonatal jaundice occurs during days 2 and 3 of life and may worsen after discharge from birthing facilities, the period when such neonates are most at risk of kernicterus. The severity of the jaundice ranges from subclinical to levels compatible with kernicterus; the associated anemia is rarely severe. Episodes of acute hemolytic anemia usually begin within hours of an oxidative stress and end when G6PD-deficient erythrocytes have hemolyzed; therefore, the severity of the anemia associated with these acute hemolytic episodes is proportionate to the deficiency of G6PD and the oxidative stress. Viral and bacterial infections are the most common triggers, but many drugs and toxins can also precipitate hemolysis. Paradoxically, primaquine, the 8-aminoquinoline antimalarial agent, has a strong association with induction of hemolytic anemia among individuals with G6PD deficiency, particularly

the more severe forms. The disorder called favism results from hemolysis secondary to the ingestion of fava beans – which contain β-glycosides, naturally occurring oxidants – by individuals with more severe forms of G6PD deficiency, such as *G6PD* Med.

In addition to neonatal jaundice and acute hemolytic anemia, G6PD deficiency can (rarely) cause congenital or chronic nonspherocytic hemolytic anemia. Such patients generally have a profound deficiency of G6PD that causes chronic anemia and an increased susceptibility to infection, which arises because the NADPH supply within granulocytes is inadequate to sustain the oxidative burst necessary for killing phagocytosed bacteria.

Management

Although biochemical screening tests for G6PD deficiency are available, they are not routinely used in North America. Elsewhere in the world, despite high prevalence of G6PD deficiency, cost prohibits widespread testing. This is particularly problematic because the antimalarial drug, primaquine, used to cure *P. vivax* malaria, will precipitate hemolysis in individuals with G6PD deficiency; therefore, it tends to be avoided where otherwise needed, for want of information about G6PD status. Efforts toward inexpensive and effective point-of-care testing for G6PD deficiency are underway for use in malaria-endemic regions.

G6PD deficiency should be suspected in individuals of African, Mediterranean, or Asian ancestry who present with either an acute hemolytic episode or neonatal jaundice. G6PD deficiency is diagnosed by measurement of G6PD activity in erythrocytes; this activity should be measured only when the individual has had neither a recent transfusion nor a recent hemolytic episode. (Because G6PD deficiency occurs primarily in older erythrocytes, measurement during or immediately after a hemolytic episode often gives a false-negative result.)

The key to management of G6PD deficiency is prevention of hemolysis by prompt treatment of infections and avoidance of oxidant drugs (e.g., sulfonamides, sulfones, nitrofurans) and toxins (e.g., naphthalene) (see www.g6pd.org for a comprehensive listing). Although too recent for conclusive evidence, the COVID-19 pandemic has renewed attention to the possible adverse effects of certain antiviral drugs in individuals who are G6PD deficient. Given the scale of potential overlap between the current world rates of COVID-19 infection and G6PD-deficient individuals, further research is strongly warranted. Although most individuals with a hemolytic episode will not require medical intervention, those with severe anemia and hemolysis may require resuscitation and erythrocyte transfusions. Infants presenting with neonatal jaundice respond well to the same therapies as for others with neonatal jaundice (hydration, phototherapy, and exchange transfusions).

Inheritance

From a mother carrying a *G6PD* pathogenic variant, each son has a 50% chance of being affected, and each daughter has a 50% chance of being a carrier. Each daughter of an affected father will be a carrier, but sons will be unaffected. The risk that carrier daughters will have clinically significant symptoms is proportional to the residual enzyme activity, which depends on the degree of skewing of X chromosome inactivation.

QUESTIONS FOR SMALL GROUP DISCUSSION

1. The consumption of fava beans and the occurrence of G6PD deficiency are coincident in many areas. What evolutionary advantage might the consumption of fava beans give populations with G6PD deficiency?
2. Several hundred different variants have been described that cause G6PD deficiency. Presumably, most of these have persisted because of selection. Discuss heterozygote advantage in the context of G6PD deficiency.
3. What is pharmacogenetics? How does G6PD deficiency illustrate the principles of pharmacogenetics?

REFERENCES

Bunn HF: The triumph of good over evil: Protection by the sickle gene against malaria, *Blood* 121:20–25, 2013.

Howes RE, Battle KE, Satyagraha AW, *et al*: G6PD deficiency: Global distribution, genetic variants and primaquine therapy, *Adv Parasitol* 81:133–201, 2013.

Luzzatto L, Seneca E: G6PD deficiency: A classic example of pharmacogenetics with on-going clinical implications, *Br J Haematol* 164:469–480, 2014.

Luzzatto L, Arese P: Favism and Glucose-6-Phosphate Dehydrogenase Deficiency, *N Engl J Med*. 378:60–71, 2018. https://www.nejm.org/doi/10.1056/nejmra1708111

HEREDITARY HEMOCHROMATOSIS
(MIM 235200) (*HFE* Pathogenic Variants)

Autosomal Recessive

Kelsey Guthrie

PRINCIPLES

- Incomplete penetrance and variable expressivity
- Sex differences in penetrance
- Population screening versus at-risk testing
- Molecular versus biochemical testing

MAJOR PHENOTYPIC FEATURES

- Average age at onset: 40 to 60 years in males; after menopause in females
- Fatigue, hypogonadism, progressive increase in skin pigmentation, diabetes, cirrhosis, cardiomyopathy
- Elevated serum transferrin iron saturation
- Elevated serum ferritin level

HISTORY AND PHYSICAL FINDINGS

S.F. was a 30-year-old healthy male of northern European descent referred to the Genetics clinic; his 55-year-old father had just been diagnosed with cirrhosis due to hereditary hemochromatosis. History and physical examination findings were normal. S.F. had a transferrin iron saturation of 48% (normal, 20–50%), a normal serum ferritin level (<300 ng/mL), and normal liver transaminase activities. S.F. was an obligate carrier for the condition, but since his mother (also of Northern European descent) had an 11% population risk for being a carrier of a pathogenic variant in the hereditary hemochromatosis gene (*HFE*), his prior risk for having inherited a second pathogenic variant in this gene was 5.5%. S.F. chose to have his *HFE* gene examined. Molecular testing targeted to the two most common *HFE* variants revealed that he was homozygous for the p.Cys282Tyr variant, putting him at risk for development of hemochromatosis. He was referred to his primary care provider to follow serum ferritin levels annually and to institute therapy as needed.

BACKGROUND

Disease Etiology and Incidence

Hereditary hemochromatosis (MIM 235200) is a disease of iron overload that occurs in some individuals with homozygous or compound heterozygous pathogenic variants in the *HFE* gene. The majority (80–90%) of individuals with hereditary hemochromatosis are homozygous for a p.Cys282Tyr variant. Most remaining affected individuals are compound heterozygotes for the p.Cys282Tyr and p.His63Asp variants. Homozygosity for p.His63Asp does not lead to clinical hemochromatosis unless there is an additional cause of iron overload. The carrier rate in those of European ancestry is approximately 6.2% for p.Cys282Tyr and approximately 25% for p.His63Asp. Using US ancestry population definitions, approximately 1 in 225 "whites" of non-Hispanic ancestry will be p.Cys282Tyr homozygotes. The frequency of p.Cys282Tyr homozygotes is far lower in other US groups. For instance, approximately 1 in 900 Native Americans are p.Cys282Tyr homozygotes, and the frequency is even lower for those of Hispanic, African-American, Pacific Islander, and Asian ancestry.

The penetrance of hereditary hemochromatosis has been difficult to determine, as estimates vary widely. Biochemical penetrance (defined as increased transferrin saturation with or without elevated serum ferritin) has been estimated to be 75% in men and 50% in women, based on two large studies. Estimates of clinical penetrance (signs and symptoms related to iron overload) are lower; a study from Melbourne showed that 28.4% of men had documented iron overload–related disease compared with only 1.2% of women having the same. Overall, both biochemical and clinical penetrance is higher in men than in women. In addition, p.Cys282Tyr/His63Asp compound heterozygotes are at much lower risk for hereditary hemochromatosis than are p.Cys282Tyr homozygotes. The exact penetrance in p.Cys282Tyr homozygotes is unclear; however, longitudinal population-based screening studies showed that 38 to 50% of p.Cys282Tyr homozygotes develop biochemical evidence of iron overload and 10 to 33% eventually develop clinical symptoms. Penetrance is clearly incomplete.

At least four additional primary iron overload disorders with features that overlap with hemochromatosis have been identified on the basis of clinical, biochemical, and genetic characteristics. Juvenile hereditary hemochromatosis – or hemochromatosis type 2 (HFE2) – is autosomal recessive, comprising two forms: HFE2A (MIM 602390) is caused by variants in *HJV*; HFE2B (MIM 613313) is caused by variants in *HAMP*. *TFR2*-related hereditary hemochromatosis – or hemochromatosis type 3 (HFE3, MIM 604250) – is an autosomal recessive disorder caused by variants in *TFR2*. Ferroportin-associated iron overload – or hemochromatosis type 4 (HFE4, MIM 606069) – is an autosomal dominant disorder caused by variants in *SLC40A1*. At least two additional related disorders (hemochromatosis type 5 [HFE5, MIM 615517], an autosomal dominant disorder caused by variants in *FTH1*, and African iron overload disorder [MIM 601195]) have been reported but are not clearly defined at this time.

Pathogenesis

Body stores of iron are determined largely by dietary iron absorption from enterocytes of the small intestine and release of endogenous iron from macrophages that phagocytose red blood cells. Iron release from enterocytes and macrophages is regulated by a circulating iron response hormone, hepcidin,

Northern European

Hereditary hemochromatosis
with cirrhosis
p → 55 yr

c → non-expressing
HFE p.Cys282Tyr/Cys282Tyr

S.F. 30 yr

Pedigree Case 20

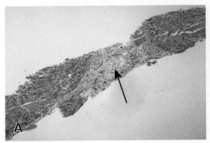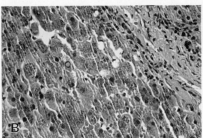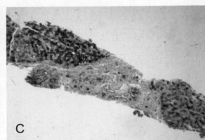

Figure C.20.1 Liver of patient with hereditary hemochromatosis showing iron deposition and cirrhosis. (A) Low-power view showing area of fibrosis (*arrow*; hematoxylin and eosin stain). (B) Higher power view showing iron deposition (*brown* pigment seen within hepatocytes) next to an area of fibrosis (hematoxylin and eosin stain). (C) Perls stain in which iron stains *dark blue*. Heavy staining in hepatocytes flanks an area of fibrosis with much less iron deposition. (Courtesy Victor Gordeuk, Howard University, Washington, DC.)

which is synthesized in the liver and released to block further iron absorption when iron supplies are adequate. Abnormal HFE interferes with hepcidin signaling, which results in the stimulation of enterocytes and macrophages to release iron. The body, therefore, continues to absorb and recycle iron, despite an iron-overloaded condition.

Ultimately, a small proportion of individuals with two variant *HFE* genes will develop symptomatic iron overload. Early symptoms include fatigue, arthralgia, decreased libido, and abdominal pain. An additional presentation is the finding of elevated transferrin iron saturation or ferritin on routine screening. Late findings of iron overload include hepatomegaly, cirrhosis (Fig. C.20.1), hepatocellular carcinoma, diabetes mellitus, cardiomyopathy, hypogonadism, arthritis, and a progressive increase in skin pigmentation. Males develop symptoms between the ages of 40 and 60 years. Women do not develop symptoms until after menopause. Prognosis is excellent in individuals diagnosed and treated before the development of cirrhosis. Those diagnosed with cirrhosis and treated effectively with phlebotomy still have a 10 to 30% risk for liver cancer years later.

Management

There are three phenotypes possible for those with *HFE*-associated hereditary hemochromatosis: clinical HFE hemochromatosis, biochemical HFE hemochromatosis, and nonexpressing p.Cys282Tyr homozygotes. Management depends on which type a patient has. Those with clinical HFE hemochromatosis (symptoms and/or end-organ damage) will start therapeutic phlebotomy and may undergo a liver biopsy. Those with biochemical HFE hemochromatosis are defined as those who do not have clinical symptoms but have an elevated transferrin-iron saturation of 45% or higher and serum ferritin concentration above the upper limit of normal (i.e., >300 ng/mL in men and >200 ng/mL in women), as well as two *HFE*-associated hereditary hemochromatosis–causing variants on confirmatory *HFE* gene testing. Those with biochemical HFE hemochromatosis should undergo therapeutic phlebotomy, in accordance with current guidelines.

Individuals with an elevated serum ferritin concentration (either clinical or biochemical hemochromatosis) undergo phlebotomy to remove a unit of blood and achieve a ferritin concentration of ≤50 ng/mL. Initial treatment usually involves a weekly removal of 500 mL of blood. Once the ferritin concentration is below 50 ng/mL, maintenance phlebotomy is performed every 3 to 4 months. Symptomatic patients with initial ferritin concentrations of more than 1000 ng/mL should undergo liver biopsy to determine whether cirrhosis is present.

Nonexpressing p.Cys282Tyr homozygotes have two variants but do not have elevated transferrin-iron saturation and/or serum ferritin concentration. These individuals do not have iron overload and therefore do not need treatment. They are monitored with serum ferritin levels annually.

Inheritance

Hereditary hemochromatosis is an autosomal recessive disorder with reduced penetrance. Each sib of an affected individual has a 25% chance of having two pathogenic alleles. The child of an affected individual will be a carrier and has a 5% risk for having two pathogenic alleles if the other parent is of European descent. Because of the apparently low penetrance of this disease, universal population screening for *HFE* variants is not indicated.

QUESTIONS FOR SMALL GROUP DISCUSSION

1. Why do women have a much lower incidence of clinical hemochromatosis?
2. Besides phlebotomy, what dietary interventions would be indicated to prevent iron overload?
3. Discuss the possible reasons for the high prevalence of the p.Cys282Tyr variant among individuals of European ancestry.

REFERENCES

Barton JC, Edwards CQ: HFE hemochromatosis. 2000 Apr 3 [Updated 2018 Dec 6]. In Adam MP, Ardinger HH, Pagon RA, editors: *GeneReviews® [Internet]*, Seattle, 1993–2022, University of Washington. https://www.ncbi.nlm.nih.gov/books/NBK1440/

Kanwar P, Kowdley KV: Diagnosis and treatment of hereditary hemochromatosis: an update, *Expert Rev Gastroenterol Hepatol* 7:517–530, 2013.

Kowdley KV, Brown KE, Ahn J, Sundaram V: ACG clinical guideline: Hereditary hemochromatosis [published correction appears in *Am J Gastroenterol* 114(12):1927, 2019], *Am J Gastroenterol* 114(8):1202–1218, 2019. https://doi.org/10.14309/ajg.0000000000000315

Wallace DF, Subramaniam VN: The global prevalence of HFE and non-HFE hemochromatosis estimated from analysis of next-generation sequencing data, *Genet Med* 18(6):618–626, 2016. https://doi.org/10.1038/gim.2015.140

HEMOPHILIA (MIM 306700 and MIM 306900)
(*F8* or *F9* Pathogenic Variants)

X-Linked

David Lillicrap

PRINCIPLES

- Intrachromosomal recombination
- Transposable element insertion
- Variable expressivity
- Protein replacement therapy

MAJOR PHENOTYPIC FEATURES

- Age at onset: infancy to adulthood
- Bleeding diathesis
- Hemarthroses
- Hematomas

HISTORY AND PHYSICAL FINDINGS

S.T., a healthy 38-year-old woman, scheduled an appointment for counseling regarding her risk for having a child with hemophilia. She had a maternal uncle who had died in childhood from hemophilia and a brother (B.T.) who had had bleeding problems as a child, but these had resolved during adolescence. No other family members had bleeding disorders. The geneticist explained to S.T. that her family history was suggestive of an X-linked abnormality of coagulation such as hemophilia A or B and that her brother's improvement was particularly suggestive of the hemophilia B variant: factor IX Leyden. To confirm the diagnosis of hemophilia, the geneticist told S.T. that B.T. should be evaluated first, because identification of an isolated carrier is difficult. S.T. talked to B.T., and he agreed to an evaluation. Review of his records showed that he had been diagnosed with factor IX deficiency as a child, but now had nearly normal plasma levels of factor IX. DNA sequence analysis confirmed that he had a variant in the *F9* gene promoter (c.-20A>T), consistent with factor IX Leyden. Subsequent testing of S.T. showed that she did not carry the variant identified in her brother.

BACKGROUND

Disease Etiology and Incidence

Hemophilia A (MIM 306700) and hemophilia B (MIM 306900) are X-linked disorders of coagulation caused by pathogenic variants in the *F8* and *F9* genes, respectively. Such variants of *F8* cause deficiency or dysfunction of clotting factor VIII; those of *F9* cause deficiency or dysfunction of clotting factor IX.

Hemophilia is found in all population groups. Hemophilia A has an incidence of 1 in 5000 to 10,000 newborn males. Hemophilia B is less common, with an incidence of 1 in 30,000 males.

Pathogenesis

The coagulation system maintains the integrity of the vasculature through a delicate balance of clot formation, remodeling, and inhibition. The proteases and protein cofactors composing the clotting cascade are present in the circulation as inactive precursors and must be sequentially activated at the site of injury to form a fibrin clot. Timely and efficient formation of a clot requires exponential activation and amplification of the protease cascade. Clotting factors VIII and IX that, along with the substrate factor X, form the "intrinsic tenase" complex are key to this amplification. They activate clotting factor X, which, in turn, converts prothrombin to thrombin in the prothrombinase complex and also activates more factor VIII (see Fig. 9.10). Activated factor IX functions as a protease and factor VIII as a cofactor. Deficiency or dysfunction of either factor IX or factor VIII causes hemophilia.

Pathogenic variants of *F8* include deletions, insertions, inversions, and single nucleotide variants. The most common is a structural rearrangement involving inversion of the first 22 exons of the *F8* gene. It accounts for 25% of all hemophilia A variants and for 45% of severe hemophilia A variants. This inversion results from an intrachromosomal recombination between sequences in intron 22 of *F8* and homologous

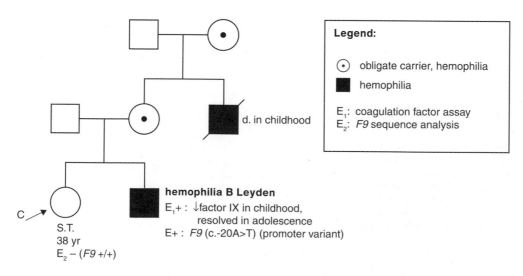

Legend:

⊙ obligate carrier, hemophilia

■ hemophilia

E_1: coagulation factor assay
E_2: *F9* sequence analysis

d. in childhood

hemophilia B Leyden
E_1+ : ↓factor IX in childhood,
resolved in adolescence
E+ : *F9* (c.-20A>T) (promoter variant)

C →
S.T.
38 yr
E_2 − (*F9* +/+)

TABLE C.21.1 Clinical Classification and Clotting Factor Levels

Classification	% Activity (Factor VIII or IX)
Severe	<1
Moderate	1–5
Mild	5–40

sequences telomeric to *F8*. Another intriguing class of *F8* alteration involves the retrotransposition of L1 repeats into the gene. For all *F8* pathogenic variants, the residual enzymatic activity of the "intrinsic tenase" complex correlates with the severity of clinical disease (see Table C.21.1).

Many different *F9* variants have been identified in individuals with hemophilia B. In contrast to the frequent partial inversion of *F8* in hemophilia A, no common *F9* variant has been identified for hemophilia B. Factor IX Leyden is an unusual *F9* variant caused by single nucleotide variants in the *F9* promoter. It is associated with very low levels of factor IX and severe hemophilia during childhood, but spontaneous resolution of hemophilia occurs at puberty, as factor IX levels nearly normalize. For each *F9* variant, the residual enzymatic activity of the factor VIII–factor IX complex correlates with the severity of clinical disease (see Table C.21.1).

Phenotype and Natural History

Hemophilia is classically a male disease, although females can be affected because of skewed X chromosome inactivation. Indeed, approximately 25% of females heterozygous for a hemophilic variant manifest some form of increased bleeding tendency. Clinically, hemophilia A and hemophilia B are indistinguishable. Both are characterized by bleeding into soft tissues, muscles, and weight-bearing joints (Fig. C.21.1). Bleeding occurs within hours after trauma and often continues for a prolonged time. Those with severe disease are often diagnosed as newborns because of excessive cephalohematomas or prolonged bleeding from umbilical or circumcision wounds. Patients with moderate disease often do not develop hematomas or hemarthroses until they begin to crawl or walk and, therefore, escape diagnosis until that time. Those with mild disease most often present in adolescence or adulthood with traumatic hemarthroses or prolonged bleeding after surgery or trauma.

Hemophilia A and hemophilia B are diagnosed and distinguished by measurement of factor VIII and IX activity levels. For both hemophilia A and hemophilia B, the level of factor VIII or IX activity predicts the clinical severity.

Management

The diagnosis of hemophilia A is established by identifying low factor VIII clotting activity in the presence of a normal von Willebrand factor level. Molecular genetic testing of *F8*, the gene encoding factor VIII, identifies disease-causing variants in as many as 98% of individuals with hemophilia A. The diagnosis of hemophilia B is established by identifying low factor IX clotting activity. Molecular genetic testing of *F9*, the gene encoding factor IX, identifies disease-causing variants in more than 99% of individuals with hemophilia B. Both tests are available clinically.

Gene therapy trials for both hemophilia A and B have shown promise, and the first licensed gene therapy product for these disorders may shortly arrive in clinics. Currently, the standard of care is intravenous replacement of the deficient factor—a therapy that has increased life expectancy from an average of 1.4 years in the early 1900s to approximately 65 years today. In addition, novel hemophilia therapies have recently entered

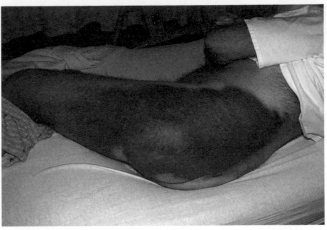

Figure C.21.1 Large soft tissue hematoma in a patient with mild hemophilia A, 4 days after an episode of minor trauma. (Courtesy David Lillicrap.)

the clinic, including replacement therapies with extended half-lives and an FVIII mimetic bispecific antibody that can be administered subcutaneously every 2 to 4 weeks.

Inheritance

If a woman has a family history of hemophilia, her carrier status can be determined by identification of the *F8* or *F9* variant segregating in the family. Routine identification of pathogenic variants using targeted exome sequencing is now widely available and is the preferred approach for definitive carrier detection. Functional plasma clotting factor levels (FVIII:C and FIX:C) will be reduced in ~50% of carriers, and this measurement will be a better indicator of the woman's likelihood of manifesting a bleeding tendency.

If a mother is a carrier, each son has a 50% risk for hemophilia, and each daughter has a 50% risk for inheriting the *F8* or *F9* variant allele. Approximately 25% of women heterozygous for a hemophilia variant will show evidence of increased bleeding, most often in the form of menorrhagia.

If a mother has a son with hemophilia but no other affected relatives, her *a priori* risk for being a carrier depends on the type of variant. Single nucleotide variants and the common *F8* inversions almost always arise in male meiosis. As a result, 98% of mothers of a male with such a variant are carriers – the consequence of a new paternal variant (i.e., in the affected male's maternal grandfather). In contrast, deletions usually arise during female meiosis. If there is no knowledge of the variant type (such as if the proband is unavailable for testing), then approximately one-third of affected cases are assumed to result from a *de novo* variant in *F8* or *F9*. Through the application of Bayes' theorem, this risk can be modified by considering the number of unaffected sons in the family (see Chapter 17).

QUESTIONS FOR SMALL GROUP DISCUSSION

1. What other diseases are caused by recombination between repeated genome sequences? Compare and contrast the recombination mechanism observed with hemophilia A with that observed with Smith-Magenis syndrome and with familial hypercholesterolemia.

2. One of the more unusual variants in *F8* is insertion of an L1 element into exon 14. What are transposable elements? How do transposable elements move within a genome? Name another disease caused by movement of transposable elements.

3. In individuals with hemophilia B due to factor IX Leyden, why does the deficiency of factor IX resolve during puberty?

4. Compare and contrast protein replacement for hemophilia to that for Gaucher disease. Approximately 30% of individuals with severe hemophilia A, and 5% of patients with severe hemophilia B develop a clinically significant immune response against factor VIII or IX. Why? Is there a genetic predisposition to development of antibodies against the replacement factors? How could this immune reaction be circumvented? Would gene therapy be helpful for patients with antibodies?

5. Discuss current approaches to gene therapy in hemophilia.

REFERENCES

Johnsen JM, Fletcher SN, Huston H, *et al.* Novel approach to genetic analysis and results in 3000 hemophilia patients enrolled in the My Life, Our Future initiative, *Blood Adv* 1(13):824–834, 2017.

Konkle BA, Josephson NC, Nakaya Fletcher S: Hemophilia A. http://www.ncbi.nlm.nih.gov/books/NBK1404/

Konkle BA, Josephson NC, Nakaya Fletcher S: Hemophilia B. http://www.ncbi.nlm.nih.gov/books/NBK1495/

Santagostino E, Fasulo MR: Hemophilia A and hemophilia B: Different types of diseases? *Semin Thromb Hemost* 39:697–701, 2013.

Miller CH: The clinical genetics of hemophilia B (factor IX deficiency), *Appl Clin Genet* 14:445–454, 2021.

22Q11.2 DELETION SYNDROME (MIM 188400 DiGeorge Syndrome or MIM 192430 Velocardiofacial Syndrome)

Autosomal Dominant or De Novo

Jacob A.S. Vorstman

PRINCIPLES

- Recurrent copy number variant
- Variable penetrance and variable expressivity
- Pleiotropy
- Factors modifying phenotypic outcome

MAJOR PHENOTYPIC FEATURES

- Congenital cardiac anomalies
- Congenital palatal anomalies and velopharyngeal insufficiency
- Immunodeficiency
- Hypoparathyroidism and hypocalcemia
- Developmental disorders including global developmental delay, language disorder, intellectual disability, specific learning disorders, autism spectrum disorder (ASD), and attention deficit hyperactivity disorder (ADHD)
- Neuropsychiatric disorders; in particular, anxiety disorders and schizophrenia spectrum disorders

HISTORY AND PHYSICAL FINDINGS

A.C., a 6-year-old girl, was referred to a developmental pediatrician because of possible learning issues. Mother reported no significant complications around pregnancy and birth; however, both breastfeeding and bottle-feeding had been a struggle, with difficulty sucking and frequent nasal regurgitations, leading to a diagnosis of gastrointestinal reflux. At age 3 years, A.C. was referred to a cardiologist after her pediatrician detected a heart murmur; subsequent testing revealed a ventricular septal defect (VSD), which was surgically repaired a few months later. Her recovery from cardiac surgery was complicated by several seizure episodes, which were caused by low serum calcium levels, attributed to the physical stress of the surgery. Seizures receded after starting calcium/vitamin D supplement. Following her protracted hospital stay, her parents expressed concerns about A.C.'s lagging language development. While initially reassured that she would "catch up" given her improved cardiac condition postsurgery, eventually, her parents were referred to the developmental pediatrician. At that point, A.C. was 6 years old and her grade 1 teacher had expressed concerns about her behavior in the classroom, citing difficulties with learning to count, problems in communication, social interaction, and attention and discussed the possible need for educational support. Given her presentation, the pediatrician ordered a chromosome microarray (including parental samples), which revealed a de novo ~3 Mb deletion of 22q11.2 in A.C. As parents were considering family expansion, they were counseled that the 22q11.2 deletion was likely the cause of the heart condition, the velopharyngeal insufficiency, the hypocalcemia, and subsequent seizures in their daughter. In addition, they were advised that the a priori probability of any next child to also have this deletion was low (<~5%, taking into account the possibility of germline mosaicism).

Developmental assessment by the pediatrician revealed a mild overall delay in milestones, with her expressive language most affected relative to the other domains, and some features consistent with possible ASD. After reading up on the information provided on the internet, parents were increasingly worried about the reported 25% risk of schizophrenia in individuals with 22q11DS.

BACKGROUND

Prior to the discovery in the early 1980s of this recurrent deletion on the long arm of chromosome 22, several clinical entities were recognized, including DiGeorge syndrome, velocardiofacial syndrome, and conotruncal anomaly face syndrome. Subsequent cytogenetic studies revealed the 22q11.2 deletion as the unifying etiology of these clinically defined conditions. In the general population, 22q11DS is among the most commonly identified genetic causes of developmental delay, congenital heart defects, and cleft palate. In approximately 0.5% of patients with schizophrenia, the underlying cause is the 22q11.2 deletion.

Disease Etiology and Incidence

The 22q11.2 deletion syndrome (22q11DS; MIM 188400 and 192430) is caused by a ~3 Mb deletion of the 22q11.2 locus, affecting approximately 50 protein-coding genes. In about 15% of cases, the deletion is mediated by low copy repeats nested within this typical region, leading to smaller-sized (~0.7–2 Mb) deletions associated with similar phenotypic manifestations, albeit less penetrant for the distal nested atypical deletions. The deletion occurs de novo in the majority (~90–95%) of cases. Among the minority of those who inherit this variant, carriership in a parent is often discovered upon parental testing, prompted by the genetic diagnosis in their offspring.

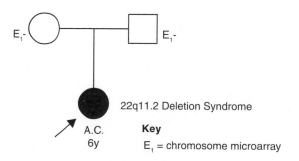

22q11.2 Deletion Syndrome

A.C.
6y

Key

E₁ = chromosome microarray

- Heart murmur
- Ventricular septal defect → repaired surgically
- Hypocalcemia
- Velopharyngeal insufficiency
- Mild global developmental delay
- Signifcant expressive language delay

E₁+: ~ 3Mb deletion of 22q11.2

22q11DS is an example of a copy number variant that is recurrent in the population, the consequence of low-copy repeat (LCR) sequences that render the flanked genomic region prone to DNA misalignment during meiosis. The result of this nonallelic homologous recombination (NAHR) is a deletion (or duplication) of DNA sequence in the resulting gamete. Indeed, duplications of the same region can lead to the 22q11.2 duplication syndrome (MIM 608363), which has overlapping phenotypic features with the 22q11.2 deletion, involving the palate, the immune system, the heart, and neuropsychiatric outcomes. The nature and severity of phenotypic outcomes with the 22q11.2 duplication is even more variable than with the reciprocal deletion, with a higher rate of unaffected or only mildly affected carriers. Of note, findings suggest that the association with ASD may be stronger for the 22q11.2 duplication than for the 22q11.2 deletion, whereas the risk for schizophrenia spectrum disorders is not increased among those with the duplication.

Pathogenesis

While the exact trajectory from haploidy to the pathophysiology of the observed phenotypes in 22q11DS remains to be

elucidated, mounting evidence implicates a role of several of the genes directly affected by the typical 22q11.2 deletion, including *TBX1, DGCR8, CRKL, COMT, RANBP1, SEPT5,* and *PRODH*. Biological consequences include abnormal development of the pharyngeal arches and of the central nervous system, mitochondrial dysfunction, disturbances in the production of small coding RNAs, and abnormal function of neurotransmitter systems.

Despite the usually strong impact of the 22q11.2 deletion, individual phenotypic expression is heterogeneous and thought to be influenced by additional genetic variants across the genome, including both rare and common, as well as environmental factors and stochastic effects that are inherent to the process of development.

Phenotype and Natural History

Phenotypic manifestations of 22q11DS are highly variable, with no associated feature present in all carriers; when present, any feature can show a wide range of severity (Fig. C.22.1). This reflects variable expressivity for the disorder. Along with pleiotropy – multiple phenotypic effects associated with the same

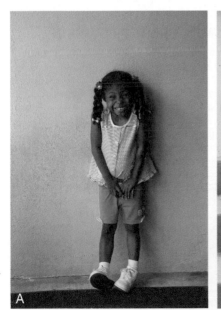
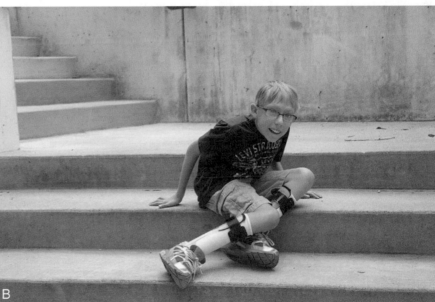
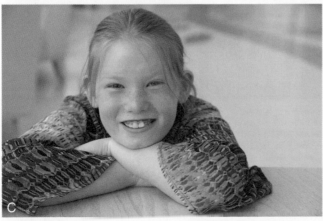
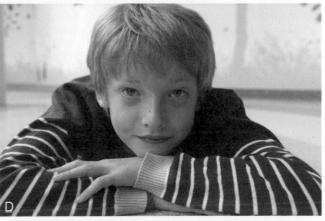

Figure C.22.1 (A) Jayda, (B) Jacob, (C) Eliza, and (D) Nathan. Each child in this figure has a molecularly confirmed 22q11.2 deletion. Even though morphological features of 22q11DS are variable and can be subtle, especially in young children, a pattern is noticeable when observing multiple children. Externally observable features include a relatively long face and almond-shaped eyes (narrow palpebral fissures); a broad nasal bridge and bulbous nose tip; small, low-set ears, often with overfolded helices; and long, tapered fingers. We acknowledge the International 22q11.2 Foundation (22q.org); photographs by Rick Guidotti, Positive Exposure (PositiveExposure.org).

variant – such aspects of phenotypic expression are now seen as typical of the 22q11.2 deletion and increasingly recognized as characteristic of many other rare pathogenic genetic variants.

The conditions most commonly associated with 22q11DS are cardiac defects – most often affecting the outflow tract – including tetralogy of Fallot, interrupted aortic arch, truncus arteriosus, and ventricular septal defects. The syndrome can also involve palatal abnormalities including overt and occult cleft palate, immune defects related to hypoplasia of the thymus and/or abnormal T cell production, hypoparathyroidism leading to hypocalcemia, and gastrointestinal abnormalities. Individuals with 22q11DS often have atypical developmental trajectories, often diagnosed early in life as global developmental delay. Subsequent assessments may reveal intellectual disability, ADHD (typically of the inattentive subtype), or autism spectrum disorder. During childhood, anxiety disorders are more prevalent. In early adulthood, the diagnosis of schizophrenia is made in ~25% of individuals carrying this deletion.

In many cases, a congenital physical defect recognized around birth triggers genetic testing, leading to diagnosis of the 22q11.2 deletion. However, as illustrated by the present case, substantial diagnostic delay occurs in a proportion of individuals, despite one or more characteristic clinical manifestations.

For 22q11DS, the breadth and respective frequency of its associated features is becoming increasingly clear; now, one of the most pressing challenges is to translate these group-level observations into reliable predictions for the individual carrier of this variant (see Chapter 19). Here, insight into the role of factors that modify phenotypic impact has proven essential. For example, findings from a large consortium study indicated that cognitive decline in the early teenage years is most prominent among individuals with 22q11DS who later develop schizophrenia. Another study showed that the cumulative effect of common variation – summarized in polygenic scores (see Chapter 9) – modified both schizophrenia and cognitive outcomes among individuals with 22q11DS. With growing study sample sizes, the explanatory power of polygenic scores is expected to increase as well, potentially bringing improved prediction of phenotypic trajectories to the individual level, within the clinical realm. From an ethical perspective, the clinical implementation of individual risk prediction requires appropriate clinical management, encompassing education, support, and monitoring or intervention for those identified as most at risk.

Management

Given the potential involvement of multiple organ systems, referral to specialist services for screening of possible defects should be considered, following the genetic diagnosis. Specialties commonly involved with 22q11DS include pediatrics, cardiology, speech pathology, plastic surgery, immunology, and endocrinology. (For a comprehensive discussion of common features and management recommendations, see practical guidelines in the reference list below). As many children with 22q11DS display atypical neurodevelopmental trajectories and behaviors, early assessment by a developmental pediatrician, psychiatrist, and/or psychologist is highly recommended. Given the increased vulnerability for psychiatric disorders – in particular, schizophrenia – it is important to offer frequent monitoring of development and behavior and to maintain an optimal balance between the profile of abilities on the one hand, and academic and social expectations on the other.

Prevention

Increasingly, researchers realize that the ability to identify genetically predisposing risk for certain phenotypic outcomes during subsequent development provides an opportunity for preventative interventions. For example, about half of individuals with 22q11DS develop scoliosis, the progression of which may be mitigated by early detection. Similarly, the emerging evidence for the benefits of early intervention programs for children with signs of autism provides a strong rationale to explore similar approaches in children with 22q11DS.

Inheritance

In most individuals with a 22q11.2 deletion, the causal event has been a *de novo* variant in the parental germline, with a low recurrence risk for sibs of the proband related to the possibility of parental germline mosaicism. Additional investigations would be needed to consider the possibility of a balanced parental chromosome rearrangement having predisposed to the copy number variant. The reciprocal 22q11.2 duplication, which is generally associated with a milder phenotype, is more frequently familial (inherited). For either form of the variant at this locus, the transmission rate from a carrier to offspring is 50%.

QUESTIONS FOR SMALL GROUP DISCUSSION

1. Compared to many other pathogenic copy number variants (CNVs), the 22q11.2 deletion stands out in several ways, including its relatively high prevalence and time since discovery, both of which have fostered the build-up of knowledge and experience with this specific variant. Discuss ways in which 22q11DS may serve as a model for other clinically relevant pathogenic rare variants.

2. Typically, the phenotypic effect of a variant such as in 22q11DS is calculated from the proportion of individuals with the genotype who express a certain phenotype (e.g., "the rate of intellectual disability in 22q11DS is ~45%"). Is there an alternative way to evaluate the phenotypic impact of a pathogenic genetic variant?

3. The phenotypic impact of a rare pathogenic variant such as in 22q11DS tends to be considered in isolation; however, these variants each occur in the context of a unique genome. Describe ways that the influence of "the rest of the genome" can be measured based on (additional) genetic testing results in 22q11DS.

REFERENCES

Óskarsdóttir S, Boot E, Crowley TB, et al: *Genet Med.* 2023 Mar;25(3):100338. doi: 10.1016/j.gim.2022.11.006. Epub 2023 Feb 2. PMID: 36729053.

Schneider M, Debbane M, Bassett AS, et al: Psychiatric disorders from childhood to adulthood in 22q11.2 deletion syndrome: Results from the International Consortium on Brain and Behavior in 22q11.2 Deletion Syndrome, *Am J Psychiatry* 171:627–639, 2014.

Davies RW, Fiksinski AM, Breetvelt EJ, et al: Using common genetic variation to examine phenotypic expression and risk prediction in 22q11.2 deletion syndrome, *Nat Med* 26:1912–1918, 2020.

McDonald-McGinn DM, Sullivan KE, Marino B, et al: 22q11.2 deletion syndrome, *Nat Rev Dis Primers* 1:15071, 2015.

23

HOLOPROSENCEPHALY (Nonsyndromic Form) (MIM 142945) (Sonic Hedgehog [*SHH*] variants)

Autosomal Dominant

Paul Kruszka

PRINCIPLES

- Developmental regulatory gene
- Genetic heterogeneity
- Position-effect variants
- Incomplete penetrance and variable expressivity

MAJOR PHENOTYPIC FEATURES

- Age at onset: prenatal
- Ventral forebrain maldevelopment
- Facial dysmorphism
- Developmental delay

HISTORY AND PHYSICAL FINDINGS

Dr. D., a 37-year-old physicist, presented to the Genetics clinic with his wife because their first child died at birth with holoprosencephaly. The pregnancy had been uncomplicated, and the child had a normal chromosome microarray. Neither he nor his wife reported any major medical problems. Dr. D. had been adopted as a child and did not know the history of his biological family. His wife's family history was not suggestive of any genetic disorders. Careful examination of Dr. D. and his wife showed that he had an absent superior labial frenulum and slight hypotelorism but no other dysmorphic findings. His physician explained to him that the holoprosencephaly in his child and his absent superior labial frenulum and slight hypotelorism were suggestive of autosomal dominant holoprosencephaly. Subsequent multigene sequencing panel testing confirmed that Dr. D. had a pathogenic variant in the sonic hedgehog gene (*SHH*). The couple was counseled regarding a 50% recurrence risk of the *SHH* variant for each subsequent pregnancy and the inability to predict severity. Reproductive options include preimplantation genetic diagnosis and others, with targeted testing for the identified *SHH* variant. (see Chapter 18).

BACKGROUND

Disease Etiology and Incidence

Holoprosencephaly (HPE, MIM 142945) has a birth incidence of 1 in 10,000 to 1 in 12,000 and is the most common human congenital brain defect. Female to male ratio is 1.4:1.

HPE results from a variety of causes, including structural genomic and single-gene disorders, environmental factors such as maternal diabetes, and possibly maternal exposure to cholesterol-lowering agents (statins). The disorder occurs both in isolation and as a feature of various syndromes, such as Smith-Lemli-Opitz syndrome. Nonsyndromic familial HPE, when inherited, is predominantly autosomal dominant, although both autosomal recessive and X-linked inheritance have been reported. Approximately 25 to 50% of all HPE is associated with a structural genomic abnormality; the nonrandom distribution of such variants predicts at least 12 different HPE loci, including 7q36, 13q32, 2p21, 18p11.3, and 21q22.3.

SHH (MIM 236100), the first gene identified with variants causing HPE, maps to 7q36. *SHH* pathogenic variants account for approximately 30 to 40% of familial nonsyndromic autosomal dominant HPE but for less than 5% of nonsyndromic HPE overall. Other genes implicated in autosomal dominant nonsyndromic HPE are *ZIC2*, accounting for 5%, and *SIX3* and *TGIF*, each accounting for 1.3%. Cohesin complex genes (*STAG2*, *SMC1A*, *SMC3*, *RAD21*) account for 1.8% of nonsyndromic HPE. *STAG3* and *SMC1A* associated with HPE are X-linked.

Pathogenesis

SHH is a secreted signaling protein required for developmental patterning in both mammals and insects (see Chapter 15).

Human *SHH* pathogenic variants are loss-of-function changes. Some of the abnormalities affecting *SHH* expression are translocations that occur 15 to 256 kb 5' to the coding region of *SHH*. These translocations are referred to as position-effect variants because they do not change the coding sequence but disrupt distant regulatory elements, chromatin structure, or both, thereby altering *SHH* expression.

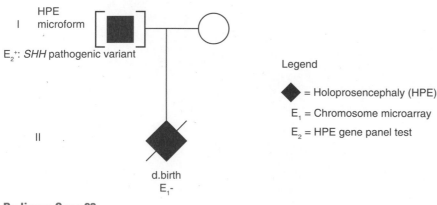

Legend

= Holoprosencephaly (HPE)

E_1 = Chromosome microarray

E_2 = HPE gene panel test

Pedigree Case 23

Phenotype and Natural History

The prosencephalic malformations of HPE follow a continuum of severity. They are usually subdivided into alobar HPE (no evidence of an interhemispheric fissure), semilobar HPE (posterior interhemispheric fissure only), and lobar HPE (ventricular separation and almost complete cortical separation) (Fig. C.23.1). Among those with HPE and a normal chromosome microarray, 63% have alobar HPE, 28% have semilobar HPE, and 9% have lobar HPE. Other commonly associated central nervous system malformations include undivided thalami, dysgenesis of the corpus callosum, hypoplastic olfactory bulbs, hypoplastic optic bulbs and tracts, and pituitary dysgenesis.

The spectrum of facial dysmorphism in HPE extends from cyclopia to normal and usually reflects the severity of the central nervous system malformations. Dysmorphic features associated with, but not diagnostic of, HPE include microcephaly or macrocephaly, anophthalmia or microphthalmia, hypotelorism or hypertelorism, dysmorphic nose, palatal anomalies, bifid uvula, a single central incisor, and absence of a superior labial frenulum.

Delayed development occurs in nearly all individuals with HPE. The severity of delay correlates with the severity of central nervous system malformation; that is, those with normal brain imaging usually have normal intelligence. In addition to delayed development, patients frequently have seizures, brainstem dysfunction, and sleep dysregulation.

Among individuals with HPE but without structural genomic abnormalities, survival varies inversely with the severity of the facial phenotype. Patients with cyclopia or ethmocephaly usually do not survive a week; approximately 50% of those with alobar HPE die before 4 to 5 months of age, and 80% before a year. Approximately 50% of those with isolated semilobar or lobar HPE survive the first year.

Management

Patients with HPE require an expeditious evaluation within the first few days of life. Treatment is symptomatic and supportive. Aside from the medical concerns of the patient, a major part of management includes counseling and supporting the parents, as well as defining the cause of HPE.

Inheritance

Etiologically, HPE is extremely heterogeneous, and the recurrence risk in a family is dependent on the identification of the underlying cause. The child of a diabetic mother has a 1% risk for having HPE. For parents of a child with a structural genomic anomaly, the recurrence risk depends on whether one of them has a genomic abnormality that gave rise to the anomaly in their child. For parents of a child with syndromic HPE, the recurrence risk depends on the recurrence risk for that syndrome. In the absence of a family history of HPE or a recognized genomic or syndromic cause of HPE, parents and siblings must be examined closely for microforms: subtle features (as outlined above) associated with HPE. For parents with a negative family history, no identifiable causes of HPE, and no microforms suggestive of autosomal dominant HPE, the empirical recurrence risk is approximately 4% to 5%. In some cases, digenic inheritance involving other HPE-associated genes may explain a proband's severe phenotype in the context of *SHH* variants with otherwise low-penetrance phenotypes.

Although autosomal recessive and X-linked HPE have been reported, most families with an established mode of inheritance exhibit autosomal dominant inheritance. The penetrance of autosomal dominant HPE is approximately 70%. Among obligate carriers of autosomal dominant HPE, the risk of a child being affected with severe HPE is 16 to 21% and of being affected with a microform 13 to 14%. The phenotype

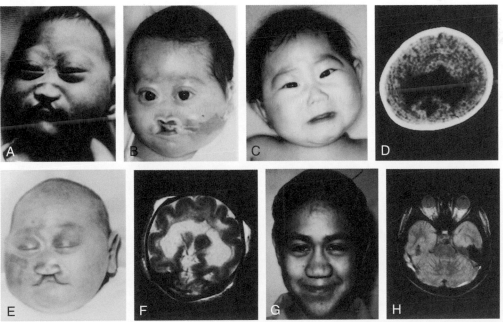

Figure C.23.1 Holoprosencephaly (HPE) in patients with *SHH* variants. (A) Microcephaly, absence of nasal bones, midline cleft palate, and semilobar HPE. (B) Semilobar HPE, premaxillary agenesis, and midline cleft lip. (C) and (D) Mild facial findings with severe semilobar HPE on magnetic resonance imaging. (E) and (F) Microcephaly, prominent optic globes, premaxillary agenesis, and cleft lip, with semilobar HPE on magnetic resonance imaging. (G) and (H) Microcephaly, ocular hypotelorism, flat nose without palpable cartilage, midface and philtrum hypoplasia, normal intelligence, and normal brain on magnetic resonance imaging. All patients have *SHH* variants. Patients (A) and (B) also have variants of *TGIF*, and patient (C) also has a variant in *ZIC2*. *TGIF* variants indirectly decrease *SHH* expression. (Courtesy M. Muenke, National Human Genome Research Institute, National Institutes of Health, Bethesda, Maryland. Modified by permission from Nanni L, Ming JE, Bocian M, et al: The mutational spectrum of the sonic hedgehog gene in holoprosencephaly: SHH mutations cause a significant proportion of autosomal dominant holoprosencephaly. *Hum Mol Genet* 8:2479–2488, 1999.)

of the carrier does not affect the risk for their offspring to be affected, nor does it predict the severity if the child is affected.

Clinical molecular testing using ever-evolving diagnostic panels for known HPE genes is currently available. If a pathogenic variant is identified, a targeted assay can be used for any further testing for the family. Severe HPE can be detected by prenatal ultrasound examination at 16 to 18 weeks of gestation.

QUESTIONS FOR SMALL GROUP DISCUSSION

1. What factors might explain the variable expressivity and penetrance of *SHH* variants among siblings?
2. Discuss genetic disorders with a sex bias and the mechanisms underlying the sex bias. As examples, consider Rett syndrome to illustrate embryonic sex-biased lethality, pyloric stenosis to illustrate a sex bias in disease frequency, and coronary heart disease in familial hypercholesterolemia to illustrate a sex bias in disease severity.
3. Considering the many loci associated with HPE, discuss why variants in different genes give rise to identical phenotypes.
4. Considering that *GLI3* is in the signal transduction cascade of SHH, discuss why *GLI3* loss-of-function variants do not give rise to the same phenotype as *SHH* loss-of-function variants.
5. Discuss the role of cholesterol in brain morphogenesis.

REFERENCES

Kauvar EF, Muenke M: Holoprosencephaly: Recommendations for diagnosis and management, *Curr Opin Pediatr* 22:687–695, 2010.

Kruszka P, Berger SI, Casa V, *et al.* Cohesin complex-associated holoprosencephaly, *Brain* 142(9):2631–2643, 2019. https://doi.org/10.1093/brain/awz210. PMID: 31334757; PMCID: PMC7245359.

Tekendo-Ngongang C, Muenke M, Kruszka P: Holoprosencephaly overview. http://www.ncbi.nlm.nih.gov/books/NBK1530/

24

HUNTINGTON DISEASE (MIM 143100)
(*HTT* Pathogenic Variant [CAG Expansion])

Autosomal Dominant

Christopher Pearson • Janet A. Buchanan

PRINCIPLES

- Tandem repeat expansion
- Dynamic variant
- Anticipation with parent-of-origin bias
- Delayed onset
- Presymptomatic counseling, predictive testing

MAJOR PHENOTYPIC FEATURES

- Age at onset: late childhood (juvenile HD) to late adulthood (infantile [extremely rare]) neurodegeneration
- Progressive movement, cognitive and psychiatric abnormalities

HISTORY AND PHYSICAL FINDINGS

M.P., a 45-year-old man, first noted declining memory and concentration, followed by involuntary movements of his fingers and toes, facial grimacing, and pouting. He was aware of his condition, became depressed, and consulted his family doctor. He had been previously healthy and was unaware of any similarly affected relatives; however, he had been raised by his single mother after his biological father abandoned them. M.P. had an older brother (B.P.) and one healthy daughter (D.P.). M.P. was referred to a neurologist who suspected Huntington disease (HD). This was confirmed by laboratory analysis of his DNA, which showed an expanded CAG repeat tract in one *HTT* gene on chromosome 4p16.3. M.P. asked the neurologist about options for treatment. He was advised that some medications are helpful for specific symptoms in some patients, that research is very active toward therapies targeting the cause of the disease, and that these might be more effective in the future. At present, no cure is possible, but there might be the option to participate in a clinical trial. M.P. was offered multidisciplinary assistance, including physical and occupational therapy, and encouraged to contact a local Huntington patient support group. M.P. was then referred to a Genetics clinic specializing in HD, along with his daughter (D.P.) and brother (B.P.). The genetics specialists helped with the shock of a diagnosis that was new to this family and explained that given a firm diagnosis in M.P., the probability that D.P. had inherited the expanded allele predisposing to HD was about 50% (reduced marginally because she was apparently unaffected at age 25). B.P. was also at somewhat less than 50% risk. They discussed the option of presymptomatic genetic testing, and both D.P. and B.P. went ahead with this after several more counseling sessions. The lab results (Fig. C.24.1) showed that B.P. had not inherited the pathogenic allele, but D.P. had inherited the CAG-expanded *HTT* allele from her father. D.P. then asked about options for her future potential children. The geneticist described the possibility of preimplantation genetic testing as a means to avoid passing her expanded allele on to future offspring, with the offer of further discussion when the situation was right.

BACKGROUND

Disease Etiology and Incidence

Huntington disease (HD) is an autosomal dominant, progressive neurodegenerative disorder caused by tandem repeat

expansions in the *HTT* gene (see Chapter 13). The prevalence of HD is at least 10-fold higher in Europe, North America, and Australia (in the range of 1/10,000 population) than in Asia. Estimates depend on the means of ascertainment, and variation in prevalence reflects population distribution of haplotypes associated with predisposition to expansion in the gene.

Pathogenesis

The *HTT* gene product – huntingtin – is ubiquitously expressed but its function remains unknown.

Pathogenic variants in *HTT* usually result from expansion of a polyglutamine-encoding CAG repeat sequence in exon 1; normal *HTT* alleles have 10 to 26 CAG repeats, whereas pathogenic HD-causing alleles have 36 or more repeats (see Chapter 13). Approximately 3% of patients develop HD as the result of a new CAG repeat expansion, but most inherit the pathogenic expanded allele from an affected parent. Newly pathogenic expanded alleles arise from further expansion of an intermediate allele (27–35 CAG repeats) (sometimes previously called a premutation). When such an event occurs, the transmitting parent is nearly always the father.

Expansion of the huntingtin polyglutamine tract appears to confer a deleterious novel property that is necessary and sufficient for the induction of an HD phenotype. In addition to the diffuse, severe atrophy of the neostriatum – the hallmark of HD – expression of mutant huntingtin causes transcriptomic dysregulation, neuronal dysfunction, generalized brain atrophy, and changes in neurotransmitter levels. Accumulating neuronal nuclear and cytoplasmic aggregates comprise mutant elongated huntingtin along with other characteristic biomarkers. Ultimately, expression of this abnormal huntingtin leads to neuronal death; however, it is likely that clinical symptoms and neuronal dysfunction precede both the development of intracellular aggregates and neuronal death. The mechanism by which expression of this expanded polyglutamine tract causes HD remains unclear.

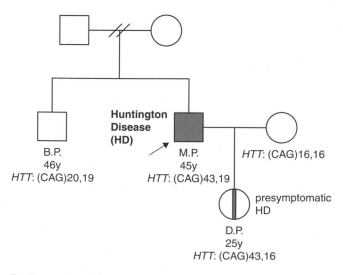

Pedigree Case 24

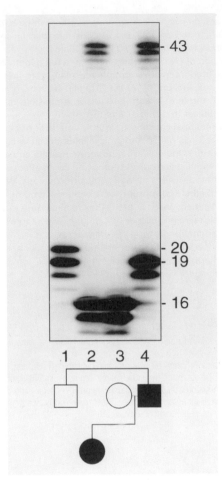

Figure C.24.1 Segregation of an *HTT* gene pathogenic allele in a family with Huntington disease; Southern blot analysis of polymerase chain reaction (*PCR*) products derived from amplification of the CAG repeats in exon 1 of *HTT*. Each allele generates a full-length fragment as well as two or more shorter fragments, because of difficulties with the PCR across a triplet repeat. Notice that the affected father and daughter both have an allele with a full penetrance HD-causing expansion (43 CAG repeats) and a normal allele (19 and 16 repeats, respectively). The daughter's unaffected mother and her unaffected paternal uncle have *HTT* alleles with a normal number of CAG repeats. (Courtesy M. R. Hayden, University of British Columbia, Vancouver, Canada.)

Phenotype and Natural History

As a group average, the age at disease onset is inversely proportional to the number of *HTT* CAG repeats. Individuals with adult-onset disease usually have 40 to 55 repeats; those with juvenile-onset disease usually have more than 60 repeats (see Fig. 7.19). Those with 36 to 39 *HTT* CAG repeats represent reduced penetrance and may or may not develop HD in their lifetime. The number of repeats does not correlate with features of HD other than age at onset.

Instability and further expansion of the CAG repeats within expanded *HTT* alleles often results in genetic anticipation: progressively earlier onset with succeeding generations. Once the number of CAG repeats is 36 or more, expansion generally continues during paternal transmission. During maternal transmission, expansions are less frequent and less extensive. Individuals with juvenile onset (before age 20) often have a massive expansion of the CAG repeat (60–350 units), of which about 75% are inherited paternally.

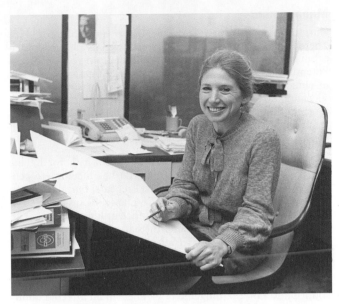

Figure C.24.2 Nancy S. Wexler at the National Institute of Neurological Disorders and Stroke (*NINDS*), Washington DC, c. 1980. Dr. Wexler's family history helped motivate her lifelong commitment to research on Huntington disease and support for those living with it. She spearheaded the initiative to work with families in communities around Lake Maracaibo in Venezuela, where the prevalence of HD is high. The landmark pedigree she and colleagues created with family members and DNA samples they collected over many yearly visits were instrumental in linking the gene associated with HD to its location on chromosome 4p16.3 in 1983, and to its full cloning and characterization a decade later. (Courtesy Huntington Disease Foundation.)

Approximately one-third of patients present with psychiatric abnormalities; two-thirds have a combination of cognitive and motor disturbances. The mean age at presentation is 35 to 44 years. Approximately 25% of cases develop HD after age 50, and 10% before age 20. The median survival after diagnosis is 15 to 18 years, and the mean age at death is approximately 55 years.

HD is characterized by progressive motor, cognitive, and psychiatric abnormalities. The motor disturbances involve both voluntary and involuntary movement, initially interfering little with daily activities but generally becoming incapacitating as HD progresses. Chorea, which is present in more than 90% of those with HD, is the most common involuntary movement, characterized by nonrepetitive, nonperiodic jerks that cannot be suppressed. Cognitive abnormalities begin early in the disease course; language is usually affected later than are other cognitive functions. Behavioral disturbances, which usually develop later in the disease course, include social disinhibition, aggression, outbursts, apathy, sexual deviation, and increased appetite. The psychiatric manifestations can develop at any time and include personality changes, affective psychosis, and schizophrenia.

Advancement of the disease coincides with ongoing somatic expansion of *HTT*, especially in vulnerable brain regions, supporting the concept that these dynamic variants drive disease progression. In the end stages of HD, individuals usually develop such severe motor impairments that they are fully dependent on others. They also experience weight loss, sleep disturbances, incontinence, and mutism. Behavioral disturbances tend to decrease as the disease advances.

Management

Currently no curative treatments are available for HD. Therapy focuses on supportive care as well as pharmacological management of the behavioral and neurological problems. Potential therapeutics are under active investigation, including in clinical trials. Some approaches involve attempts at gene silencing, targeting the expanded *HTT* allele (https://huntingtonstudygroup.org).

Inheritance

Each child of a parent with HD has a 50% risk for having inherited a pathogenic *HTT* allele. HD has incomplete penetrance with alleles of 36 to 39 CAG repeats, but all children who inherit a full penetrance *HTT* allele (40 or more CAG repeats) will develop HD, given a sufficient lifespan.

From a father with an intermediate allele, the empirical risk of a full penetrance *HTT* allele in an offspring is approximately 3%.

Presymptomatic testing and prenatal testing are forms of predictive testing (see Chapter 18) and are best interpreted after confirmation of a pathogenic *HTT* allele in an affected family member. Family members at risk can be tested using the same molecular analysis as that for diagnosis. Recommendations regarding presymptomatic genetic testing for untreatable conditions such as HD include the need for neurological and psychological evaluation before testing and for psychological support from family members or friends. Additionally, the individual should be deemed old enough (typically an adult) and competent to make an informed choice regarding such testing (see Chapter 19). The implications of such results are obviously life altering.

QUESTIONS FOR SMALL GROUP DISCUSSION

1. Individuals who are heterozygous or homozygous for pathogenic *HTT* alleles have similar clinical expression of HD. How can this be explained?
2. Some studies suggest that a father with an intermediate allele and an affected child has a higher risk of subsequently transmitting a full penetrance allele than does a father with a similar allele and no affected children. Discuss possible mechanisms for this predisposition to transmit *HTT* pathogenic alleles.
3. Expansion of *HTT* from intermediate to full penetrance alleles occurs predominantly through the male germline, whereas similar expansion of *FMR1* (fragile X syndrome) occurs through the female germline. Discuss possible mechanisms for sex biases in disease transmission.
4. By international consensus, asymptomatic at-risk children are not tested for *HTT* pathogenic alleles because such testing removes that individual's autonomy. Results could open the child to familial and social stigma and could affect educational and career decisions as well as health coverage. When might it be, nonetheless, appropriate to test an asymptomatic at-risk child? What advances in medicine are necessary to make testing of all asymptomatic at-risk children acceptable? (Consider the reasoning underlying newborn screening.)
5. What aspects of HD make it a good potential candidate for gene therapy interventions? What aspects are particularly challenging for such strategies?

REFERENCES

Bordelon YM: Clinical neurogenetics: Huntington disease, *Neurol Clin* 31:1085–1094, 2013.
Nicholas S Caron, Galen EB Wright, and Michael R Hayden. GeneReviews: Huntington Disease. http://www.ncbi.nlm.nih.gov/books/NBK1305/
Journal of Huntington's Disease Special Issue on DNA Repair and Somatic Repeat Expansion in Huntington's Disease Direct Link: https://content.iospress.com/journals/journal-of-huntingtons-disease/10/1

25

HYPERTROPHIC CARDIOMYOPATHY (MIM 192600)
(Cardiac Sarcomere Gene Variants)

Autosomal Dominant

Miriam Reuter

PRINCIPLES

- Locus heterogeneity
- Age-related penetrance
- Variable expressivity

MAJOR PHENOTYPIC FEATURES

- Age at onset: adolescence and early adulthood
- Left ventricular hypertrophy
- Outflow tract obstruction
- Diastolic dysfunction
- Systolic dysfunction/heart failure
- Sudden death

HISTORY AND PHYSICAL FINDINGS

A 30-year-old healthy man presented to a heart clinic with dyspnea, palpitation, and chest pain. His father had congestive heart failure, and his paternal uncle had sudden cardiac death at 18 years of age while practicing football. The cardiologist explained to the patient the possibility of heart disease running in his family. Cardiac examination showed double apical impulse, fourth heart sound, jugular venous pulse, and double carotid arterial pulse. Echocardiogram showed asymmetrical septal hypertrophy with no structural anomalies, diagnostic of hypertrophic cardiomyopathy. Consistent with his clinical history, physical features, and family history, multigene panel testing identified a pathogenic variant, p.Arg403Gln in *MYH7*. At-risk family members were referred for clinical evaluation and were offered molecular genetic testing for the variant.

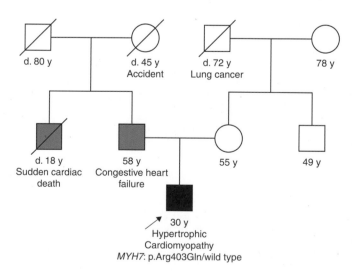

Pedigree Case 25

BACKGROUND
Disease Etiology and Incidence

Hypertrophic cardiomyopathy (HCM), the most common monogenic cardiovascular disease, is an autosomal dominant disorder caused by pathogenic variants in genes encoding structural or regulatory components of the cardiac sarcomere. Of those patients with positive genetic tests, approximately 80% are found to have variants in *MYBPC3* and *MYH7*, whereas other genes (*TNNI3*, *TNNT2*, *ACTC1*, *MYL2*, *MYL3*, *PLN*, and *TPM1*) each account for a small proportion of pathogenic variants (1–5%). An additional five genes with strong or moderate validity (*ALPK3*, *ACTN2*, *CSRP3*, *TNNC1*, *JPH2*) may account for <1% of cases.

Pathogenesis

Over 1000 pathogenic and likely pathogenic variants for nonsyndromic HCM have been reported in the various genes that encode components of the cardiac sarcomere or calcium-regulatory proteins. Variants in additional, functionally related genes (listed above) have been proposed with strong or moderate clinical validity. A pathogenic variant can be identified in approximately 50 to 60% of individuals with nonsyndromic HCM and a family history of the condition. In contrast, only about 20 to 30% of individuals without a family history have positive results.

Syndromic presentations of HCM have diverse etiologies and therapeutic strategies. Examples include Danon disease (*LAMP2*), Fabry disease (*GLA*), Friedreich ataxia (*FXN*), mitochondrial DNA depletion syndrome (e.g., *SLC25A4*), hereditary amyloidosis (*TTR*), myofibrillar myopathy (*FLNC*), and rasopathies (see Case 41).

Phenotype and Natural History

HCM is characterized by left ventricular hypertrophy (LVH) (Fig. C.25.1) in the absence of predisposing cardiovascular conditions (e.g., aortic stenosis, long-standing hypertension). The clinical manifestations of HCM range from asymptomatic to progressive heart failure to arrhythmias (atrial fibrillation as well as malignant ventricular arrhythmias) to sudden cardiac death, varying from individual to individual even within the same family. Common symptoms include shortness of breath (particularly with exertion), chest pain, palpitation, orthostasis, presyncope, and syncope. Most often, the LVH of HCM becomes apparent during adolescence or young adulthood but may manifest at any age.

Management

Genetic assessment for HCM includes a three-generation family history, genetic counseling, and molecular genetic testing using multigene panels complemented by deletion and duplication testing. In rare cases (and with low yield), genome-wide sequencing (exome or genome) can be applied if panel testing is negative. Interpretation of genetic variants is based on criteria outlined by the American College of Medical Genetics and Genomics (see Chapter 17): (1) cosegregation with the HCM phenotype in family members; (2) previously reported

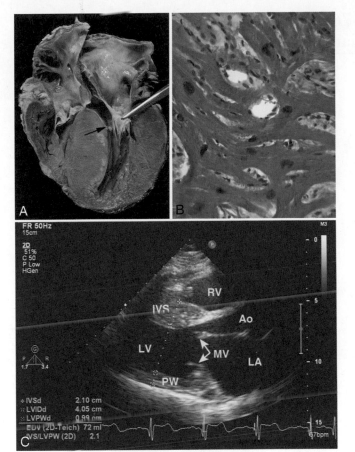

Figure C.25.1 Hypertrophic cardiomyopathy with asymmetric septal hypertrophy. (A) The septal muscle bulges into the left ventricular outflow tract, and the left atrium is enlarged. The anterior mitral leaflet has been reflected away from the septum to reveal a fibrous endocardial plaque (*arrow*) (see text). (B) Histological appearance demonstrating myocyte disarray, extreme hypertrophy, and exaggerated myocyte branching, as well as the characteristic interstitial fibrosis. (C) Echocardiographic appearance of hypertrophic cardiomyopathy. Parasternal long-axis view from a patient with hypertrophic cardiomyopathy demonstrating asymmetrical septal hypertrophy. The interventricular septum (IVS) measures 2.1 cm (normal 0.6–1.0 cm), and the posterior wall measures 0.99 cm. *Ao*, Aorta; *LA*, left atrium; *LV*, left ventricle; *MV*, mitral valve; *PW*, posterior wall; *RV*, right ventricle. (A) and (B) from Schoen FJ: The heart. In Kumar V, Abbas AK, Aster JC, editors: *Robbins and Cotran pathologic basis of disease,* Philadelphia, 2015, WB Saunders, pp 523–578. (C) from Issa ZF, Miller JM, Zipes DP: *Clinical arrhythmology and electrophysiology: a companion to Braunwald's heart disease,* Philadelphia, 2012, WB Saunders, pp 618–624.

family members (predictive testing). Clinically unaffected family members with pathogenic HCM-associated variants should undergo clinical cardiovascular screenings (every 1–2 years in children and adolescents, every 3–5 years in adults). If the causative genetic variant in an individual with HCM remains unknown or uncertain, clinical cardiovascular screenings should be performed in all first-degree family members (every 1–3 years in children and adolescents depending on the age of onset in affected relatives, every 3–5 years in adults). Screening should be initiated no later than puberty. Early childhood screening is appropriate if there is a family history of early-onset disease or other clinical concerns.

No treatments to prevent disease development or to reverse established manifestations currently exist. The treatment of manifestations includes medical management of diastolic dysfunction, medical or surgical management of ventricular outflow obstruction, restoration and maintenance of sinus rhythm in those with atrial fibrillation, implantable cardioverter-defibrillator in survivors of cardiac arrest and those at high risk for cardiac arrest, medical treatment for heart failure, and consideration for cardiac transplantation when indicated. The prevention of secondary complications includes consideration of anticoagulation in those with persistent or paroxysmal atrial fibrillation to reduce the risk for thromboembolism, and care by an experienced cardiologist and obstetrician trained in high-risk obstetrics during the pregnancy of a person with HCM. Patients should avoid dehydration, hypovolemia (i.e., use diuretics with caution), and medications that decrease afterload (e.g., angiotensin-converting enzyme [ACE] inhibitors, angiotensin receptor blockers, and direct vasodilators). Moderate-intensity recreational exercise is considered beneficial for most patients with HCM.

Inheritance

HCM follows autosomal dominant inheritance with variable expressivity and incomplete, age-related penetrance; each first-degree relative of an affected patient has a 50% chance of carrying the pathogenic variant and potentially developing HCM. Sporadic cases may be due to *de novo* variants in the proband but absent from the parents.

Preconception or prenatal genetic counseling should be offered to discuss the risk of disease transmission and reproductive options (see Chapter 18).

QUESTIONS FOR SMALL GROUP DISCUSSION

1. Name other disorders that show age-related penetrance. What are the factors that can contribute to age-related penetrance of a disease?
2. Discuss possible reasons for locus heterogeneity in HCM.
3. What are the criteria to classify a variant as benign?
4. When is genetic testing indicated in a proband with suspected HCM?

or identified as a cause of HCM; (3) low allele frequency in controls; (4) important alteration in protein structure and function; and (5) evolutionary conservation of the substituted residue or computational assessment of prediction of functional perturbation. Despite the use of these criteria, a considerable number of variants remain classified as variants of unknown significance (VUS) (see Chapter 17), and longitudinal reevaluation is recommended.

A molecular diagnosis enables cascade testing of at-risk family members. Only pathogenic/likely pathogenic variants should be used for the genetic testing of clinically unaffected

REFERENCES

Cirino AL, Ho C: Familial hypertrophic cardiomyopathy overview. http://www.ncbi.nlm.nih.gov/books/NBK1768/

Ommen SR, Mital S, Burke MA, et al: 2020 AHA/ACC guideline for the diagnosis and treatment of patients with hypertrophic cardiomyopathy. https://www.ahajournals.org/doi/10.1161/CIR.0000000000000937

Ingles J, Goldstein J, Thaxton C, et al: Evaluating the clinical validity of hypertrophic cardiomyopathy genes. https://www.ahajournals.org/doi/10.1161/CIRCGEN.119.002460

Richards S, Aziz N, Bale S, et al: Standards and guidelines for the interpretation of sequence variants: A joint consensus recommendation of the American College of Medical Genetics and Genomics and the Association for Molecular Pathology. https://www.ncbi.nlm.nih.gov/pmc/articles/PMC4544753/

26

PROTEUS SYNDROME (MIM 176920)
(*AKT1* Gene *de novo* Mosaic Variant)

Leslie G. Biesecker • Christopher A. Ours

PRINCIPLES

- Somatic mosaicism
- Sporadic occurrence
- Gain of function variant
- Phenotypic heterogeneity

MAJOR PHENOTYPIC FINDINGS

- Age at onset: early to middle childhood
- Progressive segmental overgrowth
- Cerebriform connective tissue nevus (CCTN)
- Bony overgrowth
- Dysregulated adipose tissue and lipomas
- Cystic lung disease
- Vascular malformations
- Increased risk of venous thromboembolism

HISTORY AND PHYSICAL FINDINGS

J.D. is a 6-year-old male child who presented with multiple skin lesions and asymmetric lower extremities. His parents first noticed that his left leg was larger than the right when he was 9 months old. Around the same time, the parents saw a streak of raised rough skin on the left side of his abdomen that extended to, but did not cross, his midline. The pigmentation of the raised skin has increased since onset. When he was 4 years old, he developed flesh-colored bumps on the bottom of his left foot. These have thickened over time and coalesced to form ridges resembling the surface of a brain (Fig. C.26.1). Suspecting a mosaic overgrowth disorder, the geneticist obtained a skin punch biopsy from this abnormal skin on the foot for genetic testing by a sequencing panel for genes associated with overgrowth. This showed the presence of a mosaic *AKT1* c.49 G>A p.Glu17Lys variant. This variant, along with the clinical presentation, confirmed a diagnosis of Proteus syndrome. The geneticist shared with the family a plan to monitor him for continued overgrowth, involving a multidisciplinary team to include dermatology, physical therapy, and orthopedic surgery for possible future surgical treatment of leg length discrepancy with epiphysiodesis. The family was referred to a research center for consideration of participation in a natural history study and a therapeutic trial.

Disease Etiology and Incidence

AKT1-related Proteus syndrome (MIM 176920) is an ultrarare segmental overgrowth disorder occurring in <1/1,000,000 live births. It is caused by a mutational event in the *AKT1* gene during development. This postzygotic process results in somatic mosaicism, whereby a fraction of cells become heterozygous for an activating variant of *AKT1*. *AKT1*-related Proteus syndrome is an obligate mosaic condition because (it is hypothesized) germline heterozygosity results in early embryonic death. This has been demonstrated in mouse models and there are no known individuals with Proteus syndrome who have a germline heterozygous activating variant in *AKT1*.

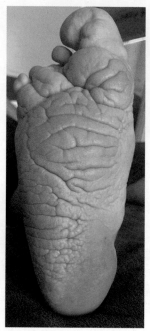

Figure C.26.1 Noah, who has Proteus syndrome, enjoys riding his scooter and playing soccer. This is a cerebriform connective tissue nevus on the right foot with associated overgrowth of the great toe. These lesions begin as small nodules that later develop a cerebriform appearance and can progress to involve the entire plantar surface. (*Courtesy Christopher Ours and Leslie Biesecker.*)

Pathophysiology

AKT1 is serine/threonine kinase that plays critical roles in the regulation of cell growth and survival. Variants in the inhibitory pleckstrin homology domain of the AKT1 protein can lead to increased phosphorylation and activate downstream effectors to promote cell growth and survival. In Proteus syndrome, this most commonly occurs through a single nucleotide transition (c.48 G>A) that predicts a glutamic acid to lysine substitution at amino acid position 17 (p.Glu17Lys). AKT1 signaling occurs in a wide range of cell types; consequently, nearly any tissue in Proteus syndrome can be affected. The dysregulation of cell growth manifests as proliferation and hyperplasia leading to overgrowth of the affected tissue. In some instances, neoplasia arises in particular tissues but is rarely malignant. This is the same *AKT1* variant as that identified in many cancers.

Phenotype

The phenotype of Proteus syndrome typifies mosaic distribution with a spectrum of clinical severity and interindividual heterogeneity. A large majority of individuals have few or no signs of the disease at birth. The overgrowth often becomes apparent during the first few years of life. The natural history of Proteus syndrome is one of relentless progression, particularly in childhood, which may result in permanent disability or need for surgical intervention including amputation.

The diagnosis of Proteus syndrome is made through a combination of molecular identification of an activating *AKT1* variant in affected tissue and clinical features of the disorder. Though Proteus syndrome may affect nearly any tissue in the body, the most common manifestations are skin and bone overgrowth, lung abnormalities, thrombosis, organ asymmetry, and tumor predisposition. The hallmark lesion of Proteus syndrome is the cerebriform connective tissue nevus that most commonly occurs on the plantar surface of the foot (see Fig. C.26.1). This initially presents as a flesh-colored confluence of papules and nodules and progresses to a cerebriform appearance. Other skin manifestations include epidermal nevi that may have increased pigmentation or increased hair growth following Blaschko's lines.

The bony overgrowth in Proteus syndrome most commonly causes elongation of the long bones leading to leg length discrepancy and angulation deformities (Fig. C.26.2). It also causes scoliosis and craniofacial asymmetry. Pulmonary manifestations include obstructive lung disease with lung cysts and restrictive lung disease caused by scoliosis and chest wall deformities. Vascular anomalies, particularly venous, and lipomatous dysregulation may be present. Asymmetry, enlargement, or cyst formation in the liver, spleen, or kidney can occur. Individuals with Proteus syndrome are at an increased risk of tumor development; these include low-grade epithelial tumors of the ovary or testis, meningioma, and parotid adenoma.

Management

Appropriate diagnosis of *AKT1*-related Proteus syndrome is paramount for care and prognostication. Because the variant occurs as a postzygotic mutational event, DNA testing must be performed on affected tissue. Most commonly, this is done by a skin punch biopsy. Testing blood is not appropriate, as it may yield a negative result when, in fact, other tissues harbor the pathogenic variant. Molecular diagnostic strategies must take into consideration the limitations imposed by mosaicism; for example, Sanger sequencing may fail to detect low levels of variant otherwise revealed by higher read-depth next-generation sequencing approaches (see Chapter 17). This diagnostic approach should also be employed in the evaluation of other segmental overgrowth disorders, such as *PIK3CA*-related overgrowth spectrum disorders. The management of *AKT1*-related Proteus syndrome should be tailored to an individual's manifestations but is primarily supportive and/or surgical. Targeted therapy with inhibitors of AKT is a potential treatment strategy under investigation.

The soft tissue and bony overgrowth in *AKT1*-related Proteus syndrome may lead to significant morbidity, pain, and functional limitations. Debulking of soft tissue overgrowth may be an option but the risk of recurrence and need for multiple surgeries should be considered. Bony overgrowth of the lower extremities and leg length discrepancy may be addressed by temporary epiphysiodesis, which halts the lengthening of the affected long bones while the contralateral leg is allowed to grow and catch up. Physeal arrest may also be needed, such as when digits have reached an adult length before skeletal maturity.

When individuals with Proteus syndrome undergo surgery, prophylactic anticoagulation is recommended, as they are at increased risk of blood clots. Thromboembolic events, particularly in the perioperative period, are the leading cause of death in Proteus syndrome.

There is no known, approved, primary medical therapy for the pulmonary manifestation of Proteus syndrome. Advanced disease may require supplemental oxygen, noninvasive ventilation, or resection of the affected lung tissue.

The role of the PI3K/AKT signaling pathway in cancer has led to the development of several small molecular inhibitors. Clinical studies that repurpose these inhibitors for segmental overgrowth are ongoing.

Inheritance

AKT1-related Proteus syndrome is sporadic and does not follow a mendelian pattern of inheritance. It is caused by a somatic, rather than germline, variant. Consistent with this is a report of monozygotic twins discordant for Proteus syndrome. It is not inherited and affected individuals have had children unaffected by the disorder.

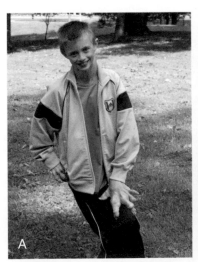 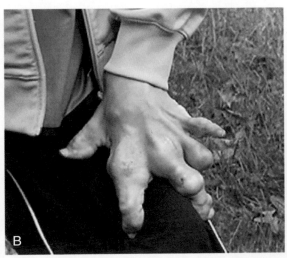 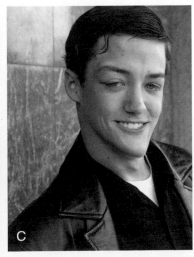

Figure C.26.2 (A) Jordan enjoys playing soccer during a gathering of the Proteus Syndrome Foundation (proteus-syndrome.org). Involvement of the lower extremity can cause leg length discrepancy and impaired mobility. (B) Detail of Jordan's hand showing soft tissue and bony overgrowth resulting in elongation of fingers, angular deformity, and decreased range of motion. (C) Brian is an adult with Proteus Syndrome and is also active in his support group. Note overgrowth of the skull. This can cause head and facial asymmetry including the shown supraorbital ridge protuberance and mandibular asymmetry. Photography by Rick Guidotti, Positive Exposure (positiveexposure.org).

QUESTIONS FOR SMALL GROUP DISCUSSION

1. Each individual with Proteus syndrome has a unique pattern of overgrowth. What about the cause of Proteus syndrome creates this phenotypic heterogeneity?
2. Why is DNA from blood or saliva not an appropriate source for genetic testing in Proteus syndrome?
3. Discuss other disorders that are caused by somatic mosaicism. Are these conditions hereditary?

REFERENCES

Biesecker LG, Sapp JC. Proteus syndrome. In Adam MP, Ardinger HH, Pagon RA, Wallace SE, Bean LJH, Gripp KW, Mirzaa GM, Amemiya A, editors: *GeneReviews®*, 1993. https://www.ncbi.nlm.nih.gov/pubmed/22876373

Lindhurst MJ, Sapp JC, Teer JK, *et al.* A mosaic activating mutation in AKT1 associated with the Proteus syndrome, *N Engl J Med* 365(7):611–619, 2011. https://doi.org/10.1056/NEJMoa1104017

Sapp JC, Buser A, Burton-Akright J, Keppler-Noreuil KM, Biesecker LG: A dyadic genotype-phenotype approach to diagnostic criteria for Proteus syndrome, *Am J Med Genet C Semin Med Genet* 181(4):565–570, 2019. https://doi.org/10.1002/ajmg.c.31744

27

FETAL GROWTH RESTRICTION (Abnormal Fetal Karyotype)

Spontaneous Chromosomal Deletion

Marisa Gilstrop Thompson

PRINCIPLES

- Prenatal diagnosis
- Ultrasound screening
- Interstitial deletion
- Cytogenetic and genome analysis
- Genetic counseling
- Pregnancy management options

MAJOR PHENOTYPIC FEATURES

- Age at onset: prenatal
- Fetal growth restriction
- Increased nuchal fold
- Dysmorphic facies

CASE DESCRIPTION

A.G. was a 26-year-old gravida 2, para 1 woman referred for ultrasonography for routine second trimester examination of fetal anatomy. A.G. denied any medication, drug, or alcohol exposure during the pregnancy, and both parents were in good health. The biometric parameters from the fetal anatomy study suggested a 17.5-week fetus. On the basis of first trimester ultrasound dating and the date of the patient's last menstrual period, however, the fetus should have been at approximately 21 weeks of gestation. This discrepancy suggested symmetrical fetal growth restriction. Further evaluation also revealed increased nuchal fold measurements of 6.1 to 7.3 mm. The couple was offered genetic counseling, considering an early diagnosis of growth restriction and a thickened nuchal fold, and were subsequently counseled on the increased risk for fetal aneuploidy. The counselor also discussed other etiologies of fetal growth restriction, including (but not limited to) fetal infection, placental disease, teratogen exposures, and maternal comorbidities. After counseling, the couple elected to have an amniocentesis for diagnostic testing. Results of infection evaluation from the amniocentesis were negative. The chromosome results revealed an interstitial chromosome 4p deletion, with karyotype 46,XX,del(4)(p15.1p15.32). The counselor

told the parents that such a finding had been previously associated with possible skeletal anomalies, neurologic abnormalities, and intellectual disability. Parental chromosomal evaluation was recommended, to determine whether either parent carried a balanced chromosomal abnormality; these test results were normal. After delivery, a detailed exam of the child revealed bilateral epicanthal folds, low-set and posteriorly rotated ears, prominent nasal bridge, and micrognathia. Redundant posterior nuchal skin was also noted. Parents were reassured that the recurrence risk was low but that testing would, nonetheless, be available for any future pregnancy.

BACKGROUND

Disease Etiology and Incidence

Fetal growth restriction (FGR) is diagnosed when the estimated fetal weight or abdominal circumference is less than the 10th percentile (Fig. C.27.1). Prenatally, a diagnosis of FGR does not take into account the individualized growth potential of each fetus. This means that a larger fetus who has not achieved their growth potential will not be identified and a constitutionally small fetus may be misdiagnosed. A newborn with a history of FGR should be distinguished from a newborn who is small for gestational age (SGA). The latter is also below the 10th percentile in size but does not reflect the antenatal growth quality. They are usually described as being small for physiological reasons, such as the size of the parents.

FGR may result from utero-placental insufficiency, exposure to drugs or alcohol, congenital infections, or intrinsic genetic limitations of growth potential. Fetuses with growth restriction due to nutritional compromise tend to have less restriction of head growth than of the rest of the body. Several chromosomal disorders are associated with FGR. A finding of early or symmetrical FGR increases the likelihood that a fetus is affected by a chromosomal abnormality, such as trisomy 18, triploidy, or maternal uniparental disomy for chromosome 7 or 14. Nuchal fold measurements of more than 3 mm in the first trimester (11–14 weeks) or of 6 mm or more in the second trimester are considered increased and are associated with a greater risk for chromosomal abnormalities. Approximately one in seven fetuses with a second-trimester nuchal thickening will have Down syndrome. The ultrasound findings in A.G.'s fetus increased the suspicion of aneuploidy, leading to identification of the small interstitial deletion in 4p, which is the likely explanation for the fetal abnormalities.

The etiology and incidence of such a rare deletion are not entirely understood, especially in light of the normal parental chromosomes. Most *de novo* deletions originate at meiosis, but they may also arise during mitosis in tissue destined to become gonadal, so that a parent has gonadal mosaicism. The latter cannot be ruled out with any certainty by fibroblast or lymphoblast testing of the parents; consequently, prenatal testing should be offered in future pregnancies.

Pathogenesis

The deletion breakpoints on the short arm of chromosome 4 in 46,XX,del(4)(p15.1p15.32) flank a 14.5-Mb segment of DNA. Forty-seven known protein-coding genes exist within

46, XY   A.G. 26y
                46, XX

P — fetal growth restriction

amiocentesis @ 21wk
46,XX,del(4)(p15.1p15.32)

Pedigree Case 27

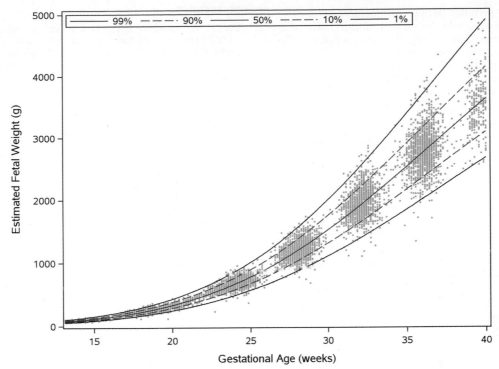

Figure C.27.1 World Health Organization fetal growth chart: estimated fetal weight percentiles. The growth chart for estimated fetal weight is based on a longitudinal study of 1387 low-risk pregnancies from 10 countries. Under optimal living and nutritional conditions, fetal growth was not uniform but exposed a substantial dispersion, which was wider among the large fetuses than the small ones. Fetal weight during pregnancy is estimated by a formula that combines ultrasound measurements of the distance between the parietal bones of the fetal skull (biparietal diameter), head circumference, abdominal circumference, and femur length. (From Kiserud T, Piaggio G, Carroli G, et al: The World Health Organization fetal growth charts: A multinational longitudinal study of ultrasound biometric measurements and estimated fetal weight, *PLoS Med* 14:e1002220, 2017.)

this deleted region; haploinsufficiency for one or more of these genes is the likely cause of the phenotype of this fetus. Chromosome microarray testing allows a more precise definition of breakpoints in deletions or duplications than does prenatal karyotype. Knowledge of which genes are involved in the deleted area may add more precise prognostic information if the involvement of critical genes is in question.

Phenotype and Natural History

All pregnancies – regardless of family, medical, or pregnancy history – are at an approximate 3 to 5% risk for developmental disabilities or a birth defect in the infant. Although this couple was not at increased risk, the routine second trimester ultrasound findings increased the suspicion of fetal aneuploidy. The finding of an interstitial deletion is likely to explain the ultrasound findings. Although this exact deletion had not been reported previously, many deletions of the short arm of chromosome 4 have been associated with birth defects. For example, Wolf-Hirschhorn syndrome (Fig. 6.8) is due to a microdeletion of 4p, resulting in severe intellectual disability and physical anomalies. FISH analysis in this fetus revealed that the sequences for the Wolf-Hirschhorn critical region at 4p16.3 were present on both copies of chromosome 4, and that the deletion in this case was more proximal, in band p15. In this case, as with any substantial loss or gain of material on an autosome not previously reported in other patients, the outcome is likely to involve both physical and neurological impairment, the severity of which cannot be predicted.

Management

No curative treatments are available for chromosome abnormalities. The overriding question for many couples regarding the outcome for their unborn child is whether the fetus is at risk for intellectual disability or a significant birth defect. In light of the already present ultrasound anomalies and the identified chromosomal abnormality, this fetus would have sequelae, the extent of which is not predictable. In such cases, the couple is counseled in detail about the limited information and the inability to predict the outcome of the pregnancy. The options include continuation of the pregnancy with expectant management, with or without adoption, or termination of pregnancy.

Follow-up ultrasound evaluations can assess fetal growth and development. Long-term progressive FGR alone suggests a poor prognosis for the fetus. By the late second trimester, the majority of cardiac lesions that would require intervention at birth can usually be identified through sonography. Consultation with neonatologists and maternal-fetal medicine specialists can provide information regarding what to expect at delivery and the types of postnatal evaluations that should be considered. There may be advantages to arranging for delivery in a tertiary facility that provides specialized neonatal intensive care and surgery.

In clinical scenarios where termination is elected for management, either an induction of labor or surgical management can be performed up to the mid–second trimester (based on local legislation). The emotional and physical benefits and disadvantages of the two procedures should be outlined in detail by a qualified obstetrician/gynecologist. The discussion should account for the option of autopsy (which can be particularly important when prenatal testing did not confirm a diagnosis) and the comparison of timing and predictability of each method (see Chapter 18). Finally, the parents can be offered the option of giving the neonate up for adoption if they decide that termination is not an option or unaffordable, or because the anomalies were identified too late in the pregnancy to allow termination.

Inheritance

De novo deletions have a low recurrence risk, accounting for the chance of undetectable gonadal mosaicism in either parent. Prenatal testing, such as chorionic villus sampling or amniocentesis, is available for future pregnancies, although the low risk for miscarriage from these procedures may be comparable to the actual empirical risk for a recurrence (see Chapter 18).

QUESTIONS FOR SMALL GROUP DISCUSSION

1. What is the difference between the terms *small for gestational age* (SGA) and *fetal growth restriction* (FGR)?
2. What would be the advantages and disadvantages of performing amniocentesis for karyotype at 24 weeks of gestation in a pregnancy thought to have FGR, even if the societal regulations and family situation preclude a pregnancy termination, if the amniocentesis demonstrates a chromosomal abnormality?

REFERENCES

Bianchi D, Crombleholme T, D'Alton M, *et al*: *Fetology: Diagnosis and management of the fetal patient*, ed 2, New York, 2010, McGraw Hill.

Gardner RJM, Amor DJ: *Gardner and Sutherland's chromosome abnormalities and genetic counseling*, ed 5, Oxford, 2018, Oxford University Press.

Kiserud T, Benachi A, Hecher K, Perez RG, Carvalho J, Piaggio G, Platt LD: The World Health Organization fetal growth charts: Concept, findings, interpretation, and application, *Am J Obstet Gynecol* 218(2S):S619–S629, 2018. https://doi.org/10.1016/j.ajog.2017.12.010. PMID: 29422204

Meler E, Sisterna S, Borrell A: Genetic syndromes associated with isolated fetal growth restriction, *Prenat Diagn* 40(4):432–446, 2020.

South ST, Corson VL, McMichael JL, *et al*: Prenatal detection of an interstitial deletion in 4p15 in a fetus with an increased nuchal skin fold measurement, *Fetal Diagn Ther* 20:58–63, 2005.

LONG QT SYNDROME (MIM 192500) (Cardiac Ion Channel Gene)

Autosomal Dominant or Recessive

Robert Hamilton

PRINCIPLES

- Locus heterogeneity
- Incomplete penetrance
- Genetic susceptibility to medications

MAJOR PHENOTYPIC FEATURES

- QTc prolongation (>470 msec in males, >480 msec in females)
- Tachyarrhythmias (torsades de pointes)
- Syncopal episodes
- Sudden death
- Pharmacogenetics

HISTORY AND PHYSICAL FINDINGS

A.B. is a 30-year-old woman with long QT (LQT) syndrome who presented to the Genetics Clinic with her husband because they are contemplating a pregnancy. The couple wanted to know the recurrence risk for this condition in their future children and the genetic testing and prenatal diagnosis options that might be available to them. She was also concerned about potential risks to her own health in carrying a pregnancy. A.B. was diagnosed with LQT syndrome in her early 20s when she was evaluated after the sudden death of her 15-year-old brother. Overall, she is a healthy individual with normal hearing, no dysmorphic features, and an otherwise negative review of systems. She has never had any fainting episodes. Electrocardiographic findings confirmed the diagnosis of the syndrome in A.B., and a paternal aunt, but not in her father, who had a normal QTc interval. Her mother's history and family history are negative for any features of LQT syndrome. Molecular testing in A.B., using a commercial LQT panel, revealed a missense variant in *KCNH2*. This had been previously seen in families with Romano-Ward syndrome, type LQT2. A.B., was initially prescribed β-blockade medication, which she is continuing,

and an implantable cardioverter-defibrillator (ICD). ICDs were previously often prescribed for LQT syndrome, based on family history of sudden death, although current guidelines no longer recommend this. The Genetics Clinic advised the couple that the recurrence risk to each of their future offspring would be 50% and answered their questions about pregnancy risks and prenatal diagnosis options, as described below.

BACKGROUND

Disease Etiology and Prevalence

The LQT syndromes are a heterogeneous group of disorders, referred to as channelopathies, because they are caused by defects in cardiac ion channels or channel-interacting proteins. The overall prevalence of LQT disorders is approximately 1 in 5000 to 7000 individuals.

The genetics underlying LQT syndromes is complex. First, there is locus heterogeneity. Variants in at least five known cardiac ion channel genes (*KCNQ1*, *KCNH2*, *SCN5A*, *KCNE1*, and *KCNE2*) are responsible for most cases of LQT. Variants in additional genes are known but are much rarer. Second, different variant alleles at the same locus can result in two distinct LQT syndromes with two different inheritance patterns: the autosomal dominant Romano-Ward syndrome and the autosomal recessive Jervell and Lange-Nielsen syndrome (MIM 220400). Digenic inheritance has been reported.

Pathogenesis

LQT syndrome is caused by repolarization defects in cardiac cells. Repolarization is a controlled process that requires a balance between inward currents of sodium and calcium and outward currents of potassium. Imbalances cause the action potential of cells to increase or decrease in duration, causing elongation or shortening, respectively, of the QT interval on electrocardiogrjaphy. Most cases of LQT syndrome are caused by loss-of-function variants in genes that encode subunits

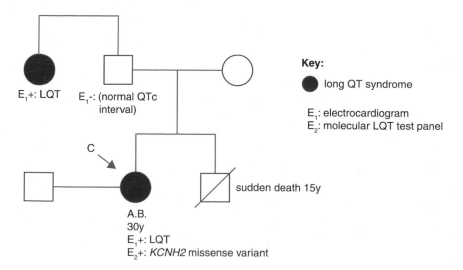

Key:

⬤ long QT syndrome

E_1: electrocardiogram
E_2: molecular LQT test panel

E_1+: LQT E_1−: (normal QTc interval)

C

A.B.
30y
E_1+: LQT
E_2+: *KCNH2* missense variant

sudden death 15y

of regulatory proteins for potassium channels (genes whose names begin with *KCN*). These variants decrease the outward, repolarization current, thereby prolonging the action potential of the cell and lowering the threshold for another depolarization. In others with LQT syndrome, gain-of-function variants in a sodium channel gene, *SCN5A*, lead to an increased influx of sodium, resulting in similar shifting of action potential and repolarization effects.

Phenotype and Natural History

The LQT syndromes are characterized by elongated QT interval and T-wave abnormalities on electrocardiography (Fig. C.28.1), including tachyarrhythmia and torsades de pointes—a ventricular tachycardia characterized by a change in amplitude and twisting of the QRS complex. Torsades de pointes is associated with a prolonged QT interval and typically stops spontaneously, but may persist and worsen to ventricular fibrillation.

In the most common LQT syndrome, Romano-Ward, syncope due to cardiac arrhythmia is the most frequent symptom; if undiagnosed or left untreated, it recurs and can be fatal in 10 to 15% of cases. However, between 30 and 50% of individuals with the syndrome never show syncopal symptoms. Cardiac episodes are most frequent from the preteen years through the

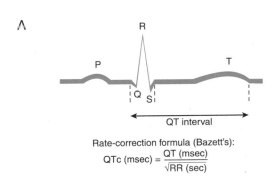

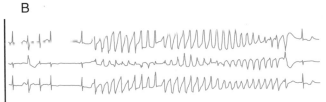

Figure C.28.1 (A) Measurement of the QT interval from the electrocardiogram. The diagram depicts the normal electrocardiogram with the P wave representing atrial activation, the QRS complex representing ventricular activation and the start of ventricular contraction, and the T wave representing ventricular repolarization. Owing to heart rate sensitivity of the QT interval, this parameter is corrected (normalized) to heart rate (as reflected by the beat-to-beat RR interval), yielding the QTc. QT and QTc can both be expressed in milliseconds or seconds. (B) Arrhythmia onset in long QT syndrome. Three simultaneous (and distinct) electrocardiographic channel recordings in a patient with QT prolongation and runs of continuously varying polymorphic ventricular tachycardia (torsades de pointes). Torsades de pointes may resolve spontaneously or progress to ventricular fibrillation and cardiac arrest. ((A) modified with permission from Liu BA, Juurlink DN: Drugs and the QT interval – Caveat doctor. *N Engl J Med* 351:1053–1056, 2004. (B) modified from Chiang C, Roden DM: The long QT syndromes: Genetic basis and clinical implications, *J Am Coll Cardiol* 36:1–12, 2000.)

20s. Risk appears to decrease over time, but is likely simply remaining stable in the face of other competing risks for mortality that rise with age. Episodes may occur at any age when triggered by QT-prolonging medications (see list at http://www.qtdrugs.org). Nonpharmacological triggers for cardiac events in the Romano-Ward syndrome differ on the basis of the gene responsible. LQT1 triggers are typically adrenergic stimuli, including exercise and sudden emotion. Individuals with LTQ2 are at risk with exercise and at rest and with auditory stimuli, such as alarm clocks and phones. LQT3 individuals have episodes with slower heart rates during rest periods and sleep. Of LQT1 cases, 40% are symptomatic before age 10 years, whereas symptoms occur this early in only 10% of those with LTQ2 and rarely with LQT3. There are at least 17 genes associated with LQT syndromes, of which 3—*KCNQ1*, *KCNH2*, and *SCN5A* – account for approximately 90% of gene-identified cases, with 20 to 40% of all cases remaining gene elusive.

The LQT syndrome exhibits reduced penetrance in terms of both electrocardiographic abnormalities and syncopal episodes. As many as 30% of affected individuals can have QT intervals that overlap with the normal range. Variable expression of the disorder can occur within and between families. Due to reduced penetrance, exercise electrocardiography is often used for diagnosis of at-risk family members but is not 100% sensitive. Genetic testing is becoming increasingly common, and treatment is often recommended with the finding of a pathogenic or likely pathogenic variant, even when no clear phenotype is present, as such individuals carry some risk for cardiac events.

LQT syndromes may be accompanied by other findings on physical examination. For example, Jervell and Lange-Nielsen syndrome (MIM 220400) is characterized by congenital, profound sensorineural hearing loss together with LQT syndrome. It is an autosomal recessive disorder caused by particular variants within the same two genes (*KCNQ1* and *KCNE1*) or pairs of genes (digenic disease) implicated in the autosomal dominant Romano-Ward syndrome. Heterozygous relatives of Jervell and Lange-Nielsen syndrome patients are not deaf but have a risk for Romano-Ward LQT syndrome.

Management

Treatment of the LQT syndrome is aimed at prevention of syncopal episodes and cardiac arrest. Optimal treatment is influenced by identification of the gene responsible in a given case. For instance, β-blocker therapy before the onset of symptoms is most effective in LQT1 and, to a somewhat lesser extent, in LQT2. Its efficacy in LQT3 is reduced, although membrane-stabilizing beta-blockers, such as Propranolol, have some efficacy in LQT3. β-Blockade therapy must be monitored closely for age-related dose adjustment, and it is imperative that doses are not missed. Some beta-blockers appear more effective than others. Pacemakers may be necessary for individuals with bradycardia; access to external defibrillators may be appropriate. After consideration of left stellate ganglionectomy, ICDs may be needed in individuals with symptomatic LQT2 or LQT3, or in others with the LQT syndrome in whom β-blocker therapy is problematic, such as those with asthma, depression, or diabetes. ICD is a class 1 recommendation for those who are survivors of a cardiac arrest, possibly except for those with LQT1 who have not been previously treated with a β-blocker. Although a family history of cardiac arrest may influence the person's decision to seek or accept an ICD, there is limited evidence that this is a risk factor for cardiac events.

Medications such as the antidepressant, amitriptyline, over-the-counter cold medications such as phenylephrine and diphenhydramine, or antifungal drugs, including fluconazole and ketoconazole, should be avoided because of their effect on prolonging the QT interval or causing increased sympathetic tone. Vigorous activities and sports were previously recommended to be avoided. Increasing evidence now shows that this is unnecessary if mitigating risk reduction strategies are in place (β-blocker therapy; accompanying responsible person aware of the patient's condition and of nearby automatic external defibrillator and emergency medical services equipment/facilities).

Management During Pregnancy

Although prenatal diagnosis for LQT syndrome can be performed genetically in many cases, few families choose to do so, perhaps because the condition is usually easily and effectively treated. Similarly, few families choose invasive genetic testing during early pregnancy. Nevertheless, these options should be discussed with families.

Mothers with LQT syndrome may be susceptible to life-threatening arrhythmias during pregnancy, labor, delivery, and postpartum. They should have close clinical assessments and monitoring, with consideration for access to a specialized cardiologist. There is evidence for increased risk of stillbirth and miscarriage. Most patients can be managed with uninterrupted β-blocker therapy during pregnancy and the postpartum period, and vaginal delivery is usually possible. Fetal LQT syndrome can often be diagnosed based on a lower observed resting fetal heart rate; fetal ventricular arrhythmias can occur. It is important to also closely assess the fetus from a paternal LQT syndrome case, as the fetus is typically not receiving β-blocker from the mother. A newborn electrocardiogram (ECG) should be performed; a pediatric heart rhythm specialist assessment should be arranged; consideration should be given for genetic testing in the newborn (for which results may take several weeks).

Inheritance

Offspring of individuals with the Romano-Ward syndrome have a 50% chance of inheriting the parental gene variant. Most affected individuals have an affected (although perhaps asymptomatic) parent, because the rate of *de novo* variants is low. A detailed family history and careful cardiac evaluation of family members are extremely important and could be lifesaving. The recurrence risk for Jervell and Lange-Nielsen syndrome in siblings of patients with this disorder is 25%, as expected with an autosomal recessive condition. However, siblings, if heterozygous, are also at risk for the Romano-Ward syndrome with 25% penetrance of LQT alone, without deafness.

QUESTIONS FOR SMALL GROUP DISCUSSION

1. Some genetic syndromes rely on clinical evaluation for diagnosis, even with the availability of molecular testing. In the case of LQT syndrome, how would you proceed with a patient thought to have LQT on family history? Why?
2. Discuss the ethics of testing minors in this condition.
3. You have just diagnosed a child with Jervell and Lange-Nielsen syndrome. What do you counsel the family in regard to recurrence risk and management for other family members?

REFERENCES

Alders M, Mannens MMAM: Romano-Ward syndrome. http://www.ncbi.nlm.nih.gov/books/NBK1129/

Guidicessi JR, Ackerman MJ: Genotype- and phenotype-guided management of congenital long QT syndrome, *Curr Probl Cardiol* 38:417–455, 2013.

Martin CA, Huang CL, Matthews GD: The role of ion channelopathies in sudden cardiac death: Implications for clinical practice, *Ann Med* 45:364–374, 2013.

Tranebjaerg L, Samson RA, Green GE: Jervell and Lange-Nielsen syndrome. http://www.ncbi.nlm.nih.gov/books/NBK1405/

29

LYNCH SYNDROME (MIM 120435)
(DNA Mismatch Repair Genes Pathogenic Variants)

Autosomal Dominant

David Malkin

PRINCIPLES

- Tumor suppressor genes
- Multistep carcinogenesis
- Somatic mutation
- Microsatellite instability
- Variable expressivity and incomplete penetrance

MAJOR PHENOTYPIC FEATURES

- Age at onset: middle adulthood
- Colorectal cancer
- Multiple primary cancers

HISTORY AND PHYSICAL FINDINGS

P.P., a 38-year-old banker and mother of three children, was referred to the cancer Genetics Clinic by her physician for counseling regarding her family history of cancer. Her father, brother, nephew, niece, and paternal uncle all developed colorectal cancer, while her paternal grandmother had been diagnosed in her 40s with pancreatic cancer. P.P. did not have a history of medical or surgical problems. The findings from her physical examination were normal. The geneticist explained to P.P. that her family history was suggestive of Lynch syndrome (also known as hereditary nonpolyposis colon cancer, HNPCC) and that the most efficient way to confirm this was through molecular genetic testing, beginning with a living affected family member. P.P.'s niece, N.P., the only surviving affected family member, agreed to be tested. Testing of an archived tumor sample from N.P.'s resected colon identified microsatellite instability (MSI); sequencing of DNA from N.P.'s blood with a multigene panel revealed a germline pathogenic variant in *MLH1*. Subsequent targeted sequence testing showed that P.P. did not carry the same pathogenic variant; therefore, the geneticist counseled that the risk to her and to her children for development of cancer was similar to that of the general population. Her unaffected brother was found to carry the *MLH1* pathogenic variant and continued with annual screening by colonoscopy (see Fig. C.29.1).

BACKGROUND
Disease Etiology and Prevalence

At least 50% of individuals in middle- and high-income countries develop a colorectal tumor by age 70 years; approximately 10% of these individuals eventually develop colorectal cancer. Lynch syndrome (MIM 120435) is a genetically heterogeneous autosomal dominant cancer predisposition syndrome that is caused by pathogenic variants in DNA mismatch repair genes. Lynch syndrome has a prevalence of 2 to 5 per 1000 and accounts for approximately 3 to 8% of colorectal cancer.

Pathogenesis

In most colorectal cancers, including in familial adenomatous polyposis, the tumor karyotype becomes progressively more aneuploid (see Chapter 16). Approximately 15% of colorectal cancers do not have such chromosomal instability but have insertions or deletions in repetitive genomic sequences. MSI occurs in 85 to 90% of Lynch syndrome tumors. Consistent with this observation, approximately 70% of Lynch syndrome families with carcinomas exhibiting MSI have pathogenic germline variants in one of four DNA mismatch repair genes: *MSH2, MSH6, MLH1,* or *PMS2.*

DNA mismatch repair reduces DNA replication errors by 1000-fold. Errors of DNA synthesis cause mispairing and deform the DNA double helix. A complex of mismatch repair proteins recruits other enzymes to excise the segment of newly synthesized mismatched DNA and resynthesize it.

As is typical for tumor suppressor genes, both alleles of a DNA mismatch repair gene must lose function to cause MSI. This somatic loss of function can occur by loss of heterozygosity, intragenic mutation, or promoter hypermethylation.

In Lynch syndrome, several microsatellite loci mutate during the progression from adenoma to carcinoma. Inactivation of genes containing microsatellite sequences could play key roles in tumor progression. For example, MSI induces frameshift mutations in the transforming growth factor receptor II gene (*TGFBR2*). Pathogenic *TGFBR2* alleles cause the loss of TGFβRII expression, which reduces the ability of TGFβ to inhibit the growth of colonic epithelial cells. *TGFBR2* mutations occur in early Lynch syndrome lesions and may contribute to the growth of adenomas. Lynch syndrome also results from epigenetic silencing of *MSH2* caused by deletion of 3′exons of *EPCAM* and intergenic regions directly upstream of *MSH2.*

MLH1 and *MSH2* germline pathogenic variants account for approximately 90% of pathogenic alleles in Lynch syndrome families. *MSH6* variants account for an additional 7 to 10%, whereas *PMS2* variants are found in fewer than 5% of cases.

Phenotype and Natural History

Although individuals with Lynch syndrome develop polyps similar in number to those of the general population, they develop them at younger ages. Their median age at diagnosis with a colorectal adenocarcinoma is younger than 50 years; that is, 10 to 15 years younger than in the general population. Individuals with a defined *MLH1* or *MSH2* germline variant have an 80% lifetime risk for development of colorectal cancer; the penetrance of *MSH6* and *PMS2* variants is much lower. About 60 to 70% of adenomas and carcinomas in Lynch syndrome occur between the splenic flexure and ileocecal junction. In contrast, most sporadic colorectal cancers (and cancer in familial adenomatous polyposis) occur in the descending colon and sigmoid. Carcinomas in Lynch syndrome are less likely to have chromosome instability and aneuploidy; they behave less aggressively than sporadic colon cancer. For this reason, individuals with Lynch syndrome have a better age- and stage-adjusted prognosis than do patients with familial adenomatous polyposis or colorectal tumors with chromosome instability.

Lynch-associated cancers also include cancer of the stomach, small bowel, pancreas, kidney, endometrium, and ovaries; cancers of the lung and breast are not associated (see Fig. C.29.1). Individuals with a defined pathogenic germline variant in a Lynch syndrome-associated gene have a more than

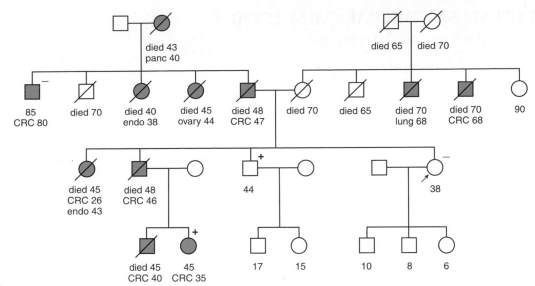

Figure C.29.1 Family segregating an *MLH1* pathogenic variant. Note the frequent occurrence of colorectal cancer as well as other Lynch syndrome-associated cancers, such as endometrial cancer, pancreatic cancer, and ovarian cancer. Note that one family member had cancers of the colorectum and endometrium and that another had sporadic colon cancer (tested negative for family variant). *Shaded symbols* indicate a diagnosis of cancer. Ages are shown directly below each symbol. A *plus sign* identifies carriers of the *MLH1* variant, and a *minus sign* identifies a noncarrier by DNA testing. Cancer diagnoses are followed by the age at diagnosis. *CRC*, colorectal cancer; *endo*, endometrial cancer; *lung*, lung cancer; *ovary*, ovarian cancer; *panc*, pancreatic cancer. (Courtesy T. Pal and S. Narod, Women's College Hospital and University of Toronto, Canada.)

90% lifetime risk for development of colorectal cancer, one of these associated cancers, or both.

Management

Lynch syndrome has no distinguishing physical features. The minimal criteria for considering Lynch syndrome are the occurrence of colorectal cancer or another Lynch syndrome-associated tumor in three members of a family, at least two of whom are first-degree relatives, across two or more generations, and the development of colorectal cancer in at least one affected individual before the age of 50 years. In individuals without a family history but with early-onset colorectal cancer, genetic testing for Lynch syndrome is ideally performed in a stepwise manner. This involves evaluation of tumor tissue for MSI through molecular MSI testing and/or immunohistochemistry of the four mismatch repair proteins. The presence of MSI in the tumor alone is not sufficient to diagnose Lynch syndrome; 10 to 15% of sporadic colorectal cancers exhibit MSI due to somatic methylation of the *MLH1* promoter. Immunohistochemistry testing helps to identify the mismatch repair gene that most likely harbors a causal germline variant.

Early recognition of Lynch syndrome is necessary for effective intervention. Begun at age 25, surveillance colonoscopy of the proximal colon or prophylactic surgical removal of the colon increases life expectancy by 13.5 years or more than 15 years, respectively. Surveillance endometrial biopsies and abdominal ultrasound scans for at-risk women have not been proven to prevent uterine or ovarian cancer seen in this condition. In families with a known pathogenic germline variant, identification of the DNA mismatch repair gene allele can focus surveillance on those family members carrying the variant allele. In Lynch syndrome families without an identified germline variant, the frequent surveillance is needed for all at-risk individuals.

Inheritance

The general population risk for development of colorectal cancer is empirically 5 to 6% but markedly modified by family history. Individuals with a first-degree relative with colorectal cancer have a 1.7 relative risk, which increases to 2.75 if two or more first-degree relatives had colorectal cancer. If an affected first-degree relative developed colorectal cancer before age 44, the relative risk increases to more than 5.

In contrast, any offspring of an individual with a DNA mismatch repair gene germline variant has a 50% risk for having inherited that variant. Anyone carrying such a variant has a lifetime cancer risk of up to 90%, considering the associated penetrance of colon and other cancers, and the background population risk. Prenatal diagnosis is highly controversial and not routine but is theoretically possible if the causal germline variant has been identified in the parent. Because of incomplete penetrance and variation in expressivity, the severity and onset of Lynch syndrome and the occurrence of associated cancers cannot be predicted.

QUESTIONS FOR SMALL GROUP DISCUSSION

1. Compare the mechanisms of tumorigenesis in disorders of nucleotide excision repair, chromosomal instability, and microsatellite instability.
2. How should someone with a family history of Lynch syndrome be counseled if testing for DNA mismatch repair gene variants is positive? Negative?
3. Discuss the ethics of testing of minors for Lynch syndrome.

REFERENCES

Brenner H, Kloor M, Pox CP: Colorectal cancer, *Lancet* 383:1490–1502, 2014.

Idos G, Valle L: Lynch syndrome. In Pagon RA, Bird TD, Dolan CR, editors: *GeneReviews*, 2004 [Updated 2021] http://www.ncbi.nlm.nih.gov/books/NBK1211/

Matloff J, Lucas A, Polydorides AD, *et al*: Molecular tumor testing for Lynch syndrome in patients with colorectal cancer, *J Natl Compr Canc Netw* 11:1380–1385, 2013.

30

MARFAN SYNDROME (MIM 154700)
(*FBN1* Pathogenic Variants)
Autosomal Dominant

Shira G. Ziegler

PRINCIPLES

- Dominant negative and haploinsufficiency
- Variable expressivity

MAJOR PHENOTYPIC FEATURES

- Age at onset: variable; from infancy to adult
- Disproportionate tall stature
- Skeletal anomalies
- Ectopia lentis
- Mitral valve prolapse
- Aortic dilation and rupture
- Spontaneous pneumothorax
- Lumbosacral dural ectasia

CASE PRESENTATION

J.L., a healthy 16-year-old high school basketball star, was referred to the genetics clinic for evaluation for Marfan syndrome. His physique was similar to that of his late father. His father, a tall, thin man, had died during a morning jog; no other family members had a history of skeletal abnormalities, sudden death, vision loss, or congenital anomalies. On physical examination, J.L. had an asthenic habitus, high arched palate, mild pectus carinatum, arachnodactyly, arm span to height ratio of 1.2, soft diastolic murmur, and stretch marks on his shoulders and thighs. He was referred for echocardiography, which showed dilation of the aortic root with moderate aortic valve regurgitation. An ophthalmological examination demonstrated bilateral iridodonesis and slight superior displacement of the lenses. On the basis of his physical examination and testing results, there was a strong clinical suspicion of Marfan syndrome. A comprehensive panel for genes associated with thoracic aortic aneurysm revealed a pathogenic variant in the *FBN1* gene, confirming the diagnosis of Marfan syndrome. J.L. was started on an angiotensin II receptor blocker (ARB) to lower blood pressure and attenuate TGFβ signaling. He continued to have annual imaging to monitor the growth of his

aorta and determine appropriate timing for prophylactic aortic root replacement. He was advised to continue recreational aerobic activities but to avoid strenuous isometric exercise or competitive sports to exhaustion.

BACKGROUND

Disease Etiology and Incidence

Marfan syndrome (MIM 154700) is an autosomal dominant connective tissue disorder that results from pathogenic variants in the fibrillin-1 gene (*FBN1*, MIM 134797). There is a reported incidence of 1 in 3000 to 5000 individuals, and approximately 25 to 35% of affected individuals have their *FBN1* variant as the result of a *de novo* disease-causing DNA mutation.

Clinical Characteristics

Marfan syndrome, a systemic disorder of connective tissue with a high degree of clinical variability, comprises a broad phenotypic continuum ranging from mild adult-onset presentations to overt, severe, and rapidly progressive neonatal multiorgan disease. Primary manifestations involve the ocular, skeletal, and cardiovascular systems. Ocular abnormalities associated with Marfan syndrome include ectopia lentis (Fig. C.30.1), flat corneas, increased globe length causing axial myopia, and a predisposition for retinal detachment. The skeletal abnormalities include disproportionate tall stature (arm span to height ratio >1.05; upper to lower segment ratio <0.85 in adults), arachnodactyly, pectus deformities,

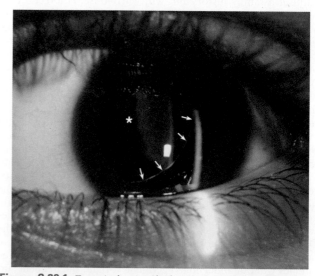

Figure C.30.1 Ectopia lentis. Slit-lamp view of the left eye of a patient with Marfan syndrome. The *asterisk* indicates the center of the lens that is displaced superior nasally; normally, the lens is in the center of the pupil. The *arrows* indicate the edge of the lens that is abnormally visible in the pupil. (Courtesy A. V. Levin, The Hospital for Sick Children and University of Toronto, Canada.)

d. age 42
(unexpected, sudden death)
tall, arachnodactyly

Marfan syndrome

J.L. 16 y.o.
tall, arachnodactyly
FBN1: pathogenic variant

Pedigree Case 30

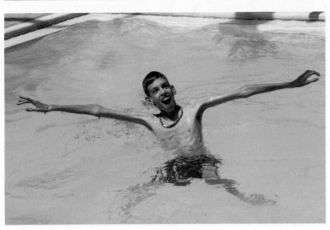

Figure C.30.2 Billy, who has Marfan syndrome, representing The Marfan Foundation (www.marfan.org). Note his disproportionately long arms for the size of his trunk (dolichostenomelia) and long fingers (arachnodactyly). Photograph by Rick Guidotti, Positive Exposure (www.positiveexposure.org).

scoliosis, flat feet, and joint laxity (Fig. C.30.2). Craniofacial manifestations include dolichocephaly, malar hypoplasia, micrognathia, retrognathia, and a high and narrow palate. Common cardiovascular abnormalities include aortic root dilation, mitral valve prolapse, mitral or aortic regurgitation, and aortic dissection. Striae atrophicae, recurrent herniae, and lumbosacral dural ectasia are common. Pulmonary predispositions include spontaneous pneumothorax, apical blebs, and sleep apnea.

Many features of Marfan syndrome develop with age. Subluxation of the lens is often present in early childhood but can progress through adolescence. Retinal detachment, glaucoma, and cataracts show increased frequency in Marfan syndrome. Skeletal anomalies such as anterior chest deformity and scoliosis worsen with bone growth. Cardiovascular complications manifest at any age and progress throughout life.

The major causes of premature death in patients with Marfan syndrome are heart failure from valve regurgitation and aortic dissection and rupture (see Fig. 14.6). As surgical and medical management of cardiovascular disease has improved, so has survival. In the early 1970s, prior to the advent of effective surgical approaches, the average age of death for a Marfan syndrome patient was 32 years; by 1993, the life expectancy of Marfan syndrome patients increased to 72 years. Now, with proper management, the life expectancy of someone with Marfan syndrome approximates that of the general population.

Diagnosis

Marfan syndrome is a diagnosis based upon the recognition of characteristic features in the ocular, skeletal, and cardiovascular systems. Aortic root dilation and ectopia lentis carry disproportionate weight in the diagnostic criteria, given their relative specificity for this disorder. The diagnosis of Marfan syndrome is established in a proband who has one of the following sets of findings:

1. An *FBN1* pathogenic variant known to be associated with Marfan syndrome AND one of the following: aortic root enlargement (Z-score ≥2.0) or ectopia lentis.
2. Demonstration of aortic root enlargement (Z-score ≥2.0) and ectopia lentis OR a defined combination of features throughout the body yielding a systemic score ≥7 per the modified Ghent criteria.

Although molecular confirmation of an *FBN1* variant is not a requirement for diagnosis, it can play a pivotal role in children with emerging clinical manifestations or in atypically mild presentations of disease.

Pathogenesis

The gene *FBN1* encodes fibrillin-1, an extracellular matrix glycoprotein, which polymerizes to form microfibrils in both elastic and nonelastic tissues, such as the aortic adventitia, ciliary zonules, and skin. During embryogenesis, microfibrils composed of fibrillin-1 and/or fibrillin-2 are deposited in the extracellular space and are thought to serve as a structural scaffold.

Disease-causing *FBN1* variants either result in the production of abnormal protein (e.g., missense variants or in-frame indels or splicing events) or lead to a premature termination codon and degradation of the mutant transcript through nonsense-mediated mRNA decay (e.g., nonsense variants or frameshifts). The former is consistent with a dominant-negative mechanism; mutant missense variants allow the production of abnormal protein that can interfere with the secretion, matrix deposition, and/or stability of normal microfibrils. The latter is an example of haploinsufficiency; decreased extracellular fibrillin-1 is insufficient to initiate effective microfibrillar assembly. Ultimately, both mechanisms lead to nonfunctional or decreased extracellular fibrillin 1.

While it was initially believed that Marfan syndrome resulted from a loss of structural integrity due to decreased extracellular fibrillin-1, it is now understood that fibrillin-1 regulates the bioavailability and activity of the multipotential cytokine transforming growth factor-β (TGFβ). When fibrillin-1 is deficient, as in Marfan syndrome, dysregulation of TGFβ signaling is a major contributor to phenotypic expression. Antagonism of TGFβ signaling in postnatal life is sufficient to mitigate multiple manifestations of disease in fibrillin-1-deficient mouse models, including progressive aortic root aneurysm, myxomatous degeneration of the mitral valve, developmental emphysema, and skeletal muscle myopathy. The same features are attenuated in mouse models of Marfan syndrome upon administration of ARBs in association with blunting of TGFβ signaling in the relevant tissue (see Chapter 14).

Management

There is presently no cure for Marfan syndrome; treatment therefore focuses on prevention and symptomatic management. Ophthalmological management includes frequent examinations, correction of the myopia, and, often, lens replacement. Orthopedic management includes bracing or surgery for scoliosis. Pectus deformity repair is largely cosmetic. Physical therapy or orthotics can compensate for joint instability.

Cardiovascular management includes a combination of medical and surgical therapy. Medical therapy attempts to prevent or to slow progression of aortic dilation by reducing heart rate, blood pressure, and ventricular ejection force with β-adrenergic blockers and/or by attenuating TGFβ signaling using ARBs. Multiple clinical trials have been performed to determine the efficacy of therapeutic interventions on Marfan syndrome patients. A recent meta-analysis of seven prospective trials and >1500 patients showed that ARB therapy is associated with slower progression of aortic dilation when compared to placebo or when added to beta-blocker therapy. Overall, many experts in the field agree that both beta-blockers and ARBs are safe and generally well tolerated in Marfan syndrome and that the earlier intervention is initiated, the better the outcome – even in very young children. Prophylactic replacement of the aortic root is recommended when aortic dilation or aortic regurgitation becomes sufficiently severe. Most patients now receive a valve-sparing aortic root replacement that eliminates the need for chronic anticoagulation. Cardiovascular protection is also achieved through restriction of participation in contact sports, competitive sports, and isometric exercise.

Pregnancy can precipitate progressive aortic enlargement or dissection. The aortic dissections are believed to be secondary to the hormonal, blood volume, and cardiac output changes associated with pregnancy and parturition. Current evidence suggests that there is a high risk for dissection in pregnancy if the aortic root measures more than 4 cm at conception. Women can elect to undergo valve-sparing aortic root replacement before pregnancy, although this will not eliminate the risk for dissection of other aortic segments, prominently including the descending thoracic aorta.

Inheritance

Offspring of individuals with Marfan syndrome have a 50% risk of having Marfan syndrome. In families with Marfan syndrome and a known *FBN1* pathogenic variant, at-risk individuals can be identified with clinical evaluation and genetic testing. Prenatal or preimplantation genetic diagnosis is also available for families with a known *FBN1* variant.

QUESTIONS FOR SMALL GROUP DISCUSSION

1. Homocystinuria has many features overlapping with those of Marfan syndrome. How can these two disorders be distinguished by medical history? By physical examination? By biochemical testing?

2. What are dominant negative variants? What are gain-of-function variants? Contrast the two. Why are dominant negative variants common in connective tissue disorders?

3. If one wished to design a curative treatment for a disorder caused by dominant negative variants, what must the therapy accomplish at a molecular level? How is this different from treatment of a disease caused by loss of function?

REFERENCES

Al-Abcha A, Saleh Y, Mujer M, Boumegouas M, Herzallah K, Charles L, Elkhatib L, Abdelkarim O, Kehdi M, Abela GS: Meta-analysis examining the usefulness of angiotensin receptor blockers for the prevention of aortic root dilation in patients with the Marfan syndrome, *Am J Cardiol* 128:101–106, 2020.

Dietz HC: Marfan syndrome, 2001 [Updated 2022]. https://www.ncbi.nlm.nih.gov/books/NBK1335/

31

MEDIUM-CHAIN ACYL-COA DEHYDROGENASE DEFICIENCY
(MIM 201450) (*ACADM* Pathogenic Variation)

Autosomal Recessive

Alexander Y. Kim

PRINCIPLES

- Loss-of-function pathogenic variants
- Newborn screening
- Early prevention

MAJOR PHENOTYPIC FEATURES

- Typical age of onset: between 3 and 24 months
- Hypoketotic hypoglycemia
- Vomiting
- Lethargy
- Hepatic encephalopathy

CASE REPORT

A.N. was a previously healthy 6-month-old girl who presented to the emergency department with vomiting and lethargy. Her initial evaluation was notable for palpable hepatomegaly, blood glucose level of 32 mg/dL, and absent urine ketones. Her hypoglycemia was complicated by a brief seizure. Recommendations from the Metabolic Genetics team included biochemical and molecular genetic testing as well as dextrose-containing intravenous (IV) fluids. Tandem mass spectrometry (MS/MS) demonstrated elevations of C8, C6, C10, and C10:1 acylcarnitine species in her plasma. She was found to have a viral infection. Her clinical condition improved with IV fluids containing 10% dextrose. Additional history revealed that her parents are healthy first cousins, that she has a healthy 2-year-old brother, and that she was born in a country without newborn screening. Consistent with her clinical findings, targeted single-gene testing revealed homozygosity for the *ACADM* c.985A>G (p.Lys329Glu) pathogenic variant. Her asymptomatic brother was subsequently found to be homozygous for the same pathogenic variant.

BACKGROUND
Disease Etiology and Incidence

Fatty acid oxidation disorders (FAODs) are potentially life-threatening but treatable inborn errors of metabolism, with a combined incidence between 0.9 and 15.2 per 100,000. Medium-chain acyl-CoA dehydrogenase (MCAD) deficiency is the most common FAOD. It is caused by homozygous or compound heterozygous pathogenic variants in the *ACADM* gene, which encodes the MCAD enzyme. Likely as a consequence of founder effects, the frequency of MCAD deficiency is highest in those of Northern European, Portuguese of Romani, and Native American of California ancestries. The number of cases expected varies across different populations. For example, an incidence of 1 in 4900 live births has been reported in northern Germany, in contrast to 1 in 263,500 live births in Taiwan.

Pathogenesis

MCAD deficiency is caused by biallelic loss-of-function variants. There are several common pathogenic variants, including c.985A>G, which results in p.Lys329Glu substitution in the MCAD protein and accounts for 56 to 91% of loss-of-function alleles in individuals with MCAD deficiency. There are no clear genotype-phenotype correlations, but specific genotypes may be considered predictive of phenotype in the future. For example, compound heterozygosity for c.985A>G and c.600-18G>A has been associated with an attenuated phenotype that may not be ascertained via newborn screening (NBS).

MCAD is one of the enzymes involved in intramitochondrial fatty acid oxidation, which is required for hepatic ketogenesis during periods of prolonged fasting and/or increased energy demand once hepatic glycogen stores have been depleted. This inborn error of metabolism is associated with hypoketotic hypoglycemia and several characteristic biochemical findings, including elevations of several acylcarnitine species (C6, C8, C10, and C10:1) in plasma, medium-chain dicarboxylic acids in urine, and medium-chain acylglycines in urine.

Phenotype and Natural History

Most individuals with MCAD deficiency are now ascertained via NBS programs. After diagnosis and with treatment, the prognosis is excellent. Historically (and in regions of the world without NBS programs), the typical age of onset is between 3 and 24 months. However, later initial presentation, including during adulthood, has been described. Individuals with MCAD deficiency are at increased risk for acute metabolic crisis, which is a medical emergency that requires immediate treatment. For individuals affected by, but undiagnosed with MCAD deficiency, the mortality rate of the first acute metabolic crisis is 18 to 25%. Potential precipitants include viral infections, prolonged fasting, and alcohol intoxication. In addition to hypoketotic hypoglycemia, acute metabolic crisis in the context of MCAD deficiency may be characterized by lethargy, seizures, hepatomegaly, hepatic dysfunction, and hyperammonemia, which can quickly progress to coma and death. Ongoing metabolic management is critical for preventing morbidity and mortality.

Biochemically, prominent elevation of octanoylcarnitine (C8) is characteristic; ratios between C8 and other acylcarnitine species (C2, C10) may be used for interpretation (see Fig. C.31.1). However, it is important to note that biochemical normalization has been described in individuals with MCAD deficiency who are not under metabolic stress.

Management

MCAD deficiency is an ideal disorder for inclusion in NBS programs, since it is common, and has a significantly improved prognosis when diagnosed and treated (see Chapter 19). As a consequence, many NBS programs incorporated MS/MS-based analysis of acylcarnitine species for MCAD deficiency and other FAODs, starting in the mid-1990s. False-negative results have been reported for individuals with MCAD deficiency, including newborns with low free carnitine levels. A few have presented with symptoms prior to the return of NBS results. Additionally, women with undiagnosed MCAD deficiency have been ascertained via NBS for their newborns. If the diagnosis of MCAD deficiency is suspected based upon an abnormal NBS result and/or symptomatic clinical presentation, then confirmation can be undertaken via molecular analysis of the *ACADM* gene. Enzyme activity testing is not typically required, since the combination of biochemical and molecular

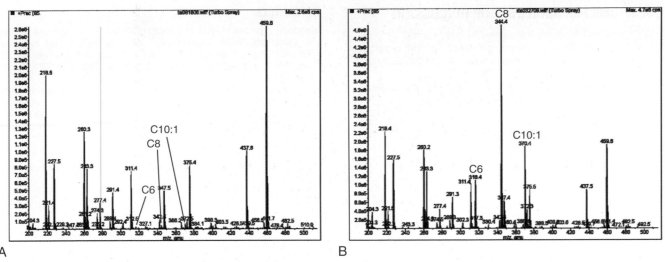

Figure C.31.1 Plasma acylcarnitine profiles obtained via flow injection electrospray ionization tandem mass spectrometry of butylated compounds. The peak heights as measured along the y-axis indicate the amounts of various acylcarnitine species, which are identified by their specific mass-to-charge ratios (m/z), as measured in atomic mass units (*amu*) along the x-axis. The 6 carbon (C6), 8 carbon (C8), and 10 carbon with an unsaturated bond (C10:1) acylcarnitine species are designated in *red*. (A) Unaffected individual: the C6, C8, and C10:1 peaks are barely detectable. (B) Individual with medium-chain acyl-CoA dehydrogenase (*MCAD*) deficiency: the C6, C8, and C10:1 peaks are markedly elevated, particularly the elevation of C8 as is characteristic of MCAD deficiency. (Courtesy of Tina Cowen, Stanford School of Medicine.)

genetic testing is capable of establishing the diagnosis, even in asymptomatic but affected individuals.

The mainstay of metabolic management for MCAD deficiency is avoidance of fasting, to prevent acute metabolic crisis. The maximum number of hours that may safely elapse between feeds is age dependent, with infants requiring the most frequent feeding. Adhering to this treatment principle allows individuals with MCAD deficiency to remain healthy and asymptomatic in the absence of metabolic stressors.

Metabolic stressors, such as intercurrent illness and surgery, increase the risk of acute metabolic crisis in individuals with MCAD deficiency. It is imperative to prevent/reverse catabolism in individuals with inadequate oral intake by treating them with IV fluids (10% dextrose with electrolytes running at 1.5–2 times maintenance rate). There is no consensus regarding the use of levocarnitine when an individual is well, but its use during acute illness is recommended at a dose of 100 mg/kg/day intravenously divided every 6 hours.

Women with MCAD deficiency who are pregnant must avoid catabolism, given their increased risk for metabolic decompensation.

Inheritance

MCAD deficiency is inherited in an autosomal recessive manner. The parents of an affected individual are considered obligate asymptomatic carriers. Any apparently unaffected siblings of an affected individual should be tested for MCAD deficiency, since diagnosis would lead to beneficial and potentially lifesaving intervention (see Chapter 19). There is a 25% chance that each sibling of an affected individual will also have MCAD deficiency, a 50% chance that the sibling will be an asymptomatic carrier, and a 25% chance that the sibling will be neither affected nor a carrier. All offspring of an affected individual will inherit an *ACADM* pathogenic variant. The recurrence risk of MCAD deficiency for such an offspring is determined by the carrier status of the reproductive partner.

Prenatal and preimplantation genetic testing is possible when the *ACADM* pathogenic variants have been identified for any at-risk couple comprising two carriers or one carrier and an affected individual.

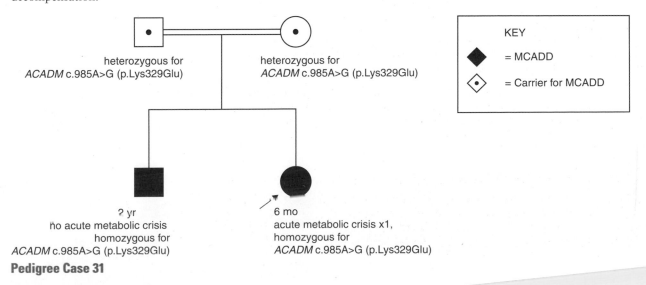

heterozygous for
ACADM c.985A>G (p.Lys329Glu)

heterozygous for
ACADM c.985A>G (p.Lys329Glu)

KEY
◆ = MCADD
◇ = Carrier for MCADD

? yr
no acute metabolic crisis
homozygous for
ACADM c.985A>G (p.Lys329Glu)

6 mo
acute metabolic crisis x1,
homozygous for
ACADM c.985A>G (p.Lys329Glu)

Pedigree Case 31

QUESTIONS FOR SMALL GROUP DISCUSSION

1. What other FAODs are included in NBS programs?
2. What are the criteria for including a disorder in NBS programs?
3. Can an individual who is heterozygous for an *ACADM* pathogenic variant be ascertained via NBS?
4. What are the false-positive and false-negative rates for MCAD deficiency NBS?

REFERENCES

Marsden D, Bedrosian CL, Vockley J: Impact of newborn screening on the reported incidence and clinical outcomes associated with medium- and long-chain fatty acid oxidation disorders, *Genet Med* 23(5):816–829, 2021. https://doi.org/10.1038/s41436-020-01070-0 Epub 2021 Jan 25. PMID: 33495527; PMCID: PMC8105167

Merritt JL 2nd, Chang IJ: Medium-chain acyl-coenzyme A dehydrogenase deficiency. 2000 Apr 20 [Updated 2019 Jun 27. In Adam MP, Ardinger HH, Pagon RA, *et al.*, editors: *GeneReviews® [Internet]*, Seattle, University of Washington, 1993–2022. GeneReviews https://www.ncbi.nlm.nih.gov/books/NBK1424/

32

MILLER-DIEKER SYNDROME (MIM 247200)
(17p13.3 Heterozygous Deletion)
Chromosomal Deletion

Kristen Miller

PRINCIPLES

- Microdeletion syndrome
- Contiguous gene disorder/genomic disorder
- Haploinsufficiency

MAJOR PHENOTYPIC FEATURES

- Age at onset: prenatal
- Lissencephaly type 1 or type 2
- Facial dysmorphisms
- Severe global developmental delay
- Seizures
- Early death

HISTORY AND PHYSICAL FINDINGS

B.B., a 5-day-old male born at 38 weeks gestation, was admitted to the neonatal intensive care unit with marked hypotonia and feeding difficulties. He was the product of an uncomplicated pregnancy: a 20-week anatomic survey was within normal limits, and noninvasive circulating cell-free DNA screening returned with normal/low-risk results. B.B. was born by spontaneous vaginal delivery with Apgar scores of 8 at 1 minute and 9 at 5 minutes. There is no known family history of genetic conditions, neurological disorders, congenital anomalies, or recurrent pregnancy loss. On physical examination, B.B. was noted to have hypotonia and mild dysmorphic facial features, including bitemporal narrowing, depressed nasal bridge, small nose with anteverted nares, and micrognathia. The findings from his examination were otherwise normal, including: serum electrolyte values, metabolic screen, and screening for congenital infections. A brain ultrasound showed hypoplastic corpus callosum, mild ventricular dilatation, and a smooth cortex. The genetics team recommended magnetic resonance imaging (MRI) of the brain, as well as a chromosomal microarray. MRI revealed a thickened cerebral cortex, complete cerebral agyria, multiple cerebral heterotopias, hypoplastic corpus callosum, normal cerebellum, and normal brainstem. Microarray identified a 1.2-Mb deletion on 17p13.3, including the *PAFAH1B1* gene (formerly known as *LIS1*). On the basis of these results, the geneticist explained to the parents that B.B. had Miller-Dieker syndrome. Following consultation with palliative care, B.B.'s parents declined aggressive intervention and elected comfort care only. B.B. died at 2 months of age. Chromosome analysis and fluorescence *in situ* hybridization (FISH) for the *PAFAH1B1* gene returned normal for both parents.

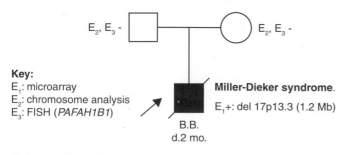

Key:
E₁: microarray
E₂: chromosome analysis
E₃: FISH (*PAFAH1B1*)

B.B.
d. 2 mo.

Miller-Dieker syndrome.
E₁+: del 17p13.3 (1.2 Mb)

Pedigree Case 32

BACKGROUND
Disease Etiology and Incidence

Miller-Dieker syndrome (MDS, MIM 247200) is a contiguous gene deletion syndrome caused by a heterozygous deletion of 17p13.3. The mechanism underlying recurrent deletion of 17p13.3 has not yet been elucidated, but it may (like other microdeletion syndromes; see Chapter 6) involve recombination between low-copy repeated DNA sequences. MDS is a rare disorder, occurring in possibly 40/1 million births in all populations. Up to 25 to 30% of classical lissencephaly may be due to MDS.

Pathogenesis

More than 50 genes have been mapped within the MDS deletion region in 17p13.3, but only the *PAFAH1B1* gene (MIM 601545) has definitively been associated with a specific phenotypic feature of MDS: heterozygous pathogenic variants in *PAFAH1B1* cause lissencephaly. *PAFAH1B1* encodes the brain isoform of the noncatalytic β subunit of platelet-activating factor acetylhydrolase (PAFAH), which hydrolyzes platelet-activating factor – an inhibitor of neuronal migration. PAFAH also binds to and stabilizes microtubules and may play a role in the microtubule reorganization required for neuronal migration.

Haploinsufficiency of *PAFAH1B1* alone, however, does not cause the other dysmorphic features associated with MDS. Pathogenic variants within *PAFAH1B1* cause isolated lissencephaly sequence (ILS) (MIM 607432); that is, lissencephaly without other dysmorphisms. Dysmorphic features are observed in essentially all patients with MDS; therefore, it is presumed that these features must result from haploinsufficiency of one or more different genes in the common MDS deletion interval. Several other candidate genes have been identified that may also contribute to the MDS phenotype, but no definitive relationship has been demonstrated.

Phenotype and Natural History

The hallmark features of MDS include brain dysgenesis (which is often severe), hypotonia, failure to thrive, epilepsy, and facial dysmorphisms. The brain dysgenesis is characterized by lissencephaly type 1 (complete agyria) or type 2 (widespread agyria with a few sulci at the frontal or occipital poles), a cerebral cortex with four instead of six layers, gray matter heterotopias, and attenuated white matter (see Chapter 15). Characteristic facial features include high forehead, bitemporal narrowing, flattened helices, hypertelorism, epicanthal folds, small nose with depressed nasal bridge and anteverted nares, vertical forehead furrow, prominent lateral nasal folds, round philtrum and upper lip with a thin, downward facing vermillion border, flat midface, and micrognathia. Some individuals also have extra-CNS anomalies, which can include cardiac defects, cleft palate, genitourinary anomalies (abnormal male genitalia, cystic or pelvic kidney[s]), polydactyly, and omphalocele.

Although the brain malformations of MDS result from incomplete migration of neurons to the cerebral cortex during the third and fourth months of gestation, lissencephaly is often not detected by fetal MRI or ultrasonography until late in gestation. In addition to structural anomalies, prenatal findings can include fetal growth restriction, polyhydramnios, and decreased fetal movement.

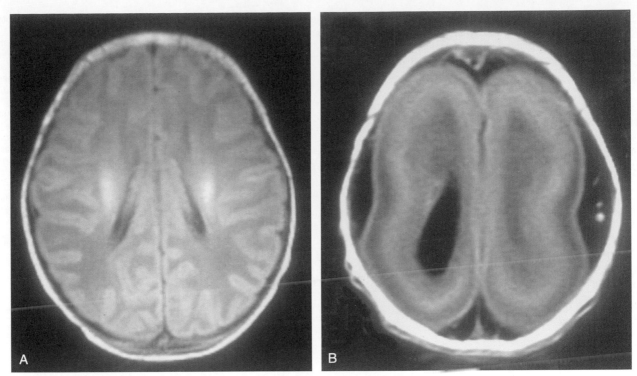

Figure C.32.1 Brain magnetic resonance images of infants without lissencephaly (A) and with Miller-Dieker syndrome (B). Note the smooth cerebral surface, the thickened cerebral cortex, and the classic "figure-8" appearance of the brain of the patient with Miller-Dieker syndrome. (Courtesy D. Chitayat, The Hospital for Sick Children and University of Toronto, Canada.)

Individuals with MDS almost universally exhibit poor feeding and growth. Smiling, brief visual fixation, and nonspecific motor responses are the only developmental skills that most acquire. In addition, opisthotonos and spasticity are frequent. Head circumference is often small to normal at birth, but microcephaly often becomes apparent in older individuals. Nearly all die by 2 years of age, although at least one individual has been reported surviving until age 17. Aspiration pneumonia and seizures are major causes of mortality.

Facial dysmorphisms in combination with lissencephaly on MRI often suggest a diagnosis of MDS (Fig. C.32.1). Confirmation of the diagnosis, however, requires detection of a 17p13.3 deletion by chromosomal microarray, since only about 60% of cases have a deletion of the MDS critical region that is cytogenetically visible. For individuals with ILS and normal microarray results, *PAFAH1B1* sequencing and deletion/duplication analysis may be indicated, as intragenic deletions and sequence variants can also result in ILS. At least nine autosomal and two X-linked genes have also been associated with ILS.

MANAGEMENT

There is no cure for MDS; therefore, treatment focuses on the management of symptoms and palliative care. Nearly all patients require pharmacological management of their seizures. Individuals with ILS may have intractable epilepsy. Many receive nasogastric or gastrostomy tube feedings to alleviate or reduce complications secondary to poor feeding and repeated aspiration.

Prenatal diagnosis of MDS requires detection of a 17p13.3 deletion in chorionic villi or amniocytes. While some laboratories offer screening of circulating cell-free DNA for certain microdeletions, the MDS critical region is not commonly included on these test panels.

Inheritance

Approximately 80% of affected individuals have microdeletion of 17p13.3 that is *de novo*, and 20% inherited the deletion from a parent who carries a balanced chromosomal rearrangement. Ring chromosomes have also been reported. Individuals with MDS as a result of a translocation may have additional clinical features resulting from a co-occurring partial trisomy. Because of the frequency of inheritance from a parent with a balanced translocation, karyotype analysis and FISH for *PAFAH1B1* (for submicroscopic cryptic translocations) should be performed for both parents of a proband. A parent with a balanced translocation involving 17p13.3 has an approximate 25% risk that a liveborn child will have either MDS or a duplication of 17p (which is often milder), and about a 20% risk for pregnancy loss. In contrast, if a patient has MDS as a result of a *de novo* deletion, the risk for recurrence is thought to be very low (but not zero) in future children. Gonadal mosaicism, though not yet reported in MDS, remains a theoretical mechanism for recurrence.

QUESTIONS FOR SMALL GROUP DISCUSSION

1. Rubenstein-Taybi syndrome is caused either by deletion of 16p13.3 or by pathogenic variants of the *CREBBP* transcription factor. Compare and contrast the relationship of *CREBBP* and Rubenstein-Taybi syndrome with the relationship of *PAFAH1B1* and MDS. Why is MDS a contiguous gene deletion syndrome, whereas Rubenstein-Taybi syndrome is not?

2. Pathogenic variants of either *PAFAH1B1* on chromosome 17 or *DCX* on the X chromosome account for approximately 75% of ILS cases. What features of the family history and brain MRI scan can be used to focus testing on *DCX* as opposed to *PAFAH1B1*?

3. At 30 weeks of gestation, a woman has a fetal ultrasound examination showing fetal lissencephaly. The pregnancy was

otherwise uncomplicated, and fetal ultrasound findings earlier in gestation had been normal. What counseling and evaluation are indicated? Discuss your counseling approach if she and her spouse wish to terminate the pregnancy at 32 weeks of gestation.

REFERENCES

Brock S, Dobyns WB, Jansen A: PAFAH1B1-related lissencephaly/subcortical band heterotopia. 2009 Mar 3 [Updated 2021 Mar 25]. In Adam MP, Ardinger HH, Pagon RA, *et al.*, editors: *GeneReviews® [Internet]*, Seattle, 1993–2022. https://www.ncbi.nlm.nih.gov/books/NBK5189/

Cardoso C, Leventer RJ, Ward HL, *et al*: Refinement of a 400-kb critical region allows genotypic differentiation between isolated lissencephaly, Miller-Dieker syndrome, and other phenotypes secondary to deletions of 17p13.3, *Am J Hum Genet* 72(4):918–930, 2003. https://doi.org/10.1086/374320

Hsieh DT, Jennesson MM, Thiele EA, *et al*: Brain and spinal manifestations of Miller-Dieker syndrome, *Neurol Clin Pract* 3:82–83, 2013.

Mishima T, Watari M, Iwaki Y, Nagai T, Kawamata-Nakamura M, Kobayashi Y, Fujieda S, Oikawa M, Takahashi N, Keira M, Yoshida H, Tonoki H: Miller-Dieker syndrome with unbalanced translocation 45, X, psu dic(17;Y)(p13;p11.32) detected by fluorescence in situ hybridization and G-banding analysis using high resolution banding technique, *Congenit Anom (Kyoto)* 57(2):61–63, 2017 Mar. https://doi.org/10.1111/cga.12193. PMID: 27644460

Pilz D: Miller-Dieker syndrome. Orphanet encyclopedia. September 2003: https://www.orpha.net/consor/cgi-bin/Disease_Search.php?lng=EN&data_id=4054&Disease_Disease_Search_diseaseGroup=Miller-Dieker&Disease_Disease_Search_diseaseType=Pat&Disease(s)/group%20of%20diseases=Miller-Dieker-syndrome&title=Miller-Dieker%20syndrome&search=Disease_Search_Simple. Expert reviewer(s): Pr Daniela PILZ. Last update: April 2005.

Wynshaw-Boris A: Lissencephaly and LIS1: Insights into molecular mechanisms of neuronal migration and development, *Clin Genet* 72:296–304, 2007.

33 MYOCLONIC EPILEPSY WITH RAGGED-RED FIBERS (MIM 545000)
(Mitochondrial tRNA^lys Variant)

Matrilineal, Mitochondrial

Eric Shoubridge

PRINCIPLES

- Mitochondrial DNA variants
- Maternal inheritance
- Genetic bottleneck in intergenerational transmission
- Heteroplasmy
- Replicative segregation
- Genotype varies in time and space
- Threshold expression

MAJOR PHENOTYPIC FEATURES

- Age at onset: childhood through adulthood
- Myopathy
- Dementia
- Myoclonic seizures
- Ataxia
- Deafness
- Multiple symmetric lipomatosis

CASE REPORT

R.S., a 15-year-old boy, was referred to the Neurogenetics clinic for myoclonic epilepsy; his electroencephalogram was characterized by bursts of slow wave and spike complexes. Before the seizures developed, he had been well and developing normally. His family history was remarkable for a maternal uncle who had died of an undiagnosed myopathic disorder at 53 years; a maternal aunt with progressive dementia who had presented with ataxia at 37 years; and an 80-year-old maternal grandmother with deafness, diabetes, and renal dysfunction. On examination, R.S. had generalized muscle wasting and weakness, myoclonus, and ataxia. Initial evaluation detected sensorineural hearing loss, slowed nerve conduction velocities, and mildly elevated blood and cerebrospinal fluid lactate levels. Results of a subsequent muscle biopsy identified abnormal mitochondria, deficient staining for cytochrome *c* oxidase, and ragged-red fibers: muscle fibers with accumulations of subsarcolemmal mitochondria that stained red with Gomori trichrome, giving the fibers a "moth-eaten" appearance on cross-section. Longitudinal sections showed that the defect was segmental, showing that muscle fibers are linear mosaics. Molecular testing of a skeletal muscle biopsy specimen for variants within the mitochondrial genome (mtDNA) identified in 80% of the muscle mtDNAs a heteroplasmic variant (c.8344 G>A, *tRNA^lys* gene), a variant known to be associated with myoclonic epilepsy with ragged-red fibers (MERRF). Subsequent testing of blood samples from R.S.'s mother, aunt, and grandmother confirmed that they also were heteroplasmic for this pathogenic variant, but each with a generally smaller proportion in mtDNAs than found in skeletal muscle of R.S. A review of the autopsy of the deceased uncle identified ragged-red fibers in some muscle groups. The physician counseled the family members (R.S.'s sibs and his mother's sibs) that they were either manifesting or nonmanifesting obligate carriers of a deleterious mtDNA variant that compromised oxidative phosphorylation. No other family members chose to be tested for the familial variant.

BACKGROUND
Disease Etiology and Incidence

MERRF (MIM 545000) is a rare disorder caused by pathogenic variants in mtDNA in the *tRNA^lys* (*MT-TK*) gene. More than 90% of affected individuals have one of three variants within this gene: c.8344 G>A accounts for 80%; c.8356T>C and c.8363 G>A together account for an additional 10% (see Fig. 13.24). The disease is inherited maternally because mitochondria are inherited almost exclusively from the mother. Individuals presenting with MERRF are always heteroplasmic for mtDNAs carrying the pathogenic variant. Homoplasmy for this variant is not compatible with survival (see Chapters 7 and 13).

Pathogenesis

Mitochondria generate energy for cellular processes by producing adenosine triphosphate (ATP) through oxidative phosphorylation. Five enzyme complexes, I to V, comprise the oxidative phosphorylation pathway. Except for complex II, each complex has some components encoded in mtDNA and some in the nuclear genome. MtDNA encodes 13 of the polypeptides in the oxidative phosphorylation complexes, as well as two ribosomal RNAs (rRNAs) and 22 transfer RNAs (tRNAs) (see Fig. 13.24).

In MERRF, the activities of complexes I and IV are usually most severely reduced. The tRNA^lys variants associated with MERRF reduce the amount of charged tRNA^lys in the mitochondria by 50 to 60% and prevent a posttranscriptional modification in the wobble U of the anticodon. The latter is essential for translation of both mitochondrial codons specifying lysine (AAA, AAG) and for the m^1A modification at position 58 that affects translation elongation and nascent chain stability. Complexes I and IV have the most components synthesized within the mitochondria, and this explains why they are the most severely affected.

Because mitochondria contain multiple mtDNAs and each cell contains multiple mitochondria (actually a network that undergoes continuous fusion and fission), a cell can contain wild-type mtDNAs and variant mtDNAs in varying proportions. The expression of the MERRF phenotype in any cell, organ, or individual ultimately depends on the relative proportions of each and the consequent reduction in oxidative phosphorylation capacity. The threshold for expression of a biochemical phenotype due to the tRNA^lys variant is quite high: about 85% variant mtDNAs. Above this threshold, there is a precipitous decline in mitochondrial translation. At 100% variant mtDNAs, mitochondrial translation is close to zero and the oxidative phosphorylation system is essentially nonfunctional. That explains why homoplasmy for the common MERRF variant is incompatible with life.

Increases in the proportion of variant mtDNA can occur by a combination of inheritance, preferential replication of variant mtDNA, and selection. First, the children of heteroplasmic mothers have widely varying proportions of mtDNA genotypes because of replicative segregation; that is, random partitioning of mitochondria during expansion of the oogonial population, particularly because of the mitochondrial "genetic bottleneck" that occurs during oogenesis. At least for the tRNA^lys variant that causes MERRF, intergenerational transmission appears to be stochastic. Second, as heteroplasmic cells in an individual undergo mitosis, the proportion of mtDNA genotypes in daughter cells changes from that of the parent cell by replicative segregation. Third, because changes in the proportion of mtDNA genotypes affect the cellular phenotype, mtDNA may be subject to selective pressures. These pressures vary among tissues and result in different mtDNA populations in different tissues of the same person. Thus, both intercellular and intergenerational mtDNA transmissions follow the principles of population genetics.

PHENOTYPE AND NATURAL HISTORY

The classic MERRF phenotype includes myoclonic epilepsy and mitochondrial myopathy with ragged-red fibers (Fig. C.33.1). Other associated findings can include abnormal brainstem evoked responses, sensorineural hearing loss, ataxia, renal dysfunction, diabetes, cardiomyopathy, and dementia. Onset of symptoms can be in childhood or adult life, and the course can be slowly progressive or rapidly downhill.

Because mtDNA genetics follows quantitative and stochastic principles, clinical features of affected relatives vary in pattern and severity and do not have an easily defined clinical course. The absence of ragged-red fibers in a muscle biopsy specimen does not exclude MERRF. Within pedigrees, phenotypes generally correlate well with the severity of the oxidative phosphorylation deficit.

MANAGEMENT

Treatment is symptomatic and palliative. No specific therapies are currently available. Some patients have been given cocktails containing coenzyme Q10, L-carnitine, and other supplements in an attempt to optimize the activity of the oxidative phosphorylation system, but it is not clear whether these have provided direct benefit to patients.

INHERITANCE

The risk to children of affected males is essentially zero because, with only one known exception, children do not inherit paternal mtDNA. The risk to children of affected or unaffected females with a MERRF variant can be estimated by prenatal testing but because of the mitochondrial genetic bottleneck, the confidence intervals for predicting a severe phenotype are very large. Preimplantation genetic testing of blastomeres in early embryos is possible. Mitochondrial replacement therapy for mothers carrying the pathogenic variant has recently become a possibility in some countries.

Similarly, molecular testing of blood samples from at-risk family members is complicated because of replicative segregation and potential tissue-specific selection; however, the available data suggest that the levels of the variant in blood are modestly lower (~10%) than those in postmitotic tissues (skeletal muscle).

QUESTIONS FOR SMALL GROUP DISCUSSION

1. How does a variant mtDNA molecule, arising *de novo* in a cell with hundreds of normal molecules, become such a significant fraction of the total that energy-generating capacity is compromised and symptoms develop?

2. In the fetus, oxygen tension is low and most energy is derived from glycolysis. How could this observation affect the prenatal expression of deleterious oxidative phosphorylation variants?

3. What is the mechanism of the mitochondrial genetic bottleneck, and why do you think it might have evolved?

4. How does genetic complementation explain the threshold behavior of this tRNA variant? Do you think a similar mechanism might exist for variants in protein-coding genes?

REFERENCES

Boulet, L., G. Karpati, and E.A. Shoubridge, Distribution and threshold expression of the tRNA(Lys) mutation in skeletal muscle of patients with myoclonic epilepsy and ragged-red fibers (MERRF). *Am J Hum Genet*, 1992. 51(6): p. 1187–200.

Larsson, N.G., *et al.*, Segregation and manifestations of the mtDNA tRNA(Lys) A-->G(8344) mutation of myoclonus epilepsy and ragged-red fibers (MERRF) syndrome. *Am J Hum Genet*, 1992. 51(6): p. 1201–12.

Richter, U., *et al.*, RNA modification landscape of the human mitochondrial tRNA(Lys) regulates protein synthesis. *Nat Commun*, 2018. 9(1): p. 3966.

Suzuki T, Nagao A, Suzuki T: Human mitochondrial tRNAs: Biogenesis, function, structural aspects and diseases, *Ann Rev Genet* 45:299–329, 2011.

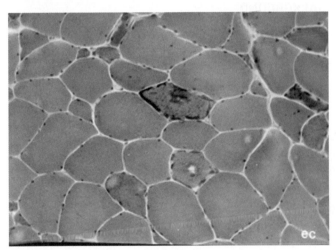

Figure C.33.1 MERRF Histochemistry. Segregation of pathogenic mtDNAs determines muscle phenotype. Courtesy, Eric Shoubridge

Key

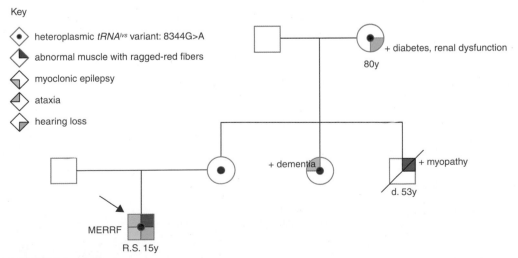

Pedigree Case 33

Autosomal Dominant

Krista Schatz

PRINCIPLES

- Variable expressivity
- Extreme pleiotropy
- Tumor-suppressor gene
- Loss-of-function variants
- Allelic heterogeneity
- *De novo* variants
- Revised diagnostic criteria in 2021

MAJOR PHENOTYPIC FEATURES

- Age at onset: prenatal to late childhood
- Café au lait spots
- Axillary and inguinal freckling
- Cutaneous neurofibromas
- Lisch nodules (iris hamartomas)
- Plexiform neurofibromas
- Optic glioma
- Choroidal abnormalities
- Specific osseous lesions

HISTORY AND PHYSICAL FINDINGS

L.M. was a 2-year-old girl referred to Genetics initially because of five café au lait spots, of which three measured larger than 5 mm in diameter. She had no axillary or inguinal freckling, no osseous malformations, and no neurofibromas. Physical examination of her parents revealed no stigmata of neurofibromatosis. The reported family history was also negative for known features of neurofibromatosis. The consulting geneticist informed the parents and referring pediatrician that L.M. did not meet the clinical criteria for neurofibromatosis type 1. They were offered the option of

molecular genetic testing or of following up in 1 to 2 years for repeat clinical evaluation. The family elected to defer Genetic testing and to follow up with Genetics.

L.M. returned to the Genetics clinic at 5 years of age. She now had Lisch nodules in both eyes and 12 café au lait spots, 8 of which measured at least 5 mm in diameter. She also had axillary freckling bilaterally. She was given a clinical diagnosis of neurofibromatosis 1 and referred to an NF1 specialist for long-term follow-up. Given their lack of features, her parents were told that L.M. likely had a *de novo* variant and the recurrence risk was therefore low, but that gonadal mosaicism could not be excluded. The family was again offered the option of molecular genetic testing in L.M. for confirmation. If the underlying variant was identified, then parental testing could be completed for recurrence information purposes. L.M.'s parents declined both molecular testing in L.M. and prenatal testing during their next pregnancy.

BACKGROUND

Disease Etiology and Incidence

Neurofibromatosis 1 (NF1, MIM 162200) is an autosomal dominant condition with symptoms most frequently expressed in the skin, eye, skeleton, and nervous system. NF1 results from pathogenic variants in the neurofibromin gene (*NF1*). The disease has an incidence of approximately 1 in 3000 persons, making it one of the most common autosomal dominant genetic conditions. Approximately half of the people with NF1 have *de novo* variants. The mutation rate for the *NF1* gene is one of the highest known for any human gene, at approximately 1/10,000 live births. Approximately 80% of the *de novo* variants are paternal in origin, and there is some evidence for a paternal age effect increasing the mutation rate (see Chapter 4).

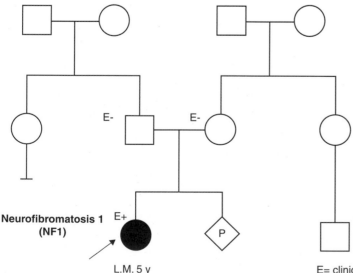

Neurofibromatosis 1
(NF1)

L.M. 5 y

E= clinically examined for NF1 stigmata

Pedigree Case 34

Pathogenesis

NF1 is a large gene (350 kb and 60 exons) that encodes neurofibromin. This protein is widely expressed in almost all tissues but most abundantly in the brain, spinal cord, and peripheral nervous system. Neurofibromin is thought to regulate several intracellular processes, including the activation of Ras GTPase, thereby controlling cellular proliferation and acting as a tumor suppressor.

More than 3000 pathogenic variants in the *NF1* gene have been identified; most are unique to an individual family. The clinical manifestations result from a loss of function of the gene product. A pathogenic variant can be identified for more than 95% of individuals who meet clinical diagnostic criteria for NF1.

NF1 is characterized by extreme clinical variability, both between and within families. This variability is probably caused by a combination of genetic, nongenetic, and stochastic factors. The vast majority of variants do not show genotype-phenotype correlations; however, large deletions that include the entire *NF1* gene and surrounding genes ("NF1 microdeletions") are more common in those with a higher tumor burden, intellectual disability, and coarse facies. Additionally, several variants have been associated with a "Noonan-like" phenotype (see Case 41), with a seemingly lower risk for tumors and an increased risk for cardiovascular features; however, even the variants with some genotype-phenotype correlations show variable expressivity.

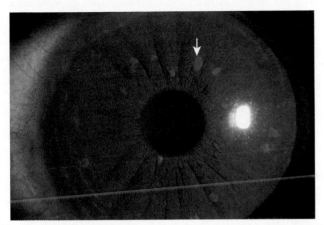

Figure C.34.1 Iris showing numerous Lisch nodules (one typical nodule is indicated by the *arrow*). (Courtesy K. Yohay, Johns Hopkins School of Medicine, Baltimore, Maryland.)

PHENOTYPE AND NATURAL HISTORY

NF1 is a multisystem disorder with neurological, musculoskeletal, ophthalmological, and skin abnormalities and a predisposition to neoplasia (Figs. C.34.1 and C.34.2). The clinical

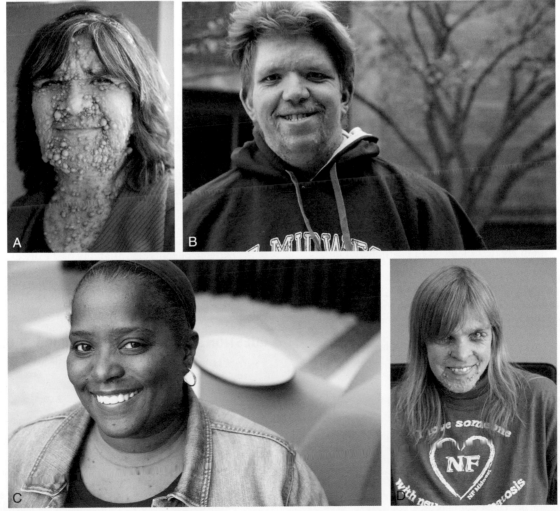

Figure C.34.2 (A) Lorena, (B) Jon, (C) Evita, and (D) Jeanette are representing the Neurofibromatosis Network (nfnetwork.org). Photograph by Rick Guidotti, Positive Exposure (www.PositiveExposure.com).

diagnostic criteria for NF1 were originally published in 1998 and revised in 2021 (Box C.34.1). It is important to note that per the revised criteria, a pathogenic variant in the *NF1* gene alone is not enough to meet clinical diagnostic criteria; a second feature is still needed. Nearly all individuals with NF1 but no family history will meet clinical criteria by age 8 years. Children who have inherited NF1 can usually be identified clinically within the first year of life, requiring only one other feature of the disease for diagnosis.

Although NF1 has essentially complete penetrance, manifestations are extremely variable. Multiple café au lait spots and cutaneous neurofibromas are present in nearly all affected individuals, with freckling seen in 90% of cases. Many individuals with NF1 have only cutaneous manifestations and iris Lisch nodules (Fig. C.34.1). Numerous neurofibromas are usually present in adults. Plexiform neurofibromas are less common, though they occur in about 30 to 50% of individuals with NF1. Ocular manifestations include optic gliomas (which may lead to blindness), iris Lisch nodules, and choroidal abnormalities. The most serious bone complications are scoliosis, vertebral dysplasia, pseudarthrosis, and overgrowth. Stenosis of pulmonic, renal, and cerebral vessels and hypertension are also frequent. Vitamin D deficiency is more common. Neurofibromas are at risk for malignant transformation to malignant peripheral nerve sheath tumors (MPNSTs), the most frequent malignancy in individuals with NF1. The most common neoplasms for children with NF1 (other than neurofibromas) are optic nerve gliomas, brain tumors, and malignant myeloid disorders. Other tumors may also occur, including early-onset breast cancer, pheochromocytoma, and gastrointestinal stromal tumors. Early screening for breast cancer is recommended in women with NF1. Approximately half of the children with NF1 have a learning disability or attention deficits, which can persist into adulthood.

Individuals with features of NF1 limited to one region of the body, and who have unaffected parents, may be diagnosed with segmental (or regional) NF1. Segmental NF1 may represent an unusual distribution of clinical features by chance, or somatic mosaicism for an *NF1* gene variant. In those who are suspected to have segmental or mosaic disease, molecular genetic testing on affected tissue has the highest sensitivity.

MANAGEMENT

NF1 has classically been a clinical diagnosis. Genetic testing was not routinely performed because of the ability to make a clinical diagnosis, the size of the gene, and the allelic heterogeneity. Molecular genetic testing is available, however, typically using a combination of sequence and copy number analyses to search for pathogenic variants. This is useful for those in whom the diagnosis is less obvious. As more disorders are identified that have features overlapping with NF1, and test costs decline, molecular genetic testing is becoming more frequent. For people with NF1 who wish to undergo reproductive testing – such as through prenatal diagnosis or preimplantation genetic testing – a molecular diagnosis is required. Treatments are not curative, but focus on symptomatic management. Ongoing surveillance in an individual with NF1 should include an annual physical examination conducted by someone familiar with NF1, annual ophthalmological evaluation in childhood (less frequent for adults), regular developmental assessments in childhood, annual scoliosis screening in childhood, and regular blood pressure measurements. Imaging studies should be performed based on clinical features.

The physical features caused by NF1 can be the most distressing manifestation for affected individuals. Discrete cutaneous and subcutaneous neurofibromas can be surgically removed if they are disfiguring or inconveniently located. Plexiform neurofibromas causing disfigurement or impingement can also be surgically managed. However, surgical intervention for these neoplasms can be problematic because they are often intimately involved with nerves and tend to grow back at the site of removal.

INHERITANCE

NF1 is inherited in an autosomal dominant manner. This means that each child of an affected individual has a 50% chance to inherit the condition, although the features of an affected child may be different and cannot be accurately predicted. Prenatal and preconception testing is often available for those families in whom a causative *NF1* gene variant has been identified (see Chapter 18). Although prenatal diagnosis is accurate, it will not provide prognostic information because of the extreme phenotypic variability of the disease. Parents of an affected child who themselves do not have NF1 still have an increased chance that additional children would have NF1 because of the possibility of gonadal mosaicism. While this chance is relatively low, it has been documented with NF1.

BOX C.34.1 2021 REVISED DIAGNOSTIC CRITERIA FOR NEUROFIBROMATOSIS TYPE 1

A diagnosis of NF1 can be given if an individual has two or more of the following manifestations:
- ≥6 café-au-lait-macules[1]
  - >5 mm in greatest diameter in prepubertal children
  - >15 mm in greatest diameter in postpubertal individuals
- Freckling in axillary or inguinal region[1]
- ≥2 neurofibroma tumors of any type *or* one plexiform neurofibroma
- ≥2 Lisch nodules *or* ≥2 choroidal abnormalities
- Optic pathway glioma
- A distinctive osseous lesion such as: sphenoid dysplasia[2]; anterolateral bowing of tibia (tibial dysplasia); or pseudarthrosis of a long bone
- A pathogenic *NF1* gene variant
- A parent with NF1 by the above criteria

QUESTIONS FOR SMALL GROUP DISCUSSION

1. Why is there such clinical variability in NF1? What factors could be influencing this phenotype?
2. Why is a positive family history of NF1 one of the major diagnostic criteria for this condition and not for other autosomal dominant conditions?
3. Review the major points of discussion with a family that requests prenatal testing for NF1 based on a known variant in one of the parents.
4. Given that loss of function is the mechanism of disease in NF1, how would a treatment of NF1 need to be targeted at the molecular level to specifically address this? How is that different from a disease caused by a dominant negative mutation?

---

[1]If only café-au-lait macules and freckling are present, the diagnosis is most likely NF1 but (exceptionally) the person might have another diagnosis, such as Legius syndrome. At least one of the two pigmentary findings (café-au-lait macules or freckling) should be bilateral.

[2]Sphenoid wing dysplasia is not a separate criterion in the case of an ipsilateral orbital plexiform neurofibroma.

REFERENCES

Friedman JM: Neurofibromatosis 1. http://www.ncbi.nlm.nih.gov/books/NBK1109/.

Kehrer-Sawatzki H, Mautner VF, Cooper DN: Emerging genotype-phenotype relationships in patients with large NF1 deletions, *Hum Genet* 136(4):349–376, 2017. https://doi.org/10.1007/s00439-017-1766-y

Koczkowska M, Callens T, Chen Y, *et al*: Clinical spectrum of individuals with pathogenic NF1 missense variants affecting p.Met1149, p.Arg1276, and p.Lys1423: genotype-phenotype study in neurofibromatosis type 1, *Hum Mutat* 41(1):299–315, 2020. https://doi.org/10.1002/humu.23929

Legius E, Messiaen L, Wolkenstein P, *et al*: Revised diagnostic criteria for neurofibromatosis type 1 and Legius syndrome: An international consensus recommendation, *Genet Med* 23(8):1506–1513, 2021. https://doi.org/10.1038/s41436-021-01170-5. Epub 2021 May 19.

Trevisson E, Morbidoni V, Forzan M, *et al*: The Arg1038Gly missense variant in the NF1 gene causes a mild phenotype without neurofibromas, *Mol Genet Genomic Med* 7(5):e616, 2019. https://doi.org/10.1002/mgg3.616

ROIFMAN SYNDROME (MIM 616651)
RNU4ATAC Noncoding RNA Gene Pathogenic Variants

Autosomal Recessive

Maian Roifman • Chaim M. Roifman

PRINCIPLES

- Genotypic specificity
- Compound heterozygosity
- Allelic disorders
- Splicing defect
- Treatable condition
- Noncoding gene

MAJOR PHENOTYPIC FINDINGS

- Immune deficiency
- Spondyloepiphyseal dysplasia
- Growth restriction
- Retinal dystrophy
- Distinctive facial features
- Intellectual disability

HISTORY AND PHYSICAL FINDINGS

The patient is a 3-year-old male, born at term to nonconsanguineous healthy parents. The family history was unremarkable. There was a prenatal history of intrauterine growth restriction. At birth, his weight and length plotted below the 3rd centile. Since birth, he was noticed to have hypotonia and delayed developmental milestones. Since the age of 6 months, he had suffered repeated episodes of otitis media and had so far three documented episodes of pneumonia. At the age of 18 months, he was diagnosed with eczema affecting the face, arms, and legs. On examination, he was found to have hypoplastic alae nasi, a long philtrum, and a thin upper lip. He had short stature, brachydactyly, bilateral single palmar creases, and 5th-digit clinodactyly.

On immunological evaluation, which included quantitative immunoglobulins, specific antibodies to vaccines, in vitro lymphocyte mitogenic responses, and lymphocyte subset phenotype, there were low antibody titers in response to the tetanus toxoid, pertussis, and polio vaccines. Skeletal survey showed signs of spondyloepiphyseal dysplasia. Microarray analysis revealed normal chromosomes and whole exome sequencing was negative. Molecular genetic testing with a primary immune deficiency gene panel revealed compound heterozygous variants in the *RNU4ATAC* gene. Parental testing showed that each parent is a carrier of one of the variants.

BACKGROUND
Disease Etiology and Incidence

Roifman syndrome is caused by biallelic pathogenic variants in the noncoding *RNU4ATAC* gene (within intron 2 of the *CLASP1* gene on chromosome 2). For Roifman syndrome specifically, at least one pathogenic variant must be in the stem II region of the gene. The incidence of Roifman syndrome is unknown, with 16 cases described thus far.

Pathogenesis

RNU4ATAC is a noncoding small nuclear RNA (snRNA) gene, a component of the minor spliceosome complex, responsible for properly splicing approximately 800 genes. *RNU4ATAC* has four domains that are thought to be highly important for the function of the spliceosome:
- stem II (at the 5′ end of the gene)
- 5′ stem-loop critical region
- stem I
- Sm protein-binding site

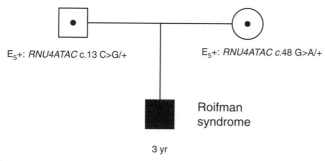

E_5+: *RNU4ATAC* c.13 C>G/+ E_5+: *RNU4ATAC* c.48 G>A/+

Roifman syndrome

3 yr

intrauterine growth restriction
b. → weight, length <3rd %ile, hypotonia, delayed milestones
6 mo. → repeated otitis media, pneumonia (x3)
18 mo. → eczema, distinctive facial features

E_1+: low vaccine Ab titres
E_2+. spondyloepiphyseal dysplasia
E_3 -
E_4 -
E_5+: *RNU4ATAC* c.13 C>G; c.48 G>A

Legend

E_1 = immunology evaluation
E_2 = skeletal survey
E_3 = chromosomal microarray analysis
E_4 = exome sequencing
E_5 = sequencing panel:
    primary immune deficiency genes

The variants in *RNU4ATAC* identified in individuals with Roifman syndrome impair minor intron splicing, suggesting that impaired splicing of multiple genes causes the features of Roifman syndrome.

Roifman syndrome is associated with high genotypic specificity in *RNU4ATAC*. All cases exhibit a variant in the highly conserved stem II region of the gene; thus termed the obligatory variants in Roifman syndrome. From the cases described thus far, it appears that Roifman syndrome is caused by biallelic variants: both in the stem II region, or a combination of one obligatory variant (in the stem II region) and another elsewhere in the alternate allele.

Other Allelic Disorders

A disorder allelic to Roifman syndrome is microcephalic osteodysplastic primordial dwarfism type I (MOPD1) – or Taybi-Linder syndrome – (MIM 210710). It is almost invariably lethal and is characterized by severe and progressive prenatal onset growth restriction, most strikingly affecting the head and causing a sloping forehead from birth. Other features are proptotic eyes, bulbous nose, micrognathia, sparse hair and dysplastic nails, and metaphyseal dysplasia with short, bowed limbs. Neurological impairment is severe, in the context of major brain malformations and intractable seizures. These children also have hearing loss and neuroendocrine dysfunction. The condition is very rare, with approximately 50 cases reported, and is typically lethal by age 3 years. Recent reports of adults with MOPD1 show their phenotype to be milder, but consistent with the more severe forms. Survival may be related to specific genotypes. This condition, involving the same gene as Roifman syndrome, has an interesting genotypic relationship, with no documented cases bearing alterations in the stem II region of *RNU4ATAC* (seen as critical to the Roifman phenotype); rather, missense variants are found in other domains, especially the 5′ stem-loop region. This may explain the distinct phenotypes, especially relating to immune deficiency.

Lowry-Wood syndrome (MIM 226960) is another rare allelic disorder, distinguished from Roifman syndrome by the presence of congenital nystagmus and lack of clinically significant immune deficiency.

These three disorders with some overlapping features are all caused by biallelic variants in *RNU4ATAC* (MIM 601428). As more combinations of pathogenic variants are identified, genotype-phenotype correlations may more clearly account for the distinct phenotypes. Confusion may arise from assigning a clinical diagnosis of Lowry-Wood syndrome or Roifman syndrome to someone who does not have the distinguishing features of congenital nystagmus or immune deficiency, respectively. Careful phenotyping to maintain this distinction would be beneficial for clinicians to accurately clarify genotype-phenotype correlation moving forward.

PHENOTYPE AND NATURAL HISTORY

Most individuals with Roifman syndrome present in infancy or early childhood with recurrent infections. Rarely, this history may not be severe and thus may not prompt referral for immunologic consultation, leading to undiagnosed treatable immune deficiency. In cases where an immune deficiency was not recognized in early childhood, retrospective reviews of medical histories have revealed features typical of immune deficiency. Generalized mild hypotonia is also an early sign. Later in childhood, these patients may present to a pediatric specialist or geneticist with intellectual disability, short stature, and/or symmetrical growth deficiency.

All individuals with Roifman syndrome exhibit humoral immune deficiency manifesting as recurrent sinopulmonary infections, and an inability to produce specific antibodies, reflected in low antibody titers to vaccines. Almost half of them also exhibit features of T-cell abnormalities, such as recurrent viral and fungal infections, atopy, and autoimmune disorders, correlated with abnormal T-cell function on immunological investigations.

Facial features of Roifman syndrome may not be immediately recognizable in the neonatal period. The most striking features include a long, tubular nose with hypoplastic alae nasi, long philtrum with a thin upper lip, and down-turned corners of the mouth (Fig. C.35.1). Palpebral fissures are also long, appearing as relatively large eyes.

Newborns with Roifman syndrome typically have mild symmetrical growth restriction, with weight, length, and head circumference plotting at the lower normal range, or just below the 2nd centile. With age, height becomes the most severely impacted growth parameter, and final adult height typically plots 2 to 4 standard deviations below the mean. Head circumference remains around the 2nd centile for age into adulthood. Weight is proportionally low in childhood but can vary in adulthood.

Clinical features of this skeletal dysplasia include short stature, short trunk, brachydactyly, and 5th-digit clinodactyly. Radiographic findings include delayed ossification, flattened and irregular epiphyses, vertebral notching, loss of lumbar lordosis, and short metacarpals (Fig. C.35.1).

Early hypotonia contributes to mild motor developmental delay. At school age, psychoeducational testing reveals lower IQ with deficiencies in several domains, including attention, processing speed, perceptual reasoning, visual perceptual organization, memory, and computation and math skills. Retinal dystrophy presents as night blindness in early to mid childhood.

Occasional additional findings in Roifman syndrome include partial agenesis of the corpus callosum, hippocampal atrophy, mild ventriculomegaly, cardiac abnormality, sensorineural hearing loss, and hypogonadotropic hypogonadism.

Molecular diagnosis of Roifman syndrome can be made via primary immune deficiency gene panel testing or targeted Sanger sequencing of the *RNU4ATAC* gene. Note that genetic diagnostic findings will be missed by current standard nontargeted molecular approaches, such as exome sequencing, that focus only on coding sequence. Whole genome sequencing would be able to detect *RNU4ATAC* variants and will likely replace exome sequencing as the standard molecular test for genetic diagnosis in the future.

MANAGEMENT

Following the initial diagnosis of Roifman syndrome, to establish the extent of disease and needs in the affected individual, consultation should be arranged with an immunologist for detailed B- and T-cell investigations and initiation of intravenous immunoglobulin (IVIG) treatment. In addition, the individual should undergo skeletal survey, developmental assessment (especially during school age), eye examination, echocardiogram, audiology assessment if there is a suspicion of hearing loss, and consultation with a clinical geneticist and/or genetic counselor.

IVIG is provided to reduce the number of infections and improve clinical outcomes in individuals with Roifman syndrome. Immune function should be reassessed every year.

Retinal dystrophy and congenital heart defects are treated as needed and managed by the respective specialists.

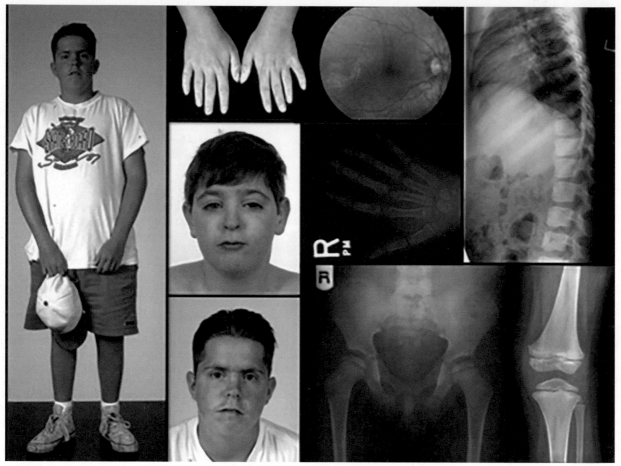

Figure C.35.1 Clinical and radiographic features of Roifman syndrome. (Modified from Merico D, Roifman M, Braunschweig U, et al: Compound heterozygous mutations in the noncoding *RNU4ATAC* cause Roifman syndrome by disrupting minor intron splicing, *Nat Commun* 6:8718, 2015. https://doi.org/10.1038/ncomms9718)

The sequelae of bone dysplasia, such as joint or bone pain, should be managed by orthopedic surgery and/or rheumatology specialists.

INHERITANCE

Roifman syndrome is inherited in an autosomal recessive manner. The parents of an affected child are presumed heterozygote carriers, and their genotype can be readily confirmed through targeted sequence analysis. Carriers of Roifman syndrome are asymptomatic. At conception, each sibling of an affected individual has a 25% chance of being affected, a 50% chance of being an asymptomatic carrier, and a 25% chance of being unaffected and not a carrier. Once a genotype has been established for the proband, prenatal or preimplantation genetic diagnosis is feasible.

Unless an individual with Roifman syndrome has children with an affected individual or a carrier, his/her offspring will be obligate heterozygotes (carriers) for a pathogenic variant in *RNU4ATAC*. To date, no individual with Roifman syndrome has been known to reproduce.

QUESTIONS FOR SMALL GROUP DISCUSSION

1. You have just seen a 2-year-old girl with a history of growth restriction, hypotonia, mild motor developmental delay, and facial features consistent with Roifman syndrome. When you ask the parents about the frequency of infections, they tell you she has had two episodes of pneumonia in the past year. What tests would you order? Why?
2. Discuss the importance of early diagnosis in this condition.
3. You have just identified an individual to be a carrier of a pathogenic variant in the stem II region of *RNU4ATAC*. How would you counsel the individual regarding reproductive risk?

REFERENCES

Merico D, Roifman M, Braunschweig U, Yeun RKC, Alexandrova R, Bates A, Reid B, Nalpathamkalam T, Wang Z, Thiruvahindrapuram B, Gray P, Kakakios A, Peake J, Hogarth S, Manson D, Buncic R, Pereira SL, Herbrick J, Blencowe B, Roifman CM, Scherer SW: Compound heterozygous mutations in the noncoding RNU4ATAC gene cause Roifman syndrome by disrupting minor intron splicing, *Nat Commun* 6:8718–8728, 2015.

Helihan I, Ehresmann S, Magnani C, Forzano F, Baldo C, Brunetti-Pierri N, Campeau PM. Lowry-Wood syndrome: further evidence of association with RNU4ATAC, and correlation between genotype and phenotype. *Hum Genet*. 2018 Dec;137(11–12):905–909.

Roifman CM: Antibody deficiency, growth retardation, spondyloepiphyseal dysplasia and retinal dystrophy: A novel syndrome, *Clin Genet* 55:103–109, 1999.

ORNITHINE TRANSCARBAMYLASE DEFICIENCY (MIM 311250)
(OTC Pathogenic Variant)

X-Linked

Ada Hamosh

PRINCIPLES

- Inborn error of metabolism
- X-linked inheritance
- X chromosome inactivation
- Manifesting heterozygotes
- Asymptomatic carriers
- Germline mutation rate much greater in spermatogenesis than in oogenesis

MAJOR PHENOTYPIC FINDINGS

- Age at onset: hemizygous male with null variant – neonatal; heterozygous female – with severe intercurrent illness, post-partum, or never
- Hyperammonemia
- Coma

HISTORY AND PHYSICAL FINDINGS

J.S. is a 4-day-old male infant brought to the emergency department because he could not be aroused. The parents reported a history of 24 hours of decreased intake, vomiting, and increasing lethargy. He was the 3-kg, full-term product of an uncomplicated gestation born to a healthy 26-year-old primiparous woman. Physical examination showed a comatose, hyperpneic, nondysmorphic male newborn. Initial laboratory evaluation revealed a blood NH_3 concentration of 900 μM (normal in a newborn is <75) and elevated venous pH of 7.48, with a normal bicarbonate concentration and anion gap. A urea cycle disorder was suspected, so plasma amino acid levels were determined on an emergency basis. Glutamine was elevated at 1700 μM (normal, <700 μM), and citrulline was undetectable (normal is 7–34 μM) (Fig. C.36.1). Analysis of urine for organic acids was normal; urinary orotic acid was extremely elevated. Elevated urine orotic acid levels with low citrulline indicate a diagnosis of ornithine transcarbamylase deficiency, pending confirmation by DNA sequencing.

Further questioning of J.S.'s mother revealed that she had a lifelong aversion to protein and a brother who died in the first week of life of unknown causes. J.S. was started on intravenous sodium benzoate and sodium phenylacetate (Ammonul®) and arginine hydrochloride. The child was transported by air to a tertiary care center equipped for neonatal hemodialysis. On arrival, his plasma NH_3 level had dropped to 700 μM. The parents were counseled about the high risk for brain damage from this degree of hyperammonemia. They elected to proceed with hemodialysis, which was well tolerated and resulted in the decline of the blood NH_3 to less than 200 μM after 4 hours. The child was maintained on Ammonul® and high calories from intravenous dextrose and intralipids until the NH_3 level was normal, at which point he was slowly started on a protein-restricted diet and continued on oral nitrogen scavengers, initially sodium phenylbutyrate and then transitioned to glycerol phenylbutyrate. He will be monitored for hyperammonemia, especially during intercurrent illnesses. His prognosis remains guarded. Once a pathogenic variant is identified by sequencing of the *OTC* gene, either alone or as part of a urea cycle gene panel, J.S.'s mother and maternal grandmother should be offered testing to confirm the presence of the variant. If they are found to be carriers, additional at-risk family members should be offered testing (e.g., proband's maternal aunt and her three children).

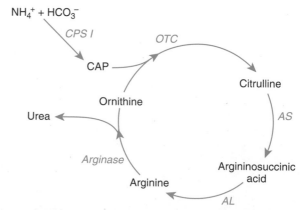

Pedigree Case 36

BACKGROUND

Disease Etiology and Incidence

Ornithine transcarbamylase (OTC) deficiency (MIM 311250) is an X-linked disorder of urea cycle metabolism caused by pathogenic variants of the gene encoding ornithine transcarbamylase (*OTC*). It has an incidence of 1 in 30,000 males. The exact incidence of manifesting females is unknown.

Pathogenesis

Ornithine transcarbamylase is an enzyme in the urea cycle (see Fig. C.36.1). The urea cycle is the mechanism by which

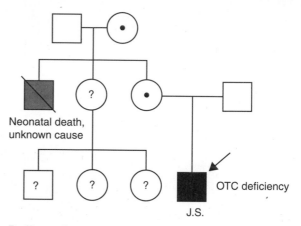

Figure C.36.1 The urea cycle. *AL*, argininosuccinate lyase; *AS*, argininosuccinate synthetase; *CAP*, carbamoyl phosphate; *CPS I*, carbamoyl phosphate synthetase I; *OTC*, ornithine transcarbamylase.

waste nitrogen is detoxified and excreted. Complete deficiency of any enzyme within the cycle (except arginase) leads to severe hyperammonemia in the neonatal period. For patients with urea cycle defects, arginine becomes an essential amino acid (see Fig. C.36.1). In utero, excess nitrogen is metabolized by the mother. Postnatally, however, accumulation of waste nitrogen in the extremely catabolic period after birth leads to elevation of glutamine and alanine, the body's natural pools for nitrogen, and ultimately to elevated levels of NH_4. Plasma NH_4 levels above 200 micromolar may cause brain damage; the degree of brain damage is related to peak blood concentrations of NH_4 and glutamine and the duration of the elevations. Thus, early detection and treatment of hyperammonemia are critical to outcome, both from the neonatal hyperammonemia and expected subsequent ammonia elevations with catabolism due to illness.

Males are hemizygous for the *OTC* gene and more severely affected by its pathogenic variants. Because *OTC* undergoes random X chromosome inactivation (see Chapter 6), females are mosaic for expression of the variant and can demonstrate a wide range of enzyme functions and clinical severity. Female heterozygotes can be completely asymptomatic and able to eat as much protein as they wish. Alternatively, if their loss of OTC activity is more significant, they may find themselves avoiding dietary protein and subject to recurrent, symptomatic hyperammonemia.

PHENOTYPE AND NATURAL HISTORY

Males with complete OTC deficiency are asymptomatic at birth, but begin vomiting, become lethargic, and eventually lapse into coma within 48 to 72 hours. Because they have been vomiting, they are usually dehydrated as well. Untreated males with null variants usually die in the first week of life. Even if the patient with OTC deficiency is promptly and successfully treated in the neonatal period, the risk remains high for recurrent bouts of hyperammonemia, particularly during intercurrent illnesses, because complete control of severe OTC deficiency is difficult, even with dietary protein restriction and medications that divert the NH_3 to nontoxic pathways (see Chapter 14). With each episode of hyperammonemia, the patient may suffer brain damage or die in a matter of only a few hours.

Girls (or boys with partial OTC deficiency) are usually asymptomatic in the neonatal period but may develop hyperammonemia during intercurrent febrile illnesses, such as influenza, or with excessive dietary protein intake. Other catabolic stresses, such as surgery, pregnancy, long bone fracture, or the use of steroids, may also precipitate hyperammonemia. As with affected males, symptomatic females are at risk for brain damage and intellectual disability, but these serious complications can usually be anticipated and prevented by instituting aggressive interventions to prevent catabolism.

OTC deficiency and carbamoyl phosphate synthetase deficiency (see Fig. C.36.1) cannot be detected reliably by newborn screening. Citrulline is routinely included in newborn screening by tandem mass spectrometry of serum amino acids. A high citrulline is suggestive of citrullinemia, argininosuccinase deficiency, or citrin deficiency. It is more difficult to detect a low citrulline level, since the lower limit of normal is 7 μM. As the most common of the urea cycle defects, OTC deficiency should be considered in any hyperammonemic newborn.

MANAGEMENT

Plasma NH_3 concentration should be measured in any sick neonate. For most urea cycle defects, the pattern of abnormalities on quantitative amino acid determination is diagnostic.

Measurement of urine orotic acid will distinguish between OTC deficiency (in which it is elevated) and carbamoyl phosphate synthetase deficiency – both of which are characterized by very low or absent citrulline. Determination of urine organic acids is also important to rule out an organic aciduria, which can also present with hyperammonemia in the newborn period. Gene panel sequencing is available to confirm the diagnosis.

Acutely hyperammonemic urea cycle patients should be treated with a four-pronged approach: (1) 10% dextrose at twice the maintenance rate to provide calories in the form of sugar for gluconeogenesis and thereby reduce catabolism of endogenous proteins, and elimination of dietary protein intake; (2) intravenous Ammonul®, which is a solution of sodium benzoate and sodium phenylacetate, both of which provide diversion therapy by driving the excretion of nitrogen independently of the urea cycle (see Chapter 14); (3) intravenous arginine hydrochloride to provide adequate amounts of arginine, an essential amino acid for these patients, and to drive any residual enzyme activity by ensuring adequate substrate to the urea cycle; and (4) if a patient does not respond to the initial bolus of these medications, hemodialysis.

Chronic management entails careful control of dietary calories and protein as well as oral phenylbutyrate. Maintenance of a high carbohydrate intake spares endogenous protein from being catabolized for gluconeogenesis; dietary protein restriction reduces the load of NH_3 requiring detoxification through the urea cycle. Phenylbutyrate is readily converted to phenylacetate, which permits non–urea-cycle-dependent nitrogen excretion.

The family must be carefully trained to look for early signs of hyperammonemia, such as irritability, vomiting, and sleepiness, so that the patient can be promptly taken to the hospital for intravenous treatment.

There is great difficulty in achieving metabolic control and substantial risk for brain damage or death within hours of the onset of metabolic decompensation. Once a patient has grown sufficiently (>10 kg) to tolerate the procedure, liver transplantation should be presented as an option, to provide a functioning urea cycle. Gene therapy clinical trials are currently underway, using either an adeno-associated virus vector or lipid nanoparticles to deliver mRNA.

INHERITANCE

OTC deficiency is inherited as an X-linked trait. Because OTC deficiency is nearly always a genetic lethal disorder, approximately 67% of the mothers of affected infants would be expected to be carriers, as discussed in Chapters 7 and 17. In fact, 90% of the mothers of affected infants are carriers. The reason for this discrepancy is the incorrect underlying assumption of equal male and female mutation rates used for the theoretical calculation, as mutations in the *OTC* gene are much more frequent (~50-fold) in the male germline than in the female germline. Most mothers of an isolated boy with OTC deficiency are carriers, resulting from a new mutation inherited on their paternal X chromosome.

From a woman who is a carrier of an OTC deficiency allele, her sons who receive the pathogenic allele will be affected with OTC deficiency; her daughters will be carriers who may or may not be symptomatic, depending on random X inactivation in the liver. Males with partial OTC deficiency who reproduce will have all carrier daughters and no affected sons. When the variant in the family is known, prenatal or preimplantation genetic testing by sequencing is available. Prenatal diagnosis using an assay of the OTC enzyme is not practical because the enzyme is not expressed in chorionic villi or amniotic fluid cells.

QUESTIONS FOR SMALL GROUP DISCUSSION

1. Discuss Lyon's Law and explain the variability of disease manifestations in females.
2. Why is arginine an essential amino acid in this disorder? Arginine is ordinarily not an essential amino acid in humans.
3. What organic acidurias cause hyperammonemia?
4. What are some reasons for and against performing a liver transplant for OTC deficiency? Is this procedure more helpful here than for other inborn errors of metabolism, or less so?

REFERENCE

Uta L-K, Ljubica C, Hiroki M, Kara S, Nicholas AM, Erin M: Ornithine transcarbamylase deficiency. http://www.ncbi.nlm.nih.gov/books/NBK154378/.

POLYCYSTIC KIDNEY DISEASE (MIM 173900 and MIM 613095) (*PKD1* or *PKD2* Pathogenic Variants)

Autosomal Dominant

Terry J. Watnick • Ashima Gulati

PRINCIPLES

- Variable expressivity
- Genetic and allelic heterogeneity
- Highly penetrant
- Two-hit hypothesis

MAJOR PHENOTYPIC FINDINGS

- Age at onset: childhood through adulthood
- Progressive chronic kidney disease
- Kidney cysts
- Extrarenal cysts most commonly hepatic
- Intracranial saccular aneurysms
- Other less common associations: mitral valve prolapse, colonic diverticula

CASE EXAMPLE

P.J., a 35-year-old man with a 4-month history of intermittent right-sided flank pain, presented to his local emergency department with severe pain and hematuria. A renal ultrasound scan showed right-sided nephrolithiasis with pelvicalyceal dilatation and numerous scattered cysts in large-sized kidneys bilaterally, consistent with polycystic kidney disease. The findings from his physical examination were normal except for mild hypertension and a systolic murmur consistent with a history of mitral valve prolapse. Labs demonstrated normal electrolytes and an estimated glomerular filtration rate of 96 mL/min/1.73 m² (CKD-EPI Creatinine Equation 2021). Urine dipstick and microscopic analysis showed 2+ proteinuria and 7 RBC/hpf (red blood cells per high-powered field). P.J.'s father had received a kidney transplant at age 58 for end-stage kidney disease due to polycystic kidney disease. P.J.'s paternal grandmother was reported to have kidney disease, but she died of a ruptured intracranial aneurysm at 42 years. P.J.'s son, B.J., was born prematurely at 26 weeks gestation due to complications of maternal oligohydramnios; prenatal ultrasound showed large diffusely echogenic fetal kidneys. He died in the immediate postnatal period and an autopsy showed bilateral glomerulocystic kidney disease. At the time of B.J.'s death, the physicians had suggested that P.J. and his wife, W.J., be evaluated to see whether either of them had polycystic kidney disease; however, they elected not to pursue this evaluation because of guilt and grief about their son's death. P.J. was admitted for pain control and management of his obstructive nephrolithiasis. During this admission, the nephrologists told P.J. that he had autosomal dominant polycystic kidney disease. P.J. and W.J. then requested a genetics evaluation in preparation for a future pregnancy; testing involved a next-generation targeted sequencing panel, including the genes most implicated in polycystic kidney disease. Results for P.J. showed that he was heterozygous for a pathogenic truncating allele in *PKD1*, which was consistent with his clinical diagnosis and family history. W.J. was found to be heterozygous for a hypomorphic variant allele in the same gene, providing a plausible explanation for their late son's severe phenotype. With this information, prenatal testing could be considered.

BACKGROUND

Disease Incidence and Etiology

Autosomal dominant polycystic kidney disease (ADPKD) is the most common inherited form of kidney failure, with an incidence of 1 in 400 to 1 in 1000 live births. ADPKD constitutes 5% of US cases of end-stage kidney disease, with about

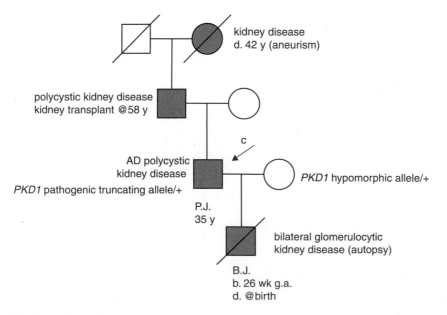

polycystic kidney disease
kidney transplant @58 y

AD polycystic
kidney disease

PKD1 pathogenic truncating allele/+

P.J.
35 y

c

PKD1 hypomorphic allele/+

kidney disease
d. 42 y (aneurism)

bilateral glomerulocytic
kidney disease (autopsy)

B.J.
b. 26 wk g.a.
d. @birth

12 million affected individuals worldwide. ADPKD is caused by pathogenic variants in either of two genes – *PKD1* (MIM 601313, #173900) and *PKD2* (MIM 173910, #613095) – occurring in ~77% and ~15% of cases, respectively. About 8% of cases in genetically investigated ADPKD cohorts remain unresolved as "no variant detected" in either *PKD1* or *PKD2*. These cases may be due to the technical challenges of *PKD1* sequencing because it is GC rich and has at least six nearly identical pseudogenes (with high sequence homology to *PKD1* exons 1–32) also on chromosome 16.

In addition, variants in newly discovered genes may present similarly, with bilateral polycystic kidneys but with a variable kidney disease course. These genes include *GANAB*, *DNAJB11*, *ALG9*, and *HNF1B*. Though there may be a phenotypic overlap with the polycystic kidney presentation, a thorough clinical and radiological assessment is often able to distinguish classical APDKD due to *PKD1* or *PKD2* from these phenocopy genes.

Genotype-phenotype correlations have been studied in large prospective ADPKD cohorts; *PKD1*-related kidney disease is more severe than that of *PKD2* (genic influence). Individuals with a *PKD1* variant develop end-stage kidney disease at an average age of 54 years, compared with 74 years for *PKD2*. Among individuals with altered *PKD1* alleles, those with truncating variants tend to have more severe disease than those with missense alterations (allelic influence). No single pathogenic variant in *PKD1* or *PKD2* accounts for >2% of families in a large database (http://pkdb.pkdcure.org).

Pathogenesis

PKD1 encodes polycystin 1, a transmembrane receptor-like protein of unknown function. *PKD2* encodes polycystin 2, an integral membrane protein with homology to the transient receptor potential (TRP) family of ion channels. Polycystins 1 and 2 interact as part of a heteromultimeric complex in the primary cilium, endoplasmic reticulum, exosomes, and the plasma membrane. Numerous cellular signaling pathways are dysregulated in ADPKD kidneys, with metabolic reprogramming emerging as a key consequence of polycystin loss. One hypothesis is that the polycystin complex in the primary cilium restrains a proproliferative pathway and that inhibition is released upon loss of polycystin signaling or in the absence of cilia. How this relates to a potential role for the polycystins as a receptor-activated calcium channel complex is hotly debated. Identifying the upstream and downstream cellular signaling pathways that are modulated by polycystins continues to be intensively investigated.

Cyst formation in ADPKD appears to follow a "two-hit" mechanism, similar to that observed with tumor suppressor genes and neoplasia (see Chapter 16). Despite heterozygous inheritance of the pathogenic allele, somatic hits in the alternate allele result in clonal expansion of a renal tubular epithelial cell with consequent cystic transformation of kidney tubules. Each renal epithelial cell thus contains a unique combination of germ line and somatic variants, resulting in reduced polycystin signaling.

PHENOTYPE AND NATURAL HISTORY

ADPKD may manifest at any age, but symptoms or signs most frequently appear in the third or fourth decade. Patients can present with urinary tract infections, hematuria, urinary tract obstruction (clots or nephrolithiasis), nocturia, hemorrhage into a renal cyst, or complaints of flank pain from the mass effect of enlarged kidneys (Fig. C.37.1). Now, with the frequent use of imaging, cysts may be detected incidentally. Hypertension affects 20 to 30% of children and nearly 75% of adults with ADPKD and is thought to be a secondary effect of

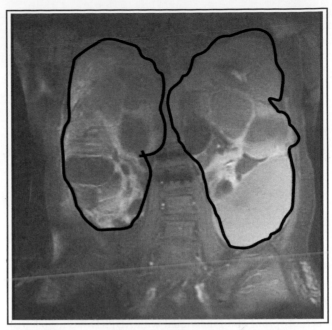

Figure C.37.1 MRI from an individual with autosomal dominant polycystic kidney disease showing bilaterally enlarged cystic kidneys (*outlined in black*) extending into the pelvis.

intrarenal ischemia and activation of the renin-angiotensin system. Nearly half of patients develop end-stage kidney disease by age 60. Hypertension, recurrent urinary tract infections, male sex, and early age of clinical onset are most predictive of early renal failure.

ADPKD exhibits both inter- and intrafamilial variability for age at onset and severity. Part of the interfamilial variation is secondary to locus heterogeneity, as ADPKD2 is a milder disease than ADPKD1. Intrafamilial variation is more marked between generations than among siblings, suggesting an interaction of environment and genetic background. The rate of somatic mutation may vary among family members, with impact on disease severity.

ADPKD is a systemic disease. In addition to renal cysts, individuals may develop hepatic (the most common extrarenal manifestation), pancreatic, splenic, and seminal vesicle and epididymal cysts. There is increased propensity to develop an intracranial aneurysm and this risk shows familial clustering. Colonic diverticula and cardiac valvular abnormalities are less commonly associated, and there is increased risk for aortic and tricuspid valve insufficiency, and mitral valve prolapse.

MANAGEMENT

In general, ADPKD is diagnosed by family history and renal ultrasound examination. By age 20 years, 80 to 90% of individuals have detectable cysts; nearly 100% have them by 30 years. However, these ultrasound-based imaging estimates are mostly validated for *PKD1* disease and are less reliable with *PKD2*-associated milder phenotype. If necessary for prenatal diagnosis or identification of a related kidney donor, the diagnosis can be confirmed by gene sequencing in most families.

The management and treatment of patients with ADPKD focuses on slowing the progression of renal disease and minimizing its symptoms. Hypertension and urinary tract infections are treated aggressively to preserve renal function. Pain from the mass effect of the enlarged kidneys can sometimes be managed by drainage and sclerosis of the cysts.

Individuals with larger kidneys are at risk for more rapid decline in renal function; total kidney volume (most accurately measured by magnetic resonance imaging [MRI]) is a useful predictive marker of kidney disease progression. Tolvaptan, a vasopressin V_2-receptor antagonist, is FDA approved in the United States for use in selected patients ≥18 years at risk for rapid ADPKD progression.

INDICATIONS FOR ADPKD MOLECULAR TESTING

There is currently no clinical utility in distinguishing *PKD1* from *PKD2* disease; however, molecular genetic confirmation may be considered for:

1. atypical clinical presentations, especially in the absence of a family history
2. preconception and prenatal genetic counseling
3. assessing treatment candidacy with specific therapies or clinical trials
4. screening for a living related kidney donor

INHERITANCE

Each offspring of an individual with ADPKD has a 50% risk of being affected. Sporadic cases and patients with no family history constitute a substantial proportion: up to 10 to 15%. These can be due to *de novo* gene variants or rare cases of parental germline mosaicism. Someone with a *de novo* variant can be a mosaic of normal and variant cells, and the contribution of variant cells correlates with disease severity. Such somatic mosaicism accounts for ~1% of those with ADPKD.

About 2% of individuals with ADPKD present with a severe perinatal to early childhood form.

For parents of a child with disease onset *in utero*, the risk that a subsequent child will be severely affected is approximately 25%.

Biallelic inheritance of partially functional *PKD1* pathogenic alleles can result in very-early-onset ADPKD, providing one explanation for severe perinatal disease. Such disease usually manifests in homozygotes or compound heterozygotes as large kidneys with multiple small cysts, or as diffusely echogenic kidneys, mimicking the autosomal recessive form of polycystic kidney disease. Histopathology of this very-early-onset ADPKD is often consistent with glomerulocystic kidney disease. Digenic inheritance – the combination of heterozygous variants in two genes, such as *PKD 1* or *2* and *HNF1B* or *PKHD1* (the gene causing an autosomal recessive form of polycystic kidney disease) – may also lead to very-early-onset disease. In general, however, variable expressivity precludes prediction of the severity of disease. For families in whom the pathogenic variant is known, preimplantation or prenatal genetic diagnosis is available.

QUESTIONS FOR SMALL GROUP DISCUSSION

1. Compare the molecular mechanism of cyst development in ADPKD with the development of neurofibromas in neurofibromatosis type 1.
2. Many mendelian diseases have variable expressivity that might be accounted for by modifier loci. How would one identify such loci?
3. Why is ADPKD occasionally associated with tuberous sclerosis? How might this illustrate a contiguous gene deletion syndrome?
4. How can ADPKD be distinguished from autosomal recessive polycystic kidney disease?
5. What factors underlie the genetic complexity of variant detection in *PKD1*? What is the most suitable methodology for molecular genetic testing in ADPKD?

REFERENCES

Harris PC, Torres VE: Polycystic kidney disease, autosomal dominant, *Gene Reviews®*. https://www.ncbi.nlm.nih.gov/books/NBK1246/.

Inker LA, Eneanya ND, Coresh J, *et al.*, Chronic Kidney Disease Epidemiology Collaboration, *New England Journal of Medicine* 385 (19):1737–1749, 2021.

Lanktree MB, Haghighi A, di Bari I, Song X, Pei Y: Insights into autosomal dominant polycystic kidney disease from genetic studies, *Clin J Am Soc Nephrol* 16(5):790–799, 2021. https://doi.org/10.2215/CJN.02320220. Epub 2020 Jul 20. PMID: 32690722; PMCID: PMC8259493.

Ma M, Gallagher AR, Somlo S: Ciliary mechanisms of cyst formation in polycystic kidney disease, *Cold Spring Harb Perspect Biol* 9(11):a028209, 2017. https://doi.org/10.1101/cshperspect.a028209. PMID: 28320755; Free PMC article.

Podrini C, Cassina L, Boletta A: Metabolic reprogramming and the role of mitochondria in polycystic kidney disease, *Cell Signal* 67:109495, 2020. https://doi.org/10.1016/j.cellsig.2019.109495. Epub 2019 Dec 6. PMID: 31816397.

Torres VE, Harris PC: Progress in the understanding of polycystic kidney disease, *Nat Rev Nephrol* 15(2):70–72, 2019. https://doi.org/10.1038/s41581-018-0108-1. PMID: 30607031; PMCID: PMC6543819.

PRADER-WILLI SYNDROME (MIM 176270)
(Absence of Paternally Derived 15q11-q13)
Chromosomal Deletion, Uniparental Disomy

Jill A. Fahrner

PRINCIPLES

- Imprinting
- Uniparental disomy (UPD)
- Microdeletion
- Recombination between repeated DNA sequences

MAJOR PHENOTYPIC FINDINGS

- Age at onset: infancy
- Hypotonia
- Infantile feeding difficulties
- Hyperphagia
- Obesity
- Cognitive impairment
- Behavioral differences
- Short stature
- Dysmorphism

HISTORY AND PHYSICAL FINDINGS

C.V. was born at 37 weeks gestation by cesarian section due to breech presentation. Shortly after birth, he was noted to be hypotonic and feeding poorly. His three older siblings and nonconsanguineous parents were in good health; there was no family history of neuromuscular, developmental, genetic, or feeding disorders. Review of the medical record did not reveal a history of overt seizures, hypoxic insults, infection, cardiac abnormalities, or blood glucose or electrolyte abnormalities. On examination, C.V. was severely hypotonic with lethargy, weak cry, decreased reflexes, and a poor suck, and he had scrotal hypoplasia and cryptorchidism. Subsequent evaluation included high-resolution SNP microarray testing, which revealed long continuous stretches of apparent homozygosity on the long arm of chromosome 15, suggestive of uniparental isodisomy (UPD) for chromosome 15. Subsequent methylation testing of the Prader-Willi/Angelman region on 15q11-q13 (see Chapter 6) revealed methylation of the Prader-Willi syndrome (PWS) imprinting control region just upstream of *SNRPN* on

both copies of chromosome 15. This represents an abnormal methylation pattern and is consistent with a diagnosis of PWS. Chromosome analysis revealed a 46,XY karyotype. The geneticist explained to the parents that their son had Prader-Willi syndrome. He continued to be followed in the Epigenetics and Chromatin Clinic. At age 1 year, he was noted to have dysmorphisms, including a narrow bitemporal diameter, almond-shaped eyes, a thin upper lip, downturned corners of the mouth, and small hands and feet. He had developed growth failure resulting in short stature; his height was beyond 2 standard deviations (SDs) below the mean for age. Growth hormone therapy was subsequently initiated, and at 3.5 years, his height had normalized to average for this age. However, he had developed obesity: his weight and body mass index (BMI) of 26 were 3.5 and 5 SDs above the mean for age, respectively.

BACKGROUND

Disease Etiology and Incidence

Prader-Willi syndrome (MIM 176270) has an incidence of 1 in 10,000 to 15,000 live births. It is a neurodevelopmental disorder caused by loss of expression of genes on paternally derived chromosome 15q11-q13. Such loss can arise by several mechanisms; recent data suggest that approximately 60% of patients have a deletion of 15q11-q13, 36% have maternal uniparental disomy, 3 to 4% have imprinting defects, and less than 1% have another chromosomal abnormality involving this region (see Chapter 6).

Pathogenesis

PWS is an imprinting disorder. Whereas most genes are expressed equally from both alleles, imprinting refers to the phenomenon of differential expression of a gene depending on the parent of origin (see Chapters 3, 6 and 8). Many genes within 15q11-q13 are imprinted. Some imprinted genes are expressed exclusively by the paternal allele, and others are expressed exclusively by the maternal allele (Fig. C.38.1). Imprints, and thus correct expression of imprinted genes, are maintained in somatic lineage cells throughout the life of the organism. However, during gametogenesis, erasure and reestablishment of the imprint is required so that egg cells acquire maternal imprints and sperm cells acquire paternal imprints. Attainment of proper imprints in the germline is regulated by an imprinting control region (ICR). At the molecular level, imprints consist of DNA methylation and other chromatin marks that regulate gene expression.

Deletion of 15q11-q13 on the paternal chromosome gives rise to PWS because individuals formed from sperm carrying the deletion will be missing genes that are active only when paternally derived. The mechanism underlying recurrent deletions is aberrant recombination between low-copy repeat sequences flanking the deletion interval (see Chapter 6). Most of these large interstitial deletions have one of two common proximal breakpoints (BP1 or BP2) and a common distal breakpoint (BP3). Type 1 deletions are larger (~5.7 Mb) and extend from BP1 to BP3; type 2 deletions are smaller (~4.8 Mb) and extend from BP2 to BP3. Some affected individuals have atypical deletions.

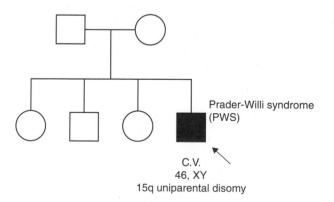

Prader-Willi syndrome
(PWS)

C.V.
46, XY
15q uniparental disomy

Pedigree Case 38

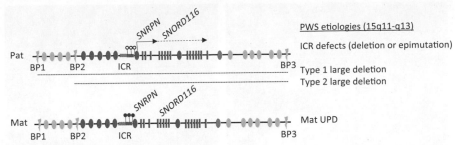

Figure C.38.1 Genomic structure of 15q11-q13 and etiologies of PWS. Imprinted genes are regulated by DNA methylation of the imprinting control region (ICR). The PWS ICR (blue) is normally unmethylated (unfilled lollipops) on the paternal allele (pat), allowing for exclusive expression of blue imprinted genes (ovals, protein-coding genes; vertical bars, small nucleolar RNAs), including SNRPN and SNORD116. The PWS ICR (blue) is normally methylated (filled red lollipops) on the maternal allele (mat), silencing blue imprinted genes. The pink Angelman syndrome ICR is oppositely imprinted in brain, leading to exclusive expression of UBE3A (pink oval) from the mat. Green genes are nonimprinted and biallelically expressed. BP, breakpoint.

Maternal uniparental disomy gives rise to PWS because the individual has two maternal chromosomes 15 and no paternal chromosome 15. Imprinted genes that are only expressed from a paternal copy cannot be expressed. Maternal uniparental disomy is thought to develop secondary to trisomy rescue, that is, loss of the paternal chromosome 15 from a conceptus with chromosome 15 trisomy that had resulted from maternal nondisjunction.

ICR defects can also give rise to PWS: individuals with only maternally imprinted 15q11-q13 do not express genes active only on a paternally imprinted 15q11-q13. ICR defects arise from DNA methylation abnormalities called *epimutations* or from microdeletions limited to the PWS-ICR (distinct from the larger type 1 and 2 deletions mentioned above).

Rarely, an individual has a chromosomal rearrangement (e.g., a translocation or inversion) spanning this region and giving rise to PWS, sometimes inherited from a parent with a balanced rearrangement.

Despite the fact that loss of a paternally imprinted 15q11-q13 gives rise to PWS, and despite the identification of many imprinted genes within this region, the precise cause of PWS is still unknown. Genomic imprinting in the region is controlled by the PWS-ICR, which has a CpG island that is unmethylated on the paternal allele and methylated on the maternal allele. This results in genes under its control being expressed from the paternal allele and silenced on the maternal allele. The PWS-ICR overlaps with and regulates *SNRPN*, among other genes. Also called *SNURF-SNRPN*, the gene encodes two proteins and hosts multiple noncoding small nucleolar RNA (snoRNA) genes – including the *SNORD116* cluster – and regulates their expression. The full PWS phenotype may be due to loss of multiple genes within the region, but all known cases of PWS are thought to lack expression of paternally derived *SNORD116*.

PHENOTYPE AND NATURAL HISTORY

In early infancy, PWS is characterized by severe hypotonia, feeding difficulties, and hypogonadism with cryptorchidism in males. The hypotonia improves over time, although adults remain mildly hypotonic. The hypogonadism, which is mostly of hypothalamic origin, does not improve with age and usually causes delayed and incomplete pubertal development as well as infertility. Central hypothyroidism and central adrenal insufficiency have been documented. Feeding difficulties usually resolve by 9 months, and subsequently there is a period of improved feeding and typical growth. However, between 2 and 4.5 years of age, weight increases in the absence of increased appetite or food intake. Between 4.5 and 8 years, appetite and caloric intake increase, though affected individuals can feel full. Subsequently, these individuals develop extreme hyperphagia and lack of satiety. Accompanying food-seeking behaviors (hoarding, foraging, stealing, and eating nonfood items) often require that food be locked up. This behavior and a low metabolic rate cause marked obesity – a major cause of morbidity due largely to cardiopulmonary disease and type 2 diabetes mellitus.

Most children with PWS have delayed motor and language development as well as mild intellectual disability (mean IQ, 60–80). They also have behavioral problems, including temper tantrums, stubbornness, manipulative behavior, poor adaptation to changes in routine, and obsessive-compulsive disorders, such as skin picking. These behaviors continue into adulthood and remain disabling. Affected individuals often experience sleep disturbance and may develop psychosis during adolescence or early adulthood.

Other anomalies associated with PWS include short stature, scoliosis, strabismus, osteoporosis, and dysmorphism. Dysmorphic features include a narrow bifrontal diameter, almond-shaped eyes, small mouth with down-turned corners, and small hands and feet (Fig. C.38.2). A subset of patients has hypopigmentation of the hair, eyes, and skin.

Longevity can be nearly normal if obesity is avoided. Causes of death in children are mostly respiratory and other febrile illnesses. Obesity-related cardiovascular problems and complications from diabetes, sleep apnea, and gastrointestinal problems are more common in adults. While there are concerns regarding increased rates of unexpected death among individuals with PWS on growth hormone therapy, the general consensus is that the benefits of growth hormone therapy outweigh the risks (see below).

MANAGEMENT

Although often suspected from history and physical features, a diagnosis of PWS is defined genetically by the absence of a paternally imprinted 15q11-q13. Absence of the paternal imprint is detected by DNA methylation analysis showing that the 5' end of *SNRPN* has only a maternal methylation pattern (Fig. C.38.3). If the DNA methylation analysis confirms PWS, the molecular etiology should be sought, so as to aid in genetic counseling for recurrence risk. A high-resolution SNP microarray can identify a deletion or maternal uniparental isodisomy. Alternatively, FISH analysis for 15q11-q13 can be used to look for a deletion. In addition, chromosome analysis should be done to determine the presence of a translocation or inversion. Only uniparental isodisomy would be detected on SNP microarray, and neither form of UPD would be detected

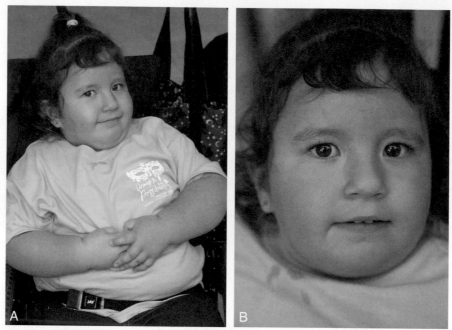

Figure C.38.2 (A), (B) Ley Lanie has Prader-Willi syndrome (Prader-Willi Syndrome Association USA [pwsausa.org]). Photograph by Rick Guidotti, Positive Exposure (www.positiveexposure.org).

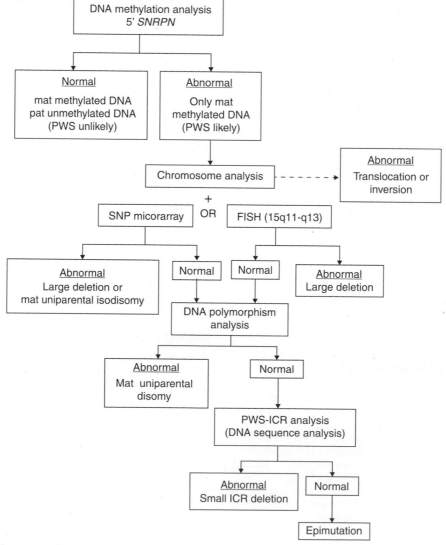

Figure C.38.3 Molecular testing algorithm for Prader-Willi syndrome. See text for details. FISH, fluorescence *in situ* hybridization; ICR, imprinting control region; mat, maternal; pat, paternal.

with chromosome analysis and FISH without SNP array. Thus if normal, DNA polymorphism analysis should follow. Finally, when other molecular tests are negative, DNA sequence analysis of the ICR is warranted, to seek microdeletions causing an imprinting defect. If no microdeletion is identified, an epimutation should be suspected.

No pharmacological therapies are currently available to treat the underlying cause of PWS. Developmental services, including physical, occupational, and speech therapies, should be started early. Specialized educational settings are also important to maximize developmental and cognitive potential. A very low-calorie and restrictive diet and exercise are the mainstays for controlling obesity. Growth hormone replacement can normalize height, improve lean body mass, and improve cognitive functioning. Behavioral management is most effective with strict limit setting and serotonin reuptake inhibitors. Adults usually perform best in sheltered living and employment environments. Group homes specifically for individuals with PWS in which access to food is tightly controlled and exercise programs are in place are optimal. An ongoing multidisciplinary approach for evaluation and management of the above manifestations is recommended.

INHERITANCE

The recurrence risk for PWS is related to the molecular cause. For *de novo* deletions, maternal uniparental disomy, and epimutations, the recurrence risk is less than 1%. For ICR deletions, the risk can be as high as 50% if paternally inherited. The risk for recurrence may also be increased if the proband has a predisposing unbalanced chromosome rearrangement. This is often due to a balanced parental chromosome rearrangement; thus, parental chromosome analyses should be considered.

QUESTIONS FOR SMALL GROUP DISCUSSION

1. Angelman syndrome also arises from imprinting defects of 15q11-q13. Compare and contrast the phenotypes and causative molecular mechanisms of Prader-Willi syndrome and Angelman syndrome.
2. How might imprinting explain the phenotypes associated with triploidy?
3. Beckwith-Wiedemann syndrome and Russell-Silver syndrome also appear to be caused by abnormal expression of imprinted genes. Explain.

REFERENCES

Butler MG, Hartin SN, Hossain WA, *et al*: Molecular genetic classification in Prader-Willi syndrome: A multisite cohort study, *J Med Genet* 2019;56:149–153.

Driscoll DJ, Miller JL, Schwartz S, *et al*: Prader-Willi syndrome, *GeneReviews®*. http://www.ncbi.nlm.nih.gov/books/NBK1330/.

Mendiola AJP, LaSalle JM: Epigenetics in Prader-Willi syndrome, *Front in Genet*, 2021;12:624581. https://doi.org/10.3389/fgene.2021.624581

Autosomal Dominant or Sporadic

Janet A. Buchanan • Ashwin Mallipatna

PRINCIPLES

- Tumor suppressor gene
- Two-hit hypothesis
- Somatic mutation
- Tumor predisposition
- Cell-cycle regulation
- Variable expressivity

MAJOR PHENOTYPIC FINDINGS

- Age at onset: childhood
- Leukocoria
- Strabismus
- Visual deterioration
- Conjunctival congestion or chemosis

HISTORY AND PHYSICAL FINDINGS

J.V., a 1-year-old girl, was referred by her pediatrician for evaluation of right strabismus and leukocoria: a reflection from a white mass within the eye giving the appearance of a white pupil (see Fig. 16.7). Her mother reported that she had developed progressive right esotropia in the month before seeing her pediatrician. There was no evidence of pain, swelling, or redness in her right eye. She was otherwise healthy, as were her parents and a 4-year-old sister (R.V.); no other family members had had ocular disease. Findings from her physical examination were otherwise normal. Her ophthalmological examination defined a solitary retinal tumor of 8 disc diameters arising near the macula of her right eye. Her left eye was found to be unaffected during examination in the eye clinic. A magnetic resonance imaging of the head and orbits did not show extension of the tumor outside the globe nor within the optic nerve. There was also no independent midline tumor of the brain ("trilateral" retinoblastoma) noted, especially looking around the pineal region. An exam under anesthesia confirmed the diagnosis and allowed for staging of the cancer, in addition to confirming that the left eye was indeed unaffected. She received intraarterial chemotherapy followed by multiple sessions of laser photocoagulation to retain the affected eye and preserve vision. DNA analysis of her blood, by gene sequencing, showed that she had a germline nonsense variant (C to T transition) in one allele of

her retinoblastoma (*RB1*) gene on chromosome 13q14, which was not found in the germline of either parent. They were advised that J.V.'s germline variant put her at high risk for additional retinal tumors in both eyes and that frequent monitoring under general anesthesia would be required for early detection and intervention. She would be at risk throughout her life for sarcomas and other cancers. Due to the small risk of undetected mosaicism for the apparently *de novo* variant in one or the other parent, blood DNA from R.V. was also tested and the *RB* variant was ruled out.

BACKGROUND

Disease Etiology and Incidence

Retinoblastoma (MIM 180200) is a rare embryonic neoplasm of retinal origin (Fig. C.39.1) that results from pathogenic germline and/or somatic variants in both alleles of the *RB1* gene. It occurs worldwide with an incidence of 1 in 18,000 to 1 in 30,000.

Pathogenesis

The retinoblastoma protein (pRb or RB or RB1) is a tumor suppressor that plays an important role in regulating the progression of proliferating cells through the cell cycle and the exit of differentiating cells from the cell cycle. This protein affects these two functions by sequestration of other transcription factors and by promoting deacetylation of histones, a chromatin modification associated with gene silencing.

Retinoblastoma-associated *RB1* variants occur throughout the coding region and promoter of the gene. Those within the coding region either destabilize pRb or compromise its association with enzymes necessary for histone deacetylation. Variants within the promoter reduce expression of otherwise normal pRb. Both types of genetic variants result in a loss of functional pRb.

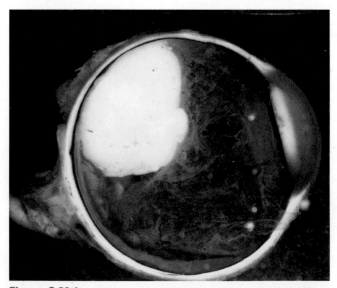

Figure C.39.1 Midline cross-section of an enucleated eye from a patient with retinoblastoma. Note the large primary tumor in the posterior third of the globe and a few white vitreous seeds. (The brown discoloration of the vitreous is a fixation artifact.) (Courtesy R. A. Lewis, Baylor College of Medicine, Houston.)

Key:
E: *RB1* sequence analysis (blood)

E - ☐——○ E -

retinoblastoma

E - ○   ● R.V.   J.V.
4 y   1 y

E+ : *RB1* pathogenic variant / +

Pedigree Case 39

An *RB1* germline pathogenic variant is found in close to 50% of all children with retinoblastoma (including all those with bilateral retinoblastoma and about 20% of those with unilateral disease), but less than 10% of all children have a positive family history. *RB1* variants include genomic structural abnormalities of chromosome 13q14, single-base substitutions, and small insertions or deletions. Evidence suggests that most new germline variants arise on the paternal allele, whereas somatic variants arise with equal frequency on the maternal and paternal alleles. Nearly half occur at CpG dinucleotides. After either the inheritance of a pathogenic allele or a first somatic mutation event on one allele, the other *RB1* allele must also lose function (the second "hit" of the two-hit hypothesis; see Chapter 16) for a cell to proliferate unchecked and develop into a retinoblastoma. Loss of a functional second allele occurs by a novel mutation event, loss of heterozygosity, or promoter CpG island hypermethylation. Deletion or the development of isodisomy occurs most frequently, and promoter hypermethylation occurs least frequently.

Heritable retinoblastoma usually segregates as an autosomal dominant disorder with full penetrance, although a few families have been described with reduced penetrance. The *RB1* variants identified in these latter families include missense variants, in-frame deletions, and promoter variants. In contrast to the more common null *RB1* alleles, these are believed to represent alleles with some residual function.

PHENOTYPE AND NATURAL HISTORY

Approximately 60% of affected children have unilateral retinoblastoma and 40% bilateral retinoblastoma. Children with bilateral retinoblastoma generally present during the first year of life, whereas those with unilateral disease present somewhat later, with a peak between 24 and 30 months. All children with bilateral disease have germline *RB1* variants, but not all children with germline variants develop bilateral disease. The disease is diagnosed before 5 years of age in 80 to 95% of affected children. Retinoblastoma is fatal if untreated, but with appropriate therapy, more than 80 to 90% of children are free of disease 5 years after diagnosis.

As expected with involvement of a key cell-cycle regulator, those with germline *RB1* variants have a markedly increased risk for secondary neoplasms. This risk is increased by environmental factors, such as treatment of the initial retinoblastoma with radiotherapy. The most common secondary neoplasms are osteosarcomas, soft tissue sarcomas, and melanomas. There is no increase in second malignant neoplasms in those with nonhereditary retinoblastoma.

MANAGEMENT

Early detection and treatment are essential for optimal outcome. The goals of therapy are to cure the disease and to preserve as much vision as possible. Treatment is tailored to the stage of tumor and involvement of adjacent tissues. Treatment options for intraocular retinoblastoma involve enucleation or eye salvage. Eye salvage of intraocular tumors commonly involves multiple sessions of chemotherapy delivered through various modalities, including direct infusion into the ophthalmic artery of the affected eye. This is followed by multiple examinations under anesthesia to identify and treat residual or recurrent tumor activity with laser photocoagulation and/or cryotherapy.

Children with unilateral disease at the time of the presentation are offered genetic tests to determine their germline risk. If available, tumor DNA from an enucleated eye is tested, making it more efficient to look for one of the two identified tumor variants in other tissues, such as in blood. If a germline variant can be ruled out, the patient does not require frequent follow-up. In those children who are found to carry a germline RB1 variant, frequent examinations are recommended to detect any new retinoblastomas in the unaffected eye, because 10% of apparently sporadic cases result from a new parental germline mutation. Such frequent examinations continue until at least 3 years of age under anesthesia, and to at least 7 years of age with retinal examinations at the ophthalmologist's office.

INHERITANCE

The *Cancer Staging Manual* (8th edition) from the American Joint Committee on Cancer (AJCC) includes a prognosticating stage "H" that defines heritable retinoblastoma, in view of the significant role of hereditability in its disease prognosis. A stage of "H0" is assigned to patients with unilateral retinoblastoma (or retinoma) with no germline *RB1* pathogenic variant identified on molecular genetic testing, or where the residual risk of mosaicism is <1%. A stage of "H1" is assigned to those with bilateral retinoblastoma, trilateral retinoblastoma, retinoblastoma with positive family history, or identification of a germline *RB1* pathogenic variant.

For all survivors of AJCC Stage H1 retinoblastoma, the empirical risk for their offspring to be affected is close to 50%; this risk reflects the high likelihood of a second, somatic mutation (or "hit") in the second *RB1* allele of a retinal cell in the offspring. On the other hand, if the parent had unilateral disease, the empirical risk for a child to be affected is 19%; this reflects the proportion of "first hit" events that are germline, rather than somatic, in children with unilateral disease. Nearly 90% of children who develop retinoblastoma are the first individuals affected within the family. Interestingly, 1% of unaffected parents of an affected child have evidence of a retinoma (the benign precursor of retinoblastoma) on retinal examination; for these families, therefore, the risk for a child to be affected is about 50%. Except for the rare situation in which one parent is a non-expressing carrier of an *RB1* pathogenic variant, families in which neither parent had retinoblastoma have a risk for recurrence equivalent to that of the general population.

A parent with H1 retinoblastoma who has a known germline RB1 variant may be offered prenatal testing to determine the risk of their unborn offspring having retinoblastoma. Determining this risk provides the opportunity for the pregnancy to be induced at 36 weeks gestation and immediately followed by screening to detect and treat small tumors. This improves this child's chance for avoiding chemotherapy and retaining maximum vision.

QUESTIONS FOR SMALL GROUP DISCUSSION

1. What other diseases develop as a result of a high frequency of variants in CpG dinucleotides? What is the mechanism of mutation at CpG dinucleotides? What could explain the increased frequency of CpG dinucleotide mutations with increasing paternal age?

2. Compare and contrast the type and frequency of tumors observed in Li-Fraumeni syndrome with those observed in retinoblastoma. Both Rb and p53 are tumor suppressors; why are *TP53* variants associated with a different phenotype than *RB1* variants?

3. Discuss four diseases that arise as a result of somatic mutations. Examples should illustrate chromosomal recombination, loss of heterozygosity, gene amplification, and accumulation of single nucleotide variants.

4. Both SRY (see Chapter 6) and Rb regulate development by modulating gene expression through the modification of chromatin structure. Compare and contrast the two different mechanisms that each uses to modify chromatin structure.

REFERENCES

Lohmann DR, Gallie BL: Retinoblastoma. http://www.ncbi.nlm.nih.gov/books/NBK1452/.

Mallipatna AC, Gallie BL, Chévez-Barrios P, Lumbroso-Le Rouic L, Chantada GL, Doz F, Brisse HJ, Munier FL, Albert DM, Català-Mora J, Finger P: *Retinoblastoma*. *AJCC cancer staging manual*, ed 8, New York, 2017, Springer, pp 819–831.

Villegas VM, Hess DJ, Wildner A, *et al*: Retinoblastoma, *Curr Opin Ophthalmol* 24:581–588, 2013.

X-Linked Dominant

John Christodoulou

PRINCIPLES

- Loss-of-function variant
- Variable expressivity
- Sex-dependent phenotype

MAJOR PHENOTYPIC FINDINGS

- Age at onset: neonatal to early childhood
- Acquired microcephaly
- Neurodevelopmental regression
- Repetitive stereotypic hand movements

HISTORY AND PHYSICAL FINDINGS

P.J. had normal growth and development until 12 months of age. At 24 months, she was referred to Neurology Clinic because of decelerating head growth and progressive loss of language and motor skills. She had lost purposeful hand movements and developed repetitive hand wringing by 30 months. She also had mild microcephaly, truncal ataxia, gait apraxia, and severely impaired expressive and receptive language. No other family members had any neurological diseases. On the basis of these findings, the neurologist suggested that P.J. might have Rett syndrome. The physician explained that Rett syndrome is a result of variants in the methyl-CpG–binding protein 2 gene (*MECP2*) in most individuals and that testing for such variants could help confirm the diagnosis. Subsequent gene-targeted testing of P.J.'s DNA identified a known pathogenic heterozygous *MECP2* variant: she carried the transition c.763C>T, which causes a truncation of the MeCP2 protein [p.(Arg255*)]. Neither parent carried the variant.

BACKGROUND

Disease Etiology and Prevalence

Rett syndrome (RTT; MIM 312750) is an X-linked dominant disorder with a female prevalence of 1 in 10,000 to 1 in 23,000. It is caused by loss-of-function variants in the *MECP2*

gene. With the advent of array comparative genomic hybridization (array CGH) technology, males with duplications on the X chromosome in the region of *MECP2* have been identified; these males typically have severe intellectual disability. Males with a pathogenic variant in *MECP2* and 47,XXY genotype can also have Rett syndrome with a phenotype similar to that of females. Two other genes – *CDKL5* and *FOXG1* – can lead to phenotypes that overlap with Rett syndrome but are now recognized as distinct clinical entities. CDKL5 is an X-linked serine/threonine kinase that regulates neuronal proliferation and differentiation. Pathogenic variants in this gene cause microcephaly, severe seizures (typically infantile-onset epileptic encephalopathy), and severe intellectual disability. FOXG1 is a transcription factor that plays a key role in the development of the anterior brain. Pathogenic variants in *FOXG1* cause an autosomal dominant disorder with similar features but also cause brain malformations, such as forebrain abnormalities, and defects in the corpus callosum.

Pathogenesis

MECP2 encodes a nuclear protein that binds methylated DNA and recruits histone deacetylases to regions of methylated DNA. The precise function of MeCP2 has not been fully defined, but it does mediate transcriptional silencing and epigenetic regulation of genes in these regions of methylated DNA. Accordingly, dysfunction or loss of MeCP2, as observed in Rett syndrome, would be predicted to cause inappropriate activation of target genes. MeCP2 may be a transcriptional activator and may play a role in long-range chromatin remodeling and in gene splicing.

The brains of individuals with Rett syndrome are small and have a normal gross morphology without neuronal loss. Rett syndrome is, therefore, not a typical neurodegenerative disease. Within much of the cortex and hippocampus, the neurons from RTT individuals are smaller and more densely packed than normal and have a simplified dendritic branching pattern. These observations suggest that MeCP2 is important for establishing and maintaining neuronal interactions, rather than for neuronal precursor proliferation or neuronal determination.

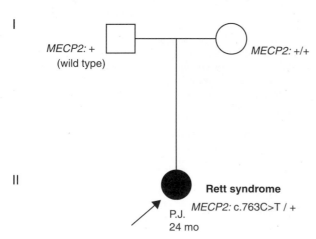

I

MECP2: +
(wild type)

MECP2: +/+

II

Rett syndrome

P.J.
24 mo

MECP2: c.763C>T / +

Pedigree Case 40

Figure C.40.1 Holly is exhibiting hand wringing, which is an easily recognizable clinical clue to the Rett syndrome diagnosis. (Photo courtesy of International Rett Syndrome Foundation.)

PHENOTYPE AND NATURAL HISTORY

Classic Rett syndrome is a progressive neurodevelopmental disorder occurring almost exclusively in girls (Fig. C.40.1). After apparently normal development until 6 to 18 months of age, individuals enter a short period of developmental slowing and stagnation with decelerating head growth. Subsequently, they rapidly lose speech and acquired motor skills, particularly purposeful hand use. During this time, social interaction is also lost, and affected individuals are often misdiagnosed as having autism. With continued disease progression, they develop stereotypic hand movements, breathing irregularities, ataxia, and seizures. After a brief period of apparent stabilization, usually during the preschool to early school years, they deteriorate further to become severely intellectually disabled and develop progressive spasticity, rigidity, and scoliosis. Individuals usually live into adulthood, but their life span is shortened due to an increased incidence of unexplained sudden death, which, in some cases, may be a consequence of having a prolonged QTc ECG abnormality.

Besides Rett syndrome, pathogenic *MECP2* variants may cause a broad spectrum of diseases affecting both boys and girls. Among girls, the range extends from severely affected individuals who never learn to speak, turn, sit, or walk and develop severe epilepsy, to mildly affected individuals who speak and have good gross motor function as well as relatively well-preserved hand function. Among boys, the range of phenotypes encompasses congenital encephalopathy, intellectual disability with various neurological symptoms, and mild intellectual disability only. It has been suggested that the lower prevalence of males with pathogenic *MECP2* variants may be due to increased intrauterine death, but this remains to be established.

MANAGEMENT

Suspected on the basis of clinical features, the diagnosis of Rett syndrome is usually confirmed by DNA testing (including single gene or gene panel testing or genomic sequencing with analysis as part of an intellectual disability panel); current testing detects pathogenic *MECP2* variants in up to 98% of individuals with classic/typical Rett syndrome and 86% of individuals with atypical/variant Rett syndrome. The clinical diagnostic criteria for typical Rett syndrome include normal prenatal and perinatal periods followed by a period of regression and four other main findings: partial or complete loss of acquired purposeful hand skills, partial or complete loss of acquired language skills, gait abnormalities, and stereotypic hand movements. A number of features may present (breathing disturbances when awake, bruxism when awake, sleep disturbances, abnormal muscle tone, peripheral vasomotor abnormalities, scoliosis or kyphosis, growth retardation, small cold hands and feet, inappropriate laughing/screaming spells, diminished response to pain and intense eye communication). These features are not necessary to establish a clinical diagnosis of typical Rett syndrome but may help in establishing a clinical diagnosis of atypical Rett syndrome.

Currently there are no curative treatments for Rett syndrome and management focuses on supportive and symptomatic therapy, including individually tailored physical and occupational therapy programs. Current medical therapy includes anticonvulsants for seizures, serotonin uptake inhibitors for agitation, carbidopa or levodopa for rigidity, and melatonin to ameliorate sleep disturbances. There are currently a number of clinical trials underway (see https://clinicaltrials.gov/ct2/results?cond=rett+syndrome&term=&cntry=&state=&city=&dist=), and preclinical gene therapy trials are also showing promise. Families often face major challenges with social adjustment and coping and should therefore be provided with the opportunity to interact with similarly affected families through support groups and be referred for professional counseling as needed.

INHERITANCE

Approximately 99% of Rett syndrome is sporadic. Most *MECP2* variants are *de novo*, although in rare cases they can be inherited from an unaffected or mildly affected mother with skewed X chromosome inactivation. At least 70% of *de novo* variants arise in the paternal germline.

If a couple has an affected child with a pathogenic *MECP2* variant but the *MECP2* variant is not identified in either parent, the risk to future siblings is low, although it is higher than among the general population because of the possibility of undetected germline mosaicism. In contrast, if the mother carries a disease-causing *MECP2* variant, each daughter and son has a 50% risk for inheriting the variant. However, poor genotype-phenotype correlations (with some exceptions) among individuals with *MECP2* variants generally prohibit prediction of whether a female fetus with a *MECP2* variant will develop classic Rett syndrome or another *MECP2*-associated disease. Similarly, identification of a *MECP2* variant in a male fetus does not predict intrauterine demise, the development of congenital encephalopathy, or another *MECP2*-associated disease.

QUESTIONS FOR SMALL GROUP DISCUSSION

1. *MECP2* is on the X chromosome. Discuss how this could affect the phenotypic variability observed among females with *MECP2* variants. Discuss how this might account for the fewer numbers of males with *MECP2* variants and the differences in disease severity observed generally between males and females.

2. Given that MeCP2 is an epigenetic mediator of gene expression, discuss possible molecular mechanisms by which genetic background, environment, and stochastic factors could cause the phenotypic variability observed among males with *MECP2* variants.

3. Rett syndrome is a neurodevelopmental disorder without neurodegeneration. Why might the absence of neurodegeneration make this disease more amenable to treatment than Alzheimer disease or Parkinson disease? Why less amenable? In this context, also discuss possible molecular mechanisms for the neurodevelopmental regression observed with Rett syndrome.

4. What defines a disease: the molecular variant or the clinical phenotype?

REFERENCES

Kaur S, Christodoulou J: *MECP2* disorders. In Adam MP, Ardinger HH, Pagon RA, Wallace SE, Bean LJH, Gripp KW, Mirzaa GM, Amemiya A, editors: *GeneReviews® [Internet]*, Seattle (WA), 2001 Oct 3, University of Washington, Seattle, pp 1993–2021. [updated 2019 Sep 19]. PMID: 20301670. https://pubmed.ncbi.nlm.nih.gov/20301670/

Marano D, Fioriniello S, D'Esposito M, Della: Ragione F: Transcriptomic and epigenomic landscape in Rett syndrome, *Biomolecules* 11(7):967, 2021. https://doi.org/10.3390/biom11070967. PMID: 34209228; PMCID: PMC8301932.

Neul JL, Kaufmann WE, Glaze DG, Christodoulou J, Clarke AJ, Bahi Buisson N, Leonard H, Bailey ME, Schanen NC, Zappella M, Renieri A, Huppke P, Percy AK: RettSearch Consortium: Rett syndrome: revised diagnostic criteria and nomenclature, *Ann Neurol* 68(6):944–950, 2010. https://doi.org/10.1002/ana.22124. PMID: 21154482; PMCID: PMC3058521.

Autosomal Dominant, Autosomal Recessive

Miriam Reuter

PRINCIPLES

- Genetic heterogeneity
- Gain of function
- Pleiotropy
- Variable expressivity

MAJOR PHENOTYPIC FINDINGS

- Characteristic facial features
- Heart defects, hypertrophic cardiomyopathy
- Short stature
- Developmental delay
- Coagulation defects
- Lymphatic dysplasias

HISTORY AND PHYSICAL FINDINGS

C.M., a 38-year-old gravida 1, para 0, presented for a routine ultrasound examination at 13 weeks of gestation. Fetal crown-rump length was consistent with the gestational age; nuchal translucency was 4.6 mm (>99th centile). The couple was counseled regarding an increased risk for fetal aneuploidy and other disorders but decided against further diagnostic workup or prenatal genetic testing. A male baby L.M. was born at term by spontaneous vaginal delivery; his weight, length, and head circumference were normal. Postnatally, he was found to have a heart murmur, and echocardiography revealed pulmonary valve stenosis. Because of feeding difficulties, he was admitted to a neonatal intensive care unit. A clinical geneticist noticed down-slanting palpebral fissures, ptosis, pectus excavatum, cryptorchidism, and muscular hypotonia. Due to the combination of physical features, she suspected a RASopathy. Multigene panel sequencing identified a pathogenic variant: p.Tyr62Asp in *PTPN11*. Parental testing by Sanger sequencing for the variant in question confirmed it to be de novo in L.M. The parents were counseled that the recurrence risk for future children was low but higher than for the general population due to potential gonadal mosaicism. Early motor and speech development were delayed; he spoke his first single words at 15 months and walked unaided at 17 months. Individualized educational support and physical therapy were initiated. At 3 years of age, his height and weight were below the 3rd centile, and the option of growth hormone treatment was discussed with the parents. IQ testing at the age of 6 years was normal; Wechsler Intelligence Scale for Children revealed a full-scale IQ of 91.

BACKGROUND

Disease Etiology and Incidence

Noonan syndrome is most commonly an autosomal dominant condition, caused by pathogenic variants in genes related to the Ras-mitogen-activated protein kinase (Ras-MAPK) pathway. Approximately 50% of individuals with Noonan syndrome are found to have a pathogenic variant in *PTPN11*, and 10 to 13% have a pathogenic variant in *SOS1*. Other genes account for a smaller proportion of patients, including *RAF1* (~5%), *RIT1* (~5%), and *KRAS* (<5%), while pathogenic variants in *BRAF*, *LZTR1*, *MAP2K1*, and *NRAS* are found in <1% of patients with Noonan syndrome.

The estimated birth prevalence of Noonan syndrome is 1:1000 to 1:2500, but mild manifestations may be underdiagnosed.

Pathogenesis

Pathogenic variants for Noonan syndrome are associated with enhanced signaling of the Ras-MAPK (Ras-Raf-MEK-ERK) pathway and therefore a gain-of-function mechanism. This protein kinase cascade regulates various proteins, including transcription factors involved in cell proliferation and other developmental processes. Autosomal dominant Noonan syndrome is caused by pathogenic variants in *PTPN11*, *SOS1*, *RAF1*, *RIT1*, *KRAS*, *BRAF*, *LZTR1*, *MAP2K1*, or *NRAS*, most of which are missense; many are recurrent and/or cluster in well-established protein domains. Autosomal recessive Noonan syndrome is caused by biallelic loss-of-function variants in *LZTR1*.

Differential diagnoses or allelic disorders include Turner syndrome (Monosomy X) (Case 47), cardiofaciocutaneous syndrome (*BRAF*, *MAP2K1*, *MAP2K1*, *KRAS*, *MEK1*), Costello syndrome (*HRAS*), Noonan syndrome with multiple lentigines (*PTPN11*, *RAF1*), Noonan syndrome-like disorder with loose anagen hair (*SHOC2*), Noonan syndrome-like disorder with or without juvenile myelomonocytic leukemia (*CBL*), neurofibromatosis (*NF1*) (Case 34), and Legius syndrome (*SPRED1*). Due to phenotypic overlaps, many RASopathy multigene diagnostic panels include testing for a variety of related disorders.

PHENOTYPE AND NATURAL HISTORY

Noonan syndrome is a developmental disorder that affects different parts of the body. Affected children can have distinctive facial features, congenital heart defects, short stature, variable degrees of developmental delay, and other physical manifestations.

Facial features (Fig. C.41.1) can be subtle or characteristic – partly dependent on age – including wide-spaced down-slanting palpebral fissures, ptosis and fullness of the eyelids, wide-based nose with depressed root, low-set, posteriorly rotated ears with fleshy helices, grooved philtrum, short neck with excess nuchal skin, and low posterior hairline. Congenital heart disease is reported in 50-80% of individuals with Noonan syndrome. The most common defects are right-sided lesions (pulmonic stenosis) and/or hypertrophic cardiomyopathy. Hypertrophic cardiomyopathy affects ~20% of all individuals with Noonan syndrome and is often diagnosed in the first 6 months of life. Other cardiac defects include septal defects, tetralogy of

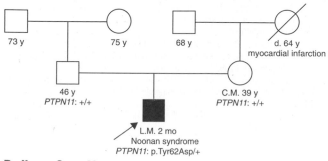

Pedigree Case 41

73 y

75 y

68 y

d. 64 y
myocardial infarction

46 y
PTPN11: +/+

C.M. 39 y
PTPN11: +/+

L.M. 2 mo
Noonan syndrome
PTPN11: p.Tyr62Asp/+

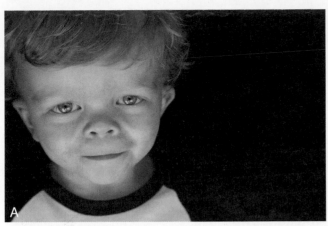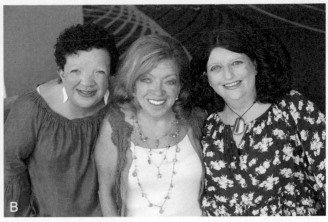

Figure C.41.1 Distinctive facial features of individuals with Noonan syndrome (www.rasopathiesnet.org) can change with age and often become more subtle in adulthood. (A) Ezra is an adorable boy, here at age 4 years. Facial features of the syndrome that are apparent to a geneticist are: broad forehead, small chin, widely spaced, down-slanting palpebral fissures, full upper eyelids, and short broad nose with depressed root and bulbous, upturned tip. (B) April, Martha, and Michelle present with curly hair, high anterior hairline, widely spaced, down-slanting palpebral fissures, blue green irises, ptosis, and Cupid's bow appearance of the upper lip. Photographs by Rick Guidotti, Positive Exposure (www.positiveexposure.org).

Fallot, and coarctation of the aorta. ECG abnormalities are found in ~90% of individuals with Noonan syndrome. While ~40 to 50% of adults with Noonan syndrome have short stature, birth weight and length are usually in the normal range. A growth failure often becomes obvious after the first year of life, and feeding difficulties are common. Delays in motor development can be associated with muscular hypotonia. Neurocognitive outcomes and behavioral anomalies (including attention/hyperactivity disorder, depression, or anxiety) are very variable; intellectual disability (IQ below 70) is found in 6 to 23% of individuals with Noonan syndrome. Other common features include coagulation defects or bleeding disorders and anomalies of the urinary tract, eyes, skin, or cryptorchidism in males. Lymphatic dysplasia can affect internal organs or limbs and can manifest prenatally as increased nuchal translucency or cystic hygroma. An elevated risk for a spectrum of different cancers and malignancies has been reported.

Genotype-phenotype correlations have been reported for Noonan syndrome; for example, pathogenic variants in *RAF1* or *RIT1* are more frequently associated with hypertrophic cardiomyopathy, whereas *KRAS* variants are associated with lower cognitive skills. Broader genetic testing will help to define the phenotypic spectrum of different genes and variants.

MANAGEMENT

If Noonan syndrome is suspected, a thorough clinical evaluation is warranted, including complete physical and neurologic examination, growth monitoring, cardiac evaluation, ophthalmologic and hearing evaluation, coagulation screen, renal ultrasound, imaging of brain and spine only if there are neurological abnormalities, radiographs of spine and rib cage, a formal neuropsychological assessment, and genetics consultation. Most manifestations of Noonan syndrome are treated as for others in the general population. Growth hormone treatment can increase the growth rate in children with short stature.

INHERITANCE

Pathogenic variants in *PTPN11*, *SOS1*, *RAF1*, *RIT1*, *KRAS*, *BRAF*, *MAP2K1*, and *NRAS* cause autosomal dominant Noonan syndrome. Those variants can be de novo (in 25–70% of individuals) or can be inherited from either parent. Recurrence risk for siblings depends on the genetic status of the parents: low in the case of a de novo variant, taking into account the risk for gonadal mosaicism, or 50% in the case of an inherited variant. Offspring of affected individuals have a 50% probability of inheriting the pathogenic variant.

Pathogenic variants in *LZTR1* can cause autosomal dominant or recessive forms of Noonan syndrome: Missense variants within the Kelch domain act in a dominant manner (with recurrence risks as above), whereas hypomorphic or loss-of-function variants act in a recessive manner. For autosomal recessive Noonan syndrome, the recurrence risk for siblings is 25%; offspring of affected individuals inherit one pathogenic allele and are obligate carriers.

QUESTIONS FOR SMALL GROUP DISCUSSION

1. What are the reasons why, for certain diseases, pathogenic variants cluster at so-called "mutation hotspots"?
2. Sporadic tumors can also harbor somatic variants that activate the Ras-MAPK pathway (e.g., in *PTPN11*, *KRAS*, *NRAS*, and *BRAF*; https://cancer.sanger.ac.uk/cosmic). Why are many of those variants different from the ones found in the germline of individuals with Noonan syndrome?
3. How can variants in the same gene cause both autosomal dominant and recessive forms of a disease?

REFERENCES

Allanson JE, Roberts AE: Noonan syndrome, *GeneReviews® [Internet].* Seattle (WA): University of Washington, Seattle; 1993–2021. https://www.ncbi.nlm.nih.gov/books/NBK1124/.

Motta M, Fidan M, Bellacchio E, *et al*: Dominant Noonan syndrome-causing LZTR1 mutations specifically affect the Kelch domain substrate-recognition surface and enhance RAS-MAPK signaling, *Hum Mol Genet* 15;28(6):1007–1022, 2019.

Noonan Syndrome Guideline Development Group: Management of Noonan syndrome—a clinical guideline 2010. https://rasopathiesnet.org/wp-content/uploads/2014/01/265_Noonan_Guidelines.pdf.

SICKLE CELL DISEASE (MIM 603903)

Autosomal Recessive (for Disease)

Isaac Odame

Detectable carrier state (sickle cell trait)

PRINCIPLES

- Heterozygote advantage
- Homozygote or compound heterozygote genotypes
- Geographic variation in allele frequencies

MAJOR PHENOTYPIC FINDINGS

- Age of onset: childhood
- Hyposplenia/asplenia
- Hemolytic anemia
- Acute pain episodes
- Acute chest syndrome
- Cerebrovascular disease
- End-organ damage

CASE REPORT

A Nigerian couple brought their 9-month-old son, K.O., to the emergency department because he was crying inconsolably with swelling of his hands and feet. His parents had noticed the swelling before bedtime the night before, but K.O. had been unable to sleep, crying throughout the night. He had been well the day before and did not have fever. K.O. was diagnosed with sickle cell disease through newborn screening in California, where the family had traveled for the father's graduate studies. At age 2 weeks, a blood sample from K.O., analyzed using high-performance liquid chromatography (HPLC), had revealed HbF 88.5%, HbS 9.4%, and HbA$_2$ 2.1%, confirming that he had sickle cell disease. Hemoglobin analysis done on K.O.'s parents via HPLC confirmed that they both had sickle cell trait. K.O.'s older sister, 3 years old and born in Nigeria, also has sickle cell trait.

K.O. was hospitalized for 3 days, receiving aggressive pain management with morphine infusion and ibuprofen. The parents were offered hydroxyurea therapy as disease modifying therapy, as it is proven to reduce vasoocclusive pain episodes, acute chest syndrome, need for blood transfusions, and hospitalization. In addition, the parents were referred for genetic counseling

to explore avenues of preventing sickle cell disease in their future offspring. During the genetic counseling session, prenatal diagnosis and preimplantation genetic diagnosis were discussed as options for the parents to consider (see Chapter 17).

BACKGROUND

Disease Etiology and Incidence

Sickle hemoglobin (HbS) is a structural variant of normal adult hemoglobin (HbA) caused by a missense variant in the β-globin gene (*HBB*) that causes substitution of valine for glutamic acid at position 6 of the β-globin subunit (β^S) of the hemoglobin molecule. Sickle cell disease (SCD) refers to a group of disorders characterized by the presence of at least one β^S allele and a second *HBB* variant that results in the predominant production of HbS. Its most common form is due to homozygosity for the β^S allele (SS); however, compound heterozygosity for the β^S allele with other *HBB* variants – including hemoglobin C or a β-thalassemia allele – can also cause SCD. The prevalence of SCD varies widely among populations, in proportion to past and present exposure to malaria, and is being influenced by world migration. The sickle cell variant appears to confer some resistance to malaria and thus a survival advantage to individuals heterozygous for the variant. (See Chapters 10, 12).

Pathogenesis

Hemoglobin is composed of four subunits: two α subunits encoded by *HBA* (MIM 141800) on chromosome 16 and two β subunits encoded by *HBB* (MIM 141900) on chromosome 11. The p.Glu6Val variant in β-globin decreases the solubility of deoxygenated hemoglobin and causes it to form a gelatinous network of stiff fibrous polymers (polymerization), distorting the red blood cell, giving it a sickle shape. These sickled erythrocytes occlude capillaries and postcapillary venules and cause vasoocclusion and infarctions. Initially, oxygenation causes the hemoglobin polymer to dissolve and the erythrocyte to regain its normal shape; however, repeated sickling and unsickling produce irreversibly sickled cells that are removed from the

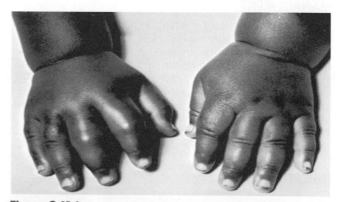

Figure C.42.1 A photo of SCD dactylitis – one of the earliest manifestations of sickle cell anemia. (From Lichtman MA, Shafer MS, Felgar RE, Wang N: *Lichtman's atlas of hematology 2016, 2017,* McGraw Hill. https://accessmedicine.mhmedical.com/)

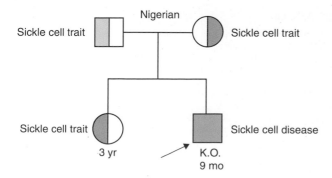

Nigerian
Sickle cell trait — Sickle cell trait

Sickle cell trait
3 yr

K.O.
9 mo
Sickle cell disease

Pedigree Case 42

circulation by the spleen. The rate of removal exceeds the production capacity of the marrow and causes a hemolytic anemia.

PHENOTYPE AND NATURAL HISTORY

Patients with SCD generally present in the first two years of life with anemia, splenomegaly, repeated infections, and dactylitis (painful swelling of the hands or feet from the occlusion of the capillaries in small bones) (Fig. C.42.1). Vasoocclusive infarctions occur in many tissues, causing strokes, acute chest syndrome, renal papillary necrosis, autosplenectomy, leg ulcers, priapism, bone aseptic necrosis, and visual loss. Bone vasoocclusion causes painful "crises" and, if untreated, these painful episodes can persist for days or weeks. The functional asplenia, from infarction and other poorly understood factors, increases susceptibility to bacterial infections, such as pneumococcal sepsis. Infection is a major cause of death at all ages, although progressive renal failure and pulmonary failure are also common causes of death in the fourth and fifth decades. These individuals also have a high risk for the development of life-threatening aplastic anemia after parvovirus infection, which causes a temporary cessation of erythrocyte production.

Heterozygotes for the variant (who are said to have sickle cell trait) do not have anemia and are usually clinically normal. Under nonphysiologic conditions of severe hypoxia, however, erythrocytes of individuals with sickle cell trait may sickle and cause symptoms similar to those observed with SCD. With extreme exertion and dehydration, there is increased risk for rhabdomyolysis in sickle cell heterozygotes.

MANAGEMENT

When early diagnosis through newborn screening is followed by interventions such as penicillin prophylaxis through 5 years of age, pneumococcal vaccinations, prompt management of febrile illness, and parental education, over 95% of children born with SCD survive beyond 18 years of age. Persistence of fetal hemoglobin greatly ameliorates disease severity (see Chapter 14). Hydroxyurea therapy – an oral medication that induces fetal hemoglobin production – has proven efficacy (laboratory and clinical benefits) in both adults and children with SCD. Transcranial Doppler screening is an effective way to identify SCD children at risk of stroke (velocities ≥ 200 cm/s). In such children, chronic blood transfusion reduces the risk of stroke by over 90%. Hydroxyurea therapy can substitute for chronic blood transfusion to prevent first or recurrent stroke. Recently, other disease-modifying therapies for SCD have been approved in certain countries: L-glutamine, crizanlizumab (a P-selectin binding humanized monoclonal antibody), and voxelotor (binds to HbS and reduces polymerization).

Allogeneic bone marrow transplantation is the only treatment currently available that can cure SCD, but access is limited by the availability of suitable donors (see Chapter 14). Recently, clinical trials of lentiviral-mediated gene therapy, and CRISPR/Cas9-mediated genome editing approaches involving *ex vivo* gene modification of autologous hematopoietic stem cells, are showing promising results.

INHERITANCE

Because SCD is an autosomal recessive disorder, future siblings of an affected child whose parents both have sickle cell trait have a 25% risk for SCD and a 50% risk for sickle cell trait. When other pathogenic *HBB* alleles are involved in combination with a β^S allele, the recurrence risks for sibs are 25% for a phenotype similar to that of the proband, 25% for sickle cell trait, and 25% for the phenotype associated with the other pathogenic allele. With the use of fetal DNA derived from chorionic villi or amniocytes, prenatal diagnosis is available by molecular analysis for the variant alleles as identified in parental samples.

QUESTIONS FOR SMALL GROUP DISCUSSION

1. Name two other diseases that may have become prevalent because of a heterozygote survival advantage. What is the rationale for hypothesizing a heterozygote advantage for those diseases?
2. How is the geographical distribution of the sickle gene variant explained by the heterozygous advantage against falciparum malaria?
3. Although it is always a severe disease, the severity of sickle cell disease is determined partially by the haplotype on which the variant occurs. How could the haplotype affect disease severity?
4. What is the expected clinical severity of SCD in the offspring of a couple receiving genetic counseling if:
   a. Mother is heterozygous for the S allele and partner heterozygous for a β^+-thalassemia allele?
   b. Mother is heterozygous for a β^0-thalassemia allele and partner heterozygous for the S allele?
   c. Mother is heterozygous for the C allele and partner heterozygous for the S allele?
   d. Mother heterozygous for the S allele and partner heterozygous for a hereditary persistence of fetal hemoglobin (HPFH) allele?
5. What issues would apply to the consideration of either germline or somatic cell gene therapy for this disorder?

REFERENCES

Brandow AM, Liem RI: Advances in the diagnosis and treatment of sickle cell disease, *J Hematol Oncol* 15(1):20, 2022. https://doi.org/10.1186/s13045-022-01237-z. PMID: 35241123.
GeneReviews®. https://www.ncbi.nlm.nih.gov/books/NBK1377/.

Autosomal Recessive

Changrui Xiao • Cynthia J. Tifft

PRINCIPLES

- Lysosomal storage disease
- Population variation in allele frequencies
- Genetic drift
- Pseudodeficiency
- Population screening

MAJOR PHENOTYPIC FINDINGS

- Age at onset: infancy through adulthood
- Neurodegeneration
- Macrocephaly
- Retinal cherry-red macula
- Psychiatric illness

CASE REPORT

R.T. and S.T., a couple of Ashkenazi Jewish ancestry, were referred to the Genetics clinic for evaluation of their risk for having a child with Tay-Sachs disease. S.T. had a sister who died of Tay-Sachs disease as a child. R.T. had a paternal uncle living in a psychiatric home, but he did not know what disease his uncle had. Both R.T. and S.T. recalled getting enzymatic carrier testing done as teenagers and were told they had reduced hexosaminidase A activity in the carrier range. Exon sequencing of *HEXA* confirmed that S.T. is heterozygous for a pathogenic variant, whereas R.T. has a pseudodeficiency allele with no other variant. The counselor discussed with the couple that the risk of any potential children to be a carrier for Tay-Sachs disease would be 1 in 2 (or 50%). She reassured them that their offspring would not be at risk for Tay-Sachs disease.

BACKGROUND

Disease Etiology and Incidence

Tay-Sachs disease (MIM 272800), or GM_2 gangliosidosis type I, is an autosomal recessive disorder of ganglioside catabolism that is caused by a deficiency of hexosaminidase A (see Chapter 13). In addition to severe infantile-onset disease, there are juvenile- and adult-onset forms of Tay-Sachs disease.

The incidence of Tay-Sachs disease varies widely among populations, ranging from 1 in 3600 births within Ashkenazi Jewish populations (prior to widespread carrier screening) to 1 in 360,000 among other North American births. Persons of French Canadian, Louisiana Cajun, and Pennsylvania Amish ancestry have a carrier frequency comparable to that of Ashkenazi populations. The increased carrier frequency in these four populations appears to be due to genetic drift, although heterozygote advantage cannot be excluded (see Chapter 10). Screening of high-risk populations for carriers and subsequent prevention has reduced the incidence of Tay-Sachs disease among Ashkenazi Jewish populations in the United States by nearly 90% (see Chapters 13 and 18).

Pathogenesis

Gangliosides are ceramide-based glycosphingolipids present in all cell surface membranes, but most abundant in the brain, where they are concentrated in neuronal surface membranes, particularly in dendrites and axon termini. They function as receptors for various glycoprotein hormones and bacterial toxins and are involved in cell differentiation and cell-cell interaction.

Hexosaminidase A is a lysosomal enzyme composed of two subunits. (see Fig. 13.4) The α subunit is encoded by the *HEXA* gene, and the β subunit is encoded by the *HEXB* gene. In the presence of GM_2 activator protein, hexosaminidase A removes the terminal *N*-acetylgalactosamine from the ganglioside GM_2. Pathogenic variants in *HEXA* can lead to the accumulation of GM_2 in the lysosome and therefore Tay-Sachs disease of the infantile, juvenile, or adult type. Biallelic variants in *HEXB* or *GM2A* can cause the related Sandhoff disease (MIM 268800) or GM_2 activator deficiency (MIM272750), respectively, through the accumulation of GM_2. The mechanism by which the accumulation of GM_2 ganglioside causes neuronal death has not been fully defined, although, by analogy with Gaucher disease (see Chapter 13, Case 18), accumulations of toxic byproducts of GM_2 ganglioside lead to neuropathology.

The level of residual hexosaminidase A activity correlates inversely with the severity of the disease. In general, those with infantile-onset GM_2 gangliosidosis have two null alleles; that is, no hexosaminidase A enzymatic activity. Those with juvenile- or adult-onset forms of GM_2 gangliosidosis are usually compound heterozygotes, either for a null *HEXA* allele and an allele with low residual hexosaminidase A activity, or for two alleles with low residual activity.

PHENOTYPE AND NATURAL HISTORY

Acute infantile Tay-Sachs disease is characterized by neurological deterioration beginning between the ages of 3 and 6 months and progressing to death by 2 to 4 years. Motor development usually plateaus or begins to regress by 8 to 10 months and progresses to loss of voluntary movement within the second year of life. Visual loss begins within the first year and progresses rapidly; it is almost uniformly associated with a cherry-red macula on funduscopic examination (Fig. C.43.1). Seizures usually begin near the end of the first year and progressively worsen. Progressive macrocephaly is usually seen beginning at 18 months. Further deterioration in the second year of life results in decerebrate posturing, swallowing difficulties, worse seizures, and finally, an unresponsive, vegetative state.

Juvenile-onset Tay-Sachs disease manifests between 2 and 4 years and is characterized by plateauing of motor and speech development followed by neurological deterioration. Dysarthria and abnormal gait are common presenting features. By the end of the first decade, most affected individuals experience spasticity, dysphagia, and seizures. By 10 to 15 years, most develop decerebrate posturing and enter a vegetative state, with death generally occurring in the second decade. Vision is lost, but cherry-red maculae are not always present. Optic atrophy and retinitis pigmentosa often occur late in the disease course.

Adult-onset Tay-Sachs disease manifests in late teens to early adulthood as a slowly progressive neurological and psychiatric condition. Common features include motor neuron disease, cerebellar ataxia, dysarthria, executive dysfunction,

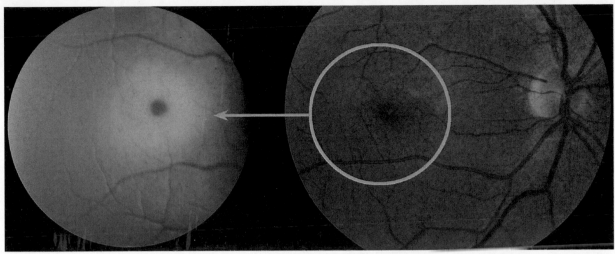

Figure C.43 1 *Cherry red* macula in Tay-Sachs disease. *Right*, Normal retina. The *circle* surrounds the macula, lateral to the optic nerve. *Left*, The macula of a child with Tay-Sachs disease. The *cherry-red* center is the normal retina of the fovea at the center of the macula that is surrounded by a macular retina made white by abnormal storage of GM_2 in retinal neurons. (Courtesy A. V. Levin, The Hospital for Sick Children and University of Toronto, Canada.)

and psychiatric manifestations such as depression, anxiety and, occasionally, psychosis. Vision is rarely affected, and results of the ophthalmological examination are generally normal.

DIAGNOSIS AND MANAGEMENT

The diagnosis of Tay-Sachs disease relies on the demonstration of both absent to nearly absent hexosaminidase A activity and normal to elevated activity of hexosaminidase B, in addition to the identification of biallelic pathogenic variants in *HEXA* on molecular testing.

Tay-Sachs disease is currently an incurable disorder; therefore, treatment focuses on the management of symptoms and palliative care. Nearly all patients require pharmacological management of their seizures. Physical and occupational therapy may be helpful for motor development or maintenance of motor function. Speech and swallow therapy can help maintain language skills and detect potential aspiration risk. For late-onset cases, psychiatric symptoms should be assessed regularly, and medications may be indicated. Some medications are contraindicated in late-onset individuals due to the worsening of symptoms.

CARRIER SCREENING

Tay-Sachs is the hallmark example of carrier screening in at-risk populations. Traditionally, such screening has been performed by determining the serum activity of hexosaminidase A with an artificial substrate. In the setting of pregnancy or oral contraceptive use, leukocytes are preferred over serum for testing, due to a high false-positive rate in the latter. While enzymatic analysis is a reliable method for carrier screening, results may be confounded by the presence of pseudodeficiency alleles or the rare pathogenic B1 variant that shows normal enzyme activity in vitro; therefore, carrier status, when determined enzymatically, is usually confirmed by molecular

analysis of *HEXA*. Exon sequencing of the *HEXA* gene on a next-generation sequencing platform is a sensitive method for carrier detection and is increasingly being used as the first line screening test for persons of all ancestral backgrounds. Two pseudodeficiency alleles and more than 170 pathogenic variants have been identified in the *HEXA* gene. Among persons of Ashkenazi Jewish background who are found to be positive through enzymatic carrier screening, 2% are heterozygous for a pseudodeficiency allele and 95 to 98% are heterozygous for one of three pathogenic variants: two causing infantile-onset and one causing adult-onset disease (see Chapter 13). In contrast, among other North Americans who are found to be positive via enzymatic carrier screening, 35% are heterozygous for a pseudodeficiency allele.

Recent recommendations from the American College of Medical Genetics and Genomics (ACMG) note that carrier screening paradigms should be agnostic to race, ethnicity, and ancestry (see Chapters 10 and 17).

Exon sequencing of *HEXA* is a sensitive method for carrier screening for Tay-Sachs, though ambiguous screening results should be confirmed via enzymatic analysis.

INHERITANCE

For potential parents without a family history of Tay-Sachs disease, the empirical risk for having an affected child depends on the frequency of pathogenic *HEXA* variants in their respective ancestral groups. For most North Americans, the empirical risk for being a carrier is approximately 1 in 250 to 1 in 300, whereas individuals of Ashkenazi Jewish descent (and others, as above) have an empirical carrier risk of 1 in 30. For couples who are both carriers, the risk of any offspring of theirs to have Tay-Sachs disease is 25% for each pregnancy.

Prenatal and preimplantation diagnosis rely on identification of the *HEXA* variants and require that the disease-causing *HEXA* variant(s) in a family have already been identified.

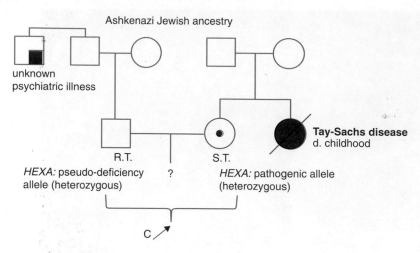

Pedigree Case 43

QUESTIONS FOR SMALL GROUP DISCUSSION

1. Screening for what other diseases are complicated by pseudodeficiency?
2. What is genetic drift? What are its causes? Name two other diseases that seem to be associated with genetic drift.
3. Should population screening be instituted to identify carriers of other diseases?
4. What diseases are phenocopies of adult-onset hexosaminidase A deficiency? Consider psychiatric disorders and adult-onset neuronal ceroid-lipofuscinosis. What diseases are genocopies of infantile-onset hexosaminidase A deficiency? Consider GM$_2$ activator mutations. How would you distinguish between a phenocopy and hexosaminidase A deficiency?

REFERENCES

Bley AE, Giannikopoulos OA, Hayden D, *et al*: Natural history of infantile GM$_2$ gangliosidosis, *Pediatrics* 128:e1233–e1241, 2011.

Shapiro BE, Hatters-Friedman S, Fernandes-Filho JA, Anthony K, Natowicz MR: Late-onset Tay-Sachs disease: Adverse effects of medications and implications for treatment, *Neurology* 67(5):875–877, 2006. https://doi.org/10.1212/01.wnl.0000233847.72349.b6. PMID: 1696655.

Toro C, Shirvan L, Tifft C: *HEXA* disorders. http://www.ncbi.nlm.nih.gov/books/NBK1218/.

Toro C, Zainab M, Tifft CJ: The GM2 gangliosidoses: unlocking the mysteries of pathogenesis and treatment, *Neurosci Lett* 764:136195, 2021. https://doi.org/10.1016/j.neulet.2021.136195. Epub 2021 Aug 25. PMID: 34450229; PMCID: PMC8572160.

α-THALASSEMIA (α-Globin Deficiency) (MIM 604131)

Isaac Odame

PRINCIPLES

- Heterozygote advantage
- Population variation in allele frequencies
- Gene deletions versus single nucleotide variants
- Homozygote; compound heterozygote
- Gene dosage

MAJOR PHENOTYPIC FINDINGS

- Age at onset: intrauterine (fetus), at birth
- Microcytic hypochromic anemia
- Fetal anemia and hypoxia
- Fetal hydrops
- Death in utero or shortly after birth
- High-risk pregnancy
- Transfusion dependency

CASE REPORT

J.Z., a 25-year-old healthy Canadian woman, presented to her obstetrician for routine prenatal care. Results of her complete blood count showed mild microcytic hypochromic anemia (hemoglobin 96 g/L, mean corpuscular volume [MCV] 69.6 fL, mean corpuscular hemoglobin [MCH] 23.1 pg). She was of Chinese ancestry and her spouse, T.C., of Thai ancestry. J.Z. was unaware of any blood disorders in her or T.C.'s family. Nonetheless, hemoglobin analysis via high-performance liquid chromatography (HPLC) showed slightly decreased HbA_2 ($\alpha 2\delta 2$) and normal HbF ($\alpha 2\gamma 2$). Her serum ferritin and transferrin saturation were normal – ruling out iron deficiency anemia – all suggesting that J.Z. likely had α-thalassemia trait. Blood tests on T.C. showed similar features to those of J.Z.: microcytic (MCV 70.1 fL), hypochromic (MCH 23.5 pg) anemia (Hb 99 g/L) with no evidence of iron deficiency, and normal HbA_2 ($\alpha 2\delta 2$) and HbF ($\alpha 2\gamma 2$) on hemoglobin analysis. Molecular genetic testing by a multiplex gap-PCR assay on J.Z. and T.C. showed that they were both heterozygotes for α^0-thalassemia deletion of the South-East Asian type (--^{SEA}/$\alpha\alpha$). After referral to the Genetics clinic, the geneticist explained to this couple that the risk for this pregnancy (or any child of theirs) to have homozygous α^0-thalassemia major (Hb Bart hydrops fetalis) was 25%. Hb Bart hydrops

fetalis can have serious consequences for the fetus, including severe anemia and hypoxia, resulting in fetal death (stillbirth) or death soon after delivery. Complications can also occur in mothers who carry pregnancies with Hb Bart hydrops fetalis. To prevent these outcomes in an affected fetus, intrauterine blood transfusions would be required to treat the severe fetal anemia.

The couple elected to undergo prenatal diagnosis by amniocentesis, since J.Z. was already 18 weeks into the pregnancy. Molecular laboratory results showed that the fetus was a homozygote for the South-East Asian deletion (--^{SEA}/--^{SEA}) and predicted to develop signs of Hb Bart hydrops fetalis with possible maternal complications. J.Z. and T.C. were referred to the Fetal Medicine Unit at the teaching hospital, where interventional pathways were discussed, including close monitoring of fetus and mother with regular intrauterine blood transfusions to treat fetal anemia or termination of pregnancy.

BACKGROUND

Disease Etiology and Prevalence

Thalassemias are autosomal recessive anemias caused by deficient synthesis of α-globin or β-globin. A relative deficiency of α-globin causes α-thalassemia, and a relative deficiency of β-globin causes β-thalassemia (see Chapter 12).

Thalassemia is most common among persons of Mediterranean, Africa, Middle Eastern, Indian, Chinese, and South-East Asian descent. Thalassemias appear to have evolved because they confer heterozygote advantage by providing some resistance against malaria; the prevalence of thalassemia in a defined population therefore reflects past and present exposure of the population to malaria (see Chapter 10). The prevalence of α-thalassemia trait (i.e., asymptomatic heterozygous carriers) ranges from less than 0.01% in natives of nonmalarial areas – such as the United Kingdom, Iceland, and Japan – to approximately 70% among natives of some Southwest Pacific islands; Hb H disease and Hb Bart hydrops fetalis are restricted to Mediterranean and South-East Asian regions. (The prevalence of β-thalassemia trait ranges from approximately 1–2% among Africans and African Americans to 30% in some villages of Sardinia.)

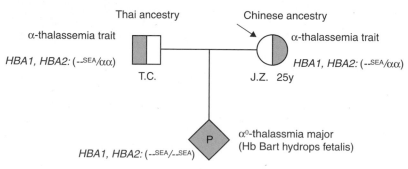

Thai ancestry — α-thalassemia trait
HBA1, HBA2: (--^{SEA}/$\alpha\alpha$)
T.C.

Chinese ancestry — α-thalassemia trait
HBA1, HBA2: (--^{SEA}/$\alpha\alpha$)
J.Z. 25y

P — α^0-thalassemia major (Hb Bart hydrops fetalis)
HBA1, HBA2: (--^{SEA}/--^{SEA})
amniocentesis 18 wks

Pedigree Case 44

Pathogenesis

Thalassemia arises from inadequate production and unbalanced accumulation of globin subunits. Inadequate hemoglobin production causes hypochromia and microcytosis. The severity of thalassemia is proportionate to the severity of the imbalance between α-globin and β-globin production. Because α-globin is produced throughout gestation, fetuses without α-globin genes (--/--) suffer from severe anemia leading to hypoxia, heart failure, and hydrops; they are incapable of producing normal HbF ($\alpha_2\gamma_2$) and primarily produce Hb Bart (γ_4), which is nonfunctional. This disorder is known as Hb Bart hydrops fetalis. Without intrauterine blood transfusions, the expected outcome is intrauterine fetal death, stillbirth, or death soon after birth. Where resources are available for intrauterine blood transfusions, increasing numbers of babies born with Hb Bart hydrops fetalis are surviving to adulthood. These survivors predominantly produce Hb H (β_4), since they do not produce any α-globin. Hb H is nonfunctional and causes hypoxia and hemolytic anemia; therefore, regular blood transfusions are needed for survival.

Deletion of α-globin genes accounts for 80 to 85% of α-thalassemia; the rest are caused by nondeletional variants. In contrast, approximately 15 pathogenic single nucleotide variants account for more than 90% of β-thalassemia. Molecular studies of both α-globin and β-globin gene variants strongly suggest that these have arisen independently in different populations and then achieved their high frequency by selection

PHENOTYPE AND NATURAL HISTORY

The α-globin variant alleles are separated into four clinical groups, reflecting the impairment of α-globin production due to α-globin gene deletions or pathogenic small variants. The phenotypes observed in a population reflect the nature of α-globin alleles in that population. Chromosomes with deletions of both tandem α-globin genes are observed in South-East Asia and the Mediterranean basin; therefore, Hb H disease and Hb Bart hydrops fetalis usually occur in these populations and not in Africans, whose chromosome deletions typically involve only one α-globin gene. Individuals missing only one or two α-globin genes have α-thalassemia trait, with mild hypochromic microcytic anemia, and are asymptomatic. Hb H disease is associated with moderate anemia with a mild course. Hb Bart hydrops fetalis was previously considered a universally fatal condition; however, with recent advances in prenatal care and the availability of intrauterine blood transfusions, an increasing number of individuals now survive into adulthood, albeit being transfusion dependent. Blood transfusions alone lead to iron overload, which causes cardiac, hepatic, and endocrine complications. Where resources are available, regular monitoring for iron overload and the use of iron chelation therapies can prevent or minimize the complications of iron overload.

MANAGEMENT

Initial screening for α- or β-thalassemia trait is usually done by determination of red cell indices on blood samples. For individuals without iron deficiency anemia, the diagnosis of β-thalassemia trait is usually confirmed by finding increased levels of HbA$_2$ ($\alpha_2\delta_2$) and HbF ($\alpha_2\gamma_2$) (which contain other β-like globin chains from the β-globin cluster) by hemoglobin analysis or by DNA analysis, or both. In contrast, α-thalassemia trait is not associated with significant changes in HbA$_2$ (normal or slightly reduced); HbF and is confirmed by DNA analysis.

Treatment of Hb H is primarily supportive. Therapy includes folate supplementation, avoidance of oxidant drugs and iron, prompt treatment of infection, and judicious blood transfusion.

Fetuses with Hb Bart hydrops fetalis suffer severe hypoxia in utero during the third trimester or shortly after birth. Therefore, identifying couples at risk – in order to provide them with timely genetic counseling and prenatal diagnosis early in the pregnancy – should be a major goal. Termination of pregnancy can be offered, as the untreated condition could be associated with maternal morbidity and mortality. For couples who choose to carry on the pregnancy with an affected fetus, fetal monitoring for hydrops and intrauterine blood transfusions is increasingly leading to successful delivery of babies with Hb Bart hydrops fetalis, who subsequently require lifelong transfusions. Bone marrow transplantation is an established and available curative treatment, while gene therapy and genome editing are emerging curative approaches.

INHERITANCE

For parents who both have α-thalassemia trait, the risk for their child to have Hb H disease or Hb Bart hydrops fetalis depends on the nature of their α-globin gene deletions. Parents with α-thalassemia trait can have either the -α/-α or --/αα genotype (i.e., deletions in *cis* or in *trans*). Depending on their respective genotypes, all their children could have α-thalassemia trait (-α/-α) or be at risk for Hb H disease (-α/--) or Hb Bart hydrops fetalis (--/--).

For both α- and β-thalassemia, prenatal diagnosis is possible by molecular analysis of fetal DNA from either chorionic villi or amniocytes. Molecular prenatal diagnosis of thalassemia is most efficient if the variants have already been identified in the carrier parents. Preimplantation diagnosis has been achieved based on similar genetic analyses.

QUESTIONS FOR SMALL GROUP DISCUSSION

1. Compare and contrast the genetic counseling of a woman in early pregnancy with confirmed α-thalassemia trait (--/αα) if she is found to have a partner with confirmed.
   a. α-thalassemia trait (-α/-α)
   b. α-thalassemia trait (--/αα)
2. What are the molecular mechanisms for α-globin gene deletion and α-globin gene triplication?
3. Describe carrier screening for α-thalassemia. What demographic and clinical factors should be considered in determining when carrier screening for α-thalassemia should be applied? Should individuals from classically low-risk ancestry groups be screened if their partner has α-thalassemia or β-thalassemia trait? Consider population admixture.
4. α-Thalassemia is the most common single-gene disorder in the world. Three mechanisms can increase the frequency of a gene variant in a population: selection, genetic drift, and founder effects. Describe each mechanism and the reason why selection is likely to account for the high frequency of α-thalassemia.

REFERENCE

Hannah T, Orly D: GeneReviews®. Alpha-thalassemia, 2020. https://www.ncbi.nlm.nih.gov/books/NBK1435/.

Autosomal Semidominant

Iris Cohn

PRINCIPLES

- Pharmacogenetics
- Precision medicine
- Cancer and immunosuppression chemotherapy
- Population variation

MAJOR PHENOTYPIC FINDINGS

- Age at onset: deficiency is present at birth, manifestation requires drug exposure
- Myelosuppression
- Increased risk for brain tumor in thiopurine methyltransferase–deficient patients with acute lymphoblastic leukemia receiving brain irradiation

HISTORY AND PHYSICAL FINDINGS

J.B. is a 19-year-old man with long-standing ulcerative colitis. Because he has been refractory to steroid treatment, his physician prescribed azathioprine at a standard dose of 2.5 mg/kg/day. After a few weeks, J.B. developed severe leukopenia. The physician measured thiopurine methyltransferase (*TPMT*) activity in the red cells and found it to be normal. The physician remembered that J.B. had received a red blood cell transfusion 3 weeks previously and decided to determine his *TPMT* metabolizer status by genotyping. J.B. was found to be a compound heterozygote for the *TPMT*2 and -*3A* alleles. Consequently, he should have been started and maintained on 6 to 10% of the standard dose of azathioprine.

BACKGROUND
Disease Etiology and Incidence

Thiopurine methyltransferase (TPMT) is the enzyme responsible for phase II metabolism of thiopurines (azathioprine, 6-mercaptopurine [6MP], thioguanine) by catalyzing *S*-methylation and thus inactivating these compounds. Azathioprine, a commonly used immunosuppressant, is activated by conversion to 6-MP; its metabolism is thus also affected by TPMT activity. These agents are used as immunosuppressants for various systemic inflammatory diseases, such as inflammatory bowel disease, rheumatoid arthritis, and lupus, and for preventing the rejection of solid tumor transplants as a second line therapy. Thiopurines such as 6-MP and thioguanine are also components in the standard treatment of acute lymphoblastic leukemia. Approximately 3 to 14% of the general population carry at least one nonfunctional *TPMT* allele that causes accumulation of higher levels of toxic thiopurine metabolites. These individuals are at increased risk of moderate to severe bone marrow suppression (Fig. C.45.1). Of individuals of European or African ancestry, 0.3% have two nonfunctional *TPMT* alleles and are considered TPMT-poor metabolizers. When treated with standard doses of thiopurines, these individuals will experience life-threatening hematopoietic toxicities. Deficiency is much less common in other population groups.

PHENOTYPE AND NATURAL HISTORY

Toxicity from thiopurines was first recognized in patients receiving 6-MP for acute lymphoblastic leukemia. Although patients with 6-MP toxicity had a risk for life-threatening leukopenia, those who survived were noted to have longer periods of leukemia-free survival. Among TPMT-deficient patients with acute lymphoblastic leukemia, there was an increased risk for radiation-induced brain tumors and chemotherapy-induced acute myelogenous leukemia. The *TPMT* gene is highly polymorphic, with over 40 reported variant (*) alleles. *TPMT*1 allele is associated with normal enzyme activity and is considered the wild-type allele. Three variant *TPMT* alleles account for over 90% of the *TPMT* alleles with reduced or absent activity.

*TPMT*2 was the first variant allele described and has a missense variant (c.238 G>C) that results in an alanine to proline substitution at codon 80 (p.Ala80Pro). *TPMT* *2 is much less commonly seen than either *TPMT*3A or *3 C. *TPMT*3A allele is the most common variant, with a 5% frequency in individuals of European ancestry; it involves two variants in *cis*: c.460 G>A (p.Tyr240Cys) and c.719 A>G (p.Ala154Thr). The *TPMT*3 C allele contains only the Tyr240Cys variant and is more common in East Asian, African-American, and some African populations with a 2% frequency. The Ala154Thr variant has not been seen in isolation and presumably occurred on a chromosome that already carried the Tyr240Cys allele after European migration.

TPMT testing can prevent thiopurine toxicity by allowing dose adjustment before starting therapy. It is the standard of care for acute lymphoblastic leukemia (ALL) and has a favorable cost-benefit analysis for inflammatory bowel disease.

There are different technologies available that determine an individual's TPMT activity level: TPMT activity test (phenotype) and TPMT genetic test (genotype).

TPMT phenotype is measured in red blood cells by radiochemical or chromatographic techniques. False negatives are common in patients who have received blood transfusions as long as 3 months before. Additionally, in children with ALL, disease and treatment related reasons that may influence the TPMT enzyme activity in the red blood cells.

TPMT genotype is done using a polymerase chain reaction (PCR) platform and identifies the most common TPMT variants. Rare variants leading to reduced or lack of enzyme activity may be omitted from a standard platform.

Currently, neither TPMT genotype nor phenotype can guarantee a 100% identification of a TPMT deficient individual.

MANAGEMENT

Patients with complete TPMT deficiency should receive 6 to 10% of the standard dose of thiopurine medications. Heterozygous patients may start at the full dose but should have a dose reduction to half within 6 months or as soon as any myelosuppression is observed. The effect of *TPMT* common variants is an instructive example of the clinical importance of pharmacogenetics in individualized medicine (see Chapter 19).

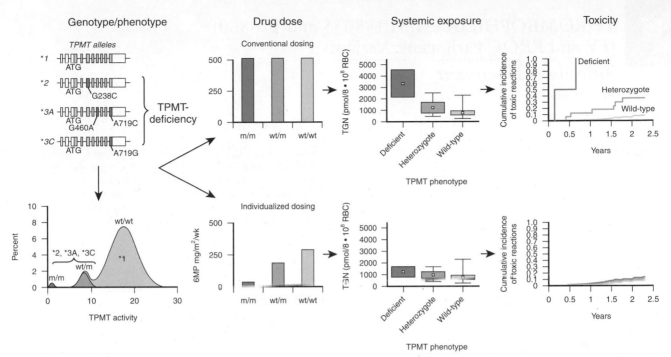

Figure C.45.1 Genetic polymorphism of thiopurine *S*-methyltransferase (*TPMT*) and its role in determining response to thiopurine medications (azathioprine, mercaptopurine, and thioguanine). The *upper left panel* depicts the predominant *TPMT* variant alleles causing autosomal semidominant inheritance of TPMT activity in humans. As depicted in the adjacent *top three panels*, when uniform (conventional) dosages of thiopurine medications are given to all patients, *TPMT* homozygous variant patients accumulate 10-fold higher cellular concentrations of the active thioguanine nucleotides (*TGNs*); heterozygous patients accumulate approximately 2-fold higher TGN concentrations. These differences translate into a significantly higher frequency of toxicity (*far right panels*). As depicted in the *bottom left three panels*, when genotype-specific dosing is used, similar cellular TGN concentrations are achieved, and all three TPMT phenotypes can be treated without acute toxicity. 6MP, 6-Mercaptopurine; RBC, red blood cell. (From Eichelbaum M, Ingelman-Sundberg M, Evans WE: Pharmacogenomics and individualized drug therapy. *Annu Rev Med* 57:119–137, 2006.)

INHERITANCE

The *a priori* risk of an individual of European ancestry carrying a *TPMT* deficiency allele is approximately 10%. In other populations, it is 2 to 5%.

QUESTIONS FOR SMALL GROUP DISCUSSION

1. *TPMT* polymorphisms account for significant variation in the metabolism of thiopurines such as azathioprine, 6-mercaptopurine, and thioguanine. Name several conditions in which thiopurines therapy is commonly used.
2. Does poor metabolism in the *TPMT* gene result in toxicity or decreased effect?
3. Why do humans have genes for drug metabolism?
4. Suggest explanations for ethnic variation in these genes.

REFERENCES

Dean L: Azathioprine therapy and TPMT and NUDT15 genotype. In Pratt VM, Scott SA, Pirmohamed M, Esquivel B, Kane MS, Kattman BL, Malheiro AJ, editors: *Medical Genetics Summaries [Internet]*, Bethesda (MD), 2012, National Center for Biotechnology Information (US). 2012 Sep 20 [updated 2020 Aug 5]. PMID: 28520349.

Relling MV, Gardner EE, Sandborn WJ, *et al*: Clinical pharmacogenetics implementation consortium guidelines for thiopurine methyltransferase genotype and thiopurine dosing, *Clin Pharmacol Ther* 89:387–391, 2011.

Scott SA: Personalizing medicine with clinical pharmacogenetics, *Genet Med* 13:987–995, 2011.

46

THROMBOPHILIA (MIM 188055 and 176860)
(*FV* and *PROC* Pathogenic Variants)

Autosomal Dominant

Manuel Carcao

PRINCIPLES

- Gain of function (factor V Leiden)
- Loss of function (protein C)
- Dosage effect
- Digenic inheritance
- Incomplete penetrance
- Genetic and environmental modifiers
- Heterozygote advantage
- Founder effect

MAJOR PHENOTYPIC FINDINGS

- Age at onset: adulthood
- Deep venous thrombosis

HISTORY AND PHYSICAL FINDINGS

J.J., a 45-year-old businessman of French and Swedish descent, suddenly developed shortness of breath the day after a trans–Pacific Ocean flight. His right leg was swollen and warm. Subsequent studies identified a thrombus in the popliteal and iliac veins and a pulmonary embolus. Both of his parents had had leg venous thromboses, and a sister (S.J.) had died of a pulmonary embolism during pregnancy. DNA panel screening for inherited causes of thrombophilia identified that J.J. was heterozygous for the factor *(F)* factor (F) V Leiden missense variant (c.1691G>A) and heterozygous for a frameshift variant (c.3363insC) in *PROC*, the gene encoding protein C. Studies of other family members (see family tree) identified S.J. (from archival tissue), J.J.'s father, and older brother (not known to have had thrombotic disease) as heterozygotes for FV Leiden. They identified the *PROC* variant (in a heterozygous

state) in S.J., J.J.'s mother, and older sister (not known to have had thrombotic disease). Thus J.J. and S.J. were double heterozygotes for variants—in two unlinked genes—that predispose to thrombosis. Other family members (J.J.'s parents, brother, and older sister) were each heterozygous for one of these variants. All were counseled as to how to mitigate their personal risk of future thrombotic events and about thrombophilia risks for potential offspring.

BACKGROUND
Disease Etiology and Prevalence

Venous thrombosis (MIM 188050) is a multifactorial disorder (see Chapter 9). Its prevalence is thought to be lower among Asian and African populations than among those of European ancestry. Predisposing influences are a variety of genetic and nongenetic factors that lead to blood flow stasis, endothelial damage/trauma, and/or hypercoagulability. Identifiable genetic hypercoagulable states include variants that lead to (1) deficiencies of natural anticoagulants (e.g., protein C, protein S, antithrombin or tissue factor pathway inhibitor [TFPI]), (2) production of abnormal procoagulant factors with increased resistance to natural anticoagulants (FV Leiden), (3) excessive production of procoagulants (e.g., prothrombin G20210A), or (4) impaired clot lysis (e.g., dysfibrinogenemias).

While population prevalence of these disorders is about 4 to 6% (FV Leiden), 2% (prothrombin variants), or <1% (protein C and S variants), the prevalence among persons with venous thromboembolism is much higher: 12 to 14% (FV Leiden), 6 to 18% (prothrombin variant), 5 to 15% (protein C or S variants), and 25% overall.

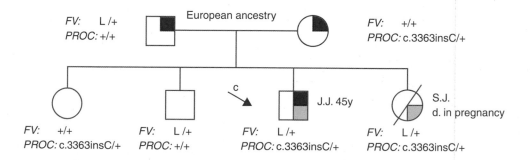

FV: L /+
PROC: +/+

European ancestry

FV: +/+
PROC: c.3363insC/+

FV: +/+
PROC: c.3363insC/+

FV: L /+
PROC: +/+

c

FV: L /+
PROC: c.3363insC/+

J.J. 45y

FV: L /+
PROC: c.3363insC/+

S.J.
d. in pregnancy

Thrombophilia **Key:**

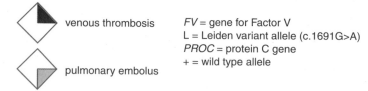

venous thrombosis

pulmonary embolus

FV = gene for Factor V
L = Leiden variant allele (c.1691G>A)
PROC = protein C gene
+ = wild type allele

Pedigree Case 46

FV Leiden, a missense variant in the FV gene (c.1691G>A leading to an amino acid change p.Arg506Gln), has a (heterozygous) prevalence among healthy European populations of about 4 to 6%. In select groups – some Roma clusters in Eastern Europe and some regions in Scandinavia – the prevalence may be as high as 15%. In contrast, among non-European populations (Asian or African), the variant is extremely rare. It is thought that FV Leiden arose from a mutation in a European founder about 21,000 years ago; it likely conveyed a survival advantage to female carriers by lessening bleeding from menstruation and childbirth. Homozygosity for FV Leiden occurs in approximately 1 in 5000 individuals.

Protein C (PROC) deficiency (MIM 176860) has a prevalence of 0.2 to 0.4%, with no major population differences. Inherited deficiency of PROC arises from variants in the *PROC* coding and regulatory sequences. Many are sporadic, although some – such as the French-Canadian variant, c.3363insC – entered populations through founder effects. Unlike the gain-of-function FV Leiden, *PROC* variants impair PROC production (85–90% of cases) or produce abnormal PROC with reduced function (10–15% of cases). All cause reduced PROC activity (levels generally less than 55% of normal), leading to reduced inactivation of activated clotting factors V and VIII, thus predisposing to increased clot formation.

Pathogenesis

The coagulation system maintains a delicate balance of clot formation – arising from a coordinated sequence of procoagulants (enzymes [FVII, FXI, FIX, FX, and FII] and cofactors [FV and FVIII]) – and clot inhibition caused by several natural anticoagulants that dampen fibrin production to prevent overwhelming clot formation (thrombosis) and disseminated intravascular coagulation (see Fig. 9.10). This fine balance can be undone, leading either to bleeding – usually from insufficient procoagulant activity (e.g., deficiency of FVIII [hemophilia A]) – or to excessive clotting, usually from insufficient anticoagulant activity or increased procoagulant activity (high levels or procoagulants with increased resistance to anticoagulation, e.g., FV Leiden) (Fig. C.46.1).

Activated FV – a cofactor for activated FX – accelerates the conversion of prothrombin (FII) to thrombin (activated FII). Membrane-bound FV (as well as FVIII) is inactivated by activated PROC, which cleaves activated factor V at three sites (Arg306, Arg506, and Arg679). Protein S – a cofactor for protein C – accelerates the inactivation of activated FV by PROC. Consequently, a lower amount of either protein C or S will result in insufficient dampening of FV cofactor function, resulting in excessive conversion of prothrombin to thrombin, leading to excessive clot formation.

The FV Leiden variant removes the preferred site for PROC proteolysis of activated FV, thereby slowing inactivation of activated FV, predisposing to excess thrombin formation and ultimately to clot formation. The lifetime risks for venous thrombosis due to FV Leiden heterozygosity or homozygosity are approximately 10 to 40% and 80%, respectively. In both cases, most thromboses occur in adulthood, particularly after 40 years of age. This can occur much earlier in women taking conventional oral contraceptives.

Heterozygous *PROC* pathogenic variants predispose to thrombophilia and carry a 20 to 75% lifetime risk for venous thrombosis. This is much higher than with heterozygous FV Leiden. Inheritance of two pathogenic *PROC* alleles usually

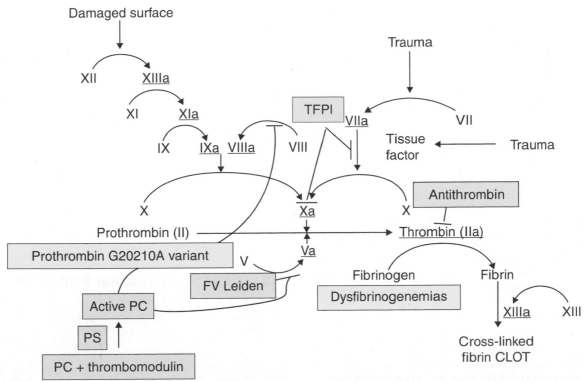

Figure C.46.1 Coagulation cascade showing both natural procoagulants (*black*) and anticoagulants (*red*). Natural procoagulants are shown in *black* and natural anticoagulants in *red* (in *yellow boxes*: antithrombin, *TFPI* [tissue factor pathway inhibitor], and activated protein C/protein S and thrombomodulin). The negative feedback provided by these is shown in *red lines*. Additionally, variants in natural procoagulants (factor V Leiden, prothrombin, dysfibrinogenemia) leading to thrombophilias are shown in *green boxes*. Note that high levels of certain procoagulants (e.g., FVIII) have also been shown to cause thrombophilia. Activated factors are denoted by a little "a" and are underlined. *PC*, protein C; *PS*, protein S, *TFPI*, tissue factor pathway inhibitor. (Courtesy Dr. Manuel Carcao, SickKids Hospital.)

results in purpura fulminans: a form of disseminated intravascular coagulation presenting in neonates/infants, which is often fatal if not treated promptly.

Being heterozygous for FV Leiden or for a *PROC* pathogenic variant makes a person genetically more susceptible to a venous clot. However, such individuals may never experience a blood clot (e.g., J.J.'s brother and older sister), depending on other genetic and nongenetic risk modifiers. Factors that increase such risk include anything that causes (1) increased blood stasis (immobility, obesity and/or pregnancy) resulting in compressed veins, (2) endothelial damage/trauma (surgery, trauma, cardiac disease, presence of central venous lines), or (3) increased thrombophilia (hypercoagulable state). The latter can result from acquired conditions that further increase thrombophilic potential: being on oral contraceptives (triples risk of thrombosis), pregnancy, antiphospholipid antibodies (e.g., in systemic lupus erythematosus), advanced age, and tobacco smoking. Additional genetic factors include non–O blood type or mild bleeding disorders, which may reduce the risk of clots in heterozygotes for FV Leiden or *PROC* variants. The interplay of various genetic and nongenetic factors ultimately determines the likelihood of thrombosis. Note that J.J. developed a blood clot only at age 45, following a long-distance flight, despite his digenic heterozygosity for variants in two thrombophilia genes. By then, he had the additional risks of older age and blood stasis from immobility during the flight. Compared to the general population, women heterozygous for FV Leiden have a 3- to 5-fold increased risk of venous thrombosis, but this increases to 20- to 30-fold if they are also on oral contraceptives.

PHENOTYPE AND NATURAL HISTORY

Although thrombi can develop in any vein, most arise at sites of injury or in the large venous sinuses or valve cusp pockets of the legs. Leg thrombi are usually confined to the distal veins of the calf, but approximately 20% extend into more proximal vessels (i.e., in the thigh and possibly pelvis) leading to proximal deep venous thrombosis (DVT). This can cause swelling, warmth, erythema, tenderness, distention of superficial veins, and prominent venous collaterals, although (if the clot is small) individuals may be asymptomatic.

Once formed, a thrombus can propagate along the vein, eventually giving rise to an embolism (a piece of thrombus that detaches itself and moves – usually to the lungs), or gradually being removed by fibrinolysis, or becoming organized and possibly recanalized. A pulmonary embolism is serious and can be acutely fatal if it obstructs the pulmonary arterial system, which occurs in 5–20% of those presenting initially with DVT. In contrast, thrombi that persist can chronically impede venous return and cause postthrombotic syndrome: a condition of venous hypertension and valvular insufficiency leading to chronic leg edema and pain and (less commonly) to skin breakdown and ulceration. Individuals with proximal DVT have a 40% risk for recurrent venous thrombosis if not placed on long-term anticoagulation.

MANAGEMENT

The diagnosis of DVT of the calf is difficult because individuals are often asymptomatic, and most tests are relatively insensitive until the thrombus extends proximally into larger veins in the thigh. Doppler ultrasonography is used most often to diagnose DVT as it detects flow abnormalities in the veins.

FV Leiden can be identified directly by DNA analysis or can be suspected based on activated PROC resistance. Protein C deficiency is diagnosed by measuring PROC activity; *PROC*

variants are identified by molecular genetic analysis. One caveat when testing PROC levels is that, as for all vitamin K-dependent factors (FII, FVII, FIX, FX, protein C and S), levels are reduced in neonates and infants, only achieving normal adult levels in adolescence. Hence a slightly "reduced" PROC in early life is likely normal.

FV Leiden is one of the most requested tests in clinical genetics laboratories. The matter is controversial, but also evolving. The American College of Medical Genetics and Genomics revised its guidance in 2018, saying, "testing is recommended for certain targeted populations/circumstances; it is not recommended indiscriminately for all patients with VTE [venous thromboembolism] or for the general population. Testing indications from different professional organizations vary."

Acute treatment focuses on minimizing thrombus propagation and associated complications – particularly pulmonary embolism – usually with anticoagulation and elevation of the affected extremity. Subsequent therapy focuses on prevention of recurrent venous thrombosis through identification and reduction/amelioration of acquired risk factors (e.g., oral contraceptives, obesity) and short-term anticoagulant use (in settings of surgery, trauma) or long-term continuous anticoagulant prophylaxis. Treatment recommendations for patients with PROC deficiency and FV Leiden are still evolving. All should receive standard initial therapy followed by at least 3 to 6 months of anticoagulant therapy. It is unclear which individuals with a single pathogenic allele should receive prolonged therapy, but this is generally prescribed for those with a second episode of DVT. In contrast, individuals homozygous for FV Leiden or other thrombophilia variants, or who are doubly heterozygous for digenic thrombophilia variants (such as J.J. and his deceased sister) are usually placed on long-term anticoagulation after their initial episode.

INHERITANCE

Each child of a couple in which one parent is heterozygous for a thrombophilic variant has a 50% risk of inheriting the thrombophilic allele. This, in turn, is associated with about a 50% lifetime risk for blood clot (compared to about 5% in the general population).

Being heterozygous for any inherited thrombophilia allele is reasonably common: estimated at 6 to 8% of the population. Among such individuals, it cannot be predicted who will develop a blood clot, but if they do occur, it is rare in childhood. Consequently, testing young children for these conditions is controversial. Prenatal testing is not routine; however, it may be useful when there is the possibility of homozygous or compound heterozygous *PROC* variants, because of the severity of the disease (purpura fulminans) and the need for prompt neonatal treatment. Similarly, testing of girls in families with known thrombophilias is advised prior to prescribing oral contraceptives.

QUESTIONS FOR SMALL GROUP DISCUSSION

1. Some studies of oral contraceptives suggest that such drugs decrease the blood levels of protein S. How would this predispose to thrombosis? At a molecular level, why would this be expected to enhance the development of venous thromboses in women with an FV Leiden variant? Should such women avoid the use of oral contraceptives? Should all or only selected women be tested for FV Leiden before being prescribed oral contraceptives?

2. Testing of asymptomatic relatives for FV Leiden is controversial. To be of clear utility, what should presymptomatic testing allow?

3. Synergism is the multiplication of risk with the cooccurrence of risk factors. Illustrate this with FV Leiden and protein C deficiency (the family of J.J. is an example), FV Leiden and oral contraceptive use, and FV Leiden and surgery/immobility.

4. FV Leiden is thought to reduce intrapartum bleeding. How would this lead to a heterozygote advantage and maintenance of a high allele frequency in the population?

REFERENCES

Kujovich JL: Factor V Leiden thrombophilia. http://www.ncbi.nlm.nih.gov/books/NBK1368/.

Lindqvist PG, Dahlbäck B: Carriership of Factor V Leiden and evolutionary selection advantage, *Curr Med Chem* 15:1541–1544, 2008.

Sode BF, Allin KH, Dahl M, Gyntelberg F, Nordestgaard BG: Risk of venous thromboembolism and myocardial infarction associated with factor V Leiden and prothrombin mutations and blood type, *CMAJ* 185(5):E229–37, 2013.

Zhang S, Taylor AK, Huang X, Luo B, Spector EB, Fang P, Richards CS; ACMG Laboratory Quality Assurance Committee. Venous thromboembolism laboratory testing (factor V Leiden and factor II c.*97G>A), 2018 update: a technical standard of the American College of Medical Genetics and Genomics (ACMG). *Genet Med.* 2018 Dec;20(12):1489–1498. https://pubmed.ncbi.nlm.nih.gov/30297698/. Epub 2018 Oct 5. PMID: 30297698.

TURNER SYNDROME (Female Monosomy X)
Chromosomal

Jeanne Wolstencroft • David Skuse

PRINCIPLES
- Nondisjunction
- Prenatal selection
- Haploinsufficiency

MAJOR PHENOTYPIC FEATURES
- Age at onset: prenatal
- Short stature
- Ovarian dysgenesis
- Sexual immaturity

HISTORY AND PHYSICAL FINDINGS

L.W., a 14-year-old girl, was referred to the endocrinology clinic for evaluation of absent secondary sexual characteristics (menses and breast development). Although born small for gestational age, she had been in good health and had normal intellect. No other family members had similar problems. Her examination was normal except for short stature, Tanner stage I sexual development, and broad chest with widely spaced nipples. After briefly discussing causes of short stature and delayed or absent sexual development, her physician requested follicle-stimulating hormone (FSH) level, growth hormone (GH) level, bone age study, and chromosome analysis. These tests showed a normal GH level, an elevated FSH level, and an abnormal karyotype (45,X). The physician explained that L.W. had Turner syndrome. L.W. was treated with GH supplements to maximize her linear growth; one year later, she started estrogen and progesterone therapy to induce the development of secondary sexual characteristics.

BACKGROUND
Disease Etiology and Incidence

Turner syndrome is a disorder caused by complete or partial absence of a second X chromosome in females. It has an incidence of between 1 in 2000 and 1 in 5000 liveborn girls. Approximately 50% of Turner syndrome cases are associated with a 45,X karyotype, 25% with a structural abnormality of the second X chromosome, and 25% with 45,X mosaicism (see Chapter 6).

Monosomy for the X chromosome can arise either by the failure to transmit a sex chromosome to one of the gametes or by loss of a sex chromosome from the zygote or early embryo. Failure to transmit a paternal sex chromosome to a gamete is the most common cause of a 45,X karyotype; 70 to 80% of girls with a 45,X karyotype are conceived from a sperm lacking a sex chromosome. Loss of a sex chromosome from a cell in the early embryo is the likely cause of 45,X mosaicism.

Pathogenesis

The mechanism by which X chromosome monosomy causes Turner syndrome in girls is poorly understood. The X chromosome contains many loci that do not undergo complete X inactivation (see Chapter 6), several of which appear to be necessary for ovarian maintenance and female fertility.

Although oocyte development requires only a single X chromosome, oocyte maintenance requires two X chromosomes. In the absence of a second X chromosome, therefore, oocytes in fetuses and neonates with Turner syndrome degenerate, and their ovaries atrophy into streaks of fibrous tissue. The genetic bases for the other features of the syndrome – such as the cystic hygroma, lymphedema, broad chest, cardiac anomalies, renal anomalies, and sensorineural hearing deficit – have not been defined but presumably reflect haploinsufficiency for one or more X-linked genes that do not normally undergo inactivation in the female.

PHENOTYPE AND NATURAL HISTORY

Although 45,X conceptuses account for 1 to 2% of all pregnancies, less than 1% of 45,X conceptions result in a liveborn infant. In view of the mild phenotype in individuals with Turner syndrome, this high rate of miscarriage and its timing are remarkable, suggesting that a second sex chromosome is required for intrauterine survival, particularly at the beginning of the second trimester.

All individuals with Turner syndrome have short stature, and more than 90% have ovarian dysgenesis. The latter is sufficiently severe that only 10 to 20% of these girls have spontaneous pubertal development (breast budding and pubic hair growth), and only 2 to 5% have spontaneous menses. Many also have physical anomalies, such as webbed neck, low nuchal hairline, broad chest, cardiac anomalies, renal anomalies, sensorineural hearing deficit, edema of the hands and feet, or dysplastic nails (Fig. C.47.1). Nearly 50% have a bicuspid aortic valve and therefore an increased risk for aortic root dilatation and dissection. Nearly 60% have renal anomalies and an increased risk for renal dysfunction.

Most of these girls and women have normal intellectual development; verbal intelligence is usually within the average range, but performance intelligence is typically half a standard deviation lower. Those with intellectual impairment usually have an X chromosome structural abnormality. Individuals with Turner syndrome have a higher risk of developing psychiatric or neurodevelopmental disorders, including a fourfold increase in risk of autism spectrum disorder. Most of those with Turner syndrome report difficulties in making and keeping friends in adolescence and report social isolation in adulthood.

In addition to the complications resulting from their congenital anomalies, women with Turner syndrome have an increased incidence of osteoporotic fractures, thyroiditis, diabetes mellitus type 1 and type 2, inflammatory bowel disease, and cardiovascular disease. The causes of the diabetes mellitus, thyroid disorders, and inflammatory bowel disease are unclear. Estrogen deficiency is probably largely responsible for the osteoporosis and the increased incidence of atherosclerosis, ischemic heart disease, and stroke; diabetes mellitus probably accentuates the cardiovascular effects of the estrogen deficiency.

MANAGEMENT

When stature in an individual with Turner syndrome falls below the 5th percentile, she is usually treated with GH

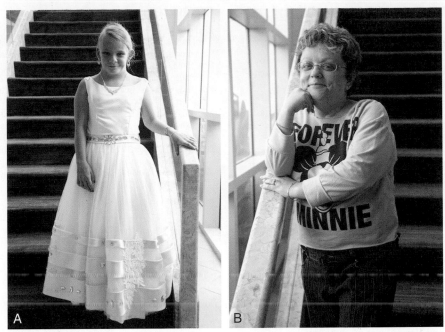

Figure C.47.1 (A) Hannah and (B) Connie representing their support group (Turner Syndrome Society of the United States [turner-syndrome.org]). (Photos by Rick Guidotti, Positive Exposure [positiveexposure.org].)

supplements until her bone age reaches 15 years (Fig. C.47.2). On average, this treatment results in a gain of 6 to 8 cm in predicted height; the improvement in final height is less, however, the later GH therapy is started. Concurrent estrogen therapy decreases the effectiveness of GH.

Estrogen therapy is usually initiated at approximately 14 to 15 years of age to promote development of secondary sexual characteristics and reduce the risk for osteoporosis. Progesterone therapy is added to the regimen to induce menses, either at the time of the first vaginal breakthrough bleeding or in the second year of estrogen therapy. Both are associated with an increased risk for thrombosis, and case reports indicate that there may be a risk in those with Turner syndrome above that for the general population of hormone therapy users.

In addition, medical management usually includes serial echocardiography to evaluate aortic root dilatation and valvar heart disease, renal ultrasonography to find congenital renal anomalies, and a glucose tolerance test to detect diabetes.

Women who have complete ovarian dysgenesis do not ovulate spontaneously or conceive children. If they have adequate cardiovascular and renal function, women with Turner syndrome can have children via in vitro fertilization and ovum donation. They do, however, have a significantly increased risk for aortic dissection and rupture with pregnancy.

INHERITANCE

Turner syndrome is not associated with advanced maternal or paternal age. Although there have been a few familial recurrences, it is usually sporadic, and the empirical recurrence risk for future pregnancies is not increased above that of the general population. If Turner syndrome is suspected on the basis of fetal ultrasound findings, such as a cystic hygroma, the diagnosis should be confirmed by chromosome analysis of chorionic villi or amniocytes.

Only a few pregnancies have been reported among spontaneously menstruating patients with Turner syndrome. Among the resulting offspring, one in three has had congenital anomalies, such as congenital heart disease, Down syndrome, or spina bifida. The apparently increased risk for congenital anomalies

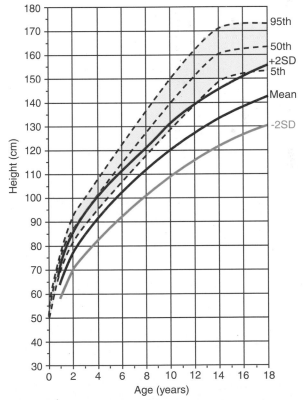

Figure C.47.2 Growth curves for normal (*shaded dotted lines*) and approximately 350 Turner syndrome girls (*solid lines*). None of the subjects received hormone treatment. (Modified from Lyon AJ, Preece MA, Grant DB: Growth curve for girls with Turner syndrome. *Arch Dis Child* 60:932, 1985, by permission.)

may be due to ascertainment bias in reporting, because pregnancy is unusual in these women. If the increased risk is a real finding, the cause is unknown.

QUESTIONS FOR SMALL GROUP DISCUSSION

1. Some observations have suggested that patients with Turner syndrome who inherit a paternal X chromosome are more outgoing and have better social adaptation than those who inherit a maternal X chromosome. What molecular mechanisms could explain this?
2. X-chromosome monosomy is the only viable human monosomy (other than the Y in males). Discuss possible reasons.
3. Discuss possible reasons for the high rate of birth defects among the children of women with Turner syndrome.
4. Maternal meiotic nondisjunction gives rise more frequently to Down syndrome and paternal meiotic nondisjunction to Turner syndrome. Discuss possible reasons.
5. Discuss the psychosocial support and counseling that are appropriate and necessary for individuals with Turner syndrome.

REFERENCES

Björlin Avdic H, Butwicka A, Nordenström A, Almqvist C, Nordenskjöld A, Engberg H, Frisén L: Neurodevelopmental and psychiatric disorders in females with Turner syndrome: A population-based study, *J Neurodev Disord* 13(1):1–9, 2021.

Gonzalez L, Witchel SF: The patient with Turner syndrome: Puberty and medical management concerns, *Fertil Steril* 98:780–786, 2012.

Hong DS, Reiss AL: Cognitive and neurological aspects of sex chromosome aneuploidies, *Lancet Neurol* 13:306–318, 2014.

Hook EB, Warburton D: Turner syndrome revisited: Review of new data supports the hypothesis that all viable 45,X cases are cryptic mosaics with a rescue cell line, implying an origin by mitotic loss, *Hum Genet* 133:417–424, 2014.

Legro RS: Turner syndrome: New insights into an old disorder, *Fertil Steril* 98:773–774, 2012.

Wolstencroft J, Skuse D: Social skills and relationships in Turner syndrome, *Curr Opin Psychiatry* 32(2):85–91, 2019.

48 XERODERMA PIGMENTOSUM (MIM 278700)
(Defect of Nucleotide Excision Repair, *XPA* Pathogenic Variants)

Autosomal Recessive

Ada Hamosh

PRINCIPLES

- Variable expressivity
- Genetic heterogeneity
- Genetic complementation
- Caretaker tumor-suppressor genes

MAJOR PHENOTYPIC FINDINGS

- Age at onset: childhood
- Ultraviolet light sensitivity
- Skin cancer
- Neurological dysfunction

HISTORY AND PHYSICAL FINDINGS

W.S., a 3-year-old girl, was referred to the dermatology clinic for evaluation of severe sun sensitivity and freckling. On physical examination, she was photophobic and had conjunctivitis and prominent freckled hyperpigmentation in sun-exposed areas; her development and physical examination were otherwise normal. W.S. was the child of nonconsanguineous Japanese parents; no one else in the family was similarly affected. The dermatologist explained that W.S. had classic features of xeroderma pigmentosum, that is, "parchment-like, pigmented skin." To confirm the diagnosis, W.S. was referred to genetics for testing and counseling. The results of single variant analysis testing of *XPA* confirmed the diagnosis of xeroderma pigmentosum due to homozygous splice site variant, c.390-1 G>C, which is very common in the Japanese population (see below). Despite appropriate preventive measures, W.S. developed metastatic melanoma at 15 years of age and died 2 years later. Her parents had two other children; neither was affected with xeroderma pigmentosum.

BACKGROUND
Disease Etiology and Incidence

Xeroderma pigmentosum (XP) is a genetically heterogeneous autosomal recessive disorder of DNA repair that causes marked sensitivity to UV irradiation (see Table C.48.1). In the United

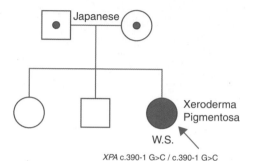

Pedigree Case 48

States and Europe, the prevalence is approximately 1 in 1 million, but in Japan, the prevalence is 1 in 22,000. Over 55% of XP patients in Japan have XPA and, among these individuals, more than 90% are homozygous for the *XPA* c.390-1 G>C variant at the splice acceptor site of intron 3. Approximately 1% of the Japanese population carries this allele, presumably due to founder effect.

Pathogenesis

Repair of DNA damaged by UV irradiation occurs via three mechanisms: excision repair, postreplication repair, and photoreactivation. Excision repair mends DNA damage via nucleotide excision repair or base excision repair. Postreplication repair is a damage tolerance mechanism that allows replication of DNA across a damaged template. Photoreactivation reverts damaged DNA to the normal chemical state without removing or exchanging any genetic material.

Nucleotide excision repair is a complex but versatile process involving at least 30 proteins. The basic principle is the removal of a small single-stranded DNA segment containing a lesion by incision to either side of the damaged segment and subsequent gap-filling repair synthesis with the use of the intact complementary strand as a template. Within transcribed genes, DNA damage blocks RNA polymerase II progression. The stalled RNA polymerase II initiates nucleotide excision

TABLE C.48.1 Complementation Groups in Xeroderma Pigmentosum and Related Disorders

Complementation Group	MIM	Gene	Process Affected	Phenotype
XPA	278700	*XPA*	Recognition of DNA damage	XP
XPB	133510	*ERCC3*	DNA unwinding	XP-CS, TTD
XPC	278720	*XPC*	Recognition of DNA damage	XP
XPD	278730	*ERCC2*	DNA unwinding	XP, TTD, XP-CS
XPE	278740	*DDB2*	Recognition of DNA damage	XP
XPF	278760	*ERCC4*	Endonuclease	XP, sometimes with late-onset neurologic abnormalities
XPG	278780	*ERCC5*	Endonuclease	XP, XP-CS
XPV	278750	*POLH*	Translesional DNA synthesis	XP
CSA	216400	*ERCC8*	Transcription-coupled repair	CS
CSB	133540	*ERCC6*	Transcription-coupled repair	CS

CS, Cockayne syndrome; *TTD*, trichothiodystrophy; *XP*, xeroderma pigmentosum; *XP-CS*, combined XP and Cockayne syndrome phenotype.

repair (transcription-coupled repair). In the rest of the genome and on nontranscribed strands of genes, a nucleotide excision repair complex identifies DNA damage by detection of helical distortions within the DNA (global genome repair).

On occasion, nucleotide excision repair will not have repaired a lesion before DNA replication. Because such lesions inhibit the progression of DNA replication, postreplication repair bypasses the lesion, allowing DNA synthesis to continue. DNA polymerase η mediates translesional DNA synthesis; it efficiently and accurately catalyzes synthesis past dithymidine lesions.

XP is caused by pathogenic variants in genes involved in the global genome repair subpathway of nucleotide excision repair or those affecting postreplication repair. In contrast, Cockayne syndrome, a related disorder, is caused by pathogenic variants affecting the transcription-coupled repair subpathway of nucleotide excision repair. XP and Cockayne syndrome have been separated into 10 biochemical complementation groups; each group reflects dysfunction of a different component of nucleotide excision repair or postreplication repair (see Table C.48.1).

The reduced or absent capacity for global genome repair or postreplication repair represents a loss of caretaker functions required for the maintenance of genome integrity, causing accumulation of oncogenic mutations (see Chapter 16). Cutaneous neoplasms from individuals with XP have a higher level of oncogene and tumor suppressor gene mutations than do tumors from others without XP, and the XP mutations appear to be highly UV specific.

PHENOTYPE AND NATURAL HISTORY

Individuals with XP develop symptoms at a median age of 1 to 2 years, although about 5% have onset after 14 years. Initial symptoms commonly include easy sunburning, acute photosensitivity, freckling, and photophobia. Continued cutaneous damage causes premature skin aging (thinning, wrinkling, solar lentigines, telangiectasias), premalignant actinic keratoses, and benign and malignant neoplasms (Fig. C.48.1). Nearly 65% of individuals develop basal cell or squamous cell carcinomas, or both, and approximately 5% develop melanomas. Approximately 90% of the carcinomas occur at the sites of

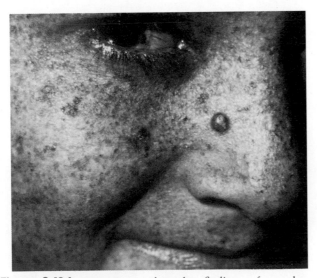

Figure C.48.1 Cutaneous and ocular findings of xeroderma pigmentosum. Note the freckled hyperpigmentation, the papillomatous and verrucous lesions on the skin, and the conjunctivitis. (Courtesy M. L. Levy, Baylor College of Medicine and Texas Children's Hospital, Houston.)

greatest UV exposure – the face, neck, head, and tip of the tongue. Individuals with XP have a 10- to 20-fold increased risk of other neoplasias, including brain and other central nervous system tumors, hematologic malignancies, breast cancer, papillary thyroid cancer, and kidney cancer. Before the introduction of preventive measures, the median age for development of cutaneous neoplasms was 8 years – 50 years younger than in the general population – and the frequency of such neoplasms was more than 1000-fold greater than that of the general population.

In addition to cutaneous signs, 60 to 90% of affected individuals experience ocular abnormalities, including photophobia, conjunctivitis, blepharitis, ectropion, and neoplasia. Again, the distribution of ocular damage and neoplasms corresponds to the sites of greatest UV exposure.

Approximately 25% of affected individuals experience progressive neurologic degeneration. Features include sensorineural deafness, intellectual disability, spasticity, hyporeflexia or areflexia, segmental demyelination, ataxia, choreoathetosis, and supranuclear ophthalmoplegia. The severity of neurological symptoms is usually proportionate to the severity of the nucleotide excision repair deficit. The neurodegeneration may result from an inability to repair DNA damaged by endogenously generated oxygen free radicals. The Japanese *XPA* variant results in absent XPA protein and, in addition to the skin and eye manifestation, leads to significant neurologic deterioration.

Nucleotide excision repair also corrects DNA damage from many chemical carcinogens, such as cigarette smoke, charred food, and cisplatin. Consequently, affected individuals have a 10- to 20-fold increase in the incidence of internal neoplasms, such as brain tumors, leukemia, lung tumors, and gastric carcinomas.

Without preventive protection, individuals with XP have a life span shortened by approximately 30 years. Metastatic melanoma and squamous cell skin carcinoma are the most common causes of death.

Cockayne syndrome and trichothiodystrophy are also caused by defects in components of the cellular mechanism for repair of UV-induced DNA damage. Both are characterized by poor postnatal growth, diminished subcutaneous tissue, joint contractures, thin papery skin with photosensitivity, intellectual disability, and neurological deterioration. Children with Cockayne syndrome also have retinal degeneration and deafness; those with trichothiodystrophy have ichthyosis and brittle hair and nails. Individuals with either syndrome rarely live past the second decade but do not have an increase in the frequency of skin cancers. However, defects in some repair genes (*ERCC2*, *ERCC3*, and *ERCC5*) produce phenotypes that combine characteristics of XP and either Cockayne syndrome or both Cockayne syndrome and trichothiodystrophy (see Table C.48.1).

MANAGEMENT

Diagnosis of XP is established using panel gene sequencing or exome sequencing by identification of biallelic pathogenic variants in one of the known XP genes. When these results are inconclusive, a clinical diagnosis relies on functional tests of DNA repair and UV sensitivity; such tests are usually performed on cultured skin fibroblasts.

The management of individuals with XP includes avoidance of exposure to sunlight, protective clothing, physical and chemical sunscreens, and careful surveillance for and excision of cutaneous malignant neoplasms. Measurement of head circumference, neurological assessment, hearing tests, and routine ophthalmologic examination are indicated. While no curative treatments are currently available, oral isotretinoin or acitretin can prevent development of additional skin cancers in those who have had multiple lesions excised. Systemic retinoids have side effects and are absolutely contraindicated in pregnancy; thus effective contraception is necessary in sexually active women of childbearing age who take these agents.

INHERITANCE

Because XP is an autosomal recessive disease, many affected individuals have no family history of the disorder. For parents of a child affected with XP, the likelihood for future children to have XP is 25%. Prenatal and preimplantation genetic diagnosis is possible by molecular testing if both pathogenic variants have been identified, or by functional testing of DNA repair and UV sensitivity in cultured amniocytes or chorionic villi.

QUESTIONS FOR SMALL GROUP DISCUSSION

1. Define complementation groups and explain their use for defining the biochemical basis of disease.
2. Compare and contrast XP and Cockayne syndrome. Why is Cockayne syndrome not associated with an increased risk for neoplasia?
3. Individuals with XP have a defect of cutaneous cellular immunity. How could the sensitivity of those with XP to UV irradiation explain this immunodeficiency? How could this immunodeficiency contribute to cancer susceptibility?
4. Werner syndrome, Bloom syndrome, XP, ataxia-telangiectasia, and Fanconi anemia are inherited diseases of genomic instability. What are the molecular mechanisms underlying each of these disorders? What types of genomic instability are associated with each disorder?

REFERENCES

DiGiovanna JJ, Kraemer KH: Shining a light on xeroderma pigmentosum, *J Invest Dermatol* 132:785–796, 2012.

Imoto K, Nadem C, Moriwaki S, *et al*: Ancient origin of a Japanese xeroderma pigmentosum founder mutation, *J Dermatol Sci* 69(2):175–176, 2013. https://doi.org/10.1016/j.jdermsci.2012.10.008

Kraemer KH, DiGiovanna JJ, Tamura D: Xeroderma pigmentosum. In Adam MP, Mirzaa GM, Pagon RA, editors: *GeneReviews® [Internet]*, Seattle (WA), 2003 Jun 20, University of Washington, Seattle, pp 1993–2022. [Updated 2022 Mar 24]. https://www.ncbi.nlm.nih.gov/books/NBK1397/

Leung AKC, Barankin B, Lam JM, Leong KF, Hon KL: Xeroderma pigmentosum: an updated review, *Drugs Context* 11, 2022. https://doi.org/10.7573/dic.2022-2-5

Menck CF, Munford V: DNA repair diseases: What do they tell us about cancer and aging? *Genet Mol Biol* 37:220–233, 2014.

Autosomal Dominant

Carolyn Dinsmore Applegate

PRINCIPLES

- Anticipation
- Short telomere syndromes
- Telomerase
- Telomere length

MAJOR PHENOTYPIC FEATURES

- Idiopathic pulmonary fibrosis
- Aplastic anemia with or without immunodeficiency
- Genetic anticipation
- Short telomere length for age

HISTORY AND PHYSICAL FINDINGS

C.A., an 11-year-old female, was recently diagnosed with aplastic anemia upon evaluation for increased bruising. Her medical history is otherwise significant for mild failure to thrive in infancy and borderline short stature. She reached her developmental milestones appropriately and is above grade level academically. Her father and 9-year-old brother are healthy. Her family history (see pedigree) is significant for thrombocytopenia in her 34-year-old mother and early graying in her 31-year-old maternal aunt. Her maternal grandfather died at age 61 from pulmonary fibrosis and his brother died in his late 50s from lung disease and liver cirrhosis in the setting of moderate alcohol and tobacco use. Based on C.A.'s family history, a short telomere syndrome (STS) was suspected after

hematology referred her to a medical geneticist and genetic counselor. Telomere length measured by flow cytometry and fluorescence in situ hybridization (FlowFISH) showed a telomere length significantly below the 1st percentile. Sequencing for a panel of genes associated with the STSs identified a heterozygous pathogenic variant in the *TERT* gene in C.A. The family was counseled that C.A. has an STS and that, as an autosomal dominant condition likely inherited from her mother, her brother has a 50% chance to also have an STS. Cascade-targeted testing for the pathogenic *TERT* variant showed that her mother and brother are also heterozygous for the pathogenic variant. After reduced-intensity chemotherapy, C.A. underwent haploidentical bone marrow transplant using her father as a donor.

BACKGROUND
Disease Etiology and Incidence

The short telomere syndromes (STSs) are caused by pathogenic variants in the genes encoding the enzyme, telomerase, and other components of the telomere-maintenance complex. The organ systems most commonly affected are the bone marrow, liver, lungs, and immune system. Age of onset and clinical presentation correlates with telomere length. Among individuals diagnosed with idiopathic pulmonary fibrosis, a pathogenic variant in *TERT* or *TERC* – which code for the two components of telomerase – can be identified in 8% to 15% of familial cases and 1% to 3% of sporadic cases.

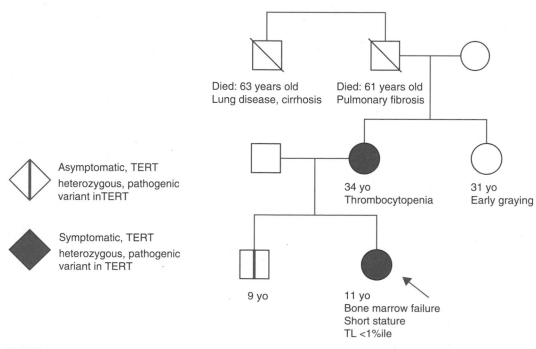

Died: 63 years old
Lung disease, cirrhosis

Died: 61 years old
Pulmonary fibrosis

Asymptomatic, TERT heterozygous, pathogenic variant in TERT

Symptomatic, TERT heterozygous, pathogenic variant in TERT

34 yo
Thrombocytopenia

31 yo
Early graying

9 yo

11 yo
Bone marrow failure
Short stature
TL <1%ile

TL, Telomere length; yo, years old.

Pedigree Case 49

Pathogenesis

Telomeres are repetitive sequences of DNA (TTACCG) present in 300 to 8000 copies at the ends of each chromosome. Shortening of the telomere occurs with each cell division, eventually leading to a DNA damage response that limits the capacity of stem cells to divide, because of apoptosis or senescence. Telomerase maintains telomere length by synthesizing new telomere DNA. The telomerase reverse transcriptase component, encoded by the *TERT* gene, is most commonly altered among STSs, accounting for 40% of cases across age groups. Pathogenic variants in the RNA component of telomerase, *TERC* (also known as *hTR*), along with those in 12 other genes, explain the remaining known subsets. In about 20 to 30% of cases, the gene responsible remains unrecognized.

The pathophysiology of STS has two main mechanisms. In high cell turnover compartments, such as the bone marrow and immune system, short telomere length limits the replicative potential and induces bone marrow failure. These organs are primarily affected in infants and children with severe short telomere defects. In adults, short telomere length may cause mild bone marrow failure and myelodysplastic syndrome – a clonal disorder of the bone marrow – but far more often manifests as pulmonary disease, with 70% of cases appearing as idiopathic pulmonary fibrosis (IPF). Short telomere length alone is not enough to induce stem cell failure in the lung, because this is a slow turnover compartment. Instead, it lowers the threshold for "second hits" from smoking or other exogenous (or endogenous) damage that provokes lung scarring. Up to 10% of adults with STSs may also develop liver disease, usually manifesting as cirrhosis.

Testing

Average telomere length follows a normal distribution pattern and can be plotted on a nomogram based on age; length decreases with age. Telomere length testing is recommended as the first line of investigation for the STSs in children and young adults. Telomere length below the 1st percentile has a high specificity for an STS, although other inherited bone marrow failure syndromes may be also associated with short telomeres. The specificity in adults is lower; adults highly suspected to have a related disease should have both telomere length and gene evaluation. Since telomere lengths above the 50th percentile have essentially a 100% negative predictive value, such testing is useful to rule out an STS across age groups. Genetic testing for telomere conditions is best done using a panel of genes known to cause the STSs; currently published genes account for about 70% of cases. Testing on exome-based platforms should be used with caution since *TERC*, as an RNA component, may not be captured by technologies using exome capture. Gene panel sequencing of an individual with telomere lengths below the 1st percentile is used to identify the disease-causing variant in the family. Subsequently, targeted variant testing can be offered for predictive or confirmatory testing in family members. Individuals with telomere lengths of 1% to 10% for age can also benefit from gene panel sequencing. Negative genetic test results do not eliminate the possibility of an STS, since not all causal genes have been identified.

Phenotype and Natural History

The phenotypic presentations of the STSs lie on a spectrum and are directly related to the severity of telomere shortening (Fig. C.49.1). Disease manifestations are age and telomere length dependent. Individuals with the most significant telomere shortening present in infancy with primary immune deficiency, most commonly manifesting as enterocolitis or aplastic anemia. Hoyeraal-Hreidarsson syndrome (HHS) presents with prenatal onset and syndromic manifestations of short telomeres, including fetal growth restriction (FGR), cerebellar hypoplasia, and microcephaly, in addition to severe immunodeficiency. Dyskeratosis congenita (DKC) is characterized by a triad of abnormal skin pigmentation, nail dystrophy, and leukoplakia (white patches) of the oral mucosa, along with short telomeres. DKC portends a high risk of bone marrow failure (up to 80%) in addition to an increased risk to develop pulmonary fibrosis, liver cirrhosis and/or certain malignancies. Pulmonary fibrosis is the most frequent manifestation of the STSs and represents the milder end of the spectrum. The age of

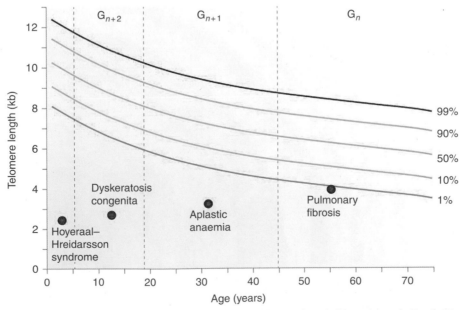

Figure C.49.1 Age-dependent manifestations of telomere syndromes. Telomere length has a normal distribution across all ages. The percentile *lines* show the typical age-related telomere length. The red *circles* show the age and phenotypic presentation of short telomere syndromes associated with the severity of telomere shortening. (Armanios M, Blackburn EH: The telomere syndromes, *Nat Rev Genet* 13(10):693–704, 2012 Oct. https://doi.org/10.1038/nrg3246. Epub 2012 Sep 11. Erratum in *Nat Rev Genet*, 14(3):235, 2013 Mar. PMID: 22965356; PMCID: PMC3548426.)

onset of short telomere-related pulmonary fibrosis ranges from the 50s to 80s, which significantly overlaps that of idiopathic pulmonary fibrosis in the general population but with a slight skew toward earlier onset. Women with STSs – particularly those with a history of smoking – may present with emphysema, independent of or in addition to pulmonary fibrosis.

Management

Treatment of STSs predominantly involves symptom management. Diagnosis of an STS informs treatment choice: immune-modulating drugs do not mitigate the symptoms or prevent progression of IPF or bone marrow failure and increase the risk for adverse effects. Individuals undergoing bone marrow and/or lung transplantation require reduced-intensity chemotherapy. Telomere length and targeted variant testing of asymptomatic family members can be useful to guide donor selection for individuals undergoing haploidentical bone marrow transplant.

INHERITANCE

The STSs follow the rules of Mendelian inheritance. Most STS disorders are inherited in an autosomal dominant pattern; *DKC1* variants are X-linked. HHS is typically caused by biallelic pathogenic variants in the telomere maintenance genes or in males with loss-of-function variants in the *DKC1* gene.

Individuals inherit their chromosomes, including their telomere length, from each parent. In some families with these disorders, telomere length becomes progressively shorter in successive generations, resulting in earlier ages of onset and differences in phenotypic expression of the condition (see Pedigree). Although mechanistically different than trinucleotide repeat expansion disorders, progressive shortening of telomeres in successive generations is another example of genetic anticipation.

QUESTIONS FOR SMALL GROUP DISCUSSION

1. Explain the involvement of different organ systems in the short telomere syndromes. In this pedigree, describe the risk to other family members and the most likely phenotypic presentation.
2. What might be the possible ill effects of long telomeres? How could this affect treatment of short telomere syndromes?
3. Compare and contrast the reasons for anticipation in short telomere syndromes and trinucleotide repeats.

REFERENCES

Alder JK, Hanumanthu VS, Strong MA, DeZern AE, Stanley SE, Takemoto CM, Danilova L, Applegate CD, Bolton SG, Mohr DW, Brodsky RA, Casella JF, Greider CW, Jackson JB, Armanios M: Diagnostic utility of telomere length testing in a hospital-based setting, *Proc Natl Acad Sci U S A* 115(10):E2358–E2365, 2018. https://doi.org/10.1073/pnas.1720427115

Armanios M, Blackburn EH: The telomere syndromes, *Nat Rev Genet* 13(10):693–704, 2012. https://doi.org/10.1038/nrg3246

Armanios MY, Chen JJ, Cogan JD, Alder JK, Ingersoll RG, Markin C, Lawson WE, Xie M, Vulto I, Phillips JA 3rd, Lansdorp PM, Greider CW, Loyd JE: Telomerase mutations in families with idiopathic pulmonary fibrosis, *N Engl J Med* 356(13):1317–1326, 2007. https://doi.org/10.1056/NEJMoa066157

Savage SA, Niewisch MR: Dyskeratosis congenita and related telomere biology disorders. In Adam MP, Mirzaa GM, Pagon RA, *et al.*, editors: *GeneReviews® [Internet]*, Seattle, 2009 Nov 12, University of Washington, pp 1993–2022. [Updated 2022 Mar 31]. https://www.ncbi.nlm.nih.gov/books/NBK22301/

Glossary

5′-Cap A modified nucleotide at the 5′ end of a growing mRNA chain, required for normal processing, stability, and translation of mRNA.

Acceptor splice site The boundary between the 3′ end of an intron and the 5′ end of the following exon. Also called the *3′ splice site*.

Acrocentric Refers to a chromosome with the centromere near one end. The human acrocentric chromosomes (13, 14, 15, 21, and 22) have satellite-bearing short arms that carry genes for ribosomal RNA. See *Chromosomal satellite*.

Active chromatin hub Nuclear domain where the proteins bound to the locus control region colocalize to permit gene expression.

Adjacent segregation During meiosis in a cell with a balanced reciprocal translocation, chromosomes form a *quadrivalent* and segregate in one of three ways: alternate, adjacent-1, or (rarely) adjacent 2. With adjacent segregation, unbalanced gametes are formed, causing zygotic lethality (see *Alternate segregation*; Fig. 5.11).

Adverse selection A term used in the insurance industry to describe the situation in which individuals with private knowledge of having an increased risk for illness, disability, or death buy disproportionately more coverage than those at a lower risk.

Allele One of the alternative versions of a gene or DNA sequence at a given locus.

Allele-specific oligonucleotide (ASO) A short DNA probe synthesized to match a particular DNA sequence precisely, allowing the discrimination of alleles that differ by only a single base.

Allelic heterogeneity In a population, different alleles at a single locus. Among individuals, different variant alleles at the same genetic locus associated with the same or similar phenotypes.

Allelic imbalance Unequal expression of the two alleles of a gene, which is monoallelic in the extreme. It can be random – as in *X-inactivation* – influenced by cellular selection pressure, or determined by parent of origin of the allele (*genomic imprinting*). It is a feature of neoplastic cells; for example, reflected as loss of heterozygosity.

Allogenic In transplantation, denotes individuals (or tissues) that are of the same species but that have different antigens (alternative spelling: allogeneic).

α-fetoprotein (AFP) A fetal glycoprotein excreted into the amniotic fluid. When the fetus has certain abnormalities – especially an open neural tube defect – AFP reaches abnormally high concentration in amniotic fluid (and maternal serum).

Alternate segregation During meiosis in a cell with a balanced reciprocal translocation, chromosomes form a quadrivalent; if subsequent segregation is "alternate," balanced gametes are formed that have either a normal chromosome complement or contain the two reciprocal balanced translocation chromosomes (see *Adjacent segregation*; Fig. 5.11).

***Alu* family of repetitive DNA** One class of repetitive sequences dispersed in the human genome, resulting from *retrotransposition*, so named because they are cleaved by the restriction enzyme AluI. Each sequence is approximately 280 bp. About 1 million copies exist per genome (see *Repetitive DNA, LINE sequences*).

Amniocentesis A procedure used in prenatal diagnosis to obtain amniotic fluid, which contains proteins and cells of fetal origin that can be analyzed prenatally. Amniotic fluid is withdrawn from the amniotic sac by syringe after needle insertion through the abdominal and uterine wall.

Analytic validity In reference to a clinical laboratory test, the accuracy with which a given characteristic is identified. Standards for clinical use are established by professional and federal regulators such as CLIA (Clinical Laboratory Improvement Amendments) (see *Clinical utility, Clinical validity*).

Anaphase Stages in mitosis or meiosis (Anaphase I, II) when chromosomes separate and move to opposite poles of the dividing cell. In mitosis and anaphase II of meiosis, centromeres divide, and sister chromatids become daughter chromosomes. In anaphase I, homologous paired chromosomes move to opposite poles.

Ancestry informative markers Loci with alleles that show large differences in frequency among populations originating in different parts of the world.

Aneuploidy A form of *heteroploidy* where the chromosome number is not an exact multiple of the haploid number. (Note that absence or presence of complete sets is still considered euploidy.) Aneuploid karyotypes in humans have the suffix "-somy"; for example, *trisomy* (the presence of an extra chromosome) and *monosomy* (the absence of a single chromosome).

Anomalies Birth defects resulting from malformations, deformations, or disruptions.

Anticipation The progressively earlier onset and increased severity of certain diseases in successive generations of a family. The phenomenon is a feature of diseases (e.g., myotonic dystrophy or Huntington disease (Case 24) associated with genomic repeat expansions that are dynamic and continue to expand through generations.

Anticodon A three-base segment of transfer RNA (tRNA) complementary to a codon in messenger RNA (mRNA).

Antisense oligonucleotide (ASO) Synthetic short single-stranded DNA or RNA molecule that can hybridize specifically to its complementary RNA sequence in a specific target to alter function. Antisense binding to pre-mRNA or microRNA triggers effects by causing its degradation, inhibiting its translation, or modulating its splicing. ASO-based strategies have strong therapeutic potential, notably for conditions such as Duchenne muscular dystrophy and spinal muscular atrophy. (Note that ASO is also used as an abbreviation for allele-specific oligonucleotide.)

Antisense strand of DNA The noncoding DNA strand, which is complementary to mRNA and serves as the template for RNA synthesis. Also called the *transcribed strand*.

Apoenzyme The protein component of an enzyme that also requires a cofactor to become active. The apoenzyme with the cofactor is termed the *holoenzyme*.

Apoptosis Programmed natural cell death that is highly regulated and can confer advantages to the organism. (Distinguished from necrosis.) Various disease states occur when apoptosis is either inhibited (e.g., cancers or inflammatory conditions) or hyperactive (e.g., neurodegenerative or hematological disorders).

Array CGH Comparative genome hybridization performed by hybridizing a test DNA sample to a wafer ("chip") onto which a large number of specified reference nucleic acid fragments ("probes") have been arrayed in a matrix pattern. It detects genomic copy number variation at high resolution with high throughput. See *Microarray*.

Ascertainment The selection of individuals for inclusion in a genetic study.

Ascertainment bias Sampling bias in a medical context, such that measurement of the true frequency of a phenomenon is distorted by how a study population is ascertained. Care is needed in family studies to account for such bias.

Association (1) In genetic epidemiology, the occurrence of a particular genotype significantly more or less frequently among individuals with a given trait than among the general population. (Contrast with *linkage*, which refers to nonrandom association between genotypes.) (2) In dysmorphology, a group of abnormalities of unknown etiology and pathogenesis that is seen together more often than would be expected by chance.

Assortative mating Selection of a mate with preference for a particular genotype; that is, nonrandom mating. More often positive (preference for a mate of the same genotype) than negative.

Assortment The random separation of homologous chromosomes to the gametes during meiosis. Alleles of different genes assort independently, unless they are linked.

Autologous Refers to cells or tissues obtained from the same individual, such as in transplantation.

Autosome Any nuclear chromosome other than the sex chromosomes; 22 pairs in the human karyotype. A trait involving an autosomal gene or gene pair shows *autosomal inheritance*.

Balanced polymorphism (or balanced polymorphic alleles) The result of balancing selection. A variant allele may be maintained at relatively high frequency in the population despite being deleterious in the homozygous state, usually due to heterozygote advantage.

Barr body The sex chromatin as seen in female somatic cells, representing an inactive X chromosome.

Base pair (bp) A pair of complementary nucleotide bases, as in double-stranded DNA. Used as the unit of length of a DNA sequence.

Bayesian analysis A mathematical method widely used in genetics to calculate recurrence risks. The method combines information from several sources (genetics, pedigree information, and test results) to determine the probability that an individual will develop or transmit a certain disorder.

Beneficence The ethical principle of behaving in a way that promotes the well-being of others. Contrast with *Maleficence*.

Binomial expansion When there are two alternative classes, one with probability p and the other with probability $1 - p = q$, the frequencies of the possible combinations of p and q in a series of n trials is $(p + q)^n$.

Biochemical genetics The study of the genetic basis for phenotype focused on biochemical pathways and metabolism.

Bioinformatics Computational analysis and storage of biological and experimental data, widely applied to genomic and proteomic studies.

Birth defect An abnormality present at birth, not necessarily genetic.

Bivalent A pair of homologous chromosomes in association, as seen at metaphase of the first meiotic division.

Blastocyst See Chapter 15 Box 15.1.

Blood group The phenotype produced by genetically determined antigens on a red blood cell. The antigens formed by a set of allelic genes make up a blood group system.

Body mass index (BMI) A measure of weight corrected for height, used to classify weight status. Calculated as weight divided by square of the height (kg/m^2).

Caretaker genes Tumor-suppressor genes that are indirectly involved in controlling cellular proliferation by repairing DNA damage and maintaining genomic integrity, thereby protecting protooncogenes and gatekeeper tumor-suppressor genes from mutations that could lead to cancer.

Carrier An individual heterozygous for a particular variant allele. The term is used for a heterozygote for an autosomal recessive trait, or for a heterozygous female for an X-linked recessive trait. Also used to describe an individual with a chromosomal alteration, such as a translocation. In reference to dominant traits, "heterozygous for…" is clearer terminology.

Case-control study An epidemiological method in which individuals with a condition (the cases) are compared with suitably chosen individuals without the condition (the controls) with respect to the relative frequency of various putative risk factors.

Cell cycle The series of stages through which a cell progresses as it prepares for and undergoes a mitotic division. Consists of the G_1, S, G_2, and M stages.

Cell-free DNA DNA detectable in body fluids that is not packaged as chromatin inside the nucleus of a cell.

Centimorgan (cM) A unit of distance between loci along chromosomes, named for Thomas Hunt Morgan, reflecting recombination frequency. One cM corresponds to recombination between loci in 1% of meiotic events.

Centromere The primary constriction on the chromosome, where sister chromatids are held together and at which the kinetochore is formed. Required for normal segregation in mitosis and meiosis.

Centrosomes A pair of centers that organize the growth of the microtubules of the mitotic spindle; visible at the poles of the dividing cell in late prophase.

CGH See *Comparative genome hybridization*.

Chain termination codon See *Termination codon*.

Checkpoints Positions in the *cell cycle*, usually at the junction between the G_1 and S or the G_2 and M stages, at which the cell determines whether to proceed to the next stage of the cycle.

Chemical individuality A term coined by Archibald Garrod to describe the naturally occurring differences in the genetic and biochemical makeup of individuals that makes each one unique.

Chemical library An annotated collection of hundreds to tens of thousands of small molecules, increasingly used in drug discovery. High-throughput screening may identify a compound that interacts with a target; for example, to restore activity to an altered protein. Such chemicals or their derivatives may then be developed into drugs.

Chimera An individual composed of cells derived from two genetically different zygotes. In humans, *blood group chimeras* result from exchange of hematopoietic stem cells by dizygotic twins in utero; *dispermic chi-*

meras, which are very rare, result from fusion of two zygotes into one individual. Chimerism is also an inevitable result of transplantation. Contrast with *mosaic* (see *Mosaicism*).

Chorionic villus sampling (CVS) A procedure used for prenatal diagnosis between 11 and 14 weeks of gestation. Fetal tissue for analysis is withdrawn from the villous area of the chorion either trans-cervically or transabdominally under ultrasonographic guidance.

Chromatids After DNA replication, chromosomes consist of two parallel strands of chromatin (referred to as *sister chromatids*), connected at the centromere.

Chromatin The complex of DNA and proteins of which chromosomes are composed. See *Nucleosome*.

Chromatin remodeling DNA packaged in nucleosomes is subject to remodeling between chromatin states through the activity of enzymatic chromatin remodeling complexes. Packaged DNA can thereby be made accessible to facilitate the regulation of transcription, DNA repair, recombination, and replication.

Chromosomal satellite At the end of each short arm of acrocentric chromosomes, a small mass of chromatin containing genes for ribosomal RNA; not to be confused with *satellite DNA*.

Chromosome A thread-like structure in the cell nucleus consisting of chromatin.

Chromosome arm The portion of a chromosome from the centromere to the telomere. Each chromosome has two arms of varying sizes. See *p* (arm) and *q* (arm).

Chromosome disorder A clinical condition in which there is duplication, loss, or rearrangement of chromosomal material comprising a whole chromosome or significant portion thereof.

Chromosome instability syndrome Hereditary condition that predisposes to a high frequency of chromosome breakage and rearrangements. Often associated with markedly increased risk for a variety of cancers.

Chromosome segregation The separation of chromosomes or chromatids in cell division, yielding an equal number of chromosomes in each daughter cell.

Chromosome shattering (chromothripsis) In some cancer cells, novel and complex chromosome rearrangements occur due to breakage and rejoining. The mechanism is unknown.

Chromosome spread As seen under the microscope, chromosomes halted for viewing in metaphase or prometaphase.

Cis Refers to the relationship between two sequences that are on the same chromosome; literally meaning "on the near side of." Contrast with *trans*.

Clinical heterogeneity Occurrence of clinically different phenotypes resulting from variants in the same gene.

Clinical utility In reference to a clinical laboratory test, the ability of that test to improve the medical care that an individual receives.

Clinical validity In reference to a clinical laboratory test, the ability of that test to detect the disease that the test was designed to detect.

Clonal evolution The process of successive genetic changes that occur in a developing tumor cell population.

Clone (1) (n) A cell line derived from a single ancestral diploid cell; (v) the act of generating such a cell line or clone. (2) In molecular biology, a recombinant DNA molecule containing a gene or other DNA sequence that has been isolated and inserted into a vector for propagation.

Coding strand In double-stranded DNA, the strand that has the same 5′ to 3′ sense and sequence as mRNA, except that in mRNA, U substitutes for T. The coding strand is *not* transcribed by RNA polymerase. Also called the *sense strand*.

Codominant If both alleles of a heterozygous pair are expressed, then the traits determined by them are codominant.

Codon A triplet of three bases in a DNA or RNA molecule, specifying a single amino acid.

Cohort study A longitudinal study of a random sample of a population with shared characteristics to study outcomes. They do not involve intervention or control groups.

Colinearity The parallel relationship between the sequence of DNA bases (or the RNA transcribed from it) and the amino acid sequence of the corresponding polypeptide.

Commitment The transition of an embryonic cell from pluripotency to its particular fate. See pluripotent.

Comparative genome hybridization (CGH) A technique used to compare two different DNA samples with respect to relative content of a particular DNA segment or segments, to detect copy number variations (CNVs). CGH can be used with fluorescence in situ hybridization (FISH) of metaphase chromosomes or with DNA fragments arrayed on a solid support (array CGH (a*CGH*)).

Complementary DNA (cDNA) DNA synthesized from a messenger RNA template with the enzyme reverse transcriptase. See *Genomic DNA* for comparison.

Complex inheritance Also called nonmendelian inheritance. A trait with complex inheritance usually results from alleles at more than one locus interacting, along with environmental and/or epigenetic factors.

Compound heterozygote (or genetic compound) An individual or a genotype with two different variant alleles at the same locus. In contrast, a *homozygote* has two identical variant alleles.

Concordant Sharing a certain qualitative trait or having values of a quantitative trait that are similar in magnitude. Contrast with *Discordant*.

Conditional probability In Bayesian analysis, the chance of an observed outcome, given that another event has already occurred. The product of the prior and conditional probabilities is the joint probability.

Confined placental mosaicism Mosaicism in a *chorionic villus sampling* (CVS) specimen obtained from the placenta that is not present in the fetus itself.

Congenital Present at birth; not necessarily genetic.

Consanguinity The state of being related by descent from a common ancestor (the adjective is *consanguineous*).

Consensus (or canonical) sequence In genes or proteins, a sequence in which each base or amino acid residue represents the one most frequently found at that position.

Consultand An individual who consults a genetic counselor for genetic information.

Contiguous gene syndrome A syndrome resulting from a *deletion* or duplication of chromosomal DNA extending over two or more contiguous genes.

Copy number variant (CNV) An unbalanced variation in DNA sequence defined by the loss or addition of a segment of DNA, typically defined as larger than 1 kb and ranging up to 3 Mb. CNVs may be alleles that are tandem replications involving two or more copies of a DNA segment. See *Structural variant*.

Cordocentesis (percutaneous umbilical cord blood sampling [PUBS]) An invasive procedure to obtain a sample of fetal blood directly from the umbilical cord.

Correlation A statistical term describing the degree to which two variables move in relation to one another. Correlation does not imply cause. Represented by the correlation coefficient *r*.

Coupling (*cis*) The phase of two alleles at syntenic loci when both are on the same chromosome. See *Phase* and *Repulsion*.

CpG island Segments of genomic DNA that are particularly rich in the dinucleotide 5′-CG-3′, found in the promoters of many housekeeping genes. The "p" in CpG refers to the phosphate of the DNA backbone connecting the cytidine and guanidine nucleosides.

Crossover (crossing over) The reciprocal exchange of segments between chromatids of homologous chromosomes, characteristic of prophase of the first meiotic division. See also *Recombination*. Unequal crossing over between misaligned chromatids can lead to duplication of the involved segment on one chromatid and deletion on the other.

Cryptic splice site A coding or noncoding DNA sequence similar to a consensus splice site but not normally used. Alterations in the normal or in the cryptic splice site may increase its use by the splicing apparatus.

Cytogenetics The study of chromosomes.

Cytokinesis Cleavage of cytoplasm at the end of mitosis, resulting in two separate cells, each with a full complement of chromosomes.

Cytotrophoblast The fetal cells of the chorionic villi that are sampled for prenatal analysis by CVS. See Chorionic villus sampling.

Daughter chromosomes The two individual chromosomes formed when a single chromosome composed of paired chromatids separates at the centromere in anaphase of cell division.

Deformation syndrome A recognizable pattern of dysmorphic features caused by extrinsic factors that affect the fetus in utero.

Degeneracy (or redundancy) of the code The genetic code is described as degenerate because most amino acids are specified by more than 1 of the 64 codons. The degeneracy usually involves the third base of a codon and can mitigate the impact of common base substitutions.

Degree of relationship The distance between two individuals in a pedigree. First-degree relatives include parents, siblings, and children. Second-degree relatives are aunts and uncles, nephews and nieces, grandparents and grandchildren.

Deletion The loss of a sequence of DNA, of any size, from a chromosome. A chromosome deletion may occur from the end of a chromosome (terminal deletion) or within a chromosome arm (interstitial). See *Copy number variation* (CNV).

Deoxyribonucleic acid See *DNA*.

Determination See Chapter 15 Box 15.1.

Developmental disorder A broad construct referring to the outcome of disruption of the normal developmental program for any organ system. Usually prenatal in onset but can first present postnatally. Often applied more narrowly to mean neurodevelopmental disorder, having origins in early brain development, with delays or deficits in one or more areas of development including motor, language, socialization, and cognition.

Developmental program The process by which a cell in an embryo achieves its fate.

Deviation (D) In linkage analysis, a measure of difference between an observed haplotype frequency and that expected based on the individual allele frequencies. A measure of linkage disequilibrium, usually normalized to allele frequencies using the D' metric.

Dicentric Referring to a structurally abnormal chromosome with two centromeres. If a dicentric chromosome segregates as if it has only one centromere, it is referred to as *pseudodicentric*.

Dictyotene The stage of the first meiotic division in which a human oocyte remains from late fetal life until ovulation. See meiosis.

Differentiation The acquisition by a cell of novel characteristics specific for a particular cell type or tissue. See Chapter 15.

Digenic inheritance A situation in which a phenotype is explained by a combination of genotypes at two independent loci (in contrast to monogenic or *polygenic inheritance*). Oligogenic refers to involvement of a few genes.

Diploid Describing the presence of two sets of chromosomes, as in most somatic cells (i.e., double the *haploid* number found in the gametes). In humans, the diploid chromosome number is 46.

Discordant Not sharing a certain qualitative trait or having values of a quantitative trait that are at opposite ends of the distribution. Contrast with *Concordant*.

Disorder of sex development (DSD) (previously called intersex) A range of conditions that lead to abnormal development of the sex organs and atypical genitalia – genitalia that are not clearly male or female. Also includes a phenotype reflecting a mismatch between chromosomal sex and phenotypic sex.

Dispermy The fertilization of one ovum by two spermatozoa.

Disruption The cause of a birth defect due to destruction of tissue, such as by vascular occlusion, a teratogen, or rupture of the amniotic sac with entrapment.

Dizygotic (DZ) twins Twins produced by two separate ova, separately fertilized. Also called *fraternal twins*.

DNA (deoxyribonucleic acid) The molecule that encodes the genes responsible for the structure and function of living organisms and allows the transmission of genetic information from generation to generation.

DNA (genetic) fingerprint (profile) A genotypic profile used to unambiguously and uniquely specify the individual from which the DNA was obtained (except for monozygotic twins), especially for forensics and ancestry testing.

DNA methylation In eukaryotes, the addition of a methyl residue to the 5-position of the pyrimidine ring of a cytosine base in DNA to form 5-methylcytosine.

DNA polymerase An enzyme that can synthesize a new DNA strand using a previously synthesized DNA strand as a template.

DNA proofreading Recognition and removal of a noncomplementary DNA base inserted during replication, followed by its replacement with the correct complementary base.

Dominant A trait is dominant if it is phenotypically expressed in heterozygotes. If heterozygotes and homozygotes for a variant allele have the same phenotype, the disorder is a *pure dominant* (rare in human genetics). If homozygotes have a more severe phenotype than do heterozygotes, the disorder is termed *semidominant* or *incompletely dominant*.

Dominant negative The effect of a variant allele whose protein product disrupts the function of a wild-type allele in the same cell. Contrast with *haploinsufficiency*.

Donor splice site The boundary between the 3′ end of an exon and the 5′ end of the next intron. Also called *5′ splice site*.

Dosage compensation A mechanism to make the amount of product transcribed from X-linked genes in females equivalent to that in males. Humans accomplish this through X *inactivation*.

Double heterozygote An individual who is heterozygous at each of two different loci. Contrast with *compound heterozygote*.

Double minutes Very small accessory chromosomes, a form of gene amplification.

Driver gene A gene that has been found repeatedly to carry somatic variants in many samples of the same type of cancer or even in different cancers – too frequently to be the product of random events. These altered genes are thus presumed to be involved in the development or progression of the cancer itself. See *Passenger gene*.

Dynamic variant An unstable heritable element in DNA, typically an expanded trinucleotide repeat sequence. These tend to increase in size from one generation to the next, thus the term *dynamic*. Examples include CAG in Huntington disease (Case 24) or CGG in fragile X syndrome (Case 17). See Chapters 7 and 13.

Dysmorphic features Morphological developmental abnormalities, as seen in many syndromes of genetic or environmental origin.

Ecogenetic disorder A disorder resulting from the interaction of a genetic predisposition with an environmental factor.

Ectoderm One of the three primary *germ layers* of the early embryo, that farthest from the yolk sac. It gives rise to the nervous system, the skin, and neural crest derivatives such as craniofacial structures and melanocytes.

Ectopic expression Expression of a gene in places where it is not normally expressed.

Embryonic stem cell See *Stem cell* and Chapter 15 Box 15.1.

Empirical risk Based on observed numbers rather than on knowledge or theory of the cause, in human genetics, the probability that a trait will occur in an individual.

ENCODE Project Acronym for *Encyclopedia of DNA Elements*; a public consortium to identify the functional elements of human and mouse genomes.

Endoderm One of the three primary *germ layers* of the early embryo. Ultimately gives rise to the gut, liver, and portions of the urogenital system.

Endophenotype (intermediate phenotype) In genetic epidemiology, particularly in psychiatric genetics, a heritable biological trait that is a marker of risk for a genetically complex disorder.

Enhancer A DNA sequence that acts in *cis* (i.e., on the same chromosome) to increase transcription of a gene. The enhancer may be upstream or downstream of the gene, in the same or the reverse orientation. Contrast with *silencer*.

Enzymopathy A metabolic disorder resulting from deficiency or abnormality of a specific enzyme.

Epigenetic Referring to any factor that can affect gene function without change in the primary DNA sequence. Some typical epigenetic factors involve alterations in DNA methylation, chromatin structure, histone modifications, and transcription factor binding that change genome structure and affect gene expression.

Episome A DNA element that exists as an autonomously replicating sequence in a eukaryotic cell or can integrate into chromosomal DNA. Adeno-associated viral vectors, used in gene therapy, are episomes.

Euchromatin The major component of chromatin, relatively uncondensed and transcriptionally active. It stains lightly with G banding. Contrast with *heterochromatin*.

Eugenics The study (now considered unethical) of how to increase prevalence of desirable traits in a population through selective breeding. The opposite is *dysgenics*.

Eukaryote A unicellular or multicellular organism in which the cells have a nucleus with a nuclear membrane and other specialized characteristics.

Euploid Any chromosome number that is an exact multiple of the number in a haploid gamete (n). Most human somatic cells are diploid (2n). Contrast with *aneuploid*.

Exome The part of genome that consists of exons. In humans this is about 1.5% of the genome.

Exon A region of a gene that is represented in mature messenger RNA after removal of introns. It may code for a protein or be noncoding.

Exon skipping Bypassing an exon in a pre-mRNA due to a splice-site or other variant. Therapeutically, a molecular intervention to exclude a faulty or misaligned exon from a pre-mRNA, thereby rescuing expression of the altered gene.

Expression profile A quantitative assessment of the mRNAs present in a cell type, tissue, or tumor. Often used for comparative characterizations.

Expressivity The extent to which a genetic trait is expressed. If there is variable expressivity, the trait may vary in expression from mild to severe. Contrast with *Penetrance*.

Familial Referring to a trait that is more common in relatives of an affected individual than in the general population, whether the cause is genetic, environmental, or both.

Fate See Chapter 15 Box 15.1.

Fetal cells Any cells derived from a fetus: placental cells, obtained by *chorionic villus sampling*; skin, respiratory, and urinary tract cells obtained from amniotic fluid by *amniocentesis*; or fetal blood cells obtained by *cordocentesis*.

Fetal phase Stage of intrauterine development from weeks 9 to 40.

Fibroblasts An easily accessible mesenchymal cell type obtained from skin and commonly used in tissue culture experiments.

Fitness The probability (f) of transmitting one's genes to the next generation compared with the population average.

Flanking sequence A region of DNA preceding or following any other segment of DNA; usually in reference to a gene or exon.

Fluorescence in situ hybridization (FISH) See *In situ hybridization*.

Founder effect A high frequency of a variant allele in a population founded by a small ancestral group when one or more of the founders was a carrier of the allele.

Fragile site Nonstaining gap in the chromatin of a metaphase chromosome, such as the fragile site at Xq27 in fragile X syndrome (Case 17).

Frameshift mutation/variant A deletion or insertion of DNA that is not an exact multiple of three base pairs, thus changing the reading frame of the gene downstream of the alteration.

G-banding (Giemsa staining) Method of staining chromosomes to generate reproducible alternating light and dark bands.

Gain-of-function mutation/variant A genetic change associated with an increase in one or more of the normal functions of a protein (also called hypermorphic) or a new function for the protein (also called neomorphic). See also *Novel property mutation/variant*.

Gamete A mature reproductive cell (ovum or sperm) with the haploid chromosome number.

Gene A hereditary unit; in molecular terms, a sequence of chromosomal DNA that is required to produce a functional product.

Gene dosage The number of copies of a particular gene in the genome.

Gene family A set of genes containing highly similar DNA sequences, indicating that the genes have evolved from an ancestral gene by duplication and subsequent divergence.

Gene flow Gradual diffusion of genes from one population to another across a barrier. The barrier may be physical or cultural and may be breached by migration or mixing.

Gene map Representation of the characteristic arrangement of genes on the chromosomes.

Gene mutation Alteration of the sequence of DNA in a gene. The change may or may not create any phenotypic effect.

Gene pool The sum of all genes, including variant alleles, in a population.

Gene transfer therapy (gene therapy) Treatment of a genetic disease by introduction of DNA sequences or alteration of existing sequences, for therapeutic benefit. Distinction is made between *somatic cell* and *germline* gene therapy; the latter being prohibited in most jurisdictions.

Genetic Determined by genes; not to be confused with *congenital*.

Genetic admixture The outcome of the merging of previously isolated ancestral populations with genetic exchange through mating.

Genetic code The 64 triplets of nucleotide bases that specify the 20 amino acids found in proteins (see Table 3.1).

Genetic counseling The provision of information and assistance to individuals and/or family members affected by or at risk for a disorder that may be genetic; specifically, concerning the consequences of the disorder, the probability of developing or transmitting it, and the ways in which it may be prevented or ameliorated.

Genetic disorder A condition wholly or partly caused by a gene abnormality.

Genetic drift Random fluctuation of allele frequencies in small populations.

Genetic epidemiology A branch of public health research concerned with characterizing and quantifying the influence of genetic variation in the population on the incidence, prevalence, and causation of disease.

Genetic heterogeneity The same or similar phenotypes resulting from variants in different genes; commonly used interchangeably with *locus heterogeneity*. See *Allelic heterogeneity*, *Clinical heterogeneity*, and *Locus heterogeneity*.

Genetic lethal A variant allele or genetically determined trait that leads to failure to reproduce (not necessarily to death before reproduction).

Genetic load The reduction of mean genetic fitness of a population or an individual.

Genetic marker A locus that has readily classifiable alleles and can be used in genetic studies. See *Polymorphism*.

Genetic screening Testing of family members of an affected proband or of the population as a whole to identify individuals at risk for developing or transmitting a specific disorder.

Genocopy A trait is a genocopy when a similar phenotype is determined by a genotype at a different locus.

Genome The complete DNA sequence, containing the entire genetic information of a gamete, an individual, a population, or a species.

Genome editing A technology that uses proteins adapted from bacteria or plants (e.g., CRISPR/Cas9) to target a particular site within the genome of a cell with high efficiency and specificity. Once the site is targeted, it can be changed, undergo repair of a preexisting mutation, or undergo alteration of an epigenetic imprint.

Genome sequencing The process of determining the sequence of DNA bases in the genome, including coding and noncoding. Also called *whole genome sequencing*, although some parts of the genome continue to resist access by current technologies. For methods, see *Sanger sequencing* and *Massively parallel sequencing* (noting that other new methods are evolving rapidly). Differentiate from *gene sequencing* or *targeted sequencing*. Complete RNA transcriptome sequencing is also a form of genome sequencing.

Genome-wide association study (GWAS) A genetic association study using hundreds of thousands to millions of variants at polymorphic loci distributed throughout the genome to identify genes associated with a particular trait.

Genome-wide testing Evaluation of the entire genome. May include *microarray (comparative genomic hybridization), exome sequencing,* or *whole genome sequencing.* Requires pretest counseling, and the method should be specified.

Genomic disorder A condition that results from loss or gain of a relatively large segment of DNA *(copy number variation [CNV])* or sometimes rearrangement. The disease mechanism may be due to a *contiguous gene syndrome,* when genes clustered together in the genome are affected by the CNV. For examples, see Case 8 (Charcot-Marie-Tooth syndrome) and Case 22 (22q11.2 deletion syndrome). Typically, the deleted or duplicated region is flanked by *segmental duplications.*

Genomic DNA The chromosomal DNA sequence of a genome, gene or segment of a gene that includes noncoding as well as coding regions. Also, DNA that has been isolated directly from cells or chromosomes or the cloned copies of all or part of such DNA.

Genomic imprinting An epigenetic phenomenon creating monoallelic expression in which the allele to be expressed is determined by the parental origin of each allele. See Case 38 (Prader-Willi syndrome), for example.

Genomic medicine The practice of medicine based on large-scale genomic information, such as sequencing of large gene panels, exomes, or whole genomes; expression profiling to characterize tumors or to define prognosis in cancer; genotyping of variants in genes involved in drug metabolism or action to determine an individual's correct therapeutic dosage; or analysis of multiple protein biomarkers to monitor therapy or to provide predictive information in presymptomatic individuals.

Genomics The field of genetics concerned with structural and functional studies of the genome.

Genotype (1) The genetic constitution of an individual, as distinguished from the *phenotype.* (2) More specifically, the alleles present at one or more loci.

Germ layer See Chapter 15 Box 15.1.

Germline The cell line from which gametes are derived.

Germline mosaicism Presence of two or more genetically different germlines in one organism, resulting from somatic mutation during cellular proliferation and differentiation.

Gonadal dysgenesis A *disorder of sex development* in which the gonads fail to develop normally. In complete gonadal dysgenesis, external genitalia are normal, whereas in incomplete gonadal dysgenesis, the external genitalia are ambiguous.

Haploid The chromosome number of a normal gamete, which has one member of each chromosome pair; referring to a cell or nucleus with one set of chromosomes. In humans, the haploid number is 23.

Haploinsufficiency The situation in which dosage matters: the contribution from a wild-type allele is insufficient to compensate for loss at the other allele – due to deletion or a *loss-of-function variant* – resulting in an abnormal phenotype.

Haplotype A group of alleles in coupling at closely linked loci, usually inherited as a unit.

Hardy-Weinberg law A mathematical equation that relates allele frequency to genotype frequency, for a population that meets certain criteria (i.e., is in Hardy-Weinberg equilibrium [see Chapter 10]). Its major application in medical genetics is in counseling for recessive disorders.

Hemizygous A term for the genotype of an individual with only one representative of a chromosome or chromosome segment, rather than the usual two; refers especially (but not exclusively) to X-linked genes in the male.

Hemoglobin switching Change in expression of the various globin genes during developmental stages of hematopoiesis.

Heritability (h2) The fraction of total phenotypic variance in a population that is due to genotypic differences; a statistical estimate of the hereditary contribution to a quantitative trait.

Heterochromatin Condensed DNA that stains darkly. Regions such as centromeres, acrocentric short arms, and portions of human chromosomes 1, 9, 16, and Y constitute *constitutive heterochromatin* and are relatively genetically inactive in all cells. *Facultative heterochromatin* is a variable feature, exemplified by the inactive X chromosome. Contrast with *euchromatin.*

Heterodisomy See *Uniparental disomy.*

Heterogeneity See *Allelic heterogeneity, Clinical heterogeneity, Genetic heterogeneity,* and *Locus heterogeneity.*

Heteroplasmy The presence, due to variant(s), of more than one type of mitochondrial DNA among the mitochondria of a single individual. Contrast with *homoplasmy.*

Heteroploidy Any chromosome number other than the normal, such as triploidy, tetraploidy, or aneuploidy.

Heterozygote (heterozygous) An individual or genotype with two different alleles, one of which is wild-type, at a given locus on a pair of homologous chromosomes. Contrast with *compound heterozygote.*

Heterozygote advantage Increased fitness of a *heterozygote* for a pathogenic variant allele and the wild-type allele, relative to both homozygotes. The classic example is heterozygosity for the sickle cell variant in the *HBB* gene, which confers resistance to malaria. See *Balanced polymorphism.*

Histocompatibility The situation in which a graft contains no antigens that the host lacks.

Histones Proteins associated with DNA in the chromosomes; they are rich in basic amino acids (lysine or arginine) and virtually invariant throughout eukaryote evolution. Covalent modifications of histones are important *epigenetic* regulators of gene expression.

The pattern of histones and their modifications constitute the epigenetic "histone code."

Holandric inheritance See *Male-to-male transmission*.

Holoenzyme The functional compound formed by the binding of an apoenzyme with its appropriate coenzyme.

Homeobox gene A gene that contains a conserved 180 base-pair homeobox sequence, encoding a protein motif known as the homeodomain. This comprises a DNA-binding motif, which has a role in transcriptional regulation of genes involved in development.

Homogeneously staining regions (HSRs) Chromosome regions that stain uniformly and represent amplified copies of a DNA segment.

Homologous A term used in genetics with different meanings in different contexts. (1) In bioinformatics, referring to similar nucleotide or amino acid sequences, as seen between *orthologous* or *paralogous* genes. (2) In cytogenetics, a pair of chromosomes, one inherited paternally, the other maternally. Sex chromosomes in males (X and Y) are only partially homologous. (3) In evolution, structures in different organisms are termed *homologous* if they evolved from a structure present in a common ancestor.

Homologue Something that is homologous.

Homoplasmy The presence of only one type of mitochondrial DNA in the mitochondria of a single individual. Contrast with *heteroplasmy*.

Homozygote (homozygous) An individual or genotype with identical alleles at a given locus.

Housekeeping genes Genes expressed in most or all cells because their products provide basic functions in the maintenance of cell structure and function.

Human Genome Project A major research project, international in scope, that took place from 1990 to 2003 and resulted in the mapping, sequencing, and assembly of a representative human genome and the genomes of many model organisms.

Human leukocyte antigen (HLA) See *Major histocompatibility complex*.

Hybridization In molecular biology, the bonding of two complementary single-stranded nucleic acid molecules according to the rules of base pairing. See *Comparative genome hybridization* and *Fluorescence in situ hybridization*.

Hydatidiform mole An abnormality of the placenta associated with very abnormal fetal development. In a *complete mole*, the karyotype is usually 46,XX, but can be 46,XY, representing duplication of the chromosomes of the sperm with no maternal contribution. A *partial mole* is triploid, usually with an extra paternal chromosome set.

Immunoglobulin gene superfamily A family of evolutionarily related genes composed of human leukocyte antigen (HLA) class I and class II genes, immunoglobulin genes, T-cell receptor genes, and other genes encoding cell surface molecules.

Imprinting See *Genomic imprinting*.

Imprinting center A regulatory region in the germline that acts as a master cis-regulatory element to local regions of imprinted genes. Also called imprinting control region.

In situ hybridization Use of a labeled DNA sequence as a probe corresponding to a gene or DNA segment to be mapped, applied to a slide-mounted cell spread. With a fluorescent probe, it is *fluorescence in situ hybridization (FISH)*.

In vitro fertilization A reproductive technology by which sperm fertilizes an egg in tissue culture and the fertilized egg is introduced back into the uterus for implantation.

Inborn error of metabolism A genetically determined biochemical disorder in which a specific protein defect disturbs a metabolic pathway.

Inbreeding The mating of closely related individuals. The progeny of such mating is said to be inbred. (Note that some consider the term *inbred* to be pejorative when it is applied to human populations.)

Inbreeding, coefficient of (F) The probability that a child of a consanguineous mating will be homozygous at a given locus for an allele inherited through each parent from a common ancestor.

Incompletely dominant A trait that is inherited in a dominant manner but is more severe in a homozygote than in a heterozygote (synonym: *semi-dominant*).

Indel Abbreviation for insertion/deletion: a small structural variant defined by the presence or absence of a segment of DNA, ranging from one base to a few hundred base pairs. Includes simple indels, microsatellites, and minisatellite variants.

Index case The family member affected with a genetic disorder who is the first to draw attention to a pedigree. See *Proband*.

Induced pluripotent stem cells (iPS cells) *Pluripotent stem cells* derived from differentiated somatic cells that have been induced to lose their differentiated state and revert to pluripotency by artificially expressing a small number of specific transcription factors.

Induction The process by which the fate of one region of an embryo is influenced by extracellular signals from a second, usually neighboring, region.

In-frame deletion A deletion that does not destroy the normal reading frame of the gene.

Initiator codon The codon for methionine (AUG) that signals the start of translation in *Messenger RNA*.

Inner cell mass See Chapter 15 Box 15.1.

Insertion A structural variation in which a DNA segment from a chromosome, or from an exogenous source such as a retrovirus, is inserted into the genome.

Intergenic DNA The mostly untranscribed DNA from between genes that makes up a large proportion of the total DNA in the genome.

Intermediate repeat expansion In genes associated with unstable nucleotide repeats (e.g., *HTT, FMR1*), expanded alleles in the range between normal and full Penetrance are not themselves pathogenic but are at risk for further expansion during meiosis. Offspring of individuals with intermediate expansion alleles are thus at increased risk for the disorder. Terminology is evolving. See also *Premutation,* dynamic variant and Case 24 (Huntington disease) and Case 17 (Fragile X syndrome).

Interphase The stage of the *cell cycle* between two successive mitoses.

Intervening sequence See *Intron.*

Intron A segment of a gene that is initially transcribed but then removed from within the primary RNA transcript by splicing together the sequences (exons) on either side of it.

Inversion A balanced chromosomal rearrangement in which a segment of a chromosome is reversed end to end. If the centromere is included in the inversion, the inversion is *pericentric*; if not, it is *paracentric.*

Isochromosome An abnormal chromosome in which one arm is duplicated (forming two arms of equal length, with the same loci in reverse sequence) and the other arm is missing.

Isodisomy See *Uniparental disomy.*

Isolate A subpopulation in which mating takes place largely or exclusively within the subpopulation.

Isolated case An individual who is the only member of his or her kindred affected by a genetic disorder, either by chance or due to new mutation. See also *Sporadic.*

Karyotype The chromosome constitution of an individual. Also (n) a photomicrograph of the chromosomes of an individual systematically arranged, and (v) the process of preparing such a photomicrograph.

kb (kilobase or kilobase pair) A unit of 1000 bases in a DNA or RNA sequence.

Kindred An extended family.

Kinetochore A structure at the centromere to which the spindle fibers are attached.

LINE sequences Long interspersed nuclear elements, a class of repetitive DNA up to 6 kb in length, occurring in several hundred thousand copies in the genome, some of which are capable of *retrotransposition.* Also called L1 elements.

Linkage analysis A statistical method to determine whether two or more loci are assorting independently or are transmitted together during meiosis because of proximity on the chromosome.

Linkage disequilibrium (LD) The occurrence of combinations of alleles in coupling phase at two or more linked loci (haplotypes) more frequently than expected from the frequency of the alleles in the population. Opposite is linkage equilibrium.

Linkage map A chromosome map showing the relative positions of genes and other DNA markers on the chromosomes, as determined by linkage analysis.

lncRNA See *Noncoding RNA.*

Locus The position occupied by a gene on a chromosome. Different forms of the gene (*alleles*) may occupy the locus. Plural: loci.

Locus control region (LCR) A DNA domain, situated outside a cluster of structural genes, responsible for the appropriate expression of the genes within the cluster.

Locus heterogeneity Identical phenotypes resulting from variants at two or more different loci.

LOD score The *l*ogarithm of the *od*ds in favor of linkage of two gene loci. By convention, a LOD score of 3 (odds of 1000:1 in favor) is proof of linkage, and a LOD score of −2 (100:1 against) is proof that the loci are unlinked. See Linkage analysis.

Loops Three-dimensional arrangements of chromatin, packaged as solenoids, attached to the chromosome scaffold. Thought to be structural or functional units of chromosomes.

Loss-of-function mutation/variant A change in DNA associated with a reduction or a complete loss of one or more of the normal functions of a protein.

Loss of heterozygosity (LOH) Functional loss of a normal allele from one chromosome, allowing a defective allele on the homologous chromosome to be clinically manifest. A feature of many cases of retinoblastoma, breast cancer, and other tumors due to mutation in a tumor-suppressor gene.

Lymphoblastoid cells B-lymphocytes immortalized in culture by infection with Epstein-Barr virus.

Lyon's law (or hypothesis) Basic features of the phenomenon of X inactivation, which was first described by the late British geneticist Mary Lyon. Upgraded from the Lyon hypothesis to a law at the 50th anniversary of her discovery. Silencing of gene expression is sometimes referred to as *lyonization.*

Major histocompatibility complex (MHC) The complex locus on human chromosome 6p that includes the highly polymorphic human leukocyte antigen (HLA) genes.

Male-to-male transmission A pattern of inheritance of a trait from a father to any of his sons, establishes autosomal dominant inheritance. When from a father to all of his sons and none of his daughters, it is indicative of Y-linked inheritance, also referred to as *holandric inheritance.*

Maleficence Behavior that harms others. Avoidance of maleficence is one of the cardinal principles of ethics. Contrast with *Beneficence.*

Malformation syndrome A recognizable pattern of congenital anomalies that are known or thought to be causally related (may be genetic or environmental, e.g., CHARGE syndrome (Case 9) or phenytoin or warfarin embryopathy).

Manhattan plot A graph of all of the *P* values for an association between a trait and all of the markers used in a genome-wide association study (GWAS) study, displayed along the chromosomes. It is called a *Manhattan plot* because the peaks of strong association resemble the tips of skyscrapers (see Fig. 9.4 for example).

Manifesting heterozygote A female heterozygous for an X-linked recessive disorder in whom nonrandom X inactivation makes the trait manifest to some degree.

Map distance A theoretical concept based on recombination frequency. Measured in units of centimorgans, defined as the genetic length over which recombination occurs in 1% of meioses.

Marker chromosome A small unidentified chromosome seen in a chromosome preparation. Also referred to as a *supernumerary chromosome* or *extra structurally abnormal chromosome*.

Massively parallel sequencing Various highly automated, high-throughput technologies that allow simultaneous sequence analysis of millions of DNA fragments. Such *next generation sequencing* (NGS) can detect variations, including single-base substitution and *copy number variants* (CNVs), and is used primarily for multigene panels and genome, exome, and transcriptome sequencing.

Maternal inheritance The transmission of genetic information only through the mother. See *Mitochondrial inheritance*.

Maternal serum screening Laboratory test that measures levels of substances such as α-fetoprotein, human chorionic gonadotropin, and unconjugated estriol in a pregnant woman's blood to screen for fetuses at increased risk of certain trisomies or neural tube defects.

Mb (megabase or megabase pair) A unit of 1,000,000 bases or base pairs in genomic DNA.

Meiosis Cell division occurring in the diploid germ cells, yielding gametes containing the haploid chromosome number. Two meiotic divisions occur: meiosis I (when homologous pairs separate and the chromosome number is reduced) and meiosis II (when sister chromatids separate).

Mendelian Patterns of inheritance that follow the classic laws of Mendel: autosomal dominant, autosomal recessive, and X-linked. See *Single-gene disorder*.

Mesoderm See Chapter 15 Box 15.1.

Mesonephric duct Structure in the genital ridges of the early embryo that will develop into male internal sexual organs. Also called the *Wolffian duct*.

Messenger RNA (mRNA) An RNA, transcribed from the DNA of a gene, that directs the sequence of amino acids of the encoded polypeptide. Contrast with *noncoding RNA*.

Metacentric Refers to a chromosome with a central centromere and arms of apparently equal length.

Metaphase Following prometaphase, the stage of mitosis or meiosis in which chromosomes are maximally condensed, attached to spindle fibers, and lined up on the cell's equatorial plane. The stage at which chromosomes are most easily examined.

Metastasis Spread of malignant cells to other sites in the body.

Methemoglobin The oxidized form of hemoglobin, containing ferric rather than ferrous iron, which is incapable of binding oxygen.

Microarray Miniaturized wafer ("chip") made of glass, plastic, or silicon onto which nucleic acids have been arrayed, used for hybridization studies. See also *Comparative genome hybridization and Expression profile*.

Microdeletion A chromosomal deletion that is too small to be seen under the microscope. See also *Copy number variation*.

MicroRNAs (miRNAs) An abundant class of several thousand small (approximately 22 bases) single-stranded RNAs that are gene regulatory elements. They suppress gene expression posttranscriptionally by targeting specific mRNAs for cleavage or by suppressing mRNA translation.

Microsatellite See *Short tandem repeat*.

Microsatellite instability (MSI) A phenotype of cancer cells in which loss of function of mismatch repair genes causes errors such as slipped mispairing to go unrepaired when microsatellite sequences are replicated. These errors lead to tissue Mosaicism so that the cancer appears to contain more than two alleles at many short tandem repeat polymorphic loci.

Minor allele frequency The frequency of the second most common allele at a locus. Used in population genetics to differentiate between common and rare variants.

Missense mutation/variant A mutation that changes a codon for one amino acid to that of another amino acid.

Mitochondrial bottleneck In oogenesis, only a small portion of mitochondria in a germ cell is transmitted to each oocyte, thereby allowing significant variation in the degree of heteroplasmy between offspring and rapid evolution between generations.

Mitochondrial DNA (mtDNA) The DNA in the circular chromosome of the mitochondria; in humans, containing 37 genes. Mitochondrial DNA is present in many copies per cell, is maternally inherited, and evolves 5 to 10 times as rapidly as genomic DNA.

Mitochondrial inheritance Inheritance of a trait encoded in the mitochondrial genome. The mitochondria are contributed almost exclusively by the egg, not sperm; therefore, mitochondrial inheritance is through the maternal line.

Mitosis The process of ordinary cell division, resulting in two cells genetically identical (barring any process error) to the parent cell.

Mitotic spindle In a mitotic cell, an arrangement of microtubules attached to the kinetochores of centromeres and to opposite cell poles. These guide the separation of sister chromatids during anaphase.

Modifier gene A gene whose alleles alter the phenotype associated with a nonallelic gene. Often applied to the effect on the expressivity of mendelian disorders caused by variants at other loci.

Monosomy A chromosome constitution in which one member of a chromosome pair is missing, as in 45,X Turner syndrome (Case 47).

Monozygotic (MZ) twins Twins derived from a single zygote. Sometimes termed identical twins; however, they may have genetic differences that have arisen post fertilization.

Morphogen See Chapter 15 Box 15.1.

Morphogenesis See Chapter 15 Box 15.1.

Mosaic development See Chapter 15 Box 15.1.

Mosaicism A condition in which an organism is composed of two or more genetically distinct tissues or cell lines, that were derived from a single zygote. Contrast with *chimera*.

Multifactorial disease A disorder resulting from a combination of multiple factors, typically multigenetic, epigenetic, and environmental. Demonstrates *complex inheritance* rather than mendelian inheritance patterns.

Multiple hypothesis testing A concept in statistics referring to a cause of false-positive significance. Applied to *GWAS* testing, the likelihood of finding apparent association with a trait of interest – due to chance alone – increases with the number of marker alleles (i.e., hypotheses) being tested. More stringent thresholds of significance must be applied.

Multiplex ligation-dependent probe amplification (MLPA) A robust and accurate laboratory technique used to detect copy number variations in multiple samples.

Mutagen An agent that increases the spontaneous mutation rate by causing changes in DNA.

Mutant (adj) Resulting from or showing the effects of *mutation*. (n) A form altered by *mutation*. See *variant* as preferred nomenclature to avoid implication of negative outcome.

Mutation Genetic change that gives rise to heritable variation; the process by which such changes arise. See *Variant*.

Mutation rate (μ) The frequency of mutation at a given locus, expressed as mutations per locus per gamete (or per generation, which is the same).

Natural selection As first expounded by Charles Darwin in *On the Origin of Species*, the theory that individuals with adaptive traits are more likely to survive and reproduce, such that these traits become more common in the population. A driving force of evolution.

Negative predictive value The probability that subjects with a negative test result will truly not have or develop the trait being tested or screened for. Contrast with *positive predictive value*.

Neoplasia An abnormal growth produced by imbalance between normal cellular proliferation and normal cellular attrition. May be benign or malignant (cancer).

Next generation sequencing To avoid ambiguity as technology evolves, greater specificity is preferred. See *Massively parallel sequencing*.

Noncoding gene See *Noncoding RNA*.

Noncoding RNA (ncRNA) After transcription, an RNA product that will not be translated to a protein product. Sometimes referred to as *long noncoding RNAs* or *lncRNAs* to avoid confusion with short ncRNAs such as *miRNAs* or *siRNAs*. For example, see *XIST* RNA, under *X inactivation*. Contrast with *messenger RNA*.

Noncoding strand See *antisense strand of DNA*.

Nondisjunction The failure of two members of a chromosome pair to disjoin during meiosis I, or of paired chromatids to disjoin during meiosis II or mitosis, resulting in one daughter cell with both and the other with neither.

Noninvasive prenatal screening (NIPS) or testing (NIPT) Use of cell-free DNA of fetal origin in maternal blood to screen for fetal aneuploidy.

Nonsense-mediated mRNA decay A cellular mechanism to prevent translation into truncated proteins by recognizing and degrading mRNAs carrying premature translation termination (nonsense) codons.

Nonsense mutation/variant A single-base substitution in DNA resulting in a *termination codon*.

Nonsynonymous Describes a single nucleotide variant (SNV) that alters a codon and therefore the resulting amino acid sequence of the encoded peptide.

Normal distribution The symmetrical, bell-shaped curve describing the frequency of particular values of a measured quantity in a population.

Novel property mutation/variant A genetic change that confers a new property on the protein. Also called gain-of-function or neomorphic mutation/variant.

Nuchal translucency An ultrasonographic finding of an echo-free space between the skin line and the soft tissue overlying the cervical spine in the fetal neck. Associated with fetal aneuploidy.

Nucleoside A structural subunit of nucleic acids, made up of a purine or pyrimidine base and a ribose or deoxyribose sugar. Adenosine, cytosine, guanosine, and thymidine (in DNA) or uridine (in RNA).

Nucleosome The primary structural unit of eukaryotic chromatin, consisting of 146 base pairs of DNA wrapped twice around a core of eight histone molecules.

Nucleotide A *nucleoside* with a phosphate group attached to the 5′ carbon of the sugar molecule. A nucleic acid is a polymer of many nucleotides.

Null allele An allele that results either in total absence of the gene product or total loss of function of the product.

Obligate heterozygote An individual who may be clinically unaffected but, on the basis of pedigree analysis, must carry a specific variant allele.

Odds A ratio of probabilities or risks, often to assess the relative chance of an event occurring. Odds can vary in value from 0 to infinity.

Odds ratio (OR) A comparison of the odds that individuals who share a particular feature or factor (e.g., a genotype, an environmental exposure, or a drug) will have a disease or trait versus the odds for individuals who lack the factor. An OR that differs from 1 means there is an association of disease risk with the genetic marker, whereas OR = 1 means there is no association (see Chapter 11). see *Relative risk*.

Oligonucleotide A short DNA or RNA molecule found in nature (such as *microRNA*) or synthesized for use in laboratory applications – such as polymerase chain reaction or DNA sequencing – or therapies (see *Antisense oligonucleotide [ASO]*).

Oncogene A dominantly acting *driver gene* responsible for tumor development. When a *protooncogene* is activated by mutation, overexpression, or amplification, the oncogene in somatic cells may lead to neoplastic transformation. See also *Tumor-suppressor gene*.

Oogonia Cells derived from primordial germ cells in females that develop into primary oocytes at the end of the third month of fetal life. Primary oocytes enter prophase of meiosis I and then stop, completing meiosis and differentiation into mature ova at the time of ovulation and fertilization.

Open reading frame The interval between a start codon and a downstream stop codon, which may or may not be translated.

Origin of replication One of the hundreds of thousands of sites along each chromosome at which DNA replication begins during the S phase of the cell cycle.

Orthologous Refers to genes in different species that are similar in DNA sequence and usually retain the same function in each species. Orthologous genes originate from the same gene in a common ancestor. Contrast with *paralogous*.

p (1) In cytogenetics, the short arm of a chromosome (from the French *petit*). (2) In population genetics, the frequency of the more common allele of a pair. (3) In biochemistry, abbreviation of *protein* (e.g., p53 is a 53-kD protein).

Pachytene Substage of prophase I in meiosis I following synapsis of homologous chromosomes to form tetrads (bivalents); the stage when meiotic recombination takes place.

Paralogous Refers to two or more genes in a single species that are similar in DNA sequence and function, related through a gene duplication event. Examples are α- and β-globin genes. Contrast with *orthologous*.

Paramesonephric duct Structure in the genital ridges of the early embryo that will develop into female internal sexual organs in the female. Also called the müllerian duct.

Parental transmission bias A phenomenon seen with the inheritance of unstable repeat expansion variants, in which further expansions of the repeat are more likely to occur when transmitted by the parent of one sex than by the other (see Case 17 [Fragile X syndrome], dynamic variants.).

Partial aneusomy Subchromosomal mutation leading to loss of one copy of a segment of a chromosome (partial monosomy) or to gain of a third, extra copy of a segment of a chromosome (partial trisomy).

Passenger gene variant Most genetic variants in tumors appear to be random, are not recurrent in particular cancer types, and probably occur as the cancer develops, rather than directly causing the cancer to develop or progress. Compare with *driver gene*.

Pathogenic variant A genetic variant that causes a disease, either alone (for dominant or X-linked disorders) or in combination with a pathogenic variant on the other allele for recessive conditions.

Pedigree In medical genetics, the diagram of a family history of a hereditary condition(s), indicating the family members, their relationship to the proband and each other, and their status with respect to a particular hereditary condition(s).

Penetrance The fraction of individuals with a genotype known to cause a trait who have any signs or symptoms of the trait. It may be age related. Contrast with *expressivity*.

Pharmacogenetics The area of biochemical genetics concerned with the impact of variation in individual genes on drug response and metabolism.

Pharmacogenomics The application of genomic information or methods to pharmacological interventions.

Pharmacokinetics The study of the rate at which the body absorbs, transports, metabolizes, or excretes a drug or its metabolites.

Phase In an individual heterozygous at two syntenic loci, phase refers to the chromosomal relationship of the pairs of alleles as being in *coupling* and *repulsion*.

Phenocopy A mimic of a genetically determined phenotype, produced instead by an environmental factor.

Phenotype The observed biochemical, physiological, and morphological characteristics of an individual, as determined by genotype and the environment in which it is expressed. Also, the constellation of features that can be recognized as a disease, disorder, or complex trait (e.g., hair, eye, and skin pigment).

Phenotypic threshold effect Primarily as applied for *mtDNA*, a threshold proportion of *heteroplasmy* for a given variant mitochondrial gene may determine when phenotypic expression or disease occurs.

Philadelphia chromosome A seminal discovery in cancer cytogenetics, this abnormally small chromosome 22 is the hallmark of chronic myelogenous leukemia. It is the outcome of a specific reciprocal translocation between chromosomes 9 and 22 (details in Case 10 [Chronic myelogenous leukemia] and Chapter 16).

Pleiotropy (n) The effects of a single gene on multiple unrelated phenotypic features (usually in different organ systems).

Pleiotropic (v) Describes such a gene.

Pluripotent Describes the ability to give rise to different types of differentiated tissues or structures. See *Stem cell* and Chapter 15.

Point mutation See *Single nucleotide variant (SNV)*.

Polar bodies During oogenesis, meiosis I and II divisions each generate a haploid daughter cell with very little cytoplasm; these are not functional ova.

Polyadenylation In the synthesis of mature mRNA, a sequence of 20 to 200 adenosine residues (the polyA tail) is added to the 3′ end of an RNA transcript, aiding its transport out of the nucleus and, usually, its stability.

Polygenic Involving many genes, typically with small additive effects. When epigenetic or environmental factors are recognized, polygenic inheritance is called *complex or multifactorial inheritance*.

Polygenic (risk) score A number that summarizes the estimated effect of many genetic variants on a phenotype or trait. The score, which is typically calculated as a weighted sum of trait-associated alleles, is usually comprised of common variants but can also include rare variants.

Polymerase chain reaction (PCR) The molecular genetic technique by which a short DNA or RNA sequence is amplified enormously by means of two flanking oligonucleotide primers used in repeated cycles of primer extension and DNA synthesis with DNA polymerase.

Polymorphism The occurrence together in a population of two or more alternative alleles, each at a frequency greater than that which could be maintained by recurrent mutation alone. A locus is arbitrarily considered to be polymorphic if a rarer allele (minor allele) has a frequency of at least 0.01, so that the heterozygote frequency is at least 0.02. By convention, any allele rarer than this is a *rare variant*. Despite common usage of polymorphism to mean an allele at a polymorphic locus, or (mistakenly) to benign changes, the terms "common variant," "single-nucleotide variant," and "nonpathogenic variant" are more accurate.

Population genetics The study of genetic variants in populations and of how their frequencies change over time in response to forces such as mutation, selection, genetic drift, and gene flow. (See Chapter 10.)

Positive predictive value The probability that individuals with a positive test result actually have or will develop the trait in question. Contrast with *negative predictive value*.

Preimplantation diagnosis A type of prenatal diagnosis undertaken following in vitro fertilization and before implantation to the uterus. From a multicellular embryo, now usually at the trophoblast stage, one or more cells are removed to be tested for the presence of a disease-causing genetic variant. An embryo that does not have the variant of concern can then be implanted to establish a pregnancy.

Premature ovarian insufficiency Loss of normal ovarian function before age 40.

Premutation Evolving terminology – see *Intermediate repeat expansion*. In disorders associated with unstable repeats (e.g., fragile X syndrome [see Case 17], Huntington disease [see Case 24]), a moderate expansion of the number of repeats, with increased risk for further expansion during meiosis. This may cause the full disorder in offspring due to a full-penetrance expansion variant. With Huntington disease (*HTT* gene), an intermediate expansion allele is not itself pathogenic. With fragile X syndrome (*FMR1* gene), currently, a distinction is made between intermediate alleles and premutation alleles; the latter being associated with a distinct syndrome, such as the fragile X–associated tremor/ataxia syndrome (FXTAS) or premature ovarian insufficiency.

Primary constriction See *Centromere*.

Primary transcript The initial, unprocessed RNA transcript of a gene that is collinear with the genomic DNA, containing introns as well as exons.

Proband The affected family member through whom the family is ascertained. Also called the *propositus* or *index case*.

Prometaphase The stage of mitosis between *prophase* and *metaphase* in which the nuclear membrane dissolves and chromosomes attach to the mitotic spindle.

Promoter A regulatory DNA sequence of 100 to 1000 base pairs located at the 5′ end of a gene, to which proteins bind to initiate transcription.

Pronuclei Immediately following fertilization, chromosomes of sperm and egg are enclosed in separate nuclear membranes, each a haploid pronucleus. These migrate within the egg, fuse, and the two sets of chromosomes join into a single diploid nucleus.

Prophase The first stage of cell division, during which the chromosomes become visible as discrete structures and subsequently thicken and shorten. Prophase of the first meiotic division is further characterized by pairing (*synapsis*) of homologous chromosomes.

Propositus See *Proband*.

Proteome The collection of all proteins in a cell, tissue, or organism at a particular time. Contrast with *transcriptome* and *genome*.

Proteomics The comprehensive analysis and cataloguing of proteins and *proteomes*. Parallels *genomics*.

Protooncogene A gene involved in normal cell division or proliferation that may become activated by mutation or other mechanism to become an *oncogene*.

Pseudoautosomal regions (PAR1, PAR2) Homologous segments of the X and Y chromosomes, at the most distal portion of their respective p and q arms, at which crossing over occurs during male meiosis. Genes in these regions escape X inactivation in females; they are inherited in an autosomal rather than strictly sex-linked manner.

Pseudodeficiency allele A clinically benign allele causing reduced functional activity, as detected by in vitro assays, but sufficient in vivo activity to prevent clinical manifestation.

Pseudogene (1) An inactive gene within a gene family, derived by mutation of an ancestral active gene and frequently located in the same region of the chromosome as its functional counterpart (nonprocessed pseudogene). (2) A DNA copy of an mRNA, created by *retrotransposition* and inserted randomly in the genome (processed pseudogene). Processed pseudogenes are probably never functional.

Pseudomosaicism A cell culture artifact that may arise in karyotype preparation.

Purine One of the two types of nitrogen-containing bases (the other being pyrimidine) in DNA and RNA (adenine and guanine).

Pyrimidine One of the two types of nitrogen-containing bases (the other being purine) in DNA and RNA (cytosine and thymine in DNA, cytosine and uracil in RNA).

q (1) In cytogenetics, the long arm of a chromosome. (2) In population genetics, the frequency of the less common allele of a pair. Compare with *p*.

Quadrivalent In a cell with a balanced translocation, the complex of four chromosomes that forms in meiosis I synapsis, consisting of the two translocated chromosomes paired with the two corresponding normal chromosomes.

Qualitative trait A trait that is descriptive in nature. Contrast with *quantitative trait*.

Quantitative trait A trait based on information that can be measured or counted. Differences among individuals often follow a normal distribution in the population. Contrast with *qualitative trait*.

Random mating Selection for procreation without regard to the genotype of the mate. In a randomly mating population, the probability that a parent transmits a given allele is equal to the population allele frequency. Random mating is a prerequisite for *Hardy-Weinberg* equilibrium.

Reading frame One of the three possible ways of reading a nucleotide sequence as a series of triplets for potential translation into a protein sequence. See *Open reading frame*.

Rearrangement Chromosome breakage followed by reconstitution into an abnormal combination. The outcome may be balanced or unbalanced, depending on whether any genetic material is gained or lost.

Recessive Refers to a trait that is expressed only in homozygotes, compound heterozygotes, or hemizygotes for the allele(s).

Reciprocal translocation See *Translocation*.

Recombinant Describes an individual, organism, cell, protein, chromosome, or DNA with a new combination of genetic material.

Recombinant chromosome A chromosome that results from exchange of reciprocal segments by crossing over between a homologous pair of parental chromosomes during meiosis.

Recombination fraction (θ) In genetic linkage analysis, the fraction of offspring in which a recombination (crossing over) has occurred between two genetic loci.

Recurrence risk The probability that a genetic trait present in a family will recur in another member of the same or a subsequent generation.

Reduction division The first meiotic division, so-called because at this stage the chromosome number per cell is reduced from diploid to haploid.

Redundancy The situation in which genes (often *paralogous*) have overlapping functions. Also, in reference to the *genetic code*, see *Degeneracy*.

Regulative development See Chapter 15 Box 15.1.

Regulatory element A DNA segment, such as a promoter, insulator, enhancer, or locus control region, within or near a gene that regulates the expression of the gene.

Regulatory gene A gene that codes for an RNA or protein molecule that regulates the expression of other genes.

Relative risk (RR) A comparison of the *risk* for a disease or trait in individuals who share a particular factor (e.g., genotype, an environmental exposure, or a drug) versus the *risk* among individuals who lack the factor. An RR that differs from 1 means there is an association of disease risk with the genetic marker, whereas RR = 1 means there is no association. When a disease event is rare, there is little difference between RRs and *odds ratios* (ORs) (see Chapters 11 and 19).

Relative risk ratio (λ_r) (subscript refers to "relatives") In complex disorders, the frequency of a trait in close relatives of an affected person over the prevalence in the general population (see Chapter 9). Compare to *standardized incidence ratio*.

Repetitive (repeat) DNA DNA sequences that are present in multiple copies in the genome.

Replicative segregation Replication of *mtDNA* takes place throughout the cell cycle. At cell division, copies of *mtDNA* in each of the mitochondria in each cell segregate (assort) randomly into the daughter cells.

Repulsion (*trans*) The phase of two alleles at syntenic loci when they are *not* on the same chromosome. See *Phase* and *Coupling*.

Retrotransposition A process by which a molecule of RNA, often derived from transcription of a repetitive element such as *Alu* or *LINE*, is transcribed by *reverse transcriptase* into a molecule of DNA, which is then inserted into another site in the genome.

Retrovirus An RNA virus that, upon infection, uses *reverse transcriptase* to transcribe its RNA into DNA, which can integrate into the host genome. Exploited as vectors for gene therapy.

Reverse transcriptase An RNA-dependent DNA polymerase that catalyzes the synthesis of DNA on an RNA template.

Ribonucleic acid See *RNA*.

Ribosome A cytoplasmic organelle composed of ribosomal RNA and protein, on which polypeptides are synthesized based on the sequences of messenger RNA.

Ring chromosome A structurally abnormal chromosome in which the telomeres have been deleted and the broken arms have reunited in ring formation.

Risk The probability of a particular occurrence, especially as applied to an adverse outcome, such as disease.

RNA (ribonucleic acid) A ribose-containing nucleic acid formed on a DNA template; the template on which polypeptides are synthesized. *Transfer RNA (tRNA)*, in cooperation with the ribosomes, brings amino acids into position along the mRNA template. *Ribosomal RNA (rRNA)*, a component of the ribosomes, functions as a nonspecific site of polypeptide synthesis. See also *Messenger RNA (mRNA) and Noncoding RNAs (ncRNAs)*.

RNA editing Posttranscriptional modification of any type of RNA transcript, including base changes and other modifications that can affect function or stability of the molecule; also called RNA epigenetics. Associated with functions such as neuronal regulation and immune defense. See Chapter 3.

RNA interference (RNAi) A system for regulating gene expression; *microRNA* molecules form double-stranded structures with mRNA, either targeting it for destruction or blocking its translation. Scientists have taken advantage of this normal, endogenous system of gene regulation to design new and powerful technologies for gene silencing by use of exogenously supplied RNAi sequences. See Chapter 14.

RNA polymerase An enzyme that synthesizes RNA on a DNA template. Multiple RNA polymerases each synthesize different RNA molecules; the best studied is RNA polymerase II, responsible for primary transcription of mRNA.

RNA splicing The excision of introns from primary RNA transcripts and splicing together of exons, to generate mature mRNA from the primary transcript.

Robertsonian translocation A translocation between two acrocentric chromosomes by fusion at or near the centromere, with loss of the short arms.

Sanger sequencing Developed in the laboratory of Fred Sanger in 1977, it remains the gold standard for accuracy of DNA sequence determination. Though impractical for large-scale analyses, it is still used for some targeted sequencing or confirmation analysis. It is also called the chain termination method.

Satellite DNA DNA containing many tandem repeats of a short basic repeating unit. The name derives from the tendency of such repetitive DNA to separate from bulk DNA on density gradients. See Chapter 2. Not to be confused with *chromosomal satellite*.

Scaffold (1) In chromosome structure, the protein backbone observed after histones are depleted. (2) In genome sequence assemblies, an intermediate between contig and chromosome.

Segmental duplication Blocks of nearly identical sequences distributed across the genome that predispose to duplication and deletion of the segments of DNA located between them.

Segregation In genetics, the distribution of genetic material into daughter cells. For chromosomes, it is the orderly disjunction of the haploid set of homologous chromosomes at meiosis I or sister chromatids at meiosis II. For mitochondria, refers to the distribution of newly formed mitochondria into daughter cells during mitosis. See *Nondisjunction* and *Replicative segregation*.

Segregation distortion Deviation of genotype frequencies from expected mendelian segregation ratios.

Selection In population genetics, the operation of forces that determine the relative fitness of a genotype in the population, thus affecting the frequency of particular alleles. The coefficient of selection, s, is a measure of the proportion of variant alleles at a locus that are not passed on to the next generation and is given by 1-f, where f is the coefficient of fitness. See Chapter 10.

Sense strand See *Coding strand*.

Sensitivity (true positive rate) In diagnostic tests, the frequency with which the test result is positive when the condition is present. Not to be confused with *positive predictive value*.

Sequence (1) In genomics and molecular genetics, the order of nucleotides in a segment of DNA or RNA. (2) In clinical genetics, a recognizable pattern of dysmorphic features due to various causes; to be distinguished from *malformation syndrome*.

Sex chromatin See *Barr body*.

Sex chromosomes The X and Y chromosomes.

Sex-influenced Referring to a trait that is not X-linked in its pattern of inheritance but is expressed differently, either in degree or in frequency, between males and females.

Sex-limited Referring to a trait that is expressed in only one sex, although the gene that determines the trait is autosomal.

Sex-linked A general term referring to genes on either of the sex chromosomes. In human and medical genetics, the term is typically replaced by *X-linked* or *Y-linked*.

Short tandem repeat At a polymorphic locus, a variable number of tandemly repeated dinucleotide, trinucleotide, or tetranucleotide units, such as $(TG)_n$, $(CAA)_n$, or $(GATA)_n$; different numbers of units constitute the different alleles. Also termed a *microsatellite marker*.

Sib, sibling A brother or sister.

Sibship All the sibs in a family.

Silencer A DNA sequence that acts in *cis* (i.e., on the same chromosome) to decrease transcription of a nearby gene. The silencer may be upstream or downstream of the gene, in the same or the reverse orientation (contrast with *enhancer*).

Single nucleotide variant (SNV) An altered sequence at a single base pair in DNA. The term single nucleotide polymorphism (*SNP*) is used widely to imply a relatively common variant (present in >1%), and although entrenched, more precise terminology (such as "common SNV") is now encouraged.

Single-copy DNA DNA whose linear order of specific nucleotides is represented once (or at most a few times) in the haploid genome.

Single-gene disorder A disorder due to one or a pair of pathogenic alleles at a single locus. Also called monogenic disorder or mendelian disorder.

Slipped strand mispairing A mutational mechanism that occurs during DNA replication of sequences with tandem nucleotide repeats. A nascent DNA strand can temporarily dissociate and reanneal, becoming misaligned due to the repeats, generating a deletion or expansion.

Small (or short) interfering RNAs (siRNAs) A class of naturally occurring or synthesized 20- to 25-nucleotide–long, double-stranded RNA molecules that regulate gene expression by inducing the degradation of complementary mRNA, by the process of RNA interference. They have substantial therapeutic potential against targets that otherwise cannot be treated by drugs.

SNP array A type of microarray that uses *oligonucleotides* corresponding to high-frequency genomic single nucleotide variants from polymorphic loci to detect a chromosomal or subchromosomal deletion or duplication (i.e., CNV). Alternative to *comparative genome hybridization;* used for *GWAS* and *LOH* studies.

Solenoid A 30 nm helical secondary structure in chromatin organization, functioning to package DNA in the nucleus.

Somatic cell Any cell of the body, excluding the *germline.*

Somatic mutation A mutation that occurs in a somatic cell rather than in the germline.

Somatic recombination Rearrangement of DNA sequences in the chromosomes of lymphocyte precursor cells, thus generating antibody and T-cell receptor diversity.

Southern blot A molecular technique to detect specific DNA sequences. Following restriction enzyme digestion and gel electrophoresis to separate DNA molecules by size, DNA is transferred from the gel to a membrane and hybridized with a labeled probe of interest. For radioactively labeled probes, the membrane is exposed to X-ray film and the size of specific DNA restriction fragments can then be determined by their position on the blot, in relation to size standards. This eponym for the British scientist, Ed Southern, was followed somewhat tongue-in-cheek by terms, northern blot and western blot for similar approaches applied for RNA and protein detection, respectively.

Specialty proteins Proteins with unique functions contributing to the individuality of the limited types of cells in which they are expressed. Contrast with *Housekeeping proteins.*

Specification A step in the differentiation pathway. See Chapter 15 Box 15.1.

Specificity (true negative rate) In diagnostic tests, the frequency with which a test result is negative when the condition is absent. Not to be confused with *negative predictive value.*

Spermatogonia Diploid cells derived from early germ cells in the male. They divide to replenish their population and, at puberty, undergo a series of developmental steps, including meiosis, leading to terminal differentiation into mature spermatozoa.

Splicing See *RNA splicing.*

Sporadic In medical genetics, referring to a trait that has occurred in isolation, without evidence of family history. This may be due to a nongenetic or a complex multifactorial cause, or a new germline or somatic mutation. Compare to *familial.*

Standardized incidence ratio (SIR) The ratio of the observed incidence of cancer during a given time period in a specific group divided by the number expected over that same time period in age-matched controls. See Chapter 16.

Stem cell A cell capable of (1) self-renewal or proliferation while in an undifferentiated state and (2) differentiation into specialized cell types. Some classes include embryonic, fetal, adult, or induced pluripotent stem cells.

Stop codon See *Termination codon.*

Stratification The situation in which a population contains subgroups whose members are not freely and randomly mating with the members of other subgroups.

Structural gene A gene coding for any RNA or protein product other than a regulatory factor.

Structural protein A protein, such as collagen or elastin, that serves a structural role in a tissue.

Structural rearrangement/variant A change in the structure of one or more chromosomes. The alteration may be balanced if there is no change in genomic content (e.g., balanced translocation or inversion), or unbalanced, if genomic content is abnormal (e.g., duplication or deletion).

Submetacentric Refers to a chromosome with its centromere off-center, creating arms of different lengths. Compare to *metacentric* and *acrocentric.*

Synapsis Close pairing of homologous chromosomes in prophase of the first meiotic division.

Synaptonemal complex During meiosis I, the protein complex that forms between homologous chromosomes and mediates synapsis and recombination.

Syndrome A characteristic pattern of anomalies found together, presumed to be due to a single underlying cause (genetic or teratogenic). See Chapter 15.

Synonymous Describes a single nucleotide variant (SNV) that does not alter the resulting amino acid sequence of the encoded peptide (because of *redundancy [degeneracy]* of the genetic code).

Synteny The physical presence together on the same chromosome of two or more genetic loci, whether or not they are close enough together for linkage to be demonstrated (the adjective is *syntenic*).

Tandem repeats Two or more copies of the same (or similar) DNA sequence arranged in a direct head-to-tail succession along a chromosome.

TATA box In the promoter region of many genes, a DNA sequence that is most commonly TATAAA; it indicates both the direction and strand of transcription and is usually located 25 to 35 base pairs upstream from the transcription start site.

T-cell antigen receptor (TCR) Genetically coded receptor on the surface of T lymphocytes that specifically recognizes antigen molecules.

Telocentric Refers to a chromosome form, abnormal in humans, in which the centromere is at one end and there is only a single arm.

Telomerase (Terminal transferase) A ribonucleoprotein reverse transcriptase (i.e., RNA + protein + enzyme) that maintains telomere length to protect chromosome ends in proliferating cells. With its own RNA template for synthesizing species-specific hexamers it adds them to the ends of telomeres. See Case 49 (Telomere-related pulmonary fibrosis) and Chapter 15.

Telomere A region of repetitive nucleotide sequence at the end of each chromosome arm, which protects the end from progressive degradation (shortening). Human telomeres end with tandem copies of the sequence (TTAGGG)$_n$. They have roles in cancers and in age-related disorders where they may show different manifestations and *anticipation* due to progressive telomere shortening. (See Case 49 [Telomere-related pulmonary fibrosis] and Chapter 15.)

Telophase The final stage of meiotic or mitotic cell division that begins when the daughter chromosomes reach the poles of the dividing cell and that lasts until the two daughter cells take on the appearance of interphase cells.

Teratogen An agent that produces or increases the incidence of prenatal/congenital malformations.

Termination codon One of the three codons (UAG, UAA, and UGA) that terminate synthesis of a polypeptide. Also called a *stop codon* or *chain-termination codon*.

Tertiary structure Three-dimensional configuration of a molecule.

Tetraploid Describing a cell with four (4n) copies of each chromosome, or an individual made up of such cells.

The Cancer Genome Atlas (TCGA) A public database of mutations, epigenomic modifications, and abnormal gene expression profiles found in a wide variety of cancers.

Trans (1) Refers to the relationship between two genomic sequences located on opposite homologous chromosomes. Literally means "across from." (2) Trans effects are those mediated by a molecule from outside the target, such as diffusible factors acting throughout the genome. Contrast with *cis*.

Transcription The synthesis of a single-stranded RNA molecule from a DNA template in the cell nucleus, catalyzed by RNA polymerase. Applies not only to mRNA but also to tRNA, rRNA, and various noncoding RNAs.

Transcription factor A protein that regulates the rate of transcription by binding to the regulatory region of a gene. Its defining feature is a specific DNA-binding domain. It may work alone or with other proteins in a complex.

Transcriptome The collection of all RNA transcripts made in a cell.

Transfer RNA (tRNA) See *RNA*.

Transformation In cancer biology, the in vivo process by which a normal cell becomes malignant.

Translation The synthesis of a polypeptide from its mRNA template.

Translocation The transfer of a segment of one chromosome to another chromosome. If two nonhomologous chromosomes exchange pieces, the translocation is *reciprocal*. See also *Robertsonian translocation*.

Triploid Refers to a cell with three copies of each chromosome (3n), or an individual made up of such cells.

Trisomy The state of having three representatives of a given chromosome instead of the usual pair, such as trisomy 21 (Down syndrome).

tRNA Transfer RNA; see *RNA*.

Tumor-suppressor gene A type of *driver gene* where the wild-type is involved in the regulation of cell proliferation. Loss-of-function variants in both alleles can lead to tumor development, as with the retinoblastoma (*RB1*) gene (Case 39) or the *TP53* gene. Contrast with *oncogene*.

Two-hit theory In cancer biology, the theory that some forms of cancer can be initiated when both alleles of a tumor-suppressor gene become inactivated in the same cell.

Unbalanced (skewed) X inactivation A substantial deviation from the expected equal distribution of inactivation between the two X chromosomes in a female.

Uniparental disomy (UPD) The presence of two copies of a given chromosome (or part thereof), both inherited from one parent, with no copy from the other parent. If both homologues of the parental pair are present, the situation is *heterodisomy*; if one parental homologue is present in duplicate, the situation is *isodisomy*. See Chapter 6 and Case 38.

Unstable repeat expansion See *Dynamic variant*.

Untranslated region (UTR) The segment of a gene and corresponding mRNA either that precedes the initiator codon (5'-UTR) or follows the stop codon (3'-UTR).

Variant (n) An allele that differs from *wild-type*. (adj) Referring to an altered allele. To specify the consequence of a variant allele, modifiers such as "disease-causing," "loss-of-function," "single nucleotide," "common," "rare," "copy number," "pathogenic," "benign," "of uncertain significance," etc. are used.

Variant of uncertain significance (VUS) A genomic sequence variant detected whose pathogenetic significance is currently unknown. This consequence of relatively untargeted screening by sequencing or microarrays has created challenges for diagnostics – particularly prenatal – but it is not a static designation. Further knowledge and experience can move the designation in the direction of "benign" or "pathogenic." See Chapter 17.

Vector In gene transfer therapy, a DNA molecule, such as a virus, whose genome has been engineered to contain and express a therapeutic DNA sequence of interest. It is used to deliver the DNA sequence into a cell.

VNTR (variable number of tandem repeats) A type of DNA variant created by a tandem arrangement of varying numbers of copies of short DNA sequences. These highly polymorphic loci were exploited in early linkage studies and in DNA "fingerprinting" for paternity testing and forensic medicine. See *Satellite DNA*.

Whole exome sequencing (WES) Also called exome sequencing (ES). Use of high-throughput methods to sequence all the exons of protein-coding genes (the *exome*), which comprise about 1.5% of the genome. See *Whole genome sequencing* and Chapter 5.

Whole genome sequencing (WGS) Use of high-throughput methods to determine the sequence of an individual's entire genome (minus the few percent that current technologies are not capable of sequencing). See Chapter 5.

Wild type A term from classical genetics used to indicate the "normal" allele (often symbolized as + or wt) or the normal phenotype, that is, as it occurs commonly in nature. It is sometimes applied to the most frequent allele in a population.

X chromosome The larger of the two sex chromosomes; in humans, normally present in two copies in females and one copy in males.

X inactivation Inactivation of genes on one X chromosome in somatic cells of female mammals, generally occurring randomly, early in embryonic life. See *Lyon's law (hypothesis)* and Chapters 3 and 6.

X linkage The presence of alleles at loci on the X chromosome and/or the characteristic inheritance patterns that they engender. Genes on the X chromosome, or traits determined by such genes, are X-linked.

Y chromosome The smaller of the two sex chromosomes, normally present in one copy in males only.

Y linkage Genes on the Y chromosome, or traits (e.g., the male sex) determined by such genes, are Y-linked.

Zone of polarizing activity Region in a developing limb bud that secretes morphogens to specify the posterior side of the developing limb bud. See Chapter 15.

Zygosity The number of zygotes from which a multiple birth is derived. See *Monozygotic (MZ) twins* and *Dizygotic (DZ) twins*. Also, the status of an allele in a gene or region: homozygous, heterozygous, hemizygous.

Zygote The first diploid cell resulting from fertilization between two *gametes*; a fertilized ovum.

Zygotene Stage in meiosis I when homologous chromosomes align along their entire length to permit *synapsis*.

Answers to Problems

CHAPTER 2 *Ada Hamosh and Stephen W. Scherer*

1. (a) *A* or *a*.
   (b) i. At meiosis I. ii. At meiosis II.
2. Meiotic nondisjunction.
3. $(1/2)^{23} \times (1/2)^{23}$; you would be female.
4. (a) 23; 46.
   (b) 23; 23.
   (c) At fertilization; at S phase of the next cell cycle.
5. Genes/Mb estimates: chromosome 1, ≈9; chromosome 13, ≈3-4; chromosome 18, ≈4; chromosome 19, ≈19; chromosome 21, ≈5; chromosome 22, ≈10.

   Because of the higher density of genes, a chromosome abnormality of chromosome 19 would more likely impact phenotype than one of similar size on chromosome 18. Similarly, a chromosome 22 structural variant would more likely have a clinical impact than one for chromosome 21. Of course, these are generalizations, since the degree of clinical impact may depend on the function of the genes involved (e.g., developmental vs. metabolic).

CHAPTER 3 *Stephen W. Scherer*

1. There are several possible sequences because of the degeneracy of the genetic code. One possible sequence of the double-stranded DNA is:

   | 5′ | AAA | AGA | CAT | CAT | TAT | CTA | 3′ |
   | 3′ | TTT | TCT | GTA | GTA | ATA | GAT | 5′ |

   RNA polymerase "reads" the bottom (3′ to 5′) strand. The sequence of the resulting mRNA would be 5′ AAA AGA CAU CAU UAU CUA 3′.

   The variants represent the following kinds of mutations:
   - Mutant 1: single-nucleotide substitution in fifth codon; e.g., UAU → UGU (from TAT → TGA at the DNA level).
   - Mutant 2: frameshift mutation, deletion in first nucleotide of third codon.
   - Mutant 3: frameshift mutation, insertion of G between first and second codons.
   - Mutant 4: in-frame deletion of three codons (nine nucleotides), beginning at the third base.

2. Chromosomes contain chromatin, consisting of nucleosomes, which are DNA coiled around histone proteins. Chromosomes contain several thousand kilobase pairs of DNA (or several million base pairs), coding for hundreds of genes, each containing (usually) both introns and exons. The exons comprise a series of three-nucleotide codons, each specifying an amino acid. Each gene has a promoter at its 5′ end that directs transcription of the gene under appropriate conditions.

3. An altered promoter could interfere with or eliminate transcription of the gene. A variant of the initiator codon would prevent normal translation of the mRNA. Variants at splice sites can interfere with the normal process of RNA splicing, leading to abnormal mRNAs. A 1-bp deletion in the coding sequence would lead to a frameshift variant, thus changing the frame in which the genetic code is read downstream from the deletion; this would alter the encoded amino acids and change the sequence of the protein. (See examples in Chapter 11.) A nonsynonymous variant in the stop codon would allow translation to continue beyond its normal stopping point, thus adding new amino acids to the end of the encoded protein. Altered splicing or frameshifts can also introduce a premature stop codon, which in the last exon or last ~50 bp of the penultimate exon usually leads to nonsense mediated mRNA decay and complete absence of protein product.

4. Sequence changes in introns can influence RNA splicing, thus leading to an abnormally spliced mRNA (see Chapter 11). *Alu* or LINE sequences can be involved in abnormal recombination events between different copies of the repeat, thus deleting or rearranging genes. LINE repeats can also actively transpose around the genome, potentially inserting into a functional gene and disrupting its normal function. Locus control regions influence the proper expression of genes in time and space; deletion or alteration of a locus control region can thus disrupt normal expression of a gene (see Chapter 12). Pseudogenes are, generally, nonfunctional copies of genes; thus in most instances, variants in a pseudogene would not be expected to contribute to disease, although there are rare exceptions.

5. RNA splicing generates a mature RNA from the primary RNA transcript by combining segments of exonic RNA and eliminating intronic RNA. RNA splicing is a critical step in normal gene expression in all tissues and operates at the level of RNA. Genomic DNA remains unchanged. In contrast, somatic rearrangement, as part of the normal

process of generating immunoglobulin and T-cell receptor diversity during lymphocyte development, involves segments of genomic DNA rearranged to eliminate certain sequences and generate mature genes. Normal somatic rearrangement is highly specific to only these genes and cell types. Abnormal nonspecific somatic rearrangement is a feature of tumor cells.

6. Genomic imprinting involves epigenetic silencing of an allele (or alleles at closely located genes) due to epigenetic marks inherited through the germline, based on parental origin of the chromosome. X inactivation also involves epigenetic silencing of alleles along much of an entire chromosome, but reflecting a random choice of one or the other X chromosome at the time of initiation of the inactivation process in early embryonic development.

CHAPTER 4   *Stephen W. Scherer and Ada Hamosh*

1. (a) Copy number variant (CNV).
   (b) Insertion/deletion (Indel).
   (c) A variant in a splice site.
   (d) An inversion.
   (e) A single-nucleotide variant (or in/del) in a noncoding region or intron, or one that leads to a synonymous substitution.
2. Each birth involves 2 alleles for a given locus. One generation is ~20 years. Thus 41 mutations / 9 million alleles / 2 generations = $\approx 2.3 \times 10^{-6}$ mutations / generation at the aniridia locus. The estimate is based on assumptions that ascertained cases from parents with normal vision result from new mutations, that the disease is fully penetrant, that all new affected individuals are liveborn (and ascertained), and that there is only a single locus responsible for aniridia.
3. A microsatellite, because these typically have more alleles, providing greater capacity to distinguish genomes.
4. Different types of mutations are sensitive to maternal or paternal age. Both single nucleotide mutations and new copy number variants (CNVs) show an increase in frequency with increasing age of the father. In contrast, meiotic nondisjunction for many chromosomes (including chromosome 21) shows an increase with increasing age of the mother. The rate of mutation (per bp) varies greatly among different locations around the genome, including hot spots, although the basis for this is poorly understood. Intrachromosomal homologous recombination can lead to copy number variation in gene families or to deletion/duplications for regions flanked by homologous sequences (e.g., segmental duplications). Overall, the rate of mutation can be influenced by genetic variation, both at a population level and in specific parental genomes.

CHAPTER 5   *Dimitri J. Stavropoulos*

1. (a) The infant has an unbalanced male karyotype with 46 chromosomes in which one chromosome 18 has been replaced by a derivative chromosome 18. The der(18) chromosome is the result of a translocation between one chromosome 7 and one chromosome 18 with breakpoints in the long arms at bands 7q33 and 18q12.3, respectively. The microarray results characterize the karyotypic imbalance to be a terminal gain (trisomy) of chromosome region 7q33 to 7qter spanning genomic coordinates 136240808 to 159345973, and a terminal loss (monosomy) of chromosome region 18q12.3 to 18qter with genomic coordinates 45466214 to 80373285. The genomic coordinates are based on human genome build GRCh38.
   (b) To determine whether the abnormality is *de novo* or inherited from a balanced carrier parent, thus influencing the predicted recurrence risk for a subsequent offspring.
   (c) Forty-six chromosomes, male; there is one normal 7 and one normal 18, plus a reciprocal translocation between chromosomes 7 (with breakpoint in band 7q33) and 18 (with breakpoint in band 18q12.3). This is a balanced karyotype. See Fig. 5.11 as an example of meiotic pairing and segregation for balanced reciprocal translocations. The father can produce gametes that are normal, chromosomally balanced translocation, or unbalanced translocation.
2. (a) ~95%.
   (b) No increased risk based on this result alone, but prenatal diagnosis may be offered.
3. Postzygotic nondisjunction, in an early mitotic division. Although the clinical course cannot be predicted with complete accuracy, it is possible that she will be somewhat less severely affected than would a child with nonmosaic trisomy 21.
4. (a) If the supernumerary marker contains euchromatic material with dosage-sensitive genes, the proband is expected to be clinically affected, whereas a small marker restricted to the centromeric and other repetitive sequences is not expected to cause an abnormal phenotype.
   (b) Abnormal phenotype (trisomy 13; see Chapter 6).
   (c) Normal phenotype, but risk for chromosomally unbalanced offspring.
   (d) Normal phenotype, but risk for chromosomally unbalanced offspring depending on the size of the inverted segment.
5. (a) Not indicated.
   (b) Fetal chromosome analysis by noninvasive prenatal screening (e.g., cell-free fetal DNA in maternal serum) or rapid aneuploidy testing following chorionic villus sampling or amniocentesis; at risk for trisomy 21, in particular.

(c) Karyotype is indicated for the child to investigate whether the extra copy of chromosome 21 is part of a Robertsonian translocation. If a Robertsonian translocation is identified in the proband, parental karyotypes are indicated. If a balanced Robertsonian translocation is identified in one of the parents, there is a risk of having offspring with trisomy of the chromosomes involved in the robertsonian translocation.

(d) Chromosome/genome analysis is not indicated. Targeted genetic analysis for the causative *CFTR* variants in the parents is indicated (see Chapter 7).

(e) Chromosome microarray analysis is indicated for the boys to test for genome-wide copy number variants. Alternatively, genome sequencing may be considered to identify genome-wide copy number as well as sequence level variants. If clinical findings indicate the possibility of fragile X syndrome, a specific DNA diagnostic test would be indicated.

6. (a) Paracentric inversion of the X chromosome in a female, between bands Xq21 and Xq26, determined by karyotyping.

(b) Terminal deletion of 1p36.2 to 1pter in a female, determined by karyotyping.

(c) Female with interstitial deletion within band q11.2 of chromosome 15, determined by fluorescence *in situ* hybridization (FISH) with probes for the *SNRPN* gene and D15S10 locus.

(d) Female with interstitial deletion of chromosome 15, between bands q11.2 and q13, determined by karyotyping. FISH analysis confirmed the deletion using probes for the *SNRPN* gene and D15S10 locus

(e) Female karyotype appeared normal by G-banding, but chromosome microarray analysis identified a duplication within chromosome 1 from genomic position 1755688 to 2633531 using genome build GRCh38. This duplication involves bands 1p36.33 and 1p36.32.

(f) Male with a supernumerary marker chromosome, determined by karyotyping. The marker was identified by FISH as originating from chromosome 8 using probe D8Z1 targeted to chromosome 8 centromere sequences.

(g) Female with Down syndrome, with a 13q;21q Robertsonian translocation containing the long arms of chromosomes 13 and 21, in addition to two normal chromosomes 21, and one normal chromosome 13 determined by karyotyping.

(h) Chromosomally balanced male carrier of a 13q;21q Robertsonian translocation, in addition to a single normal chromosome 21 and a single normal chromosome 13, as determined by karyotyping.

7. arr[GRCh38] 22q11.21(18874431_20348930)x1

CHAPTER 6   *Feyza Yilmaz, Christine R. Beck, Charles Lee*

1. Theoretically, X and XX gametes in equal proportions; expected XX, XY, XXX, and XXY offspring (25% each). In actuality, XXX women have virtually all chromosomally normal offspring, (XX or XY), implying that XX gametes are at a significant disadvantage or are lost.

2. The inversion is balanced, and it is possible that the relevant region of chromosome 9 has very few genes and that the inversion does not interfere with gene structure or function. As with other pericentric inversions, the risk is to their offspring. However, the flanking regions of 9p and 9q are so large (i.e., most of those chromosome arms) that duplication or deletion resulting from meiotic crossing over may be incompatible with life. Alternatively, centromeric regions of chromosomes are relatively poor in recombination; thus there may be very few crossovers in this region, and the inv(9) could pass to the next generation unchanged.

3. No. XYY can result only from meiosis II nondisjunction in the male, whereas XXY can result from nondisjunction at meiosis I in the male or at either division in the female.

4. Translocation of Y chromosome material containing the sex-determining region (and the *SRY* gene) to the X chromosome or to an autosome.

5. The small r(X) may contain genes that normally would undergo X inactivation but fail to do so for lack of an X inactivation center. Such genes would show biallelic expression at higher levels than in typical males or females. This abnormal gene expression may underlie the intellectual disability, or it could be due to an incidental unrelated genetic issue.

   In the second family, the larger r(X) contains the X inactivation center. Thus one predicts that X inactivation should proceed normally and the r(X) would be the inactive X in all cells (due to secondary cell selection; see Fig. 6.13B). The phenotype is somewhat uncertain, however, because this individual may be deficient for genes that would typically escape X inactivation and be expressed biallelically; some features of Turner syndrome may therefore be present.

6. Expected karyotype: 46,XX; Disorder: congenital adrenal hyperplasia. Counseling: autosomal recessive; prenatal diagnosis possible; need for clinical attention in neonatal period to determine gender issues and to forestall salt-losing crises.

7. (a) None; the short arms of all acrocentric chromosomes are believed to be identical and contain multiple copies of rRNA genes.

(b) None if the deletion involves only heterochromatin (Yq12). A more proximal deletion might delete genes important in spermatogenesis (see Fig. 6.14).

(c) Cri du chat syndrome, severity depending on the amount of DNA deleted (see Fig. 6.8).

(d) Some features of Turner syndrome, but with normal stature; the Xq– chromosome is preferentially inactivated in all cells (provided that the X inactivation center is not deleted), thus reducing the potential severity of such a deletion. Deletion of the same amount of DNA on different chromosomes might delete a vastly different number of genes, thus leading to different phenotypic expectations (see Fig. 2.7)

8. (a) A 1% risk is often quoted, but the risk is probably not greater than the population age-related risk.

(b) Age-related risk is >1%.

(c) No increased risk if the niece with Down syndrome has trisomy 21, but if the niece carries a Robertsonian translocation, the consultand may be a carrier and at high risk.

(d) 10–15%; see text.

(e) Empirically, only a few percent. The woman's age-related risk is relevant.

9. 46,XX,rob(21;21)(q10;q10) or 46,XX,der(21;21)(q10;q10). (There is no need to add +21 to the karyotype.)

10. Crossing over leads to either balanced gametes or nonviable gametes (see Fig. 5.12). Thus liveborn offspring are genomically balanced.

CHAPTER 7 *Neal Sondheimer*

1. (b) Calvin and Cathy are obligate heterozygotes. Given that Calvin and Cathy are first cousins, it is also very likely that they inherited their variant allele through Betty and Barbara from the same grandparent. Thus Betty and Barbara are likely but not obligate carriers. DNA-based carrier testing will answer the question definitively.

2. (a) Heterozygous at each of two loci (e.g., A/a B/b).

(b) George and Grace are likely carriers for one autosomal recessive form of hearing loss; Horace is either a homozygote or compound heterozygote at this same locus. Gilbert and Gisele are both homozygotes or compound heterozygotes for hearing loss due to pathogenic variants at a hearing loss locus as well. The fact that all of Horace and Hedy's children are hearing impaired suggests that the same locus is involved in both families.

3. Variable expressivity—d
Consanguinity—c
X-linked dominant inheritance—g
New mutation—e
Allelic heterogeneity—h
Locus heterogeneity—a
Homozygosity for an autosomal dominant trait—b
Pleiotropy—f

4. (b) They are homozygous for the family's hemophilia A pathogenic variant.

(c) 100% for a son of Elise; virtually zero for a daughter unless Elise's partner has hemophilia A.

(d) Enid is an obligate carrier (heterozygote for hemophilia A variant); the chance a son will be affected is 50%. The probability a daughter will be affected is virtually zero unless Enid's partner has hemophilia A.

5. (a) New variant or germline mosaicism in one of the parents.

(b) Mutation rate at the NF1 locus if truly a new mutation; if one of the parents is a germline mosaic, the risk in the next pregnancy is a function of the fraction of gametes carrying the variant, which is unknown.

(c) Mutation rate at the NF1 locus if truly a new mutation; if the father is a germline mosaic for NF1, the risk in the next pregnancy is a function of the fraction of sperm carrying the variant, which is unknown.

(d) 50%.

6. The chance of inheriting the pathogenic allele through both parents from the shared female ancestor is 1/128. This can only occur if the allele is inherited in every generation; the odds multiply. The probability that the allele descends the father's side is $1/2 \times 1/2 \times 1/2 = 1/8$. The odds that it descends the mother's side is $1/2 \times 1/2 \times 1/2 \times 1/2 = 1/16$ since there is one additional transmission required. The odds of it transmitting down both branches are $1/8 \times 1/16 = 1/128$.

7. Autosomal dominant is most likely. We see vertical transmission, including male to male, from generation to generation, males and females affected. Autosomal recessive and X-linked recessive are possible but unlikely. Autosomal recessive would require that both spouses of the two affected individuals in generations I and II be carriers, which is unlikely unless the pedigree comes from a genetic isolate. X-linked recessive would require that the same two women be carriers for the same condition as their affected partners. Mitochondrial and X-linked dominant inheritance patterns are incompatible with male-to-male transmission. In addition, there are female offspring of affected males who are not affected, which doesn't occur in X-linked dominant inheritance.

CHAPTER 8 *Sarah Goodman, Cheryl Cytrynbaum, Rosanna Weksberg*

1. (a) The first wave of epigenetic erasure occurs in all cells of the preimplantation embryo at ~8 days. The second occurs at ~5 weeks but only in primordial germ cells. Imprinted loci are protected in the first wave but undergo epigenetic reprogramming in the second.

(b) In the first wave of epigenetic reprogramming, embryonic cells undergo genome-wide demethylation in a passive manner in the maternal genome—that is, methylation marks are not maintained following cell division—and in an active manner in the paternal genome, enzymatically driven by TET proteins.

2. Higher levels of DNA methylation at the IAP retrotransposon insertion result in transcriptional repression and lower constitutive expression of the Agouti gene. The corresponding phenotype is healthy, brown mice, as opposed to obese, yellow mice. In pregnant dams, diets high in methyl donors are more likely to produce healthy, brown offspring, while diets supplemented with bisphenol A have the opposite outcome.

3. Imprinting disorders occur with increased frequency following ART, i.e., disorders characterized by epigenetic aberrations at imprinted regions and genes. Imprinting disorders associated with ART include Beckwith-Wiedemann, Russell-Silver, Angelman, and Prader-Willi syndromes. Furthermore, individuals who present with one of these disorders following ART may demonstrate imprint deregulation at multiple imprinting loci.

4. (a) Neurodevelopmental disorders (including intellectual disability) and growth dysregulation are the most common features of mendelian disorders of the epigenetic machinery. Other common features include seizures, facial dysmorphism, and heart abnormalities.

(b) Epigenetic regulators commonly function as writers, readers, and erasers of epigenetic marks. These proteins may be further subclassified based on whether they regulate DNA methylation or histone modifications (e.g., histone acetylation or methylation). However, some epigenetic regulators do not fit neatly into these groups, such as chromatin remodelers, which can have multiple functions, including the regulation of histone modifications.

5. With respect to constitutional disorders of the epigenetic machinery, a DNA methylation signature is a set of CpGs across the genome that exhibit differential methylation in the blood of individuals carrying variants in a specific gene, as compared to healthy controls. DNA methylation signatures may serve as diagnostic tests by identifying individuals with the same DNA methylation patterns as those known to have a specific disorder caused by pathogenic variants in a specific gene. Signatures can also be used to classify sequence variants of uncertain significance in epigenetic regulator genes as either pathogenic or benign.

Within the cancer field, DNA methylation signatures can be used to classify different tumor subtypes, which impacts the prognosis and selection of optimal treatment. DNA methylation signatures can also be used to identify the origin of metastatic tumors.

6. A histone deacetylase inhibitor (HDACi) is an epigenetic regulator that increases levels of histone acetylation and, thereby, the levels of open chromatin. Such drugs are currently used in the treatment of various cancers and autoimmune diseases.

CHAPTER 9 *Cristen J. Willer and Gonçalo R. Abecasisa*

1. Because the MZ twin concordance is not 100%, there is likely to be at least some component of susceptibility due to environmental factors. Because the concordance in MZ twins is more than double the concordance in DZ twins, the inheritance is likely to be multifactorial (more than a single gene involved in risk).

2. Answer a->ii, b->i, c->iii.

3. A self-learning exercise.

CHAPTER 10 *Alice B. Popejoy*

1. (a) The probability of having any 1 of the 5 variants is 0.2; then, the expected proportion of homozygotes for any 1 of the 5 alleles would be $0.2 \times 0.2 = 0.04$. Since there are 5 possible variants for which one could be homozygous, the total proportion of expected homozygous individuals is $0.04 \times 5 = 0.2$.

(b) Heterozygotes would thus constitute $1 - 0.2 = 0.8$ (80%) of the population.

(c) The frequency of homozygotes for the first allele would be $0.40 \times 0.40 = 0.16$; $0.30 \times 0.30 = 0.09$ for the second allele; $0.15 \times 0.15 = 0.0225$, $0.1 \times 0.1 = .01$, and $0.05 \times 0.05 = .0025$ for the remaining alleles. The probability that an individual would be homozygous for any allele is then the sum of all homozygous genotype probabilities as calculated above:

$$0.16 + 0.09 + 0.0225 + 0.01 + 0.0025 = 0.285.$$

This means that 28.5% of individuals would be homozygous at this locus; the rest (71.5%) would be heterozygous.

2. (a) Assume there are 100 individuals in the population, carrying 200 alleles at a particular locus. The frequency of A is $(2 \times {}^{81}\!/_{200}) + ({}^{18}\!/_{200}) = 0.9$ and frequency of $a = 0.1$

(b) The allele and genotype frequencies will be the same as in this generation, assuming Hardy-Weinberg equilibrium.

3. (a) When q is small, $p \approx 1$, and so $2pq \approx 2q$. Therefore, if $2pq = 0.04$, the frequency of the pathogenic allele $q \approx .02$. (One can also calculate q precisely by letting $2pq = 2(1-q)q = 0.04$, or $q^2 - q + 0.02 = 0$ and solve the quadratic equation.)

(b) Assuming only heterozygotes (unaffected carriers) are likely to reproduce, then $0.04 \times 0.04 = 0.0016$ (0.16%) of reproductive pairings will be between heterozygotes, with the potential to produce affected offspring.

(c) Prevalence of carriers among the offspring of couples in which both partners are heterozygous is 50%. This may be discovered mathematically or visually using a Punnett Square showing that half the offspring of two heterozygotes are also heterozygous.

(d) When the mode of inheritance is autosomal dominant with full penetrance, the presence of the pathogenic allele confers the condition, so there would be no unaffected adult carriers (0%). If the mode of inheritance were X-linked dominant, the answer is the same; males and females with the allele would have the condition. However, if the mode of inheritance were X-linked recessive, males would be affected but female carriers would remain unaffected due to their (presumably healthy) additional X chromosome. Thus, assuming an equal ratio of male to female individuals in this population, the prevalence of unaffected adult carriers would be half the carrier frequency for an autosomal recessive mode of inheritance = $2pq/2 = 0.04/2 = 0.02$.

4. Only c. is in equilibrium. Possible explanations for deviation from Hardy-Weinberg equilibrium include natural selection (for or against particular genotypes), nonrandom mating, gene flow or recent migration, population substructure due to different ancestral populations, or founder effects.

5. (a) Assuming Arjun has no family history of the condition due to its rarity in the population, his risk of having a heterozygous genotype ($2pq$) can be calculated using the Hardy-Weinberg formula, where p is the frequency of the non-pathogenic allele and q is the frequency of the pathogenic allele. The prevalence of the condition is 1/90,000; since it is an autosomal recessive trait, that means this is the frequency of the homozygous genotype for the pathogenic allele: q^2. To obtain the allele frequency, we take the square root of the prevalence: $\sqrt{1/90000} = 0.00333$. Then, we can obtain the allele frequency for the non-pathogenic allele by subtraction : $1 - 0.00333 = 0.9666$. To obtain the carrier frequency, or the proportion of heterozygous individuals in the population, we calculate $2pq = 2*0.00333*0.9666 = 0.00664$. Converted to a fraction, this is roughly a 1/150 chance of being an unaffected carrier.

(b) Meera has a 2/3 chance of being a carrier because her sister has the trait. Both their parents must have one copy of the pathogenic allele and Meera has a ½ chance of having inherited the pathogenic allele from either parent. The chance she inherited both pathogenic alleles is 0, because she is unaffected. There are 3 possible genotypes for Meera: heterozygous (in 2 different ways;

depending on which parent passed down their pathogenic allele) and homozygous for the non-pathogenic allele. Thus, 2 of these 3 possibilities would translate to Meera being an unaffected carrier.

(c) In order for Meera and Arjun's child to have this syndrome, they would both need to be unaffected carriers, and both pass on the Hurler allele. As calculated above, Meera and Arjun's carrier risks are 2/3 and approximately 1/150, respectively. Thus, the likelihood that their first child would have Hurler syndrome is approximately 2/3 × 1/150 × ¼ = 1/900.

(d) The chance is exactly the same, regardless of whether or not Meera and Arjun have similar results on a commercial test for continental-level estimated genetic ancestry proportions.

6. (a) Facioscapulohumeral muscular dystrophy: $q = \frac{1}{50,000}$. [$2pq \approx 1/25000 = .00004$; $p^2 = 1 - .00004 = .99996$; $p = \sqrt{.99996} = .99998$; $q = 1 - q = .00002$ (= 1/50,000)]. Friedreich Ataxia (AR): $q = 1/158$. [$q^2 = 1/25000$; $q^2 = \sqrt{1/25000} = 1/158$]. Duchenne Muscular Dystrophy (XLR): $q = 1/12,500$. [Almost all affected individuals are male; half the population is male; each male has one X chromosome; incidence in males represents the pathogenic allele frequency].

(b) When affected individuals can suddenly have children, the incidence of autosomal dominant and X-linked conditions would increase rapidly because only 1 copy of the pathogenic allele is required to cause the autosomal dominant condition; 1 pathogenic allele for the X-linked condition is required for male children to be affected. The incidence of an autosomal recessive condition would also increase, but very slowly, because 2 copies of the pathogenic allele are required to produce an affected offspring.

7. Pathogenic allele frequencies are approximately $\sqrt{1/685} = 0.038$ in the region of Quebec and $\sqrt{1/100000} = 1/316 = 0.003$ elsewhere. The difference in allele frequencies could be (1) founder effect (or more generally, genetic drift) in the early Quebec population when it was very small, followed by expansion of the population (bottleneck) resulting in a higher relative frequency of the pathogenic allele, or (2) environmental conditions of unknown type that provided a heterozygote advantage in the Quebec region for the pathogenic allele.

CHAPTER 11 *Christian R. Marshall*

1. The HD and MNSs loci map far enough apart on chromosome 4 to be unlinked, even though they are syntenic.

2. The LOD scores indicate that this variant in the α-globin gene locus is closely linked to the polycystic

kidney disease gene. The peak LOD score, 25.85, occurs at 5 cM. The odds in favor of linkage at this distance compared with no linkage at all are $10^{25.85}:1$ (i.e., almost $10^{26}:1$). The data in the second study indicate that there is no linkage between the disease gene and the variant in this family. Thus there is genetic heterogeneity in this disorder.

3. Every parent who passed on the cataract and was genotyped was also informative at the *CRYGD* locus; that is, was heterozygous for the alleles at this gene locus. The phase is known by inspecting the pedigree in individuals IV-7 and IV-8 because they received both the cataract allele and the *A* allele in the *CRYGD* gene from their father (but note, we do not know what the phase was in the father simply by inspection). Individual IV-10 received the B allele from his father and does not have cataracts. We do not know the phase in individuals IV-3 or IV-4 because information from their deceased father is missing. Phase is also known in individuals V-1, V-2, V-6, and V-7. The cataract seems to co-segregate with the A allele here with no obligate crossovers in this family. A complete LOD score analysis could be performed, including additional families, or one could sequence the *CRYGD* gene itself for pathogenic variants in affected persons.

4. (a) Whole exome sequencing is the sequencing of the exome or the coding portion of the genome. To perform exome sequencing, the exons or targets need to be captured either through amplification or by using baits that can hybridize to the coding sequence and pull down the intended targets. The final product is a library that is enriched for exons that can then be sequenced.

   (b) Advantages to GS over ES include:
      (i) Better technical coverage of the coding sequence of the genome since there is no enrichment step that can introduce bias.
      (ii) Can detect pathogenic variation beyond the scope of targeted exome analysis, including deep intronic and intergenic regions.
      (iii) Can detect a broader spectrum of variant classes, including structural variation (either balanced changes or unbalanced copy number variation), mitochondrial variation (if not targeted in the exome kit), and some repeat expansions.
      (iv) Ability to detect copy number variation at a higher resolution and resolve more complex rearrangements when the breakpoints are sequenced.

   Disadvantages of GS over ES include:
      (i) Computationally more challenging analyze.
      (ii) Difficult to interpret noncoding changes.
      (iii) Cost of sequencing is higher.
      (iv) Less sensitive for the detection of mosaic coding changes since the average cover age of a GS(30X) is lower than that for ES(~100X).

5. No, because you would not know if II-2 inherited the variant allele D along with the A from her father or the A from her mother. Phase becomes unknown again, as in Fig. 11.10A.

6. Yes, phase is known in the mother of the two affected boys because she must have received the variant factor VIII allele (h) and the M allele at the polymorphic locus on the X from her father.

7. Odds ratio for the variant and disease = (a/b)/(c/d) = ad/bc.

   Relative risk = [a/(a + b)]/[c/(c + d)] = a(c + d)/c(a + b).

   With three times as many controls, the odds ratio = a(3b)/c(3d) = 3ad/3bc = ad/bc, which is unchanged from the previous odds ratio.

   Relative risk = [a/(a + 3b)]/[c/(c + 3d)] = a(c + 3d)/c(a + 3b), which is not the same as the previously calculated relative risk.

CHAPTER 12 *Gregory Costain*

1. The pedigree should contain the following information: Hydrops fetalis is due to a total absence of α chains. The parents each must have the genotype αα/−−. The α− genotype is common in some populations, including Melanesians. Parents with this genotype cannot transmit a −−/−− genotype to their offspring.

2. Individuals with β-thalassemia will often be compound heterozygotes because there is high allelic heterogeneity (i.e., many different pathogenic variants) in most populations in which β-thalassemia is common. In isolated populations, the chance that an individual is a true homozygote of a single allele is greater than it would be in an admixed population. True homozygosity is more likely in an isolate with a high frequency of a single allele or a few alleles, or if parents are consanguineous. See text in Chapter 7.

3. Three bands on the RNA blot could indicate, among other possibilities, that (a) one allele is producing two mRNAs, one normal in size and the other abnormal, and the other allele is producing one mRNA of abnormal size; (b) both alleles are making a normal-sized transcript and an abnormal transcript, but the aberrant ones are of different sizes; or (c) one allele is producing three mRNAs of different sizes, and the other allele is making no transcripts.

   Scenario (c) is highly improbable. Two mRNAs from a single allele could result from a splicing defect that allows the normal mRNA to be made, but at reduced efficiency; abnormal splicing yields another transcript of abnormal size. This results from either intron sequences not removed from the mRNA or the loss of exon sequences from the mRNA. In this case, the other abnormal band comes from the other allele. A larger band from the other allele could result from a splicing defect or an insertion, whereas a smaller band could be due to a splicing defect or a deletion. Hb E is caused by an allele from which both a normal and a shortened transcript are made (see Fig. 12.10); the normal mRNA makes up 40% of the total β-globin mRNA, producing only a mild anemia.

4. These two variants affect different globin chains. The expected offspring are normal, Hb M Saskatoon heterozygotes with methemoglobinemia, Hb M Boston heterozygotes with methemoglobinemia, and double heterozygotes with four hemoglobin types: normal, each type of Hb M, and a type with abnormalities in both chains. In the double heterozygotes, the clinical consequences are unknown—probably more severe methemoglobinemia.

5. $\frac{2}{3} \times \frac{2}{3} \times \frac{1}{4} = \frac{1}{9}$

6. ¼

7. 8, 1, 2, 7, 10, 4, 9, 5, 6, and 3.

8. Reasons for failure to detect the second allele in the gene responsible for an autosomal recessive condition by exome sequencing include but are not limited to:
   - Nonexonic (e.g., intronic) variant affecting exon splicing or gene expression.
   - Copy number or structural variation beyond the limit of detection of exome sequencing.
   - Poor coverage of the exonic region that contains the variant of interest.

9. Approximately two-thirds of the couples to whom such infants were born did not know about thalassemia or the prevention programs. Approximately 20% chose to continue the pregnancy after prenatal diagnosis, and false paternity was identified in 13% of cases.

CHAPTER 13 *Ada Hamosh*

1. Mechanisms to create an elongated protein:
   - A variant in the normal stop codon that allows translation to continue.
   - A splice variant that results in the inclusion of intron sequences in the coding region. The intron sequences would have to be free of stop codons for sufficient length to allow the extra 50 kD of translation.
   - An insertion, with an open reading frame, into the coding sequence.

   Approximately 500 extra residues would be added to the protein if the average molecular weight of an amino acid is ~100, encoded by 1500 nucleotides.

2. Variants in either gene can cause familial hypercholesterolemia; these are thus genocopies of one another (for comparison, see Glossary for the definition of phenocopy).

3. A nucleotide substitution that changes one amino acid residue to another should be termed a putative pathogenic variant, unless a functional assay of the protein demonstrates that the change impairs the function to a degree consistent with the phenotype of the patient. Lack of population prevalence is an argument in support of pathogenicity in autosomal dominant (monoallelic variant) disease, but it is not necessarily helpful in recessive disease where unaffected carriers will be identified in the general population.

4. (a) DNA analysis would be useful. A blood sample would be a source of DNA to assay using a targeted variant assay, *CFTR* genotyping panel, or perhaps next-generation sequencing to look for pathogenic variants.

   (b) If Johnny has CF, the chances are ~0.95 × 0.95, or 90%, that he has a pair of variants that could be readily identified by DNA analysis. The probability that he is homozygous for the p.Phe508del variant is 0.7 × 0.7, or 49%. However, given his normal sweat chloride concentration, the likelihood of being homozygous for the p.Phe508del variant is very low as this variant is known to be associated with high sweat chloride concentrations.

   (c) If he does not have this variant, he could certainly still have CF, involving other pathogenic alleles in *CFTR*.

5. James may have a new variant on the X chromosome. If this is the case, there is no risk for recurrence. Alternatively, the mother may be a mosaic, and the mosaicism includes her germline. In this case, there is a definite risk that the variant X could be inherited by another son or passed to a carrier daughter. Approximately 5% to 15% of cases of this type are due to maternal germline mosaicism. Thus the risk of recurrence for her male offspring is half of this, or 2.5 to 7.5%.

6. For DMD, as a classic X-linked recessive disease that is lethal in males, one-third of cases are predicted to be new mutations. The large size of the gene likely accounts for the high mutation rate at this locus. There is no reason to believe that ancestry impacts any of these factors.

7. A female like T.N. might have the disease because she carries a *DMD* pathogenic variant on the X chromosome inherited from her mother. T.N. could show clinical symptoms if her paternal X (carrying a normal allele at this locus) was subject to nonrandom inactivation in most or all cells. Alternatively, she could have Turner syndrome and her only X chromosome (inherited from her mother) carries a *DMD* pathogenic variant. A third explanation would be that she has a balanced X;autosome translocation that disrupts the *DMD* gene on the translocated X chromosome. Balanced X;autosome translocations show nonrandom inactivation of the structurally normal X due to secondary cell selection (see Chapter 6).

8. The limited number of amino acids that substitute for glycine in altered collagen reflects the nature of the genetic code. Single-nucleotide substitutions at the third positions of the glycine codons allow only a limited number of missense mutations (see Table 3.1).

9. The box in Chapter 13 entitled "Mutant Enzymes and Disease: General Concepts" lists the possible causes of loss of multiple enzyme activities: They may share a cofactor whose synthesis or transport is defective; they may share a subunit encoded by the abnormal gene; they may be processed by a common enzyme whose activity is critical to their becoming active; or they may normally be located in the same organelle, and a defect in biologic processes of the organelle can affect all four enzymes. For example, they may not be imported normally into the organelle and may be degraded in the cytoplasm. Almost all enzymopathies are recessive (see text), and most genes are autosomal. The likelihood of autosomal recessive inheritance is increased, given the consanguinity.

10. Dominance effects with multimeric proteins can be the result of perturbed interactions between subunits of protein complexes, or to stoichiometric imbalances. Dominant negative effects occur when altered subunits disrupt the activity of the wild-type protein complex. Haploinsufficiency is one source of imbalance that can cause stoichiometric problems in protein complexes, with a dominant effect on a phenotype. Some collagen disorders, such as osteogenesis imperfects, exemplify this characteristic.

11. This situation is well illustrated by diseases due to variants in mtDNA or in the nuclear genome that impair the function of the oxidative phosphorylation complex. Nearly all cells have mitochondria; therefore oxidative phosphorylation occurs in nearly all cells. Nonetheless, phenotypes associated with defects in oxidative phosphorylation involve damage to only a subset of organs, particularly the neurologic and muscular systems with their high energy requirements.

12. One example is phenylketonuria, in which intellectual disability is the only significant pathologic effect of deficiency of phenylalanine hydroxylase. The enzyme is found, not in the brain, but solely in the liver and kidneys—organs that are unaffected by this biochemical defect. Hypercholesterolemia due to deficiency of the LDL receptor is another example. Although the LDL receptor is found in many cell types, its hepatic deficiency is primarily responsible for the increase in LDL cholesterol levels in blood.

13. There are two defining characteristics of these alleles: (1) The Hex A activity that they encode is sufficiently reduced to allow their detection in screening assays (when the other allele is a common Tay-Sachs variant with virtually no activity), and (2) their Hex A activity is nevertheless adequate to prevent the accumulation of the natural substrate (GM2 ganglioside). There are probably only a few substitutions in the Hex A protein that would reduce activity only modestly. The region of residues 247 to 249 appears to be relatively tolerant of substitutions, at least of Trp for Arg.

14. A gain-of-function variant leads to an abnormal increase in the activities performed relative to the wild-type protein. Consequently, the overall integrity of the altered protein and each of its functional domains must remain. In addition, of course, the variant must confer the gain of function. Variants other than missense variants (e.g., deletions, insertions, premature stops) are almost uniformly highly disruptive to protein structure.

15. The presence of three common alleles for Tay-Sachs disease in the Ashkenazi population seems likely due to a heterozygote advantage, or to genetic drift (one form of which is the founder effect, as explained in Chapter 10) or to a combination of these. The high frequency of these alleles might also be due to gene flow, although the population of origin of the three common variants is not apparent, making this explanation seem less likely (in contrast, say, to the evidence indicating that the most common PKU alleles in many populations around the world are of Celtic origin).

16. As with any genetically complex disorder, the other sources of genetic variation in Alzheimer disease (AD) may include (1) additional AD loci, with lower effect sizes, that have not yet been identified; (2) synergistic effects between known AD genes (or between known genes and environmental risks); (3) genes that harbor multiple very rare variants of large effect, but which are undetectable by genome-wide association studies because each occurs on a different background.

17. According to this model, the increased number of CUG repeats binds an abnormally large fraction of RNA-binding proteins, including, for example, splice regulators, thereby depleting the cell of these critical proteins. One approach to therapy might be to prevent this binding. This might be achieved by introducing, perhaps by gene transfer (see Chapter 14), a viral vector that expresses a GAC trinucleotide repeat. This would bind to the CUG repeat sequences in the RNA and block the binding of the RNA-binding proteins to the expanded CUG repeats. Expression of excess GAC repeat–containing molecules might itself have undesirable side effects, however, such as binding to CUG codons that encode leucine, blocking their translation.

CHAPTER 14 *Ronald Doron Cohn and Ada Hamosh*

1. Unresponsive patients may have variants that drastically impair the synthesis of a functional gene product, whereas responsive patients may have variants in the regulatory region of the gene that can be counteracted by the administration of IFN-γ. Alternatively, responsive patients may produce a defective cytochrome b

polypeptide with some residual function, such that increased production in response to IFN-γ increases the oxidase activity enough to be significant.

2. An enzyme that is normally intracellular can function extracellularly if the substrate is in equilibrium between the intracellular and extracellular fluids and if the product is either nonessential inside the cell or in a similar equilibrium state. Thus enzymes with substrates and products that do not fit these criteria would not be suitable for this strategy. This approach does not work for phenylalanine hydroxylase because of its intracellular location and need for tetrahydrobiopterin as cofactor. This strategy would not work for storage diseases such as Tay-Sachs because the substrate of the enzyme is trapped inside the lysosome. In Lesch-Nyhan syndrome, the most important pathologic process is in the brain, and the enzyme in the extracellular fluid would not be able to cross the blood-brain barrier.

3. Rhonda is homozygous for an allele that prevents the production of any LDL receptor. Thus the combination of a bile acid–binding resin and a drug (e.g., lovastatin) to inhibit cholesterol synthesis would have no effect on increasing the synthesis of LDL receptors. The boy receiving such treatment must have one or two variant alleles that produce a receptor with some residual function, capable of increased expression.

4. Unresponsive individuals probably have variant alleles, most commonly in the *CBS* gene, that do not make any enzyme protein, that decrease its cellular abundance in some other way (e.g., make an unstable protein), or that disrupt the conformation of the protein so extensively that its pyridoxal-phosphate binding site has no affinity for the cofactor, even at high concentrations. Tom is likely to have two *CBS* alleles that are responsive. As first cousins with the same recessive disease, Tom and Allan are likely to share one pathogenic (but responsive) allele. Allan is likely to have a second allele that is either unresponsive or less responsive to the cofactor that that of his cousin.

5. (a) You need both a promoter that will allow the synthesis of sufficient levels of the mRNA in the target tissue of choice and the *PAH* cDNA. You also need a vector to deliver the "gene" into the cell.

(b) A *PAH* "gene" will probably be effective in any tissue that has a good blood supply for the delivery of phenylalanine and an adequate source of the cofactor of the enzyme, tetrahydrobiopterin. The promoter would have to be capable of driving transcription in the target tissue chosen for the treatment.

(c) Any variant that severely reduces the abundance of the protein in the cell but has no effect on transcription. This group includes those that impair translation or that render the protein highly unstable. The thalassemias include examples of all these types.

(d) Liver cells are capable of making tetrahydrobiopterin, whereas other cells may not be. The target cell for the gene transfer should thus be capable of making this cofactor; otherwise, the enzyme will not function unless the cofactor is administered in large amounts.

(e) Human PAH probably exists as a homodimer or homotrimer. In individuals whose alleles produce an abnormal polypeptide (vs. none at all), these alleles may manifest a dominant negative effect on the product of the transferred gene. This effect could be overcome by making a gene construct that produces more of the normal enzyme protein (thus diluting the effect of the mutant polypeptide) or by transferring the gene into a cell type that does not normally express PAH and that would therefore not be subject to the dominant negative effect.

6. One must consider the kinds of variants that decrease the abundance of a protein but are associated with residual function. One such class includes those that decrease the abundance of the mRNA but do not alter the protein sequence. This type might include enhancer or promoter variants, splice variants, or others that destabilize the mRNA. In this case, one could consider strategies to increase expression from the altered alleles. A second class includes variants within the coding sequence that destabilize the protein but still allow some residual function. Here, a strategy to increase the stability or the function of the altered protein should be considered. For example, if the affected protein has a cofactor, one could administer increased amounts of the cofactor, provided such an approach would not have unacceptable side effects.

7. The drug can facilitate the skipping of a premature stop codon, allowing the translational apparatus to misincorporate an amino acid that has a codon comparable to that of the termination codon. This treatment might allow the synthesis of a protein of normal size in both individuals, but with different characteristics. In the responsive individual, the nonsense codon may be in a functionally neutral part of the protein, and the substituted amino acid allowed normal folding, processing, and function of the corrected protein. In the nonresponsive individual, however, the nonsense variant might have been located (for example) in codon 117, which in wild-type *CFTR* is an Arg residue (see Fig. 13.14). This Arg residue contributes to the Cl− channel of *CFTR*. Despite bypassing the stop codon, the drug would not lead to incorporation of Arg at this critical position.

CHAPTER 15 *Anthony Wynshaw-Boris and Ophir Klein*

1. Before determination, an embryo can lose one or more cells, and the remaining cells can undergo

specification and ultimately develop into a complete embryo. Once cells are determined, however, mosaic development takes place—an embryonic tissue will follow its developmental program regardless of what happens elsewhere in the embryo. Regulative development means that an embryonic cell can be removed by blastomere biopsy for the purpose of preimplantation diagnosis without harming the rest of the embryo.

2. a–3, b–2, c–4, d–1.

3. a–4, b–3, c–5, d–2, e–1.

4. Mature T or B cells that have somatically rearranged their T-cell receptor or immunoglobulin loci would not be appropriate. This change is not epigenetic; it is a permanent alteration of the DNA sequence itself. Animals derived from a single nucleus from a mature T or B cell are incapable of mounting an appropriately broad immune response.

5. Consider issues of regulation versus simple capacity to carry out a biochemical reaction. Also, consider dominant negative effects of transcription factors, taking into account the frequent binary nature of such factors (DNA-binding and activation domains).

CHAPTER 16 *Michael F. Walsh*

1. Approximately 15% of unilateral retinoblastoma is the heritable form but affecting only one eye. You need family history and careful examination of both parents' retinas, looking for signs of a scar that could have been a spontaneously regressed retinoblastoma. Genome analysis may be indicated if the tumor is associated with other malformations. Targeted sequence and deletion/duplication analysis of the child's *RB1* gene may reveal a germline pathogenic variant, in which case, it is a heritable retinoblastoma, and the child is at risk for tumors in the other eye, in the pineal gland, and for sarcomas later in life, particularly associated with radiation therapy. Knowing the *RB1* variant, the parents can be tested to see if one or the other is a nonpenetrant carrier; if so, future offspring are each at 50% risk for retinoblastoma. Prenatal diagnosis could be offered for future pregnancies whether the variant is obvious in a parent, since gonadal mosaicism cannot be ruled out. If prenatal diagnosis is not used or if the fetus carries a pathogenic variant and the parents choose to allow the pregnancy to go to term, the newborn would need examination under anesthesia as soon as possible after birth and then at frequent intervals to ensure timely intervention.

   If the blood test does not show the child to be clearly heterozygous for a pathogenic variant, somatic mosaicism in the child is still possible, with increased risk for tumor in the other eye or for sarcomas later in life; therefore, monitoring is still needed. Sequencing of the tumor itself may show a change that could be specifically assayed using next-generation sequencing of the peripheral blood DNA to look for evidence of low-level mosaicism.

2. Colorectal cancer seems to require a number of sequential mutations in several genes, which can take many years, whereas retinoblastoma results from one (in hereditary) or two (in sporadic) pathogenic changes in the retinoblastoma gene. Age dependence may also reflect the number, timing, and rate of cell divisions in colon cells and in retinoblasts. Colon cells are constantly dividing and dying (and acquiring mutations that may or not be properly repaired) throughout a person's lifetime, whereas once the retinoblasts have matured into retinal cells, they are pretty much nondividing so have no accumulation of proliferative, neoplastic lesions.

   Pediatric syndromes with colon cancer: familial adenomatous polyposis *(APC)*, Li-Fraumeni syndrome *(TP53)*, constitutional microsatellite mismatch repair deficiency (CMMRD) *(MSH2, MSH6, MLH1, PMS2)*, juvenile polyposis *(BMPR1A, SMAD4)*, *MUTYH*-associated polyposis.

3. A cell line with i(17q) is monosomic for 17p and trisomic for 17q. Thus formation of the isochromosome leads to loss of heterozygosity for genes on 17p. This may be particularly important because one or more tumor suppressor genes (such as *TP53*) are present on 17p; a "second hit" on the other copy of *TP53* would lead to complete loss of the p53 protein function. In addition, a number of proto-oncogenes map to 17q. It is possible that increasing their dosage may confer a growth advantage on cells containing the i(17q).

4. The chief concern is the need to reduce radiation exposure to the lowest possible level because of the risk for cancer in children with this genetic defect.

5. Although most (>95%) breast cancer appears to follow multifactorial inheritance, there are two known genes (*BRCA1* and *BRCA2*) in which pathogenic variants confer a substantial increased lifetime risk for breast cancer (five- to seven-fold), inherited in an autosomal dominant manner. Certain variants in other genes, such as *ATM, BARD1, BRIP1, CDH1, CHEK2, PALB2, PTEN,* and *TP53*, increase the lifetime breast cancer risk significantly beyond the 12% background population risk, but generally not to the extent seen with variants in *BRCA1* or *BRCA2*. In the absence of a pathogenic variant in a hereditary breast cancer gene, the empirical risk figures are consistent with an overall multifactorial model; there is an approximately two-fold increased risk for breast cancer in any woman with a first-degree female relative with breast cancer.

   Sequence analysis could be performed for probands in Margaret's and Wilma's families, and if a relevant variant were found in *BRCA1, BRCA2*, or one of the other genes as above, a direct variant test could be offered to their relatives. As sisters, each would be at 50% risk of having inherited the same variant; their lifetime cancer risk would vary somewhat with the penetrance associated with the respective genes involved. If no pathogenic variant were found in the probands, their ancestry and age at tumor discovery, as well as the unilaterality or bilaterality would be considered for adjusting the relative empirical risk of their sisters (see Case 7 (*BRCA1/BRCA2*). With respect to Elizabeth, one leading breast cancer researcher, Nadine Tung, suggested that population-wide screening for disease-causing variants in *BRCA1* or *BRCA2* should be initiated independent of family history. Screening recommendations for genes associated with moderately penetrant breast cancer *CHEK2*, *ATM* and *PALB2* differ from those for *BRCA1*, *BRCA2* and *TP53* (https://www.ncbi.nlm.nih.gov/pmc/articles/PMC5513673/pdf/nihms877760.pdf)

6. It is likely that many activated oncogenes, if inherited in the germline, would disrupt normal development and be incompatible with survival. There are a few exceptions, such as activating *RET* variants in MEN2 and activating *MET* variants in hereditary papillary kidney cancer. These activated oncogenes must have tissue-specific oncogenic effects without affecting development. Although it is not known why such specific types of cancers occur in individuals who inherit germline activating variants in these oncogenes, one plausible theory is that other genes expressed in most of the tissues of the body counteract their effect, thereby allowing normal development and suppressing oncogenic effects in most of the tissues in heterozygotes.

Activating genes, as opposed to tumor suppressors, enable cells to continue proliferating rather than impacting cell cycle regulators that keep cells in check.

CHAPTER 17   *Carolyn Dinsmore Applegate and Jodie Marie Vento*

1. (a) Prior risk, $\frac{1}{4}$; posterior risk (given two normal brothers), $\frac{1}{10}$.

   (b) CSNB is genetically heterogeneous, with at least 17 different genes implicated. If an autosomal dominant form with reduced penetrance is the cause in this family, there is a small probability that Rosemary, Meera, and Elsie are all be nonpenetrant carriers. If an autosomal recessive gene variant is involved, then Rosemary was an obligate carrier and Elsie's probability would be ¼. The risk that her offspring would be affected with CSNB then depends on the population-based likelihood that her partner is a carrier of a pathogenic variant in the same gene.

2. (a) In A, Nathan has a new mutation with probability μ.

   In B, Molly has the new mutation; her prior probability is 2μ because the new mutation could have occurred on either her paternal or her maternal X chromosome.

   In C, Lucy is a carrier. As shown earlier in this chapter in the Box describing the calculation for the probability that any female is a carrier of an X-linked lethal disorder, Lucy's prior probability is 4μ. Molly inherited the variant gene; Martha did not, so the probability that her two sons would be unaffected is essentially 1.

   In D, Lucy is a carrier, as are Molly, and Martha who did not pass the variant gene to her two sons.

   (We ignore the other highly unlikely combinations of carrier states.) The conditional probabilities can then be calculated from these various joint probabilities.

   Molly is a carrier in situations B, C, and D, so her probability of being a carrier is $\frac{13}{21}$.

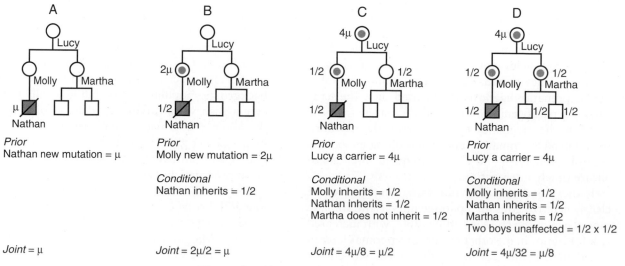

Figure for Chapter 17, question 2.

Similarly, Molly's mother, Lucy: 5/21; Norma and Nancy, 13/42; Olive and Odette, 13/84; Martha, 1/21; Nora and Nellie, 1/42; Maud, 5/42; Naomi, 5/84.

(b) To have a 2% risk for having an affected son, a woman must have an 8% chance of being a carrier; thus, Martha, Nora, and Nellie would not be obvious candidates for prenatal diagnosis by DNA analysis because their carrier risk is less than 8%.

3. $(\frac{1}{2})^{13}$ for 13 successive male births.
$(\frac{1}{2})^{13} \times 2$ for 13 consecutive births of the same sex. The probability of a boy is $\frac{1}{2}$ for each pregnancy.

4. (a) Use the first equation, $I = \mu + \frac{1}{2}H$. To solve for H and substitute it for H in the second equation, $H = 2\mu + \frac{1}{2}H + If$. Solve for I, $I = 3\mu/(1 - f)$. Substituting 0.7 for f gives:
The incidence of affected males $I = 10\mu$.
The incidence of carrier females $H = 18\mu$.
Chance next son of the mother of an isolated case will be affected is $\frac{1}{2}H \times 0.9 = 0.45$.

(b) Substitute $f = 0$ into the equations and you get $I = 3\mu$ and $H = 4\mu$.

(c) 0.147.

Prior	18μ ⊙	$1-18\mu = \sim1$ ◯
Conditional	1/2 ■	μ ■
Joint	9μ	μ
Posterior	0.9	0.1

Figure for Chapter 17, question 4.

5. (a) The prior risk that either Ira or Margie is a cystic fibrosis carrier is $\frac{2}{3}$; therefore, the probability that both are carriers is $\frac{2}{3} \times \frac{2}{3} = \frac{4}{9}$.

(b) Their risk for having an affected child in any pregnancy is $\frac{1}{4} \times \frac{4}{9} = \frac{1}{9}$.

(c) Bayesian analysis determines that the revised probability of them both being carriers with 3 unaffected children is approximately 1/4.

Thus the chance that a next child will be affected is $\frac{1}{4} \times \frac{1}{4} = \frac{1}{16}$.

	Both Carriers	Not Both Carriers
Prior	$\frac{4}{9}$	$\frac{5}{9}$
Conditional (3 unaffected children)	$(\frac{3}{4})^3$	1
Joint	$\frac{4}{9} \times (\frac{3}{4})^3 = 0.19$	$\frac{5}{9} = 0.56$
Posterior	$0.19/(0.19 + 0.56)$ $= \frac{1}{4}$	$0.56/0.75 = \approx \frac{3}{4}$

6. The child's prior probability of carrying an abnormal myotonic dystrophy gene is $\frac{1}{2}$. If he has a $\frac{1}{2}$ chance of being asymptomatic at age 14 despite carrying a variant, then his chance of being a carrier given that he is asymptomatic at age 14 is $\frac{1}{3}$. Testing for the expanded allele would be informative; however, in an asymptomatic child, such testing should wait until the individual is mature enough to decide for himself. At age 14, this might be considered (see Chapter 19).

7. (a) Yes; autosomal recessive, autosomal dominant (new mutation), X-linked recessive, multifactorial inheritance, structural variation, and a chromosome disorder all need to be considered, as would nongenetic factors such as prenatal teratogen exposure and intrauterine infection. A careful physical examination and laboratory testing are required for a proper assessment of risks for this couple.

(b) This increases suspicion that the disorder is autosomal recessive, but all other causes must still be investigated thoroughly.

(c) This fact certainly supports the likelihood that the problem has a genetic explanation. The pedigree pattern would be consistent with autosomal recessive inheritance only if all sisters' partners were carrying abnormal alleles of the same gene. An X-linked recessive pattern (particularly if the affected children are all male) or a chromosome defect (e.g., the mothers of the affected children having balanced translocations with unbalanced karyotypes in the affected children) ought to be considered. The mother and her son should receive a genetic evaluation appropriate to the clinical findings, such as chromosomal microarray, exome (sometimes whole genome), and fragile X analysis. The number and order of how these tests are used can vary depending on the health system and on the clinical presentation.

8. Tay Sachs disease is an autosomal recessive condition. Sequencing revealed one pathogenic variant and one variant of unknown significance (VUS). Parental testing was an important step to help determine the phase of these variants. Since both variants are maternally inherited, we know that they are in cis, meaning on the same gene, rather than one in the maternally inherited *HEXA* and one in the paternally inherited *HEXA*. This means that Ananya could have another variant that has not been identified through the sequencing analysis. Although intragenic deletions and duplications are rare, it would be important to ensure that deletion/duplication analysis is done on Ananya.

CHAPTER 18 *Angie Child Jelin and Ignatia B. Van den Veyver*

1. c, e, f, i, d, h, g, b, a.

2. Any conception will either be Down syndrome or rarely monosomy 21, with the latter being almost

always lethal. Thus they should receive counseling and consider other alternatives for having children.

3. No, not necessarily (e.g., the problem could be maternal cell contamination or a vanishing twin).

4. The level of maternal serum α-fetoprotein (MSAFP) is typically elevated when the fetus has an open neural tube defect. The levels of MSAFP and unconjugated estriol are usually reduced and the human chorionic gonadotropin level is usually elevated when the fetus has Down syndrome. The levels of MSAFP, human chorionic gonadotrophin, and unconjugated estriol are reduced in trisomy 18.

5. (a) Given that her CPK levels indicate she is a carrier of DMD and she had an affected brother, she must have inherited the *DMD* variant allele from her mother. Sequence analysis with deletion/duplication analysis would be the most direct means to find the variant *DMD* allele. If this does not reveal the variant, it would be possible to use genetic markers to distinguish her maternal and paternal alleles, if one or both parents are available for testing.

   (b) Either direct or indirect analysis could be used for prenatal diagnosis for future pregnancies of this woman.

6. Question for discussion. Consider issues of sensitivity and specificity of each of the different forms of testing, the psychosocial issues of prenatal diagnosis and termination at different stages of pregnancy, and risk for complications of the two invasive methods.

7. (a) Panel testing or whole exome sequencing are additional options. Trio whole exome sequencing has a diagnostic yield of 31 to 33%. Risks associated with exome testing, including the risk of detecting a variant of unknown significance, false paternity, disclosure of homozygosity indicating the parents are related, as well as risks associated with insurance coverage.

   (b) The patient should be counseled in regard to options for fetal endotracheal occlusion. The genetic diagnosis should be considered prior to proceeding with fetal intervention as it is important for prognostic counseling.

CHAPTER 19 *Ronald Doran Cohn and Iris Cohn*

1. You would expect 625 FVL homozygotes and 48,750 heterozygotes.

   (a)

Genotype	iCVT		
	Affected	Unaffected	Total
Homozygous FVL	1	624	625
Heterozygous FVL	2	48,748	48,750
Wild type	15	950,610	950,625
Total	18	999,982	1,000,000

FVL, Factor V Leiden; *iCVT*, idiopathic cerebral vein thrombosis.

(b) Relative risk for iCVT in FVL heterozygotes = $(2/48{,}750)/(15/950{,}625) = {\approx}3$.

(c) Relative risk for iCVT in FVL homozygotes = $(1/625)/(15/950{,}625) = {\approx}101$.

(d) Sensitivity of testing positive for either one or two FVL alleles = $3/18 = 17\%$.

(e) Positive predictive value for homozygotes = $1/625 = 0.16\%$.

   Positive predictive value for heterozygotes = $2/48{,}748 = 0.004\%$.

   Although the relative risks are elevated with FVL, particularly when the individual is homozygous for the allele, the disorder itself is very rare and thus the PPV is low.

   This example highlights the concept that a relative risk is always a comparison to people who do not carry a particular marker whereas a PPV is the actual (or absolute) risk for someone who carries the marker.

2. You would expect ≈62 FVL homozygotes and 4875 heterozygotes.

Genotype	DVT		
	Affected	Unaffected	Total
Homozygous FVL	3	59	62
Heterozygous FVL	58	4825	4875
Wild-type	39	95,025	95,063
Total	100	99,000	100,000

DVT, Deep venous thrombosis; *FVL*, factor V Leiden.

Relative risk for DVT in FVL heterozygotes taking OCs = ≈30.

Relative risk for DVT in FVL homozygotes taking oral contraceptives (OCs) = ≈118.

Sensitivity of testing positive for either one or two FVL alleles = 62%.

Positive predictive value for homozygotes = $3/62 = {\approx}5\%$.

Positive predictive value for heterozygotes = $58/4875 = 1.2\%$.

   Note that DVT is more common than the example of idiopathic cerebral vein thrombosis given in question 1, whereas the relative risks for homozygotes are of similar magnitude (101 vs. 118); thus the PPV of testing homozygotes is accordingly much higher but is still only 5%.

3. You should first explain to the parents that the test is routinely performed on all newborns and that, as in many screening tests, results are often falsely positive. Further, the test result may be a true positive, and if it is, a more accurate and definitive test needs to be done to know the child's condition and what treatment will be required. The child should be brought in as soon as possible for examination. Appropriate samples will be used to confirm phenylalanine level, to determine if the child has classic or variant PKU or hyperphenylalaninemia, and to test for abnormalities

in biopterin metabolism. Once a diagnosis is made, dietary phenylalanine restriction is instituted to bring blood phenylalanine levels to below the toxic threshold (>360 μmol/L). The child must then be monitored regularly, and dietary adjustments made to manage the blood phenylalanine levels.

4. Issues to consider in formulating your response: Consider the benefits of preventing disease by knowing a newborn's genotype at the β-globin locus. Knowing the genotype can help prevent pneumococcal sepsis or other complications of sickle cell anemia with timely administration of antibiotics.

   Distinguish between SS homozygotes and AS heterozygotes. What harm might accrue from the identification of AS individuals by newborn screening? What does identification of a newborn with SS or AS tell you about the genotypes of the parents and genetic risks for future offspring to the parents?

5.

HLA-B*1502 allele present	TEN or SJS		
	Affected	Unaffected	Total
+	44	3	47
−	0	98	98
Total	44	101	145

SJS, Stevens-Johnson syndrome; *TEN,* toxic epidermal necrolysis.

Sensitivity = 44/44 = 100%.
Specificity = 98/101 = 97%.
Positive predictive value = 44/47 = 94%.

6. The two most common *CYP2C9* variants in people of European ancestry are known as *CYP2C9*2* and *CYP2C9*3*. Both of these lead to a decrease in warfarin metabolism to such degrees that prescription doses are typically reduced by one-third and one-fifth, respectively. In individuals with African ancestry, the four most common *CYP2C9* variants associated with warfarin sensitivity are *CYP2C9*5*, *CYP2C9*6*, *CYP2C9*8*, and *CYP2C9*11*. These lead to a decrease in warfarin metabolism that would necessitate a reduction in prescription doses by one-third to one-sixth. In other populations, the effects of these variants are less certain but are an active area of research.

7. Multiple variations in the polymorphic *CYP2C19* gene have been associated with clopidogrel resistance—a condition in which the drug clopidogrel is less effective than normal in people who are treated with it. The variants associated with clopidogrel resistance decrease the enzyme's ability to convert the drug to its active form.

   The normal version of the gene, *CYP2C19*1*, provides instructions for producing a normally functioning CYP2C19 enzyme. With two copies of the *CYP2C19*1* version of the gene in each cell, one can convert clopidogrel normally. The two most common *CYP2C19* gene polymorphisms associated with clopidogrel resistance (known as *CYP2C19*2* and *CYP2C19*3*) result in the production of a nonfunctional CYP2C19 enzyme that is unable to activate clopidogrel.

CHAPTER 20 *Bartha Maria Knoppers and Ma'n H. Zawati*

1. The first consideration is testing the boy for an incurable disease. Because the boy has symptoms and the family is seeking a diagnosis, this is not the same as an asymptomatic child being considered for predictive testing for an adult-onset disorder. Huntington disease in a child is the result of an increased expansion of an enlarged trinucleotide repeat in one of the parents (usually the father). If DNA reveals such a finding in the child, it will automatically raise the likelihood that one of the parents—probably the father—has an expanded allele that will cause adult-onset Huntington disease in him. Diagnostic testing in the child should therefore be carried out only with informed consent from the parents. Other issues: If one of the parents carries the *HTT* expanded allele, what do you do about testing the asymptomatic older sib?

2. To justify screening, one must show that the good to come from screening—the beneficence of the testing—outweighs the harm. Consider the issue of autonomy: Implicit in the act of informing families that their child has a chromosomal abnormality is that the child cannot decide about such testing later in life. How predictive is the test? Will it diagnose a possible chronic disability that may or may not develop or may vary in severity or have little possible intervention? One might ask whether there are effective interventions for the abnormalities in learning and behavior that occur in some individuals with sex chromosome anomalies. Informing the parents and providing educational and psychological intervention before major problems arise may prove beneficial. On the other hand, telling parents there might be a problem may create a self-fulfilling prophecy by altering parental attitudes toward the child. (See, for instance: Howell R: Ethical issues surrounding newborn screening, *Int. J. Neonatal Screen* 7:3, 2021.)

3. You must consider the extent to which withholding information constitutes "a serious threat to another person's health or safety." In these different disorders, consider how serious the threat is and whether there is any effective intervention if the relative were informed of the risk.

4. Give your rationale for picking the disorders you choose. Consider such factors as how great a threat to health is the disorder; whether the disorder is likely to remain undiscovered and a potential cause of serious illness if not found before symptoms develop by

sequencing; how predictive is finding a gene mutation for the disease; and how effective, how invasive, and how risky are any interventions.

A framework for considering potentially pathogenic sequence variants detected by whole exome or whole genome sequencing can be found in the following resources:

Richards S, Aziz N, Bale S, et al: Standards and guidelines for the interpretation of sequence variants: a joint consensus recommendation of the American College of Medical Genetics and Genomics and the Association for Molecular Pathology. *Genet Med*. doi:10.1038/gim.2015.30, 2015.

American College of Medical Genetics and Genomics: ACMG SF v3.1 list for reporting of secondary findings in clinical exome and genome sequencing: a policy statement of the ACMG.

Miller DT, Lee K, Abul-Husn NS, et al: ACMG Secondary Findings Working Group. Electronic address: documents@acmg.net. *Genet Med* 24:1407–1414, 2022. doi:10.1016/j.gim.2022.04.006.

Index